HANDBOOK OF
DISEASES

Springhouse Corporation
Springhouse, Pennsylvania

STAFF

Senior Publisher: Matthew Cahill

Clinical Manager: Cindy Tryniszewski, RN, MSN

Art Director: John Hubbard

Senior Editor: June Norris

Clinical Editors: Maryann Foley, RN, BSN; Judith Schilling McCann, RN, BSN; Beverly Ann Tscheschlog, RN

Editors: Marylou Webster Ambrose, Kathleen Angone, Margaret Eckman, Peter Johnson

Copy Editors: Cynthia C. Breuninger (manager), Lynette High, Mary Durkin, Christina Ponczek, Doris Weinstock

Designers: Stephanie Peters (senior associate art director), Darcy Faralio, Linda Franklin

Typographers: Diane Paluba (manager), Elizabeth Bergman, Joyce Rossi Biletz, Phyllis Marron, Valerie Rosenberger

Manufacturing: Deborah Meiris (director), Pat Dorshaw (manager), T.A. Landis

Production Coordinator: Margaret A. Rastiello

Editorial Assistants: Beverly Lane, Mary Madden

Indexer: Robin Hipple

©1996 by Springhouse Corporation. All rights reserved. No part of this publication may be used or reproduced in any manner whatsoever without written permission except for brief quotations embodied in critical articles and reviews. For information, write Springhouse Corporation, 1111 Bethlehem Pike, P.O. Box 908, Springhouse, PA 19477-0908. Authorization to photocopy items for internal or personal use, or for the internal or personal use of specific clients, is granted by Springhouse Corporation for users registered with the Copyright Clearance Center (CCC) Transactional Reporting Service, provided that the fee of $.75 per page is paid directly to CCC, 222 Rosewood Dr., Danvers, MA 01923. For those organizations that have been granted a license by CCC, a separate system of payment has been arranged. The fee code for users of the Transactional Reporting Service is 0874348382/96 $00.00 + $.75.
Printed in the United States of America.
HDIS-051198

 A member of the Reed Elsevier plc group

Library of Congress Cataloging-in-Publication Data
Handbook of diseases.
  p. cm.
  Includes bibliographical references and index.
  1. Diseases — Handbooks, manuals, etc.
I. Springhouse Corporation.
  [DNLM: 1. Diseases — handbooks.
2. Diagnosis — handbooks.
3. Therapeutics — handbooks. QZ 39 H2358 1996]
RC55.H265 1996
616—dc20   95-4485
DNLM/DIC   CIP
ISBN 0-87434-838-2 (alk paper)

CONTENTS

Contributors and Consultants

Brian P. Burlew, MD, FCCP,
Pulmonologist, St. Luke's Hospital,
Bethlehem, Pa.

Gerald A. Charnogursky, MD, Medical
Director, Joslin Center for Diabetes at
MacNeal Hospital, Berwyn, Ill.

JoAnn Coleman, RN, MS, CS, OCN,
Clinical Nurse Specialist, Gastrointestinal
Surgery, The Johns Hopkins Hospital,
Baltimore

Rae L. Conley, RN, MSN, Clinical Nurse
Specialist, Thomas Jefferson University
Hospital, Philadelphia

Brian B. Doyle, MD, Clinical Professor of
Psychiatry; Director, Anxiety Disorders
Program, Georgetown University Medical
School, Washington, D.C.

**Phyllis Dubendorf, RN, MSN, CCRN,
CNRN,** Clinical Nurse Specialist, Thomas
Jefferson University Hospital, Philadelphia

Michael D. Ellis, MD, FACOG, Attending
Physician, Abington (Pa.) Memorial
Hospital

Lori S. Farmer, RN, MS, ARNP, Director of
Genetic and Perinatal Counseling,
Fayetteville (N.C.) Diagnostic Center

Arnold W. Gurevitch, MD, Chief, Division
of Dermatology; Professor of Clinical
Medicine, Harbor–U.C.L.A. Medical
Center, Torrance, Calif.

Sundaram Hariharan, MD, Assistant
Professor of Internal Medicine
(Nephrology), University of Cincinnati

Mary L. Harris, MD, Assistant Professor
of Medicine, The Johns Hopkins Medical
Institutions, Baltimore

Karen Jantzi, RN, MSN, Psychiatric
Coordinator, Indian Creek Foundation,
Harleysville, Pa.

Mark E. Johnson, MD, Assistant
Professor of Surgery, Orthopedic
Oncology Section, M.D. Anderson
Cancer Center, Houston

Nancy N. Konstantinides, RN,C, MS,
Nurse Practitioner, University of
Minnesota Hospital and Clinics,
Minneapolis

Karen E. Michael, RN, MSN, Case
Manager, Greater Atlantic Health Service,
Philadelphia

Attila Nakeeb, MD, Senior Resident,
Department of Surgery, The Johns
Hopkins Hospital, Baltimore

Judith L. Nerad, MD, Assistant Professor
of Medicine, Loyola University Medical
Center, Maywood, Ill.

Thaddeus S. Nowinski, MD, Clinical
Associate Professor, Thomas Jefferson
University, Philadelphia; Associate
Surgeon, Wills Eye Hospital, Philadelphia

John J. O'Shea, MD, Chief, Lymphocyte
Cell Biology Section, Arthritis and
Rheumatism Branch, National Institute of
Arthritis and Musculoskeletal and Skin
Diseases, National Institutes of Health,
Bethesda, Md.

Mary Pasdur, RN, MSN, OCN, Clinical
Nurse Specialist, M.D. Anderson Cancer
Center, Houston

Iris M. Reyes, MD, Assistant Professor,
Department of Emergency Medicine,
Hospital of the University of
Pennsylvania, Philadelphia

Allan Ronald, MD, FRCPS, Professor of
Internal Medicine, University of Manitoba,
Winnipeg, Canada

Ellamarie Russo-De Mara, DO, FACOG,
Associate Professor of OB/GYN, New
York College of Osteopathic Medicine,
Old Westbury, N.Y.

Lawrence E. Schilder, DO, Assistant
Professor, Loyola University Stritch
School of Medicine, Division of
Hematology/Oncology, Berwyn, Ill.

Kristine A. Scordo, RN, PhD, Clinical
Director, Clinical Nurse Specialist, The
Cardiology Center of Cincinnati

Alan L. Silverberg, MD, Infectious
Disease Consultant, Philadelphia

Warren Summer, MD, Section Chief,
Pulmonary–Critical Care Medicine,
Louisiana State University Medical
Center, New Orleans

Maureen R. Tierney, MD, MSc, Fellowship
Director and Attending Physician,
Infectious Disease Unit, Massachusetts
General Hospital, Boston

Patricia D. Weiskittel, RN, MSN, CNN,
Clinical Nurse Specialist, University
Hospital, Cincinnati

FOREWORD

As a health care professional, you must have a vast fund of knowledge at your command. But regardless of how much information you absorb—from textbooks and journals, from patient charts, and from discussions with colleagues— you never really know what to expect until you reach a patient's bedside. Maybe you'll find that the admission diagnosis was incorrect or that the patient has developed an unexpected complication or a new illness. To complicate matters further, standards of care for various illnesses are constantly changing.

How can you cope with constant change and the immense database that underlies modern medical care? The answer, of course, is constant education, a substantial part of which is to read, read, read. Unfortunately, you can't possibly digest the shear amount of information out there—or get it quickly enough. That's why you need the pocket-sized *Handbook of Diseases.* You may not always have time to seek out and pour through textbooks. Consult this handbook before walking into a patient's room to rapidly refresh your memory about the important considerations of his illness. Quickly skim an entry afterward to clarify any point you're unsure of; then, if necessary, go back and ask the patient more questions or even repeat part of your exam.

This portable, indispensable reference contains the latest information on more than 435 diseases, conveniently arranged in alphabetical order. Every entry has been reviewed and updated by clinical experts. The book also covers *DSM-IV* criteria for psychiatric disorders and newly recognized diseases, such as hantavirus pulmonary syndrome. The easy-to-follow format—featuring short paragraphs and bulleted lists—allows you to quickly scan an entire entry or instantly pinpoint the specific information you need.

Each disease entry begins with a brief definition. Next follows a discussion of causes; a description of characteristic signs and symptoms; an outline of laboratory tests and other diagnostic procedures, including typical results; and a summary of treatment options. A special considerations section at the end of each entry outlines specific care measures for the hospital and home, including guidelines for giving preoperative and postoperative care, administering medications, and ensuring patient comfort.

Two special features — *Teaching checklist* and *Hazard* — zero in on what to teach your patient about his disease and any unusual dangers to watch for. Where appropriate, the phrase *Life-threatening disorder* (another special feature) precedes the disease name at the start of designated entries. Many illustrations and charts, including staging charts for cancer, also supplement the text.

Using the *Handbook of Diseases* makes the task of keeping current a little less daunting. Make it your constant companion, and you'll wonder how you ever functioned without it.

JOHN J. O'SHEA, MD
Chief, Lymphocyte Cell Biology Section
Arthritis and Rheumatism Branch
National Institute of Arthritis and
Musculoskeletal and Skin Diseases
National Institutes of Health
Bethesda, Maryland

ABDOMINAL INJURIES

Blunt and penetrating abdominal injuries may damage major blood vessels as well as internal organs. Their most immediate life-threatening consequences are hemorrhage and hypovolemic shock; later threats include infection. The prognosis depends on the extent of injury and on which organs are damaged, but it's generally improved by prompt diagnosis and surgical repair.

Causes

Blunt (nonpenetrating) abdominal injuries usually result from automobile accidents, falls from heights, or athletic injuries; penetrating abdominal injuries, from stab and gunshot wounds.

Signs and symptoms

Depending on the degree of injury and the organs involved, symptoms will vary, as follows:

• Penetrating abdominal injuries cause obvious wounds. For example, gunshots often produce both entrance and exit wounds, with variable blood loss, pain, and tenderness. These injuries often cause pallor, cyanosis, tachycardia, shortness of breath, and hypotension.

• Blunt abdominal injuries cause severe pain (such pain may radiate beyond the abdomen, for instance, to the shoulders), bruises, abrasions, contusions, or distention. They may also result in tenderness, abdominal splinting or rigidity, nausea, vomiting, pallor, cyanosis, tachycardia, and shortness of breath. Rib fractures often accompany blunt injuries.

In both blunt and penetrating injuries, massive blood loss may cause hypovolemic shock. In general, damage to solid abdominal organs (liver, spleen, pancreas, and kidneys) causes hemorrhage; damage to hollow organs (stomach, intestine, gallbladder, and bladder) causes rupture and release of the organs' contents (including bacteria) into the abdomen, which, in turn, produces inflammation.

Diagnosis

A history of abdominal trauma, clinical features, and laboratory results confirm the diagnosis and determine organ damage. Consider any upper abdominal injury a thoracicoabdominal injury until proven otherwise. Laboratory studies vary with the patient's condition but usually include:

• *chest X-rays* (preferably done with the patient upright, to show free air)

• *abdominal films*

• *examination of stools and stomach aspirate* for blood

• *blood studies* (decreased hematocrit and hemoglobin levels point to blood loss; coagulation studies evaluate hemostasis; white blood cell count is usually elevated but doesn't necessarily point to infection; type and crossmatch to prepare for blood transfusion)

• *arterial blood gas analysis* to evaluate respiratory status

• *serum amylase levels,* which often may be elevated in pancreatic injury

• *aspartate aminotransferase and alanine aminotransferase levels,* which increase with tissue injury and cell death

• *excretory urography* and *cystourethrography* to detect renal and urinary tract damage

• *radioisotope scanning* and *ultrasound* to detect liver, kidney, or spleen injury

• *angiography* to detect specific injuries, especially to the kidneys

• *peritoneal lavage,* with insertion of a lavage catheter to check for blood, urine, pus, ascitic fluid, bile, and chyle (a milky fluid absorbed by the intestinal lymph vessels during digestion). In blunt trauma with equivocal abdominal findings, this procedure helps establish the need for exploratory surgery.

• *computed tomography scan* to detect abdominal, head, or other injuries

• *exploratory laparotomy* to detect specific injuries when other clinical evidence is incomplete

• other laboratory studies to rule out associated injuries.

Treatment
Abdominal injuries require emergency treatment to control hemorrhage and prevent hypovolemic shock, by infusion of I.V. fluids and blood components. After stabilization, most abdominal injuries require surgical repair; some patients, however, require immediate surgery. Analgesics and antibiotics increase patient comfort and prevent infection. Most patients require hospitalization; if they're asymptomatic, they may require observation for only 6 to 24 hours.

Special considerations
• Emergency care in patients with abdominal injuries supports vital functions by maintaining airway, breathing, and circulation. At admission, immediately evaluate respiratory and circulatory status and, if possible, obtain a history.

• To maintain airway and breathing, intubate the patient and provide mechanical ventilation as necessary; otherwise, provide supplemental oxygen.

• Using a large-bore needle, start two or more I.V. lines for monitoring and rapid fluid infusion, using a normal saline solution. Then draw a blood sample for laboratory studies. Also, insert a nasogastric tube and, if necessary, an indwelling urinary catheter; monitor stomach aspirate and urine for blood.

• Obtain vital signs for baseline data; continue to monitor them every 15 minutes.

• Apply a sterile dressing to open wounds. After assessing the patient, splint a suspected pelvic injury by tying the patient's legs together with a pillow between them. Try not to move the patient.

• Give analgesics for pain. Usually, narcotics aren't recommended; but if the pain is severe, give narcotics in small titrated I.V. doses.

• If necessary, give tetanus prophylaxis and prophylactic I.V. antibiotics.

• Prepare the patient for surgery. Get a consent form signed by the patient or a responsible relative. Remove the patient's dentures. Type and cross-match blood.

• If the injury was caused by a motor vehicle accident, find out if the police were notified, and if not, notify them. If the patient suffered a gunshot or stab wound, notify the police, place all his clothes in a bag, and retain them for the police. Document the number and sites of the wounds. Contact the patient's family and offer them reassurance.

ACHILLES TENDON CONTRACTURE

This condition is a shortening of the Achilles tendon (tendo calcaneus or heel cord), which causes foot pain and strain, with limited ankle dorsiflexion.

Causes

Achilles tendon contracture may reflect a congenital structural anomaly or a muscular reaction to chronic poor posture, especially in women who wear high-heeled shoes or joggers who land on the balls of their feet instead of their heels. Other causes include paralytic conditions of the legs, such as poliomyelitis or cerebral palsy.

Signs and symptoms

Sharp, spasmodic pain during dorsiflexion of the foot characterizes the reflex type of Achilles tendon contracture. In footdrop (fixed equinus), contracture of the flexor foot muscle prevents placing the heel on the ground.

Diagnosis

Physical examination and patient history suggest Achilles tendon contracture. A simple test confirms the condition: While the patient keeps his knee flexed, the examiner places the foot in dorsiflexion; gradual knee extension forces the foot into plantar flexion.

Treatment

Achilles tendon contracture is treated conservatively by raising the inside heel of the shoe (in the reflex type); gradually lowering the heels of shoes (sudden lowering can aggravate the problem), and stretching exercises, if the cause is high heels; or using support braces or casting to prevent footdrop in a paralyzed patient. Alternative therapy includes using wedged plaster casts or stretching the tendon by manipulation. Analgesics may be given to relieve pain.

With fixed footdrop, treatment may include surgery (z-tenotomy), although this procedure may weaken the tendon. Z-tenotomy allows further stretching by cutting the tendon. After surgery, a short leg cast maintains the foot in 90-degree dorsiflexion for 6 weeks. Some surgeons allow partial weight-bearing on a walking cast after 2 weeks.

Special considerations

• After surgery to lengthen the Achilles tendon, elevate the casted foot to decrease venous pressure and edema by raising the foot of the bed or supporting the foot with pillows.

• Record the neurovascular status of the toes (temperature, color, sensation, capillary refill time, toe mobility) every hour for the first 24 hours, then every 4 hours. If any changes are detected, increase the elevation of the patient's legs and notify the surgeon immediately.

• Prepare the patient for ambulation by having him dangle his foot over the side of the bed for short periods (5 to 15 minutes) before he gets out of bed, allowing for gradual increase of venous pressure.

• Assist the patient in walking (usually within 24 hours of surgery), using crutches and a non-weight-bearing or touch-down gait.

• Protect the patient's skin with moleskin or by "petaling" the edges of the cast.

• Before discharge, teach the patient how to care for the cast, and advise him to elevate his foot regularly when sitting or whenever the foot throbs or becomes edematous.

• Make sure the patient understands how much exercise and walking are recommended after discharge.

• To prevent Achilles tendon contracture in paralyzed patients, apply support braces, universal splints, casts, or high-topped sneakers. Make sure the weight of the sheets doesn't keep paralyzed feet in plantar flexion.

• For other patients, teach good foot care, and urge them to seek immediate medical care for foot problems. Warn women against wearing high heels constantly, and suggest regular foot (dorsiflexion) exercises.

ACNE VULGARIS

An inflammatory disease of the sebaceous follicles, acne vulgaris primarily affects adolescents, although lesions can appear as early as age 8. Although acne strikes boys more often and more severely, it usually occurs in girls at an earlier age and tends to last longer, sometimes into adulthood. The prognosis is good with treatment.

Causes

The cause of acne is multifactoral, but theories regarding dietary influences appear to be groundless. Research now centers on follicular occlusion, androgen-stimulated sebum production, and *Propionibacterium acnes* as possible primary causes.

Predisposing factors include heredity; oral contraceptives (many females experience an acne flare-up during their first few menstrual cycles after starting or discontinuing oral contraceptives); androgen stimulation; certain drugs, including corticosteroids, adrenocorticotropic hormone, androgens, iodides, bromides, trimethadione, phenytoin, isoniazid, lithium, and halothane; cobalt irradiation; or hyperalimentation.

Other precipitating factors include exposure to heavy oils, greases, or tars; trauma or rubbing from tight clothing; cosmetics; emotional stress; or unfavorable climate.

More is known about the pathogenesis of acne. Androgens stimulate sebaceous gland growth and production of sebum, which is secreted into dilated hair follicles that contain bacteria. The bacteria, usually *Propionibacterium acnes* and *Staphylococcus epidermidis*—which are normal skin flora—secrete lipase. This enzyme interacts with sebum to produce free fatty acids, which provoke inflammation. Also the hair follicles produce more keratin, which joins with the sebum to form a plug in the dilated follicle.

Signs and symptoms

The acne plug may appear as a closed comedo, or whitehead (if it doesn't protrude from the follicle and is covered by the epidermis), or as an open comedo, or blackhead (if it does protrude and isn't covered by the epidermis). The black coloration is caused by the melanin or pigment of the follicle.

Rupture or leakage of an enlarged plug into the dermis produces inflammation and characteristic acne pustules, papules, or, in severe forms, acne cysts or abscesses. Chronic, recurring lesions produce acne scars.

Diagnosis

The appearance of characteristic acne lesions, especially in an adolescent patient, confirms the presence of acne vulgaris.

Treatment

Commonly, acne is treated topically with benzoyl peroxide, a powerful antibacterial, alone or in combination with tretinoin, a keratolytic (retinoic acid). Both agents may irritate the skin.

Systemic therapy consists primarily of antibiotics, usually tetracycline, to decrease bacterial growth until the

HAZARD

RISKS OF ISOTRETINOIN THERAPY

Because isotretinoin is known to cause birth defects, the manufacturer, with approval of the Food and Drug Administration, recommends the following precautions:
• pregnancy testing before dispensing
• dispensing only a 30-day supply

• repeat pregnancy testing throughout the treatment period
• effective contraception during treatment
• informed consent of the patient or parents regarding the drug's adverse effects.

---

patient is in remission; then a lower dosage is used for long-term maintenance. Tetracycline is contraindicated during pregnancy because it discolors the teeth of the fetus. Erythromycin is an alternate for these patients. Exacerbation of pustules or abscesses during either type of antibiotic therapy requires a culture to identify a possible secondary bacterial infection.

Oral isotretinoin combats acne by inhibiting sebaceous gland function and keratinization. But because of its severe adverse effects, the 16- to 20-week course of isotretinoin is limited to those with severe papulopustular or cystic acne who don't respond to conventional therapy. (See *Risks of isotretinoin therapy.*)

Females may benefit from the administration of estrogens to inhibit androgen activity. Improvement rarely occurs before 2 to 4 months and exacerbations may follow its discontinuation. Unfortunately, the high estrogen doses that are required present a major risk of severe adverse effects.

Other treatments for acne vulgaris include intralesional corticosteroid injections, exposure to ultraviolet light (but never when a photosensitizing agent, such as tretinoin, is being used), cryotherapy, or surgery.

Special considerations
• Check the patient's drug history because certain medications, such as oral contraceptives, may cause an acne flare-up.
• Try to identify predisposing factors that may be eliminated or modified.
• Explain the causes of acne to the patient and family. Make sure they understand the prescribed treatment is more likely to improve acne than a strict diet and fanatic scrubbing with soap and water. Provide written instructions regarding treatment.
• Instruct the patient receiving tretinoin to apply it at least 30 minutes after washing the face and at least 1 hour before bedtime. Warn against using it around the eyes or lips. After treatments, the skin should look pink and dry. If it appears red or starts to peel, the preparation may have to be weakened or applied less often.
• Advise the patient to avoid exposure to sunlight or to use a sunscreen. If the prescribed regimen includes tretinoin and benzoyl peroxide, avoid skin irritation by using one preparation in the morning and the other at night.
• Instruct the patient to take tetracycline on an empty stomach and not to take it with antacids or milk since it interacts with their metallic ions and is then poorly absorbed.
• Tell the patient who is taking isotretinoin to avoid vitamin A supplements,

which can worsen any adverse effects. Also discuss how to deal with the dry skin and mucous membranes that usually occur during treatment. Warn the female patient about the severe risk of teratogenicity. Monitor liver function and lipid levels.

• Inform the patient that acne takes a long time to clear—even years for complete resolution. Encourage continued local skin care even after acne clears. Explain the adverse effects of all drugs.

• Pay special attention to the patient's perception of his physical appearance, and offer emotional support.

LIFE-THREATENING DISORDER

ACQUIRED IMMUNODEFICIENCY SYNDROME

Currently one of the most widely publicized diseases, acquired immunodeficiency syndrome (AIDS) is marked by progressive failure of the immune system. Though it's characterized by gradual destruction of cell-mediated (T-cell) immunity, it also affects humoral immunity and even autoimmunity because of the central role of the CD4$^+$ T lymphocyte in immune reactions. The resultant immunodeficiency makes the patient susceptible to opportunistic infections, unusual cancers, and other abnormalities that define AIDS.

This syndrome was first described by the Centers for Disease Control and Prevention (CDC) in 1981. Since then, the CDC has declared a case surveillance definition for AIDS and modified it several times, most recently in 1993.

A retrovirus—the human immunodeficiency virus (HIV) Type I—is the primary etiologic agent. Transmission of HIV occurs by contact with infected blood or body fluids and is associated with identifiable high-risk behaviors. It's therefore disproportionately represented in homosexual and bisexual men, I.V. drug users, neonates of HIV-infected women, recipients of contaminated blood or blood products (dramatically decreased since mid-1985), and heterosexual partners of persons in the former groups. Because of similar routes of transmission, AIDS shares epidemiologic patterns with hepatitis B and sexually transmitted diseases.

The natural history of AIDS infection begins with infection by the HIV retrovirus, which is detectable only by laboratory tests, and ends with the severely immunocompromised, terminal stage of this disease. Depending on individual variations and the presence of cofactors that influence progression, the time elapsed from acute HIV infection to the appearance of symptoms (mild to severe) to the diagnosis of AIDS and, eventually, to death varies greatly. Current antiretroviral therapy (for example, with zidovudine) and treatment and prophylaxis of common opportunistic infections can delay the natural progression of HIV disease and prolong survival.

Causes

AIDS results from infection with HIV, which strikes cells bearing the CD4$^+$ antigen; the latter (normally a receptor for major histocompatibility complex molecules) serves as a receptor for the retrovirus and lets it enter the cell. HIV prefers to infect the CD4$^+$ lymphocyte but may also infect other CD4$^+$ antigen-bearing cells of the GI tract, uterine cervical cells, and neuroglial cells. After invading a cell, HIV replicates, leading to cell death, or becomes latent. HIV infection leads to profound pathology, either directly, through destruction of CD4+ cells, other immune cells, and neuroglial cells, or indirectly, through the secondary effects of CD4+ T-cell dysfunction and resultant immunosuppression.

The infection process takes three forms:
• immunodeficiency (opportunistic infections and unusual cancers)
• autoimmunity (lymphoid interstitial pneumonitis, arthritis, hypergammaglobulinemia, and production of autoimmune antibodies)
• neurologic dysfunction (AIDS dementia complex, HIV encephalopathy, and peripheral neuropathies).

Transmission
HIV is transmitted by direct inoculation during intimate sexual contact, especially associated with the mucosal trauma of receptive rectal intercourse; transfusion of contaminated blood or blood products (a risk diminished by routine testing of all blood products); sharing of contaminated needles; or transplacental or postpartum transmission from infected mother to fetus (by cervical or blood contact at delivery and in breast milk).

Accumulating evidence suggests that HIV is not transmitted by casual household or social contact. The average time between exposure to the virus and diagnosis of AIDS is 8 to 10 years, but shorter and longer incubation times have also been recorded.

Signs and symptoms
HIV infection manifests itself in many different ways. After a high-risk exposure and inoculation, the infected person usually experiences a mononucleosis-like syndrome, which may be attributed to a flu or other virus and then may remain asymptomatic for years. In this latent stage, the only sign of HIV infection is laboratory evidence of seroconversion. When symptoms appear, they may take many forms:
• persistent generalized adenopathy
• nonspecific symptoms (weight loss, fatigue, night sweats, fevers)
• neurologic symptoms resulting from HIV encephalopathy
• opportunistic infection or cancer.

The clinical course varies slightly in children with AIDS. Apparently, their incubation time is shorter with a mean of 17 months. Signs and symptoms resemble those in adults, except for findings related to sexually transmitted disease. Children show virtually all of the opportunistic infections observed in adults, with a higher incidence of bacterial infections: otitis media, pneumonias other than *Pneumocystis carinii,* sepsis, chronic salivary gland enlargement, and lymphoid interstitial pneumonia.

Diagnosis
The CDC defines AIDS as an illness characterized by one or more "indicator" diseases coexisting with laboratory evidence of HIV infection and other possible causes of immunosuppression. The CDC's current AIDS surveillance case definition requires laboratory confirmation of HIV infection in people who have a CD4+ T-cell count of 200 cells/µl or who have an associated clinical condition or disease.

Antibody tests
The most commonly performed tests, antibody tests indicate HIV infection indirectly by revealing HIV antibodies. The recommended protocol requires initial screening of individuals and blood products with an enzyme-linked immunosorbent assay (ELISA) test. A positive ELISA test should be repeated and then confirmed by an alternate method, usually the Western

blot or an immunofluorescence assay. However, antibody testing isn't always reliable. Because the body takes a variable amount of time to produce a detectable level of antibodies, a "window" varying from a few weeks to as long as 35 months in one documented case allows an HIV-infected person to test negative for HIV antibodies.

Antibody tests are also unreliable in neonates because transferred maternal antibodies persist for 6 to 10 months. To overcome these problems, direct testing is performed to detect HIV. Direct tests include antigen tests (p24 antigen), HIV cultures, nucleic acid probes of peripheral blood lymphocytes, and the polymerase chain reaction.

Other tests

Additional tests to support the diagnosis and help evaluate the severity of immunosuppression include $CD4^+$ and $CD8^+$ T-lymphocyte subset counts, erythrocyte sedimentation rate (ESR), complete blood cell count, serum beta$_2$-microglobulin, p24 antigen, neopterin levels, and anergy testing. Because many opportunistic infections in AIDS patients are reactivations of previous infections, patients are also tested for syphilis, hepatitis B, tuberculosis, toxoplasmosis and, in some areas, histoplasmosis.

Treatment

No cure has yet been found for AIDS; however, at least three beneficial forms of treatment are available for HIV disease:

• Antiretroviral treatments are designed to inhibit or inactivate the HIV virus.

• Immunomodulatory agents are designed to boost the weakened immune system.

• Anti-infective and antineoplastic agents combat opportunistic infections and associated cancers; some are used prophylactically to help patients resist opportunistic infections.

Current treatment protocols combine two or more agents in an effort to gain the maximum benefit with the fewest adverse reactions. Combination therapy also helps inhibit the production of resistant, mutant strains. Supportive treatments help maintain nutritional status and relieve pain and other distressing physical and psychological symptoms.

Many pathogens in AIDS respond to anti-infective drugs but tend to recur after treatment ends. For this reason, most patients need continuous anti-infective treatment, presumably for life or until the drug is no longer tolerated or effective.

Zidovudine

Treatment with zidovudine has proved effective in slowing the progression of HIV infection, decreasing opportunistic infections, and prolonging survival. However, it often produces serious adverse reactions and toxicities. Initially zidovudine may be prescribed to be taken as 200 mg every 4 hours for a total daily dose of 1,200 mg (or a total daily dose of 1,000 mg in patients who did not want to interrupt sleep for the sixth dose). This dosage schedule — called high-dose zidovudine — is being replaced by lower dosage schedules that are proving effective and significantly less toxic.

The current recommendation is to take 100 mg every 4 hours for a total daily dose of 600 mg, or 500 mg if the patient does not want to interrupt sleep. Didanosine (DDI) may be recommended for patients who can't tolerate, or who no longer respond to, zidovudine therapy. Zalcitabine (DDC) is used in combination with zidovudine in advanced AIDS to enhance the return of $CD4^+$ T-lymphocyte levels.

Special considerations

• Health care workers and the public are advised to use precautions in all situations that risk exposure to blood, bodily fluids, and secretions. Diligently practicing universal precautions can prevent the inadvertent transmission of AIDS, hepatitis B, and other infectious diseases that are transmitted by similar routes.

• Recognize that a diagnosis of AIDS is profoundly distressing because of the disease's social impact and the discouraging prognosis. The patient may lose his job and financial security as well as the support of family and friends. Coping with an altered body image, the emotional burden of serious illness, and the threat of death may overwhelm the patient.

ACROMEGALY AND GIGANTISM

Chronic, progressive diseases, acromegaly and gigantism are marked by hormonal dysfunction and startling skeletal overgrowth. Acromegaly occurs after epiphyseal closure, causing bone thickening and transverse growth and visceromegaly. Gigantism begins before epiphyseal closure and causes proportional overgrowth of all body tissues. Although the prognosis depends on the causative factor, these disorders usually reduce life expectancy unless treated in a timely way.

Causes

Typically, oversecretion of human growth hormone (HGH) produces changes throughout the entire body, resulting in acromegaly and, when oversecretion occurs before puberty, gigantism. Eosinophilic or mixed-cell adenomas of the anterior pituitary gland may cause this oversecretion, but the etiology of the tumors themselves remains unclear. Occasionally, HGH levels are elevated in more than one family member, which suggests the possibility of a genetic cause.

The earliest clinical sign of acromegaly is soft-tissue swelling of the extremities, which causes coarsening of the facial features. This rare form of hyperpituitarism occurs equally among men and women, usually between ages 30 and 50.

In gigantism, proportional overgrowth of all body tissues starts before epiphyseal closure. This causes remarkable height increases of as much as 6″ (15 cm) a year. Gigantism affects infants and children, causing them to attain as much as three times the normal height for their age. As adults, they may ultimately reach a height of more than 80″ (203 cm).

Signs and symptoms

Acromegaly develops slowly, whereas gigantism develops abruptly.

Acromegaly

This disorder typically produces diaphoresis, oily skin, hypermetabolism, and hypertrichosis. Severe headache, central nervous system impairment, bitemporal hemianopia, loss of visual acuity, and blindness may result from the intrasellar tumor compressing the optic chiasm or nerves.

Hypersecretion of HGH produces cartilaginous and connective tissue overgrowth, resulting in a characteristic hulking appearance, with an enlarged supraorbital ridge and thickened ears and nose. Prognathism, projection of the jaw, becomes marked and may interfere with chewing. Laryngeal hypertrophy, paranasal sinus enlargement, and thickening of the tongue cause the voice to sound deep and hollow. Distal phalanges display an arrowhead appearance on X-rays, and the fingers are thickened. Irritability, hostility, and various psychological disturbances may occur.

Prolonged effects of excessive HGH secretion include bowlegs, barrel chest, arthritis, osteoporosis, kyphosis, hypertension, and arteriosclerosis. Both gigantism and acromegaly may also cause signs of glucose intolerance and clinically apparent diabetes mellitus because of the insulin-antagonistic character of HGH.

Gigantism

This disorder produces some of the same skeletal abnormalities seen in acromegaly. As the disease progresses, the pituitary tumor enlarges and invades normal tissue, resulting in the loss of other trophic hormones, such as thyroid-stimulating hormone, luteinizing hormone, follicle-stimulating hormone, and corticotropin, thus causing the target organ to stop functioning.

Diagnosis

Plasma HGH levels measured by radioimmunoassay typically are elevated. However, because HGH secretion is pulsatile, the results of random sampling may be misleading.

The glucose suppression test offers more reliable information. Glucose normally suppresses HGH secretion; therefore, a glucose infusion that does not suppress the hormone level to below the accepted normal value of 5 ng/ml, when combined with characteristic clinical features, strongly suggests hyperpituitarism.

In addition, skull X-rays, a computed tomography scan, arteriography, and magnetic resonance imaging determine the presence and extent of the pituitary lesion. Bone X-rays showing a thickening of the cranium (especially of frontal, occipital, and parietal bones) and of the long bones, as well as os-

teoarthritis in the spine, support this diagnosis.

Treatment

Overproduction of HGH is curbed through removal of the underlying tumor by cranial or transsphenoidal hypophysectomy or pituitary radiation therapy. In acromegaly, surgery is mandatory when a tumor causes blindness or other severe neurologic disturbances.

Postoperative therapy often requires replacement of thyroid, cortisone, and gonadal hormones. Adjunctive treatment may include administration of bromocriptine and octreotide, which inhibit HGH synthesis.

Special considerations

• Grotesque body changes characteristic of this disorder can cause severe psychological stress. Provide emotional support to help the patient cope with an altered body image.

• Examine the patient for skeletal manifestations, such as arthritis of the hands and osteoarthritis of the spine. Administer prescribed medications. To promote maximum joint mobility, perform or assist with range-of-motion exercises.

• Evaluate muscular weakness, especially in the patient with late-stage acromegaly. Check the strength of his handclasp. If it's very weak, help with tasks such as cutting food.

• Keep the skin dry. Avoid using an oily lotion, since the skin is already oily.

• Test blood for glucose. Check for signs of hyperglycemia (sweating, fatigue, polyuria, polydipsia).

• Be aware that the tumor may cause visual problems. If the patient has hemianopia, stand where he can see you.

• Keep in mind that this disease can also cause inexplicable mood changes. Reassure the family that these mood changes result from the disease and can be modified with treatment.

• Before surgery, reinforce what the surgeon has told the patient, if possible, and try to allay the patient's fear with a clear and honest explanation of the scheduled operation. If the patient is a child, explain to his parents that such surgery prevents permanent soft-tissue deformities but won't correct bone changes that have already taken place. Arrange for counseling, if necessary, to help the child and parents cope with these permanent defects.

• After surgery, diligently monitor vital signs and neurologic status. Be alert for any alteration in level of consciousness, pupil equality, or visual acuity as well as vomiting, falling pulse rate, or rising blood pressure. These changes may signal an increase in intracranial pressure due to intracranial bleeding or cerebral edema.

• Check blood glucose often. Remember, HGH levels usually fall rapidly after surgery, removing an insulin-antagonist effect in many patients and possibly precipitating hypoglycemia.

• Measure intake and output hourly, and watch for large increases. Transient diabetes insipidus, which sometimes occurs after surgery for hyperpituitarism, can cause such increases in urine output.

• If the transsphenoidal approach is used, a large nasal pack is kept in place for several days. Because the patient must breathe through his mouth, give good mouth care.

• Pay special attention to the mucous membranes — which usually become very dry — and the incision site under the upper lip, at the top of the gum line.

• The surgical site is packed with a piece of tissue generally taken from a midthigh donor site. Watch for cerebrospinal fluid (CSF) leaks from the packed site. Look for increased external nasal drainage or drainage into the nasopharynx. CSF leaks may necessitate additional surgery to repair the leak.

• Encourage the patient to ambulate on the first or second day after surgery.

• If necessary, before the patient is discharged, emphasize the importance of continuing hormone replacement therapy. Make sure the patient and his family understand which hormones are to be taken and why, as well as the correct times and dosages. Warn against stopping the hormones suddenly.

• Advise the patient to wear a medical identification bracelet at all times and to bring his hormone replacement schedule with him whenever he returns to the hospital.

• Instruct the patient to have followup check-ups for the rest of his life because there's a slight chance that the tumor which caused his condition could recur.

ACTINOMYCOSIS

An infection primarily caused by the gram-positive anaerobic bacillus *Actinomyces israelii,* actinomycosis produces granulomatous, suppurative lesions with abscesses. Common infection sites are the head, neck, thorax, and abdomen, but it can spread to contiguous tissues, causing multiple draining sinuses.

Sporadic and infrequent, actinomycosis affects twice as many males — especially those ages 15 to 35 — as females. It's likely to infect people with dental disease.

Causes
A. israelii occurs as part of the normal flora of the throat, tonsillar crypts, and mouth (particularly around carious

teeth); infection results from its traumatic introduction into body tissues.

Signs and symptoms

Symptoms appear from days to months after injury and may vary, depending on the site of infection.

In *cervicofacial actinomycosis* (lumpy jaw), painful, indurated swellings appear in the mouth or neck up to several weeks following dental extraction or trauma. They gradually enlarge and form fistulas that open onto the skin. Sulfur granules (yellowish gray masses that are actually colonies of *A. israelii*) appear in the exudate.

In *pulmonary actinomycosis,* aspiration of bacteria from the mouth into areas of the lungs already anaerobic from infection or atelectasis produces a fever and a cough that becomes productive and occasionally causes hemoptysis. Eventually, empyema follows, a sinus forms through the chest wall, and septicemia may occur.

In *gastrointestinal actinomycosis,* ileocecal lesions are caused by swallowed bacteria, which produce abdominal discomfort, fever, sometimes a palpable mass, and an external sinus. This follows intestinal mucosa disruption, usually by surgery or an inflammatory bowel condition such as appendicitis.

Rare sites of actinomycotic infection are the bones, brain, liver, kidneys, and female reproductive organs. Symptoms reflect the organ involved.

Diagnosis

Isolation of *A. israelii* in exudate or tissue confirms actinomycosis. Other tests that help identify it are:

• *microscopic examination* of sulfur granules

• *Gram staining* of excised tissue or exudate to reveal branching gram-positive organisms

• *chest X-ray* to show lesions in unusual locations such as the shaft of a rib.

Treatment

High-dose I.V. penicillin or tetracycline therapy precedes surgical excision and drainage of abscesses in all forms of the disease and continues for 3 to 6 weeks. Following parenteral therapy, treatment with oral penicillin or tetracycline may continue for 1 to 6 months.

Special considerations

• Dispose of all dressings in a sealed plastic bag.

• After surgery, provide proper aseptic wound management.

• Administer prescribed antibiotics. Before giving the first dose, ask the patient if he has any allergies. Watch for a hypersensitivity reaction (rash, fever, itching, and signs of anaphylaxis). If the patient has a history of any allergies, keep epinephrine 1:1,000 and resuscitative equipment available.

• Stress the importance of good oral hygiene and proper dental care.

LIFE-THREATENING DISORDER

ACUTE RESPIRATORY FAILURE IN COPD

In patients with essentially normal lung tissue, acute respiratory failure (ARF) usually means a partial pressure of carbon dioxide ($PaCO_2$) greater than 50 mm Hg and a partial pressure of oxygen (PaO_2) less than 50 mm Hg. These limits, however, don't apply to patients with chronic obstructive pulmonary disease (COPD), who often have a consistently high $PaCO_2$ and low PaO_2. In patients with COPD, only acute deterioration in arterial blood gas (ABG) values, with corresponding clinical deterioration, indicates ARF.

Causes

ARF may develop in COPD patients from any condition that increases the work of breathing and decreases the respiratory drive. Such conditions include respiratory tract infection (such as bronchitis or pneumonia) — the most common precipitating factor — bronchospasm, or accumulating secretions secondary to cough suppression. Other causes of ARF in COPD include:

• *central nervous system (CNS) depression* — head trauma or injudicious use of sedatives, narcotics, tranquilizers, or oxygen

• *cardiovascular disorders* — myocardial infarction, congestive heart failure, or pulmonary emboli

• *airway irritants* — smoke or fumes

• *endocrine and metabolic disorders* — myxedema or metabolic alkalosis

• *thoracic abnormalities* — chest trauma, pneumothorax, or thoracic or abdominal surgery.

Signs and symptoms

In COPD patients with ARF, increased ventilation-perfusion mismatching and reduced alveolar ventilation decrease arterial PaO_2 (hypoxemia) and increase arterial $PaCO_2$ (hypercapnia). This rise in carbon dioxide tension lowers the pH. The resulting hypoxemia and acidemia affect all body organs, especially the central nervous, respiratory, and cardiovascular systems. Specific symptoms vary with the underlying cause of ARF but may include:

• *Respiratory symptoms.* Rate may be increased, decreased, or normal, depending on the cause; respirations may be shallow, deep, or alternate between the two; air hunger may occur. Cyanosis may or may not be present, depending on the hemoglobin level and

arterial oxygenation. Auscultation of the chest may reveal crackles, rhonchi, wheezes, or diminished breath sounds.

• *CNS symptoms.* The patient shows evidence of restlessness, confusion, loss of concentration, irritability, tremulousness, diminished tendon reflexes, and papilledema; he may slip into a coma.

• *Cardiovascular symptoms.* Tachycardia, with increased cardiac output and mildly elevated blood pressure secondary to adrenal release of catecholamines, occurs early in response to a low PaO_2. With myocardial hypoxia, arrhythmias may develop. Pulmonary hypertension also occurs.

Diagnosis

Progressive deterioration of ABG levels and pH, when compared to the patient's "normal" values, strongly suggests ARF in COPD. (In patients with essentially normal lung tissue, pH below 7.35 usually indicates ARF, but COPD patients display an even greater deviation from this normal value, as they do with blood $PaCO_2$ and PaO_2.) The following findings are also supportive:

• *Bicarbonate levels* are increased, reflecting metabolic alkalosis or metabolic compensation for chronic respiratory acidosis.

• *Hematocrit and hemoglobin levels* are abnormally low, which may be due to blood loss, indicating decreased oxygen-carrying capacity.

• *Serum electrolyte levels* may indicate hypokalemia, which may result from compensatory hyperventilation — an attempt to correct alkalosis; hypochloremia often occurs in metabolic alkalosis.

• *White blood cell count* is elevated if ARF is due to bacterial infection; Gram stain and sputum culture can identify pathogens.

• *Chest X-ray findings* identify pulmonary pathology, such as emphysema, atelectasis, lesions, pneumothorax, infiltrates, or effusions.

• *Electrocardiogram* reveals arrhythmias, which commonly suggest cor pulmonale and myocardial hypoxia.

Treatment

ARF in COPD patients is an emergency that requires cautious oxygen therapy (using nasal prongs or Venturi mask) to raise the patient's PO_2. If significant respiratory acidosis persists, mechanical ventilation through an endotracheal or a tracheostomy tube may be necessary. High-frequency ventilation may be used if the patient doesn't respond to conventional mechanical ventilation. (See *Understanding high-frequency ventilation.*) Treatment routinely includes antibiotics for infection, bronchodilators and, possibly, steroids.

Special considerations

• Because most ARF patients are treated in the intensive care unit (ICU), orient them to the environment, procedures, and routines to minimize their anxiety.

• To reverse hypoxemia, administer oxygen at concentrations to maintain PO_2 of at least 50 to 60 mm Hg. Patients with COPD usually require only small amounts of supplemental oxygen. Watch for a positive response, such as improvement in the patient's breathing and color and in ABG results.

• Maintain a patent airway. If the patient is retaining carbon dioxide, encourage him to cough and to breathe deeply with pursed lips. If the patient is alert, have him use an incentive spirometer; if he's intubated and lethargic, turn him every 1 to 2 hours.

• Use postural drainage and chest physiotherapy to help clear secretions.

• In an intubated patient, suction the trachea, as needed, after hyperoxygenation. Observe for a change in the quantity, consistency, and color of the sputum. Provide humidification to liquefy secretions.

• Observe the patient closely for respiratory arrest. Auscultate for chest sounds. Monitor ABGs, and be alert for any changes.

• Monitor and record serum electrolytes carefully, and correct imbalances; monitor fluid balance by recording intake and output or daily weights.

• Check the cardiac monitor for arrhythmias.

If the patient requires mechanical ventilation:

• Check ventilator settings, cuff pressures, and ABG values often since the fraction of inspired oxygen (FIO_2) setting depends on ABG levels. Draw specimens for ABG analysis 20 to 30 minutes after every FIO_2 change or check ABG levels with oximetry.

• Prevent infection by using sterile technique while suctioning and by changing ventilator circuits every 24 to 48 hours.

• Because stress ulcers are common in intubated ICU patients, check gastric secretions for evidence of bleeding if the patient has a nasogastric tube or complains of epigastric tenderness, nausea, or vomiting. Monitor hemoglobin and hematocrit levels, and check all stools for occult blood. Administer antacids, histamine$_2$ receptor antagonists, or sucralfate.

• Prevent tracheal erosion that can result from artificial airway cuff overinflation, which compresses tracheal wall vasculature. Use minimal leak technique and a cuffed tube with high residual volume (low-pressure cuff), a foam cuff, or a pressure-regulating valve on the cuff.

• To prevent nasal necrosis, keep the nasotracheal tube midline within the nostrils and provide good hygiene. Loosen tape periodically to prevent skin breakdown. Avoid excessive

UNDERSTANDING HIGH-FREQUENCY VENTILATION

Used to treat a patient with respiratory failure, high-frequency ventilation (HFV) is a mechanical ventilation technique that uses high ventilation rates (60 to 3,000 breaths/minute, depending on the type of HFV), low tidal volumes, brief inspiratory time, and low peak airway pressures. HFV has three different delivery forms — high-frequency jet ventilation (HFJV), high-frequency positive-pressure ventilation, and high-frequency oscillation. Here's a brief summary of how HFJV works.

Mechanics of HFJV

• A humidified, high-pressure gas jet pulses through the narrow-lumen gas jet valve on inspiration and accelerates as it flows through the port's narrow lumen and into the patient's endotracheal tube.
• The pressure and velocity of the jet stream cause a drag effect that entrains low-pressure gases into the patient's airway.
• These gas flows combine to deliver 100 to 200 breaths/minute to the patient.
• The gas stream moves down the airway in a progressively broader wave front of decreasing velocity.
• Tidal volume is delivered to airways under constant pressure.
• The gas stream creates turbulence, which causes the gas to vibrate in the airways. Alveolar ventilation increases without raising mean airway pressure or peak inflation pressure.

Uses

• Treatment of bronchopleural fistulas
• Rigid or fiber-optic bronchoscopy
• Laryngeal surgery
• Thoracic surgical procedures
• Treatment of infant and adult respiratory distress syndrome (limited clinical experience)

Benefits

• Improved venous return
• Decreased airway pressures and (possibly) improved pulmonary artery pressure
• Improved arterial gas exchange
• Decreased right ventricular afterload
• Reduced chance of pulmonary barotrauma and decreased cardiac output

Special considerations

• Regularly check the mechanical setup, parameter alarms, and tubing connections.
• Assess the patient's respiratory status regularly.
• Assess airway secretions. If they're extremely viscous, you may need to increase humidification to prevent formation of mucus plugs.

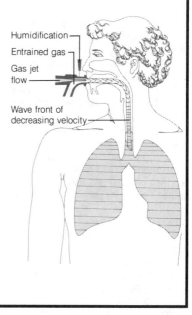

Humidification
Entrained gas
Gas jet flow
Wave front of decreasing velocity

movement of any tubes and make sure the ventilator tubing is adequately supported.

ACUTE TUBULAR NECROSIS

Also known as *acute tubulointerstitial nephritis,* acute tubular necrosis (ATN) accounts for about 75% of all cases of acute renal failure. It's the most common cause of acute renal failure in critically ill patients. ATN injures the tubular segment of the nephron, causing renal failure and uremic syndrome. Mortality ranges from 40% to 70%, depending on complications from underlying diseases. Nonoliguric forms of ATN have a better prognosis.

Causes
ATN results from ischemic or nephrotoxic injury, most commonly in debilitated patients, such as the critically ill or those who have undergone extensive surgery.

In ischemic injury, disruption of blood flow to the kidneys may result from circulatory collapse, severe hypotension, trauma, hemorrhage, dehydration, cardiogenic or septic shock, surgery, anesthetics, or reactions to transfusions. Ischemic ATN can damage the epithelial and basement membranes and can cause lesions in the renal interstitium.

In nephrotoxic injury, damage may follow ingestion of certain chemical agents or result from a hypersensitive reaction of the kidneys. Because nephrotoxic ATN doesn't damage the basement membrane of the nephron, it's potentially reversible.

ATN may result from:

• diseased tubular epithelium that allows leakage of glomerular filtrate across the membranes and reabsorption of filtrate into the blood.
• obstruction of urine flow by the collection of damaged cells, casts, red blood cells (RBCs), and other cellular debris within the tubular walls.
• ischemic injury to glomerular epithelial cells, resulting in cellular collapse and decreased glomerular capillary permeability.
• ischemic injury to vascular endothelium, eventually resulting in cellular swelling and obstruction.

Signs and symptoms
ATN is usually difficult to recognize in its early stages because effects of the critically ill patient's primary disease may mask the symptoms of ATN. The first recognizable effect may be decreased urine output. Generally, hyperkalemia and the characteristic uremic syndrome soon follow, with oliguria (or, rarely, anuria) and confusion, which may progress to uremic coma. Other possible complications may include congestive heart failure, uremic pericarditis, pulmonary edema, uremic lung, anemia, anorexia, intractable vomiting, and poor wound healing due to debilitation.

Fever and chills are ominous signs of infection, the leading cause of death in ATN.

Diagnosis
This disorder is hard to diagnose accurately until it has progressed to an advanced stage. The most significant laboratory clues are urinary sediment containing RBCs and casts, and diluted urine of a low specific gravity (1.010), low osmolality (less than 400 mOsm/kg), and high sodium level (40 to 60 mEq/L).

Blood studies reveal elevated blood urea nitrogen and serum creatinine levels, anemia, defects in platelet adherence, metabolic acidosis, and hyperkalemia. An electrocardiogram may show arrhythmias (from electrolyte imbalances) and, with hyperkalemia, a widening QRS segment, disappearing P waves, and tall, peaked T waves.

Treatment

Vigorous supportive measures are required during the acute phase of ATN until normal kidney function resumes.

Initial treatment may include administration of diuretics and infusion of a large volume of fluids to flush tubules of cellular casts and debris and to replace fluid loss. However, this treatment carries a risk of fluid overload. Long-term fluid management requires daily replacement of projected and calculated losses (including insensible loss).

Other appropriate measures to control complications include transfusion of packed RBCs for anemia and administration of antibiotics for infection. Hyperkalemia may require emergency I.V. administration of 50% glucose, regular insulin, and sodium bicarbonate. Sodium polystyrene sulfonate with sorbitol may be given orally or by enema to reduce extracellular potassium levels. Peritoneal dialysis or hemodialysis may be needed if the patient is catabolic.

Special considerations

• Maintain fluid balance. Watch for fluid overload, a common complication of therapy. Accurately record intake and output, including wound drainage, nasogastric output, and peritoneal dialysis and hemodialysis balances. Weigh the patient daily.
• Monitor hemoglobin and hematocrit, and administer blood products as needed. Use fresh packed cells instead of whole blood to prevent fluid overload and congestive heart failure.
• Maintain electrolyte balance. Monitor laboratory results, and be alert for

evidence of imbalances. Enforce dietary restriction of foods containing sodium and potassium, such as bananas, orange juice, and baked potatoes. Check for potassium content in prescribed medications (for example, potassium penicillin).
• To maintain an anabolic state, provide adequate calories and essential amino acids, while restricting protein intake. Total parenteral nutrition may be indicated in the severely debilitated or catabolic patient.
• Use aseptic technique, particularly when handling catheters, because the debilitated patient is vulnerable to infection. Watch for fever, chills, delayed wound healing, or flank pain if the patient has an indwelling urinary catheter in place.
• Be alert for complications. If anemia worsens (pallor, weakness, lethargy with decreased hemoglobin), administer RBCs. For acidosis, give sodium bicarbonate or assist with dialysis in severe cases as needed. Watch for signs of diminishing renal perfusion (hypotension and decreased urine output). Encourage coughing and deep breathing to prevent pulmonary complications.
• Perform passive range-of-motion exercises. Provide good skin care; apply lotion or bath oil for dry skin. Help the patient to walk as soon as possible, but guard against exhaustion.
• Provide reassurance and emotional support. Encourage the patient and family to express their fears.
• Fully explain each procedure; repeat the explanation each time the procedure is done. Help the patient and family set realistic goals based on the patient's prognosis.
• To prevent ATN, make sure all patients are well hydrated before surgery or after X-rays that use a contrast medium. Mannitol is administered to high-risk patients before and during these procedures.

• Carefully monitor patients receiving blood transfusions to detect early signs of a transfusion reaction (fever, rash, chills), and discontinue such transfusions immediately.

ADENOID HYPERPLASIA

A fairly common childhood condition, adenoid hyperplasia or hypertrophy is the enlargement of the lymphoid tissue of the nasopharynx. Normally, adenoidal tissue is small at birth (¾" to 1¼" [2 to 3 cm]), grows until the child reaches adolescence, and then begins to slowly atrophy. In adenoid hyperplasia, however, this tissue continues to grow.

Causes
Adenoid hyperplasia has an unknown cause, but contributing factors may include heredity, chronic infection, chronic nasal congestion, persistent allergy, insufficient aeration, and inefficient nasal breathing. Inflammation resulting from repeated infection increases the patient's risk of respiratory obstruction.

Signs and symptoms
Typically, adenoid hyperplasia produces symptoms of respiratory obstruction, especially mouth breathing, snoring at night, and frequent, prolonged nasal congestion. Persistent mouth breathing during the formative years produces voice alteration and distinctive changes in facial features — a slightly elongated face, open mouth, highly arched palate, shortened upper lip, and a vacant expression.

Occasionally, the child is incapable of mouth breathing, snores loudly at night, and may eventually show effects of nocturnal respiratory insufficiency, such as intercostal retractions and na-

sal flaring. This may lead to pulmonary hypertension and cor pulmonale. Adenoid hyperplasia can also obstruct the eustachian tube and predispose to otitis media, which in turn can lead to fluctuating conductive hearing loss. Stasis of nasal secretions from adenoidal inflammation can lead to sinusitis.

Diagnosis
Nasopharyngoscopy or rhinoscopy confirms adenoid hyperplasia by visualizing an abnormal tissue mass. Lateral pharyngeal X-rays show an obliterated nasopharyngeal air column.

Treatment
Adenoidectomy is the treatment of choice for adenoid hyperplasia and is commonly recommended for the patient with prolonged mouth breathing, nasal speech, adenoid facies, recurrent otitis media, constant nasopharyngitis, and nocturnal respiratory distress. This procedure usually eliminates recurrent nasal infections and ear complications and reverses any secondary hearing loss.

Special considerations
• Before surgery, describe the hospital routine and arrange for the patient and parents to tour relevant areas of the hospital.
• Explain adenoidectomy to the child, using illustrations if necessary, and detail the recovery process. Reassure him that he'll probably need to be hospitalized. If hospital protocol allows, encourage one parent to stay with the child and participate in his care.
• After surgery, maintain a patent airway. Position the child on his side, head down, to prevent aspiration of draining secretions. Frequently check the throat for bleeding. Be alert for vomiting of old, partially digested blood (coffee-ground vomitus).

• Closely monitor vital signs, and be alert for excessive bleeding, a rise in pulse rate, a drop in blood pressure, tachypnea, and restlessness.

• If no bleeding occurs, offer cracked ice or water when the patient is fully awake.

• Tell the parents that their child may temporarily have a nasal voice.

ADENOVIRAL INFECTIONS

These viruses cause acute self-limiting febrile infections, with inflammation of the respiratory or ocular mucous membranes, or both.

Causes

Adenovirus has 35 known serotypes; it causes five major infections, all of which occur in epidemics. These organisms are common and can remain latent for years. They infect almost everyone early in life (though maternal antibodies offer some protection during the first 6 months of life).

Transmission of adenovirus can occur by direct inoculation into the eye, by the oral-fecal route (adenovirus may persist in the GI tract for years after infection), or by inhalation of an infected droplet. The incubation period is usually less than 1 week; acute illness lasts less than 5 days and can be followed by prolonged asymptomatic reinfection.

Signs and symptoms

Clinical features vary. (See *Major adenoviral infections,* page 20.)

Diagnosis

A definitive diagnosis requires isolation of the virus from respiratory or ocular secretions, or fecal smears.

During epidemics, however, typical symptoms alone can confirm the diagnosis. Because adenoviral illnesses resolve rapidly, serum antibody titers aren't useful for diagnosis.

Adenoviral diseases cause lymphocytosis in children. When they cause respiratory disease, a chest X-ray may show pneumonitis.

Treatment

Supportive treatment includes bed rest, antipyretics, and analgesics. Ocular infections may require corticosteroids and direct supervision by an ophthalmologist. Hospitalization is required in cases of pneumonia (in infants) to prevent death and in epidemic keratoconjunctivitis (EKC) to prevent blindness.

Special considerations

• During the acute illness, monitor respiratory status, and intake and output.

• Give analgesics and antipyretics as needed. Stress the need for bed rest.

• To help minimize the incidence of adenoviral disease, instruct all patients in proper handwashing to reduce fecaloral transmission. EKC can be prevented by sterilization of ophthalmic instruments, adequate chlorination in swimming pools, and avoidance of swimming pools during EKC epidemics. Killed virus vaccine (not widely available) and a live oral virus vaccine can prevent adenoviral infection and are recommended for high-risk groups.

ADRENAL HYPOFUNCTION

Primary adrenal hypofunction or insufficiency (Addison's disease) originates within the adrenal gland itself and is characterized by decreased

MAJOR ADENOVIRAL INFECTIONS

DISEASE	AGE-GROUP	CLINICAL FEATURES
Acute febrile respiratory illness	Children	Nonspecific coldlike symptoms, similar to those of other viral respiratory illnesses: fever, pharyngitis, tracheitis, bronchitis, pneumonitis
Acute respiratory disease	Adults (usually military recruits)	Malaise, fever, chills, headache, pharyngitis, hoarseness, and dry cough
Viral pneumonia	Children and adults	Sudden onset of high fever, rapid infection of upper and lower respiratory tracts, skin rash, diarrhea, intestinal intussusception
Acute pharyngoconjunctival fever	Children (particularly after swimming in pools or lakes)	Spiking fever lasting several days, headache, pharyngitis, conjunctivitis, rhinitis, cervical adenitis
Acute follicular conjunctivitis	Adults	Unilateral tearing and mucoid discharge; later, milder symptoms in other eye
Epidemic keratoconjunctivitis	Adults	Unilateral or bilateral ocular redness and edema, preorbital swelling, local discomfort, superficial opacity of the cornea without ulceration
Hemorrhagic cystitis	Children (boys)	Adenoviruria, hematuria, dysuria, urinary frequency

mineralocorticoid, glucocorticoid, and androgen secretion. Adrenal hypofunction can also occur secondary to a disorder outside the gland (such as a pituitary tumor with corticotropin deficiency), but aldosterone secretion frequently continues intact.

A relatively uncommon disorder, Addison's disease can occur at any age and in both sexes. Secondary adrenal hypofunction occurs when a patient abruptly stops taking long-term exogenous steroid therapy. With an early diagnosis and adequate replacement therapy, the prognosis for adrenal hypofunction is good.

Adrenal crisis (addisonian crisis), a critical deficiency of mineralocorticoids and glucocorticoids, generally follows acute stress, sepsis, trauma, surgery, or omission of steroid therapy in patients who have chronic adrenal insufficiency. A medical emergency, adrenal crisis necessitates immediate, vigorous treatment.

Causes
The following are causes of primary and secondary adrenal hypofunction and adrenal crisis.

Primary hypofunction
Addison's disease occurs when more than 90% of both adrenal glands are destroyed. Such destruction usually results from an autoimmune process

in which circulating antibodies react specifically against the adrenal tissue.

Other causes include tuberculosis (once the chief cause; now responsible for less than 10% of adult cases), bilateral adrenalectomy, hemorrhage into the adrenal gland, neoplasms, and infections (histoplasmosis, cytomegalovirus). Rarely, a family history of autoimmune disease predisposes the patient to Addison's disease and other endocrinopathies.

Secondary hypofunction

This type of hypofunction, which results in glucocorticoid deficiency, can stem from hypopituitarism (causing decreased corticotropin secretion), abrupt withdrawal of long-term corticosteroid therapy (long-term exogenous corticosteroid stimulation suppresses pituitary corticotropin secretion and results in adrenal gland atrophy), or the removal of a nonendocrine, corticotropin-secreting tumor.

Adrenal crisis

Following trauma, surgery, or other physiologic stress, adrenal crisis exhausts the body's stores of glucocorticoids in a person with adrenal hypofunction.

Signs and symptoms

Clinical features vary with the type of adrenal hypofunction.

Primary hypofunction

Addison's disease typically produces such effects as weakness, fatigue, weight loss, and various GI disturbances, such as nausea, vomiting, anorexia, and chronic diarrhea.

The disorder also usually causes a conspicuous bronze coloration of the skin. The patient appears to be deeply suntanned, especially in the creases of the hands and over the metacarpophalangeal joints, the elbows, and the knees. He also may exhibit a darkening of scars, areas of vitiligo (absence of pigmentation), and increased pigmentation of the mucous membranes, especially the buccal mucosa. Such abnormal skin and mucous membrane coloration results from decreased secretion of cortisol (one of the glucocorticoids), which causes the pituitary gland to simultaneously secrete excessive amounts of corticotropin and melanocyte-stimulating hormone (MSH).

Associated cardiovascular abnormalities in Addison's disease include orthostatic hypotension, decreased cardiac size and output, and a weak, irregular pulse.

Other clinical effects include decreased tolerance for even minor stress, poor coordination, fasting hypoglycemia (due to decreased gluconeogenesis), and a craving for salty food. Addison's disease may also retard axillary and pubic hair growth in females, decrease the libido (from decreased androgen production) and, in severe cases, cause amenorrhea.

Secondary hypofunction

This form of hypofunction produces similar clinical effects to primary hypofunction, but without hyperpigmentation because corticotropin and MSH levels are low. Because aldosterone secretion may continue at fairly normal levels in secondary adrenal hypofunction, this condition doesn't necessarily cause accompanying hypotension and electrolyte abnormalities.

Adrenal crisis

Producing profound weakness, adrenal crisis also causes fatigue, nausea, vomiting, hypotension, dehydration, and occasionally, high fever followed by hypothermia. If untreated, this condition can ultimately lead to vascular collapse, renal shutdown, coma, and death.

Diagnosis

Measurement of plasma cortisol levels confirms adrenal insufficiency. If secondary adrenal hypofunction is suspected, the metyrapone test is indicated.

The *metyrapone test* requires oral or I.V. administration of metyrapone, which blocks cortisol production and should stimulate the release of corticotropin from the hypothalamic-pituitary system. In Addison's disease, the hypothalamic-pituitary system responds normally, and plasma reveals high levels of corticotropin; however, plasma levels of cortisol precursor and urinary concentrations of 17-hydroxycorticosteroids don't rise. If either primary or secondary adrenal hypofunction is suspected, a corticotropin stimulation test is indicated.

The *corticotropin stimulation test* involves I.V. administration of corticotropin over 6 to 8 hours, after samples have been obtained to determine baseline plasma cortisol and 24-hour urine cortisol levels. In Addison's disease, plasma and urine cortisol levels fail to rise normally in response to corticotropin; in secondary hypofunction, repeated doses of corticotropin over successive days produce a gradual increase in cortisol levels until normal values are reached.

In a patient with typical addisonian symptoms, the following laboratory findings strongly suggest acute adrenal insufficiency:

• decreased cortisol levels in plasma (less than 10 μg/dl in the morning, with lower levels in the evening); however, this test is time-consuming, and emergency therapy shouldn't be postponed for test results

• decreased serum sodium and fasting blood glucose levels

• increased serum potassium and blood urea nitrogen levels

• elevated hematocrit levels and lymphocyte and eosinophil counts

• X-rays showing a small heart and adrenal calcification.

Treatment

For all patients with primary or secondary adrenal hypofunction, lifelong corticosteroid replacement, usually with cortisone or hydrocortisone (both of which also have a mineralocorticoid effect), is the primary treatment.

Addison's disease may also necessitate treatment with I.V. desoxycorticosterone, a pure mineralocorticoid, or oral fludrocortisone, a synthetic mineralocorticoid; both prevent dangerous dehydration and hypotension. (See *Avoiding adrenal crisis.*)

Adrenal crisis requires prompt I.V. bolus administration of 100 mg hydrocortisone. Later, 50- to 100-mg doses are given I.M. or are diluted with dextrose in saline solution and given I.V. until the patient's condition stabilizes; up to 300 mg/day of hydrocortisone and 3 to 5 L of I.V. saline solution may be required during the acute stage of adrenal crisis.

With proper treatment, adrenal crisis usually subsides quickly; the patient's blood pressure should stabilize, and water and sodium levels should return to normal. After the crisis, maintenance doses of hydrocortisone preserve physiologic stability.

Special considerations

• In adrenal crisis, monitor vital signs carefully, especially for hypotension, volume depletion, and other signs of shock (decreased level of consciousness and urine output). Watch for hyperkalemia before treatment and for hypokalemia after treatment (from excessive mineralocorticoid effect).

• If the patient also has diabetes, check blood glucose periodically because steroid replacement may necessitate adjustment of insulin dosage.

• Record weight and intake and output carefully because the patient may have volume depletion. Until onset of mineralocorticoid effect, force fluids to replace excessive fluid loss.

To manage the patient receiving maintenance therapy:

• Advise the patient to watch for symptoms of adrenal crisis and tell how to provide the necessary self-care upon discharge from the hospital.

• Arrange for a diet that maintains sodium and potassium balances.

• If the patient is anorectic, suggest six small meals a day to increase caloric intake. Ask the dietitian to provide a diet high in protein and carbohy-

drates. Keep a late-morning snack available in case the patient becomes hypoglycemic.

• Observe the patient receiving steroids for cushingoid signs, such as fluid retention around the eyes and face. Watch for fluid and electrolyte imbalance, especially if the patient is receiving mineralocorticoids. Monitor weight and check blood pressure to assess body fluid status. Be aware that steroids administered in the late afternoon or evening may cause stimulation of the central nervous system and insomnia in some patients. Check for petechiae because the patient bruises easily.

• If the patient receives glucocorticoids alone, observe for orthostatic hypotension or electrolyte abnormalities, which may indicate a need for mineralocorticoid therapy.

ADRENOGENITAL SYNDROME

Dysfunctional biosynthesis of adrenocortical steroids leads to adrenogenital syndrome. This syndrome may be inherited (congenital adrenal hyperplasia [CAH]) or acquired, usually as a result of an adrenal tumor (adrenal virilism). Salt-losing CAH may cause fatal adrenal crisis in neonates.

Causes

CAH is the most prevalent adrenal disorder in infants and children; simple virilizing CAH and salt-losing CAH are the most common forms. Acquired adrenal virilism is rare and affects females twice as often as males.

CAH is transmitted as an autosomal recessive trait that causes deficiencies in the enzymes needed for adrenocortical secretion of cortisol and, possibly, aldosterone. Compensatory secretion of corticotropin produces varying degrees of adrenal hyperplasia.

Simple virilizing CAH

In simple virilizing CAH, deficiency of the enzyme 21-hydroxylase results in underproduction of cortisol. In turn, this cortisol deficiency stimulates increased secretion of corticotropin, producing large amounts of cortisol precursors and androgens that don't require 21-hydroxylase for synthesis.

Salt-losing CAH

In salt-losing CAH, 21-hydroxylase is almost completely absent. Corticotropin secretion increases, causing excessive production of cortisol precursors, including salt-wasting compounds. However, plasma cortisol levels and aldosterone — both dependent on 21-hydroxylase — fall precipitously and, in combination with the excessive production of salt-wasting compounds, precipitate acute adrenal crisis. Corticotropin hypersecretion stimulates adrenal androgens, possibly even more than in simple virilizing CAH, and produces masculinization.

Other rare CAH enzyme deficiencies exist and lead to increased or decreased production of affected hormones.

Signs and symptoms

The following features characterize simple virilizing CAH and salt-losing CAH.

Simple virilizing CAH

The newborn female with this condition has ambiguous genitalia (an enlarged clitoris, with the urethral opening at the base, and some labioscrotal fusion) but a normal genital tract and gonads. As she grows older, signs of progressive virilization develop: early appearance of pubic and axillary hair, deep voice, acne, and facial hair.

The newborn male with this condition has no obvious abnormality; however, at prepuberty he shows accentuated masculine characteristics, such as deepened voice and an enlarged phallus, with frequent erections.

At puberty, females fail to begin menstruation, and males have small testes. Both males and females with this condition may be taller than other children their age due to rapid bone and muscle growth, but since excessive androgen levels hasten epiphyseal closure, abnormally short adult stature results.

Salt-losing CAH

In females, this condition causes more complete virilization than the simple form and results in development of male external genitalia without testes. Because males with this condition have no external genital abnormalities, immediate neonatal diagnosis is difficult, and is commonly delayed until the infant develops severe systemic symptoms. Characteristically, such an infant is apathetic, fails to eat, and has diarrhea; he develops symptoms of adrenal crisis in the first week of life (vomiting, dehydration from hyponatremia, hyperkalemia).

Unless CAH is treated promptly, dehydration and hyperkalemia may lead to cardiovascular collapse and cardiac arrest.

Diagnosis

A physical examination that reveals pseudohermaphroditism in females or precocious puberty in both sexes strongly suggests CAH.

The following laboratory findings confirm the diagnosis:
• elevated plasma 17-ketosteroid (17-KS) levels, which can be suppressed by administering oral dexamethasone

• elevated urinary metabolites of hormones, particularly pregnanetriol
• elevated plasma 17-hydroxyprogesterone levels
• normal or decreased urinary levels of 17-hydroxycorticosteroids.

Adrenal hypofunction or adrenal crisis in the first week of life suggests salt-losing CAH. Hyperkalemia, hyponatremia, and hypochloremia with excessive urinary 17-KS and pregnanetriol and decreased urinary aldosterone levels confirm it.

Treatment
In adrenogenital syndrome, treatment depends on the form of the disease.

Simple virilizing CAH
Effective treatment for simple virilizing CAH requires correction of the cortisol deficiency and inhibition of excessive pituitary corticotropin production by daily administration of cortisone or hydrocortisone. Such treatment returns androgen production to normal levels. Measurement of urinary 17-KS levels determines the initial dose of cortisone or hydrocortisone; this dose is usually large and is given I.M. Later, dosage is modified according to decreasing urinary 17-KS levels. Infants must continue to receive cortisone or hydrocortisone I.M. until age 18 months; after that, they may take it orally.

Salt-losing CAH
The infant with salt-losing CAH in adrenal crisis requires an immediate I.V. infusion of sodium chloride and glucose to maintain fluid and electrolyte balance and to stabilize vital signs. If the saline and glucose infusion doesn't control symptoms while the diagnosis is being established, desoxycorticosterone I.M. and hydrocortisone I.V. are necessary. Later, maintenance includes mineralocorticoid (desoxycorticosterone, fludrocortisone, or both) and glucocorticoid (cortisone or hydrocortisone) replacement.

Sex chromatin and karyotype studies determine the genetic sex of patients with ambiguous external genitalia. Females with masculine external genitalia require reconstructive surgery. Such surgery is usually scheduled between ages 1 and 3, after the effect of cortisone therapy has been assessed.

Special considerations
• Suspect CAH in infants hospitalized for failure to thrive, dehydration, or diarrhea, as well as in tall, sturdy-looking children with a record of numerous episodic illnesses.
• When caring for an infant with adrenal crisis, keep the I.V. line patent, infuse fluids, and give steroids.
• Carefully monitor the patient's body weight, blood pressure, and serum electrolyte levels, especially sodium and potassium levels.
• Watch for cyanosis, hypotension, tachycardia, tachypnea, and signs of shock. Keep external stress to a minimum.
• If the child is receiving maintenance therapy with steroid injections, rotate I.M. injection sites to prevent atrophy; tell parents to do the same. Teach them the possible side effects (cushingoid symptoms) of long-term therapy.
• Explain that maintenance therapy with hydrocortisone, cortisone, or the mineralocorticoid fludrocortisone is essential for life. Warn parents not to withdraw these drugs suddenly because potentially fatal adrenal insufficiency will result.
• Instruct parents to report stress and infection, which require increased steroid dosages.
• Monitor the patient receiving desoxycorticosterone or fludrocortisone for edema, weakness, and hypertension. Be alert for significant weight gain and rapid changes in height because

normal growth is an important indicator of adequate therapy.

• Instruct the patient to wear a medical identification bracelet indicating that he's on prolonged steroid therapy and providing information about dosage.

• Help parents of a female infant with male genitalia to understand that the child is physiologically a female and that this abnormality can be surgically corrected. Arrange for counseling if necessary.

LIFE-THREATENING DISORDER

ADULT RESPIRATORY DISTRESS SYNDROME

A form of pulmonary edema that causes acute respiratory failure, adult respiratory distress syndrome (ARDS, shock lung, stiff lung) results from increased permeability of the alveolar capillary membrane. Fluid accumulates in the lung interstitium, alveolar spaces, and small airways, causing the lung to stiffen. Effective ventilation is thus impaired, prohibiting adequate oxygenation of pulmonary capillary blood. Severe ARDS can cause intractable and fatal hypoxemia; however, patients who recover may have little or no permanent lung damage.

Causes
ARDS results from a variety of respiratory and nonrespiratory insults, such as:

• aspiration of gastric contents
• sepsis (primarily gram-negative), trauma (lung contusion, head injury, long bone fracture with fat emboli) or oxygen toxicity
• viral, bacterial, or fungal pneumonia or microemboli (fat or air emboli or disseminated intravascular coagulation)
• drug overdose (barbiturates, glutethimide, narcotics) or blood transfusion
• smoke or chemical inhalation (nitrous oxide, chlorine, ammonia)
• hydrocarbon and paraquat ingestion
• pancreatitis, uremia, or miliary tuberculosis (rare)
• near-drowning.

Altered permeability of the alveolar capillary membranes causes fluid to accumulate in the interstitial space. If the pulmonary lymphatics can't remove this fluid, interstitial edema develops. The fluid collects in the peribronchial and peribronchiolar spaces, producing bronchiolar narrowing.

Hypoxemia occurs as a result of fluid accumulation in alveoli and subsequent alveolar collapse, causing the shunting of blood through nonventilated lung regions. In addition, regional differences in compliance and airway narrowing cause regions of low ventilation and inadequate perfusion, which also contribute to hypoxemia.

Signs and symptoms
ARDS initially produces rapid, shallow breathing and dyspnea within hours to days of the initial injury (sometimes after the patient's condition appears stable). Hypoxemia develops, causing an increased drive for ventilation. Because of the effort required to expand the stiff lung, intercostal and suprasternal retractions result. Fluid accumulation produces crackles and rhonchi, and worsening hypoxemia causes restlessness, apprehension, mental sluggishness, motor dysfunction, and tachycardia (possibly with transient increased arterial blood pressure).

Severe ARDS causes overwhelming hypoxemia which, if uncorrected, results in hypotension, decreasing urine output, respiratory and metabolic acidosis and, eventually, ventricular fibrillation or standstill.

Diagnosis

• On room air, *arterial blood gas (ABG) analysis* initially shows a decreased partial pressure of arterial oxygen (PaO_2) — less than 60 mm Hg — and a decreased partial pressure of arterial carbon dioxide ($PaCO_2$) — less than 35 mm Hg. The resulting pH usually reflects respiratory alkalosis. As ARDS becomes more severe, ABG levels indicate respiratory acidosis (a $PaCO_2$ above 45 mm Hg) and metabolic acidosis (a bicarbonate level less than 22 mEq/L) and a decreasing PaO_2 despite oxygen therapy.

• *Pulmonary artery catheterization* helps identify the cause of pulmonary edema by evaluating pulmonary artery wedge pressure (PAWP); allows collection of pulmonary artery blood, which shows decreased oxygen saturation, reflecting tissue hypoxia; measures pulmonary artery pressure; and measures cardiac output by thermodilution techniques.

• *Serial chest X-rays* initially show bilateral infiltrates; in later stages, ground-glass appearance, and eventually (as hypoxemia becomes irreversible), "whiteouts" of both lung fields.

A differential diagnosis must rule out cardiogenic pulmonary edema, pulmonary vasculitis, and diffuse pulmonary hemorrhage. To establish etiology, laboratory work should include a sputum Gram stain, culture and sensitivity tests, and blood cultures to detect infections; a toxicology screen for drug ingestion; and, when pancreatitis is a consideration, a serum amylase determination.

Treatment

When possible, treatment is designed to correct the underlying cause of ARDS and to prevent progression and potentially fatal complications of hypoxemia and respiratory acidosis. Supportive medical care consists of administering humidified oxygen by a tight-fitting mask, which allows for use of continuous positive airway pressure (CPAP). Hypoxemia that doesn't respond adequately to these measures requires ventilatory support with intubation, volume ventilation, and positive end-expiratory pressure (PEEP). Other supportive measures include fluid restriction, diuretics, and correction of electrolyte and acid-base abnormalities.

When ARDS requires mechanical ventilation, sedatives, narcotics, or neuromuscular blocking agents, such as tubocurarine or pancuronium bromide, may be ordered to minimize restlessness and thereby oxygen consumption and carbon dioxide production, and to facilitate ventilation.

If ARDS results from fat emboli or chemical injuries to the lungs, a short course of high-dose steroids may help if given early. Treatment to reverse severe metabolic acidosis with sodium bicarbonate may be necessary, and use of fluids and vasopressors may be required to maintain blood pressure. Infections require antimicrobial drugs, if treatable.

Special considerations

• Frequently assess the patient's respiratory status. Be alert for retractions on inspiration. Note rate, rhythm, and depth of respirations, and watch for dyspnea and the use of accessory muscles of respiration. On auscultation, listen for adventitious or diminished breath sounds. Check for clear, frothy sputum that may indicate pulmonary edema.

• Observe and document the hypoxemic patient's neurologic status (level of consciousness, mental sluggishness).

• Maintain a patent airway by suctioning, using sterile, nontraumatic technique. Ensure adequate humidification to help liquefy tenacious secretions.

• Closely monitor heart rate and blood pressure. Watch for arrhythmias that may result from hypoxemia, acid-base disturbances, or electrolyte imbalance.

• With pulmonary artery catheterization, know the desired PAWP level; check readings often and watch for decreasing mixed venous oxygen saturation.

• Monitor serum electrolyte levels and correct any imbalances. Measure intake and output, and weigh the patient daily.

• Check ventilator settings frequently, and empty condensate from tubing promptly to ensure maximum oxygen delivery. Monitor ABG studies; check for metabolic and respiratory acidosis and PaO_2 changes.

• The patient with severe hypoxemia may need controlled mechanical ventilation with PEEP. Give sedatives, as needed, to reduce restlessness.

• Because PEEP may decrease cardiac output, check for hypotension, tachycardia, and decreased urine output. Suction only as needed so that PEEP is maintained, or use an in-line suctioning apparatus.

• Reposition the patient often and note any increase in secretions, temperature, or hypotension that may indicate a deteriorating condition.

• Accurately record caloric intake. Give tube feedings and parenteral nutrition, if required.

• Perform passive range-of-motion exercises, or help the patient perform active exercises, if possible. Provide meticulous skin care. Allow periods of uninterrupted sleep.

• Provide emotional support. Warn the patient who's recovering from ARDS that recovery will take some time and that he will feel weak for a while.

• Watch for all respiratory changes in the patient who has suffered injuries that may adversely affect the lungs, especially during the 2- to 3-day period after the injury, when he may appear to be improving.

ALCOHOLISM

A chronic disorder, alcoholism is usually described as an uncontrolled intake of alcoholic beverages that interferes with physical and mental health, social and familial relationships, and occupational responsibilities. Alcoholism cuts across all social and economic groups, involves both sexes, and occurs at all stages of the life cycle, beginning as early as elementary school age. About 13% of all adults over age 18 have suffered from alcohol abuse or dependence at some time in their lives.

Drinking is most prevalent between the ages of 21 and 34, but current statistics show that up to 19% of 12- to 17-year-olds have a serious drinking problem. Males are two to five times more likely to abuse alcohol than are females. According to some statistics, alcohol abuse is a factor in 60% of all automobile accidents.

Causes
Numerous biological, psychological, and sociocultural factors appear to be involved in alcohol addiction. An offspring of one alcoholic parent is seven to eight times more likely to become an alcoholic than is a peer without such a parent. Biological factors may include genetic or biochemical abnormalities, nutritional deficiencies, endocrine imbalances, and allergic responses.

Psychological factors may include the urge to drink alcohol to reduce anxiety or symptoms of mental illness; the desire to avoid responsibility in familial, social, and work relationships; and the need to bolster self-esteem.

Sociocultural factors include the availability of alcoholic beverages, group or peer pressure, an excessively stressful lifestyle, and social attitudes that approve of frequent drinking.

Signs and symptoms

Because people with alcohol dependence may hide or deny their addiction and may temporarily manage to maintain a functional life, assessing for alcoholism can be difficult.

Physical and psychosocial symptoms

• The patient's history may suggest a need for daily or episodic alcohol use to maintain adequate functioning, an inability to discontinue or reduce alcohol intake, episodes of anesthesia or amnesia (blackouts) during intoxication, episodes of violence during intoxication, and interference with social and familial relationships and occupational responsibilities.

• Many minor complaints may be alcohol-related. The patient may mention malaise, dyspepsia, mood swings or depression, and an increased incidence of infection. Observe the patient for poor personal hygiene and untreated injuries, such as cigarette burns, fractures, and bruises, that he can't fully explain. Note any evidence of an unusually high tolerance for sedatives and narcotics.

• Watch for secretive behavior. Suspect alcoholism if the patient uses inordinate amounts of after-shave lotion or mouthwash. When confronted, the patient may deny or rationalize the problem. Alternatively, he may be guarded or hostile in his response and may even sign out of the hospital against medical advice. He also may project his anger or feelings of guilt or inadequacy onto others to avoid confronting his illness.

• Chronic alcohol abuse brings with it an array of physical complications, including malnutrition, cirrhosis of the liver, peripheral neuropathy, brain damage, and cardiomyopathy. Watch for these complications in a patient with an alcohol-related disorder.

• After abstinence or reduction of alcohol intake, signs and symptoms of withdrawal—which begin shortly after drinking has stopped and last for 5 to 7 days—may vary. The patient initially experiences anorexia, nausea, anxiety, fever, insomnia, diaphoresis, and tremor, progressing to severe tremulousness, agitation and, possibly, hallucinations and violent behavior. Major motor seizures (known as "rum fits") can occur during withdrawal. Suspect alcoholism in any patient with unexplained seizures.

Diagnosis

For characteristic findings in patients with alcoholism, see *Diagnosing substance dependence and related disorders,* page 296.

Clinical findings may help support the diagnosis of alcoholism. For example, laboratory tests can confirm alcohol use and complications and document recent alcohol ingestion, as follows:

• *Blood alcohol level* of 0.10% weight/ volume (200 mg/dl) is accepted as the level of intoxication.

• *Blood urea nitrogen level* rises in severe hepatic disease.

• *Serum glucose level* is decreased.

• *Serum ammonia and amylase levels* are increased.

• *Urine toxicology studies* may help detect other types of drug abuse in patients with alcohol withdrawal delirium or another acute complication.

• *Liver function studies* reveal increased levels of serum cholesterol, lactate dehydrogenase, alanine aminotransferase, aspartate aminotransferase, and creatine kinase, which in-

HAZARD

AVOIDING THE RISKS OF DISULFIRAM THERAPY

Disulfiram acts by interfering with alcohol metabolism, which allows toxic levels of acetaldehyde to accumulate in the patient's blood.

Disulfiram can produce immediate and potentially fatal distress if the patient consumes alcohol up to 2 weeks after taking it.

Disulfiram is contraindicated during pregnancy and in patients with diabetes, heart disease, severe hepatic disease, or any disorder in which such a reaction could be especially dangerous.

---

dicate liver damage, and elevated serum amylase and lipase levels, which point to acute pancreatitis.

• *Blood studies* may identify anemia, thrombocytopenia, increased prothrombin time, and increased partial thromboplastin time.

Treatment

Total abstinence from alcohol is the only effective treatment. Supportive programs that offer detoxification, rehabilitation, and aftercare, including continued involvement in Alcoholics Anonymous (AA), may produce good long-term results.

Acute intoxication is treated symptomatically by supporting respiration, preventing aspiration of vomitus, replacing fluids, administering I.V. glucose to prevent hypoglycemia, correcting hypothermia or acidosis, and initiating emergency treatment for trauma, infection, or GI bleeding.

Treatment of chronic alcoholism relies on medications to deter alcohol use and treat effects of withdrawal; psychotherapy, consisting of behavior modification techniques, group therapy, and family therapy; and appropriate measures to relieve associated physical problems.

Aversion, or deterrent, therapy involves a daily oral dose of disulfiram to prevent compulsive drinking. (See *Avoiding the risks of disulfiram therapy.*)

Another form of aversion therapy attempts to induce aversion by administering alcohol with an emetic.

Aversion therapy with disulfiram may only substitute one drug dependence for another, so it should be used prudently. For long-term success, the recovering individual must learn to fill the place alcohol once occupied in his life with something constructive.

Tranquilizers, particularly the benzodiazepines, occasionally are used to relieve overwhelming anxiety during rehabilitation. However, these drugs have addictive potential (substituting one substance abuse problem for another), and they can precipitate a coma or even death when combined with alcohol.

Phenothiazines and other antipsychotics are prescribed to control hyperactivity and psychosis. Anticonvulsants, antiemetics, and antidiarrheals also are used to treat symptoms of alcohol withdrawal.

Supportive counseling or individual, group, or family psychotherapy may help. Ongoing support groups are also helpful. In AA, a self-help group with more than a million members worldwide, the alcoholic finds emotional support from others with similar problems. About 40% of AA's members stay sober as long as 5 years, and 30% stay sober longer than 5 years.

Special considerations
• During acute intoxication or withdrawal, carefully monitor the patient's mental status, heart rate, breath sounds, blood pressure, and temperature every 30 minutes to 6 hours.
• Examine the patient for signs of inadequate nutrition and dehydration. Institute seizure precautions and administer drugs prescribed to treat the signs and symptoms of withdrawal in chronic alcohol abuse.
• During withdrawal, orient the patient to reality because he may have hallucinations and may try to harm himself or others. Maintain a calm environment, minimizing noise and shadows to reduce the incidence of delusions and hallucinations. Avoid restraining the patient unless necessary to protect him or others.
• Approach the patient in a nonthreatening way. Limit sustained eye contact. Even if he's verbally abusive, listen attentively and respond with empathy. Explain all procedures.
• Monitor the patient for signs of depression or impending suicide.
• In chronic alcoholism, help the patient accept his drinking problem and the necessity for abstinence. Confront him about his behavior, urging him to examine his actions more realistically.
• If the patient is taking disulfiram (or has taken it within the past 2 weeks), warn him of the effects of alcohol ingestion, which may last from 30 minutes to 3 hours or longer. The reaction includes nausea, vomiting, facial flushing, headache, shortness of breath, red eyes, blurred vision, sweating, tachycardia, hypotension, and fainting. Emphasize that even a small amount of alcohol will induce this adverse reaction and that the longer he takes the drug, the greater his sensitivity to alcohol will be. Because of this, he must avoid even medicinal sources of alcohol, such as mouthwash, cough syrups, liquid vitamins, and cold remedies.
• Refer the patient to AA and offer to arrange a visit from an AA member. Stress the effectiveness of this organization.
• For individuals who have lost all contact with family and friends and who have a long history of unemployment, trouble with the law, or other problems associated with alcohol abuse, rehabilitation may involve job training, sheltered workshops, halfway houses, and other supervised facilities.
• Refer spouses of alcoholics to Al-Anon and children of alcoholics to Alateen. By participating in these self-help groups, family members learn to relinquish responsibility for the individual's drinking. Point out that family involvement in rehabilitation can reduce family tensions.
• Refer adult children of alcoholics to the National Association for Children of Alcoholics.

ALLERGIC PURPURA

A type of nonthrombocytopenic purpura, allergic purpura is an acute or chronic vascular inflammation affecting the skin, joints, and GI and genitourinary (GU) tracts in association with allergy symptoms. When allergic purpura primarily affects the GI tract, with accompanying joint pain, it is called Henoch-Schönlein syndrome or anaphylactoid purpura. However, the term *allergic purpura* applies to purpura associated with many other conditions, such as erythema nodosum. An acute attack of allergic purpura can last for several weeks and is potentially fatal (usually from renal failure); however, most patients do recover.

Fully developed allergic purpura is persistent and debilitating, possibly leading to chronic glomerulonephritis (especially following a streptococcal infection). Allergic purpura affects males more often than females and is most prevalent in children ages 3 to 7 years. The prognosis is more favorable for children than adults.

Causes

The most common identifiable cause of allergic purpura is probably an autoimmune reaction directed against vascular walls, triggered by a bacterial infection (particularly streptococcal infection). Typically, upper respiratory infection occurs 1 to 3 weeks before the onset of symptoms. Other possible causes include allergic reactions to some drugs and vaccines; allergic reactions to insect bites; and allergic reactions to some foods (such as wheat, eggs, milk, chocolate).

Signs and symptoms

Allergic purpura produces characteristic purple skin lesions that are macular, ecchymotic, and of varying size and are caused by vascular leakage into the skin and mucous membranes. The lesions usually appear in symmetrical patterns on the arms and legs and are accompanied by pruritus, paresthesia and, occasionally, angioneurotic edema. In children, skin lesions are generally urticarial and expand and become hemorrhagic. Scattered petechiae may appear on the legs, buttocks, and perineum.

Henoch-Schönlein syndrome commonly produces transient or severe colic, tenesmus and constipation, vomiting, and edema or hemorrhage of the mucous membranes of the bowel, resulting in GI bleeding, occult blood in the stools and, possibly, intussusception. Such GI abnormalities may *precede* overt, cutaneous signs of purpura. Musculoskeletal symptoms, such as rheumatoid pains and periarticular effusions, mostly affect the legs and feet.

In 25% to 50% of patients, allergic purpura is associated with GU symptoms: nephritis; renal hemorrhages that may cause microscopic hematuria and disturb renal function; bleeding from the mucosal surfaces of the ureters, bladder, or urethra; and, occasionally, glomerulonephritis. Also possible are moderate and irregular fever, headache, anorexia, and localized edema of the hands, feet, or scalp.

Diagnosis

No laboratory test clearly identifies allergic purpura (although the white blood cell count and erythrocyte sedimentation rate are elevated). Diagnosis therefore requires careful clinical observation, often during the second or third attack. Except for a positive tourniquet test, coagulation and platelet function tests are usually normal. Small-bowel X-rays may reveal areas of transient edema; tests for blood in the urine and stools are often positive. Increased blood urea nitrogen and serum creatinine levels may indicate renal involvement. The diagnosis must rule out other forms of nonthrombocytopenic purpura.

Treatment

In allergic purpura, treatment is generally aimed at relieving symptoms; for example, severe allergic purpura may require steroids to relieve edema and analgesics to relieve joint and abdominal pain. Some patients with chronic renal disease may benefit from immunosuppression with azathioprine, along with identification of the provocative allergen. An accurate allergy history is essential.

Special considerations

• Encourage the patient to maintain an elimination diet to help identify specific allergenic foods so that these foods can be eliminated from the patient's diet.

• Monitor skin lesions and level of pain. Provide analgesics as needed.

• Watch carefully for complications: GI and GU tract bleeding, edema, nausea, vomiting, headache, hypertension (with nephritis), abdominal rigidity and tenderness, and absence of stools (with intussusception).

• To prevent muscle atrophy in the bedridden patient, provide passive or active range-of-motion exercises.

• Provide emotional support and reassurance, especially if the patient is temporarily disfigured by florid skin lesions.

• After the acute stage, stress the need for the patient to *immediately* tell the doctor of *any* recurrence of symptoms (recurrence is most common about 6 weeks after initial onset) and to return for follow-up urinalysis as scheduled.

ALLERGIC RHINITIS

This immune disorder is a reaction to airborne (inhaled) allergens. Depending on the allergen, the resulting rhinitis and conjunctivitis may be seasonal (hay fever) or occur year-round (perennial allergic rhinitis). Allergic rhinitis is the most common atopic allergic reaction, affecting over 20 million Americans. It's most prevalent in young children and adolescents but can occur in all age-groups.

Causes
Hay fever reflects an immunoglobulin E (IgE)–mediated, Type I hypersensitivity response to an environmental antigen (allergen) in a genetically susceptible individual. In most cases, it's induced by wind-borne pollens: in the spring by tree pollens (oak, elm, maple, alder, birch, cottonwood); in the summer by grass pollens (sheep sorrel, English plantain); and in the fall by weed pollens (ragweed). Occasionally, hay fever is induced by allergy to fungal spores.

In perennial allergic rhinitis, inhaled allergens provoke antigen responses that produce recurring symptoms year-round.

The major perennial allergens and irritants include dust mites, feather pillows, mold, cigarette smoke, upholstery, and animal danders. Seasonal pollen allergy may exacerbate symptoms of perennial rhinitis.

Signs and symptoms
In seasonal allergic rhinitis, the key signs and symptoms are paroxysmal sneezing, profuse watery rhinorrhea, nasal obstruction or congestion, and pruritus of the nose and eyes, usually accompanied by pale, cyanotic, edematous nasal mucosa; red and edematous eyelids and conjunctivae; excessive lacrimation; and headache or sinus pain. Some patients also complain of itching in the throat and malaise.

In perennial allergic rhinitis, conjunctivitis and other extranasal effects are rare, but chronic nasal obstruction is common and often extends to eustachian tube obstruction, particularly in children.

In both types of allergic rhinitis, dark circles may appear under the patient's eyes ("allergic shiners") because of venous congestion in the maxillary sinuses. The severity of signs and symptoms may vary from season to season and from year to year.

Some patients may develop chronic complications, including sinusitis and nasal polyps.

Diagnosis
Microscopic examination of sputum and nasal secretions reveals large numbers of eosinophils. Blood chemistry studies show normal or elevated

IgE levels. A firm diagnosis rests on the patient's personal and family history of allergies and on physical findings during a symptomatic phase. Skin testing, paired with tested responses to environmental stimuli, can pinpoint the responsible allergens when interpreted in light of the patient's history.

To distinguish between allergic rhinitis and other disorders of the nasal mucosa, remember these differences:

• In chronic vasomotor rhinitis, eye symptoms are absent, rhinorrhea is mucoid, and seasonal variation is absent.

• In infectious rhinitis (the common cold), the nasal mucosa is beet red; nasal secretions contain polymorphonuclear, not eosinophilic, exudate; and signs and symptoms include fever and sore throat. This condition is not a recurrent seasonal phenomenon.

• In rhinitis medicamentosa, which results from excessive use of nasal sprays or drops, nasal drainage and mucosal redness and swelling disappear when such medication is withheld.

• In children, a differential diagnosis should rule out a nasal foreign body, such as a bean or a button.

Treatment
Symptoms are controlled by eliminating the environmental antigen, if possible, and by drug therapy and immunotherapy.

Antihistamines block histamine effects but commonly produce anticholinergic adverse effects (sedation, dry mouth, nausea, dizziness, blurred vision, and nervousness).

New antihistamines, such as terfenadine, produce fewer adverse effects and are much less likely to cause sedation. However, cardiac arrhythmias may occur with an overdose.

Inhaled intranasal steroids produce local anti-inflammatory effects with minimal systemic adverse effects. The most commonly used intranasal steroids are flunisolide and beclomethasone. These drugs usually aren't effective for acute exacerbations; nasal decongestants and oral antihistamines may be needed instead.

Advise the patient to use intranasal steroids regularly, as prescribed, for optimal effectiveness. Cromolyn sodium may be helpful in preventing allergic rhinitis. But this drug may take up to 4 weeks to produce a satisfactory effect and must be taken regularly during allergy season.

Long-term management includes immunotherapy or desensitization with injections of extracted allergens administered before or during allergy season or perennially. Seasonal allergies require particularly close dosage regulation.

Special considerations
• When caring for the patient with allergic rhinitis, monitor his compliance with prescribed drug treatment regimen. Also carefully note any changes in the control of his symptoms or any signs of drug misuse.

• Before giving allergen injections, assess the patient's symptom status. Afterward, watch for adverse reactions, including anaphylaxis and severe localized erythema.

• Keep epinephrine and emergency resuscitation equipment available, and observe the patient for 30 minutes after the injection.

• Instruct the patient to call the doctor if a delayed reaction should occur.

• Advise patients to reduce environmental exposure to airborne allergens by sleeping with the windows closed, avoiding the countryside during pollination seasons, using air conditioning to filter allergens and minimize moisture and dust, and eliminating dust-collecting items, such as wool blankets, deep-pile carpets, and heavy drapes, from the home.

• In severe and resistant cases, patients may have to consider drastic changes in lifestyle, such as relocation to a pollen-free area either seasonally or year-round.

ALOPECIA

Hair loss or alopecia usually occurs on the scalp; hair loss elsewhere on the body is less common and less conspicuous. In the nonscarring form of this disorder (noncicatricial alopecia), the hair follicle can generally regrow hair. But scarring alopecia usually destroys the hair follicle, making hair loss irreversible.

Causes
The most common form of nonscarring alopecia is male-pattern alopecia, which appears to be related to androgen levels and to aging. Genetic predisposition commonly influences the time of onset, degree of baldness, speed with which it spreads, and pattern of hair loss. Women may experience diffuse thinning over the top of the scalp.

Other forms of nonscarring alopecia include:
• *physiologic alopecia* (usually temporary): sudden hair loss in infants, loss of straight hairline in adolescents, and diffuse hair loss after childbirth
• *alopecia areata* (idiopathic form): generally reversible and self-limiting; occurs most frequently in young and middle-aged adults of both sexes
• *trichotillomania:* compulsive pulling out of one's own hair; most common in children.

Predisposing factors of nonscarring alopecia also include radiation, many types of drug therapies and drug reactions, bacterial and fungal infections, psoriasis, seborrhea, and endocrine disorders, such as thyroid, parathyroid, and pituitary dysfunctions.

Scarring alopecia causes irreversible hair loss. It may result from physical or chemical trauma or chronic tension on a hair shaft, as occurs in braiding. Diseases that produce alopecia include destructive skin tumors; granulomas; lupus erythematosus; scleroderma; follicular lichen planus; and severe fungal, bacterial, or viral infections, such as kerion, folliculitis, or herpes simplex.

Signs and symptoms
In male-pattern alopecia, hair loss is gradual and usually affects the thinner, shorter, and less pigmented hairs of the frontal and parietal portions of the scalp. In women, hair loss is generally more diffuse; completely bald areas are uncommon but may occur.

Alopecia areata affects small patches of the scalp but may also occur as alopecia totalis, which involves the entire scalp, or as alopecia universalis, which involves the entire body. Although mild erythema may occur initially, affected areas of scalp or skin appear normal. "Exclamation point" hairs (loose hairs with dark, rough, brushlike tips on narrow, less pigmented shafts) occur at the periphery of new patches. Regrowth initially appears as fine, white, downy hair, which is replaced by normal hair. (See *Alopecia areata,* page 36.)

In trichotillomania, patchy, incomplete areas of hair loss with many broken hairs appear on the scalp but may occur on other areas such as the eyebrows.

Diagnosis
Physical examination is usually sufficient to confirm alopecia. In trichotillomania, an occlusive dressing can establish a diagnosis by allowing new hair to grow, revealing that the hair is being

ALOPECIA AREATA

"Exclamation point" hairs often border new patches of alopecia areata. Not seen in any other type of alopecia, these hairs indicate the patch is expanding.

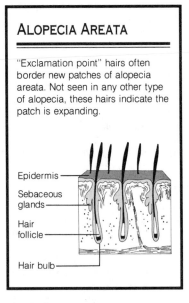

Epidermis

Sebaceous glands

Hair follicle

Hair bulb

pulled out. The diagnosis must also identify any underlying disorder.

Treatment

Topical application of minoxidil, a peripheral vasodilator more typically used as an oral antihypertensive, has had limited success in treating male-pattern alopecia. An alternate treatment is surgical redistribution of hair follicles by autografting.

In alopecia areata, minoxidil is more effective, although treatment is often unnecessary because spontaneous regrowth is common. Intralesional corticosteroid injections are beneficial for small patches and may produce regrowth in 4 to 6 weeks. Hair loss that persists for over a year has a poor prognosis for regrowth.

In trichotillomania, an occlusive dressing encourages normal hair growth simply by identifying the cause of hair loss. Treatment of other types of alopecia varies according to the underlying cause.

Special considerations

• Reassure a woman with female-pattern alopecia that it doesn't lead to total baldness. Suggest that she wear a wig.

• If the patient has alopecia areata, explain the disorder and give reassurance that complete regrowth is possible.

ALZHEIMER'S DISEASE

Also known as *primary degenerative dementia,* Alzheimer's disease accounts for over half of all dementias. An estimated 5% of people over age 65 have a severe form of this disease, and 12% suffer from mild to moderate dementia. Because this is a primary progressive dementia, the prognosis for a patient with this disease is poor.

Causes

Alzheimer's disease is thought to be related to several causal factors. These include *neurochemical factors,* such as deficiencies in acetylcholine, (a neurotransmitter), somatostatin, substance P, and norepinephrine; *environmental factors,* such as aluminum and manganese; *viral factors,* such as slow-growing central nervous system viruses; *trauma;* and *genetic immunologic factors.*

The brain tissue of patients with Alzheimer's disease has three hallmark features: neurofibrillary tangles, neuritic plaques, and granulovascular degeneration.

Signs and symptoms

Onset is insidious. Initially, the patient experiences almost imperceptible changes, such as forgetfulness, recent memory loss, difficulty learning and remembering new information, deterioration in personal hygiene and appearance, and an inability to concentrate. Gradually, tasks that require abstract thinking and activities that require judgment become more difficult. Progressive and severe deterioration in memory, language, and motor function results in a loss of coordination and an inability to write or speak.

Personality changes (restlessness, irritability) and nocturnal awakenings are common. Eventually, the patient becomes disoriented, and physical and intellectual lability and physical and intellectual disability progress. The patient becomes very susceptible to infection and accidents. Usually, death results from infection.

Diagnosis

Early diagnosis of Alzheimer's disease is difficult because the patient's signs and symptoms are subtle. A positive diagnosis is based on an accurate history from a reliable family member, mental status and neurologic examinations, and psychometric testing.

A positron emission tomography scan measures the metabolic activity of the cerebral cortex and may help in reaching an early diagnosis. An EEG and a computed tomography scan may help in later diagnosis.

Currently, the disease is diagnosed by exclusion: Various tests are performed to rule out other disorders. It cannot be confirmed until death, when an autopsy reveals pathologic findings.

Treatment

Cerebral vasodilators, such as ergoloid mesylates, isoxsuprine, and cyclandelate, are prescribed to enhance the brain's circulation; hyperbaric oxygen to increase oxygenation to the brain; psychostimulators, such as methylphenidate, to enhance the patient's mood; and antidepressants, if depression seems to exacerbate the patient's dementia. Tacrine, a centrally acting an-

ticholinesterase agent, is given to treat memory deficits.

Most drug therapies currently being used are experimental. These include choline salts, lecithin, physostigmine, deanol, enkephalins, and naloxone, which may slow the disease process. Another approach to treatment includes avoiding antacids, use of aluminum cooking utensils, and aluminum-containing deodorants to help decrease aluminum intake.

Special considerations

• Overall care focuses on supporting the patient's abilities and compensating for those abilities he has lost.
• Establish an effective communication system with the patient and his family to help them adjust to the patient's altered cognitive abilities.
• Offer emotional support to the patient and family. Teach them about the disease, and refer them to social service and community resources for legal and financial advice and support.
• Provide the patient with a a safe environment. Encourage him to exercise to help maintain mobility.

LIFE-THREATENING DISORDER

AMPUTATION, TRAUMATIC

This type of injury involves accidental loss of a body part, usually a finger, toe, arm, or leg. In complete amputation, the member is totally severed; in partial amputation, some soft-tissue connection remains.

The prognosis has improved as a result of early improved emergency and critical care management, new surgical techniques, early rehabilitation, prosthesis fitting, and new prosthesis design. New limb reimplantation techniques have been moderately successful, but incomplete nerve regeneration remains a major limiting factor.

Causes
Traumatic amputations usually result directly from accidents at the factory or farm, or from power tools or motor vehicle accidents.

Assessment
Every traumatic amputee requires careful monitoring of vital signs. If amputation involves more than just a finger or toe, assessment of airway, breathing, and circulation is also required. Because profuse bleeding is likely, watch for signs of hypovolemic shock, and draw blood for hemoglobin, hematocrit, and typing and crossmatching. In partial amputation, check for pulses distal to the amputation. After any traumatic amputation, assess for other traumatic injuries as well.

Treatment
Because the greatest immediate threat after traumatic amputation is blood loss and hypovolemic shock, emergency treatment consists of local measures to control bleeding, fluid replacement with normal saline solution and colloids, and blood replacement as needed.

Reimplantation remains controversial, but it's becoming more common and successful because of advances in microsurgery. If reconstruction or reimplantation is possible, surgical intervention attempts to preserve usable joints. When arm or leg amputations are done, the surgeon creates a stump to be fitted with a prosthesis. A rigid dressing permits early prosthesis fitting and rehabilitation.

Special considerations
• During emergency treatment, monitor vital signs (especially in hypovolemic shock); cleanse the wound; and give tetanus prophylaxis, analgesics, and antibiotics as needed.
• After complete amputation, wrap the amputated part in a dry sterile towel, and put it in a plastic bag. Keep the bag cool but not cold enough to damage or freeze the amputated part. Flush the wound with sterile saline solution, apply a sterile pressure dressing, and elevate the limb. Notify the reimplantation team.
• After partial amputation, position the limb in normal alignment, and drape it with towels or dressings soaked in sterile normal saline solution.
• Preoperative care includes thorough wound irrigation and debridement (using a local nerve block).
• Postoperative dressing changes using sterile technique help prevent skin infection and ensure skin graft viability.
• Help the amputee cope with his altered body image. Reinforce exercises and prevent stump trauma.

AMYLOIDOSIS

A rare, chronic disease, amyloidosis results in the accumulation of an abnormal fibrillar scleroprotein (amyloid), which infiltrates body organs and soft tissues. Amyloidosis is classified in two ways, based on histologic findings: the *perireticular type,* which affects the inner coats of blood vessels, and the *pericollagen type,* which affects the outer coats of blood vessels and also involves the parenchyma.

Although the prognosis varies with type and with the site and extent of involvement, amyloidosis sometimes results in permanent — usually even life-threatening — organ damage.

Causes

Amyloidosis is sometimes familial, especially in people of Portuguese ancestry. It may occur in conjunction with tuberculosis, chronic infection, rheumatoid arthritis, multiple myeloma, Hodgkin's disease, paraplegia, and brucellosis. It may also accompany Alzheimer's disease.

In amyloidosis, accumulation and infiltration of amyloid produces pressure and causes atrophy of nearby cells. Reticuloendothelial cell dysfunction and abnormal immunoglobulin synthesis occur in some types of amyloidosis. In the United States, evidence of amyloidosis on autopsy is 0.5%, but true incidence is difficult to determine.

Signs and symptoms

Amyloidosis produces dysfunction of the kidneys, heart, GI tract, peripheral nerves, and liver.

• *Kidneys.* The primary sign of renal involvement is proteinuria, leading to nephrotic syndrome and eventual renal failure.

• *Heart.* Amyloidosis often causes intractable congestive heart failure due to amyloid deposits in the subendocardium, endocardium, and myocardium.

• *GI tract.* Amyloidosis may produce stiffness and enlargement of the tongue, hindering enunciation. In addition, it may decrease intestinal motility and produce malabsorption, bleeding, infiltration of blood vessel walls, abdominal pain, constipation, and diarrhea. Tumorlike amyloid deposits may occur in all portions of this system. Chronic malabsorption may lead to malnutrition and predispose to infection.

• *Peripheral nervous system.* The appearance of peripheral neuropathy indicates peripheral nerve involvement.

• *Liver.* Hepatic amyloidosis is rare and usually coexists with other forms of this disease. It generally produces liver enlargement, often with azotemia, anemia, albuminuria and, rarely, jaundice.

Diagnosis

Histologic examination of a tissue biopsy specimen, using a polarizing or electron microscope, is often diagnostic. Rectal mucosa biopsy and abdominal fat pad aspiration are the best screening tests because they are less hazardous than a kidney or liver biopsy. Other biopsy sites include the gingiva, skin, and nerves.

In cardiac amyloidosis, other findings include faint heart sounds and an electrocardiogram showing low voltage and conduction or rhythm abnormalities resembling those characteristic of myocardial infarction. In hepatic amyloidosis, liver function studies are generally normal except for slightly elevated serum alkaline phosphatase levels.

Treatment

Kidney transplantation may be useful for amyloidosis-induced renal failure, although the donor kidney may also develop amyloidosis. Patients with cardiac amyloidosis require conservative treatment to prevent dangerous arrhythmias. Malnutrition caused by malabsorption in end-stage GI involvement may require total parenteral nutrition.

Special considerations

• Maintain nutrition and fluid balance; give analgesics to relieve intestinal pain; control constipation or diarrhea; and take steps to control infection and fever.

• Provide good mouth care for the patient with tongue involvement. Refer him for speech therapy, if needed; provide an alternate method of communication if he can't talk.

• Regularly assess airway patency when the tongue is involved, and prevent respiratory tract compromise by gentle and adequate suctioning, when indicated. Keep a tracheostomy tray available.

• When long-term bed rest is necessary, properly position the patient, and turn him often to prevent pressure ulcers. Perform range-of-motion exercises to prevent contractures.

• Provide psychological support to help the patient cope with this chronic illness.

AMYOTROPHIC LATERAL SCLEROSIS

Commonly called *Lou Gehrig's disease,* after the New York Yankees first baseman who died of this disorder, amyotrophic lateral sclerosis (ALS) is the most common of the motor neuron diseases causing muscular atrophy. Other motor neuron diseases include progressive muscular atrophy and progressive bulbar palsy. Onset occurs between ages 40 and 70. A chronic, progressively debilitating disease, ALS is rapidly fatal.

Causes

More than 30,000 Americans have ALS; about 5,000 new cases are diagnosed each year, with men affected three times more often than women. The exact cause of ALS is unknown, but about 5% to 10% of ALS cases have a genetic component. In these, it is an autosomal dominant trait and affects men and women equally.

ALS and other motor neuron diseases may result from:

• a slow-acting virus
• nutritional deficiency related to a disturbance in enzyme metabolism

• metabolic interference in nucleic acid production by the nerve fibers
• autoimmune disorders that affect immune complexes in the renal glomerulus and basement membrane.

Precipitating factors for acute deterioration include trauma, viral infections, and physical exhaustion. Disorders that must be differentiated from ALS include central nervous system syphilis, multiple sclerosis, spinal cord tumors, and syringomyelia.

Signs and symptoms

Patients with ALS develop fasciculations, accompanied by atrophy and weakness, especially in the muscles of the forearms and the hands. Other signs include impaired speech; difficulty chewing, swallowing, and breathing, particularly if the brain stem is affected; and, occasionally, choking and excessive drooling.

Mental deterioration doesn't usually occur, but patients may become depressed as a reaction to the disease. Progressive bulbar palsy may cause crying spells or inappropriate laughter.

Diagnosis

Characteristic clinical features indicate a combination of upper and lower motor neuron involvement without sensory impairment. Electromyography and a muscle biopsy help show nerve, rather than muscle, disease. The protein content of cerebrospinal fluid is increased in one-third of patients, but this finding alone doesn't confirm ALS.

Diagnosis must rule out multiple sclerosis, spinal cord neoplasm, polyarteritis, syringomyelia, myasthenia gravis, and progressive muscular dystrophy.

Treatment

ALS is untreatable. Management aims to control symptoms and provide emotional, psychological, and physical support.

Special considerations

• Care begins with a complete neurologic assessment, a baseline for future evaluations of progressing disease.

• Implement a rehabilitation program designed to maintain independence as long as possible.

• Help the patient obtain equipment, such as a walker and a wheelchair. Arrange for a visiting nurse to monitor the patient's status, to provide support, and to teach the family about the illness.

• Depending on the patient's muscular capacity, assist with bathing, personal hygiene, and transfers from wheelchair to bed. Help establish a regular bowel and bladder routine.

• To help the patient handle increased accumulation of secretions and dysphagia, teach him to suction himself. He should have a suctioning machine handy at home to reduce his fear of choking.

• To prevent skin breakdown, provide good skin care when the patient is bedridden. Turn him often, keep his skin clean and dry, and use sheepskins or pressure-relieving devices.

• If the patient has trouble swallowing, give him soft, solid foods and position him upright during meals. Gastrostomy and nasogastric tube feedings may be necessary if he can no longer swallow. Teach the patient (if he's still able to feed himself) or family members how to administer gastrostomy feedings.

• Provide emotional support. Prepare the patient and family for his eventual death, and encourage the start of the grieving process. Patients with ALS may benefit from a hospice program.

ANAL FISSURE

This conditon is a laceration or crack in the lining of the anus that extends to the circular muscle. A posterior fissure, the most common type, is equally prevalent in males and females. An anterior fissure, the rarer type, is 10 times more common in females. The prognosis is very good, especially with a fissurectomy and good anal hygiene.

Causes

A posterior fissure results from passage of large, hard stools that stretch the lining beyond its limits. An anterior fissure usually results from strain on the perineum during childbirth and, rarely, from scar stenosis. Occasionally, an oral fissure is secondary to proctitis, anal tuberculosis, or carcinoma.

Signs and symptoms

Onset of an acute anal fissure is characterized by tearing, cutting, or burning pain during or immediately after bowel movement. A few drops of blood may streak toilet paper or underclothes. Painful anal sphincter spasms result from ulceration of a "sentinel pile" (swelling at the lower end of the fissure).

A fissure may heal spontaneously and completely, or it may partially heal and break open again. A chronic fissure produces scar tissue that hampers normal bowel evacuation.

Diagnosis

Anoscopy showing a longitudinal tear and typical clinical features help establish the diagnosis. A digital examination that elicits pain and bleeding supports this diagnosis. Also, gentle traction on perianal skin can create sufficient eversion to visualize the fissure directly.

Treatment
For superficial fissures without hemorrhoids, forcible digital dilation of the anal sphincter under local anesthesia stretches the lower portion of the anal sphincter. For complicated fissures, treatment includes surgical excision of tissue, adjacent skin, and mucosal tags and division of internal sphincter muscle from external.

Special considerations
• Prepare the patient for a rectal examination; explain the necessity for the procedure.
• Provide hot sitz baths, warm soaks, and local anesthetic ointment to relieve pain.
• Tell the patient that a low-residue diet, adequate fluid intake, and stool softeners prevent straining during defecation.
• Control diarrhea with diphenoxylate or other antidiarrheals.

LIFE-THREATENING DISORDER

ANAPHYLAXIS

This condition is a dramatic, acute atopic reaction marked by the sudden onset of rapidly progressive urticaria and respiratory distress. A severe anaphylactic reaction may precipitate vascular collapse, leading to systemic shock and, sometimes, death.

Causes
The source of anaphylactic reactions is ingestion of, or other systemic exposure to, sensitizing drugs or other substances. (See *Teaching patients how to use an anaphylaxis kit,* page 44.)

Sensitizing substances
Such sensitizing substances may include serums (usually horse serum), vaccines, allergen extracts, enzymes (such as L-asparaginase), hormones, penicillin and other antibiotics, sulfonamides, local anesthetics, salicylates, polysaccharides, diagnostic chemicals (sulfobromophthalein, sodium dehydrocholate, and radiographic contrast media), foods (legumes, nuts, berries, seafoods, and egg albumin) and sulfite-containing food additives, insect venom (honeybees, wasps, hornets, yellow jackets, fire ants, mosquitoes, and certain spiders) and, rarely, ruptured hydatid cyst.

A common cause of anaphylaxis is penicillin, which induces anaphylaxis in 1 to 4 of every 10,000 patients treated with it. Penicillin is most likely to induce anaphylaxis after parenteral administration or prolonged therapy and in atopic patients with an allergy to other drugs or foods.

Pathophysiology
An anaphylactic reaction requires previous sensitization or exposure to the specific antigen, resulting in the production of specific immunoglobulin E (IgE) antibodies by plasma cells. This antibody production takes place in the lymph nodes and is enhanced by helper T cells. IgE antibodies then bind to membrane receptors on mast cells (found throughout connective tissue) and basophils.

On reexposure, the antigen binds to adjacent IgE antibodies or cross-linked IgE receptors, activating a series of cellular reactions that trigger degranulation — the release of powerful chemical mediators (such as histamine, ECF-A, and PAF) from mast cell stores. IgG or IgM enters into the reaction and activates the release of complement fractions.

At the same time, two other chemical mediators, bradykinin and leukotrienes, induce vascular collapse by stimulating contraction of certain groups of smooth muscles and by increasing vascular permeability. In turn, increased vascular permeability leads to decreased peripheral resistance and plasma leakage from the circulation to extravascular tissues (which lowers blood volume, causing hypotension, hypovolemic shock, and cardiac dysfunction).

Signs and symptoms
An anaphylactic reaction produces sudden physical distress within seconds or minutes (although a delayed or persistent reaction may occur for up to 24 hours) after exposure to an allergen. Severity of the reaction is inversely related to the interval between exposure to the allergen and the onset of symptoms. Usually, the first symptoms include a feeling of impending doom or fright, weakness, sweating, sneezing, shortness of breath, nasal pruritus, urticaria, and angioedema, followed rapidly by symptoms in one or more target organs.

Systemic effects
Cardiovascular symptoms include hypotension, shock, and sometimes cardiac arrhythmias, which, if untreated, may precipitate circulatory collapse.

Respiratory symptoms can occur at any level in the respiratory tract and commonly include nasal mucosal edema, profuse watery rhinorrhea, itching, nasal congestion, and sudden sneezing attacks. Edema of the upper respiratory tract, resulting in hypopharyngeal and laryngeal obstruction (hoarseness, stridor, and dyspnea), is an early sign of acute respiratory failure, which can be fatal.

GI and genitourinary symptoms include severe stomach cramps, nausea, diarrhea, and urinary urgency and incontinence.

Diagnosis
Anaphylaxis can be diagnosed by the rapid onset of severe respiratory or cardiovascular symptoms after ingestion or injection of a drug, vaccine, diagnostic agent, food, or food additive or after an insect sting. If these symptoms occur without a known allergic stimulus, rule out other possible causes of shock (such as acute myocardial infarction, status asthmaticus, or congestive heart failure).

Treatment and special considerations
• Anaphylaxis is always an emergency. It requires an *immediate* injection of epinephrine 1:1,000 aqueous solution, 0.1 to 0.5 ml, repeated every 5 to 20 minutes as necessary.
• In the early stages of anaphylaxis, when the patient has not yet lost consciousness and is still normotensive, give epinephrine I.M. or S.C., and help it move into the circulation faster by massaging the injection site. In severe reactions, when the patient has lost consciousness and is hypotensive, give epinephrine I.V.
• Maintain airway patency. Observe for early signs of laryngeal edema (stridor, hoarseness, and dyspnea), which will probably necessitate endotracheal tube insertion or a tracheotomy and oxygen therapy.
• In case of cardiac arrest, begin cardiopulmonary resuscitation, including closed-chest heart massage, assisted ventilation, and sodium bicarbonate; other therapy is indicated by clinical response.
• Watch for hypotension and shock, and maintain circulatory volume with volume expanders (plasma, plasma expanders, saline solution, and albumin) as needed. Stabilize blood pressure with the I.V. vasopressors norepinephrine and dopamine. Monitor blood pressure, central venous pressure, and urine output as a response index.

TEACHING PATIENTS HOW TO USE AN ANAPHYLAXIS KIT

If the doctor has prescribed an ana-phylaxis kit for your patient to use in an emergency, explain that the kit contains everything that he needs to treat an allergic reaction: a prefilled syringe containing two doses of epi-nephrine, alcohol swabs, a tourni-quet, and antihistamine tablets.

Instruct the patient to notify the doctor at once if anaphylaxis occurs (or to ask someone else to call him) and to use the anaphylaxis kit as follows.

Getting ready
• Take the prefilled syringe from the kit and remove the needle cap. Hold the syringe with the needle pointing up. Expel air from the syringe by pushing in the plunger until it stops.
• Next, clean about 4" (10 cm) of the skin on your arm or thigh with an al-cohol swab. (If you're right-handed, clean your left arm or thigh. If you're left-handed, clean your right arm or thigh.)

Injecting the epinephrine
• Rotate the plunger one-quarter turn to the right so that it's aligned with the slot. Insert the entire needle—like a dart—into the skin.
• Push down on the plunger until it stops. It will inject 0.3 ml of the drug for persons over age 12. Withdraw the needle.
Note: The dosage and administra-tion for babies and for children under age 12 must be directed by a doctor.

Removing the insect's stinger
• Quickly remove the insect's stinger if it's visible. Use a dull object, such as a fingernail or tweezers, to pull it

straight out. If the stinger can't be re-moved quickly, stop trying. Go on to the next step.

Applying the tourniquet
• If you were stung on an arm or a leg, apply a tourniquet between the sting site and your heart. Tighten the tourniquet by pulling the string.
• After 10 minutes, release the tourni-quet by pulling on the metal ring.

Taking the antihistamine tablets
• Chew and swallow the antihista-mine tablets. (Children age 12 and under should follow the directions supplied by the doctor or provided in the kit.)

Following up
• Apply ice packs—if available—to the sting site. Avoid exertion, keep warm, and see a doctor or go to a hospital immediately.
• *Important:* If you don't notice an im-provement within 10 minutes, give yourself a second injection by follow-ing the directions in the kit. If the sy-ringe has a preset second dose, don't depress the plunger until you're ready to give the second injection. Proceed as before, following the in-jection instructions.

Special instructions
• Keep the kit handy for emergency treatment at all times.
• Ask the pharmacist for storage guidelines.
• Periodically check the epinephrine in the preloaded syringe. A pinkish brown solution needs to be replaced.
• Note the kit's expiration date and replace the kit before that date.

• After the initial emergency, administer other medications, such as S.C. epinephrine, longer-acting epinephrine, corticosteroids, and diphenhydramine I.V. for long-term management; and aminophylline I.V. over 10 to 20 minutes for bronchospasm.

Caution: Rapid infusion of aminophylline may cause or aggravate severe hypotension.

• To prevent anaphylaxis, teach the patient to avoid exposure to known allergens. In a food or drug allergy, the sensitized person must learn to avoid the offending food or drug in all its forms. In an allergy to insect stings, he should avoid open fields and wooded areas during the insect season and should carry an anaphylaxis kit (containing epinephrine, an antihistamine, and a tourniquet) whenever he goes outdoors. Instruct him in the use of the kit. In addition, every patient prone to anaphylaxis should wear a medical identification bracelet identifying his allergies.

• If a patient must receive a drug to which he is allergic, prevent a severe reaction by making sure he receives careful desensitization with gradually increasing doses of the antigen or advance administration of steroids.

• A person with a known history of allergies should receive a drug with a high anaphylactic potential only after cautious pretesting for sensitivity. Closely monitor the patient during testing, and make sure you have resuscitative equipment and epinephrine ready.

• When any patient needs a drug with a high anaphylactic potential (particularly parenteral drugs), make sure he receives each dose under close medical observation.

• Closely monitor a patient undergoing diagnostic tests that use radiographic contrast dyes, such as cardiac catheterization, excretory urography, and angiography.

LIFE-THREATENING DISORDER

ANEURYSM, ABDOMINAL

In this condition, an abnormal dilation in the arterial wall generally occurs in the aorta between the renal arteries and iliac branches. Such aneurysms are four times more common in men than in women and are most prevalent in whites ages 50 to 80. Over 50% of all people with untreated abdominal aneurysms die within 2 years of diagnosis, primarily from aneurysmal rupture; over 85%, within 5 years.

Causes
About 95% of abdominal aortic aneurysms result from arteriosclerosis; the rest, from cystic medial necrosis, trauma, syphilis, and other infections. These aneurysms develop slowly.

First, a focal weakness in the muscular layer of the aorta (tunica media), due to degenerative changes, allows the inner layer (tunica intima) and outer layer (tunica adventitia) to stretch outward. Blood pressure within the aorta progressively weakens the vessel walls and enlarges the aneurysm.

Signs and symptoms
Although abdominal aneurysms usually don't produce symptoms, most are evident (unless the patient is obese) as a pulsating mass in the periumbilical area, accompanied by a systolic bruit over the aorta. Some tenderness may be present on deep palpation. A large aneurysm may produce symptoms that mimic renal calculi, lumbar disk disease, and duodenal compression. Abdominal aneurysms rarely cause diminished peripheral pulses or claudication unless embolization occurs.

Pain, rupture, and hemorrhage
Lumbar pain that radiates to the flank and groin from pressure on lumbar nerves may signify enlargement and imminent rupture. If the aneurysm ruptures into the peritoneal cavity, it causes severe, persistent abdominal and back pain, mimicking renal or ureteral colic.

Signs of hemorrhage — such as weakness, sweating, tachycardia, and hypotension — may be subtle because rupture into the retroperitoneal space produces a tamponade effect that prevents continued hemorrhage. Patients with such rupture may remain stable for hours before shock and death occur, although 20% die immediately.

Diagnosis
Because an abdominal aneurysm rarely produces symptoms, it's often detected accidentally as the result of an X-ray or a routine physical examination. Several tests can confirm suspected abdominal aneurysm:

• *Serial ultrasonography* allows accurate determination of aneurysm size, shape, and location.

• *Anteroposterior and lateral X-rays* of the abdomen can detect aortic calcification, which outlines the mass, at least 75% of the time.

• *Aortography* shows the condition of vessels proximal and distal to the aneurysm and the extent of the aneurysm but may underestimate the aneurysm's diameter, because it visualizes only the flow channel and not the surrounding clot.

Treatment
Usually, an abdominal aneurysm requires resection of the aneurysm and replacement of the damaged aortic section with a Dacron graft. If the aneurysm is small and produces no symptoms, surgery may be delayed; however, small aneurysms may also rupture. Regular physical examinations and ultrasound checks are necessary to detect enlargement, which may presage a rupture. Large aneurysms or those that produce symptoms pose a significant risk of rupture and require immediate repair. In patients with poor distal runoff, external grafting may be done.

Special considerations
• Monitor vital signs, and type and crossmatch blood.

• Obtain renal function tests (blood urea nitrogen, creatinine, electrolytes), blood samples (complete blood count with differential), an electrocardiogram and cardiac evaluation, baseline pulmonary function tests, and arterial blood gas (ABG) analysis.

• Be alert for signs of rupture, which may be immediately fatal. Watch closely for any signs of acute blood loss (decreasing blood pressure; increasing pulse and respiratory rate; cool, clammy skin; restlessness; and decreased sensorium).

• If rupture does occur, the first priority is to get the patient to surgery *immediately*. A pneumatic antishock garment may be used while transporting him to surgery. Surgery allows direct compression of the aorta to control hemorrhage. Large amounts of blood may be needed during the resuscitative period to replace blood loss. In such a patient, renal failure due to ischemia is a major postoperative complication, possibly requiring hemodialysis.

• Before elective surgery, weigh the patient, insert an indwelling urinary catheter and an I.V. line, and assist with insertion of an arterial line and a pulmonary artery catheter to monitor fluid and hemodynamic balance. Give prophylactic antibiotics.

• Explain the surgical procedure and the expected postoperative care in the intensive care unit (ICU) to patients undergoing complex abdominal surgery (I.V. lines, endotracheal [ET] and nasogastric [NG] intubation, mechanical ventilation).

• After surgery, closely monitor vital signs, intake and hourly output, neurologic status (level of consciousness, pupil size, sensation in arms and legs), and ABG levels.

• Assess the depth, rate, and character of respirations and breath sounds at least every hour.

• Watch for signs of bleeding (such as increased pulse and respiratory rate, hypotension), which may occur retroperitoneally from the graft site. Check abdominal dressings for excessive bleeding or drainage.

• Be alert for fever and other signs of infection.

• After NG intubation for intestinal decompression, irrigate the tube frequently to ensure patency. Record the amount and type of drainage.

• Suction the ET tube often. If the patient can breathe unassisted and has good breath sounds and adequate ABG levels, tidal volume, and vital capacity 24 hours after surgery, he will be extubated and will require oxygen by mask. Weigh the patient daily to evaluate fluid balance.

• Help the patient walk as soon as he's able (generally the second day after surgery).

• Provide psychological support for the patient and family. Help ease their fears about the ICU, the threat of impending rupture, and surgery by providing appropriate explanations and answering all questions.

ANEURYSM, CEREBRAL

In this type of aneurysm, localized dilation of a cerebral artery results from a weakness in the arterial wall. Its most common form is the berry aneurysm, a saclike outpouching in a cerebral artery. Cerebral aneurysms usually arise at an arterial junction in the circle of Willis, the circular anastomosis forming the major cerebral arteries at the base of the brain. Cerebral aneurysms often rupture and cause subarachnoid hemorrhage.

The prognosis is guarded. About half of all patients who suffer a subarachnoid hemorrhage die immediately; of those who survive untreated, 40% die from the effects of hemorrhage and another 20% die later from recurring hemorrhage. With new and better treatment, the prognosis is improving.

Causes

Cerebral aneurysms may result from a congenital defect, a degenerative process, or a combination of both. For example, hypertension and atherosclerosis may disrupt blood flow and exert pressure against a congenitally weak arterial wall, stretching it like an overblown balloon and making it likely to rupture.

Such a rupture is followed by subarachnoid hemorrhage, in which blood spills into the space normally occupied by cerebrospinal fluid (CSF). Sometimes, blood also spills into brain tissue and subsequently forms a clot. This may result in potentially fatal increased intracranial pressure (ICP) and brain tissue damage.

Incidence is slightly higher in women than in men, especially those in their late 40s or early to mid-50s, but a cerebral aneurysm may occur at any age, in both women and men.

Signs and symptoms

Occasionally, rupture of a cerebral aneurysm causes premonitory symptoms that last several days, such as headache, nuchal rigidity, stiff back and legs, and intermittent nausea. Usually, however, the rupture occurs abruptly and without warning, causing a sudden severe headache, nausea, vomiting and, depending on the severity and location of bleeding, altered level of consciousness (LOC), including a deep coma.

Bleeding causes meningeal irritation, resulting in nuchal rigidity, back and leg pain, fever, restlessness, irritability, occasional seizures, and blurred vision. Bleeding into the brain tissues causes hemiparesis, hemisensory defects, dysphagia, and visual defects. If the aneurysm is near the internal carotid artery, it compresses the oculomotor nerve and causes diplopia, ptosis, dilated pupil, and inability to rotate the eye.

Degrees of severity

The severity of symptoms varies from patient to patient, depending on the site and amount of bleeding. To better describe their conditions, patients with ruptured cerebral aneurysms are grouped as follows:

• *grade I: minimal bleeding.* The patient is alert with no neurologic deficit; he may have a slight headache and nuchal rigidity.

• *grade II: mild bleeding.* The patient is alert, with a mild to severe headache, nuchal rigidity and, possibly, third-nerve palsy.

• *grade III: moderate bleeding.* The patient is confused or drowsy, with nuchal rigidity and, possibly, a mild focal deficit.

• *grade IV: severe bleeding.* The patient is stuporous, with nuchal rigidity and, possibly, mild to severe hemiparesis.

• *grade V: moribund (often fatal).* If the rupture is nonfatal, the patient is in a deep coma or decerebrate.

Life-threatening factors

Generally, a cerebral aneurysm poses three major threats:

• *death from increased ICP.* Increased ICP may push the brain downward, impair brain stem function, and cut off blood supply to the part of the brain that supports vital functions.

• *Bleeding episode.* Generally, after the initial bleeding episode, a clot forms and seals the rupture, which reinforces the wall of the aneurysm for 7 to 10 days. However, after the seventh day, fibrinolysis begins to dissolve the clot and increases the risk of rebleeding. This rebleeding produces signs and symptoms similar to those accompanying the initial hemorrhage. Rebleeding episodes during the first 24 hours after the initial hemorrhage aren't uncommon, and they contribute to cerebral aneurysm's high mortality.

• *vasospasm.* The reason for this complication isn't clearly understood. Usually, vasospasm occurs in blood vessels adjacent to the cerebral aneurysm, but it may extend to major vessels of the brain, causing ischemia and altered brain function.

Other complications of a cerebral aneurysm include acute hydrocephalus (due to abnormal accumulation of CSF within the cranial cavity because of CSF blockage by blood or adhesions) and pulmonary embolism (a possible adverse effect of deep vein thrombosis or aneurysm treatment). (See *Danger signals in cerebral aneurysm.*)

Diagnosis

In cerebral aneurysm, diagnosis is based on the patient history; a neurologic examination; a computed tomography scan, which reveals subarachnoid or ventricular blood; and magnetic resonance imaging or mag-

---

HAZARD

DANGER SIGNALS IN CEREBRAL ANEURYSM

Watch for an enlarging aneurysm, rebleeding, intracranial clot, vasospasm, or other complications. These complications may be heralded by:
- decreased level of consciousness
- unilateral enlarged pupil
- onset or worsening of hemiparesis or motor deficit
- increased blood pressure
- slowed pulse
- worsening of headache or sudden onset of a headache
- renewed or worsened nuchal rigidity
- renewed or persistent vomiting.
  Intermittent signs, such as restlessness, extremity weakness, and speech alterations, can also indicate increasing intracranial pressure.

---

netic resonant angiography, which can identify a cerebral aneurysm as a "flow void" or by computer reconstruction of cerebral vessels.

Cerebral angiography remains the procedure of choice for diagnosing a cerebral aneurysm. Lumbar puncture may be used to identify blood in CSF if other studies are negative and the patient has no signs of increased ICP.

Other baseline laboratory studies include a complete blood count, urinalysis, arterial blood gas (ABG) analysis, coagulation studies, serum osmolality, and electrolyte and glucose levels.

Treatment

The risk of vasospasm and cerebral infarction is reduced by repairing the aneurysm. Usually, surgical repair (by clipping, ligation, or wrapping the aneurysm neck with muscle) takes place 7 to 10 days after the initial hemorrhage; however, surgery performed within 1 to 2 days after the hemorrhage has also shown promise in grade I and II aneurysms.

When surgical correction is risky, when the aneurysm is in a dangerous location, or when surgery is delayed because of vasospasm, treatment includes:

- bed rest in a quiet, darkened room; if immediate surgery isn't possible, such bed rest may continue for 4 to 6 weeks
- avoidance of coffee, other stimulants, and aspirin
- codeine or another analgesic as needed
- hydralazine or another antihypertensive agent if the patient is hypertensive
- calcium channel blockers to decrease spasm
- corticosteroids to reduce edema
- phenytoin or another anticonvulsant
- phenobarbital or another sedative
- aminocaproic acid, a fibrinolytic inhibitor, to minimize the risk of rebleeding by delaying blood clot lysis. However, this drug's effectiveness has been disputed.

After surgical repair, the patient's condition depends on the extent of damage from the initial hemorrhage and the degree of success of the treatment of resulting complications. Surgery can't improve the patient's neurologic condition unless it removes a hematoma or reduces the compression effect.

Special considerations

• During initial treatment after a hemorrhage, establish and maintain a patent airway because the patient may need supplemental oxygen. Position the patient to promote pulmonary drainage and prevent upper airway obstruction. If he's intubated, preoxygenation with 100% oxygen before suctioning to remove secretions will prevent hypoxia and vasodilation from carbon dioxide accumulation.

• Provide frequent nose and mouth care.

• Institute aneurysm precautions to minimize the risk of rebleeding and to avoid increased ICP. Such precautions include bed rest in a quiet, darkened room (keeping the head of the bed flat or under 30 degrees); limiting visitors; avoidance of caffeine, other stimulants, and strenuous physical activity; and restricted fluid intake. Be sure to explain why these restrictive measures are necessary.

• Turn the patient often. Encourage deep breathing and leg movement. Warn the patient to avoid all unnecessary physical activity. Assist with active range-of-motion (ROM) exercises (unless the doctor has forbidden them); if the patient is paralyzed, perform regular passive ROM exercises.

• Monitor ABG levels, LOC, and vital signs often, and accurately measure intake and output. Avoid taking temperature rectally because vagus nerve stimulation may cause cardiac arrest.

• Watch for ominous signs of life-threatening complications.

• Give fluids, and monitor I.V. infusions to avoid increased ICP.

• If the patient has facial weakness, assist him during meals, placing food in the unaffected side of his mouth. If he can't swallow, insert a nasogastric (NG) tube and give all tube feedings slowly.

• Prevent skin breakdown by taping the NG tube so it doesn't press against the nostril.

• If the patient can eat, provide a high-bulk diet (bran, salads, and fruit) to prevent straining during defecation, which can increase ICP.

• Administer a stool softener, such as dioctyl sodium sulfosuccinate, or a mild laxative as needed. *Don't* force fluids. Implement a bowel elimination program based on previous habits. If the patient is receiving steroids, check the stools for blood.

• With third-nerve or facial nerve palsy, administer artificial tears to the affected eye, and tape the eye shut at night to prevent corneal damage.

• To minimize stress, give a sedative. Be alert for signs of oversedation. Raise the side rails to help protect the patient from injury. If possible, avoid using restraints because these can cause agitation and raise ICP.

• Administer hydralazine or another antihypertensive if necessary. Carefully monitor blood pressure and be alert for *any* significant change, especially a rise in systolic pressure.

• Administer aminocaproic acid I.V. in dextrose 5% in water or orally at least every 2 hours to maintain therapeutic blood levels. (Renal insufficiency may require a dosage adjustment.) Monitor the patient for adverse reactions, such as nausea and diarrhea (most common with oral administration) and phlebitis (most common with I.V. administration).

• Reduce deep vein thrombosis by applying antiembolism stockings or sequential compression sleeves.

• If the patient can't speak, establish a simple means of communication, or use cards or a slate. Try to limit conversation to topics that won't further frustrate him. Encourage his family to speak to him in a normal tone, even if he doesn't seem to respond.

• Provide emotional support, and include the patient's family in his care as much as possible. Encourage family members to adopt a realistic attitude, but don't discourage hope.

• Before discharge, refer the patient to a visiting nurse or a rehabilitation center if necessary, and teach the patient and family how to recognize signs of rebleeding.

ANEURYSMS, FEMORAL AND POPLITEAL

These forms of aneurysm result from progressive atherosclerotic changes occurring in the walls (medial layer) of the major peripheral arteries. Aneurysmal formations may be *fusiform* (spindle-shaped) or *saccular* (pouchlike), with fusiform occurring three times more frequently. They may be singular or multiple segmental lesions, often affecting both legs, and may accompany other arterial aneurysms located in the abdominal aorta or iliac arteries.

This condition occurs most frequently in men over age 50. The clinical course is usually progressive, eventually ending in thrombosis, embolization, and gangrene. Elective surgery before complications arise greatly improves the prognosis.

Causes

Femoral and popliteal aneurysms are usually secondary to atherosclerosis. Rarely, they result from congenital weakness in the arterial wall. They may also result from trauma (blunt or penetrating), bacterial infection, or peripheral vascular reconstructive surgery (which causes "suture line" aneurysms, whereby a blood clot forms a second lumen, also called false aneurysms).

Signs and symptoms

Popliteal aneurysms may cause pain in the popliteal space when they're large enough to compress the medial popliteal nerve, and edema and venous distention if the vein is compressed. Femoral and popliteal aneurysms can produce symptoms of severe ischemia in the leg or foot, due to acute thrombosis within the aneurysmal sac, embolization of mural thrombus fragments, and, rarely, rupture.

Symptoms of acute aneurysmal thrombosis include severe pain, loss of pulse and color, coldness in the affected leg or foot, and gangrene. Distal petechial hemorrhages may develop from aneurysmal emboli.

Diagnosis

In femoral aneurysm, the diagnosis is usually confirmed by bilateral palpation that reveals a pulsating mass above or below the inguinal ligament. When thrombosis has occurred, palpation detects a firm, nonpulsating mass.

Arteriography or ultrasound may be indicated in doubtful situations. Arteriography may also detect associated aneurysms, especially those in the abdominal aorta and the iliac arteries. Ultrasound may be helpful in determining the size of the popliteal or femoral artery.

Treatment

Femoral and popliteal aneurysms require surgical bypass and reconstruction of the artery, usually with an autogenous saphenous vein graft replacement. Arterial occlusion that causes severe ischemia and gangrene may require leg amputation.

Special considerations

Before corrective surgery:

• Evaluate the patient's circulatory status, noting the location and quality of peripheral pulses in the affected arm or leg.

• Administer prophylactic antibiotics or anticoagulants as needed.

• Discuss expected postoperative procedures with the patient, and review the surgical procedure.

After arterial surgery:

• Monitor carefully for early signs of thrombosis or graft occlusion (loss of pulse, decreased skin temperature and sensation, severe pain) and infection (fever).

• Palpate distal pulses at least every hour for the first 24 hours, then as frequently as needed. Correlate these findings with preoperative circulatory assessment. Mark the sites on the patient's skin where pulses are palpable, to facilitate repeated checks.

• Help the patient walk soon after surgery, to prevent venostasis and possible thrombus formation.

To prepare the patient for discharge:

• Tell the patient to immediately inform the doctor of any recurrence of symptoms, since the saphenous vein graft replacement can fail or another aneurysm may develop.

• Explain to the patient with popliteal artery resection that swelling may persist for some time. If antiembolism stockings are ordered, make sure they fit properly, and teach the patient how to apply them. Warn against wearing constrictive apparel.

• If the patient is receiving anticoagulants, suggest measures to prevent bleeding, such as using an electric razor. Tell the patient to report any signs of bleeding immediately (bleeding gums; black, tarry stools; easy bruising).

• Explain the importance of follow-up blood studies to monitor anticoagulant therapy. Warn the patient to avoid trauma, tobacco, and aspirin.

====================

LIFE-THREATENING DISORDER

ANEURYSM, THORACIC AORTIC

====================

This condition is characterized by an abnormal widening of the ascending, transverse, or descending part of the aorta. Aneurysm of the ascending aorta is most common and most often fatal.

The aneurysm may be *dissecting,* a hemorrhagic separation in the aortic wall, usually within the medial layer; *saccular,* an outpouching of the arterial wall, with a narrow neck; or *fusiform,* a spindle-shaped enlargement encompassing the entire aortic circumference.

Some aneurysms progress to serious and, eventually, lethal complications, such as rupture of an untreated thoracic dissecting aneurysm into the pericardium, with resulting tamponade.

Causes

Commonly, a thoracic aortic aneurysm results from atherosclerosis, which weakens the aortic wall and gradually distends the lumen. An intimal tear in the ascending aorta initiates a dissecting aneurysm in about 60% of the patients.

An ascending aortic aneurysm, the most common type, is usually seen in hypertensive men under age 60. A descending aortic aneurysm, usually found just below the origin of the subclavian artery, is most common in elderly hypertensive men. It's also seen in younger patients with a history of traumatic chest injury; less often in those with infection. A transverse aortic aneurysm is the least common.

Other causes include:
• fungal infection (mycotic aneurysms) of the aortic arch and descending segments
• congenital disorders, such as coarctation of the aorta
• trauma, usually of the descending thoracic aorta, from an accident that shears the aorta transversely (acceleration-deceleration injuries)
• syphilis, usually of the ascending aorta (uncommon because of antibiotics)
• hypertension (in dissecting aneurysm).

Signs and symptoms

Pain most commonly accompanies a thoracic aortic aneurysm. (See *Clinical characteristics of thoracic dissection,* page 54.) In an ascending aneurysm, the pain is described as severe, boring, and ripping and extends to the neck, shoulders, lower back, or abdomen, but rarely radiates to the jaw and arms. Pain is more severe on the right side.

Other signs of an ascending aneurysm may include bradycardia, aortic insufficiency, pericardial friction rub caused by a hemopericardium, unequal intensities of the right carotid and left radial pulses, and a difference in blood pressure between the right and left arms. These signs are absent in a descending aneurysm. If dissection involves the carotid arteries, an abrupt onset of neurologic deficits may occur.

In a descending aneurysm, pain usually starts suddenly between the shoulder blades and may radiate to the chest; it's described as sharp and tearing.

A transverse aneurysm causes sudden, sharp, tearing pain radiating to the shoulders. It may also cause hoarseness, dyspnea, dysphagia, and dry cough because of compression of surrounding structures in this area.

Diagnosis

The patient history, clinical features, and appropriate tests provide diagnostic information. In an asymptomatic patient, diagnosis often occurs accidentally when chest X-rays show widening of the aorta. The following other tests help confirm an aneurysm:
• *Aortography,* the most definitive test, shows the lumen of the aneurysm, its size and location, and the false lumen in a dissecting aneurysm.
• *Electrocardiography (ECG)* helps distinguish a thoracic aneurysm from myocardial infarction.
• *Echocardiography* may help identify a dissecting aneurysm of the aortic root.
• *Hemoglobin* may be normal or low because of blood loss from a leaking aneurysm.
• *Computed tomography scan* can confirm and locate the aneurysm and may be used to monitor its progression.
• *Magnetic resonance imaging* may aid diagnosis.
• *Transesophageal echocardiography* is used to measure the aneurysm in both the ascending and the descending aorta.

Treatment

A dissecting aortic aneurysm is an emergency that requires prompt surgery and stabilizing measures: antihypertensives such as nitroprusside; negative inotropic agents that decrease contractility force, such as propranolol; oxygen for respiratory distress; narcotics for pain; I.V. fluids; and, possibly, whole blood transfusions.

Surgery consists of resecting the aneurysm, restoring normal blood flow through a Dacron or Teflon graft replacement and, with aortic valve insufficiency, replacing the aortic valve.

Postoperative measures include careful monitoring and continuous assessment in the intensive care unit, antibiotics, endotracheal (ET) and

CLINICAL CHARACTERISTICS OF THORACIC DISSECTION

ASCENDING AORTA	DESCENDING AORTA	TRANSVERSE
CHARACTER OF PAIN		
Severe, boring, ripping; extending to neck, shoulders, lower back, or abdomen (rarely to jaw and arms); more severe on right side	Sudden onset, sharp, tearing, usually between the shoulder blades; may radiate to the chest; most diagnostic feature	Sudden onset, sharp, boring, tearing; radiates to shoulders
OTHER SYMPTOMS AND EFFECTS		
If dissection involves carotid arteries, abrupt onset of neurologic deficit (usually intermittent); bradycardia, aortic insufficiency, and hemopericardium detected by pericardial friction rub; unequal intensity of right and left carotid pulses and radial pulses; difference in blood pressure, especially systolic, between right and left arms	Aortic insufficiency without murmur, hemopericardium, or pleural friction rub; carotid and radial pulses and blood pressure in both arms typically equal	Hoarseness, dyspnea, pain, dysphagia, and dry cough due to compression of surrounding structures
DIAGNOSTIC FEATURES		
Chest X-ray Best diagnostic tool; shows widening of mediastinum, enlargement of ascending aorta	Widening of mediastinum; descending aorta larger than ascending	Shows widening of mediastinum; descending aorta larger than ascending; widened transverse arch
Aortography False lumen; narrowing of lumen of aorta in ascending section	False lumen; narrowing of lumen of aorta in descending section	False lumen; narrowing of lumen of aorta in transverse arch
TREATMENT		
A medical emergency that requires immediate, aggressive treatment to reduce blood pressure (usually with nitroprusside or trimethaphan); surgical repair required	Surgical repair required but less urgent than for the ascending dissection; to control hypertension, nitroprusside and propranolol may be used if bradycardia and congestive heart failure are absent	Immediate surgical repair (mortality as high as 50%); control of hypertension

chest tubes, ECG monitoring, and pulmonary artery catheterization.

Special considerations
• Monitor the patient's blood pressure, pulmonary artery wedge pressure, and central venous pressure. Also evaluate pain, breathing, and carotid, radial, and femoral pulses.
• Review laboratory test results, which must include a complete blood count, differential, electrolytes, typing and crossmatching for whole blood, arterial blood gas studies, and urinalysis.
• Insert an indwelling urinary catheter. Administer dextrose 5% in water or lactated Ringer's solution and antibiotics as needed. Carefully monitor nitroprusside I.V. infusion rate; use a separate I.V. line for infusion. Adjust the dose by slowly increasing the infusion rate. Meanwhile, check blood pressure every 5 minutes until it stabilizes.
• With suspected bleeding from an aneurysm, give a whole-blood transfusion.
• Explain diagnostic tests. If surgery is scheduled, explain the procedure and expected postoperative care (I.V. lines, ET and drainage tubes, cardiac monitoring, ventilation).

After repair of a thoracic aneurysm:
• Evaluate the patient's level of consciousness. Monitor vital signs; pulmonary artery pressure, pulmonary artery wedge pressure, and central venous pressure; pulse rate; urine output; and pain.
• Check respiratory function. Carefully observe and record type and amount of chest tube drainage, and frequently assess heart and breath sounds.
• Monitor I.V. therapy.
• Give medications as appropriate.
• Watch for signs of infection, especially fever, and excessive wound drainage.

• Assist with range-of-motion exercises of legs to prevent thromboembolism due to venostasis during prolonged bed rest.
• After stabilization of vital signs and respiration, encourage and assist the patient in turning, coughing, and deep breathing. If necessary, provide intermittent positive pressure breathing to promote lung expansion.
• Help the patient walk as soon as he's able.
• Before discharge, ensure compliance with antihypertensive therapy by explaining the need for such drugs and the expected adverse effects. Teach the patient how to monitor his blood pressure. Refer him to community agencies for continued support and assistance as needed.
• Throughout hospitalization, offer the patient and family psychological support.

LIFE-THREATENING DISORDER

ANEURYSM, VENTRICULAR

This type of aneurysm is marked by an outpouching, almost always of the left ventricle, that produces ventricular wall dysfunction in about 20% of patients after myocardial infarction (MI). A ventricular aneurysm may develop within weeks after MI.

An untreated ventricular aneurysm can lead to arrhythmias, systemic embolization, or congestive heart failure (CHF) and may cause sudden death. Resection improves the prognosis in CHF or refractory patients who have developed ventricular arrhythmias.

Causes

When MI destroys a large muscular section of the left ventricle, necrosis reduces the ventricular wall to a thin sheath of fibrous tissue. Under intracardiac pressure, this thin layer stretches and forms a separate noncontractile sac (aneurysm).

Abnormal muscle wall movement

Accompanying ventricular aneurysm, abnormal muscle wall movement includes akinesia (lack of movement), dyskinesia (paradoxical movement), asynergia (decreased and inadequate movement), and asynchrony (uncoordinated movement).

During systolic ejection, the abnormal muscle wall movements associated with the aneurysm cause the remaining normally functioning myocardial fibers to increase the force of contraction in order to maintain stroke volume and cardiac output. At the same time, a portion of the stroke volume is lost to passive distention of the noncontractile sac.

Signs and symptoms

A ventricular aneurysm may cause arrhythmias — such as premature ventricular contractions or ventricular tachycardia — palpitations, signs of cardiac dysfunction (weakness on exertion, fatigue, angina) and, occasionally, a visible or palpable systolic precordial bulge.

This condition may also lead to left ventricular dysfunction, with chronic CHF (dyspnea, fatigue, edema, rales, gallop rhythm, neck vein distention); pulmonary edema; systemic embolization; and with left ventricular failure, pulsus alternans. Ventricular aneurysms enlarge but rarely rupture.

Diagnosis

Persistent ventricular arrhythmias, onset of heart failure, or systemic embolization in a patient with left ventricular failure and a history of MI strongly suggests a ventricular aneurysm. Indicative tests include the following:

• *Left ventriculography* reveals left ventricular enlargement with an area of akinesia or dyskinesia (during cineangiography) and diminished cardiac function.

• *Electrocardiography* may show persistent ST-T wave elevations after MI.

• *Chest X-ray* may demonstrate an abnormal bulge distorting the heart's contour if the aneurysm is large; the X-ray may be normal if the aneurysm is small.

• *Noninvasive nuclear cardiology scan* may indicate the site of infarction and suggest the area of aneurysm.

• *Echocardiography* shows abnormal motion in the left ventricular wall.

Treatment

Depending on the size of the aneurysm and the complications, treatment may require only routine medical examination to follow the patient's condition or aggressive measures for intractable ventricular arrhythmias, CHF, and emboli.

Emergency treatment of ventricular arrhythmias consists of antiarrhythmics I.V. or cardioversion. Preventive treatment continues with oral antiarrhythmics, such as procainamide, quinidine, or disopyramide.

Emergency treatment for CHF with pulmonary edema includes oxygen, digitalis glycosides I.V., furosemide I.V., morphine sulfate I.V. and, when necessary, nitroprusside I.V. and intubation. Maintenance therapy may include oral nitrates, prazosin, and hydralazine.

Systemic embolization requires anticoagulation therapy or embolectomy.

Refractory ventricular tachycardia, heart failure, recurrent arterial embolization, and persistent angina with coronary artery occlusion may require surgery; the most effective procedure is aneurysmectomy with myocardial revascularization.

Special considerations
• If ventricular tachycardia occurs, monitor blood pressure and heart rate.
• If cardiac arrest develops, initiate cardiopulmonary resuscitation (CPR) and call for assistance, resuscitative equipment, and medication.
• In a patient with CHF, closely monitor vital signs, heart sounds, intake and output, fluid and electrolyte balances, and blood urea nitrogen and creatinine levels.
• Because of the threat of systemic embolization, frequently check peripheral pulses and the color and temperature of extremities. Be alert for sudden changes in sensorium that indicate cerebral embolization and for any signs that suggest renal failure or progressive MI.
• If arrhythmias require cardioversion, use a sufficient amount of conductive gel to prevent chest burns. If the patient is conscious, give diazepam I.V., as needed, before cardioversion. Explain that cardioversion is a lifesaving procedure that provides brief electric shocks to the heart.
• If the patient is receiving antiarrhythmics, check appropriate laboratory tests. For instance, if the patient takes procainamide, check antinuclear antibodies because this drug may induce symptoms that mimic those of lupus erythematosus.

If the patient is scheduled to undergo resection:
• Before surgery, explain expected postoperative care in the intensive care unit (including use of such things as endotracheal tube, ventilator, hemo-dynamic monitoring, chest tubes, and drainage bottle).
• After surgery, monitor vital signs, intake and output, heart sounds, and pulmonary artery pressures. Watch for signs of infection, such as fever and drainage.
• To prepare the patient for discharge, teach him how to check for pulse irregularity and rate changes. Encourage him to follow his prescribed medication regimen — even during the night — and to watch for adverse reactions.
• Because arrhythmias can cause sudden death, refer the family to a community-based CPR training program.
• Provide psychological support for the patient and his family.

ANKYLOSING SPONDYLITIS

A chronic, usually progressive inflammatory disease, ankylosing or rheumatoid spondylitis primarily affects the sacroiliac, apophyseal, and costovertebral joints and adjacent soft tissue. Generally, the disease begins in the sacroiliac joints and gradually progresses to the lumbar, thoracic, and cervical regions of the spine. Deterioration of bone and cartilage can lead to fibrous tissue formation and eventual fusion of the spine or peripheral joints.

Ankylosing spondylitis may be equally prevalent in both sexes. Progressive disease is well recognized in men, but the diagnosis is often overlooked or missed in women, who tend to have more peripheral joint involvement.

Causes

Recent evidence strongly suggests a familial tendency in ankylosing spondylitis. The presence of histocompatibility antigen HLA-B27 (positive in over 90% of patients with this disease) and circulating immune complexes suggests immunologic activity.

Signs and symptoms

The first indication is intermittent low back pain that's usually most severe in the morning or after a period of inactivity. Other symptoms depend on the disease stage and may include:

- stiffness and limited motion of the lumbar spine
- pain and limited expansion of the chest due to involvement of the costovertebral joints
- peripheral arthritis involving shoulders, hips, and knees
- kyphosis in advanced stages, caused by chronic stooping to relieve symptoms
- hip deformity and associated limited range of motion (ROM)
- tenderness over the site of inflammation
- mild fatigue, fever, anorexia, or loss of weight; occasional iritis; aortic insufficiency and cardiomegaly; upper lobe pulmonary fibrosis (mimics tuberculosis).

These symptoms progress unpredictably, and the disease can go into remission, exacerbation, or arrest at any stage.

Diagnosis

Typical symptoms, a family history, and the presence of HLA-B27 strongly suggest ankylosing spondylitis. However, confirmation requires these characteristic X-ray findings:

- blurring of the bony margins of joints in the early stage
- bilateral sacroiliac involvement
- patchy sclerosis with superficial bony erosions

- eventual squaring of vertebral bodies
- "bamboo spine" with complete ankylosis.

Erythrocyte sedimentation rate and alkaline phosphatase and creatine kinase levels may be slightly elevated. A negative rheumatoid factor helps rule out rheumatoid arthritis, which produces similar symptoms.

Treatment

Because this disease's progression can't be stopped, treatment aims to delay further deformity by good posture, stretching and deep-breathing exercises and, in some patients, braces and lightweight supports. Anti-inflammatory analgesics, such as aspirin, indomethacin, sulfasalazine, and sulindac, control pain and inflammation.

Severe hip involvement usually necessitates surgical hip replacement. Severe spinal involvement may require a spinal wedge osteotomy to separate and reposition the vertebrae. This surgery is performed only on selected patients because of the risk of spinal cord damage and the long convalescence involved.

Special considerations

- Ankylosing spondylitis can be an extremely painful and crippling disease, so your main responsibility is to promote the patient's comfort. Keep in mind that his limited ROM makes simple tasks difficult. Offer support and reassurance.
- Administer medications as needed.
- Apply local heat and provide massage to relieve pain. Assess mobility and degree of discomfort frequently.
- Teach and assist with daily exercises, as needed, to maintain strength and function. Stress the importance of maintaining good posture.
- If treatment includes surgery, provide good postoperative care.
- Because ankylosing spondylitis is a chronic, progressively crippling con-

dition, comprehensive treatment should also reflect counsel from a social worker, visiting nurse, and dietitian.

To minimize deformities, advise the patient to:
• avoid any physical activity that places undue stress on the back, such as lifting heavy objects
• stand upright; sit upright in a high, straight chair; and avoid leaning over a desk
• sleep in a prone position on a hard mattress and avoid using pillows under neck or knees
• avoid prolonged walking, standing, sitting, or driving
• perform regular stretching and deep-breathing exercises and swim regularly, if possible
• have height measured every 3 to 4 months to detect any tendency toward kyphosis
• seek vocational counseling if his work requires standing or prolonged sitting at a desk
• contact the local Arthritis Foundation chapter for a support group.

ANORECTAL ABSCESS AND FISTULA

An anorectal abscess is a localized collection of pus caused by inflammation of the soft tissue near the rectum or anus. Such inflammation may produce an anal fistula — an abnormal opening in the anal skin — that may communicate with the rectum.

These disorders develop four times as often in men as in women, possibly because men wear rougher clothing that produces friction on the perianal skin and interferes with air circulation.

Causes

The inflammatory process that leads to abscess may begin with an abrasion or tear in the lining of the anal canal, rectum, or perianal skin, and subsequent infection by *Escherichia coli,* staphylococci, or streptococci. Such trauma may result from injections for treatment of internal hemorrhoids, enema-tip abrasions, puncture wounds from ingested eggshells or fishbones, or insertion of foreign objects.

Other preexisting lesions include infected anal fissure, infections from the anal crypt through the anal gland, ruptured anal hematoma, prolapsed thrombotic internal hemorrhoids, and septic lesions in the pelvis, such as acute appendicitis, acute salpingitis, and diverticulitis. Systemic illnesses that may cause abscesses include ulcerative colitis and Crohn's disease. However, many abscesses develop without preexisting lesions.

As the abscess produces more pus, a fistula may form in the soft tissue beneath the muscle fibers of the sphincters (especially the external sphincter), usually extending into the perianal skin. The internal (primary) opening of the abscess or fistula is usually near the anal glands and crypts; the external (secondary) opening, in the perianal skin.

Signs and symptoms

Characteristics are throbbing pain and tenderness at the site of the abscess. A hard, painful lump develops on one side, preventing comfortable sitting.

Diagnosis

Anorectal abscess is detectable on physical examination:
• *Perianal abscess* (80% of patients) is a red, tender, localized, oval swelling close to the anus. Sitting or coughing increases pain, and pus may drain from the abscess. Digital examination reveals no abnormalities.

• *Ischiorectal abscess* (15% of patients) involves the entire perianal region on the affected side of the anus. It's tender but may not produce drainage. Digital examination reveals a tender induration bulging into the anal canal.

• *Submucous or high intermuscular abscess* (5% of patients) may produce a dull, aching pain in the rectum, tenderness and, occasionally, induration. Digital examination reveals a smooth swelling of the upper part of the anal canal or lower rectum.

• *Pelvirectal abscess* (rare) produces fever, malaise, and myalgia but no local anal or external rectal signs or pain. Digital examination reveals a tender mass high in the pelvis, perhaps extending into one of the ischiorectal fossae.

If the abscess drains by forming a fistula, the pain usually subsides and the major signs become pruritic drainage and subsequent perianal irritation. The external opening of a fistula generally appears as a pink or red, elevated, discharging sinus or ulcer on the skin near the anus. Depending on the infection's severity, the patient may have chills, fever, nausea, vomiting, and malaise. Digital examination may reveal a palpable indurated tract and a drop or two of pus on palpation. The internal opening may be palpated as a depression or ulcer in the midline anteriorly or at the dentate line posteriorly. Examination with a probe may require an anesthetic.

Sigmoidoscopy, barium studies, and colonoscopy may be done to rule out other conditions.

Treatment
Anorectal abscesses require surgical incision under caudal anesthesia to promote drainage. Fistulas require a fistulotomy — removal of the fistula and associated granulation tissue — under caudal anesthesia. If the fistula tract is epithelialized, treatment requires fistulectomy — removal of the fistulous tract — followed by insertion of drains, which remain in place for 48 hours.

Special considerations
After incision to drain an anorectal abscess:

• Provide adequate medication for pain relief.

• Examine the wound frequently to assess proper healing, which should progress from the inside out. Healing should be complete in 4 to 5 weeks for perianal fistulas; in 12 to 16 weeks, for deeper wounds.

• Inform the patient that complete recovery takes time. Offer encouragement.

• Stress the importance of perianal cleanliness.

• Dispose of soiled dressings properly.

• Be alert for the first postoperative bowel movement. The patient may suppress the urge to defecate because of anticipated pain; the resulting constipation increases pressure at the wound site. Such a patient may benefit from a stool-softening laxative.

ANORECTAL STRICTURE

In anorectal stricture (stenosis, contracture), anorectal lumen size decreases; stenosis prevents dilation of the sphincter.

Causes
Anorectal stricture results from scarring after anorectal surgery or inflammation, inadequate postoperative care, or laxative abuse.

Signs and symptoms
The patient with anorectal stricture strains excessively when defecating and is unable to completely evacuate his

bowel. Other clinical effects include pain, bleeding, and pruritus ani.

Diagnosis
Visual inspection reveals narrowing of the anal canal. Digital examination reveals tenderness and tightness.

Treatment
Surgical removal of scar tissue is the most effective treatment. Digital or instrumental dilation may be beneficial but may cause additional tears and splits. If the cause of stricture is inflammation, correction of the underlying inflammatory process is necessary.

Special considerations
• Prepare the patient for the digital examination and testing by explaining procedures thoroughly.
• After surgery, check vital signs often until the patient is stable. Watch for signs of hemorrhage (excessive bleeding on rectal dressing).
• If surgery was performed under spinal anesthesia, record the patient's ability to move his legs, and keep the patient lying flat for 6 to 8 hours after surgery.
• When the patient's condition is stable, resume his normal diet, and record the time of his first bowel movement. Administer stool softeners as needed. Give analgesics, provide sitz baths, and change perianal dressings.

ANOREXIA NERVOSA

The key feature of anorexia nervosa is self-imposed starvation resulting from a distorted body image and an intense and irrational fear of gaining weight, even when the patient is obviously emaciated. An anorexic patient is preoccupied with her body size, describes herself as "fat," and commonly expresses dissatisfaction with a particular aspect of her physical appearance.

Although the term *anorexia* suggests that the patient's weight loss is associated with a loss of appetite, this is rare. Anorexia nervosa and bulimia nervosa can occur simultaneously. In anorexia nervosa, the refusal to eat may be accompanied by compulsive exercising, self-induced vomiting, or abuse of laxatives or diuretics.

Anorexia occurs in 5% to 10% of the population; about 95% of those affected are women. This disorder occurs primarily in adolescents and young adults but also may affect older women. The occurrence among males is rising.

The prognosis varies but improves if the patient is diagnosed early or if she wants to overcome the disorder and seeks help voluntarily. Mortality ranges from 5% to 15% — the highest mortality associated with a psychiatric disturbance. One-third of these deaths can be attributed to suicide.

Causes
No one knows what causes anorexia nervosa. Researchers in neuroendocrinology are seeking a physiologic cause but have found nothing definite. Clearly, social attitudes that equate slimness with beauty play some role in provoking this disorder; family factors also are implicated. Most theorists believe that refusing to eat is a subconscious effort to exert personal control over one's life.

Signs and symptoms
The patient's history usually reveals a 25% or greater weight loss for no organic reason, coupled with a morbid dread of being fat and a compulsion to be thin. Such a patient tends to be angry and ritualistic. She may report amenorrhea, infertility, loss of libido, fatigue, sleep alterations, intolerance to cold, and constipation.

DIAGNOSING ANOREXIA NERVOSA

A diagnosis of anorexia nervosa is made when the patient meets the following criteria from the *Diagnostic and Statistical Manual of Mental Disorders,* 4th ed.:
• refusal to maintain body weight over a minimal normal weight for age and height (for instance, weight loss leading to maintenance of body weight 15% below that expected); or failure to achieve expected weight gain during a growth period, leading to a body weight 15% below that expected
• intense fear of gaining weight or becoming fat, despite her underweight status
• a distorted perception of body weight, size, or shape (that is, the person claims to feel fat even when emaciated or believes that one body area is too fat even when it's obviously underweight)
• in women, absence of at least three consecutive menstrual cycles when otherwise expected to occur.

Hypotension and bradycardia may be present. Inspection may reveal an emaciated appearance, with skeletal muscle atrophy, loss of fatty tissue, atrophy of breast tissue, blotchy or sallow skin, lanugo on the face and body, and dryness or loss of scalp hair. Calluses on the knuckles and abrasions and scars on the dorsum of the hand may result from tooth injury during self-induced vomiting. Other signs of vomiting include dental caries and oral or pharyngeal abrasions.

Palpation may disclose painless salivary gland enlargement and bowel distention. Slowed reflexes may occur on percussion. Oddly, the patient usually demonstrates hyperactivity and vigor (despite malnourishment) and may exercise avidly without apparent fatigue.

Psychosocial assessment

During psychosocial assessment, the anorexic patient may express a morbid fear of gaining weight and an obsession with her physical appearance. Paradoxically, she also may be obsessed with food, preparing elaborate meals for others. Social regression, including poor sexual adjustment and fear of failure, is common. Like bulimia nervosa, anorexia nervosa often is associated with depression. The patient may report feelings of despair, hopelessness, and worthlessness as well as suicidal thoughts.

Diagnosis

For characteristic findings in patients with this condition, see *Diagnosing anorexia nervosa.*

In addition, laboratory tests help to identify various disorders and deficiencies and help to rule out endocrine, metabolic, and central nervous system abnormalities; cancer; malabsorption syndrome; and other disorders that cause physical wasting.

Abnormal findings that may accompany a weight loss exceeding 30% of normal body weight include:
• low hemoglobin level, platelet count, and white blood cell count
• prolonged bleeding time due to thrombocytopenia
• decreased erythrocyte sedimentation rate
• decreased levels of serum creatinine, blood urea nitrogen, uric acid, cholesterol, total protein, albumin, sodium, potassium, chloride, calcium, and fasting blood glucose (resulting from malnutrition)
• elevated levels of alanine aminotransferase and aspartate aminotransferase in severe starvation states

• elevated serum amylase levels when pancreatitis is not present

• in females, decreased levels of serum luteinizing hormone and follicle-stimulating hormone

• decreased triiodothyronine levels resulting from a lower basal metabolic rate

• dilute urine caused by the kidneys' impaired ability to concentrate urine

• nonspecific ST interval, prolonged PR interval, and T-wave changes on the electrocardiogram. Ventricular arrhythmias also may be present.

Treatment

Appropriate treatment aims to promote weight gain or control the patient's compulsive binge eating and purging and to correct malnutrition and the underlying psychological dysfunction. Hospitalization in a medical or psychiatric unit may be required to improve the patient's precarious physical condition. The hospital stay may be as brief as 2 weeks or may stretch from a few months to 2 years or longer.

A team approach

The most effective treatment in anorexia combines aggressive medical management, nutritional counseling, and individual, group, or family psychotherapy or behavior modification therapy. Treatment results may be discouraging. Many clinical centers are now developing inpatient and outpatient programs specifically aimed at managing eating disorders.

Treatment may include behavior modification (privileges depend on weight gain); curtailed activity for physical reasons (such as arrhythmias); vitamin and mineral supplements; a reasonable diet with or without liquid supplements; subclavian, peripheral, or enteral hyperalimentation

(enteral and peripheral routes carry less risk of infection); and group, family, or individual psychotherapy.

All forms of psychotherapy, from psychoanalysis to hypnotherapy, have been used in treating anorexia nervosa, with varying success. To be successful, psychotherapy should address the underlying problems of low self-esteem, guilt, anxiety, feelings of hopelessness and helplessness, and depression.

Special considerations

• During hospitalization, regularly monitor vital signs, nutritional status, and intake and output. Weigh the patient daily—before breakfast if possible. Because the patient fears being weighed, vary the weighing routine. Keep in mind that weight should increase from morning to night.

• Help the patient establish a target weight, and support her efforts to achieve this goal.

• Negotiate an adequate food intake with the patient. Make sure she understands that she'll need to comply with this contract or lose privileges. Frequently offer small portions of food or drinks if the patient wants them. Allow the patient to maintain control over the types and amounts of food she eats, if possible.

• Maintain one-on-one supervision of the patient during meals and for 1 hour afterward to ensure compliance with the dietary treatment program. For the hospitalized anorexic patient, food is considered a medication.

• During an acute anorexic episode, nutritionally complete liquids are more acceptable than solid food because they eliminate the need to choose between foods—something the anorexic patient often finds difficult.

• If tube feedings or other special feeding measures become necessary, fully explain these measures to the patient and be ready to discuss her fears or reluctance; limit the discussion about food itself.

• Anticipate a weight gain of about 1 lb (0.5 kg) per week.

• If edema or bloating occurs after the patient has returned to normal eating behavior, reassure her that this phenomenon is temporary. She may fear that she is becoming fat and stop complying with the prescribed treatment.

• Encourage the patient to recognize and express her feelings freely. If she understands that she can be assertive, she gradually may learn that expressing her true feelings will not result in her losing control or love.

• If a patient receiving outpatient treatment must be hospitalized, maintain contact with her treatment team to facilitate a smooth return to the outpatient setting.

• Remember that the anorexic patient uses exercise, preoccupation with food, ritualism, manipulation, and lying as mechanisms to preserve the only control she thinks that she has in her life.

• Because the patient and her family may need therapy to uncover and correct dysfunctional patterns, refer them to Anorexia Nervosa and Related Eating Disorders, a national information and support organization. This organization may help them understand what anorexia is, convince them that they need help, and help them find a psychotherapist or medical doctor who is experienced in treating this disorder.

• Teach the patient how to keep a food journal, including the types of food eaten, eating frequency, and feelings associated with eating and exercise.

• Advise family members to avoid discussing food with the patient.

ANXIETY DISORDER, GENERALIZED

Anxiety is a feeling of apprehension that some describe as an exaggerated feeling of impending doom, dread, or uneasiness. Unlike fear — a reaction to danger from a specific external source — anxiety is a reaction to an internal threat, such as an unacceptable impulse or a repressed thought that's straining to reach a conscious level.

A rational response to a real threat, occasional anxiety is a normal part of life. Overwhelming anxiety, however, can result in generalized anxiety disorder — uncontrollable, unreasonable worry that persists for at least 6 months and narrows perceptions or interferes with normal functioning. Recent evidence indicates that the prevalence of generalized anxiety disorder is greater than previously thought and may be even greater than that of depression.

Causes
Theorists share a common premise: Conflict, whether intrapsychic, sociopersonal, or interpersonal, promotes an anxiety state.

Signs and symptoms
Generalized anxiety disorder can begin at any age but typically has an onset in the 20s and 30s. It's equally common in men and women. Psychological or physiologic symptoms of anxiety states vary with the degree of anxiety. Mild anxiety mainly causes psychological symptoms, with unusual self-awareness and alertness to the environment. Moderate anxiety leads to selective inattention but with the ability to concentrate on a single task. Severe anxiety causes an inability to concentrate on more than scattered

details of a task. A panic state with acute anxiety causes a complete loss of concentration, often with unintelligible speech.

Physical examination of the patient with generalized anxiety disorder may reveal symptoms of motor tension, including trembling, muscle aches and spasms, headaches, and an inability to relax. Autonomic signs and symptoms include shortness of breath, tachycardia, sweating, and abdominal complaints.

In addition, the patient may startle easily and complain of feeling apprehensive, fearful, or angry and of having difficulty concentrating, eating, and sleeping. The medical, psychiatric, and psychosocial histories fail to identify a specific physical or environmental cause of the anxiety.

Diagnosis

For characteristic findings in patients with this condition, see *Diagnosing generalized anxiety disorder.*

In addition, laboratory tests must exclude organic causes of the patient's signs and symptoms, such as hyperthyroidism, pheochromocytoma, coronary artery disease, supraventricular tachycardia, and Ménière's disease. For example, an electrocardiogram can rule out myocardial ischemia in a patient who complains of chest pain. Blood tests, including a complete blood count, white blood cell count and differential, and serum lactate and calcium levels, can rule out hypocalcemia.

Because anxiety is the central feature of other mental disorders, psychiatric evaluation must rule out phobias, obsessive-compulsive disorders, depression, and acute schizophrenia.

Treatment

A combination of drug therapy and psychotherapy may help a patient with.

DIAGNOSING GENERALIZED ANXIETY DISORDER

When the patient's symptoms match criteria documented in the *Diagnostic and Statistical Manual of Mental Disorders,* 4th ed., the diagnosis of generalized anxiety disorder is confirmed. The criteria include the following:
• Excessive anxiety and worry about a number of events or activities occur more days than not for at least 6 months.
• The patient has difficulty in controlling the worry.
• The anxiety and worry are associated with at least three of the following six symptoms:
— restlessness or feeling keyed up or on edge
— being easily fatigued
— difficulty concentrating or mind going blank
— irritability
— muscle tension
— sleep disturbances (difficulty falling or staying asleep, or restless, unsatisfying sleep).
• The focus of the anxiety and worry isn't confined to features of an Axis I disorder.
• The anxiety, worry, or physical symptoms cause clinically significant distress or impairment in social, occupational, or other important areas of functioning.
• The disturbance is not due to the direct physiologic effects of a substance or a general medical condition and does not occur exclusively during a mood disorder, a psychotic disorder, or a pervasive developmental disorder.

generalized anxiety disorder. The benzodiazepine antianxiety drugs may relieve mild anxiety and improve the patient's ability to cope. Tricyclic antidepressants or higher doses of benzodiazepines may relieve the patient of severe anxiety and panic attacks. Buspirone, which is an antianxiety drug, causes the patient less sedation and poses less risk of physical and psychological dependence than the benzodiazepines.

Psychotherapy for generalized anxiety disorder has two goals: helping the patient identify and deal with the cause of the anxiety and eliminating environmental factors that precipitate an anxious reaction. In addition, the patient can learn relaxation techniques, such as deep breathing, progressive muscle relaxation, focused relaxation, and visualization.

Special considerations
• Stay with the patient when he's anxious, and encourage him to discuss his feelings. Reduce environmental stimuli and remain calm.
• Administer antianxiety drugs or tricyclic antidepressants as prescribed, and evaluate the patient's response to these drugs.
• Teach the patient about prescribed medications, including the need for compliance with the medication regimen. Review potential adverse reactions with the patient.
• Teach the patient effective coping strategies and relaxation techniques.
• Help the patient identify stressful situations that trigger his anxiety, and provide him with positive reinforcement when he uses alternative coping strategies.

APLASTIC AND HYPOPLASTIC ANEMIAS

These conditions result from injury to or destruction of stem cells in bone marrow or the bone marrow matrix, causing pancytopenia (anemia, granulocytopenia, thrombocytopenia) and bone marrow hypoplasia. Although often used interchangeably with other terms for bone marrow failure, aplastic anemias properly refer to pancytopenia resulting from the decreased functional capacity of a hypoplastic, fatty bone marrow.

These disorders generally produce fatal bleeding or infection, particularly when they're idiopathic or stem from chloramphenicol or from infectious hepatitis. Mortality for aplastic anemias with severe pancytopenia is 80% to 90%.

Causes
Aplastic anemias usually develop when damaged or destroyed stem cells inhibit red blood cell (RBC) production. Less commonly, they develop when damaged bone marrow microvasculature creates an unfavorable environment for cell growth and maturation. About half of such anemias result from drugs (antibiotics, anticonvulsants), toxic agents (such as benzene and chloramphenicol), or radiation. The rest may result from immunologic factors (unconfirmed), severe disease (especially hepatitis), or preleukemic and neoplastic infiltration of bone marrow. (See *Understanding bone marrow transplantation.*)

Idiopathic anemias may be congenital. Two such forms of aplastic anemia have been identified: congenital hypoplastic anemia (anemia of Blackfan

UNDERSTANDING BONE MARROW TRANSPLANTATION

In bone marrow transplantation, usually 500 to 700 ml of marrow are aspirated from the pelvic bones of a human leukocyte antigen (HLA)–compatible donor (allogeneic) or of the recipient himself during periods of complete remission (autologous). The aspirated marrow is filtered and then infused into the recipient in an attempt to repopulate the patient's marrow with normal cells.

This procedure has effected long-term, healthy survivals in about half of the patients with severe aplastic anemia. Bone marrow transplantation may also be effective in treating patients with acute leukemia, certain immunodeficiency diseases, and solid-tumor cancers.

Because bone marrow transplantation carries serious risks, it requires strict adherence to infection protection techniques and strict aseptic technique, and a primary caregiver to provide consistent care and continuous monitoring of the patient's status.

Before bone marrow infusion
• Explain that the success rate depends on the stage of the disease and on finding an HLA-identical sibling match.
• After bone marrow aspiration is completed under local anesthetic, apply pressure dressings to the *donor's* aspiration sites. Observe the sites for bleeding. Relieve pain with analgesics and ice packs as needed.
• Assess the patient's understanding of bone marrow transplantation. If necessary, correct any misconceptions about this procedure, and provide additional information Prepare the patient to expect an extended hospital stay. Explain that chemother-

apy and possibly radiation treatments are necessary to remove cells that may cause the body to reject the transplant.
• Various treatment protocols are used. For example, I.V. cyclophosphamide may be used with additional chemotherapeutic agents or total body irradiation and requires aggressive hydration to prevent hemorrhagic cystitis. Control nausea and vomiting with an antiemetic, such as ondansetron, prochlorperazine, metoclopramide, or lorazepam, as needed. Give allopurinol, as prescribed, to prevent hyperuricemia resulting from tumor breakdown products. Because alopecia is a common side effect of high-dose cyclophosphamide therapy, encourage the patient to choose a wig or scarf before treatment begins.
• Total body radiation (in one dose or several daily doses) follows chemotherapy, inducing total marrow aplasia. Warn the patient that cataracts, GI disturbances, and sterility are possible side effects.

During bone marrow infusion
• Monitor vital signs every 15 minutes.
• Watch for complications of marrow infusion, such as pulmonary embolus and volume overload.
• Reassure the patient throughout the procedure.

After bone marrow infusion
Continue to monitor the patient's vital signs every 15 minutes for 2 hours after infusion, then every 4 hours. Watch for fever and chills, which may be the only signs of infection. Give prophylactic antibiotics, as prescribed. To reduce the possibility

(continued)

UNDERSTANDING BONE MARROW TRANSPLANTATION *(continued)*

After bone marrow infusion
(continued)
of bleeding, don't administer medications rectally or I.M.
• Administer methotrexate or cyclosporine, as prescribed, to prevent graft-versus-host (GVH) reaction, a potentially fatal complication of allogeneic transplantation. Watch for signs of GVH reaction, such as maculopapular rash, pancytopenia, jaundice, joint pain, and anasarca.
• Administer vitamins, steroids, and iron and folic acid supplements as

appropriate. Administration of blood products, such as platelets and packed red blood cells, may also be indicated, depending on the results of daily blood studies.
• Provide good mouth care every 2 hours. Use hydrogen peroxide and nystatin mouthwash or oral fluconazole, for example, to prevent candidiasis and other mouth infections.
• Also provide meticulous skin care, paying special attention to pressure points and open sites, such as aspiration and I.V. sites.

---

and Diamond), which develops between ages 2 and 3 months, and Fanconi's syndrome, which develops between birth and age 10.

In Fanconi's syndrome, chromosomal abnormalities are usually associated with multiple congenital anomalies—such as dwarfism and hypoplasia of the kidneys and spleen. In the absence of a consistent familial or genetic history of aplastic anemia, researchers suspect that these congenital abnormalities result from an induced change in the development of the fetus.

Signs and symptoms
Clinical features of aplastic anemias vary with the severity of pancytopenia but often develop insidiously. Anemic symptoms include progressive weakness and fatigue, shortness of breath, headache, pallor, and, ultimately, tachycardia and congestive heart failure. Thrombocytopenia leads to ecchymosis, petechiae, and hemorrhage, especially from the mucous membranes (nose, gums, rectum, vagina) or into the retina or central nervous system. Neutropenia may lead to infec-

tion (fever, oral and rectal ulcers, sore throat) but without characteristic inflammation.

Diagnosis
Confirmation of aplastic anemia requires a series of laboratory tests:
• *RBCs* are usually normochromic and normocytic (although macrocytosis [larger-than-normal erythrocytes] and anisocytosis [excessive variation in erythrocyte size] may exist), with a total count of 1,000,000/µl or less. *Absolute reticulocyte count* is very low.
• *Serum iron* is elevated (unless bleeding occurs), but total iron-binding capacity is normal or slightly reduced. Hemosiderin is present, and tissue iron storage is visible microscopically.
• *Platelet, neutrophil,* and *white blood cell counts* fall.
• *Coagulation tests* (bleeding time), reflecting decreased platelet count, are abnormal.
• *Bone marrow aspiration* from several sites may yield a "dry tap," and a biopsy will show severely hypocellular or aplastic marrow, with varied amounts of fat, fibrous tissue, or gelatinous replacement; absence of tagged

iron (since iron is deposited in liver rather than bone marrow) and megakaryocytes; and depression of erythroid elements.

A differential diagnosis must rule out paroxysmal nocturnal hemoglobinuria and other diseases in which pancytopenia is common.

Treatment
Identifiable causes must be eliminated and vigorous supportive measures must be provided, such as transfusions of packed RBCs, platelets, and experimental human leukocyte antigen–matched leukocytes. Even after elimination of the cause, recovery can take months. Bone marrow transplantation is the treatment of choice for anemia due to severe aplasia and for patients who need constant RBC transfusions.

Preventing infection
Patients with low leukocyte counts need special measures to prevent infection. The infection itself may require specific antibiotics; however, these are not given prophylactically because they tend to encourage resistant strains of organisms. Patients with low hemoglobin counts may need respiratory support with oxygen, in addition to blood transfusions.

Other treatments
Other appropriate treatments include corticosteroids to stimulate erythroid production, marrow-stimulating agents, such as androgens (which are controversial), antilymphocyte globulin (experimental), immunosuppressive agents (if the patient doesn't respond to other therapy), and colony-stimulating factors to encourage growth of specific cellular components.

Special considerations
• If the platelet count is low (less than 20,000/μl), prevent hemorrhage by avoiding I.M. injections, suggesting the use of an electric razor and a soft toothbrush, humidifying oxygen to prevent drying of mucous membranes, and promoting regular bowel movements through the use of a stool softener and a proper diet to prevent constipation.
• Apply pressure to venipuncture sites until bleeding stops. Detect bleeding early by checking for blood in the urine and stools and assessing the skin for petechiae.
• Help prevent infection by washing your hands thoroughly before entering the patient's room, by making sure the patient is receiving a nutritious diet (high in vitamins and proteins) to improve his resistance, and by encouraging meticulous mouth and perianal care.
• Watch for life-threatening hemorrhage, infection, adverse reactions to drug therapy, and blood transfusion reaction.
• Make sure routine throat, urine, nose, rectal, and blood cultures are done regularly and correctly to check for infection. Teach the patient to recognize signs of infection, and tell him to report them immediately.
• If the patient has a low hemoglobin count, which causes fatigue, schedule frequent rest periods.
• Administer oxygen therapy as needed.
• If blood transfusions are necessary, be alert for a transfusion reaction by checking the patient's temperature and watching for other signs, such as rash, hives, itching, back pain, restlessness, and shaking chills.
• Reassure and support the patient and family by explaining the disease and its treatment, particularly if the patient has recurring acute episodes. Explain the purpose of all prescribed drugs, and discuss possible adverse reactions, including which ones he should report promptly.
• Encourage the patient who doesn't require hospitalization to continue his

normal lifestyle, with appropriate restrictions (such as regular rest periods), until remission occurs.

• To prevent aplastic anemia, monitor blood studies carefully in the patient receiving anemia-inducing drugs.

• Support efforts to educate the public about the hazards of toxic agents. Tell parents to keep toxic agents out of the reach of children.

• Encourage people who work with radiation to wear protective clothing and a radiation-detecting badge and to observe plant safety precautions. Those who work with the solvent benzene should know that 10 parts/million is the highest safe environmental level and that a delayed reaction to benzene may develop.

APPENDICITIS

The most common major surgical disease, appendicitis is inflammation of the vermiform appendix due to an obstruction. Appendicitis may occur at any age and affects both sexes equally; however, between puberty and age 25, it's more prevalent in men. Since the advent of antibiotics, the incidence and the death rate of appendicitis have declined; if untreated, this disease is invariably fatal.

Causes

Appendicitis probably results from an obstruction of the intestinal lumen caused by a fecal mass, stricture, barium ingestion, or viral infection. This obstruction sets off an inflammatory process that can lead to infection, thrombosis, necrosis, and perforation. If the appendix ruptures or perforates, the infected contents spill into the abdominal cavity, causing peritonitis, the most common and most perilous complication of appendicitis.

Signs and symptoms

Typically, appendicitis begins with generalized or localized abdominal pain in the upper right abdomen, followed by anorexia, nausea, and vomiting (rarely profuse). Pain eventually localizes in the lower right abdomen (McBurney's point) with abdominal "boardlike" rigidity, retractive respirations, increasing tenderness, increasingly severe abdominal spasms, and almost invariably, rebound tenderness. (Rebound tenderness on the opposite side of the abdomen suggests peritoneal inflammation.)

Later symptoms include constipation (although diarrhea is also possible), slight fever, and tachycardia. Sudden cessation of abdominal pain indicates a perforation or infarction of the appendix.

Diagnosis

Physical findings and characteristic clinical symptoms allow diagnosis of appendicitis. Findings that support the diagnosis include a temperature of 99° to 102° F (37.2° to 38.9° C) and a moderately elevated white blood cell count (12,000 to 15,000/μl), with increased immature cells.

The diagnosis must rule out illnesses with similar symptoms: gastritis, gastroenteritis, ileitis, colitis, diverticulitis, pancreatitis, renal colic, bladder infection, ovarian cyst, and uterine disease.

Treatment

Appendectomy is the only effective treatment. Laparoscopic appendectomies, which decrease the recovery time and thus the hospital stay, are now being done. If peritonitis develops, treatment involves GI intubation, parenteral replacement of fluids and electrolytes, and administration of antibiotics.

Special considerations
• Administer I.V. fluids to prevent dehydration. *Never* administer cathartics or enemas, which may rupture the appendix.
• Provide the patient with nothing by mouth.
• Administer analgesics judiciously because they may mask symptoms.
• To lessen pain, place the patient in Fowler's position. *Never* apply heat to the patient's lower right abdomen; this may cause the appendix to rupture.
• After appendectomy, monitor vital signs and intake and output. Give analgesics as needed.
• Teach the patient and encourage him to cough, breathe deeply, and turn frequently to prevent pulmonary complications.
• Document bowel sounds, passing of flatus, and bowel movements. These signs in a patient whose nausea and abdominal rigidity have subsided indicate that he is ready to resume oral fluids.
• Watch closely for possible surgical complications. Continuing pain and fever may signal an abscess. The complaint that "something gave way" may mean wound dehiscence. If an abscess or peritonitis develops, incision and drainage may be necessary. Frequently assess the dressing for wound drainage.
• Help the patient ambulate as soon as possible after surgery.
• In appendicitis complicated by peritonitis, a nasogastric tube may be needed to decompress the stomach and reduce nausea and vomiting. If so, record drainage and give good mouth and nose care.

ARM AND LEG FRACTURES

Fractures of the arms and legs usually result from trauma, and often cause substantial muscle, nerve, and other soft-tissue damage. The prognosis varies with the extent of disablement or deformity, the amount of tissue and vascular damage, the adequacy of reduction and immobilization, and the patient's age, health, and nutritional status.

Children's bones usually heal rapidly and without deformity. Bones of adults in poor health and with impaired circulation may never heal properly. Severe open fractures, especially of the femoral shaft, may cause substantial blood loss and life-threatening hypovolemic shock.

Causes
Most arm and leg fractures result from major trauma; for example, a fall on an outstretched arm, a skiing accident, or child abuse (shown by multiple or repeated episodes of fractures). However, in a person with a pathologic bone-weakening condition, such as osteoporosis, bone tumors, or metabolic disease, a mere cough or sneeze can also produce a fracture. Prolonged standing, walking, or running can cause stress fractures of the foot and ankle — usually in nurses, postal workers, soldiers, and joggers.

Signs and symptoms
Arm and leg fractures may produce any or all of the "5 Ps": pain and point tenderness, pallor, pulse loss, paresthesia, and paralysis. (The last three are distal to the fracture site.) Other signs include deformity, swelling, discoloration, crepitus, and loss of limb

function. Numbness and tingling, mottled cyanosis, cool skin at the end of the extremity, and loss of pulses distal to the injury indicate possible arterial compromise or nerve damage. Open fractures also produce an obvious skin wound.

Complications of arm and leg fractures include:

• permanent deformity and dysfunction if bones fail to heal (nonunion) or heal improperly (malunion)

• aseptic necrosis of bone segments from impaired circulation

• hypovolemic shock as a result of blood vessel damage (this is especially likely to develop in patients with a fractured femur)

• muscle contractures

• renal calculi from decalcification (produced by prolonged immobility)

• fat embolism.

Diagnosis

A history of trauma and a physical examination, including gentle palpation and a cautious attempt by the patient to move parts distal to the injury, suggest an arm or leg fracture.

When performing the physical examination, also check for other injuries. Anteroposterior and lateral X-rays of the suspected fracture, as well as X-rays of the joints above and below it, confirm the diagnosis.

Treatment

The following treatments are performed in arm and leg fractures.

Emergency treatment

In an emergency, the limb is splinted above and below the suspected fracture, a cold pack is applied, and the limb is elevated to reduce edema and pain.

In severe fractures that cause blood loss, direct pressure should be applied to control bleeding, and fluid replacement should be administered as soon as possible to prevent or treat hypovolemic shock.

Reduction

After a fracture has been confirmed, treatment begins with reduction (which involves restoring displaced bone segments to their normal position).

• After reduction, the fractured arm or leg must be immobilized by a splint or a cast or with traction. In closed reduction (which is accomplished by manual manipulation), a local anesthetic—such as lidocaine—and an analgesic—such as morphine I.M.—help relieve pain, whereas a muscle relaxant—such as diazepam I.V.—or a sedative—such as midazolam—facilitates the muscle stretching necessary to realign the bone.

• An X-ray study is ordered to confirm that reduction has been successful and that proper bone alignment has been achieved.

• When closed reduction is impossible, open reduction during surgery reduces and immobilizes the fracture by means of rods, plates, or screws. Afterward, a plaster cast is usually applied.

• When a splint or cast fails to maintain the reduction, immobilization requires skin or skeletal traction, using a series of weights and pulleys.

• In skin traction, elastic bandages and sheepskin coverings are used to attach traction devices to the patient's skin. In skeletal traction, a pin or wire inserted through the bone distal to the fracture and attached to a weight allows more prolonged traction.

Other measures

Treatment of open fractures also requires tetanus prophylaxis, prophylactic antibiotics, surgery to repair soft-tissue damage, and thorough debridement of the wound.

Special considerations

• Watch for signs of shock in the patient with a severe open fracture of a large bone, such as the femur.

• Monitor vital signs, and be especially alert for a rapid pulse, decreased blood pressure, pallor, and cool, clammy skin—all of which may indicate that the patient is in shock.

• Administer I.V. fluids as needed.

• Offer reassurance. With any fracture, the patient is likely to be frightened and in pain.

• Ease pain with analgesics as needed.

• Help the patient set realistic goals for recovery.

• If the fracture requires long-term immobilization with traction, reposition the patient often to increase comfort and prevent pressure ulcers. Assist with active range-of-motion exercises to prevent muscle atrophy. Encourage deep breathing and coughing to avoid hypostatic pneumonia.

• Urge adequate fluid intake to prevent urinary stasis and constipation. Watch for signs of renal calculi (flank pain, nausea, and vomiting).

• Provide good cast care. Support the cast with pillows. Observe for skin irritation near cast edges; check for foul odors or discharge. Tell the patient to report signs of impaired circulation (skin coldness, numbness, tingling, or discoloration) immediately. Warn the patient not to get the cast wet, and instruct him not to insert foreign objects under the cast.

• Encourage the patient to start moving around as soon as he's able. Help him to walk. (Remember, the patient who has been bedridden for some time may be dizzy at first.) Demonstrate how to use crutches properly.

• After cast removal, refer the patient for physical therapy to restore limb mobility.

ARTERIAL OCCLUSIVE DISEASE

In this disorder, the obstruction or narrowing of the lumen of the aorta and its major branches causes an interruption of blood flow, usually to the legs and feet. Arterial occlusive disease may affect the carotid, vertebral, innominate, subclavian, mesenteric, and celiac arteries. (See *Possible sites of major artery occlusion,* page 74.) Occlusions may be acute or chronic, and often cause severe ischemia, skin ulceration, and gangrene.

Arterial occlusive disease is more common in males than in females. The prognosis depends on the location of the occlusion, the development of collateral circulation to counteract reduced blood flow, and, in acute disease, the time elapsed between occlusion and its removal.

Causes

Arterial occlusive disease is a frequent complication of atherosclerosis. The occlusive mechanism may be endogenous, due to emboli formation or thrombosis, or exogenous, due to trauma or fracture. Predisposing factors include smoking; aging; conditions such as hypertension, hyperlipemia, and diabetes; and a family history of vascular disorders, myocardial infarction, or cerebrovascular accident.

Signs and symptoms

Evidence of this disease varies widely, according to the occlusion site. (See *Clinical features of arterial occlusive disease,* page 75.)

(Text continues on page 76.)

POSSIBLE SITES OF MAJOR ARTERY OCCLUSION

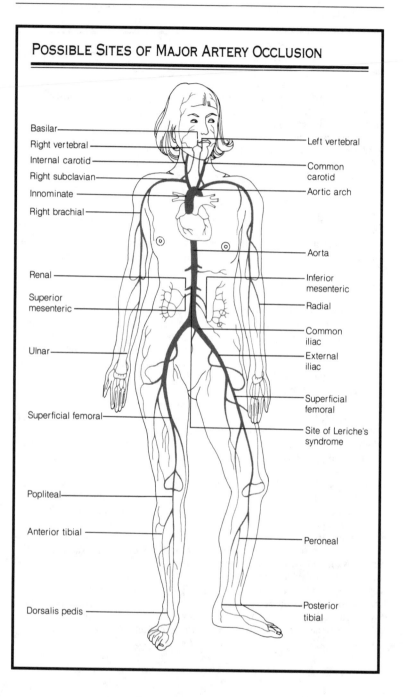

Basilar

Right vertebral

Internal carotid

Right subclavian

Innominate

Right brachial

Renal

Superior
mesenteric

Ulnar

Superficial femoral

Popliteal

Anterior tibial

Dorsalis pedis

Left vertebral

Common
carotid

Aortic arch

Aorta

Inferior
mesenteric

Radial

Common
iliac

External
iliac

Superficial
femoral

Site of Leriche's
syndrome

Peroneal

Posterior
tibial

CLINICAL FEATURES OF ARTERIAL OCCLUSIVE DISEASE

SITE OF OCCLUSION	SIGNS AND SYMPTOMS
Carotid arterial system • Internal carotid arteries • External carotid arteries	Neurologic dysfunction (transient ischemic attacks [TIAs] due to reduced cerebral circulation produce unilateral sensory or motor dysfunction [transient monocular blindness, hemiparesis], possible aphasia or dysarthria, confusion, decreased mentation, and headache; these recurrent clinical features usually last 5 to 10 minutes but may persist up to 24 hours and may herald a stroke); absent or decreased pulsation with an auscultatory bruit over the affected vessels
Vertebrobasilar system • Vertebral arteries • Basilar arteries	Neurologic dysfunction (TIAs of brain stem and cerebellum produce binocular visual disturbances, vertigo, dysarthria, and "drop attacks" [falling down without loss of consciousness]); less common than carotid TIA
Innominate Brachiocephalic artery	Neurologic dysfunction (signs and symptoms of vertebrobasilar occlusion); indications of ischemia (claudication) of right arm; possible bruit over right side of neck
Subclavian artery	Subclavian steal syndrome (characterized by the backflow of blood from the brain through the vertebral artery on the same side as the occlusion, into the subclavian artery distal to the occlusion); clinical effects of vertebrobasilar occlusion and exercise-induced arm claudication; possible gangrene, usually limited to the digits
Mesenteric artery • Superior (most commonly affected) • Celiac axis • Inferior	Bowel ischemia, infarct necrosis, and gangrene; sudden, acute abdominal pain; nausea and vomiting; diarrhea; leukocytosis; and shock due to massive intraluminal fluid and plasma loss
Aortic bifurcation (saddle block occlusion, an emergency associated with cardiac embolization)	Sensory and motor deficits (muscle weakness, numbness, paresthesia, paralysis), and signs of ischemia (sudden pain; cold, pale legs with decreased or absent peripheral pulses) in both legs
Iliac artery (Leriche's syndrome)	Intermittent claudication of lower back, buttocks, and thighs, relieved by rest; absent or reduced femoral or distal pulses; possible bruit over femoral arteries; impotence in males
Femoral and popliteal artery (associated with aneurysm formation)	Intermittent claudication of the calves on exertion, ischemic pain in feet, pretrophic pain (heralds necrosis and ulceration), leg pallor and coolness, blanching of feet on elevation, gangrene, no palpable pulses in ankles and feet

Diagnosis

In arterial occlusive disease, the diagnosis is usually based on the patient history and physical examination.

Pertinent supportive diagnostic tests include the following:

• *Arteriography* demonstrates the type (thrombus or embolus), location, and degree of obstruction, and collateral circulation. Arteriography is particularly useful in chronic disease or for evaluating candidates for reconstructive surgery.

• *Doppler ultrasonography* and *plethysmography* are noninvasive tests that, in acute disease, show decreased blood flow distal to the occlusion.

• *Ophthalmodynamometry* helps determine the degree of obstruction in the internal carotid artery by comparing ophthalmic artery pressure to brachial artery pressure on the affected side. More than a 20% difference between pressures suggests insufficiency.

• *EEG* and a *computed tomography scan* may be necessary to rule out brain lesions.

Treatment

Effective treatment depends on the cause, location, and size of the obstruction. For mild chronic disease, supportive measures include elimination of smoking, hypertension control, and walking exercise. For carotid artery occlusion, antiplatelet therapy may begin with dipyridamole and aspirin. For intermittent claudication of chronic occlusive disease, pentoxifylline may improve blood flow through the capillaries, particularly for patients who are poor candidates for surgery.

Acute arterial occlusive disease usually requires surgery to restore circulation to the affected area. Possible procedures include the following:

• *Embolectomy:* A balloon-tipped Fogarty catheter is used to remove thrombotic material from the artery. Embolectomy is used mainly for mesenteric, femoral, or popliteal artery occlusion.

• *Thromboendarterectomy:* Opening of the occluded artery and direct removal of the obstructing thrombus and the medial layer of the arterial wall; usually performed after angiography and often used with autogenous vein or Dacron bypass surgery (femoral-popliteal or aortofemoral).

• *Patch grafting:* This procedure involves removal of the thrombosed arterial segment and replacement with an autogenous vein or Dacron graft.

• *Bypass graft:* Blood flow is diverted through an anastomosed autogenous or Dacron graft past the thrombosed segment.

• *Thrombolytic therapy:* Lysis of any clot around or in the plaque by urokinase, streptokinase, or alteplase.

• *Atherectomy:* Excision of plaque using a drill or slicing mechanism.

• *Balloon angioplasty:* Compression of the obstruction using balloon inflation.

• *Laser angioplasty:* Use of excision and hot-tip lasers to vaporize the obstruction.

• *Stents:* Insertion of a mesh of wires that stretch and mold to the arterial wall to prevent reocclusion. This new adjunct follows laser angioplasty or atherectomy.

• *Combined therapy:* Concomitant use of any of the above treatments.

• *Lumbar sympathectomy:* An adjunct to surgery, depending on the condition of the sympathetic nervous system.

Amputation becomes necessary with failure of arterial reconstructive surgery or with the development of gangrene, persistent infection, or intractable pain.

Other treatments include heparin to prevent emboli (for embolic occlusion) and bowel resection after restoration of blood flow (for mesenteric artery occlusion).

Special considerations
• Provide comprehensive patient teaching, such as proper foot care. Explain all diagnostic tests and procedures. Advise the patient to stop smoking and to follow the prescribed medical regimen.

Preoperatively (during an acute episode):
• Assess the patient's circulatory status by checking for the most distal pulses and by inspecting his skin color and temperature.
• Provide pain relief as needed.
• Administer heparin by continuous I.V. drip as needed. Use an infusion monitor or pump to ensure the proper flow rate.
• Wrap the patient's affected foot in soft cotton batting, and reposition it frequently to prevent pressure on any one area. Strictly avoid elevating or applying heat to the affected leg.
• Watch for signs of fluid and electrolyte imbalance, and monitor intake and output for signs of renal failure (urine output less than 30 ml/hour).
• If the patient has a carotid, innominate, vertebral, or subclavian artery occlusion, monitor him for signs of cerebrovascular accident, such as numbness in an arm or leg and intermittent blindness.

Postoperatively:
• Monitor the patient's vital signs. Continuously assess his circulatory function by inspecting skin color and temperature and by checking for distal pulses. In charting, compare earlier assessments and observations. Watch closely for signs of hemorrhage (tachycardia, hypotension), and check dressings for excessive bleeding.
• In carotid, innominate, vertebral, or subclavian artery occlusion, assess neurologic status frequently for changes in level of consciousness or muscle strength and pupil size.
• In mesenteric artery occlusion, connect a nasogastric tube to low inter-

mittent suction. Monitor intake and output (low urine output may indicate damage to renal arteries during surgery). Check bowel sounds for the return of peristalsis. Increasing abdominal distention and tenderness may indicate extension of bowel ischemia with resulting gangrene, necessitating further excision, or they may indicate peritonitis.
• In saddle block occlusion, check distal pulses for adequate circulation. Watch for signs of renal failure and mesenteric artery occlusion (severe abdominal pain), and for cardiac arrhythmias, which may precipitate embolus formation.
• In iliac artery occlusion, monitor urine output for signs of renal failure from decreased perfusion to the kidneys as a result of surgery. Provide meticulous catheter care.
• In both femoral and popliteal artery occlusions, assist with early ambulation, but discourage prolonged sitting.
• After amputation, check the patient's stump carefully for drainage and record its color and amount, and the time. Elevate the stump, and administer adequate analgesic medication. Since phantom limb pain is common, explain this phenomenon to the patient.
• When preparing the patient for discharge, instruct him to watch for signs of recurrence (pain, pallor, numbness, paralysis, absence of pulse) that can result from graft occlusion or occlusion at another site. Warn him against wearing constrictive clothing.

ASBESTOSIS

A form of pneumoconiosis, asbestosis is characterized by diffuse interstitial fibrosis. It can develop as long as 15 to 20 years after regular exposure to asbestos has ended. A potent co-carcinogen, it aggravates the risk of lung cancer in cigarette smokers.

Causes

Asbestosis results from the inhalation of respirable asbestos fibers (50 microns or more in length, 0.5 microns or less in diameter), which assume a longitudinal orientation in the airway, move in the direction of airflow, and penetrate respiratory bronchioles and alveolar walls.

Sources include the mining and milling of asbestos, the construction industry (where asbestos is used in a prefabricated form), and the fireproofing and textile industries; asbestos is also used in the production of paints, plastics, and brake and clutch linings.

Asbestos-related diseases develop in families of asbestos workers as a result of exposure to fibrous dust shaken off workers' clothing at home. Such diseases develop in the general public as a result of exposure to fibrous dust or waste piles from nearby asbestos plants.

Pathophysiology

Inhaled fibers become encased in a brown, proteinlike sheath rich in iron (ferruginous bodies or asbestos bodies), found in sputum and lung tissue. Interstitial fibrosis develops in lower lung zones, causing obliterative changes in lung parenchyma and pleurae. Raised hyaline plaques may form in parietal pleura, diaphragm, and pleura contiguous with the pericardium.

Signs and symptoms

Clinical features may appear before chest X-ray changes. The first symptom is usually dyspnea on exertion, typically after 10 years' exposure. As fibrosis extends, dyspnea on exertion increases, until eventually, dyspnea occurs even at rest; advanced disease also causes a dry cough (may be productive in smokers), chest pain (often pleuritic), recurrent respiratory infections, and tachypnea.

Cardiovascular complications include pulmonary hypertension, right ventricular hypertrophy, and cor pulmonale. Finger clubbing commonly occurs.

Diagnosis

The patient history reveals occupational, family, or neighborhood exposure to asbestos fibers. Physical examination reveals characteristic dry crackles at lung bases.

Chest X-rays show fine, irregular, and linear diffuse infiltrates; extensive fibrosis results in a "honeycomb" or "ground-glass" appearance. X-rays may also show pleural thickening and pleural calcification, with bilateral obliteration of costophrenic angles and, in later stages, an enlarged heart with a classic "shaggy" heart border.

Pulmonary function studies show:
• *vital capacity, forced vital capacity,* and *total lung capacity:* decreased
• *forced expiratory volume:* decreased or normal
• *diffusing capacity of the lungs for carbon monoxide:* reduced when fibrosis destroys alveolar walls and thickens alveolar capillary membrane.

Arterial blood gas analysis reveals:
• *partial pressure of oxygen:* decreased
• *partial pressure of carbon dioxide:* low because of hyperventilation.

Treatment and special considerations

• Respiratory symptoms may be relieved by chest physical therapy techniques, such as controlled coughing and segmental bronchial drainage, with chest percussion and vibration. Aerosol therapy, inhaled mucolytics, and increased fluid intake (at least 3 qt [3 L] daily) may also help relieve respiratory symptoms.
• Diuretics, digitalis glycoside preparations, and salt restriction may be in-

dicated for patients with cor pulmonale.

• Hypoxia requires oxygen administration by cannula or mask (1 to 2 L/minute), or by mechanical ventilation if arterial oxygen can't be maintained above 40 mm Hg.

• Prompt administration of antibiotics is required for respiratory infections.

• Teach the patient to prevent infections by avoiding crowds and persons with infections and by receiving influenza and pneumococcal vaccines.

• Improve the patient's ventilatory efficiency by encouraging physical reconditioning, energy conservation in daily activities, and relaxation techniques.

ASCARIASIS

Also known as *roundworm infection,* ascariasis is caused by the parasitic worm *Ascaris lumbricoides.* It occurs worldwide but is most common in tropical areas with poor sanitation and in Asia, where farmers use human feces as fertilizer. In the United States, it's more prevalent in the South, particularly among 4- to 12-year-olds.

Causes

A. lumbricoides is a large roundworm resembling an earthworm. It's transmitted to humans by ingestion of soil contaminated with human feces that harbor *A. lumbricoides* ova. Such ingestion may occur directly (by eating contaminated soil) or indirectly (by eating poorly washed raw vegetables grown in contaminated soil).

Ascariasis never passes directly from person to person. After ingestion, *A. lumbricoides* ova hatch and release larvae, which penetrate the intestinal wall and reach the lungs through the bloodstream. After about 10 days in pulmonary capillaries and alveoli, the larvae migrate to the bronchioles, bronchi, trachea, and epiglottis. There they are swallowed and return to the intestine to mature into worms.

Signs and symptoms

Mild intestinal ascariasis may cause only vague stomach discomfort. The first clue may be vomiting a worm or passing a worm in the stools. Severe disease, however, causes stomach pain, vomiting, restlessness, disturbed sleep, and, in extreme cases, intestinal obstruction. Larvae migrating by the lymphatic and the circulatory systems cause symptoms that vary; for instance, when they invade the lungs, pneumonitis may result.

Diagnosis

Microscopic identification of ova in the stools or observation of adult worms, which may be passed rectally or by mouth, confirms the diagnosis. When migrating larvae invade the alveoli, other conclusive tests include X-rays that show characteristic bronchovascular markings: infiltrates, patchy areas of pneumonitis, and widening of hilar shadows. In a patient with ascariasis, these findings usually accompany a complete blood count that shows eosinophilia.

Treatment

Anthelminthic drug therapy, the primary treatment, consists of pyrantel or piperazine to temporarily paralyze the worms, permitting peristalsis to expel them. Mebendazole is also used to block helminth nutrition. These drugs are up to 95% effective, even after a single dose.

In multiple helminth infection, one of these drugs must be the first treatment; using some other anthelmintic first may stimulate *A. lumbricoides* perforation into other organs. No specific treatment exists for migratory infection because anthelmintics affect only mature worms.

In intestinal obstruction, nasogastric (NG) suctioning controls vomiting. When suctioning can be discontinued, instill piperazine and clamp the tube. If vomiting doesn't occur, give a second dose of piperazine orally 24 hours later. If this is ineffective, treatment probably requires surgery.

Special considerations
- Although isolation is unnecessary, properly dispose of feces and soiled linen, and carefully wash your hands after patient contact.
- If the patient is receiving NG suctioning, be sure to provide good mouth care.
- Teach the patient to prevent reinfection by washing hands thoroughly, especially before eating and after defecation, and by bathing and changing his underwear and bed linens daily.
- Inform the patient of possible drug adverse reactions. Tell him that piperazine may cause stomach upset, dizziness, and urticaria. Be aware that piperazine is contraindicated in seizure disorders. Pyrantel produces red stools and vomit and may cause stomach upset, headache, dizziness, and skin rash; and mebendazole, abdominal pain and diarrhea.

ASPERGILLOSIS

This condition is an opportunistic infection caused by fungi of the genus *Aspergillus,* usually *A. fumigatus, A. flavus,* or *A. niger.* It occurs in four major forms:

- *aspergilloma,* which produces a fungus ball in the lungs (called a mycetoma)

- *allergic aspergillosis,* a hypersensitive asthmatic reaction to *Aspergillus* antigens
- *aspergillosis endophthalmitis,* an infection of the anterior and posterior chambers of the eye that can lead to blindness
- *disseminated aspergillosis,* an acute infection that produces septicemia, thrombosis, and infarction of virtually any organ, but especially the heart, lungs, brain, and kidneys.

Aspergillus may cause infection of the ear (otomycosis), cornea (mycotic keratitis), and prosthetic heart valves (endocarditis); pneumonia (especially in persons receiving immunosuppressive drugs, such as antineoplastic agents or high-dose steroids); sinusitis; and brain abscesses.

The prognosis varies with each form. Occasionally, aspergilloma causes fatal hemoptysis.

Causes
Aspergillus is found worldwide, often in fermenting compost piles and damp hay. It's transmitted by inhalation of fungal spores or, in aspergillosis endophthalmitis, by the invasion of spores through a wound or other tissue injury. It's a common laboratory contaminant.

Aspergillus produces clinical infection only in persons who become especially vulnerable to it. Such vulnerability can result from excessive or prolonged use of antibiotics, glucocorticoids, or other immunosuppressive agents; from radiation; from such conditions as acquired immunodeficiency syndrome, Hodgkin's disease, leukemia, azotemia, alcoholism, sarcoidosis, bronchitis, or bronchiectasis; from organ transplants; and, in aspergilloma, from tuberculosis or another cavitary lung disease.

Signs and symptoms

The incubation period in aspergillosis ranges from a few days to weeks. In aspergilloma, colonization of the bronchial tree with *Aspergillus* produces plugs and atelectasis and forms a tangled ball of hyphae (fungal filaments), fibrin, and exudate in a cavity left by a previous illness such as tuberculosis. Characteristically, aspergilloma either produces no symptoms or mimics tuberculosis, causing a productive cough and purulent or blood-tinged sputum, dyspnea, empyema, and lung abscesses.

Allergic aspergillosis causes wheezing, dyspnea, cough with some sputum production, pleural pain, and fever.

Aspergillosis endophthalmitis usually appears 2 to 3 weeks after an eye injury or surgery, and accounts for half of all cases of endophthalmitis. It causes clouded vision, eye pain, and reddened conjunctivae. Eventually, *Aspergillus* infects the anterior and posterior chambers, where it produces purulent exudate.

In disseminated aspergillosis, *Aspergillus* invades blood vessels, and causes thrombosis, infarctions, and the typical signs of septicemia (chills, fever, hypotension, delirium), with azotemia, hematuria, urinary tract obstruction, headaches, seizures, bone pain and tenderness, and soft-tissue swelling. This form of the disorder is rapidly fatal.

Diagnosis

In patients with aspergilloma, a chest X-ray reveals a crescent-shaped radiolucency surrounding a circular mass, but this isn't definitive for aspergillosis. In aspergillosis endophthalmitis, a history of ocular trauma or surgery and a culture or exudate showing *Aspergillus* is diagnostic. In allergic aspergillosis, sputum examination shows eosinophils. Culture of mouth scrapings or sputum showing *Aspergillus* is inconclusive because even healthy persons harbor this fungus. In disseminated aspergillosis, culture and microscopic examination of affected tissue can confirm the diagnosis, but this form is usually diagnosed at autopsy.

Treatment and special considerations

- Aspergillosis doesn't require isolation.
- Treatment of aspergilloma necessitates local excision of the lesion and supportive therapy, such as chest physiotherapy and coughing, to improve pulmonary function.
- Allergic aspergillosis requires desensitization and, possibly, steroids.
- Disseminated aspergillosis and aspergillosis endophthalmitis require a 2- to 3-week course of I.V. amphotericin B (as well as prompt cessation of immunosuppressive therapy). However, the disseminated form of aspergillosis often resists amphotericin B therapy and rapidly progresses to death.

LIFE-THREATENING DISORDER

ASPHYXIA

A condition of insufficient oxygen and accumulating carbon dioxide in the blood and tissues due to interference with respiration, asphyxia results in cardiopulmonary arrest. Without prompt treatment it's fatal.

Causes

Asphyxia results from any condition or substance that inhibits respiration:

- hypoventilation as a result of narcotic abuse, medullary disease or hemorrhage, pneumothorax, respiratory muscle paralysis, or cardiopulmonary arrest

• intrapulmonary obstruction, as in airway obstruction, severe asthma, foreign body aspiration, pulmonary edema, pneumonia, and near-drowning
• extrapulmonary obstruction, as in tracheal compression from a tumor, strangulation, trauma, or suffocation
• inhalation of toxic agents, as in carbon monoxide poisoning, smoke inhalation, and excessive oxygen inhalation.

Signs and symptoms

Depending on the duration and degree of asphyxia, common symptoms include anxiety, dyspnea, agitation and confusion leading to coma, altered respiratory rate (apnea, bradypnea, occasional tachypnea), decreased breath sounds, central and peripheral cyanosis (cherry-red mucous membranes in late-stage carbon monoxide poisoning), seizures, and fast, slow, or absent pulse.

Diagnosis

The patient history and laboratory test results provide the diagnosis. Arterial blood gas measurement, the most important test, indicates decreased partial pressure of oxygen (less than 60 mm Hg) and increased partial pressure of carbon dioxide (more than 50 mm Hg). Chest X-rays may show a foreign body, pulmonary edema, or atelectasis. Toxicology tests may show drugs, chemicals, or abnormal hemoglobin. Pulmonary function tests may indicate respiratory muscle weakness.

Treatment

Asphyxia requires immediate respiratory support—with cardiopulmonary resuscitation, endotracheal intubation, and supplemental oxygen as needed. The underlying cause must be remedied: bronchoscopy for extraction of a foreign body; a narcotic antagonist like naloxone for narcotic overdose; gastric lavage for poisoning; and withholding of supplemental oxygen for carbon dioxide narcosis caused by excessive oxygen therapy.

Special considerations

• Respiratory distress is frightening, so reassure the patient during treatment.
• Give prescribed medications.
• Suction carefully, as needed, and encourage deep breathing.
• Closely monitor vital signs and laboratory test results.
• To prevent drug-induced asphyxia, warn patients about the danger of taking alcohol with other central nervous system depressants.

ASTHMA

A reversible lung disease, asthma is characterized by obstruction or narrowing of the airways, which are typically inflamed and hyperresponsive to a variety of stimuli. It may resolve spontaneously or with treatment. Its symptoms range from mild wheezing and dyspnea to life-threatening respiratory failure. Symptoms of bronchial airway obstruction may persist between acute episodes.

Causes

Although this common condition can strike at any age, half of all cases first occur in children under age 10; in this age-group, asthma affects twice as many boys as girls.

Extrinsic and intrinsic asthma

Asthma that results from sensitivity to specific external allergens is known as *extrinsic*. In cases in which the allergen is not obvious, asthma is referred to as *intrinsic*. Allergens that cause extrinsic asthma include pollen, animal dander, house dust or mold, kapok or feather pillows, food additives containing sulfites, and any other sensitizing substance.

Extrinsic (atopic) asthma usually begins in childhood and is accompanied by other manifestations of atopy (Type I, immunoglobulin E–mediated allergy), such as eczema and allergic rhinitis.

In intrinsic (nonatopic) asthma, no extrinsic allergen can be identified. Most cases are preceded by a severe respiratory infection. Irritants, emotional stress, fatigue, exposure to noxious fumes, and endocrine, temperature, and humidity changes may aggravate intrinsic asthma attacks. In many asthmatics, intrinsic and extrinsic asthma coexist.

Asthma triggers

Several drugs and chemicals may provoke an asthma attack without using the immunoglobulin E (IgE) pathway. Apparently, they trigger release of mast-cell mediators via prostaglandin inhibition. Examples of these substances include aspirin, various nonsteroidal anti-inflammatory drugs (such as indomethacin and mefenamic acid), and tartrazine, a yellow food dye.

Exercise may also provoke an asthma attack. In exercise-induced asthma, bronchospasm may follow heat and moisture loss in the upper airways.

Two-phase allergic response

When the patient inhales an allergenic substance, sensitized IgE antibodies trigger mast-cell degranulation in the lung interstitium, releasing histamine, cytokines, prostaglandins, thromboxanes, leukotrienes, and eosinophil chemotaxic factors. Histamine then attaches to receptor sites in the larger bronchi, causing irritation, inflammation, and edema. In the late phase, inflammatory cells flow in. The influx of eosinophils provides additional inflammatory mediators and contributes to local injury.

Signs and symptoms

An asthma attack may begin dramatically, with simultaneous onset of many severe symptoms, or insidiously, with gradually increasing respiratory distress. It typically includes progressively worsening shortness of breath, cough, wheezing, and chest tightness, or some combination of these symptoms.

During an acute attack, the cough sounds tight and dry. As the attack subsides, tenacious mucoid sputum is produced (except in young children, who don't expectorate). Characteristic wheezing may be accompanied by coarse rhonchi, but fine crackles aren't heard unless associated with a related complication. Between acute attacks, breath sounds may be normal.

The intensity of breath sounds in symptomatic asthma is typically reduced. A prolonged phase of forced expiration is typical of airflow obstruction. Evidence of lung hyperinflation (use of accessory muscles, for example) is particularly common in children. Acute attacks may be accompanied by tachycardia, tachypnea, and diaphoresis. In severe attacks, the patient may be unable to speak more than a few words without pausing for breath. Cyanosis, confusion, and lethargy indicate the onset of life-threatening status asthmaticus and respiratory failure. (See *Determining asthma's severity,* pages 84 and 85.)

Diagnosis

Laboratory studies in patients with asthma often show these abnormalities:

- *Pulmonary function studies* reveal signs of airway obstruction (decreased peak expiratory flow rates and forced expiratory volume in 1 second [FEV_1]), low-normal or decreased vital capacity, and increased total lung and residual capacity. However, pulmonary

DETERMINING ASTHMA'S SEVERITY

MILD ASTHMA	MODERATE ASTHMA	SEVERE ASTHMA	RESPIRATORY FAILURE
SIGNS AND SYMPTOMS DURING ACUTE PHASE			
Brief wheezing, coughing, dyspnea with activity • Infrequent nocturnal coughing or wheezing • Adequate air exchange • Intermittent, brief (less than 1 hour) wheezing, cough, or dyspnea once or twice a week • Asymptomatic between attacks	• Respiratory distress at rest • Hyperpnea • Marked coughing and wheezing • Air exchange normal or below normal • Exacerbations that may last several days	• Marked respiratory distress • Marked wheezing or absent breath sounds • Pulsus paradoxus greater than 10 mm Hg • Chest wall contractions • Continuous symptoms • Frequent exacerbations	• Severe respiratory distress • Impaired consciousness • Severe wheezing or silent chest • Use of accessory muscles of respiration • Prominent pulsus paradoxus (30 to 50 mm Hg)
DIAGNOSTIC TEST RESULTS			
• Forced expiratory volume in 1 second (FEV₁) or peak flow 80% of normal values • pH normal or increased • Partial pressure of arterial oxygen (Pao₂) normal or decreased • Partial pressure of arterial carbon dioxide (Paco₂) normal or decreased • Chest X-ray normal	• FEV, or peak flow 60% to 80% of normal values; may vary 20% to 30% with symptoms • pH generally elevated • Pao₂ increased • Paco₂ generally decreased • Chest X-ray that shows hyperinflation	• FEV, or peak flow less than 60% of normal values; may normally vary 20% to 30% with routine medications and up to 50% with exacerbations • pH normal or reduced • Pao₂ decreased • Paco₂ normal or increased • Chest X-ray that may show hyperinflation	• FEV₁ or peak flow less than 25% of normal values • pH decreased • Pao₂ less than 60 mm Hg • Paco₂ greater than 40 mm Hg

DETERMINING ASTHMA'S SEVERITY (continued)

MILD ASTHMA	MODERATE ASTHMA	SEVERE ASTHMA	RESPIRATORY FAILURE
OTHER ASSESSMENT FINDINGS			
• One attack per week (or none) • Positive response to bronchodilator therapy within 24 hours • No signs of asthma between episodes • No sleep interruption • No hyperventilation • Minimal evidence of airway obstruction • Minimal or no increase in lung volume	• Symptoms occur more than two times weekly • Coughing and wheezing between episodes • Diminished exercise tolerance • Possible sleep interruption • Increased lung volumes	• Frequent severe attacks • Daily wheezing • Poor exercise tolerance • Frequent sleep interruption • Bronchodilator therapy doesn't completely reverse airway obstruction • Markedly increased lung volumes	• Cyanosis • Tachycardia

function studies may be normal between attacks.

• *Pulse oximetry* may reveal decreased arterial oxygen saturation (SaO_2).

• *Arterial blood gas (ABG) analysis* provides the best indications of an attack's severity. In acutely severe asthma, the partial pressure of arterial oxygen is less than 60 mm Hg, the partial pressure of arterial carbon dioxide ($PaCO_2$) is 40 mm Hg or more, and pH is usually decreased.

• *Complete blood count with differential* reveals an increased eosinophil count.

• *Chest X-rays* may show hyperinflation with areas of focal atelectasis.

Before initiating tests for asthma, rule out other causes of airway obstruction and wheezing. In children, such causes include cystic fibrosis, tumors of the bronchi or mediastinum, and acute viral bronchitis; in adults, other causes include obstructive pulmonary disease, congestive heart failure, and epiglottitis.

Treatment

Acute asthma is treated by decreasing bronchoconstriction, reducing bronchial airway edema, and increasing pulmonary ventilation. Treatment after an acute episode includes avoiding or removing precipitating factors, such as environmental allergens or irritants.

If asthma is known to be caused by a particular antigen, it may be treated by desensitizing the patient through a series of injections of limited amounts of the antigen. The aim is to curb the patient's immune response to the antigen.

If asthma results from an infection, antibiotics are prescribed. Drug therapy, which is most effective when be-

gun soon after the onset of signs and symptoms, usually includes:
• bronchodilators to decrease bronchoconstriction, for example, the methylxanthines (theophylline and aminophylline) and the beta$_2$-adrenergic agonists (albuterol and terbutaline)
• corticosteroids (hydrocortisone sodium succinate, prednisone, methylprednisolone, and beclomethasone) for their anti-inflammatory and immunosuppressive effects, which decrease inflammation and edema of the airways
• cromolyn and nedocromil to help prevent the release of the chemical mediators (histamine and leukotrienes) that cause bronchoconstriction
• anticholinergic bronchodilators, such as ipratropium, which block acetylcholine, another chemical mediator.

For the most part, medical treatment of asthma attacks must be tailored to each patient. However, the following treatments are generally used:

Chronic mild asthma

A beta$_2$-adrenergic agonist by metered-dose inhaler is used (alone or with cromolyn) before exercise and exposure to an allergen or other stimuli to prevent symptoms. The beta$_2$-adrenergic agonist is used every 3 to 4 hours if symptoms occur.

Chronic moderate asthma

Initial treatment may include an inhaled beta-adrenergic bronchodilator, an inhaled corticosteroid, and cromolyn. If symptoms persist, inhaled corticosteroid dosage may be increased, and sustained-release theophylline or an oral beta$_2$-adrenergic agonist (or both) may be added. Short courses of oral corticosteroids may also be used.

Chronic severe asthma

Initially, around-the-clock oral bronchodilator therapy with a long-acting theophylline or a beta$_2$-adrenergic agonist may be required, supplemented with an inhaled beta$_2$-adrenergic agonist and an inhaled corticosteroid with or without cromolyn. An oral corticosteroid, such as prednisone, may be added in acute exacerbations.

Acute asthma attack

Acute attacks that don't respond to self-treatment may require hospital care, beta$_2$-adrenergic agonists by inhalation or S.C. injection (in three doses over 60 to 90 minutes) and, possibly, oxygen for hypoxemia. If the patient responds poorly, systemic corticosteroids and, possibly, S.C. epinephrine may help. Beta$_2$-adrenergic agonist inhalation continues hourly. I.V. aminophylline may be added to the regimen and I.V. fluid therapy is started. Patients who don't respond to this treatment, whose airways remain obstructed, and who have increasing respiratory difficulty are at risk for status asthmaticus and may require mechanical ventilation.

Status asthmaticus

Treatment consists of aggressive drug therapy: a beta$_2$-adrenergic agonist by nebulizer every 30 to 60 minutes, possibly supplemented with S.C. epinephrine, I.V. corticosteroids, I.V. aminophylline, oxygen administration, I.V. fluid therapy, and intubation and mechanical ventilation for hypercapnic respiratory failure (PaCO$_2$ of 40 mm Hg or more).

Special considerations

During an acute attack:
• First assess the severity of asthma.
• Administer the prescribed treatments and assess the patient's response.
• Place the patient in high Fowler's

position. Encourage pursed-lip and diaphragmatic breathing. Help him to relax.

• Monitor the patient's vital signs. Keep in mind that developing or increasing tachypnea may indicate worsening asthma and that tachycardia may indicate worsening asthma or drug toxicity. Blood pressure readings may reveal pulsus paradoxus, indicating severe asthma. Hypertension may indicate asthma-related hypoxemia.

• Administer prescribed humidified oxygen by nasal cannula at 2 L/minute to ease breathing and to increase SaO_2. Later, adjust oxygen according to the patient's vital signs and ABG levels.

• Anticipate intubation and mechanical ventilation if the patient fails to maintain adequate oxygenation.

• Monitor serum theophylline levels to ensure they're in the therapeutic range. Observe the patient for signs of theophylline toxicity (vomiting, diarrhea, and headache) as well as for signs of subtherapeutic dosage (respiratory distress and increased wheezing).

• Observe the frequency and severity of the patient's cough, and note whether it's productive. Then auscultate his lungs, noting adventitious or absent sounds. If his cough isn't productive and rhonchi are present, teach him effective coughing techniques. If the patient can tolerate postural drainage and chest percussion, perform these procedures to clear secretions. Suction an intubated patient as needed.

• Treat dehydration with I.V. fluids until the patient can tolerate oral fluids, which will help loosen secretions.

• If conservative treatment fails to improve the airway obstruction, anticipate bronchoscopy or bronchial lavage when the area of collapse is a lobe or larger.

During long-term care:

• Monitor the patient's respiratory status to detect baseline changes, to assess response to treatment, and to prevent or detect complications.

• Auscultate the lungs frequently, noting the degree of wheezing and quality of air movement.

• Review ABG levels, pulmonary function test results, and SaO_2 readings.

• If the patient is taking systemic corticosteroids, observe for complications, such as elevated blood glucose levels and friable skin and bruising.

• Cushingoid effects resulting from long-term use of corticosteroids may be minimized by alternate-day dosage or use of prescribed inhaled corticosteroids.

• If the patient is taking corticosteroids by inhaler, watch for signs of candidal infection in the mouth and pharynx. Using an extender device and rinsing the mouth afterward may prevent this.

• Observe the patient's anxiety level. Keep in mind that measures that reduce hypoxemia and breathlessness should help relieve anxiety.

• Keep the room temperature comfortable and use an air conditioner or a fan in hot, humid weather.

• Control exercise-induced asthma by instructing the patient to use a bronchodilator or cromolyn 30 minutes before exercise. Also instruct him to use pursed-lip breathing while exercising.

For all patients:

• Teach the patient and his family to avoid known allergens and irritants.

• Describe prescribed drugs, including their names, dosages, actions, adverse effects, and special instructions.

• Teach the patient how to use a metered-dose inhaler. If he has difficulty using an inhaler, he may need an extender device to optimize drug delivery and lower the risk of candidal infection with orally inhaled corticosteroids.

• If the patient has moderate to severe asthma, explain how to use a peak flow meter to measure the degree of airway obstruction. Tell him to keep a record of peak flow readings and to bring it to medical appointments. Explain the importance of calling the doctor at once if the peak flow drops suddenly. (A drop can signal severe respiratory problems.)

• Tell the patient to notify the doctor if he develops a fever higher than 100° F (37.8° C), chest pain, shortness of breath without coughing or exercising, or uncontrollable coughing. An uncontrollable asthma attack requires immediate attention.

• Teach the patient diaphragmatic and pursed-lip breathing as well as effective coughing techniques.

• Urge the patient to drink at least 3 qt (3 L) of fluids daily to help loosen secretions and maintain hydration.

ATELECTASIS

This condition is marked by incomplete expansion of lobules (clusters of alveoli) or lung segments, which may result in partial or complete lung collapse. The collapsed areas are unavailable for gas exchange; unoxygenated blood passes through these areas unchanged, thereby producing hypoxia.

Atelectasis may be chronic or acute and occurs to some degree in many patients undergoing upper abdominal or thoracic surgery. The prognosis depends on prompt removal of any airway obstruction, relief of hypoxia, and reexpansion of collapsed lung.

Causes

Atelectasis often results from bronchial occlusion by mucus plugs and is frequently a problem in patients with chronic obstructive pulmonary disease, bronchiectasis, or cystic fibrosis and in those who smoke heavily.

(Smoking increases mucus production and damages cilia.) Atelectasis may also result from occlusion by foreign bodies, bronchogenic carcinoma, and inflammatory lung disease.

Other causes include respiratory distress syndrome of the newborn (hyaline membrane disease), oxygen toxicity, and pulmonary edema, in which alveolar surfactant changes increase surface tension and permit complete alveolar deflation.

External compression, which inhibits full lung expansion, or any condition that makes deep breathing painful may also cause atelectasis. Such compression or pain may result from upper abdominal surgical incisions, rib fractures, pleuritic chest pain, tight dressings around the chest, or obesity (which elevates the diaphragm and reduces tidal volume).

Atelectasis may also result from prolonged immobility, which causes preferential ventilation of one area of the lung over another, or mechanical ventilation using constant small tidal volumes without intermittent deep breaths.

Central nervous system depression (as in drug overdose) eliminates periodic sighing and is a predisposing factor of progressive atelectasis.

Signs and symptoms

Clinical effects vary with the cause of collapse, the degree of hypoxia, and any underlying disease but generally include some dyspnea. Atelectasis of a small area of the lung may produce only minimal symptoms that subside without specific treatment.

However, massive collapse can produce severe dyspnea, anxiety, cyanosis, diaphoresis, peripheral circulatory collapse, tachycardia, and substernal or intercostal retraction. Also, atelectasis may result in compensatory hyperinflation of unaffected areas of the lung, mediastinal shift to the affected side, and elevation of the ipsilateral hemidiaphragm.

Diagnosis

An accurate patient history, a physical examination, and a chest X-ray provides baseline data for a diagnosis. Auscultation reveals diminished or bronchial breath sounds. When much of the lung is collapsed, percussion reveals dullness. However, extensive areas of "microatelectasis" may exist without abnormalities on the chest X-ray. In widespread atelectasis, the chest X-ray shows characteristic horizontal lines in the lower lung zones and, with segmental or lobar collapse, characteristic dense shadows often associated with hyperinflation of neighboring lung zones.

If the cause is unknown, diagnostic procedures may include bronchoscopy to rule out an obstructing neoplasm or a foreign body.

Treatment

Appropriate treatment includes incentive spirometry, mucolytics, chest percussion, postural drainage, and frequent coughing and deep-breathing exercises. If these measures fail, bronchoscopy may help remove secretions. Humidity and bronchodilators can improve mucociliary clearance and dilate airways; they're sometimes used with a nebulizer.

Atelectasis secondary to an obstructing neoplasm may require surgery or radiation therapy. Postoperative thoracic and abdominal surgery patients require analgesics to facilitate deep breathing, which minimizes the risk of atelectasis.

Special considerations

• To prevent atelectasis, encourage postoperative and other high-risk patients to cough and deep-breathe every 1 to 2 hours.

• To minimize pain during coughing exercises in postoperative patients, hold a pillow tightly over the incision; teach the patient this technique as well. *Gently* reposition these patients often and help them walk as soon as possible.

• Administer adequate analgesics to control pain.

• During mechanical ventilation, maintain tidal volume at 10 to 15 ml/kg of the patient's body weight to ensure adequate lung expansion. Use the sigh mechanism on the ventilator, if appropriate, to intermittently increase tidal volume at the rate of 10 to 15 sighs/hour.

• Use an incentive spirometer to encourage deep inspiration through positive reinforcement. Teach the patient how to use the spirometer and encourage him to use it every 1 to 2 hours.

• Humidify inspired air and encourage adequate fluid intake to mobilize secretions. To promote loosening and clearance of secretions, use postural drainage and chest percussion.

• If the patient is intubated or uncooperative, provide suctioning as needed. Use sedatives with discretion, since they depress respirations and the cough reflex and suppress sighing. Be aware that the patient won't cooperate with treatment if he's in pain.

• Assess breath sounds and ventilatory status frequently and be alert for any changes.

• Teach the patient about respiratory care, including postural drainage, coughing, and deep breathing.

• Encourage the patient to stop smoking, to lose weight, or both, as needed. Refer him to appropriate support groups for help.

• Provide reassurance and emotional support because the patient may be frightened by his limited breathing capacity.

ATOPIC DERMATITIS

This chronic skin disorder is characterized by superficial skin inflammation and intense itching. Although atopic dermatitis may appear at any age, it typically begins during infancy or early childhood. It may then subside spontaneously, followed by exacerbations in late childhood, adolescence, or early adulthood. Atopic dermatitis affects less than 1% of the population.

Causes

Several theories attempt to explain the pathogenesis of this disorder, which has an unknown cause. One theory suggests an underlying metabolically or biochemically induced skin disorder that's genetically linked to elevated serum immunoglobulin E (IgE) levels; another suggests defective T-cell function.

Exacerbating factors of atopic dermatitis include irritants, infections (commonly caused by *Staphylococcus aureus*), and some allergens. Although no reliable link exists between atopic dermatitis and exposure to inhalant allergens (such as house dust and animal dander), exposure to food allergens (such as soybeans, fish, or nuts) may coincide with flare-ups of atopic dermatitis.

Signs and symptoms

Scratching the skin causes vasoconstriction and intensifies pruritus, resulting in erythematous, weeping lesions. Eventually, the lesions become scaly and lichenified. Usually, they're located in areas of flexion and extension such as the neck, antecubital fossa, popliteal folds, and behind the ears. Patients with atopic dermatitis are prone to unusually severe viral infections, bacterial and fungal skin infections, ocular complications, and allergic contact dermatitis.

Diagnosis

Typically, the patient has a history of atopy, such as asthma, hay fever, or urticaria; family members may have a similar history. Laboratory tests reveal eosinophilia and elevated serum IgE levels.

Treatment

Measures to ease this chronic disorder include meticulous skin care, environmental control of offending allergens, and drug therapy. Because dry skin aggravates itching, frequent application of nonirritating topical lubricants is important, especially after bathing or showering. Minimizing exposure to allergens and irritants, such as wools and harsh detergents, also helps control symptoms.

Drug therapy involves corticosteroids and antipruritics. Active dermatitis responds well to topical corticosteroids, such as fluocinolone acetonide and flurandrenolide. These drugs should be applied immediately after bathing for optimal penetration. Oral antihistamines, especially the phenothiazine derivatives, such as methdilazine and trimeprazine, help control itching. A bedtime dose of antihistamines may reduce involuntary scratching during sleep. If a secondary infection develops, antibiotics are necessary.

Because this disorder may frustrate the patient and strain family ties, counseling may play a role in treatment.

Special considerations

• Monitor the patient's compliance with drug therapy.
• Teach the patient when and how to apply topical corticosteroids.
• Emphasize the importance of good personal hygiene.

- Be alert for signs and symptoms of secondary infection; teach the patient how to recognize them as well.
- If the patient's diet is modified to exclude food allergens, monitor his nutritional status.
- Discourage the use of laundry additives.
- Offer support to help the patient and his family cope with this chronic disorder.

ATTENTION-DEFICIT HYPERACTIVITY DISORDER

The patient with attention-deficit hyperactivity disorder has difficulty focusing his attention or engaging in quiet, passive activities, or both. Although the disorder is present at birth, diagnosis before age 4 or 5 is difficult unless the child shows severe symptoms. Some patients, though, aren't diagnosed until adulthood. Males are three times more likely to be affected than females.

Causes

Attention-deficit hyperactivity disorder is commonly thought to be a physiologic brain disorder with a familial tendency. Some studies indicate that it may result from disturbances in neurotransmitter levels in the brain.

Signs and symptoms

Typically, the patient is characterized as a fidgeter and a daydreamer. Other descriptive terms include inattentive and lazy. Although the patient may be highly intelligent, his school or work performance patterns are sporadic, and he may jump from one partly completed project, thought, or task to an-

other. Some patients have an attention deficit without hyperactivity; they're less likely to be diagnosed and treated.

In a younger child, signs and symptoms include an inability to wait in line, remain seated, wait his turn, or concentrate on one activity until its completion. An older child or an adult may be described as impulsive and easily distracted by irrelevant thoughts, sounds, or sights. He may also be characterized as emotionally labile or inattentive. His disorganization becomes apparent when he has difficulty meeting deadlines and keeping track of school or work tools and materials.

Diagnosis

Commonly, the child with attention-deficit hyperactivity disorder is referred for evaluation by the school. Diagnosis of this disorder usually begins by obtaining data from several sources, including the parents, teachers, and the child himself. Complete psychological, medical, and neurologic evaluations rule out other problems. Then the child undergoes tests that measure impulsiveness, attention, and the ability to sustain a task. The combined findings portray a clear picture of the disorder and of the areas of support the child will need.

For characteristic findings in patients with this condition, see *Diagnosing attention-deficit hyperactivity disorder*, page 92.

Treatment

Education represents the first step in effective treatment. The entire treatment team (which ideally includes parents, teachers, and therapists as well as the patient and the doctor) must understand the disorder and its effect on the individual's functioning.

Treatment varies, depending on the severity of symptoms and their effects on the ability to function. Behavior modification, coaching, external struc-

DIAGNOSING ATTENTION-DEFICIT HYPERACTIVITY DISORDER

The *Diagnostic and Statistical Manual of Mental Disorders*, 4th ed., groups a selection of symptoms into inattention and hyperactivity-impulsivity categories. The diagnosis of attention-deficit hyperactivity disorder is based on the person demonstrating at least six symptoms from the inattention group or at least six symptoms from the hyperactivity-impulsivity group. The symptoms must have persisted for at least 6 months to a degree that is maladaptive and inconsistent with the person's developmental level.

Symptoms of inattention

The person manifesting *inattention*:
• often fails to give close attention to details or makes careless mistakes in schoolwork, work, or other activities
• often has difficulty sustaining attention in tasks or play activities
• often does not seem to listen when spoken to directly
• often does not follow through on instructions and fails to finish schoolwork, chores, or duties in the workplace (not because of oppositional behavior or failure to understand instructions)
• often has difficulty organizing tasks and activities
• often avoids, dislikes, or is reluctant to engage in tasks that require sustained mental effort (such as schoolwork or homework)
• often loses things necessary for tasks or activities (for example, toys, school assignments, pencils, books, or tools)
• often becomes distracted by extraneous stimuli
• often demonstrates forgetfulness in daily activities.

Symptoms of hyperactivity-impulsivity

The person manifesting *hyperactivity*:
• often fidgets with hands or feet or squirms in seat
• often leaves his seat in the classroom or in other situations in which remaining seated is expected
• often runs about or climbs excessively in situations in which remaining seated is expected
• often has difficulty playing or engaging in leisure activities quietly
• often is characterized as "on the go" or acts as if "driven by a motor"
• often talks excessively.
   The person manifesting *impulsivity*:
• often blurts out answers before questions have been completed
• often has difficulty awaiting his turn
• often interrupts or intrudes on others.

Additional features

• Some symptoms that caused impairment were evident before age 7.
• Some impairment from the symptoms is present in two or more settings.
• Clinically significant impairment in social, academic, or occupational functioning must be clearly evident.
• The symptoms do not occur exclusively during the course of a pervasive developmental disorder, schizophrenia, or another psychotic disorder and are not better accounted for by another mental disorder.

ture, use of planning and organizing systems, and supportive psychotherapy help the patient cope with the disorder.

Some patients benefit from medication to relieve symptoms. Ideally, the treatment team identifies the symptoms to be managed, selects appropriate medication, and then tracks the patient's symptoms to determine the effectiveness of the medication. Stimulants, such as methylphenidate and dextroamphetamine, are the most commonly used agents. However, other drugs, including tricyclic antidepressants (such as desipramine and nortriptyline), mood stabilizers, and beta blockers sometimes help control symptoms.

Special considerations
• Work with the individual to develop external structure and controls.
• Set realistic expectations and limits because the patient with an attention deficit disorder is easily frustrated (which leads to decreased self-control).
• Remain calm and consistent.
• Keep instructions short and simple.
• Provide praise, rewards, and positive feedback whenever possible.

AUTISTIC DISORDER

A severe, pervasive developmental disorder, autistic disorder is marked by unresponsiveness to social contact, gross deficits in intelligence and language development, ritualistic and compulsive behaviors, restricted capacity for developmentally appropriate activities and interests, and bizarre responses to the environment. Autistic disorder may be complicated by epileptic seizures, depression and, during periods of stress, catatonic phenomena.

Autism usually becomes apparent before the child reaches age 30 months but, in some children, the actual onset is difficult to determine. Occasionally, autistic disorder isn't recognized until the child enters school. Autistic disorder is rare, affecting 4 to 5 children per 10,000 births. It affects three to four times more boys than girls, usually the firstborn boy. The prognosis is poor; most patients require a structured environment throughout life.

Causes
Autistic disorder is thought to result from a combination of psychological, physiologic, and sociological factors. The parents of an autistic child may appear distant and unaffectionate. However, because autistic children are unresponsive or respond with rigid, screaming resistance to touch and attention, parental remoteness may be merely a frustrated, helpless reaction to this disorder, not its cause.

Some autistic children show abnormal but nonspecific EEG findings that suggest brain dysfunction, possibly resulting from trauma, disease, or a structural abnormality. Autistic disorder also has been associated with maternal rubella, untreated phenylketonuria, tuberous sclerosis, anoxia during birth, encephalitis, infantile spasms, and fragile X syndrome.

Signs and symptoms
Typical features of infantile autistic disorder include unresponsiveness to people, language impairment, lack of imaginative play, bizarre behavior patterns, and abnormal reactions to sensory stimuli.

Unresponsiveness to people
Infants with this disorder won't cuddle, avoid eye contact and facial expression, and are indifferent to affection

and physical contact. Parents may report that the child becomes rigid or flaccid when held, cries when touched, and shows little or no interest in human contact.

As the infant grows older, his smiling response is delayed or absent. He doesn't lift his arms in anticipation of being picked up or form an attachment to a specific caregiver. Nor does he show the anxiety about strangers that's typical in the 8-month-old infant.

The autistic child fails to learn the usual socialization games (peek-a-boo, pat-a-cake, or bye-bye). He's likely to relate to others only to fill a physical need and then without eye contact or speech. The end result may be mutual withdrawal between parents and child.

Severe language impairment

The child may be mute or may use immature speech patterns. For example, he may use a single word to express a series of activities; he may say "ground" when referring to any step in using a playground slide.

His speech commonly shows echolalia (meaningless repetition of words or phrases addressed to him) and pronoun reversal ("you go walk" when he means "I want to go for a walk"). When answering a question, he may simply repeat the question to mean yes and remain silent to mean no.

Lack of imaginative play

The child shows little imagination, seldom acting out adult roles or engaging in fantasy play. In fact, he may insist on lining up an exact number of toys in the same manner over and over or repetitively mimic the actions of someone else.

Bizarre behavior

The autistic child shows characteristically bizarre behavior patterns, such as screaming fits, rituals, rhythmic rocking, arm flapping, crying without tears, and disturbed sleeping and eating patterns. His behavior may be self-destructive (hand biting, eye gouging, hair pulling, or head banging) or self-stimulating (playing with his own saliva, feces, and urine).

His bizarre responses to his environment include an extreme compulsion for sameness.

Abnormal response to sensory stimuli

The autistic child may underreact or overreact to sensory stimuli; he may ignore objects — dropping those he is given or not looking at them — or he may become excessively absorbed in them — continually watching the objects or the movement of his own fingers over the objects. He commonly responds to stimuli by head banging, rocking, whirling, and hand flapping. He tends to avoid using sight and hearing to interact with the environment.

Other behavioral abnormalities

Other characteristics of an autistic child may include:
• cognitive impairment (most have an IQ of 35 to 49)
• eating, drinking, and sleeping problems — for example, limiting his diet to just a few foods, excessive drinking, or repeatedly waking during the night and rocking
• mood disorders, including labile mood, giggling or crying without reason, lack of emotional responses, no fear of real danger but excessive fear of harmless objects, and generalized anxiety.

Diagnosis

For characteristic findings in patients with this condition, see *Diagnosing autistic disorder.*

Diagnosing Autistic Disorder

Autism is diagnosed when the patient meets the criteria in the *Diagnostic and Statistical Manual of Mental Disorders,* 4th ed. At least six characteristics from the following three categories must be present, including at least two from the social interaction category and one each from the communication and patterns categories.

Social interaction
Impairment in social interaction, as shown by at least two of the following:
• marked impairment in the use of multiple nonverbal behaviors, such as eye-to-eye gaze, facial expression, body postures, and gestures to regulate social interaction
• failure to develop peer relationships appropriate to developmental level
• no spontaneous sharing of enjoyment, interests, or achievements with others
• lack of social or emotional reciprocity
• gross impairment in ability to make peer friendships.

Communication
Impairment in communication, as shown by at least one of the following:
• delay in, or total lack of, spoken language development

• in individuals with adequate speech, marked impairment in initiating or sustaining a conversation with others
• stereotyped and repetitive use of language or idiosyncratic language
• lack of varied, spontaneous make-believe play or social imitative play appropriate to developmental level.

Patterns
Restricted, repetitive, and stereotyped patterns of behavior, interests, and activities, as manifested by at least one of the following:
• encompassing preoccupation with one or more stereotyped and restricted patterns of interest that is abnormal either in intensity or focus
• apparently inflexible adherence to specific nonfunctional routines or rituals
• stereotyped and repetitive motor mannerisms
• persistent preoccupation with parts of objects.

Additional criteria
Delays or abnormal functioning in at least one of the following before age 3:
• social interaction
• language as used in social communication
• symbolic or imaginative play.
  The disturbance is not better accounted for by Rett's disorder or childhood disintegrative disorder.

Treatment
The difficult and prolonged treatment of autistic disorder must begin early, continue for years (through adolescence), and coordinate efforts to encourage social adjustment and speech development and to reduce self-destructive behavior.

Behavioral techniques are used to decrease symptoms and increase the child's ability to respond. Positive reinforcement, using food and other rewards, can enhance language and social skills. Providing pleasurable sensory and motor stimulation (jogging, playing with a ball) encourages appropriate behavior and helps eliminate inappropriate behavior. Drug therapy with an agent such as haloperidol may be helpful.

Treatment may take place in a psychiatric institution, in a specialized school, or in a day-care program, but the current trend is toward home treatment. Because family members tend to feel inadequate and guilty, they may need counseling. Until the causes of infantile autism are known, prevention is not possible.

Special considerations
• Reduce self-destructive behaviors. Physically stop the child from harming himself, while firmly saying "no." When he responds to your voice, first give a primary reward (such as food); later, substitute verbal or physical reinforcement (such as saying "good" or giving the child a hug or a pat on the back).
• Foster appropriate use of language. Provide positive reinforcement when the child indicates his needs correctly. Give verbal reinforcement at first (such as "good" or "great"); later, give physical reinforcement (such as a hug or a pat on the hand or shoulder).
• Encourage development of self-esteem. Show the child that he's acceptable as a person.
• Encourage self-care. For example, place a brush in the child's hand and guide his hand to brush his hair. Similarly, teach him to wash his hands and face.
• Encourage acceptance of minor environmental changes. Prepare the child for the change by telling him about it. Make the change minor; for example, change the color of his bedspread or the placement of food on his plate. When he has accepted minor changes, move on to bigger ones.
• Provide emotional support to the parents, and refer them to the Autism Society of America.

• Teach the parents how to physically care for the child's needs.
• Teach the parents how to identify signs of excessive stress and the coping skills to use under these circumstances. Emphasize that they'll be ineffective caregivers if they don't take the time to meet their own needs in addition to those of their child.
• Help the parents understand that they aren't responsible for the child's condition.

Basal Cell Epithelioma

A slow-growing, destructive skin tumor, basal cell epithelioma or carcinoma usually occurs in persons over age 40; it's more prevalent in blond, fair-skinned males and is the most common malignant tumor affecting whites.

Causes

Prolonged sun exposure is the most common cause of basal cell epithelioma, but arsenic ingestion, radiation exposure, burns, immunosuppression, and, rarely, vaccinations are other possible causes.

Although the pathogenesis of basal cell epithelioma is uncertain, some experts now hypothesize that it originates when, under certain conditions, undifferentiated basal cells become carcinomatous instead of differentiating into sweat glands, sebum, and hair.

Signs and symptoms

Three types of basal cell epithelioma occur:

• *Noduloulcerative lesions* occur most often on the face, particularly the forehead, eyelid margins, and nasolabial folds. In early stages, these lesions are small, smooth, pinkish, and translucent papules. Telangiectatic vessels cross the surface, and the lesions are occasionally pigmented. As the lesions enlarge, their centers become depressed and their borders become firm and elevated. Ulceration and local invasion eventually occur. These ulcerated tumors, known as "rodent ulcers," rarely metastasize; however, if untreated, they can spread to vital areas and become infected. If they invade large blood vessels, they can cause massive hemorrhage.

• *Superficial basal cell epitheliomas* are often numerous and commonly occur on the chest and back. They're oval or irregularly shaped, lightly pigmented plaques, with sharply defined, slightly elevated threadlike borders. Because of superficial erosion, these lesions appear scaly and have small, atrophic areas in the center that resemble psoriasis or eczema. They're usually chronic and don't tend to invade other areas. Superficial basal cell epitheliomas are related to ingestion of or exposure to arsenic-containing compounds.

• *Sclerosing basal cell epitheliomas (morphealike epitheliomas)* are waxy, sclerotic, yellow to white plaques without distinct borders. Occurring on the head and neck, sclerosing basal cell epitheliomas often look like small patches of scleroderma.

Diagnosis

All types of basal cell epitheliomas are diagnosed by clinical appearance, an incisional or excisional biopsy, and histologic study.

Treatment

Depending on the size, location, and depth of the lesion, treatment may include curettage and electrodesiccation, chemotherapy, surgical excision, irradiation, or chemosurgery.

• Curettage and electrodesiccation offer good cosmetic results for small lesions.

• Topical fluorouracil is often used for superficial lesions. This medication produces marked local irritation or inflammation in the involved tissue but no systemic effects.

• Microscopically controlled surgical excision carefully removes recurrent lesions until a tumor-free plane is achieved. After removal of large lesions, skin grafting may be required.

• Irradiation is used if the tumor location requires it, and for elderly or debilitated patients who might not withstand surgery.

• Cryotherapy with liquid nitrogen freezes and kills the cells.

• Chemosurgery is often necessary for persistent or recurrent lesions. Chemosurgery consists of periodic applications of a fixative paste (such as zinc chloride) and subsequent removal of fixed pathologic tissue. Treatment continues until tumor removal is complete.

Special considerations

• Instruct the patient to eat frequent small meals that are high in protein. Suggest eggnog, pureed foods, or liquid protein supplements if the lesion has invaded the oral cavity and caused eating problems.

• Tell the patient that to prevent disease recurrence, he needs to avoid excessive sun exposure and use a strong sunscreen or sunshade to protect his skin from damage by ultraviolet rays.

• Advise the patient to relieve local inflammation from topical fluorouracil with cool compresses or corticosteroid ointment.

• Instruct the patient with noduloulcerative basal cell epithelioma to wash his face gently when ulcerations and crusting occur; scrubbing too vigorously may cause bleeding.

BELL'S PALSY

This neurologic disorder affects the seventh cranial (facial) nerve, producing unilateral facial weakness or paralysis. Onset is rapid. While it affects all age-groups, it occurs most often in persons under age 60. In 80% to 90% of patients, it subsides spontaneously, with complete recovery in 1 to 8 weeks; however, recovery may be delayed in older adults. If recovery is partial, contractures may develop on the paralyzed side of the face. Bell's palsy may recur on the same or opposite side of the face.

Causes

The seventh cranial nerve is responsible for motor innervation of the facial muscles. In Bell's palsy, the nerve is blocked by an inflammatory reaction around the nerve (usually at the internal auditory meatus). This is often associated with infections and can result from hemorrhage, tumor, meningitis, or local trauma.

Signs and symptoms

Bell's palsy usually produces unilateral facial weakness, occasionally with aching pain around the angle of the jaw or behind the ear. On the weak side, the mouth droops (causing the patient to drool saliva from the corner of his mouth), and taste perception is distorted over the affected anterior portion of the tongue. In addition, the forehead appears smooth, and the patient's ability to close his eye on the weak side is markedly impaired. When he tries to close this eye, it rolls upward (Bell's phenomenon) and shows excessive tearing.

Although Bell's phenomenon occurs in normal persons, it's not apparent because the eye closes completely and covers this eye motion. In Bell's palsy, incomplete eye closure makes this upward motion obvious.

Diagnosis

Clinical presentation in Bell's palsy includes distorted facial appearance and inability to raise the eyebrow, close the eyelid, smile, show the teeth, or puff out the cheek. After 10 days, electromyography helps predict the level of expected recovery by distinguishing temporary conduction defects from a pathologic interruption of nerve fibers.

Treatment

In Bell's palsy, treatment consists of prednisone, an oral corticosteroid that reduces facial nerve edema and improves nerve conduction and blood flow. After the 14th day of prednisone therapy, electrotherapy may help prevent atrophy of facial muscles.

Special considerations

• During treatment with prednisone, watch for adverse reactions, especially GI distress and fluid retention. If GI distress is troublesome, a concomitant antacid usually provides relief. If the patient has diabetes, prednisone must be used with caution and necessitates frequent monitoring of serum glucose levels.

• To reduce pain, apply moist heat to the affected side of the face, taking care not to burn the skin.

• To help maintain muscle tone, massage the patient's face with a gentle upward motion two to three times daily for 5 to 10 minutes, or have him massage his face himself. When he's ready for active exercises, teach him to exercise by grimacing in front of a mirror.

• Advise the patient to protect his eye by covering it with an eyepatch, especially when outdoors. Tell him to keep warm and avoid exposure to dust and wind. When exposure is unavoidable, instruct him to cover his face.

• To prevent excessive weight loss, help the patient cope with difficulty in eating and drinking. Instruct him to chew on the unaffected side of his mouth.

• Provide a soft, nutritionally balanced diet, eliminating hot foods and fluids.

• Arrange for privacy at mealtimes to reduce embarrassment.

• Apply a facial sling to improve lip alignment.

• Give the patient frequent and complete mouth care, being careful to remove residual food that collects between the cheeks and gums.

• Offer psychological support. Give reassurance that recovery is likely within 1 to 8 weeks.

BENIGN PROSTATIC HYPERPLASIA

Although most men over age 50 have some prostatic enlargement, in benign prostatic hyperplasia or hypertrophy (BPH), the prostate gland enlarges sufficiently to compress the urethra and cause some overt urinary obstruction. Depending on the size of the enlarged prostate, the age and health of the patient, and the extent of obstruction, BPH is treated symptomatically or surgically.

Causes

Recent evidence suggests a link between BPH and hormonal activity. As men age, production of androgenic hormones decreases, causing an imbalance in androgen and estrogen levels, and high levels of dihydrotestosterone, the main prostatic intracellular androgen. Other theoretical causes include neoplasm, arteriosclerosis, inflammation, and metabolic or nutritional disturbances.

Whatever the cause, BPH begins with changes in periurethral glandular tissue. As the prostate enlarges, it may extend into the bladder and obstruct urinary outflow by compressing or distorting the prostatic urethra. BPH may also cause a pouch to form in the bladder that retains urine when the rest of the bladder empties. This retained urine may lead to calculus formation or cystitis.

Signs and symptoms
Clinical features of BPH depend on the extent of prostatic enlargement and the lobes affected.

Urinary symptoms
Characteristically, the condition starts with a group of symptoms known as *prostatism:* reduced urinary stream caliber and force, difficulty starting micturition (straining), feeling of incomplete voiding and, occasionally, urine retention. As obstruction increases, urination becomes more frequent, with nocturia, incontinence, and possibly hematuria.

Physical examination reveals a visible midline mass (distended bladder) that represents an incompletely emptied bladder; rectal palpation discloses an enlarged prostate. The examination may also detect secondary anemia and, possibly, renal insufficiency secondary to obstruction.

Later effects
As BPH worsens, complete urinary obstruction may follow infection or ingestion of decongestants, tranquilizers, alcohol, antidepressants, or anticholinergics. Possible complications include infection, renal insufficiency, hemorrhage, and shock.

Diagnosis
Clinical features and a rectal examination are usually sufficient for a diagnosis. Other test findings help to confirm it:
• *Excretory urography* may indicate urinary tract obstruction, hydronephrosis, calculi or tumors, and filling and emptying defects in the bladder.
• *Elevated blood urea nitrogen and serum creatinine levels* suggest impaired renal function.
• *Urinalysis* and *urine culture* show hematuria, pyuria and, when the bacterial count exceeds $100,000/\mu l$, urinary tract infection.

In severe symptoms, a cystourethroscopy is definitive, but this test is performed only immediately before surgery to help determine the best procedure. It can show prostate enlargement, bladder wall changes, and a raised bladder.

Treatment
Conservative therapy includes prostate massages, sitz baths, fluid restriction for bladder distention, and antimicrobials for infection. Regular ejaculation may help relieve prostatic congestion.

Urine flow rates can be improved with $alpha_1$-adrenergic blockers, such as terazosin and prazosin. These drugs relieve bladder outlet obstruction by preventing contractions of the prostatic capsule and bladder neck. Finasteride, which may reduce the size of the prostate in some patients, is under investigation.

Surgery is the only effective therapy to relieve acute urine retention, hydronephrosis, severe hematuria, recurrent urinary tract infections, and other intolerable symptoms. (See *Combating septic shock in prostate surgery.*)

COMBATING SEPTIC SHOCK IN PROSTATE SURGERY

If the postsurgical patient develops severe chills, sudden fever, tachycardia, hypotension, or other signs of shock, do the following immediately:
• Notify other care team members.
• Start rapid infusion of I.V. antibiotics as needed.

• Watch for pulmonary embolism, heart failure, and renal shutdown.
• Monitor vital signs, central venous pressure, and arterial pressure continuously.

The patient may need supportive care in the intensive care unit.

A transurethral resection may be performed if the prostate weighs less than 2 oz (56.7 g). In this procedure, a resectoscope removes tissue with a wire loop and electric current. In high-risk patients, continuous drainage with an indwelling urinary catheter alleviates urine retention.

The following procedures involve open surgical removal:
• *suprapubic (transvesical) resection:* most common and useful when prostatic enlargement remains within the bladder
• *retropubic (extravesical) resection:* allows direct visualization; potency and continence are usually maintained.

Balloon dilatation of the prostate is still being investigated.

Special considerations
• Monitor and record the patient's vital signs, intake and output, and daily weight. Watch closely for signs of postobstructive diuresis (such as increased urine output and hypotension), which may lead to serious dehydration, lowered blood volume, shock, electrolyte loss, and anuria.
• Administer antibiotics, as needed, for urinary tract infection, urethral instrumentation, and cystoscopy.
• If urine retention is present, insert an indwelling catheter (usually difficult in a patient with BPH). If the

catheter can't be passed transurethrally, assist with suprapubic cystostomy (under local anesthetic). Watch for rapid bladder decompression.

After prostate surgery:
• Maintain patient comfort, and watch for and prevent postoperative complications.
• Observe for immediate dangers — shock and hemorrhage — of prostatic bleeding. Check the catheter frequently (every 15 minutes for the first 2 to 3 hours) for patency and urine color; check the dressings for bleeding.
• Many urologists insert a three-way catheter and establish continuous bladder irrigation. Keep the catheter open at a rate sufficient to maintain returns that are clear and light pink.
• Watch for fluid overload from absorption of the irrigating fluid into systemic circulation. If a regular catheter is being used, observe it closely. If drainage stops because of clots, irrigate the catheter, usually with 80 to 100 ml of normal saline solution, while maintaining strict aseptic technique.
• Also watch for septic shock, the most serious complication of prostate surgery.
• Administer belladonna and opium suppositories or other anticholinergics, as needed, to relieve painful

bladder spasms that often occur after transurethral resection.

• After an open procedure, provide suppositories (except after perineal prostatectomy), analgesics to control incisional pain, and frequent dressing changes.

• Continue infusing fluids I.V. until the patient can drink a sufficient amount (2 to 3 qt [2 to 3 L] a day) to maintain adequate hydration.

• Administer stool softeners and laxatives, as required, to prevent straining. *Do not* check for fecal impaction; a rectal examination could precipitate bleeding.

• After the catheter is removed, the patient may experience frequency, dribbling, and occasional hematuria. Reassure him that he will gradually regain urinary control. Explain this to the patient's family so that they can also reassure the patient.

• Reinforce prescribed limits on activity. Warn the patient against lifting, strenuous exercise, and long automobile rides because these increase bleeding tendency. Also caution him to restrict sexual activity for at least several weeks after discharge.

• Instruct the patient to follow the prescribed oral antibiotic drug regimen, and tell him the indications for using gentle laxatives. Urge him to seek medical care immediately if he can't void, if he passes bloody urine, or if he develops a fever.

BERYLLIOSIS

A form of pneumoconiosis, berylliosis, or beryllium poisoning, is a systemic granulomatous disorder with dominant pulmonary manifestations. It occurs in two forms: acute nonspecific pneumonitis and chronic noncaseating granulomatous disease with interstitial fibrosis, which may cause death from respiratory failure and cor pulmonale. Most patients with chronic interstitial disease become only slightly to moderately disabled by impaired lung function and other symptoms, but with each acute exacerbation, the prognosis worsens.

Causes
Berylliosis results from inhalation of beryllium or from its absorption through the skin. Its severity varies with the amount inhaled. The mechanism by which beryllium exerts its toxic effect is unknown.

This disease occurs among beryllium alloy workers, cathode ray tube makers, gas mantle makers, fluorescent light workers, missile technicians, and nuclear reactor workers; it's generally associated with the milling and use of beryllium and, less commonly, with the mining of beryl ore. Families of beryllium workers and people who live near plants where beryllium alloy is used are also at risk for berylliosis.

Signs and symptoms
Absorption of beryllium through broken skin produces an itchy rash that usually subsides within 2 weeks after exposure. A "beryllium ulcer" results from accidental implantation of beryllium metal in the skin.

Respiratory features
Respiratory signs and symptoms of acute berylliosis include swelling and ulceration of nasal mucosa, which may progress to septal perforation, tracheitis, and bronchitis (dry cough). Acute pulmonary disease may develop rapidly (within 3 days) or weeks later, producing a progressive dry cough, tightness in the chest, substernal pain, tachycardia, and signs of bronchitis. This form of the disease has a significant mortality related to respiratory failure.

About 10% of patients with acute berylliosis develop chronic disease 10 to 15 years after exposure. The chronic form causes increasing dyspnea that becomes progressively unremitting, along with mild chest pain, dry unproductive cough, and tachypnea. Pneumothorax may occur, with pulmonary scarring and bleb formation.

Other clinical features

Cardiovascular complications include pulmonary hypertension, right ventricular hypertrophy, and cor pulmonale. Other clinical features include hepatosplenomegaly, renal calculi, lymphadenopathy, anorexia, and fatigue.

Diagnosis

The patient history reveals occupational, family, or neighborhood exposure to beryllium dust, fumes, or mist. In *acute berylliosis,* chest X-rays may suggest pulmonary edema, showing acute miliary process or a patchy acinus filling, and diffuse infiltrates with prominent peribronchial markings. In *chronic berylliosis,* X-rays show reticulonodular infiltrates and hilar adenopathy, and large coalescent infiltrates in both lungs.

Pulmonary function studies show decreased vital capacity, forced vital capacity, residual volume and total lung capacity, and diffusing capacity of the lungs for carbon monoxide as well as decreased compliance as the lungs stiffen from fibrosis. Arterial blood gas analysis shows decreased partial pressure of arterial oxygen (PaO_2) and partial pressure of carbon dioxide.

The following additional tests may be performed:

• *In vitro lymphoblast transformation test* diagnoses berylliosis and monitors workers for occupational exposure to beryllium.

• *Beryllium patch test* establishes only hypersensitivity to beryllium, not the presence of disease.

• *Tissue biopsy* and *spectrographic analysis* are positive for most exposed workers but not absolutely diagnostic.

• *Urinalysis* may show beryllium in urine, but this only indicates exposure.

Differential diagnosis must rule out sarcoidosis and granulomatous infections.

Treatment

• Beryllium ulcer requires excision or curettage. Acute berylliosis requires prompt corticosteroid therapy.

• Hypoxia may require oxygen administration by nasal cannula or mask (1 to 2 L/minute). Severe respiratory failure requires mechanical ventilation if PaO_2 can't be maintained above 40 mm Hg.

• Chronic berylliosis is usually treated with corticosteroids, although it's not certain that steroids alter the progression of the disease. Lifelong maintenance therapy may be necessary.

• Respiratory symptoms may be treated with bronchodilators, increased fluid intake (at least 3 qt [3 L] daily), and chest physical therapy techniques. Diuretics, digitalis glycosides, and salt restriction may be useful in patients with cor pulmonale.

Special considerations

• Teach the patient to prevent infection by avoiding crowds and persons with infection, and by receiving influenza and pneumococcal vaccines.

• Encourage the patient to practice physical reconditioning, energy conservation in daily activities, and relaxation techniques.

BIPOLAR DISORDERS

Marked by severe pathologic mood swings from hyperactivity and euphoria to sadness and depression, bipolar disorders involve various symptom combinations:
• Type I bipolar disorder is characterized by alternating episodes of mania and depression.
• Type II is characterized by recurrent depressive episodes and occasional manic episodes.
• In some patients, bipolar disorder assumes a seasonal pattern, marked by a cyclic relation between the onset of the mood episode and a particular 60-day period of the year.

Incidence
The American Psychiatric Association estimates that 0.4% to 1.2% of adults experience bipolar disorder. This disorder affects women and men equally, is more common in higher socioeconomic groups, and is associated with high levels of creativity. It can begin any time after adolescence, but onset usually occurs between ages 20 and 35; about 35% of patients experience onset between ages 35 and 60.

Before the onset of overt symptoms, many patients with bipolar disorder have an energetic and outgoing personality with a history of wide mood swings. A related but less severe form of illness, called cyclothymic disorder, commonly precedes a bipolar disorder. (See *Cyclothymic disorder.*)

Bipolar disorder recurs in 80% of patients; as they grow older, the episodes recur more frequently and last longer. This illness is associated with a significant mortality; about 20% of patients commit suicide, many just as the depression lifts.

Causes
The origins of bipolar disorder are unclear, but hereditary, biological, and psychological factors may play a part.

Hereditary factors
The incidence of bipolar disorder among relatives of affected patients is higher than in the general population and highest among maternal relatives. The closer the relationship, the greater the susceptibility. A child with one affected parent has a 25% chance of developing bipolar disorder; a child with two affected parents, a 50% chance. The incidence of this illness in siblings is 20% to 25%; in identical twins, the incidence is 66% to 96%.

Biological factors
Although certain biochemical changes accompany mood swings, it's not clear whether these changes cause the mood swings or result from them. In both mania and depression, intracellular sodium concentration increases during illness and returns to normal with recovery.

Patients with mood disorders have a defect in the way the brain handles certain neurotransmitters—chemical messengers that shuttle nerve impulses between neurons. Low levels of the chemicals dopamine and norepinephrine, for example, have been linked to depression, whereas excessively high levels of these chemicals are associated with mania.

Changes in the concentration of acetylcholine and serotonin also may play a role. Although neurobiologists have yet to prove that these chemical shifts cause bipolar disorder, it's widely assumed that most antidepressant medications work by modifying these neurotransmitter systems.

New data suggest that changes in the circadian rhythms that control hormone secretion, body temperature, and appetite may contribute to the development of bipolar disorder.

Emotional and physical factors

Emotional or physical trauma, such as bereavement, disruption of an important relationship, or a serious accidental injury, may precede the onset of bipolar disorder; however, bipolar disorder often appears without identifiable predisposing factors.

Manic episodes may follow a stressful event, but they're also associated with antidepressant therapy and childbirth. Major depressive episodes may be precipitated by chronic physical illness, psychoactive drug dependence, psychosocial stressors, and childbirth. Other familial influences, especially the early loss of a parent, parental depression, incest, or abuse, may predispose a person to depressive illness.

Signs and symptoms

Clinical presentation varies widely, depending on whether the patient is experiencing a manic or depressive episode.

Manic features

The *manic* patient typically appears euphoric, expansive, or irritable with little control over his activities and responses. He may describe hyperactive or excessive behavior, including elaborate plans for numerous social events, efforts to renew old acquaintances by telephoning friends at all hours of the night, buying sprees, or promiscuous sexual activity. He seldom hesitates to start projects for which he has little aptitude.

The patient's activities may have a bizarre quality, such as dressing in colorful or strange garments, wearing excessive makeup, or giving advice to passing strangers. He often expresses an inflated sense of self-esteem, ranging from uncritical self-confidence to

---

CYCLOTHYMIC DISORDER

A chronic mood disturbance of at least 2 years' duration, cyclothymic disorder involves numerous episodes of hypomania or depression that are not of sufficient severity or duration to qualify as a major depressive episode or a bipolar disorder.

Cyclothymia commonly starts in adolescence or early adulthood. Beginning insidiously, this disorder leads to persistent social and occupational dysfunction.

Signs and symptoms

In the hypomanic phase, the patient may experience insomnia; hyperactivity; inflated self-esteem; increased productivity and creativity; overinvolvement in pleasurable activities, including an increased sexual drive; physical restlessness; and rapid speech. Depressive symptoms may include insomnia, feelings of inadequacy, decreased productivity, social withdrawal, loss of libido, loss of interest in pleasurable activities, lethargy, slow speech, and crying.

Diagnosis

A number of medical disorders (for example, cerebrovascular accident, brain tumors, head trauma, and endocrinopathies such as Cushing's disease) and a drug overdose can produce a similar pattern of mood alteration. These organic causes must be ruled out before making a diagnosis of cyclothymic disorder.

---

marked grandiosity, which may be delusional.

Common features of the manic phase are accelerated speech, frequent changes of topic, and flight of ideas. The patient is easily distracted and responds rapidly to external stimuli, such as background noise or a ringing telephone.

Physical examination of the manic patient may reveal signs of malnutrition and poor personal hygiene. He may report sleeping and eating less than usual.

Hypomania, more common than acute mania, can be recognized during the assessment interview by three classic symptoms: elated but unstable mood, pressured speech, and increased motor activity. The hypomanic patient may appear elated, hyperactive, easily distracted, talkative, irritable, impatient, impulsive, and full of energy, but seldom exhibits flight of ideas, delusions, or an absence of discretion and self-control.

Depressive features

The patient who experiences a *depressive episode* may report a loss of self-esteem, overwhelming inertia, social withdrawal, and feelings of hopelessness, apathy, or self-reproach. He may believe that he is wicked and deserves to be punished. His growing sadness, guilt, negativity, and fatigue place extraordinary burdens on his family.

During the assessment interview, the depressed patient may speak and respond slowly. He may complain of difficulty concentrating or thinking clearly but usually isn't obviously disoriented or intellectually impaired.

Physical examination may reveal reduced psychomotor activity, lethargy, low muscle tonus, weight loss, slowed gait, and constipation. The patient also may report sleep disturbances (falling asleep, staying asleep, or early morning awakening), sexual dysfunction, headaches, chest pains, and a heaviness in the limbs. Typically, symptoms are worse in the morning and gradually subside as the day goes on.

His concerns about his health may become hypochondriacal: He may worry excessively about having cancer or some other serious illness. In an elderly patient, physical symptoms may be the only clues to depression.

Suicide is an ever-present risk, especially as the depression begins to lift. At that point, a rising energy level may strengthen the patient's resolve to carry out suicidal plans.

The suicidal patient may also harbor homicidal ideas, for example, thinking of killing his family either in anger or to spare them pain and disgrace.

Diagnosis

For characteristic findings in patients with this condition, see *Diagnosing bipolar disorders.*

Physical examination and laboratory tests, such as endocrine function studies, rule out medical causes of the mood disturbances, including intra-abdominal neoplasm, hypothyroidism, heart failure, cerebral arteriosclerosis, parkinsonism, psychoactive drug abuse, brain tumor, and uremia. Moreover, a review of the medications prescribed for other disorders may point to drug-induced depression or mania.

Treatment

Widely used to treat bipolar disorder, lithium has proved to be highly effective in relieving and preventing manic episodes. It curbs the accelerated thought processes and hyperactive behavior without producing the sedating effect of antipsychotic drugs. In addition, it may prevent the recurrence of depressive episodes; however, it's ineffective in treating acute depression.

Because lithium has a narrow therapeutic range, treatment must be initiated cautiously and the dosage adjusted slowly. Therapeutic blood levels must be maintained for 7 to 10 days before the drug's beneficial effects appear; for this reason, antipsychotic drugs commonly are used in the interim to provide sedation and symptomatic relief. Because lithium is ex-

DIAGNOSING BIPOLAR DISORDERS

The diagnosis of bipolar disorder is confirmed when the patient meets the criteria documented in the *Diagnostic and Statistical Manual of Mental Disorders,* 4th ed.

For a manic episode

• A distinct period of abnormally and persistently elevated, expansive, or irritable mood lasting at least 1 week (or any duration if hospitalization is needed)

• During the mood disturbance period, at least three of the following symptoms must have persisted (four, if the mood is only irritable) and have been present to a significant degree:
— inflated self-esteem or grandiosity
— decreased need for sleep
— more talkative than usual or pressured to keep talking
— flight of ideas or subjective experience that thoughts are racing
— distractibility
— increased goal-directed activity or psychomotor agitation
— excessive involvement in pleasurable activities that have a high potential for painful consequences.

• The symptoms do not meet the criteria for a mixed episode.

• The mood disturbance is sufficiently severe to cause one of the following to occur:
— marked impairment in occupational functioning or in usual social activities or relationships with others
— hospitalization to prevent harm to self or others
— evidence of psychotic features.

• The symptoms are not due to the direct physiologic effects of a substance or a general medical condition.

For a hypomanic episode

• A distinct period of abnormally and persistently elevated, expansive, or irritable mood lasting at least 4 days

that's clearly different from the usual nondepressed mood

• During the mood disturbance period, at least three of the following symptoms must have persisted (four, if the mood is only irritable) and have been present to a significant degree:
— inflated self-esteem or grandiosity
— decreased need for sleep
— more talkative than usual or pressured to keep talking
— flight of ideas or subjective experience that thoughts are racing
— distractibility
— increased goal-directed activity or psychomotor agitation
— excessive involvement in pleasurable activities that have a high potential for painful consequences.

• The episode is associated with an unequivocal change in functioning that's uncharacteristic of the person when he's not symptomatic.

• Others can recognize the disturbance in mood and the change in functioning.

• The episode is not severe enough to markedly impair social or occupational functioning or to necessitate hospitalization to prevent harm to self or others, and no psychotic features are evident.

• The symptoms are not due to the direct physiologic effects of a substance or a general medical condition.

For a bipolar I single manic episode

• Presence of only one manic episode and no past major depressive episodes

• The manic episode is not better accounted for by schizoaffective disorder and is not superimposed on schizophrenia, schizophreniform disorder, delusional disorder, or psychotic disorder not otherwise specified.

(continued)

DIAGNOSING BIPOLAR DISORDERS *(continued)*

For a bipolar I disorder, most recent episode hypomanic

• Currently (or most recently) in a hypomanic episode

• The person previously had at least one manic episode or mixed episode.

• The mood symptoms cause clinically significant distress or impairment in social, occupational, or other important areas of functioning.

• The first two exacerbations of the mood episode (above) are not better accounted for by schizoaffective disorder and are not superimposed on schizophrenia, schizophreniform disorder, delusional disorder, or psychotic disorder not otherwise specified.

For a bipolar I disorder, most recent episode manic

• Currently (or most recently) in a manic episode

• The person previously had at least one major depressive episode, manic episode, or mixed episode.

• The first two exacerbations of mood episode (above) are not better accounted for by schizoaffective disorder and are not superimposed on schizophrenia, schizophreniform disorder, delusional disorder, or psychotic disorder not otherwise specified.

For a bipolar I disorder, most recent episode mixed

• Currently (or most recently) in a mixed episode

• The person previously had at least one major depressive episode, manic episode, or mixed episode.

• The first two exacerbations of mood episode (above) are not better accounted for by schizoaffective disorder and are not superimposed on schizophrenia, schizophreniform disorder, delusional disorder, or psychotic disorder not otherwise specified.

For a bipolar I disorder, most recent episode depressed

• Currently (or most recently) in a major depressive episode

• The person previously had at least one manic episode or mixed episode.

• The first two exacerbations of mood episode (above) aren't better accounted for by schizoaffective disorder and aren't superimposed on schizophrenia, schizophreniform disorder, delusional disorder, or psychotic disorder not otherwise specified.

For a bipolar I disorder, most recent episode unspecified

• Criteria, except for duration, are currently (or most recently) met for a manic, hypomanic, mixed, or major depressive episode.

• The person previously had at least one manic episode or mixed episode.

• The mood symptoms cause clinically significant distress or impairment in social, occupational, or other important areas of functioning.

• The first two exacerbations of mood episode (above) are not better accounted for by schizoaffective disorder and are not superimposed on schizophrenia, schizophreniform disorder, delusional disorder, or psychotic disorder not otherwise specified.

• The first two exacerbations of mood episode (above) are not due to the direct physiologic effects of a substance or a general medical condition.

Diagnosing Bipolar Disorders *(continued)*

For a bipolar II disorder
• Presence (or history) of one or more major depressive episodes
• Presence (or history) or at least one hypomanic episode
• The patient has never had a manic episode or a mixed episode.
• The first two exacerbations of mood episode (above) are not better ac-counted for by schizoaffective disorder and are not superimposed on schizo-phrenia, schizophreniform disorder, de-lusional disorder, or psychotic disorder not otherwise specified.
• The symptoms cause clinically sig-nificant distress or impairment in so-cial, occupational, or other important areas of functioning.

---

creted by the kidneys, any renal im-pairment necessitates withdrawal of the drug.

Anticonvulsants, such as carbama-zepine, valproic acid, and clonazepam, are used either alone or with lithium to treat mood disorders. Carbamaze-pine, a potent antimanic drug, is ef-fective in many lithium-resistant pa-tients.

Antidepressants are used to treat depressive symptoms, but they may trigger a manic episode.

Special considerations
For the manic patient:
• Attend to the manic patient's physi-cal needs. Encourage him to eat.
• As the patient's symptoms subside, encourage him to assume responsibil-ity for personal care.
• Provide emotional support, maintain a calm environment, and set realistic goals for behavior.
• Provide diversional activities suited to a short attention span; firmly dis-courage the patient if he tries to over-extend himself.
• When necessary, reorient the patient to reality, and tactfully divert conver-sations when they become intimately concerned with other patients or staff members.
• Set limits in a calm, clear, and self-confident manner for the manic pa-tient's demanding, hyperactive, manip-ulative, and acting-out behaviors. Set-ting limits tells the patient you'll pro-vide security and protection by refus-ing inappropriate and possibly harmful requests. Avoid leaving an opening for the patient to test you or argue with you.
• Listen to requests attentively and with a neutral attitude, but avoid power struggles if a patient tries to put you on the spot for an immediate answer. Explain that you'll seriously consider the request and will respond later.
• Collaborate with other staff mem-bers to provide consistent responses to the patient's manipulative or acting-out behaviors.
• Watch for early signs of frustration (when the patient's anger escalates from verbal threats to hitting an object). Tell the patient firmly that threats and hit-ting are unacceptable and that these behaviors show that he needs help to control his behavior. Then tell him that the staff will help him move to a quiet area and will help him control his be-havior so he won't hurt himself or others. Staff members who have prac-ticed as a team can work effectively to prevent acting-out behavior or to re-move and confine a patient.
• Alert the staff team promptly when acting-out behavior escalates. It's safer to have help available before you need

it than to try controlling an anxious or frightened patient by yourself.

• Once the incident is over and the patient is calm and in control, discuss his feelings with him and offer suggestions on how to prevent a recurrence.

• If the patient is taking lithium, tell him and his family to discontinue the drug and notify the doctor if signs of toxicity, such as diarrhea, abdominal cramps, vomiting, unsteadiness, drowsiness, muscle weakness, polyuria, and tremors, occur.

For the depressed patient:

• The depressed patient needs continual positive reinforcement to improve his self-esteem. Provide a structured routine, including activities to boost his self-confidence and promote interaction with others (for instance, group therapy), and keep reassuring him that his depression will lift.

• Encourage the patient to talk or to write down his feelings if he's having trouble expressing them. Listen attentively and respectfully, and allow him time to formulate his thoughts if he seems sluggish. Record your observations and conversations.

• To prevent possible self-injury or suicide, remove harmful objects (glass, belts, rope, bobby pins) from the patient's environment, observe him closely, and strictly supervise his medications. Institute suicide precautions as dictated by hospital policy.

• Attend to the patient's physical needs. If he's too depressed to take care of himself, help him with personal hygiene measures. Encourage him to eat, or feed him if necessary. If he's constipated, add high-fiber foods to his diet; offer small, frequent meals; and encourage physical activity. To help him sleep, give him back rubs or warm milk at bedtime.

• If the patient is taking an antidepressant, watch for signs of mania.

BLADDER CANCER

Bladder tumors can develop on the surface of the bladder wall (benign or malignant papillomas) or grow within the bladder wall (generally more virulent) and quickly invade underlying muscles. Most bladder tumors (90%) are transitional cell carcinomas, arising from the transitional epithelium of mucous membranes. Less common are adenocarcinomas, epidermoid carcinomas, squamous cell carcinomas, sarcomas, tumors in bladder diverticula, and carcinoma in situ. Bladder tumors are most prevalent in men over age 50 and are more common in densely populated industrial areas.

Causes
Certain environmental carcinogens, such as 2-naphthylamine, benzidine, tobacco, and nitrates, predispose people to transitional cell tumors. Thus, workers in certain industries—rubber workers, weavers and leather finishers, aniline dye workers, hairdressers, petroleum workers, and spray painters—are at high risk for such tumors. The period between exposure to the carcinogen and development of symptoms is about 18 years.

Squamous cell carcinoma of the bladder is most common in geographic areas where schistosomiasis is endemic. It's also associated with chronic bladder irritation and infection (for example, from kidney stones, indwelling catheters, and cystitis caused by cyclophosphamide).

Signs and symptoms
In early stages, approximately 25% of patients with bladder tumors have no symptoms. Commonly, the first sign is gross, painless, intermittent hematuria (often with clots in the urine). Patients

with invasive lesions often have suprapubic pain after voiding. Other symptoms include bladder irritability, urinary frequency, nocturia, and dribbling.

Diagnosis

Only cystoscopy and a biopsy can confirm bladder cancer. Cystoscopy should be performed when hematuria first appears. When it is performed under anesthesia, a bimanual examination is usually done to determine if the bladder is fixed to the pelvic wall. A thorough history and physical examination may help determine whether the tumor has invaded the prostate or the lymph nodes. (See *Comparing staging systems for bladder cancer,* page 112.)

The following tests can provide essential information about the tumor:

• *Urinalysis* can detect blood in the urine and malignant cytology.

• *Excretory urography* can identify a large, early-stage tumor or an infiltrating tumor, delineate functional problems in the upper urinary tract, assess hydronephrosis, and detect rigid deformity of the bladder wall.

• *Retrograde cystography* evaluates bladder structure and integrity. Test results help to confirm the diagnosis.

• *Pelvic arteriography* can reveal tumor invasion into the bladder wall.

• *Computed tomography scan* reveals the thickness of the involved bladder wall and detects enlarged retroperitoneal lymph nodes.

• *Ultrasonography* can detect metastasis beyond the bladder and can distinguish a bladder cyst from a tumor.

Treatment

Appropriate treatment for bladder cancer varies.

Superficial bladder tumors

Superficial bladder tumors are removed by transurethral (cystoscopic) resection and fulguration (electrical destruction). This procedure is adequate when the tumor has not invaded the muscle.

Intravesicular chemotherapy is also used for superficial tumors (especially those that occur in many sites) and to prevent tumor recurrence. This treatment involves washing the bladder directly with antineoplastic drugs — most commonly, thiotepa, doxorubicin, mitomycin, or bacille Calmette-Guérin.

If additional tumors develop, fulguration may have to be repeated every 3 months for years. However, if the tumors penetrate the muscle layer or recur frequently, cystoscopy with fulguration is no longer appropriate.

Tumors too large to be treated through a cystoscope require segmental bladder resection to remove a full-thickness section of the bladder. This procedure is feasible only if the tumor isn't near the bladder neck or ureteral orifices. Bladder instillations of thiotepa after transurethral resection may also help control such tumors.

Infiltrating bladder tumors

Radical cystectomy is the treatment of choice for infiltrating bladder tumors. The week before cystectomy, treatment may include external beam therapy to the bladder. Surgery involves removal of the bladder with perivesical fat, lymph nodes, urethra, the prostate and seminal vesicles (in males), and the uterus and adnexa (in females). The surgeon forms a urinary diversion, usually an ileal conduit. The patient must then wear an external pouch continuously. (See *Caring for a urinary stoma,* page 113.) Other diversions include ureterostomy, nephrostomy, vesicostomy, ileal bladder, ileal loop, and sigmoid conduit.

Males are impotent following radical cystectomy and urethrectomy because these procedures damage the sympathetic and parasympathetic nerves that control erection and ejac-

COMPARING STAGING SYSTEMS FOR BLADDER CANCER

Staging helps determine the most appropriate treatment for bladder cancer. One of two staging systems may be used: the TNM (tumor, node, metastasis) system or the JSM (Jewett-Strong-Marshall) system. The JSM system grades cancers O and A through D. Both systems distinguish superficial bladder cancers from invasive bladder cancers, which penetrate bladder muscle and may spread to other sites.

TNM	STAGE	JSM
SUPERFICIAL TUMOR		
TX	Primary tumor can't be assessed	—
T0	No tumor	0
Tis	Carcinoma in situ	0
Ta	Noninvasive papillary tumor	0
INVASIVE TUMOR		
T1	Tumor invades subepithelial connective tissue	—
T2	Tumor invades superficial muscle (inner half)	B_1
T3a	Tumor invades deep muscle	B_2
T3b	Tumor invades perivesical fat	C
T4	Tumor invades prostate, uterus, vagina, pelvic wall, or abdominal wall	D_1
NX	Regional lymph nodes can't be assessed	—
N0	No evidence of lymph node involvement	—
N1	Metastasis in a single lymph node, 2 cm or less in greatest dimension	D_1
N2	Metastasis in a single lymph node, between 2 and 5 cm in greatest dimension, or metastases to several lymph nodes, none greater than 5 cm in greatest dimension	—
N3	Metastasis in a lymph node more than 5 cm in greatest dimension	—
MX	Distant metastasis can't be assessed	—
M0	No evidence of distant metastasis	—
M	Distant metastasis	D_2

☑ CARING FOR A URINARY STOMA

If your patient has a urinary stoma, give him these instructions:

• First, show the patient how to prepare and apply the pouch, which may be reusable or disposable. If he chooses the reusable type, he'll need at least two.

• To select the right pouch size, teach the patient to measure the stoma and order a pouch with an opening that clears the stoma with a ⅛" margin. Instruct him to remeasure the stoma after he goes home, in case the size changes. The pouch should have a drainage valve at the bottom. Tell him to empty the pouch when it's one-third full or every 2 to 3 hours.

• To ensure a good skin seal, advise the patient to select a skin barrier that contains synthetics and little or no karaya (which urine tends to destroy). Check the pouch frequently to make sure that the skin seal remains intact. A good skin seal with a skin barrier may last for 3 to 6 days, so change the pouch only that often. Tell the patient that he can wear a loose-fitting elastic belt to help secure the pouch.

• The ileal conduit stoma reaches its permanent size 2 to 4 months after surgery. Because the intestine normally produces mucus, tell the patient not to be alarmed by mucus that appears in the draining urine.

• Instruct the patient to keep the skin around the stoma clean and free of irritation, as follows:

— After removing the pouch, wash the skin with water and mild soap. Rinse well with clear water to remove soap residue, and then gently pat the skin dry; don't rub.

— Place a gauze sponge soaked with vinegar-water (1 part : 3 parts) over the stoma for a few minutes to prevent uric acid crystal buildup. While preparing the skin, place a rolled-up dry sponge over the stoma to collect draining urine.

— Coat the skin with a silicone skin protector, and cover with the collection pouch. If skin irritation or breakdown occurs, apply a layer of antacid precipitate to the clean, dry skin before coating with the skin protector.

• Advise the patient that he can level uneven surfaces on his abdomen, such as gullies, scars, or wedges, with a variety of specially prepared products or skin barriers.

---

ulation. At a later date, the patient may desire a penile implant to make sexual intercourse (without ejaculation) possible.

Advanced bladder cancer

For patients with advanced bladder cancer, treatment includes cystectomy to remove the tumor, radiation therapy, and systemic chemotherapy with such drugs as cyclophosphamide, fluorouracil, doxorubicin, and cisplatin. This combination sometimes is successful in arresting bladder cancer.

Cisplatin is the most effective single agent.

Investigational treatments

Such treatments include photodynamic therapy and intravesicular administration of interferon alfa and tumor necrosis factor. Photodynamic therapy involves I.V. injection of a photosensitizing agent such as hematoporphyrin ether, which malignant cells readily absorb. Then a cystoscopic laser device introduces laser energy into the bladder, exposing the malignant cells to laser light, which kills them. Because this treatment also produces photosensitivity in normal cells, the patient must totally avoid sunlight for about 30 days.

Special considerations
• Before surgery, assist in selecting a stoma site that the patient can see (usually in the rectus muscle to minimize the risk of herniation). Do so by assessing the abdomen in various positions.
• After surgery, encourage the patient to look at the stoma. Provide a mirror to make viewing easier.
• To obtain a specimen for culture and sensitivity testing, catheterize the patient using sterile technique. Insert the lubricated tip of the catheter into the stoma about 2″ (5 cm). In many hospitals, a double telescope-type catheter is available for ileal conduit catheterization.
• Advise the patient with a urinary stoma that he may participate in most activities, except for heavy lifting and contact sports.
• When a patient with a urinary diversion is discharged, arrange for follow-up home health care or refer him to an enterostomal therapist, who will help coordinate the patient's care.
• Teach the patient about his urinary stoma. Encourage his spouse, a friend, or a relative to attend the teaching session. Advise this person beforehand that a negative reaction to the stoma can impede the patient's adjustment.
• All high-risk people — for example, chemical workers and people with a history of benign bladder tumors or persistent cystitis — should have periodic cytologic examinations and learn about the dangers of disease-causing agents.
• Refer ostomates to such resources as the American Cancer Society and the United Ostomy Association.

BLASTOMYCOSIS

Also called *Gilchrist's disease,* blastomycosis is caused by the yeastlike fungus *Blastomyces dermatitidis,* which usually infects the lungs and produces bronchopneumonia. Less frequently, this fungus may disseminate through the blood and cause osteomyelitis and central nervous system (CNS), skin, and genital disorders.

Untreated blastomycosis is slowly progressive and usually fatal; however, spontaneous remissions occasionally occur. With antifungal drug therapy and supportive treatment, the prognosis for patients with blastomycosis is good.

Causes
Blastomycosis is generally found in North America (where *B. dermatitidis* normally inhabits the soil) and is endemic to the southeastern United States. Sporadic cases have also been reported in Africa. Blastomycosis usually infects men ages 30 to 50, but no occupational link has been found. *B. dermatitidis* is probably inhaled by people who are in close contact with the soil. The incubation period may range from weeks to months.

Signs and symptoms
Initial clinical indicators of pulmonary blastomycosis mimic those of a viral upper respiratory infection. These findings typically include a dry, hacking, or productive cough (occasionally hemoptysis), pleuritic chest pain, fever, shaking, chills, night sweats, malaise, anorexia, and weight loss.
• Cutaneous blastomycosis causes small, painless, nonpruritic, and nondistinctive macules or papules on exposed body parts. These lesions become raised and reddened, and occa-

sionally progress to draining skin abscesses or fistulas.

• Skeletal involvement causes soft-tissue swelling, tenderness, and warmth over bony lesions, which generally occur in the thoracic, lumbar, and sacral regions; long bones of the legs; and, in children, the skull.

• Genital involvement produces painful swelling of the testes, the epididymis, or the prostate; deep perineal pain; pyuria; and hematuria.

• CNS involvement causes meningitis or cerebral abscesses, resulting in a decreased level of consciousness (LOC), lethargy, and change in mood or affect.

Other dissemination may result in Addison's disease (adrenal insufficiency), pericarditis, and arthritis.

Diagnosis

Various tests may be ordered to diagnose blastomycosis, including:

• *culture* of *B. dermatitidis* from skin lesions, pus, sputum, or pulmonary secretions

• *biopsy* of tissue from the skin or lungs, or of bronchial washings, sputum, or pus, as the doctor finds appropriate

• *complement fixation testing.* Although such testing isn't conclusive, a high titer in extrapulmonary disease is a poor prognostic sign.

• *immunodiffusion testing.* This specific study detects antibodies for the A and B antigen of blastomycosis.

In addition, suspected pulmonary blastomycosis requires a chest X-ray, which may show pulmonary infiltrates. Other abnormal laboratory findings include an increased white blood cell count and erythrocyte sedimentation rate, slightly increased serum globulin levels, mild normochromic anemia and, with bone lesions, an increased alkaline phosphatase level.

Treatment

All forms of blastomycosis respond to amphotericin B. Ketoconazole or fluconazole may be used as alternatives. Patient care is mainly supportive.

Special considerations

• In severe pulmonary blastomycosis, check for hemoptysis. If the patient is febrile, provide a cool room and give tepid sponge baths.

• If blastomycosis causes joint pain or swelling, elevate the joint and apply heat.

• In CNS infection, watch the patient carefully for decreasing LOC and unequal pupillary response.

• In men with disseminated disease, watch for hematuria.

• Infuse I.V. amphotericin B slowly (a too-rapid infusion may cause circulatory collapse). During the infusion, monitor vital signs. (Temperature may rise but should subside within 1 to 2 hours.) Watch for decreased urine output and monitor laboratory results for increased blood urea nitrogen and serum creatinine levels and hypokalemia, which may indicate renal toxicity. Report any hearing loss, tinnitus, or dizziness immediately.

• To relieve adverse effects of amphotericin B, give antiemetics and antipyretics as needed.

BLEPHARITIS

A common inflammation, blepharitis produces a red-rimmed appearance of the margins of the eyelids. It's frequently chronic and bilateral and can affect both upper and lower lids. Seborrheic blepharitis is characterized by waxy scales and is common in older adults and in persons with red hair. Staphylococcal (ulcerative) blepharitis is characterized by dry scales, with tiny ulcerated areas along the lid margins. Both types may coexist.

Blepharitis tends to recur and become chronic. It can be controlled if treatment begins before the onset of ocular involvement.

Causes

Seborrheic blepharitis generally results from seborrhea of the scalp, eyebrows, and ears; ulcerative blepharitis, from *Staphylococcus aureus* infection. (People with this infection may also tend to develop chalazions and styes.)

Signs and symptoms

Clinical features of blepharitis include itching, burning, foreign-body sensation, and sticky, crusted eyelids on waking. This constant irritation results in unconscious rubbing of the eyes (causing reddened rims) or continual blinking. Other signs include waxy scales in seborrheic blepharitis; flaky scales on lashes, loss of lashes, and ulcerated areas on lid margins in ulcerative blepharitis.

Diagnosis

In blepharitis, diagnosis depends on the patient history and characteristic symptoms. In ulcerative blepharitis, a culture of the ulcerated lid margin shows *S. aureus.*

Treatment

Early treatment is essential to prevent recurrence or complications. Treatment depends on the type of blepharitis:

• *seborrheic blepharitis:* daily shampooing of eyelashes (using a mild shampoo on a damp applicator stick or a washcloth) to remove scales from the lid margins; also, frequent shampooing of the scalp and eyebrows

• *ulcerative blepharitis:* warm compresses may be applied and a sulfonamide eye ointment or an appropriate antibiotic may be used.

• *blepharitis resulting from pediculosis:* removal of nits (with forceps) or application of ophthalmic physostigmine or other ointment as an insecticide. (This may cause pupil constriction and, possibly, headache, conjunctival irritation, and blurred vision from the film of ointment on the cornea.)

Special considerations

• Instruct the patient to gently remove scales from the lid margins daily with an applicator stick or a clean washcloth.

• Teach the patient the following method for applying warm compresses: First, run warm water into a clean bowl. Then immerse a clean cloth in the water and wring it out. Place the warm cloth against the closed eyelid. (Be careful not to burn the skin.) Hold the compress in place until it cools. Continue this procedure for 15 minutes.

• Antibiotic ophthalmic ointment should be applied after a 15-minute application of warm compresses.

• Treatment of seborrheic blepharitis also requires attention to the face and scalp.

BONE TUMORS, PRIMARY MALIGNANT

A rare type of bone cancer, primary malignant bone tumors (sarcomas of the bone) constitute less than 1% of all malignant tumors. Most bone tumors are secondary, caused by seeding from a primary site. Primary malignant bone tumors are more common in males, especially in children and adolescents, although some types do occur in people between ages 35 and 60.

The tumors may originate in osseous or nonosseous tissue. Osseous bone tumors arise from the bony structure itself and include osteogenic sarcoma (the most common), parosteal osteogenic sarcoma, chondrosarcoma, and malignant giant cell tumor. Together they make up 60% of all malignant bone tumors. Nonosseous tumors arise from hematopoietic, vascular, and neural tissues and include Ewing's sarcoma, fibrosarcoma, and chordoma. Osteogenic and Ewing's sarcomas are the most common bone tumors in childhood. (See *Types of primary malignant bone tumors,* pages 118 and 119.)

Causes
Primary malignant bone tumors have no known cause. Some researchers suggest that they arise in areas of rapid growth because children and young adults with such tumors seem to be much taller than average. Additional theories point to heredity, trauma, and excessive radiation therapy.

Signs and symptoms
Bone pain is the most common indication of primary malignant bone tumors. It's often more intense at night and isn't usually associated with mobility. The pain is dull and is usually localized, although it may be referred from the hip or spine and result in weakness or a limp. Another common sign is the presence of a mass or tumor.

The tumor site may be tender and may swell; the tumor itself is often palpable. Pathologic fractures are common. In late stages, the patient may be cachectic, with fever and impaired mobility.

Diagnosis
A biopsy (by incision or by aspiration) is essential for confirming primary malignant bone tumors. Bone X-rays and radioisotope bone and computed tomography scans show tumor size. Serum alkaline phosphatase is usually elevated in patients with sarcoma.

Treatment
• Excision of the tumor along with a 3″ (7.6 cm) margin is the treatment of choice. It may be combined with preoperative chemotherapy.
• In some patients, radical surgery (such as hemipelvectomy or interscapulothoracic amputation) is necessary. However, surgical resection of the tumor (often with preoperative *and* postoperative chemotherapy) has saved limbs from amputation.
• Intensive chemotherapy includes administration of doxorubicin, vincristine, cyclophosphamide, cisplatin, and dacarbazine. Chemotherapy may be infused intra-arterially into the long bones of the legs.

Special considerations
• Be sensitive to the emotional strain caused by the threat of amputation. Encourage communication and help the patient set realistic goals.
• If the surgery will affect the patient's lower extremities, have a physical therapist teach him how to use assistive devices (such as a walker) preoperatively.
• Teach the patient how to readjust his body weight so that he can get in and out of the bed and wheelchair.
• Before surgery, start I.V. infusions to maintain fluid and electrolyte balance and to have an open vein available if blood or plasma is needed during surgery.
• After surgery, check vital signs every hour for the first 4 hours, every 2 hours for the next 4 hours, and then every 4 hours if the patient is stable.
• Check the dressing periodically for oozing.
• Elevate the foot of the bed or place the stump on a pillow for the first 24 hours. (Be careful not to leave the

TYPES OF PRIMARY MALIGNANT BONE TUMORS

TYPE	CLINICAL FEATURES	TREATMENT
OSSEOUS ORIGIN		
Osteogenic sarcoma	• Osteoid tumor present in specimen. • Tumor arises from bone-forming osteoblast and bone-digesting osteoclast. • Occurs most often in femur, but also tibia and humerus; occasionally, in fibula, ileum, vertebra, or mandible • Usually occurs in males ages 10 to 30	• Surgery (tumor resection, high thigh amputation, hemipelvectomy, interscapulothoracic surgery) • Chemotherapy
Parosteal osteogenic sarcoma	• Develops on surface of bone instead of interior • Progresses slowly • Occurs most often in distal femur, but also in tibia, humerus, and ulna • Usually occurs in females ages 30 to 40	• Surgery (tumor resection, possible amputation, interscapulothoracic surgery, hemipelvectomy) • Chemotherapy • Combination of above
Chondrosarcoma	• Develops from cartilage • Painless; grows slowly, but is locally recurrent and invasive • Occurs most often in pelvis, proximal femur, ribs, and shoulder girdle • Usually occurs in males ages 30 to 50	• Hemipelvectomy, surgical resection (ribs) • Radiation (palliative) • Chemotherapy
Malignant giant cell tumor	• Arises from benign giant cell tumor • Found most often in long bones, especially in knee area • Usually occurs in females ages 18 to 50	• Curettage • Total excision • Radiation for recurrent disease
NONOSSEOUS ORIGIN		
Ewing's sarcoma	• Originates in bone marrow and invades shafts of long and flat bones • Usually affects lower extremities, most often femur, innominate bones, ribs, tibia, humerus, vertebra, and fibula; may metastasize to lungs • Pain increasingly severe and persistent • Usually occurs in males ages 10 to 20 • Prognosis poor	• High-voltage radiation (Tumor is very radiosensitive.) • Chemotherapy to slow growth • Amputation, only if there's no evidence of metastasis
Fibrosarcoma	• Relatively rare • Originates in fibrous tissue of bone • Invades long or flat bones (femur, tibia, mandible) but also involves periosteum and overlying muscle • Usually occurs in males ages 30 to 40	• Amputation • Radiation • Chemotherapy • Bone grafts (with low-grade fibrosarcoma)

TYPES OF PRIMARY MALIGNANT BONE TUMORS   *(continued)*

TYPE	CLINICAL FEATURES	TREATMENT
NONOSSEOUS ORIGIN *(continued)*		
Chordoma	• Derived from embryonic remnants of notochord • Progresses slowly • Usually found at end of spinal column and in sphenooccipital, sacrococcygeal, and vertebral areas • Characterized by constipation and visual disturbances • Usually occurs in males ages 50 to 60	• Surgical resection (often resulting in neural defects) • Radiation (palliative, or when surgery not applicable, as in occipital area)

stump elevated for more than 48 hours because this may lead to contractures.)

• To ease the patient's anxiety, administer analgesics for pain before morning care. If necessary, brace him with pillows, keeping the affected part at rest.

• Urge the patient to eat foods high in protein, vitamins, and folic acid and to get plenty of rest and sleep to promote recovery. Encourage some physical exercise. Administer laxatives, if necessary, to maintain proper elimination.

• Encourage fluids to prevent dehydration. Record intake and output accurately. After a hemipelvectomy, insert a nasogastric tube to prevent abdominal distention. Continue low gastric suction for 2 days after surgery or until the patient can tolerate a liquid diet. Administer antibiotics to prevent infection. Give transfusions, if necessary, and administer medication to control pain. Keep drains in place to facilitate wound drainage and prevent infection. Use an indwelling urinary catheter until the patient can void voluntarily.

• Keep in mind that rehabilitation programs after limb salvage surgery will vary, depending on the patient, the body part affected, and the type of surgery performed. For example, one patient may have a surgically implanted prosthesis (for example, after joint surgery), whereas another may have reconstructive surgery requiring an allograft (such as bone from a bone bank) or an autograft (bone from the patient's own body).

Encourage early rehabilitation for amputees as follows:

• Start physical therapy 24 hours postoperatively. Pain usually isn't severe after amputation. If it is, watch for a wound complication, such as hematoma, excessive stump edema, or infection.

• Be aware of the "phantom limb" syndrome, in which the patient "feels" an itch or tingling in an amputated extremity. This can last for several hours or persist for years. Explain that this sensation is normal and usually subsides.

• To avoid contractures and ensure the best conditions for wound healing, warn the patient not to hang the stump over the edge of the bed; sit in a wheelchair with the stump flexed; place a pillow under his hip, knee, or back, or between his thighs; lie with knees flexed; rest an above-the-knee stump on the crutch handle; or abduct an above-the-knee stump.

• Wash the stump, massage it gently, and keep it dry until it heals. Make sure the bandage is firm and is worn day and night. Know how to reapply the bandage to shape the stump for a prosthesis.

• To help the patient select a prosthesis, consider his needs and the types of prostheses available. The rehabilitation staff will help him make the final decision, but because most patients are uninformed about choosing a prosthesis, give some guidelines. Keep in mind the patient's age and possible vision problems. Generally, children need relatively simple devices, whereas older adults may need prostheses that provide more stability. Consider finances too. Children outgrow prostheses, so advise parents to plan accordingly.

• The same points are applicable for an interscapulothoracic amputee, but losing an arm causes a greater cosmetic problem. Consult an occupational therapist, who can teach the patient how to perform daily activities with one arm.

• Try to instill a positive attitude toward recovery. Urge the patient to resume an independent lifestyle. Refer older patients to community health services, if necessary. Suggest tutoring for children to help them keep up with schoolwork.

LIFE-THREATENING DISORDER

BOTULISM

A life-threatening paralytic illness, botulism results from an exotoxin produced by the gram-positive, anaerobic bacillus *Clostridium botulinum.* It occurs as botulism food poisoning, wound botulism, and infant botulism. Mortality from botulism is about 25%, with death most often caused by respiratory failure during the first week of illness.

Causes
Botulism is usually the result of ingesting inadequately cooked contaminated foods, especially those with low acid content, such as home-canned fruits and vegetables, sausages, and smoked or preserved fish or meat. Rarely, it results from wound infection with *C. botulinum.*

Botulism occurs worldwide and affects adults more often than children. Recently, findings have shown that an infant's GI tract can become colonized with *C. botulinum* from some unknown source, and then the exotoxin is produced within the infant's intestine. Incidence had been declining, but the current trend toward home canning has resulted in an upswing (approximately 250 cases per year in the United States) in recent years.

Signs and symptoms
The disease usually presents within 12 to 36 hours (range is 6 hours to 8 days) after the ingestion of contaminated food. The severity varies with the amount of toxin ingested and the patient's degree of immunocompetence. Generally, early onset (within 24 hours) signals critical and potentially fatal illness. Initial symptoms include dry mouth, sore throat, weakness, vomiting, and diarrhea.

The cardinal sign of botulism, though, is acute symmetrical cranial nerve impairment (ptosis, diplopia, dysarthria), followed by descending weakness or paralysis of muscles in the extremities or trunk, and dyspnea from respiratory muscle paralysis. Such impairment doesn't affect mental or sensory processes and isn't associated with fever.

Infant botulism

Usually afflicting infants between 3 and 20 weeks, infant botulism can produce hypotonic (floppy) infant syndrome. Symptoms are constipation, feeble cry, depressed gag reflex, and inability to suck. Cranial nerve deficits also occur in infants and are manifested by a flaccid facial expression, ptosis, and ophthalmoplegia. Infants also develop generalized muscle weakness, hypotonia, and areflexia. Loss of head control may be striking. Respiratory arrest is likely.

Diagnosis

Identification of the offending toxin in the patient's serum, stools, gastric content, or the suspected food confirms the diagnosis. An electromyogram showing diminished muscle action potential after a single supramaximal nerve stimulus is also diagnostic.

Diagnosis also must rule out other diseases often confused with botulism, such as Guillain-Barré syndrome, myasthenia gravis, cerebrovascular accident, staphylococcal food poisoning, tick paralysis, chemical intoxications, carbon monoxide poisoning, fish poisoning, trichinosis, and diphtheria.

Treatment

I.V. or I.M. administration of botulinum antitoxin (available through the Centers for Disease Control and Prevention) is the treatment of choice.

Special considerations

If you suspect ingestion of contaminated food:

• Obtain a careful history of the patient's food intake for the past several days. Check to see if other family members exhibit similar symptoms and share a common food history.

• Observe carefully for abnormal neurologic signs. If the patient returns home, tell his family to watch for signs of weakness, blurred vision, and slurred speech, and to return the patient to the hospital immediately if such signs appear.

• If ingestion has occurred within several hours, induce vomiting, begin gastric lavage, and give a high enema to purge any unabsorbed toxin from the bowel.

If clinical signs of botulism appear:

• Bring the patient to the intensive care unit, and monitor cardiac and respiratory function carefully.

• Administer botulinum antitoxin, as required, to neutralize any circulating toxin. Before giving antitoxin, obtain an accurate patient history of allergies, especially to horses, and perform a skin test. Afterward, watch for anaphylaxis or other hypersensitivity, and serum sickness. Keep epinephrine 1:1,000 (for S.C. administration) and emergency airway equipment available.

• Closely observe and accurately record neurologic function, including bilateral motor status (reflexes, ability to move arms and legs).

• Give I.V. fluids as needed. Turn the patient often, and encourage deep-breathing exercises. Isolation is not required.

• Because botulism is sometimes fatal, keep the patient and his family informed about the course of the disease.

• Immediately notify local public health authorities of all cases of botulism.

To help prevent botulism, encourage patients to observe proper techniques in processing and preserving foods. Warn them to avoid even *tasting* food from a bulging can or one with a peculiar odor, and to sterilize by boiling any utensil that comes in contact with suspected food. Ingestion of even a small amount of food contaminated with botulism toxin can prove fatal.

BRAIN ABSCESS

This type of intracranial abscess is a free or encapsulated collection of pus that usually occurs in the temporal lobe, cerebellum, or frontal lobes. It can vary in size and may occur singly or multilocularly. Brain abscess has a relatively low incidence. Although it can occur at any age, it's most common in people between ages 10 and 35 and is rare in older adults.

An untreated brain abscess is usually fatal; with treatment, the prognosis is only fair. About 30% of patients develop focal seizures. Multiple metastatic abscesses secondary to systemic or other infections have the poorest prognosis.

Causes

A brain abscess usually occurs secondary to some other infection, especially otitis media, sinusitis, dental abscess, and mastoiditis. Other causes include subdural empyema; bacterial endocarditis; human immunodeficiency virus infection; bacteremia; pulmonary or pleural infection; pelvic, abdominal, and skin infections; and cranial trauma, such as a penetrating head wound or compound skull fracture.

This condition also occurs in about 2% of children with congenital heart disease, possibly because the hypoxic brain is a good culture medium for bacteria. Common infecting organisms are pyogenic bacteria, such as *Staphylococcus aureus* and *Streptococcus viridans.* Penetrating head trauma or bacteremia usually leads to staphylococcal infection; pulmonary disease, to streptococcal infection.

Pathophysiology

A brain abscess usually begins with localized inflammatory necrosis and edema, septic thrombosis of vessels, and suppurative encephalitis. This is followed by thick encapsulation of accumulated pus, and adjacent meningeal infiltration by neutrophils, lymphocytes, and plasma cells.

Signs and symptoms

Onset varies according to cause, but generally, brain abscess produces clinical effects similar to those of a brain tumor. Early symptoms result from increased intracranial pressure (ICP) and include constant intractable headache, worsened by straining; nausea; vomiting; and focal or generalized seizures. Typical later symptoms include ocular disturbances, such as nystagmus, decreased vision, and inequality of pupils. Other features differ with the site of the abscess:

• *temporal lobe abscess:* auditory-receptive dysphasia, central facial weakness, hemiparesis
• *cerebellar abscess:* dizziness, coarse nystagmus, gaze weakness on lesion side, tremor, ataxia
• *frontal lobe abscess:* expressive dysphasia, hemiparesis with unilateral motor seizure, drowsiness, inattention, mental function impairment.

Signs of infection, such as fever, pallor, and bradycardia, are absent until late stages unless they result from the predisposing condition. If the abscess is encapsulated, they may never appear. Depending on abscess size and location, level of consciousness (LOC) varies from drowsiness to deep stupor.

Diagnosis

A history of infection — especially of the middle ear, mastoid, nasal sinuses, heart, or lungs — or a history of congenital heart disease, along with a physical examination showing such characteristic clinical features as increased ICP, point to a brain abscess. A computed tomography (CT) scan and, occasionally, arteriography (which highlights the abscess by a halo) help locate the site.

Examination of cerebrospinal fluid can help confirm infection, but lumbar puncture is too risky because it can release the increased ICP and provoke cerebral herniation. A CT-guided stereotactic biopsy may be performed to drain and culture the abscess. Other tests include culture and sensitivity of drainage to identify the causative organism, skull X-rays, and a radioisotope scan.

Treatment
Therapy consists of antibiotics to combat the underlying infection and surgical aspiration or drainage of the abscess. However, surgery is delayed until the abscess becomes encapsulated (a CT scan helps determine this) and is contraindicated in patients with congenital heart disease or another debilitating cardiac condition. Administration of a penicillinase-resistant antibiotic, such as nafcillin or methicillin, for at least 2 weeks before surgery can reduce the risk of spreading infection.

Other treatments during the acute phase are palliative and supportive; they include mechanical ventilation and administration of I.V. fluids with diuretics (urea, mannitol) and glucocorticoids (dexamethasone) to combat increased ICP and cerebral edema. Anticonvulsants, such as phenytoin and phenobarbital, help prevent seizures.

Special considerations
• The patient with an acute brain abscess requires intensive care monitoring.
• Frequently assess neurologic status, especially LOC, speech, and sensorimotor and cranial nerve function.

• Watch for signs of increased ICP (decreased LOC, vomiting, abnormal pupil response, and depressed respirations), which may lead to cerebral herniation with such signs as fixed and dilated pupils, widened pulse pressure, bradycardia or tachycardia, and absent respirations.
• Assess and record vital signs at least every hour.
• Monitor fluid intake and output carefully because fluid overload could contribute to cerebral edema.
• If surgery is necessary, explain the procedure to the patient and answer his questions.
• After surgery, continue frequent neurologic assessment. Monitor vital signs and intake and output.
• Watch for signs of meningitis (nuchal rigidity, headaches, chills, sweats), an ever-present threat.
• Change a damp dressing often, using aseptic technique and noting amount of drainage. *Never allow bandages to remain damp.* To promote drainage and prevent reaccumulation of the abscess, position the patient on the operative side.
• If the patient remains stuporous or comatose for an extended period, give meticulous skin care to prevent pressure ulcers, and position him to preserve function and prevent contractures.
• If the patient requires isolation because of postoperative drainage, make sure he and his family understand why.
• Ambulate the patient as soon as possible to prevent immobility and encourage independence.
• To prevent brain abscess, stress the need for treatment of otitis media, mastoiditis, dental abscess, and other infections. Give prophylactic antibiotics, as needed, after compound skull fracture or penetrating head wound.

BRAIN TUMORS, MALIGNANT

With an incidence of 4.5 per 100,000, malignant brain tumors (gliomas, meningiomas, and schwannomas) are common (slightly more so in men than in women).

Tumors may occur at any age. In adults, incidence is generally highest between ages 40 and 60. The most common tumor types in adults are gliomas and meningiomas; these tumors are usually supratentorial (above the covering of the cerebellum).

In children, incidence is generally highest before age 1 and then again between ages 2 and 12. The most common tumors in children are astrocytomas, medulloblastomas, ependymomas, and brain stem gliomas. In children, brain tumors are one of the most common causes of death from cancer.

Causes
The cause of brain tumors is unknown.

Signs and symptoms
Brain tumors cause central nervous system changes by invading and destroying tissues and by secondary effect — mainly compression of the brain, cranial nerves, and cerebral vessels; cerebral edema; and increased intracranial pressure (ICP). Generally, clinical features result from increased ICP; these features vary with the type of tumor, its location, and the degree of invasion. The onset of symptoms is usually insidious, and brain tumors are commonly misdiagnosed. (See *Clinical features of malignant brain tumors.*)

Diagnosis
In many cases, a definitive diagnosis follows a tissue biopsy performed by stereotactic surgery. In this procedure, a head ring is affixed to the skull, and an excisional device is guided to the lesion by a computed tomography (CT) scan or magnetic resonance imaging (MRI).

Other diagnostic tools include a patient history, a neurologic assessment, skull X-rays, a brain scan, a CT scan, MRI, and cerebral angiography. Lumbar puncture shows increased pressure and protein levels, decreased glucose levels and, occasionally, tumor cells in cerebrospinal fluid (CSF).

Treatment
Remedial approaches include removing a resectable tumor; reducing a nonresectable tumor; relieving cerebral edema, increased ICP, and other symptoms; and preventing further neurologic damage.

The mode of therapy depends on the tumor's histologic type, radiosensitivity, and location and may include surgery, radiation, chemotherapy, or decompression of increased ICP with diuretics, corticosteroids, or possibly ventriculoatrial or ventriculoperitoneal shunting of CSF.

• *Gliomas.* Treatment usually requires resection by craniotomy, followed by radiation therapy and chemotherapy. The combination of nitrosoureas (carmustine [BCNU], lomustine [CCNU], or procarbazine) and postoperative radiation is more effective than radiation alone.

• *Astrocytomas.* Surgical resection of low-grade cystic cerebellar astrocytomas brings long-term survival. Treatment of other astrocytomas includes repeated surgery, radiation therapy, and shunting of fluid from obstructed CSF pathways. Some astrocytomas are highly radiosensitive, but others are radioresistant.

CLINICAL FEATURES OF MALIGNANT BRAIN TUMORS

TUMOR	CLINICAL FEATURES
Glioblastoma multiforme *(spongioblastoma multiforme)* • Peak incidence between ages 50 and 60; twice as common in males; most common glioma • Unencapsulated, highly malignant; grows rapidly and infiltrates the brain extensively; may become enormous before diagnosed • Occurs most often in cerebral hemispheres, especially frontal and temporal lobes (rarely in brain stem and cerebellum) • Occupies more than one lobe of affected hemisphere; may spread to opposite hemisphere by corpus callosum; may metastasize into cerebrospinal fluid (CSF), producing tumors in distant parts of the central nervous system	*General* • Increased intracranial pressure (ICP), causing nausea, vomiting, headache, papilledema • Mental and behavioral changes • Altered vital signs (increased systolic pressure; widened pulse pressure, respiratory changes) • Speech and sensory disturbances • In children, irritability, projectile vomiting *Localized* • Midline: headache (bifrontal or biooccipital); worse in morning; intensified by coughing, straining, or sudden head movements • Temporal lobe: psychomotor seizures • Central region: focal seizures • Optic and oculomotor nerves: visual defects • Frontal lobe: abnormal reflexes, motor responses
Astrocytoma • Second most common malignant glioma (approximately 30% of all gliomas) • Occurs at any age; incidence higher in males • Occurs most often in white matter of cerebral hemispheres; may originate in any part of the central nervous system • Cerebellar astrocytomas usually confined to one hemisphere	*General* • Headache; mental activity changes • Decreased motor strength and coordination • Seizures; scanning speech • Altered vital signs *Localized* • Third ventricle: changes in mental activity and level of consciousness, nausea, pupillary dilation and sluggish light reflex; later—paresis or ataxia • Brain stem and pons: early—ipsilateral trigeminal, abducens, and facial nerve palsies; later—cerebellar ataxia, tremors, other cranial nerve deficits • Third or fourth ventricle or aqueduct of Sylvius: secondary hydrocephalus • Thalamus or hypothalamus: variety of endocrine, metabolic, autonomic, and behavioral changes

(continued)

CLINICAL FEATURES OF MALIGNANT BRAIN TUMORS *(continued)*

TUMOR	CLINICAL FEATURES
Oligodendroglioma • Third most common glioma • Occurs in middle adult years; more common in women • Slow-growing	*General* • Mental and behavioral changes • Decreased visual acuity and other visual disturbances • Increased ICP *Localized* • Temporal lobe: hallucinations, psychomotor seizures • Central region: seizures (confined to one muscle group or unilateral) • Midbrain or third ventricle: pyramidal tract symptoms (dizziness, ataxia, paresthesias of the face) • Brain stem and cerebrum: nystagmus, hearing loss, dizziness, ataxia, paresthesias of face, cranial nerve palsies, hemiparesis, suboccipital tenderness, loss of balance
Ependymoma • Rare glioma • Most common in children and young adults • Locates most often in fourth and lateral ventricles	*General* • Similar to oligodendroglioma • Increased ICP and obstructive hydrocephalus, depending on tumor size
Medulloblastoma • Rare glioma • Incidence highest in children ages 4 to 6 • Affects males more than females • Frequently metastasizes via CSF	*General* • Increased ICP *Localized* • Brain stem and cerebrum: papilledema, nystagmus, hearing loss, flashing lights, dizziness, ataxia, paresthesias of face, cranial nerve palsies (V, VI, VII, IX, X, primarily sensory), hemiparesis, suboccipital tenderness; compression of supratentorial area produces other general and focal symptoms

CLINICAL FEATURES OF MALIGNANT BRAIN TUMORS (continued)

TUMOR	CLINICAL FEATURES
Meningioma • Most common nongliomatous brain tumor (15% of primary brain tumors) • Peak incidence among 50-year-olds; rare in children; more common in females than males (ratio 3:2) • Arises from the meninges • Common locations include parasagittal area, sphenoidal ridge, anterior part of the base of the skull, cerebellopontine angle, spinal canal • Benign, well-circumscribed, highly vascular tumors that compress underlying brain tissue by invading overlying skull	*General* • Headache • Seizures (in two-thirds of patients) • Vomiting • Changes in mental activity • Similar to schwannomas *Localized* • Skull changes (bony bulge) over tumor • Sphenoidal ridge, indenting optic nerve: unilateral visual changes and papilledema • Prefrontal parasagittal: personality and behavioral changes • Motor cortex: contralateral motor changes • Anterior fossa compressing both optic nerves and frontal lobes: headaches and bilateral vision loss • Pressure on cranial nerves causes varying symptoms
Schwannoma *(acoustic neurinoma, neurilemoma, cerebellopontile angle tumor)* • Accounts for approximately 10% of all intracranial tumors • Higher incidence in women • Onset of symptoms between ages 30 and 60 • Affects the craniospinal nerve sheath, usually cranial nerve VIII; also, V and VII, and, to a lesser extent, VI and X on the same side as the tumor • Benign, but often classified as malignant because of its growth patterns; slow-growing—may be present for years before symptoms occur	*General* • Unilateral hearing loss with or without tinnitus • Stiff neck and suboccipital discomfort • Secondary hydrocephalus • Ataxia and uncoordinated movements of one or both arms due to pressure on brain stem and cerebellum *Localized* • V: early—facial hypoesthesia or paresthesia on side of hearing loss; unilateral loss of corneal reflex • VI: diplopia or double vision • VII: paresis progressing to paralysis (Bell's palsy) • X: weakness of palate, tongue, and nerve muscles on same side as tumor

• *Oligodendrogliomas* and *ependymomas.* Treatment includes resection and radiation therapy.

• *Medulloblastomas.* Treatment involves resection and possibly intrathecal infusion of methotrexate or another antineoplastic drug.

• *Meningiomas.* Treatment requires resection, including dura mater and bone (operative mortality may reach 10% because of large tumor size).

• *Schwannomas.* Microsurgical technique allows complete resection of the tumor and preservation of facial nerves. Although schwannomas are moderately radioresistant, postoperative radiation therapy is necessary.

Chemotherapy for malignant brain tumors includes the nitrosoureas that help break down the blood-brain barrier and allow other chemotherapeutic drugs to go through as well. Intrathecal and intra-arterial administration of drugs maximizes drug actions.

Palliative measures for gliomas, astrocytomas, oligodendrogliomas, and ependymomas include dexamethasone for cerebral edema and antacids and histamine receptor antagonists for stress ulcers. These tumors and schwannomas may also require anticonvulsants.

Special considerations
• Perform a comprehensive assessment (including a complete neurologic evaluation) to provide baseline data and guide subsequent care. Obtain a thorough health history concerning onset of symptoms.
• Assist the patient and his family in coping with the treatment, potential disabilities, and changes in lifestyle resulting from his tumor.

Throughout hospitalization:
• Carefully document seizure activity (occurrence, nature, and duration).
• Maintain airway patency.
• Monitor patient safety.
• Administer anticonvulsive drugs as needed.
• Check continuously for changes in neurologic status, and watch for an increase in ICP.
• Watch for and immediately report sudden unilateral pupillary dilation with loss of light reflex; this ominous change indicates imminent transtentorial herniation.
• Monitor respiratory changes carefully (abnormal respiratory rate and depth may point to rising ICP or herniation of the cerebellar tonsils from expanding infratentorial mass).
• Monitor temperature carefully. Fever commonly follows hypothalamic anoxia but might also indicate meningitis. Use hypothermia blankets preoperatively and postoperatively to keep the patient's temperature down and minimize cerebral metabolic demands.
• Administer steroids and osmotic diuretics such as mannitol, as needed, to reduce cerebral edema. Fluids may be restricted to 1,500 ml/24 hours. Monitor fluid and electrolyte balance to avoid dehydration.
• Observe for signs of stress ulcers: abdominal distention, pain, vomiting, and black, tarry stools. Administer antacids as needed.

Surgery requires additional patient care. After craniotomy:
• Continue to monitor general neurologic status and watch for signs of increased ICP, such as an elevated bone flap and typical neurologic changes. To reduce the risk of increased ICP, restrict fluids to 1,500 ml/24 hours.
• To promote venous drainage and reduce cerebral edema after supratentorial craniotomy, elevate the head of the patient's bed about 30 degrees. Position him on his side to allow drainage of secretions and prevent aspiration.
• As appropriate, instruct the patient to avoid Valsalva's maneuver or isometric muscle contractions when moving or sitting up in bed; these can increase intrathoracic pressure and thereby increase ICP.
• Withhold oral fluids, which may provoke vomiting and consequently raise ICP.
• After infratentorial craniotomy, keep the patient flat for 48 hours, but logroll him every 2 hours to minimize complications of immobilization. Prevent other complications by paying careful attention to ventilatory status and to cardiovascular, GI, and musculoskeletal function.
• Radiation therapy is usually delayed until after the surgical wound heals, but it can induce wound breakdown even then. Observe the wound carefully for infection and sinus formation.

• Because radiation may cause brain inflammation, watch for signs of rising ICP.

• Because the nitrosoureas — carmustine (BCNU), lomustine (CCNU), and procarbazine — used as adjuncts to radiotherapy and surgery can possibly cause delayed bone marrow depression, tell the patient to watch for and immediately report any signs of infection or bleeding that appear within 4 weeks after the start of chemotherapy.

• Before chemotherapy, give prochlorperazine or another antiemetic, as needed, to minimize nausea and vomiting.

• Teach the patient signs of recurrence; urge compliance with the treatment regimen.

• Because brain tumors may cause residual neurologic deficits that handicap the patient physically or mentally, begin rehabilitation early.

• Consult with occupational and physical therapists to encourage independence in daily activities.

• As necessary, provide aids for self-care and mobilization, such as bathroom rails for wheelchair patients.

• If the patient is aphasic, arrange for consultation with a speech pathologist.

BREAST CANCER

This disorder is the most common cancer affecting women and is the number two killer (after lung cancer) of women ages 35 to 54. It occurs in men, but rarely. The 5-year survival rate has improved from 53% in the 1940s to 70% in the 1980s because of earlier diagnosis and the variety of treatment modes now available. The death rate, however, hasn't changed in the past 50 years. Lymph node involvement is the most valuable prognostic predictor. With adjuvant therapy, 70% to 75% of women with negative nodes will survive 10 years or more, compared with 20% to 25% of women with positive nodes.

Although breast cancer may develop any time after puberty, it's most common after age 50.

Causes

The cause of breast cancer isn't known, but its high incidence in women implicates estrogen. Certain predisposing factors are clear; women at *high risk* include those who:

• have a family history of breast cancer.

• have long menstrual cycles; began menses early or menopause late.

• have never been pregnant.

• were first pregnant after age 31.

• have had unilateral breast cancer.

• have had endometrial or ovarian cancer.

• were exposed to low-level ionizing radiation.

Many other possible predisposing factors have been investigated, including estrogen therapy, antihypertensives, high-fat diet, obesity, and fibrocystic disease of the breasts.

Women at *lower risk* include those who:

• were pregnant before age 20.

• have had multiple pregnancies.

• are Indian or Asian.

Pathophysiology

Breast cancer occurs more often in the left breast than the right, and more often in the upper outer quadrant. Growth rates vary. Theoretically, slow-growing breast cancer may take up to 8 years to become palpable at ⅜″ (1 cm) in size. It spreads by way of the lymphatic system and the bloodstream, through the right heart to the lungs, and eventually to the other breast, the chest wall, liver, bone, and brain.

Many refer to the estimated growth rate of breast cancer as "doubling time," or the time it takes the malignant cells to double in number. Survival time for breast cancer is based on tumor size and spread; the number of involved nodes is the single most important factor in predicting survival time.

Classified by histologic appearance and location of the lesion, breast cancer may be:

• *adenocarcinoma* — arising from the epithelium

• *intraductal* — developing within the ducts (includes Paget's disease)

• *infiltrating* — occurring in parenchymal tissue of the breast

• *inflammatory (rare)* — reflecting rapid tumor growth, in which the overlying skin becomes edematous, inflamed, and indurated

• *lobular carcinoma in situ* — reflecting tumor growth involving lobes of glandular tissue

• *medullary or circumscribed* — a large tumor with a rapid growth rate.

These histologic classifications should be coupled with a staging or nodal status classification system for a clearer understanding of the extent of the cancer. The most commonly used system for staging cancer, both before and after surgery, is the tumor-node-metastasis (TNM) system. (See *Staging breast cancer.*)

Signs and symptoms
Warning signals of possible breast cancer include:

• a lump or mass in the breast (a hard, stony mass is usually malignant).

• a change in symmetry or size of the breast.

• a change in breast skin (thickening, scaly skin around the nipple, dimpling, edema [peau d'orange], or ulceration).

• a change in skin temperature (a warm, hot, or pink area; suspect cancer in a nonlactating woman past

childbearing age until proven otherwise).

• unusual drainage or discharge (a spontaneous discharge of any kind in a non-breast-feeding, nonlactating woman warrants thorough investigation; so does any discharge produced by breast manipulation [greenish black, white, creamy, serous, or bloody]). If a breast-feeding infant rejects one breast, this may suggest possible breast cancer.

• a change in the nipple, such as itching, burning, erosion, or retraction.

• pain (not usually a symptom of breast cancer unless the tumor is advanced, but it should be investigated).

• bone metastasis, pathologic bone fractures, and hypercalcemia.

• edema of the arm.

Diagnosis
Diagnostic measures in breast cancer include the following.

Breast self-examination
The most reliable method of detecting breast cancer is the monthly breast self-examination, followed by immediate evaluation of any abnormality.

Mammography and biopsies
Other diagnostic measures include mammography, a needle biopsy, and a surgical biopsy. Mammography is indicated for any woman whose physical examination might suggest breast cancer. It should be done as a baseline on women between ages 35 and 39; every 1 to 2 years for ages 40 to 49; and annually on women over age 50, women who have a family history of breast cancer, and women who have had unilateral breast cancer, to check for new disease. However, the value of mammography is questionable for women under age 35 (because of the density of the breasts), except those who are strongly suspected of having breast cancer.

STAGING BREAST CANCER

Cancer staging helps form a prognosis and a treatment plan. For breast cancer, most clinicians use the TNM (tumor, node, metastasis) system developed by the American Joint Committee on Cancer.

Primary tumor

TX—primary tumor can't be assessed

T0—no evidence of primary tumor

Tis—carcinoma in situ: intraductal carcinoma, lobular carcinoma in situ, or Paget's disease of the nipple with no tumor

T1—tumor 2 cm or less in greatest dimension

T1a—tumor 0.5 cm or less in greatest dimension

T1b—tumor more than 0.5 cm but not more than 1 cm in greatest dimension

T1c—tumor more than 1 cm but not more than 2 cm in greatest dimension

T2—tumor more than 2 cm but not more than 5 cm in greatest dimension

T3—tumor more than 5 cm in greatest dimension

T4—tumor of any size that extends to the chest wall or skin

T4a—tumor extends to the chest wall

T4b—tumor accompanied by edema, ulcerated breast skin, or satellite skin nodules on the same breast

T4c—both T4a and T4b

T4d—inflammatory carcinoma

Regional lymph nodes

NX—regional lymph nodes can't be assessed

N0—no evidence of nodal involvement

N1—movable ipsilateral axillary nodal involvement

N2—ipsilateral axillary nodal involvement with nodes fixed to one another or to other structures

N3—ipsilateral internal mammary nodal involvement

Distant metastasis

MX—distant metastasis can't be assessed

M0—no evidence of distant metastasis

M1—distant metastasis (including metastasis to ipsilateral supraclavicular nodes)

Staging categories

Breast cancer progresses from mild to severe as follows:

Stage 0—Tis, N0, M0

Stage I—T1, N0, M0

Stage IIA—T0, N1, M0; T1, N1, M0; T2, N0, M0

Stage IIB—T2, N1, M0; T3, N0, M0

Stage IIIA—T0, N2, M0; T1, N2, M0; T2, N2, M0; T3, N1 or N2, M0

Stage IIIB—T4, any N, M0; any T, N3, M0

Stage IV—any T, any N, M1

False-negative results can occur in as many as 30% of all tests. Consequently, with a suspicious mass, a negative mammogram should be disregarded, and a fine-needle aspiration or surgical biopsy should be done. Ultrasonography, which can distinguish a fluid-filled cyst from a tumor, can also be used instead of an invasive surgical biopsy.

Other tests
Bone scan, computed tomography scan, measurement of alkaline phosphatase levels, liver function studies, and a liver biopsy can detect distant

metastasis. A hormonal receptor assay done on the tumor can determine if the tumor is estrogen- or progesterone-dependent. (This test guides decisions to use therapy that blocks the action of the estrogen hormone that supports tumor growth.)

Treatment
Much controversy exists over breast cancer treatments. In choosing therapy, the patient and doctor should consider the stage of the disease, the woman's age and menopausal status, and the disfiguring effects of the surgery. Treatment for breast cancer may include one or any combination of the following.

Surgery
In breast cancer, surgery involves either mastectomy or lumpectomy. A *lumpectomy* may be done on an outpatient basis and may be the only surgery needed, especially if the tumor is small and there's no evidence of axillary node involvement. Radiation therapy is often combined with this surgery.

A two-stage procedure, in which the surgeon removes the lump, confirms that it's malignant, and discusses treatment options with the patient, is desirable because it allows the patient to participate in her treatment plan. Sometimes, if the tumor is diagnosed as clinically malignant, such planning can be done before surgery. In *lumpectomy and dissection of the axillary lymph nodes,* the tumor and the axillary lymph nodes are removed, leaving the breast intact.

A *simple mastectomy* removes the breast but not the lymph nodes or pectoral muscles. A *modified radical mastectomy* removes the breast and the axillary lymph nodes. A *radical mastectomy,* the performance of which has declined, removes the breast, pectoralis major and minor, and the axillary lymph nodes.

After a mastectomy, reconstructive surgery can create a breast mound if the patient desires it and doesn't have evidence of advanced disease.

Chemotherapy, tamoxifen, and peripheral stem cell therapy
Various cytotoxic drug combinations are used as either adjuvant or primary therapy, depending on several factors, including the TNM staging and estrogen receptor status. The most commonly used antineoplastic drugs are cyclophosphamide, fluorouracil, methotrexate, doxorubicin, vincristine, paclitaxel, and prednisone. A common drug combination used in both premenopausal and postmenopausal women is cyclophosphamide, methotrexate, and fluorouracil (CMF).

Tamoxifen, an estrogen antagonist, is the adjuvant treatment of choice for postmenopausal patients with positive estrogen receptor status.

Peripheral stem cell therapy may be used for advanced breast cancer.

Primary radiation therapy
Used before or after tumor removal, primary radiation therapy is effective for small tumors in early stages with no evidence of distant metastasis; it's also used to prevent or treat local recurrence. Presurgical radiation to the breast in inflammatory breast cancer helps make tumors more surgically manageable.

Other drug therapy
Breast cancer patients may also receive estrogen, progesterone, androgen, or anti-androgen aminoglutethimide therapy. The success of these drug therapies with growing evidence that breast cancer is a systemic, not local, disease has led to a decline in ablative surgery.

Special considerations

• To provide good care for a breast cancer patient, begin with a history; assess the patient's feelings about her illness, and determine what she knows about it and what she expects.

Preoperative care:

• Be sure you know what kind of surgery is scheduled, so you can prepare the patient. If a mastectomy is scheduled, in addition to the usual preoperative preparation (for example, skin preparations and allowing nothing by mouth), provide the following information:

• Teach the patient how to deep-breathe and cough to prevent pulmonary complications, and how to rotate her ankles to help prevent thromboembolism.

• Tell the patient she can ease her pain by lying on the affected side, or by placing a hand or pillow on the incision. Preoperatively, show her where the incision will be. Inform her that she'll receive pain medication and that she needn't fear addiction.

• Be aware that adequate pain relief encourages coughing and turning and promotes general well-being. Positioning a small pillow under the patient's arm provides comfort.

• Encourage the patient to get out of bed as soon as possible (even as soon as the anesthesia wears off or the first evening after surgery).

• Explain that after mastectomy, an incisional drain or suction device (Hemovac) will be used to remove accumulated serous or sanguineous fluid and to keep the tension off the suture line, promoting healing.

Postoperative care:

• Inspect the dressing anteriorly and posteriorly. Be alert for bleeding.

• Measure and record the amount and note the color of drainage. Expect drainage to be bloody during the first 4 hours and afterward become serous.

• Check circulatory status (blood pressure, pulse, respirations, and bleeding).

• Monitor intake and output for at least 48 hours after general anesthesia.

• Prevent lymphedema of the arm, which may be an early complication of any breast cancer treatment that involves lymph node dissection. Help the patient prevent lymphedema by instructing her to exercise her hand and arm regularly and to avoid activities that might cause infection in this hand or arm (infection increases the chance of developing lymphedema). Such prevention is very important because lymphedema can't be treated effectively.

• Inspect the incision. Encourage the patient and her partner to look at her incision as soon as feasible, perhaps when the first dressing is removed.

• Advise the patient to ask her doctor about reconstructive surgery or to call the local or state medical society for the names of plastic reconstructive surgeons who regularly perform surgery to create breast mounds. In many cases, reconstructive surgery may be planned prior to the mastectomy.

• Instruct the patient about breast prostheses. The American Cancer Society's Reach to Recovery group can provide instruction, emotional support and counseling, and a list of area stores that sell prostheses.

• Give psychological and emotional support. Many patients fear cancer and possible disfigurement and worry about loss of sexual function. Explain that breast surgery doesn't interfere with sexual function and that the patient may resume sexual activity as soon as she desires after surgery.

• Also explain to the patient that she may experience "phantom breast syndrome" (a phenomenon in which a tingling or a pins-and-needles sensation is felt in the area of the amputated breast tissue) or depression following mastectomy. Listen to the patient's concerns, offer support, and refer her to an appropriate organization, such as the American Cancer Society's Reach to Recovery, which offers caring and sharing groups to help breast cancer patients in the hospital and at home.

BRONCHIECTASIS

A condition marked by chronic abnormal dilation of bronchi and destruction of bronchial walls, bronchiectasis can occur throughout the tracheobronchial tree or can be confined to one segment or lobe. However, it's usually bilateral and involves the basilar segments of the lower lobes. This disease has three forms: cylindrical (fusiform), varicose, and saccular (cystic).

It affects people of both sexes and all ages. Because of the availability of antibiotics to treat acute respiratory tract infections, the incidence of bronchiectasis has dramatically decreased in the past 20 years. Its incidence is highest among Eskimos and the Maoris of New Zealand. Bronchiectasis is irreversible once established.

Causes
The different forms of bronchiectasis may occur separately or simultaneously. In *cylindrical bronchiectasis,* the bronchi expand unevenly, with little change in diameter, and end suddenly in a squared-off fashion. In *varicose bronchiectasis,* abnormal, irregular dilation and narrowing of the bronchi give the appearance of varicose veins. In *saccular bronchiectasis,* many large dilations end in sacs.

This disease results from conditions associated with repeated damage to bronchial walls, and abnormal mucociliary clearance, which cause a break-down of supporting tissue adjacent to airways. Such conditions include:
• mucoviscidosis (cystic fibrosis)
• immunologic disorders (agammaglobulinemia, for example)
• recurrent, inadequately treated bacterial respiratory tract infections, such as tuberculosis, and complications of measles, pneumonia, pertussis, or influenza
• obstruction (by a foreign body, tumor, or stenosis) in association with recurrent infection
• inhalation of corrosive gas or repeated aspiration of gastric juices into the lungs
• congenital anomalies (uncommon), such as bronchomalacia, congenital bronchiectasis, immotile-cilia syndrome (ICS), and Kartagener's syndrome, a variant of ICS characterized by situs inversus, bronchiectasis, and either nasal polyps or sinusitis.

Pathophysiology
In bronchiectasis, hyperplastic squamous epithelium denuded of cilia replaces ulcerated columnar epithelium. Abscess formation involving all layers of the bronchial wall produces inflammatory cells and fibrous tissue, resulting in both dilation and narrowing of the airways. Mucous plugs or fibrous tissue obliterates smaller bronchioles, while peribronchial lymphoid tissue becomes hyperplastic. Extensive vascular proliferation of bronchial circulation occurs and produces frequent hemoptysis.

Signs and symptoms
Initially, bronchiectasis may be asymptomatic. When symptoms do arise, they're often attributed to other illnesses. The patient usually complains of frequent bouts of pneumonia or hemoptysis. The classic symptom, however, is a chronic cough that produces copious, foul-smelling, mucopurulent secretions, possibly totaling several

cupfuls daily. Characteristic findings include coarse crackles during inspiration over involved lobes or segments, occasional wheezes, dyspnea, sinusitis, weight loss, anemia, malaise, clubbing, recurrent fever, chills, and other signs of infection.

Advanced bronchiectasis may produce chronic malnutrition and amyloidosis, as well as right heart failure and cor pulmonale due to hypoxic pulmonary vasoconstriction.

Diagnosis

A history of recurrent bronchial infections, pneumonia, and hemoptysis in a patient whose chest X-rays show peribronchial thickening, areas of atelectasis, and scattered cystic changes suggests bronchiectasis.

In recent years, computed tomography scanning has supplanted bronchography as the most useful diagnostic test for bronchiectasis. It's sometimes used with high-resolution techniques to better determine anatomic changes. Bronchoscopy doesn't establish the diagnosis of bronchiectasis, but it does help to identify the source of secretions. Bronchoscopy can also be instrumental in pinpointing the site of bleeding in hemoptysis.

Other helpful laboratory tests include:

• *sputum culture* and *Gram's stain* to identify predominant organisms
• *complete blood count* to detect anemia and leukocytosis
• *pulmonary function studies* to detect decreased vital capacity, expiratory flow, and hypoxemia; these tests also help determine the physiologic severity of the disease and the effects of therapy, and help evaluate patients for surgery.

Evaluation may also include urinalysis and an electrocardiogram. (The latter is normal unless cor pulmonale develops.) When cystic fibrosis is suspected as the underlying cause of bronchiectasis, a sweat electrolyte test is useful.

Treatment

Typically, antibiotics are given orally or I.V., for 7 to 10 days or until sputum production decreases. Bronchodilators, combined with postural drainage and chest percussion, help remove secretions if the patient has bronchospasm and thick, tenacious sputum. Bronchoscopy may be used to help mobilize secretions.

Hypoxia requires oxygen therapy; severe hemoptysis often requires lobectomy, segmental resection, or bronchial artery embolization if pulmonary function is poor.

Special considerations

• Provide supportive care and help the patient adjust to the permanent changes in lifestyle that irreversible lung damage necessitates. Thorough teaching is vital.
• Administer antibiotics, as needed, and explain all diagnostic tests.
• Perform chest physiotherapy, including postural drainage and chest percussion designed for involved lobes, several times a day. The best times to do this are early morning and just before bedtime. Instruct the patient to maintain each position for 10 minutes; then perform percussion and tell him to cough.
• Show family members how to perform postural drainage and percussion.
• Teach the patient coughing and deep-breathing techniques to promote good ventilation and the removal of secretions.
• Advise the patient to stop smoking, if appropriate, to avoid stimulating secretions and irritating the airways. Refer him to a local self-help group.
• Provide a warm, quiet, comfortable environment, and urge the patient to rest as much as possible.

• Encourage balanced, high-protein meals to promote good health and tissue healing, and plenty of fluids to aid expectoration. Give frequent mouth care to remove foul-smelling sputum. Teach the patient to dispose of all secretions properly.

• Tell the patient to avoid air pollutants and people with upper respiratory tract infections.

• Instruct the patient to take medications (especially antibiotics) exactly as prescribed.

• To help prevent this disease, treat bacterial pneumonia vigorously and stress the need for immunization to prevent childhood diseases.

BUERGER'S DISEASE

Also known as *thromboangiitis obliterans,* this inflammatory, nonatheromatous occlusive condition causes segmental lesions and subsequent thrombus formation in the small and medium arteries (and sometimes the veins), resulting in decreased blood flow to the feet and legs. Buerger's disease may produce ulceration and, eventually, gangrene.

Causes

Although the cause of Buerger's disease is unknown, a definite link exists to smoking, suggesting a hypersensitivity reaction to nicotine. Incidence is highest among men of Jewish ancestry, ages 20 to 40, who smoke heavily.

Signs and symptoms

Buerger's disease typically produces intermittent claudication of the instep, which is aggravated by exercise and relieved by rest. During exposure to low temperature, the feet initially become cold, cyanotic, and numb; later, they redden, become hot, and tingle. Occasionally, Buerger's disease also affects the hands, possibly resulting in painful fingertip ulcerations.

Associated signs and symptoms may include impaired peripheral pulses, migratory superficial thrombophlebitis, and, in later stages, ulceration, muscle atrophy, and gangrene.

Diagnosis

Patient history and physical examination strongly suggest Buerger's disease. Supportive diagnostic tests include:

• *Doppler ultrasonography* to show diminished circulation in the peripheral vessels

• *plethysmography* to help detect decreased circulation in the peripheral vessels

• *arteriography* to locate lesions and rule out atherosclerosis.

Treatment

Therapy may include an exercise program that uses gravity to fill and drain the blood vessels or, in severe disease, a lumbar sympathectomy to increase blood supply to the skin. Amputation may be necessary for nonhealing ulcers, intractable pain, or gangrene.

Special considerations

• Strongly urge the patient to discontinue smoking permanently, to enhance the effectiveness of treatment. If necessary, refer him to a self-help group to stop smoking.

• Warn the patient to avoid precipitating factors, such as emotional stress, exposure to extreme temperatures, and trauma.

• Teach proper foot care, especially the importance of wearing well-fitting shoes and cotton or wool socks. Show the patient how to inspect his feet daily for cuts, abrasions, and signs of skin breakdown, such as redness and soreness. Remind him to seek medical attention immediately after any trauma.

• If the patient has ulcers and gangrene, enforce bed rest and use a padded footboard or bed cradle to prevent pressure from bed linens. Protect the feet with soft padding. Wash them gently with a mild soap and tepid water, rinse thoroughly, and pat dry with a soft towel.

• Provide emotional support. If necessary, refer the patient for psychological counseling to help him cope with restrictions imposed by this chronic disease.

• If the patient has undergone amputation, assess rehabilitative needs, especially regarding changes in body image. Refer him to physical therapists, occupational therapists, and social service agencies as needed.

BULIMIA NERVOSA

The essential features of bulimia nervosa include eating binges followed by feelings of guilt, humiliation, and self-deprecation. These feelings cause the patient to engage in self-induced vomiting, use laxatives or diuretics, follow a strict diet, or fast to overcome the effects of the binges.

Unless the patient spends an excessive amount of time binging and purging, bulimia nervosa seldom is incapacitating. However, electrolyte imbalances (metabolic alkalosis, hypochloremia, and hypokalemia) and dehydration can occur, increasing the risk of physical complications.

Bulimia nervosa usually begins in adolescence or early adulthood and can occur simultaneously with anorexia nervosa. It affects nine women for every man. Nearly 2% of adult women meet the diagnostic criteria for bulimia nervosa; 5% to 15% have some symptoms of the disorder.

Causes
This disorder has no known cause, but psychosocial factors may contribute to its development, including family disturbance or conflict, sexual abuse, maladaptive learned behavior, struggle for control or self-identity, cultural overemphasis on physical appearance, and parental obesity. Bulimia nervosa is also associated with depression.

Signs and symptoms
The history of a patient with bulimia nervosa is marked by episodes of binge eating that may occur up to several times a day. The patient commonly reports a binge-eating episode during which she continues eating until abdominal pain, sleep, or the presence of another person interrupts it. The preferred food usually is sweet, soft, and high in calories and carbohydrate content.

The bulimic patient may appear thin and emaciated. Typically, however, although her weight frequently fluctuates, it usually stays within normal limits—through the use of diuretics, laxatives, vomiting, and exercise. So, unlike the anorexic patient, the bulimic patient can usually hide her eating disorder.

Overt clues to this disorder include hyperactivity, peculiar eating habits or rituals, frequent weighing, and a distorted body image.

The patient may complain of abdominal and epigastric pain caused by acute gastric dilation. She may also have amenorrhea. Repetitive vomiting may cause painless swelling of the salivary glands, hoarseness, throat irritation or lacerations, and dental erosion. The patient may also exhibit calluses on the knuckles or abrasions and scars on the dorsum of the hand, resulting from tooth injury during self-induced vomiting.

Psychosocial factors
A bulimic patient commonly is perceived by others as a "perfect" student, mother, or career woman; an adolescent may be distinguished for participation in competitive activities such as sports. However, the patient's psychosocial history may reveal an exaggerated sense of guilt, symptoms of depression, childhood trauma (especially sexual abuse), parental obesity, or a history of unsatisfactory sexual relationships.

Diagnosis
For characteristic findings in this condition, see *Diagnosing bulimia nervosa.*

Additional diagnostic tools include the Beck Depression Inventory, which may identify coexisting depression, and laboratory tests to help determine the presence and severity of complications. Serum electrolyte studies may show elevated bicarbonate, decreased potassium, and decreased sodium levels.

A baseline electrocardiogram may be done if tricyclic antidepressants will be prescribed for the patient.

Treatment
Interrelated physical and psychological symptoms must be treated simultaneously. Therapy may continue for several years. Merely promoting weight gain isn't sufficient to guarantee long-term recovery. A patient whose physical status is severely compromised by inadequate or chaotic eating patterns is difficult to engage in the psychotherapeutic process.

Psychotherapy concentrates on interrupting the binge-purge cycle and helping the patient regain control over her eating behavior. Treatment may be provided in either an inpatient or outpatient setting and includes behavior modification therapy, which may take place in highly structured psychoeducational group meetings.

Individual psychotherapy and family therapy, which address the eating disorder as a symptom of unresolved conflict, may help the patient understand the basis of her behavior and teach her self-control strategies. Antidepressant drugs may be used as an adjunct to psychotherapy.

The patient also may benefit from participation in self-help groups, such as Overeaters Anonymous, or in a drug rehabilitation program if she has a concurrent substance abuse problem.

Special considerations
• Supervise the patient during mealtimes and for a specified period after meals (usually 1 hour). Set a time limit for each meal. Provide a pleasant, relaxed environment for eating.
• Using behavior modification techniques, reward the patient for satisfactory weight gain.

• Establish a contract with the patient, specifying the amount and type of food to be eaten at each meal.

• Encourage the patient to recognize and express her feelings about her eating behavior. Maintain an accepting and nonjudgmental attitude, controlling your reactions to her behavior and feelings.

• Encourage the patient to talk about stressful issues, such as achievement, independence, socialization, sexuality, family problems, and control.

• Identify the patient's elimination patterns.

• Assess her suicide potential.

• Refer the patient and her family to the American Anorexia/Bulimia Association and to Anorexia Nervosa and Related Eating Disorders for additional information and support.

• Teach the patient how to keep a food journal to monitor her treatment progress.

• Outline the risks of laxative, emetic, and diuretic abuse for the patient.

• Provide assertiveness training to help the patient gain control over her behavior and achieve a realistic and positive self-image.

• If the patient is taking a prescribed tricyclic antidepressant, instruct her to take the drug with food. Warn her to avoid consuming alcoholic beverages; exposing herself to sunlight, heat lamps, or tanning salons; and discontinuing the medication unless she has notified the doctor.

LIFE-THREATENING DISORDER

BURNS

A major burn is a horrifying injury, necessitating painful treatment and a long period of rehabilitation. It's often fatal or permanently disfiguring and incapacitating (both emotionally and physically). In the United States, about 2 million persons annually suffer burns. Of these, 300,000 are burned seriously and over 6,000 are fatalities, making burns this nation's third-leading cause of accidental death.

Causes
Thermal burns, the most common type, are frequently the result of residential fires, automobile accidents, playing with matches, improperly stored gasoline, space heater or electrical malfunctions, or arson. Other causes include improper handling of firecrackers, scalding accidents, and kitchen accidents (such as a child climbing on top of a stove or grabbing a hot iron). Burns in children are sometimes traced to parental abuse.

Chemical burns result from the contact, ingestion, inhalation, or injection of acids, alkalis, or vesicants. *Electrical burns* usually occur after contact with faulty electrical wiring or with high-voltage power lines, or when electric cords are chewed (by young children). *Friction* or *abrasion burns* happen when the skin is rubbed harshly against a coarse surface. *Sunburn,* of course, follows excessive exposure to sunlight.

Assessment
The depth of damage to the skin and tissue and the size of the burn are importance factors in burn assessment.

Depth of skin and tissue damage
A traditional method gauges burn depth by degrees, although most burns are a combination of different degrees and thicknesses. (See *Depth of burn,* page 140.)

• *First-degree* — Damage is limited to the epidermis, causing erythema and pain.

• *Second-degree* — The epidermis and part of the dermis are damaged, pro-

DEPTH OF BURN

This illustration shows the depth of tissue damage in partial- and full-thickness burns. A partial-thickness burn damages the epidermis and part of the dermis, whereas a full-thickness burn affects the epidermis, dermis, and subcutaneous tissue.

Epidermis

Dermis

Subcutaneous

Muscle

Normal skin | Partial thickness | Full thickness

☐ Damaged tissue   ■ Dead tissue

ducing blisters and mild to moderate edema and pain.
• *Third-degree* — Epidermis and the dermis are damaged. No blisters appear, but white, brown, or black leathery tissue and thrombosed vessels are visible.
• *Fourth-degree* — Damage extends through deeply charred subcutaneous tissue to muscle and bone.

Burn size
The size is usually expressed as the percentage of body surface area (BSA) covered by the burn. The Rule of Nines chart most commonly provides this estimate, although the Lund and Browder chart is more accurate, because it allows for BSA changes with age. A correlation of the burn's depth and size permits an estimate of its severity.

• *Major* — third-degree burns on more than 10% of BSA; second-degree burns on more than 25% of adult BSA (more than 20% in children); burns of hands, face, feet, or genitalia; burns complicated by fractures or respiratory damage; electrical burns; all burns in poor-risk patients
• *Moderate* — third-degree burns on 2% to 10% of BSA; second-degree burns on 15% to 25% of adult BSA (10% to 20% in children)
• *Minor* — third-degree burns on less than 2% of BSA; second-degree burns on less than 15% of adult BSA (10% in children).

Other considerations
• Location — Burns on the face, hands, feet, and genitalia are most serious, because of possible loss of function.

FLUID REPLACEMENT: THE FIRST 24 HOURS AFTER A BURN

Use one of these two formulas as a general guideline for the amount of fluid replacement, but vary the specific infusions according to the patient's response, especially urinary output.

Baxter formula
4 ml of lactated Ringer's solution/kg/% body surface area (BSA)/24 hours. Give one-half of total over first 8 hours postburn and the remainder over next 16 hours.

Brooke formula
Colloids (plasma, plasmanate, dextran) 0.5 ml/kg/% BSA + lactated Ringer's solution 1.5 ml/kg/% BSA + 2,000 ml dextrose 5% in water for adults (less for children). Give one-half of the total over the first 8 hours postburn and the remainder over the next 16 hours.

• Configuration — Circumferential burns can cause total occlusion of circulation in an extremity as a result of edema. Burns on the neck can produce airway obstruction, whereas burns on the chest can lead to restricted respiratory expansion.

• History of complicating medical problems — Note disorders that impair peripheral circulation, especially diabetes, peripheral vascular disease, and chronic alcohol abuse.

• Other injuries sustained at the time of the burn.

• Patient age — Victims under age 4 or over age 60 have a higher incidence of complications and, consequently, a higher mortality.

• Pulmonary injury — Smoke inhalation can cause pulmonary injury.

Treatment and special considerations
• Immediate, aggressive burn treatment increases the patient's chance for survival. Later, supportive measures and strict aseptic technique can minimize infection. Meticulous, comprehensive burn care can make the difference between life and death. (See

Fluid replacement: The first 24 hours after a burn.)

• If the patient's burns are minor, immerse the burned area in cool saline solution (55° F [12.8° C]) or apply cool compresses. Give him pain medication as needed.

• Debride the devitalized tissue, taking care not to break any blisters. Cover the wound with an antimicrobial agent and a nonstick bulky dressing, and administer tetanus prophylaxis as needed.

• Provide thorough teaching and complete aftercare instructions for the patient. Stress the importance of keeping the dressing dry and clean, elevating the burned extremity for the first 24 hours, taking prescribed analgesics, and returning for a wound check in 1 to 2 days.

• In moderate and major burns, immediately assess the patient's airway, breathing, and circulation (ABCs). Be especially alert for signs of smoke inhalation and pulmonary damage: singed nasal hairs, mucosal burns, voice changes, coughing, wheezing, soot in the mouth or nose, and darkened sputum. Assist with endotracheal intubation and administer 100% oxygen.

• Control bleeding, and remove smoldering clothing (soak it first in saline solution if it's stuck to the patient's skin), rings, and other constricting items. Be sure to cover burns with a clean, dry, sterile bed sheet. (*Never* cover large burns with saline-soaked dressings, since they can drastically lower body temperature.)

• Begin I.V. therapy immediately to prevent hypovolemic shock and maintain cardiac output. Use lactated Ringer's solution or a fluid replacement formula.

• Once the patient is stable, take a brief history of the burn.

• Draw blood samples for a complete blood count; electrolyte, glucose, blood urea nitrogen, and serum creatinine levels; arterial blood gas analysis; and typing and crossmatching.

• Closely monitor intake and output, and frequently check vital signs. Although it may make you nervous, don't be afraid to take the patient's blood pressure because of burned limbs.

• In the hospital, a central venous pressure line and additional I.V. lines (using venous cutdown, if necessary), and an indwelling urinary catheter may be inserted.

• To combat fluid evaporation through the burn and the release of fluid into interstitial spaces (possibly resulting in hypovolemic shock), continue fluid therapy as needed.

• Check vital signs every 15 minutes (an arterial line may be inserted if blood pressure is unobtainable with a cuff). Send a urine specimen to the laboratory to check for myoglobinuria and hemoglobinuria.

• Insert a nasogastric tube to decompress the stomach and avoid aspiration of stomach contents.

• Electrical and chemical burns demand special attention. Tissue damage from electrical burns is difficult to assess because internal destruction along the conduction pathway is usually greater than the surface burn would indicate. Electrical burns that ignite the patient's clothes may cause thermal burns as well. If the electric shock caused ventricular fibrillation and cardiac and respiratory arrest, begin cardiopulmonary resuscitation at once. Get an estimate of the voltage.

• In a chemical burn, irrigate the wound with copious amounts of water or normal saline solution. Using a weak base (such as sodium bicarbonate) to neutralize hydrofluoric acid, hydrochloric acid, or sulfuric acid on skin or mucous membrane is contraindicated, since the neutralizing agent can actually produce more heat and tissue damage.

• If the chemical entered the patient's eyes, flush them with large amounts of water or saline solution for at least 30 minutes; in an alkali burn, irrigate until the pH of the cul-de-sacs returns to 7. Have the patient close his eyes, and cover them with a dry, sterile dressing. Note the type of chemical causing the burn and the presence of any noxious fumes. The patient will need an emergency ophthalmologic examination.

• Don't treat the burn wound itself in the emergency department if the patient is to be transferred to a specialized burn care unit within 4 hours after the burn. Instead, prepare the patient for transport by wrapping him in a sterile sheet and a blanket for warmth and elevating the burned extremity to decrease edema. Then, transport immediately. Once at the burn unit, the patient will receive specialized treatments, including skin grafts of various types.

Calcium Imbalance

Calcium plays an indispensable role in cell permeability, formation of bones and teeth, blood coagulation, transmission of nerve impulses, and normal muscle contraction. Nearly all (99%) of the body's calcium is found in the bones. The remaining 1% exists in ionized form in serum, and it's the maintenance of the 1% of ionized calcium in the serum that's critical to healthy neurologic function.

The parathyroid glands regulate ionized calcium and determine its resorption into bone, absorption from the GI mucosa, and excretion in urine and feces. Severe calcium imbalance requires emergency treatment, because a deficiency (hypocalcemia) can lead to tetany and convulsions; an excess (hypercalcemia), to cardiac arrhythmias.

Causes

Several factors can cause calcium imbalance.

Hypocalcemia

- *Inadequate intake of calcium and vitamin D* results in inhibited intestinal absorption of calcium.
- *Hypoparathyroidism* as a result of injury, disease, or surgery decreases or eliminates secretion of parathyroid hormone (PTH), which is necessary for calcium absorption and normal serum calcium levels.

- *Malabsorption or loss of calcium from the GI tract* can result from increased intestinal motility from severe diarrhea or laxative abuse. Malabsorption of calcium from the GI tract can also result from inadequate levels of vitamin D or PTH or a reduction in gastric acidity, which decreases the solubility of calcium salts.
- *Severe infections or burns* can lead to diseased and burned tissue trapping calcium from the extracellular fluid.
- *Overcorrection of acidosis* can lead to alkalosis, which causes decreased ionized calcium and induces symptoms of hypocalcemia.
- *Pancreatic insufficiency* may cause malabsorption of calcium and subsequent calcium loss in feces. In pancreatitis, participation of calcium ions in saponification contributes to calcium loss.
- *Renal failure* results in excessive excretion of calcium secondary to increased retention of phosphate.
- *Hypomagnesemia* causes decreased PTH secretion and blocks the peripheral action of that hormone.

Hypercalcemia

- *Hyperparathyroidism* increases serum calcium levels by promoting calcium absorption from the intestine, resorption from bone, and reabsorption from the kidneys.
- *Hypervitaminosis D* can promote increased absorption of calcium from the intestine.
- *Tumors* raise serum calcium levels by destroying bone or by releasing PTH or a PTH-like substance, osteoclast-

SIGNS AND SYMPTOMS OF CALCIUM IMBALANCE

DYSFUNCTION	HYPOCALCEMIA	HYPERCALCEMIA
CNS	• Anxiety, irritability, twitching around mouth, laryngospasm, convulsions, Chvostek's sign, Trousseau's sign	• Drowsiness, lethargy, headaches, depression or apathy, irritability, confusion
Musculoskeletal	• Paresthesia (tingling and numbness of the fingers), tetany or painful tonic muscle spasms, facial spasms, abdominal cramps, muscle cramps, spasmodic contractions	• Weakness, muscle flaccidity, bone pain, pathologic fractures
Cardiovascular	• Arrhythmias, hypotension	• Signs of heart block, cardiac arrest in systole, hypertension
GI	• Increased GI motility, diarrhea	• Anorexia, nausea, vomiting, constipation, dehydration, polydipsia
Other	• Blood-clotting abnormalities	• Renal polyuria, flank pain and, eventually, azotemia

activating factor, prostaglandins, and perhaps, a vitamin D–like sterol.

• *Multiple fractures and prolonged immobilization* release bone calcium and raise the serum calcium level.

• *Multiple myeloma* promotes loss of calcium from bone.

Other causes include milk-alkali syndrome, sarcoidosis, hyperthyroidism, adrenal insufficiency, thiazide diuretics, and loss of serum albumin secondary to renal disease.

Signs and symptoms

Indications of calcium imbalance depend on the type of imbalance.

Hypocalcemia

A lack of calcium causes nerve fiber irritability and repetitive muscle spasms. Consequently, characteristic symptoms of hypocalcemia include perioral paresthesia, twitching, car-popedal spasm, tetany, seizures, and possibly, cardiac arrhythmias. Chvostek's sign and Trousseau's sign are reliable indicators of hypocalcemia.

Hypercalcemia

Clinical effects of hypercalcemia include muscle weakness, decreased muscle tone, lethargy, anorexia, constipation, nausea, vomiting, dehydration, polydipsia, and polyuria. Severe hypercalcemia (serum levels that exceed 5.7 mEq/L) may produce cardiac arrhythmias and, eventually, coma. (See *Signs and symptoms of calcium imbalance.*)

Diagnosis

A serum calcium level less than 4.5 mEq/L confirms hypocalcemia; a level above 5.5 mEq/L confirms hypercalcemia. (However, because approximately one-half of serum calcium is bound to albumin, changes in serum protein must be considered when interpreting serum calcium levels.)

The Sulkowitch urine test shows increased calcium precipitation in hypercalcemia. In hypocalcemia, an electrocardiogram (ECG) reveals a lengthened QT interval, a prolonged ST segment, and arrhythmias; in hypercalcemia, a shortened QT interval and heart block.

Treatment
An acute imbalance requires immediate correction, followed by maintenance therapy and correction of the underlying cause.

Hypocalcemia
A mild calcium deficit may require nothing more than an adjustment in diet to allow adequate intake of calcium, vitamin D, and protein, possibly with oral calcium supplements. Acute hypocalcemia is an emergency that needs immediate correction by I.V. administration of calcium gluconate or calcium chloride.

Chronic hypocalcemia also requires vitamin D supplements to facilitate gastrointestinal absorption of calcium. To correct mild deficiency states, the amounts of vitamin D in most multivitamin preparations are adequate. For severe deficiency, vitamin D is used in four forms: ergocalciferol (vitamin D_2), cholecalciferol (vitamin D_3), calcitriol, and dihydrotachysterol, a synthetic form of vitamin D_2.

Hypercalcemia
Treatment of hypercalcemia primarily eliminates excess serum calcium through hydration with normal saline solution, which promotes calcium excretion in urine. Loop diuretics, such as ethacrynic acid and furosemide, also promote calcium excretion. (Thiazide diuretics are contraindicated in hypercalcemia because they inhibit calcium excretion.)

Corticosteroids, such as prednisone and hydrocortisone, are helpful in treating sarcoidosis, hypervitaminosis D, and certain tumors. Mithramycin can also lower the serum calcium level and is especially effective against hypercalcemia secondary to certain tumors. Calcitonin may also be helpful in certain instances.

Sodium phosphate solution administered by mouth or by retention enema promotes calcium deposits in bone and inhibits its absorption from the GI tract.

Special considerations
• Watch for hypocalcemia in patients receiving massive transfusions of citrated blood and in those with chronic diarrhea, severe infections, and insufficient dietary intake of calcium and protein (especially elderly patients).

If the patient has hypocalcemia:
• Monitor serum calcium levels every 12 to 24 hours; a calcium level below 4.5 mEq/L requires immediate attention. When giving calcium supplements, frequently check the pH level; an alkalotic state that exceeds 7.45 pH inhibits calcium ionization. Check for Trousseau's and Chvostek's signs.
• Administer calcium gluconate slow I.V. in dextrose 5% in water (*never* in saline solution, which encourages renal calcium loss). Don't add calcium gluconate I.V. to solutions containing bicarbonate; it will precipitate.
• When administering calcium solutions, watch for anorexia, nausea, and vomiting; these are possible signs of overcorrection to hypercalcemia.
• If the patient is receiving calcium chloride, watch for abdominal discomfort.
• Monitor the patient closely for a possible drug interaction if he's receiving digitalis glycosides with large doses of oral calcium supplements; watch for

signs of digitalis toxicity (anorexia, nausea, vomiting, yellow vision, and cardiac arrhythmias). Administer oral calcium supplements 1 to 1½ hours after meals or with milk.

• Provide a quiet, stress-free environment for the patient with tetany. Observe seizure precautions for patients with severe hypocalcemia that may lead to convulsions.

• To prevent hypocalcemia, advise all patients (especially the elderly ones) to eat foods rich in calcium, vitamin D, and protein, such as fortified milk and cheese. Explain how important calcium is for normal bone formation and blood coagulation. Discourage chronic use of laxatives. Also, warn hypocalcemic patients not to overuse antacids because these may aggravate the condition.

If the patient has hypercalcemia:

• Monitor serum calcium levels frequently. Watch for cardiac arrhythmias if the serum calcium level exceeds 5.7 mEq/L. Increase fluid intake to dilute calcium in serum and urine and to prevent renal damage and dehydration.

• Watch for signs of congestive heart failure in patients receiving normal saline solution diuresis therapy.

• Administer loop diuretics (not thiazide diuretics). Monitor intake and output, and check the urine for renal calculi and acidity. Provide acid-ash drinks, such as cranberry or prune juice, because calcium salts are more soluble in acid than in alkali.

• Check the patient's ECG and vital signs frequently. In the patient receiving digitalis glycosides, watch for signs of toxicity, such as anorexia, nausea, vomiting, and bradycardia (often with arrhythmia).

• Help the patient walk as soon as possible. Handle the patient with chronic hypercalcemia *gently* to prevent pathologic fractures.

• If the patient is bedridden, reposition him frequently, and encourage range-of-motion exercises to promote circulation and prevent urinary stasis and calcium loss from bone.

• To prevent recurrence, suggest a low-calcium diet and increased fluid intake.

CANDIDIASIS

Also called candidosis and moniliasis, candidiasis is usually a mild, superficial fungal infection caused by the *Candida* genus. Most often, it infects the nails (onychomycosis), skin (diaper rash), or mucous membranes, especially the oropharynx (thrush), vagina (moniliasis), esophagus, and GI tract.

Rarely, these fungi enter the bloodstream and invade the kidneys, lungs, endocardium, brain, or other structures, causing serious infections. Such systemic infection is most prevalent among drug abusers and patients already hospitalized, particularly diabetics and immunosuppressed patients. The prognosis varies, depending on the patient's resistance.

Causes
Most cases of *Candida* infection result from *C. albicans.* Other infective strains include *C. parapsilosis, C. tropicalis,* and *C. guillermondii.*

These fungi are part of the normal flora of the GI tract, mouth, vagina, and skin. They cause infection when some change in the body permits their sudden proliferation—rising glucose levels from diabetes mellitus; lowered resistance from a disease (such as cancer), an immunosuppressive drug, radiation, aging, or human immunodeficiency virus (HIV) infection; or when they're introduced systemically by I.V.

or urinary catheters, drug abuse, hyperalimentation, or surgery.

However, the most common predisposing factor remains the use of broad-spectrum antibiotics, which decrease the number of normal flora and permit an increasing number of candidal organisms to proliferate. The infant of a mother with vaginal moniliasis can contract oral thrush while passing through the birth canal.

The incidence of candidiasis is rising because of wider use of I.V. therapy and a greater number of immunocompromised patients, especially those with HIV infection.

Signs and symptoms
Superficial candidiasis produces symptoms that correspond to the following sites of infection:
• skin: scaly, erythematous, papular rash, sometimes covered with exudate, appearing below the breast, between the fingers, and at the axillae, groin, and umbilicus. In diaper rash, papules appear at the edges of the rash.
• nails: red, swollen, darkened nailbed; occasionally, purulent discharge and the separation of a pruritic nail from the nailbed
• oropharyngeal mucosa (thrush): cream-colored or bluish-white patches of exudate on the tongue, mouth, or pharynx that reveal bloody engorgement when scraped. They may swell, causing respiratory distress in infants. They are only occasionally painful but cause a burning sensation in the throats and mouths of adults. (See *Identifying thrush.*)
• esophageal mucosa: dysphagia, retrosternal pain, regurgitation and, occasionally, scales in the mouth and throat
• vaginal mucosa: white or yellow discharge, with pruritus and local excoriation; white or gray raised patches on vaginal walls, with local inflammation; dyspareunia.

IDENTIFYING THRUSH

Candidiasis of the oropharyngeal mucosa (thrush) causes cream-colored or bluish-white pseudomembranous patches on the tongue, mouth, or pharynx. Fungal invasion may extend to circumoral tissues.

Systemic infection produces chills; high, spiking fever; hypotension; prostration; and occasional rash. Specific symptoms depend on the site of infection, as follows:
• pulmonary system: hemoptysis, fever, cough
• renal system: fever, flank pain, dysuria, hematuria, pyuria
• brain: headache, nuchal rigidity, seizures, focal neurologic deficits
• endocardium: systolic or diastolic murmur, fever, chest pain, embolic phenomena
• eye: endophthalmitis, blurred vision, orbital or periorbital pain, scotoma, and exudate.

Diagnosis

Identification of superficial candidiasis depends on evidence of *Candida* on a Gram stain of skin, vaginal scrapings, pus, or sputum or on skin scrapings prepared in potassium hydroxide solution. Systemic infections require obtaining a sample for blood or tissue culture.

Treatment

The first aim of treatment is to improve the underlying condition that predisposes the patient to candidiasis, such as controlling diabetes or discontinuing antibiotic therapy and catheterization, if possible.

Nystatin is an effective antifungal for superficial candidiasis. Clotrimazole, fluconazole, ketoconazole, and miconazole are effective in mucous-membrane and vaginal *Candida* infections. Ketoconazole or fluconazole is the treatment of choice for chronic candidiasis of the mucous membranes. Treatment for systemic infection consists of I.V. amphotericin B or fluconazole.

Special considerations

• Instruct a patient using nystatin solution to swish it around in his mouth for several minutes before he swallows the solution.
• Swab nystatin on the oral mucosa of an infant with thrush.
• Provide the patient with a nonirritating mouthwash to loosen tenacious secretions and a soft toothbrush to avoid irritation.
• Relieve the patient's mouth discomfort with a topical anesthetic, such as lidocaine, at least 1 hour before meals. (It may suppress the gag reflex and cause aspiration.)
• Provide a soft diet for the patient with severe dysphagia. Tell the patient with mild dysphagia to chew food thoroughly, and make sure he doesn't choke.
• Use cornstarch or dry padding in intertriginous areas of obese patients to prevent irritation.
• Note dates of insertion of I.V. catheters, and replace them according to your hospital's policy to prevent phlebitis.
• Assess the patient with candidiasis for underlying causes such as diabetes mellitus. If the patient is receiving amphotericin B for systemic candidiasis, he may have severe chills, fever, anorexia, nausea, and vomiting. Premedicate with acetaminophen, antihistamines, or antiemetics to help reduce adverse reactions.
• Frequently check vital signs of patients with systemic infections. Provide appropriate supportive care.
• In patients with renal involvement, carefully monitor intake and output and urine blood and protein.
• Check high-risk patients daily, especially those receiving antibiotics, for patchy areas, irritation, sore throat, bleeding of mouth or gums, or other signs of superinfection. Check for vaginal discharge; record the color and amount.
• Encourage women in their third trimester of pregnancy to be examined for vaginal candidiasis to protect their infants from infection at birth.

LIFE-THREATENING DISORDER

CARDIAC ARRHYTHMIAS

Abnormal electrical conduction or automaticity changes heart rate and rhythm in cardiac arrhythmias, also called cardiac dysrhythmias. (See *Types of cardiac arrhythmias.*)

Arrhythmias vary in severity, from those that are mild, asymptomatic, and require no treatment (such as sinus ar-

(Text continues on page 157.)

Types of Cardiac Arrhythmias

This chart reviews many common cardiac arrhythmias and outlines their features, causes, and treatments. Use a normal electrocardiogram strip, if available, to compare normal cardiac rhythm configurations with the rhythm strips below. Characteristics of normal rhythm include:
• ventricular and atrial rates of 60 to 100 beats/minute
• regular and uniform QRS complexes and P waves
• PR interval of 0.12 to 0.2 second
• QRS duration < 0.12 second
• identical atrial and ventricular rates, with constant PR interval.

ARRHYTHMIA AND FEATURES	CAUSES	TREATMENT
Sinus arrhythmia • Irregular atrial and ventricular rhythms • Normal P wave preceding each QRS complex	• A normal variation of normal sinus rhythm in athletes, children, and elderly people • Also seen in digitalis toxicity and inferior wall myocardial infarction (MI)	• Atropine if rate decreases below 40 beats/minute
Sinus tachycardia • Atrial and ventricular rates regular • Rate > 100 beats/minute; rarely, > 160 beats/minute • Normal P wave preceding each QRS complex	• Normal physiologic response to fever, exercise, anxiety, pain, dehydration; may also accompany shock, left ventricular failure, cardiac tamponade, hyperthyroidism, anemia, hypovolemia, pulmonary embolism, and anterior wall MI • May also occur with atropine, epinephrine, isoproterenol, quinidine, caffeine, alcohol, and nicotine use	• Correction of underlying cause • Propranolol for symptomatic patients

(continued)

TYPES OF CARDIAC ARRHYTHMIAS *(continued)*

ARRHYTHMIA AND FEATURES	CAUSES	TREATMENT
Sinus bradycardia 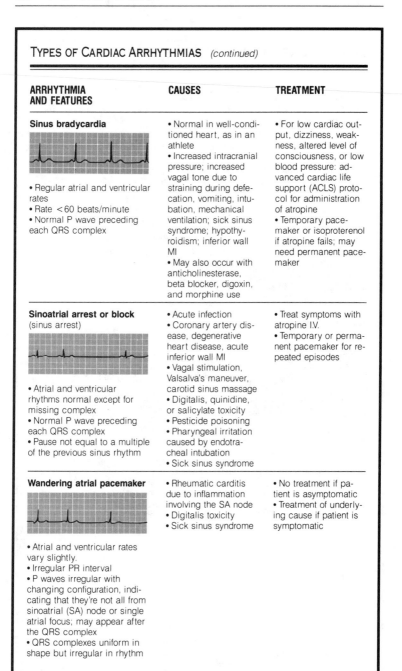 • Regular atrial and ventricular rates • Rate <60 beats/minute • Normal P wave preceding each QRS complex	• Normal in well-conditioned heart, as in an athlete • Increased intracranial pressure; increased vagal tone due to straining during defecation, vomiting, intubation, mechanical ventilation; sick sinus syndrome; hypothyroidism; inferior wall MI • May also occur with anticholinesterase, beta blocker, digoxin, and morphine use	• For low cardiac output, dizziness, weakness, altered level of consciousness, or low blood pressure: advanced cardiac life support (ACLS) protocol for administration of atropine • Temporary pacemaker or isoproterenol if atropine fails; may need permanent pacemaker
Sinoatrial arrest or block (sinus arrest) • Atrial and ventricular rhythms normal except for missing complex • Normal P wave preceding each QRS complex • Pause not equal to a multiple of the previous sinus rhythm	• Acute infection • Coronary artery disease, degenerative heart disease, acute inferior wall MI • Vagal stimulation, Valsalva's maneuver, carotid sinus massage • Digitalis, quinidine, or salicylate toxicity • Pesticide poisoning • Pharyngeal irritation caused by endotracheal intubation • Sick sinus syndrome	• Treat symptoms with atropine I.V. • Temporary or permanent pacemaker for repeated episodes
Wandering atrial pacemaker • Atrial and ventricular rates vary slightly. • Irregular PR interval • P waves irregular with changing configuration, indicating that they're not all from sinoatrial (SA) node or single atrial focus; may appear after the QRS complex • QRS complexes uniform in shape but irregular in rhythm	• Rheumatic carditis due to inflammation involving the SA node • Digitalis toxicity • Sick sinus syndrome	• No treatment if patient is asymptomatic • Treatment of underlying cause if patient is symptomatic

TYPES OF CARDIAC ARRHYTHMIAS *(continued)*

ARRHYTHMIA AND FEATURES	CAUSES	TREATMENT
Premature atrial contraction (PAC) • Premature, abnormal-looking P waves that differ in configuration from normal P waves • QRS complexes after P waves, except in very early or blocked PACs • P wave often buried in the preceding T wave or identified in the preceding T wave	• Coronary or valvular heart disease, atrial ischemia, coronary atherosclerosis, heart failure, acute respiratory failure, chronic obstructive pulmonary disease (COPD), electrolyte imbalance, and hypoxia • Digitalis toxicity; use of aminophylline, adrenergics, or caffeine • Anxiety	• If occurring more than six times per minute or increasing in frequency, digoxin, quinidine, verapamil, or propranolol; after revascularization surgery, propranolol • Treatment of underlying cause
Paroxysmal atrial tachycardia (paroxysmal supraventricular tachycardia) • Atrial and ventricular rates regular • Heart rate > 160 beats/minute; rarely exceeds 250 beats/minute • P waves regular but aberrant; difficult to differentiate from preceding T wave • P wave preceding each QRS complex • Sudden onset and termination of arrhythmia	• Intrinsic abnormality of atrioventricular (AV) conduction system • Physical or psychological stress, hypoxia, hypokalemia, cardiomyopathy, congenital heart disease, MI, valvular disease, Wolff-Parkinson-White syndrome, cor pulmonale, hyperthyroidism, and systemic hypertension • Digitalis toxicity; use of caffeine, marijuana, or central nervous system stimulants	• If patient is unstable, prepare for immediate cardioversion. • If patient is stable, vagal stimulation, Valsalva's maneuver, carotid sinus massage • Adenosine by rapid I.V. bolus injection to rapidly convert arrhythmia • If patient is stable, determine QRS complex width. For wide complex width, follow ACLS protocol for lidocaine and procainamide. For narrow complex width and normal or elevated blood pressure, follow ACLS protocol for verapamil and consider digoxin, beta blockers, and diltiazem. For narrow complex width with low or unstable blood pressure (and for ineffective drug response for others), use synchronized cardioversion.

(continued)

Types of Cardiac Arrhythmias *(continued)*

ARRHYTHMIA AND FEATURES	CAUSES	TREATMENT
Atrial flutter • Atrial rhythm at regular rate; 250 to 400 beats/minute • Ventricular rate variable, depending on degree of AV block (usually 60 to 100 beats/minute) • Sawtooth P-wave configuration possible (F waves) • QRS complexes uniform in shape, but often irregular in rate	• Heart failure, tricuspid or mitral valve disease, pulmonary embolism, cor pulmonale, inferior wall MI, and carditis • Digitalis toxicity	• If patient is unstable with a ventricular rate > 150 beats/minute, prepare for immediate cardioversion. • If patient is stable, drug therapy may include beta blockers, verapamil, digoxin, procainamide, or quinidine.
Atrial fibrillation • Atrial rhythm grossly irregular; rate > 400 beats/minute • Ventricular rate grossly irregular • QRS complexes of uniform configuration and duration • PR interval indiscernible • No P waves, or P waves that appear as erratic, irregular, baseline fibrillatory waves	• Heart failure, COPD, thyrotoxicosis, constrictive pericarditis, ischemic heart disease, sepsis, pulmonary embolus, rheumatic heart disease, hypertension, mitral stenosis, atrial irritation, complication of coronary bypass or valve replacement surgery • Nifedipine and digoxin use	• If patient is unstable with a ventricular rate > 150 beats/minute, prepare for immediate cardioversion. • If patient is stable, drug therapy may include diltiazem, beta blockers, verapamil, digoxin, procainamide, or quinidine.

Types of Cardiac Arrhythmias *(continued)*

ARRHYTHMIA AND FEATURES	CAUSES	TREATMENT

Junctional rhythm

• Atrial and ventricular rates regular: atrial rate 40 to 60 beats/minute; ventricular rate usually 40 to 60 beats/minute (60 to 100 beats/minute is accelerated junctional rhythm)
• P waves preceding, hidden within (absent), or after QRS complex; inverted if visible
• PR interval (when present) < 0.12 second
• QRS complex configuration and duration normal, except in aberrant conduction

Causes:
• Inferior wall MI or ischemia, hypoxia, vagal stimulation, sick sinus syndrome
• Acute rheumatic fever
• Valve surgery
• Digitalis toxicity

Treatment:
• Atropine for symptomatic slow rate
• Pacemaker insertion if patient doesn't respond to drugs
• Discontinuation of digoxin, if appropriate

Premature junctional contractions (junctional premature beats)

• Atrial and ventricular rhythms irregular
• P waves inverted; may precede, be hidden within, or follow QRS complex
• PR interval < 0.12 second if P wave precedes QRS complex
• QRS complex configuration and duration normal

Causes:
• MI or ischemia
• Digitalis toxicity and excessive caffeine or amphetamine use

Treatment:
• Correction of underlying cause
• Atropine
• Discontinuation of digoxin if appropriate
• May require pacemaker

First-degree AV block

• Atrial and ventricular rhythms regular
• PR interval > 0.20 second
• P wave precedes QRS complex
• QRS complex normal

Causes:
• May be seen in a healthy person
• Inferior wall MI or ischemia, hypothyroidism, hypokalemia, hyperkalemia
• Digitalis toxicity; use of quinidine, procainamide, or propranolol

Treatment:
• Cautious use of digoxin
• Correction of underlying cause
• Possibly atropine if PR interval exceeds 0.26 second or bradycardia develops

(continued)

TYPES OF CARDIAC ARRHYTHMIAS *(continued)*

ARRHYTHMIA AND FEATURES	CAUSES	TREATMENT
Second-degree AV block Mobitz I (Wenckebach) • Atrial rhythm regular • Ventricular rhythm irregular • Atrial rate exceeds ventricular rate • PR interval progressively, but only slightly, longer with each cycle until QRS complex disappears (dropped beat); PR interval shorter after dropped beat	• Inferior wall MI, cardiac surgery, acute rheumatic fever, and vagal stimulation • Digitalis toxicity; use of propranolol, quinidine, or procainamide	• Treatment of underlying cause • Atropine or temporary pacemaker for symptomatic bradycardia • Discontinuation of digoxin, if appropriate
Second-degree AV block Mobitz II • Atrial rate regular • Ventricular rhythm regular or irregular, with varying degree of block • P-P interval constant • QRS complexes periodically absent	• Severe coronary artery disease, anterior wall MI, acute myocarditis • Digitalis toxicity	• Isoproterenol for symptomatic bradycardia • Temporary or permanent pacemaker • Discontinuation of digoxin, if appropriate
Third-degree AV block (complete heart block) • Atrial rate regular • Ventricular rate slow and regular • No relation between P waves and QRS complexes • No constant PR interval • QRS interval normal (nodal pacemaker) or wide and bizarre (ventricular pacemaker)	• Inferior or anterior wall MI, congenital abnormality, rheumatic fever, hypoxia, postoperative complication of mitral valve replacement, Lev's disease (fibrosis and calcification that spreads from cardiac structures to the conductive tissue), Lenegre's disease (conductive tissue fibrosis) • Digitalis toxicity	• Atropine or isoproterenol for symptomatic bradycardia • Temporary or permanent pacemaker

TYPES OF CARDIAC ARRHYTHMIAS *(continued)*

ARRHYTHMIA AND FEATURES	CAUSES	TREATMENT
Junctional tachycardia • Atrial rate > 100 beats/minute; however, P wave may be absent, hidden in QRS complex, or preceding T wave • Ventricular rate > 100 beats/minute • P wave inverted; may occur before or after QRS complex, may be hidden in QRS complex, or may be absent • QRS complex configuration and duration normal • Onset of rhythm often sudden, occurring in bursts	• Myocarditis, cardiomyopathy, inferior wall MI or ischemia, acute rheumatic fever, complication of valve replacement surgery • Digitalis toxicity	• Temporary atrial pacemaker to override the rhythm • Carotid sinus massage, elective cardioversion • Propranolol, verapamil, or edrophonium • Discontinuation of digoxin, if appropriate
Premature ventricular contraction (PVC) • Atrial rate regular • Ventricular rate irregular • QRS complex premature, usually followed by a complete compensatory pause • QRS complex wide and distorted, usually > 0.14 second • Premature QRS complexes occurring singly, in pairs, or in threes; alternating with normal beats; focus from one or more sites • Ominous when clustered, multifocal, with R wave on T pattern	• Heart failure; old or acute MI, ischemia, or contusion; myocardial irritation by ventricular catheter or a pacemaker; hypercapnia; hypokalemia; hypocalcemia • Drug toxicity (digitalis glycosides, aminophylline, tricyclic antidepressants, beta-adrenergics [isoproterenol or dopamine]) • Caffeine, tobacco, or alcohol use • Psychological stress, anxiety, pain, exercise	• If warranted, lidocaine, procainamide, or bretylium I.V. • Treatment of underlying cause • Discontinuation of drug causing toxicity • Potassium chloride I.V. if PVC induced by hypokalemia

(continued)

TYPES OF CARDIAC ARRHYTHMIAS *(continued)*

ARRHYTHMIA AND FEATURES	CAUSES	TREATMENT
Ventricular tachycardia • Ventricular rate 140 to 220 beats/minute, regular or irregular • QRS complexes wide, bizarre, and independent of P waves • P waves not discernible • May start and stop suddenly	• Myocardial ischemia, infarction, or aneurysm; coronary artery disease; rheumatic heart disease; mitral valve prolapse; heart failure; cardiomyopathy; ventricular catheters; hypokalemia; hypercalcemia; pulmonary embolism • Digitalis, procainamide, epinephrine, or quinidine toxicity • Anxiety	• With pulse: If hemodynamically stable with ventricular rate < 150 beats/minute, follow ACLS protocol for administration of lidocaine, procainamide, or bretylium; if drugs are ineffective, initiate synchronized cardioversion. • If ventricular rate > 150 beats/minute, follow ACLS protocol for immediate synchronized cardioversion, followed by antiarrhythmic agents. • Pulseless: initiate cardiopulmonary resuscitation (CPR); follow ACLS protocol for defibrillation, endotracheal (ET) intubation, and administration of epinephrine, lidocaine, bretylium, magnesium sulfate, or procainamide.
Ventricular fibrillation • Ventricular rhythm rapid and chaotic • QRS complexes wide and irregular; no visible P waves	• Myocardial ischemia or infarction, untreated ventricular tachycardia, R-on-T phenomenon, hypokalemia, hyperkalemia, hypercalcemia, alkalosis, electric shock, hypothermia • Digitalis, epinephrine, or quinidine toxicity	• Pulseless: Initiate CPR; follow ACLS protocol for defibrillation, endotracheal intubation, and administration of epinephrine, lidocaine, bretylium, magnesium sulfate, or procainamide.

TYPES OF CARDIAC ARRHYTHMIAS   *(continued)*

ARRHYTHMIA AND FEATURES	CAUSES	TREATMENT
Asystole • No atrial or ventricular rate or rhythm • No discernible P waves, QRS complexes, or T waves	• Myocardial ischemia or infarction, aortic valve disease, heart failure, hypoxemia, hypokalemia, severe acidosis, electric shock, ventricular arrhythmias, AV block, pulmonary embolism, heart rupture, cardiac tamponade, hyperkalemia, electromechanical dissociation • Cocaine overdose	• Continue CPR; follow ACLS protocol for ET intubation, administration of epinephrine and atropine, and possible transcutaneous pacing.

rhythmia, in which heart rate increases and decreases with respiration) to catastrophic ventricular fibrillation, which necessitates immediate resuscitation.

Arrhythmias are generally classified according to their origin (ventricular or supraventricular). Their effect on cardiac output and blood pressure, partially influenced by the site of origin, determines their clinical significance.

Causes

Arrhythmias may be congenital or they may result from one of several factors, including myocardial ischemia, myocardial infarction, or organic heart disease. Drug toxicity or degeneration of the conductive tissue necessary to maintain normal heart rhythm (sick sinus syndrome) sometimes can also precipitate arrhythmias.

Special considerations

• Assess an unmonitored patient for rhythm disturbances.
• If the patient's pulse is abnormally rapid, slow, or irregular, watch for signs of hypoperfusion, such as hypotension and diminished urine output.
• Document any arrhythmias in a monitored patient, and assess for possible causes and effects.
• When life-threatening arrhythmias develop, rapidly assess the level of consciousness, respirations, and pulse.
• Initiate cardiopulmonary resuscitation, if indicated.
• Evaluate the patient for altered cardiac output resulting from arrhythmias.
• Administer medications as needed, and prepare for medical procedures (for example, cardioversion), if indicated.
• Monitor for predisposing factors — such as fluid and electrolyte imbalance — and signs of drug toxicity, especially with digoxin. Drug toxicity may require withholding the next dose.
• To prevent arrhythmias in a postoperative cardiac patient, provide adequate oxygen and reduce the heart's workload, while carefully maintaining metabolic, neurologic, respiratory, and hemodynamic status.

• To avoid temporary pacemaker malfunction, install a fresh battery before each insertion. Carefully secure the external catheter wires and the pacemaker box. Assess the threshold daily. Watch closely for premature contractions, a sign of myocardial irritation.

• To avert permanent pacemaker malfunction, restrict the patient's activity after insertion. Monitor the pulse rate regularly, and watch for signs of decreased cardiac output.

• If the patient has a permanent pacemaker, warn him about environmental hazards, as indicated by the pacemaker manufacturer. Although hazards may not present a problem, 24-hour Holter monitoring may be helpful in doubtful situations.

• Tell the patient to report lightheadedness or syncope, and stress the importance of regular checkups.

LIFE-THREATENING DISORDER

CARDIAC TAMPONADE

In this disorder, a rapid, unchecked rise in intrapericardial pressure impairs diastolic filling of the heart. The rise in pressure usually results from blood or fluid accumulation in the pericardial sac.

If fluid accumulates rapidly, this condition is commonly fatal and necessitates emergency lifesaving measures. Slow accumulation and rise in pressure, as in pericardial effusion associated with cancer, may not produce immediate symptoms because the fibrous wall of the pericardial sac can gradually stretch to accommodate as much as 1 to 2 L of fluid.

Causes

Increased intrapericardial pressure and cardiac tamponade may be idiopathic (Dressler's syndrome) or may result from the following conditions:

• effusion (in cancer, bacterial infections, tuberculosis and, rarely, acute rheumatic fever)

• hemorrhage from trauma (such as gunshot or stab wounds of the chest and perforation by a catheter during cardiac or central venous catheterization or after cardiac surgery)

• hemorrhage from nontraumatic causes (such as rupture of the heart or great vessels, or anticoagulant therapy in a patient with pericarditis)

• acute myocardial infarction (MI)

• uremia.

Signs and symptoms

Cardiac tamponade classically produces increased venous pressure with neck vein distention, reduced arterial blood pressure, muffled heart sounds on auscultation, and pulsus paradoxus (an abnormal inspiratory drop in systemic blood pressure greater than 15 mm Hg). These classic symptoms represent failure of physiologic compensatory mechanisms to override the effects of rapidly rising pericardial pressure, which limits diastolic filling of the ventricles and reduces stroke volume to a critically low level.

Generally, ventricular end-systolic volume may drop because of inadequate preload. The increasing pericardial pressure is transmitted equally across the heart cavities, producing a matching rise in intracardiac pressure, especially atrial and end-diastolic ventricular pressures.

Cardiac tamponade may also cause dyspnea, diaphoresis, pallor or cyanosis, anxiety, tachycardia, narrow pulse pressure, restlessness, and hepatomegaly, but the lung fields will be clear. The patient typically sits upright and leans forward.

Diagnosis

Classic clinical features may include the following:

• *Chest X-ray* shows slightly widened mediastinum and cardiomegaly.

• *Electrocardiography (ECG)* may reveal changes produced by acute pericarditis. This test rarely reveals tamponade but is useful to rule out other cardiac disorders.

• *Pulmonary artery catheterization* detects increased right atrial pressure, right ventricular diastolic pressure, and central venous pressure.

• *Echocardiography* records pericardial effusion with signs of right ventricular and atrial compression.

Treatment

The goal of treatment is to relieve intrapericardial pressure and cardiac compression by removing accumulated blood or fluid. Pericardiocentesis (needle aspiration of the pericardial cavity) or surgical creation of an opening dramatically improves systemic arterial pressure and cardiac output with aspiration of as little as 25 ml of fluid. Such treatment necessitates continuous hemodynamic and ECG monitoring in the intensive care unit.

Trial volume loading with temporary I.V. normal saline solution with albumin and perhaps an inotropic drug, such as isoproterenol or dopamine, is necessary to maintain cardiac output in the hypotensive patient. Although these drugs normally improve myocardial function, they may further compromise an ischemic myocardium after MI.

Depending on the cause of tamponade, additional treatment may include:

• *in traumatic injury:* blood transfusion or a thoracotomy to drain reaccumulating fluid or to repair bleeding sites

• *in heparin-induced tamponade:* the heparin antagonist protamine sulfate

• *in warfarin-induced tamponade:* vitamin K.

Special considerations

If the patient needs pericardiocentesis:

• Explain the procedure to the patient.

• Keep a pericardial aspiration needle attached to a 50 ml syringe by a three-way stopcock, an ECG machine, and an emergency cart with a defibrillator at the bedside. Make sure the equipment is turned on and ready for immediate use.

• Position the patient at a 45- to 60-degree angle. Connect the precordial ECG lead to the hub of the aspiration needle with an alligator clamp and connecting wire. When the needle touches the myocardium during fluid aspiration, you'll see an ST-segment elevation or premature ventricular contractions.

• Monitor blood pressure and central venous pressure (CVP) during and after pericardiocentesis.

• Infuse I.V. solutions to maintain blood pressure. Watch for a decrease in CVP and a concomitant rise in blood pressure, which indicate relief of cardiac compression.

• Watch for complications of pericardiocentesis, such as ventricular fibrillation, vagovagal response, or coronary artery or cardiac chamber puncture.

• Closely monitor ECG changes, blood pressure, pulse rate, level of consciousness, and urinary output.

If the patient needs thoracotomy:

• Explain the procedure to him. Tell him what to expect postoperatively (chest tubes, drainage bottles, and administration of oxygen). Teach him how to turn, deep-breathe, and cough.

• Give antibiotics, protamine sulfate, or vitamin K as needed.

• Postoperatively, monitor critical parameters, such as vital signs and arterial blood gas levels, and assess heart and breath sounds.

• Give pain medication as needed.

• Maintain the chest drainage system and be alert for complications, such as hemorrhage and arrhythmias.

LIFE-THREATENING DISORDER

CARDIOGENIC SHOCK

Sometimes called pump failure, cardiogenic shock is a condition of diminished cardiac output that severely impairs tissue perfusion. It reflects severe left ventricular failure and occurs as a serious complication in nearly 15% of all patients hospitalized with acute myocardial infarction (MI).

Cardiogenic shock typically affects patients whose area of infarction exceeds 40% of muscle mass; in such patients, the fatality rate may exceed 85%. Most patients with cardiogenic shock die within 24 hours of onset. The prognosis for those who survive is extremely poor.

Causes

Cardiogenic shock can result from any condition that causes significant left ventricular dysfunction with reduced cardiac output, such as MI (most common), myocardial ischemia, papillary muscle dysfunction, and end-stage cardiomyopathy.

Compensatory mechanisms

Regardless of the underlying cause, left ventricular dysfunction sets into motion a series of compensatory mechanisms that attempt to increase cardiac output and, in turn, maintain vital organ function.

As cardiac output falls in left ventricular dysfunction, aortic and carotid baroreceptors initiate sympathetic nervous responses. These, in turn, increase heart rate, left ventricular filling pressure, and peripheral resistance to flow to enhance venous return to the heart.

These compensatory responses initially stabilize the patient but later cause deterioration with rising oxygen demands of the already compromised myocardium. These events comprise a vicious circle of low cardiac output, sympathetic compensation, myocardial ischemia, and even lower cardiac output.

Signs and symptoms

Cardiogenic shock produces signs of poor tissue perfusion: cold, pale, clammy skin; a drop in systolic blood pressure to 30 mm Hg below baseline, or a sustained reading below 80 mm Hg not attributable to medication; tachycardia; rapid, shallow respirations; oliguria (less than 20 ml of urine/hour); restlessness and mental confusion and obtundation; narrowing pulse pressure; and cyanosis.

Although many of these clinical features also occur in congestive heart failure and other shock syndromes, they are usually more profound in cardiogenic shock.

Diagnosis

• *Auscultation* detects gallop rhythm, faint heart sounds and, possibly, if the shock results from rupture of the ventricular septum or papillary muscles, a holosystolic murmur.

• *Pulmonary artery pressure monitoring* reveals increased pulmonary artery pressure (PAP) and increased pulmonary artery wedge pressure (PAWP), reflecting a rise in left ventricular end-diastolic pressure (preload) and increased resistance to left ventricular emptying (afterload) resulting from ineffective pumping and increased peripheral vascular resistance. Thermodilution technique measures decreased cardiac output.

• *Invasive arterial pressure monitoring* shows hypotension from impaired ventricular ejection.

• *Arterial blood gas levels* may show metabolic acidosis and hypoxia.

• *Electrocardiography* may reveal evidence of acute MI, myocardial ischemia, or ventricular aneurysm.

• *Enzyme levels* show elevated creatine kinase (CK), lactate dehydrogenase (LD), aspartate aminotransferase, and alanine aminotransferase, which point to MI or myocardial ischemia and suggest heart failure or shock. CK and LD isoenzyme values may confirm acute MI.

Additional tests determine other conditions that can lead to pump dysfunction and failure, such as cardiac arrhythmias, cardiac tamponade, papillary muscle infarct or rupture, ventricular septal rupture, pulmonary emboli, venous pooling (associated with venodilators and continuous intermittent positive-pressure breathing), and hypovolemia.

Treatment
The aim of treatment is to enhance cardiovascular status by increasing cardiac output, improving myocardial perfusion, and decreasing cardiac workload. Treatment combines various cardiovascular drugs and mechanical-assist techniques.

Cardiovascular drugs
Drug therapy may include I.V. dopamine, a vasopressor that increases cardiac output, blood pressure, and renal blood flow, and I.V. amrinone or dobutamine, inotropic agents that increase myocardial contractility. When a more potent vasoconstrictor is necessary, norepinephrine is used.

I.V. nitroprusside, a vasodilator, may be used with a vasopressor to further improve cardiac output by decreasing peripheral vascular resistance (afterload) and reducing left ventricular end-diastolic pressure (preload). However, the patient's blood pressure must be adequate to support nitroprusside therapy and must be monitored closely.

Mechanical-assist techniques
The intra-aortic balloon pump (IABP) is a mechanical-assist device that attempts to improve coronary artery perfusion and decrease cardiac workload. The inflatable balloon pump is surgically inserted through the femoral artery into the descending thoracic aorta.

Once in place, the balloon inflates during diastole to increase coronary artery perfusion pressure and deflates before systole (before the aortic valve opens) to reduce resistance to ejection (afterload) and therefore lessen cardiac workload. Improved ventricular ejection, which significantly improves cardiac output, and a subsequent vasodilation in the peripheral vasculature lead to lower preload volume.

When drug therapy and IABP insertion fail, treatment may require an experimental device — the ventricular assist pump or the artificial heart.

Special considerations
• At the first sign of cardiogenic shock, check the patient's blood pressure and heart rate. If the patient is hypotensive or is having difficulty breathing, ensure a patent I.V. line and a patent airway, and provide oxygen to promote tissue oxygenation.

• Monitor arterial blood gas levels to measure oxygenation and detect acidosis from poor tissue perfusion. Increase oxygen flow as indicated by blood gas measurements. Check complete blood count and electrolyte levels.

• After diagnosis, monitor cardiac rhythm continuously. Assess skin color, temperature, and other vital signs often. Watch for a drop in systolic blood pressure to less than 80 mm Hg (usually compromising cardiac output further).

• Insert an indwelling urinary catheter to measure output. Watch for an output below 30 ml/hour.

• Using a pulmonary artery catheter, closely monitor PAP, PAWP and, if equipment is available, cardiac output. High PAWP indicates congestive heart failure and requires an immediate response.

• When a patient is on the IABP, reposition him often and perform passive range-of-motion exercises to prevent skin breakdown. However, don't flex the patient's "ballooned" leg at the hip because this may displace or fracture the catheter.

• Assess pedal pulses and skin temperature and color to make sure circulation to the leg is adequate. Check the dressing on the insertion site frequently for bleeding, and change it according to hospital protocol.

• Check the insertion site for hematoma or signs of infection, and culture any drainage.

• After the patient has become hemodynamically stable, the frequency of balloon inflation is gradually reduced to wean him from the IABP. During weaning, carefully watch for monitor changes, chest pain, and other signs of recurring cardiac ischemia and shock.

• Provide psychological support. The patient and his family may be anxious about the intensive care unit, IABP, and other tubes and devices, so offer reassurance.

• To ease emotional stress, allow frequent rest periods, and provide for as much privacy as possible.

LIFE-THREATENING DISORDER

CARDIOMYOPATHY, DILATED

Resulting from extensively damaged myocardial muscle fibers, dilated cardiomyopathy interferes with myocardial metabolism and grossly dilates all four chambers of the heart. This gives the heart a globular appearance. In this disorder, hypertrophy may be present.

Dilated cardiomyopathy leads to intractable congestive heart failure (CHF), arrhythmias, and emboli. Because this disease is usually not diagnosed until it's in the advanced stages, the patient's prognosis is generally poor.

Causes
The origin of most cardiomyopathies is unknown. Occasionally, dilated cardiomyopathy results from myocardial destruction by toxic, infectious, or metabolic agents, such as certain viruses, endocrine and electrolyte disorders, and nutritional deficiencies. Other causes include muscle disorders (myasthenia gravis, progressive muscular dystrophy, myotonic dystrophy), infiltrative disorders (hemochromatosis, amyloidosis), and sarcoidosis.

Cardiomyopathy may be a complication of alcoholism. The condition may improve with abstinence from alcohol but recurs when the patient resumes drinking.

How viruses induce cardiomyopathy is unclear, but investigators suspect a link between viral myocarditis and subsequent dilated cardiomyopathy, especially after infection with poliovirus, coxsackievirus B, influenza virus, or human immunodeficiency virus.

Metabolic cardiomyopathies are related to endocrine and electrolyte disorders and nutritional deficiencies. Thus, dilated cardiomyopathy may develop in patients with hyperthyroidism, pheochromocytoma, beriberi (thiamine deficiency), and kwashiorkor (protein deficiency). Cardiomyopathy may also result from rheumatic fever, especially among children with myocarditis.

Ante- or postpartal cardiomyopathy may develop during the last trimester or within months after delivery. Its cause is unknown, but it occurs most frequently in multiparous women over age 30, particularly those with malnutrition or preeclampsia. In these patients, cardiomegaly and CHF may reverse with treatment, allowing a subsequent normal pregnancy. If cardiomegaly persists despite treatment, the prognosis is extremely poor.

Signs and symptoms

In dilated cardiomyopathy, the heart ejects blood less efficiently than usual. Consequently, a large volume of blood remains in the left ventricle after systole, causing signs of CHF—both left-sided (shortness of breath, orthopnea, dyspnea on exertion, paroxysmal nocturnal dyspnea, fatigue, and an irritating dry cough at night) and right-sided (edema, liver engorgement, and jugular vein distention).

Dilated cardiomyopathy also produces peripheral cyanosis and sinus tachycardia or atrial fibrillation at rest in some patients, secondary to low cardiac output. Auscultation reveals diffuse apical impulses, pansystolic murmur (mitral and tricuspid regurgitation secondary to cardiomegaly and weak papillary muscles), and S_3 and S_4 gallop rhythms.

Diagnosis

No single test confirms dilated cardiomyopathy. Diagnosis requires elimination of other possible causes of CHF and arrhythmias.

• *Electrocardiography (ECG)* and *angiography* rule out ischemic heart disease; the ECG may also show biventricular hypertrophy, sinus tachycardia, atrial enlargement and, in 20% of patients, atrial fibrillation and bundle-branch heart block.

• *Chest X-ray* demonstrates cardiomegaly—usually affecting all heart chambers—and may demonstrate pulmonary congestion, pleural or pericardial effusion, or pulmonary hypertension.

• *Echocardiography* identifies left ventricular thrombi, global hypokinesia, and the degree of left ventricular dilation.

Treatment

Therapeutic goals include correcting the underlying causes and improving the heart's pumping ability with digoxin, diuretics, oxygen, and a sodium-restricted diet. Other options may involve bed rest and steroids. (See *Discharge instructions.*)

Vasodilators reduce preload and afterload, thereby decreasing congestion and increasing cardiac output. Acute heart failure requires vasodilation with nitroprusside or nitroglycerin I.V. Long-term treatment may include prazosin, hydralazine, isosorbide dinitrate, angiotensin-converting enzyme inhibitors, and anticoagulants.

When these treatments fail, therapy may require a heart transplant for carefully selected patients. Cardiomyoplasty, which wraps the latissimus dorsi muscle around the ventricles, assists the ventricle to effectively pump blood. A cardiomyostimulator delivers bursts of electrical impulses during systole, to contract the muscle.

Special considerations
• In the patient with acute failure, monitor for signs of progressive failure (decreased arterial pulses, increased neck vein distention) and compromised renal perfusion (oliguria, increased BUN and creatinine levels, and electrolyte imbalances). Weigh the patient daily.
• If the patient is receiving vasodilators, check his blood pressure and heart rate frequently. If he becomes hypotensive, stop the infusion and place him in a supine position, with his legs elevated to increase venous return and to ensure cerebral blood flow.
• If the patient is receiving diuretics, monitor for signs of resolving congestion (decreased crackles and dyspnea) or too vigorous diuresis. Check his serum potassium level for hypokalemia, especially if therapy includes digoxin.
• Before discharge, teach the patient about his illness and its treatment.
• Therapeutic restrictions and an uncertain prognosis usually cause profound anxiety and depression, so offer support and let the patient express his feelings. Be flexible with visiting hours.
• Encourage the patient's family members to learn cardiopulmonary resuscitation.

CARDIOMYOPATHY, HYPERTROPHIC

This primary disease of the cardiac muscle—also called idiopathic hypertrophic subaortic stenosis—is characterized by disproportionate, asymmetric thickening of the interventricular septum, particularly in the free wall of the left ventricle. In hypertrophic cardiomyopathy, cardiac output may be low, normal, or high, depending on whether stenosis is obstructive or nonobstructive.

If cardiac output is normal or high, the disorder may go undetected for years, but low cardiac output may lead to potentially fatal congestive heart failure (CHF). The course of the disease varies; some patients progressively deteriorate; others remain stable for years.

Causes
Despite being designated as idiopathic, in almost all cases, hypertrophic cardiomyopathy may be inherited as a non–sex-linked autosomal dominant trait. Most patients have obstructive disease, resulting from effects of ventricular septal hypertrophy and the movement of the anterior mitral valve leaflet into the outflow tract during systole. Eventually, left ventricular dysfunction, from rigidity and decreased compliance, causes pump failure.

Signs and symptoms
Clinical features of the disorder may not appear until it's well advanced, when atrial dilation and, possibly, atrial fibrillation abruptly reduce blood flow to the left ventricle. Reduced inflow

and subsequent low output may produce angina pectoris, arrhythmias, dyspnea, orthopnea, syncope, CHF, and death.

Auscultation reveals a medium-pitched systolic ejection murmur along the left sternal border and at the apex. Palpation reveals a peripheral pulse with a characteristic double impulse (pulsus biferiens) and, with atrial fibrillation, an irregular pulse.

Diagnosis

Along with typical clinical findings, the diagnosis depends on the following test results:

• *Echocardiography* (most useful) shows increased thickness of the intraventricular septum and abnormal motion of the anterior mitral leaflet during systole, occluding left ventricular outflow in obstructive disease.

• *Cardiac catheterization* reveals elevated left ventricular end-diastolic pressure and, possibly, mitral insufficiency.

• *Electrocardiography* usually demonstrates left ventricular hypertrophy, T-wave inversion, left anterior hemiblock, Q waves in precordial and inferior leads, ventricular arrhythmias, and possibly, atrial fibrillation.

• *Phonocardiography* confirms an early systolic murmur.

Treatment

The goals of treatment are to relax the ventricle and to relieve outflow tract obstruction. Propranolol, a beta-adrenergic blocking agent, slows heart rate and increases ventricular filling by relaxing the obstructing muscle, thereby reducing angina, syncope, dyspnea, and arrhythmias. However, propranolol may aggravate symptoms of cardiac decompensation. Atrial fibrillation necessitates cardioversion to treat the arrhythmia and, because of the high risk of systemic embolism, anticoagulant therapy until fibrillation subsides.

Contraindicated drugs

Vasodilators, such as nitroglycerin, reduce venous return by permitting pooling of blood in the periphery, decreasing ventricular volume and chamber size, and may cause further obstruction. They're contraindicated in patients with hypertrophic cardiomyopathy. Also contraindicated are sympathetic stimulators, such as isoproterenol, which enhance cardiac contractility and myocardial demands for oxygen, intensifying the obstruction.

Surgical alternatives

If drug therapy fails, surgery is indicated. Ventricular myotomy (resection of the hypertrophied septum) alone or combined with mitral valve replacement may ease outflow tract obstruction and relieve symptoms. However, ventricular myotomy may cause complications, such as complete heart block and ventricular septal defect, and is experimental.

Special considerations

• Because syncope or sudden death may follow well-tolerated exercise, warn such patients against any strenuous physical activity such as running.

• Administer medication as needed. *Caution:* Avoid nitroglycerin, digoxin, and diuretics because they can worsen obstruction.

• Warn the patient not to stop taking propranolol abruptly because doing so may increase myocardial demands. To determine the patient's tolerance for an increased dosage of propranolol, take his pulse to check for bradycardia and ask him to stand and walk around slowly to check for orthostatic hypotension.

• Before dental work or surgery, administer prophylaxis for subacute bacterial endocarditis.

• Provide psychologic support. If the patient is hospitalized for a long time, be flexible with visiting hours.

• Refer the patient for psychosocial counseling to help him and his family accept his restricted lifestyle and the poor prognosis.

• If the patient is a child, have his parents arrange for him to continue his studies in the hospital.

• Because sudden cardiac arrest is possible, urge the patient's family to learn cardiopulmonary resuscitation.

LIFE-THREATENING DISORDER

CARDIOMYOPATHY, RESTRICTIVE

A disorder of the myocardial musculature, restrictive cardiomyopathy is characterized by restricted ventricular filling (the result of left ventricular hypertrophy) and endocardial fibrosis and thickening. If severe, it's irreversible.

Causes

Primary restrictive cardiomyopathy is an extremely rare disorder of unknown etiology. However, restrictive cardiomyopathy syndrome, a manifestation of amyloidosis, results from infiltration of amyloid into the intracellular spaces in the myocardium, endocardium, and subendocardium.

In both forms of restrictive cardiomyopathy, the myocardium becomes rigid, with poor distention during diastole, inhibiting complete ventricular filling. It fails to contract completely during systole, resulting in low cardiac output.

Signs and symptoms

Because it lowers cardiac output and leads to congestive heart failure (CHF), restrictive cardiomyopathy produces fatigue, dyspnea, orthopnea, chest pain, generalized edema, liver engorgement, peripheral cyanosis, pallor, S_3 or S_4 gallop rhythms, and systolic murmurs of mitral and tricuspid insufficiency.

Diagnosis

• *Chest X-ray* shows massive cardiomegaly in advanced stages of this disease, affecting all four chambers of the heart; pericardial effusion; and pulmonary congestion.

• *Echocardiography* rules out constrictive pericarditis as the cause of restricted filling by detecting increased left ventricular muscle mass and differences in end-diastolic pressures between the ventricles.

• *Electrocardiography* may show low-voltage complexes, hypertrophy, atrioventricular conduction defects, or arrhythmias.

• *Arterial pulsation* reveals blunt carotid upstroke with small volume.

• *Cardiac catheterization* demonstrates increased left ventricular end-diastolic pressure and rules out constrictive pericarditis as the cause of restricted filling.

Treatment

Although no therapy currently exists for restricted ventricular filling, digitalis glycosides, diuretics, and a restricted sodium diet ease the symptoms of CHF.

Oral vasodilators—such as isosorbide dinitrate, prazosin, and hydralazine—may control intractable CHF. Anticoagulant therapy may be necessary to prevent thrombophlebitis in the patient on prolonged bed rest.

Special considerations

• In the acute phase, monitor heart rate and rhythm, blood pressure, urinary output, and pulmonary artery pressure readings to help guide treatment.

• Give psychological support. Provide appropriate diversionary activities for the patient restricted to prolonged bed rest.

• Because a poor prognosis may cause profound anxiety and depression, be especially supportive and understanding, and encourage the patient to express his fears.

• Refer the patient for psychosocial counseling, as necessary, for assistance in coping with his restricted lifestyle. Be flexible with visiting hours whenever possible.

• Before discharge, teach the patient to watch for and report signs of digoxin toxicity (anorexia, nausea, vomiting, yellow vision), to record and report weight gain and, if sodium restriction is ordered, to avoid canned foods, pickles, smoked meats, and use of table salt.

CARDIOVASCULAR DISEASE IN PREGNANCY

This disorder ranks fourth (after infection, toxemia, and hemorrhage) among the leading causes of maternal death. The physiologic stress of pregnancy and delivery is often more than a compromised heart can tolerate and often leads to maternal and fetal death.

Approximately 1% to 2% of pregnant women have cardiac disease, but the incidence is rising because medical treatment today allows more females with rheumatic heart disease and congenital defects to reach childbearing age.

With careful management, the prognosis for the pregnant patient with cardiovascular disease is good. Decompensation is the leading cause of maternal death. Infant mortality increases with decompensation because uterine congestion, insufficient oxygenation, and the elevated carbon dioxide content of the blood not only compromise the fetus, but also frequently cause premature labor and delivery.

Causes

Rheumatic heart disease is present in more than 80% of patients who develop cardiovascular complications. In the rest, these complications stem from congenital defects (10% to 15%) and coronary artery disease (2%).

The diseased heart is sometimes unable to meet the normal demands of pregnancy: a 25% increase in cardiac output, a 40% to 50% increase in plasma volume, increased oxygen requirements, retention of salt and water, weight gain, and alterations in hemodynamics during delivery. This physiologic stress often leads to the heart's failure to maintain adequate circulation (decompensation).

The degree of decompensation depends on the patient's age, the duration of cardiac disease, and the functional capacity of the heart at the outset of pregnancy.

Signs and symptoms

Typical clinical features of cardiovascular disease during pregnancy include distended neck veins, diastolic murmurs, moist basilar pulmonary crackles, cardiac enlargement (discernible on percussion or as a cardiac shadow on a chest X-ray), and cardiac arrhythmias (other than sinus or paroxysmal atrial tachycardia). Other characteristic abnormalities may include cyanosis, pericardial friction rub, pulse delay, and pulsus alternans.

Decompensation may develop suddenly or gradually, with persistent crackles at the lung bases. As it progresses, edema, increasing dyspnea on exertion, palpitations, a smothering sensation, and hemoptysis may occur.

Diagnosis

A diastolic murmur, cardiac enlargement, a systolic murmur of grade III/VI intensity, and severe arrhythmia suggest cardiovascular disease.

Determination of the extent and cause of the disease may necessitate electrocardiography, echocardiography (for valvular disorders such as rheumatic heart disease), or phonocardiography. X-rays show cardiac enlargement and pulmonary congestion. Cardiac catheterization should be postponed until after delivery, unless surgery is necessary.

Treatment

Specific treatments vary before, during, and after delivery.

Before delivery

The goal of antepartum management is to prevent complications and minimize the strain on the mother's heart, primarily through rest. This may require periodic hospitalization for patients with moderate cardiac dysfunction or with symptoms of decompensation, toxemia, or infection. Older women or those with previous decompensation may require hospitalization and bed rest throughout the pregnancy.

Drug therapy is often necessary and should always include the safest possible drug in the lowest possible dosage to minimize harmful effects to the fetus. Diuretics and drugs that increase blood pressure, blood volume, or cardiac output should be used with extreme caution.

If an anticoagulant is needed, heparin is the drug of choice. Digitalis glycosides and common antiarrhythmics, such as quinidine and procainamide, are often required. The prophylactic use of antibiotics is reserved for patients who are susceptible to endocarditis.

A therapeutic abortion may be considered for patients with severe cardiac dysfunction, especially if decompensation occurs during the first trimester. Patients hospitalized with heart failure usually follow a regimen of digitalis glycosides, oxygen, rest, sedation, diuretics, and restricted intake of sodium and fluids. Patients whose symptoms of heart failure don't improve after treatment with bed rest and digitalis glycosides may require cardiac surgery, such as valvotomy and commissurotomy.

During delivery

The patient in labor may require oxygen and an analgesic, such as meperidine or morphine, for relief of pain and apprehension without undue depression of the fetus or herself. Depending on which procedure promises to be less stressful for the patient's heart, delivery may be vaginal or by cesarean section.

After delivery

Bed rest and medications already instituted should continue for at least 1 week after delivery because of a high incidence of decompensation, cardiovascular collapse, and maternal death during the early puerperal period. These complications may result from the sudden release of intra-abdominal pressure at delivery and the mobilization of extracellular fluid for excretion, which increase the strain on the heart, especially if excessive interstitial fluid has accumulated.

Breast-feeding is undesirable for patients with severely compromised cardiac dysfunction, because it increases fluid and metabolic demands on the heart.

Special considerations

• During pregnancy, stress the importance of rest and weight control to decrease the strain on the heart. Suggest a diet of limited fluid and sodium intake to prevent vascular congestion.

• Encourage the patient to take supplementary folic acid and iron to prevent anemia.

• During labor, watch for signs of decompensation, such as dyspnea and palpitations. Monitor pulse rate, respirations, and blood pressure. Auscultate for crackles every 30 minutes during the first phase of labor and every 10 minutes during the active and transition phases. Check carefully for edema and cyanosis, and assess intake and output. Administer oxygen for respiratory difficulty.

• Use electronic fetal monitoring to watch for the earliest signs of fetal distress.

• Keep the patient in a semirecumbent position. Limit her efforts to bear down during labor, which significantly raise blood pressure and stress the heart.

• After delivery, provide reassurance, and encourage the patient to adhere to her program of treatment. Emphasize the need to rest during her hospital stay.

CARPAL TUNNEL SYNDROME

The most common of the nerve entrapment syndromes, carpal tunnel syndrome results from compression of the median nerve at the wrist, within the carpal tunnel. This nerve passes through, along with blood vessels and flexor tendons, to the fingers and thumb. The compression neuropathy causes sensory and motor changes in the median distribution of the hand.

Carpal tunnel syndrome usually occurs in women between ages 30 and 60 and poses a serious occupational health problem. Assembly-line workers and packers and persons who repeatedly use poorly designed tools are most likely to develop this disorder. Any strenuous use of the hands — sustained grasping, twisting, or flexing — aggravates this condition.

Causes

The carpal tunnel is formed by the carpal bones and the transverse carpal ligament. (See *Viewing the carpal tunnel,* page 170.) Inflammation or fibrosis of the tendon sheaths that pass through the carpal tunnel often causes edema and compression of the median nerve.

Many conditions can cause the contents or structure of the carpal tunnel to swell and press the median nerve against the transverse carpal ligament.

Such conditions include rheumatoid arthritis, flexor tenosynovitis (often associated with rheumatic disease), nerve compression, pregnancy, renal failure, menopause, diabetes mellitus, acromegaly, edema following Colles' fracture, hypothyroidism, amyloidosis, myxedema, benign tumors, tuberculosis, and other granulomatous diseases. Another source of damage to the median nerve is dislocation or acute sprain of the wrist.

Signs and symptoms

The patient with carpal tunnel syndrome usually complains of weakness, pain, burning, numbness, or tingling in one or both hands. This paresthesia affects the thumb, forefinger, middle finger, and half of the fourth finger. The patient is unable to clench his hand into a fist. The nails may be atrophic; the skin, dry and shiny.

Because of vasodilatation and venous stasis, symptoms are often worse at night and in the morning. The pain may spread to the forearm and, in severe cases, as far as the shoulder. The patient can usually relieve such pain by shaking his hands vigorously or dangling his arms at his side.

VIEWING THE CARPAL TUNNEL

The carpal tunnel is clearly visible in this palmar view and cross section of a right hand. Note the median nerve, flexor tendons of fingers, and blood vessels passing through the tunnel on their way from the forearm to the hand.

CARPAL TUNNEL

Radial nerve

Median nerve

Flexor tendons of fingers

Ulnar nerve

Flexor tendons of fingers

Transverse carpal ligament

Diagnosis

Physical examination reveals decreased sensation to light touch or pinpricks in the affected fingers. Thenar muscle atrophy occurs in about half of all cases of carpal tunnel syndrome.

The patient exhibits a positive Tinel's sign (tingling over the median nerve on light percussion). He also responds positively to Phalen's wrist-flexion test (holding the forearms vertically and allowing both hands to drop into complete flexion at the wrists for 1 minute reproduces symptoms of carpal tunnel syndrome).

A compression test supports this diagnosis: A blood pressure cuff inflated above systolic pressure on the forearm for 1 to 2 minutes provokes pain and paresthesia along the distribution of the median nerve.

Electromyography detects a median nerve motor conduction delay of more than 5 milliseconds. Other laboratory tests may identify underlying disease.

Treatment

Conservative treatment should be tried first, including resting the hands by splinting the wrist in neutral extension for 1 to 2 weeks. If a definite link has been established between the patient's occupation and the development of carpal tunnel syndrome, he may have to seek other work. Effective treatment may also require correction of an underlying disorder.

When conservative treatment fails, the only alternative is surgical decompression of the nerve by resecting the entire transverse carpal tunnel ligament or by using endoscopic surgical techniques. Neurolysis (freeing of the nerve fibers) may also be necessary.

Special considerations

• Administer mild analgesics as needed.
• Encourage the patient to use his hands as much as possible. If his dom-

inant hand has been impaired, you may have to help with eating and bathing.

• Teach the patient how to apply a splint. Tell him not to make it too tight. Show him how to remove the splint to perform gentle range-of-motion exercises, which should be done daily. Make sure the patient knows how to do these exercises before he's discharged.

• After surgery, monitor vital signs, and regularly check the color, sensation, and motion of the affected hand.

• Advise the patient who is about to be discharged to occasionally exercise his hands in warm water. If the arm is in a sling, tell him to remove the sling several times a day to do exercises for his elbow and shoulder.

• Suggest occupational counseling for the patient who has to change jobs because of carpal tunnel syndrome.

CATARACT

A common cause of vision loss, a cataract is a gradually developing opacity of the lens or lens capsule of the eye. Cataracts commonly occur bilaterally, with each progressing independently. Exceptions are traumatic cataracts, which are usually unilateral, and congenital cataracts, which may remain stationary.

Cataracts are most prevalent in persons over age 70, as part of aging. The prognosis is generally good; surgery improves vision in 95% of affected people.

Causes

Cataracts have various causes:

• *Senile cataracts* develop in elderly patients, probably because of degenerative changes in the chemical state of lens proteins.

• *Congenital cataracts* occur in neonates as genetic defects or as a sequela of maternal rubella during the first trimester.

• *Traumatic cataracts* develop after a foreign body injures the lens with sufficient force to allow aqueous or vitreous humor to enter the lens capsule.

• *Complicated cataracts* develop as secondary effects in patients with uveitis, glaucoma, retinitis pigmentosa, or a detached retina or in the course of a systemic disease, such as diabetes, hypoparathyroidism, or atopic dermatitis. They can also result from exposure to ionizing radiation or infrared rays.

• *Toxic cataracts* result from drug or chemical toxicity with prednisone, ergot alkaloids, dinitrophenol, naphthalene, or phenothiazines.

Signs and symptoms

Characteristically, a patient with a cataract experiences painless, gradual blurring and loss of vision. As the cataract progresses, the normally black pupil turns milky white.

Some patients complain of blinding glare from headlights when they drive at night; others complain of poor reading vision and an unpleasant glare and poor vision in bright sunlight. Patients with central opacities report better vision in dim light than in bright light because the cataract is nuclear and, as the pupils dilate, patients can see around the lens opacity.

Diagnosis

When shining a penlight on the pupil, observation of a white area behind the pupil suggests an advanced cataract. Ophthalmoscopy or a slit-lamp examination confirms the diagnosis by revealing a dark area in the normally homogeneous red reflex.

Treatment

Cataracts require surgical extraction of the opaque lens and postoperative correction of visual deficits. The current trend is to perform the surgery as a same day procedure.

Surgical procedures

The following procedures are used to correct cataracts:

• *Extracapsular cataract extraction* removes the anterior lens capsule and cortex, leaving the posterior capsule intact. With this procedure, a posterior chamber intraocular lens (IOL) is implanted where the patient's own lens used to be. (A posterior chamber IOL is currently the most common type used in the United States.) This procedure is appropriate for use in patients of all ages.

Some patients who have an extracapsular cataract extraction develop a secondary membrane in the posterior lens capsule (which has been left intact), and that causes decreased visual acuity. But this membrane can be removed by the Nd:YAG laser, which cuts an area out of the center of the membrane, thereby restoring vision. However, laser therapy alone can't be used to remove a cataract.

• *Phacoemulsification* fragments the lens with ultrasonic vibrations and aspirates the pieces.

• *Intracapsular cataract extraction* removes the entire lens within the intact capsule by cryoextraction (the moist lens sticks to an extremely cold metal probe for easy and safe removal with gentle traction). This procedure is rarely performed today; extracapsular cataract extraction and phacoemulsification have replaced it as the most commonly performed procedures.

• *Discission and aspiration* can still be used for children with soft cataracts, but this procedure has largely been replaced by the use of multifunction suction cutting instruments.

Possible complications of surgery include the loss of vitreous (during surgery), wound dehiscence from loosening of sutures and flat anterior chamber or iris prolapse into the wound, hyphema, pupillary block glaucoma, retinal detachment, and infection.

Correction of visual deficits

A patient with an IOL implant may experience improved vision once the eye patch is removed; however, the IOL corrects distance vision only. The patient will also need either corrective reading glasses or a corrective contact lens, which will be fitted sometime between 4 to 8 weeks after surgery.

Where no IOL has been implanted, the patient may be given temporary aphakic cataract glasses; in about 4 to 8 weeks, he'll be refracted for his own glasses.

Special considerations

• After surgery, the patient will be discharged once he recovers from anesthesia. Remind him to return for a checkup the next day and warn him to avoid activities that increase intraocular pressure such as straining.

• Urge the patient to protect his eye from accidental injury by wearing an eye shield (a plastic or metal shield with perforations) or glasses during the day and an eye shield at night.

• Administer antibiotic ointment or drops to prevent infection and steroids to reduce inflammation, or combination steroid-antibiotic eye drops.

• Watch for the development of complications, such as iris prolapse, a sharp pain in the eye, or hyphema.

• Before discharge, teach correct instillation of eye drops, and instruct the patient to immediately report any sharp eye pain. Caution him about activity restrictions, and advise him that it will take several weeks before he receives his corrective reading glasses or lenses.

CEREBRAL CONTUSION

A severe blow to the head can cause cerebral contusion, or bruising of the brain tissue. More serious than a concussion, contusion disrupts normal nerve functions in the bruised area and may cause loss of consciousness, hemorrhage, edema, and even death.

Causes
Cerebral contusion results from acceleration-deceleration or coup-contrecoup injuries. Such injuries can occur directly beneath the site of impact when the brain rebounds against the skull from the force of a blow (a beating with a blunt instrument, for example), when the force of the blow drives the brain against the opposite side of the skull, or when the head is hurled forward and stopped abruptly (as in an automobile accident when a driver's head strikes the windshield).

When these injuries occur, the brain continues moving and slaps against the skull (acceleration), then rebounds (deceleration). These injuries can also cause the brain to strike against bony prominences inside the skull (especially the sphenoidal ridges), causing intracranial hemorrhage or hematoma that may result in tentorial herniation.

Signs and symptoms
With cerebral contusion, the patient may have severe scalp wounds and labored respirations. He may lose consciousness for a few minutes or longer. If conscious, he may be drowsy, confused, disoriented, agitated, or even violent. He may display hemiparesis, decorticate or decerebrate posturing, and unequal pupillary response.

Eventually, he should return to a relatively alert state, perhaps with temporary aphasia, slight hemiparesis, or unilateral numbness. A lucid period followed by rapid deterioration suggests epidural hematoma.

Diagnosis
An accurate history of the trauma and a neurologic exam are the principal diagnostic tools. A computed tomography scan shows ischemic tissue, hematomas, and fractures. Intracranial hemorrhage contraindicates lumbar puncture.

Treatment and special considerations
• Establish a patent airway. The patient may also need a tracheotomy or endotracheal intubation.
• Perform a neurologic examination, focusing on level of consciousness (LOC), motor responses, and intracranial pressure.
• Start I.V. fluids with lactated Ringer's solution or normal saline solution. Mannitol I.V. may be given in consultation with a neurosurgeon to reduce cerebral edema. Dexamethasone I.V. or I.M. may be given for several days to control cerebral edema.
• Restrict total fluid intake to 1,200 to 1,500 ml/day to reduce volume and intracerebral swelling.
• If spinal injury is ruled out, elevate the head of the bed 30 degrees. Enforce bed rest.
• If the patient is intubated, hyperventilate him to a partial pressure of carbon dioxide level of 26 to 28 mm Hg.
• Type and crossmatch blood for a patient suspected of having intracerebral hemorrhage. A blood transfusion may be needed and possibly a craniotomy to control bleeding and to aspirate blood.
• Insert an indwelling urinary catheter. Monitor intake and output. With

unconscious patients, insert a nasogastric tube to prevent aspiration.

• Observe carefully for leakage of cerebrospinal fluid (CSF) from the nares and ear canals. If blood is in the canal and it's unclear whether CSF is mixed in, place a drop on a white sheet and check for a central spot of blood surrounded by a lighter ring (halo sign).

• If CSF leakage develops, raise the head of the bed 30 degrees. If you detect CSF leaking from the nose, place a gauze pad under the nostrils. Be sure to tell the patient not to blow his nose, but to wipe it instead. If CSF leaks from the ear, position the patient so that the ear drains naturally, and don't pack the ear or nose.

• Monitor respirations and other vital signs regularly (usually every 15 minutes). Abnormal respirations could indicate a breakdown in the respiratory center in the brain stem and a possible impending tentorial herniation — a critical neurologic emergency.

• Perform frequent checks of neurologic status. Assess for restlessness, LOC, and orientation.

• After the patient is stabilized, clean and dress any superficial scalp wounds. (If the skin has been broken, tetanus prophylaxis may be in order.) The wounds may need to be sutured.

CEREBRAL PALSY

The most common cause of crippling in children, cerebral palsy comprises a group of neuromuscular disorders resulting from prenatal, perinatal, or postnatal central nervous system (CNS) damage. Although nonprogressive, these disorders may become more obvious as an affected infant grows older.

Three major types of cerebral palsy occur — *spastic, athetoid,* and *ataxic* — sometimes in mixed forms. Motor impairment may be minimal (sometimes apparent only during physical activities such as running) or severely disabling. Associated defects, such as seizures, speech disorders, and mental retardation, are common.

The prognosis varies. In mild impairment, proper treatment may make a near-normal life possible.

Cerebral palsy occurs in an estimated 1.5 to 5:1,000 live births every year. Incidence is highest in premature infants (anoxia plays the greatest role in contributing to cerebral palsy) and in those who are small for their gestational age. Cerebral palsy is slightly more common in males than in females and occurs more often in whites.

Causes
Conditions that result in cerebral anoxia, hemorrhage, or other CNS damage are probably responsible for cerebral palsy.

Prenatal causes
Such causes include maternal infection (especially rubella), radiation, anoxia, toxemia, maternal diabetes, abnormal placental attachment, malnutrition, and isoimmunization.

Perinatal and birth difficulties
Examples of these causes include forceps delivery, breech presentation, placenta previa, abruptio placentae, depressed maternal vital signs from general or spinal anesthetic, and prolapsed cord with delay in the delivery of the head. Premature birth, prolonged or unusually rapid labor, and multiple birth (especially infants born last in a multiple birth) may also cause cerebral palsy.

Infection or trauma during infancy
Cerebral palsy may follow kernicterus resulting from erythroblastosis fetalis, brain infection, head trauma, prolonged anoxia, brain tumor, cerebral

circulatory anomalies causing blood vessel rupture, and systemic disease resulting in cerebral thrombosis or embolus.

Signs and symptoms

Each type of cerebral palsy typically produces a distinctive set of clinical features, although some children display a mixed form of the disease.

Spastic cerebral palsy

This form of the disease predominates, affecting about 70% of patients. Spastic cerebral palsy is characterized by hyperactive deep tendon reflexes, increased stretch reflexes, rapid alternating muscle contraction and relaxation, muscle weakness, underdevelopment of affected limbs, muscle contraction in response to manipulation, and a tendency toward contractures. Typically, a child with spastic cerebral palsy walks on his toes with a scissors gait, crossing one foot in front of the other.

Athetoid cerebral palsy

Affecting about 20% of patients, this form causes involuntary movements — grimacing, wormlike writhing, dystonia, and sharp jerks — that impair voluntary movement. Usually, these involuntary movements affect the arms more severely than the legs; involuntary facial movements may make speech difficult. These athetoid movements become more severe during stress, decrease with relaxation, and disappear entirely during sleep.

Ataxic cerebral palsy

Roughly 10% of patients have this form of the disease. Its characteristics include disturbed balance, incoordination (especially of the arms), hypoactive reflexes, nystagmus, muscle weakness, tremor, lack of leg movement during infancy, and a wide gait as the child begins to walk. Ataxia makes

sudden or fine movements almost impossible.

Mixed form

Some children with cerebral palsy display a combination of these signs and symptoms. In most, impaired motor function makes eating, especially swallowing, difficult and retards growth and development. Up to 40% of these children are mentally retarded, about 25% have seizure disorders, and about 80% have impaired speech. Many also have dental abnormalities, vision and hearing defects, and reading disabilities.

Diagnosis

An early diagnosis is essential for effective treatment and requires careful clinical observation during infancy and precise neurologic assessment. Suspect cerebral palsy whenever an infant:

• has difficulty sucking or keeping the nipple or food in his mouth

• seldom moves voluntarily, or has arm or leg tremors with voluntary movement

• crosses his legs when lifted from behind rather than pulling them up or "bicycling" like a normal infant

• has legs that are hard to separate, making diaper changing difficult

• persistently uses only one hand or, as he gets older, uses his hands well but not his legs.

Infants at particular risk include those with low birth weight, low Apgar scores at 5 minutes, seizures, and metabolic disturbances. However, all infants should have a screening test for cerebral palsy as a regular part of their 6-month checkup.

Treatment

Cerebral palsy can't be cured, but proper treatment can help affected children reach their full potential within the limits set by this disorder. Such treatment requires a comprehensive and cooperative effort involving doctors, nurses, teachers, psychologists, the child's family, and occupational, physical, and speech therapists. Home care is often possible. Treatment usually includes:

• braces or splints and special appliances, such as adapted eating utensils and a low toilet seat with arms, to help these children perform activities independently

• an artificial urinary sphincter for the incontinent child who can use the hand controls

• range-of-motion exercises to minimize contractures

• orthopedic surgery to correct contractures

• phenytoin, phenobarbital, or another anticonvulsant to control seizures

• sometimes muscle relaxants or neurosurgery to decrease spasticity.

Children with milder forms of cerebral palsy should attend regular school; severely afflicted children need special education classes.

Special considerations

• Speak slowly and distinctly to the child hospitalized for orthopedic surgery or treatment of complications. Encourage him to ask for things he wants. Listen patiently and don't rush him.

• Provide an adequate diet to meet the child's high energy needs.

• During meals, maintain a quiet, unhurried atmosphere with as few distractions as possible. The child may need special utensils and a chair with a solid footrest. Teach him to place food far back in his mouth to facilitate swallowing.

• Encourage the child to chew food thoroughly, drink through a straw, and suck on lollipops to develop the muscle control needed to minimize drooling.

• Allow the child to wash and dress independently, assisting only as needed.

The child may need clothing modifications.

• Give all care in an unhurried manner; otherwise, muscle spasticity may increase.

• Encourage the child and his family to participate in the patient's care so they can continue it at home.

• Care for associated hearing or visual disturbances as necessary.

• Give frequent mouth care and dental care as necessary.

• Reduce muscle spasms that increase postoperative pain by moving and turning the child carefully after surgery.

After orthopedic surgery:

• Give good cast care. Wash and dry the skin at the edge of the cast frequently, and rub it with alcohol to toughen the skin and prevent breakdown.

• Reposition the child often, check for foul odor, and ventilate under the cast with a cool air blow-dryer. Use a flashlight to check for skin breakdown beneath the cast.

• Help the child relax, perhaps by giving a warm bath, before reapplying a bivalved cast.

Help parents deal with their child's handicap:

• Set realistic individual goals.

• Assist in planning crafts and other activities.

• Stress the child's need to develop peer relationships; warn the parents against being overprotective.

• Identify and deal with family stress. Parents may feel unreasonable guilt about their child's handicap and may need psychological counseling.

• Refer parents to supportive community organizations. For more information, tell parents to contact the United Cerebral Palsy Association, Inc., or their local cerebral palsy agency.

CEREBROVASCULAR ACCIDENT

Commonly called a stroke, cerebrovascular accident (CVA) is a sudden impairment of cerebral circulation in one or more of the blood vessels supplying the brain. CVA interrupts or diminishes oxygen supply and often causes serious damage or necrosis in brain tissues.

The sooner circulation returns to normal after CVA, the better chances are for complete recovery. However, about half of those who survive a CVA remain permanently disabled and experience a recurrence within weeks, months, or years.

CVA is the third most common cause of death in the United States today and the most common cause of neurologic disability. It strikes 500,000 people each year; half of them die as a result.

Causes

Factors that increase the risk of CVA include history of transient ischemic attacks, atherosclerosis, hypertension, electrocardiogram changes, arrhythmias, rheumatic heart disease, diabetes mellitus, gout, postural hypotension, cardiac or myocardial enlargement, high serum triglyceride levels, lack of exercise, use of oral contraceptives, cigarette smoking, and family history of CVA.

The major causes of CVA are thrombosis, embolism, and hemorrhage.

Thrombosis

In middle-aged and elderly people, among whom there is a higher incidence of atherosclerosis, diabetes, and hypertension, thrombosis is the most common cause of CVA. Obstruction of a blood vessel causes the CVA. Typically, the main site of the obstruction is in extracerebral vessels, but sometimes it's intracerebral.

Thrombosis causes ischemia in brain tissue supplied by the affected vessel as well as congestion and edema. The latter may produce more clinical effects than thrombosis itself, but these symptoms subside with the edema.

Thrombosis may develop while the patient sleeps or shortly after he awakens; it can also occur during surgery or after a myocardial infarction. The risk increases with obesity, smoking, or the use of oral contraceptives. Cocaine-induced ischemic stroke is now being seen in younger patients.

Embolism

The second most common cause of CVA, embolism is an occlusion of a blood vessel caused by a fragmented clot, a tumor, fat, bacteria, or air. It can occur at any age, especially among patients with a history of rheumatic heart disease, endocarditis, posttraumatic valvular disease, myocardial fibrillation and other cardiac arrhythmias, or following open-heart surgery.

The embolus usually develops rapidly—in 10 to 20 seconds—and without warning. When it reaches the cerebral vasculature, it cuts off circulation by lodging in a narrow portion of an artery, most often the middle cerebral artery, causing necrosis and edema.

If the embolus is septic and infection extends beyond the vessel wall, an abscess or encephalitis may develop. If the infection is within the vessel wall, an aneurysm may form, which could lead to cerebral hemorrhage.

TRANSIENT ISCHEMIC ATTACK

A transient ischemic attack (TIA) is a recurrent episode of neurologic deficit, lasting from seconds to hours, that clears within 12 to 24 hours. It's usually considered a warning sign of an impending thrombotic cerebrovascular accident (CVA). In fact, TIAs have been reported in 50% to 80% of patients who have had a cerebral infarction from such thrombosis.

The age of onset varies. Incidence rises dramatically after age 50 and is highest among blacks and men.

Causes
In TIA, microemboli released from a thrombus probably temporarily interrupt blood flow, especially in the small distal branches of the arterial tree in the brain. Small spasms in those arterioles may impair blood flow and also precede TIA.

Predisposing factors are the same as for thrombotic CVAs. The most distinctive characteristics of TIAs are the transient duration of neurologic deficits and complete return of normal function.

Signs and symptoms
The clinical features of TIA easily correlate with the location of the affected artery. Signs and symptoms include double vision, speech deficits (slurring or thickness), unilateral blindness, staggering or uncoordinated gait, unilateral weakness or numbness, falling because of weakness in the legs, and dizziness.

Treatment
During an active TIA, the aim of treatment is to prevent a completed stroke and consists of aspirin or anticoagulants to minimize the risk of thrombosis. After or between attacks, preventive treatment includes carotid endarterectomy or cerebral microvascular bypass.

Hemorrhage
The third most common cause of CVA is hemorrhage. Like embolism, it may occur suddenly, at any age. Such hemorrhage results from chronic hypertension or aneurysms, which cause sudden rupture of a cerebral artery. The rupture diminishes blood supply to the area served by this artery. In addition, blood accumulates deep within the brain, further compressing neural tissue and causing even greater damage.

CVA classification
CVAs are classified according to their course of progression. The least severe is the transient ischemic attack (TIA), or "little stroke," which results from a temporary interruption of blood flow, most often in the carotid and ver-

tebrobasilar arteries. (See *Transient ischemic attack.*) A progressive stroke, or stroke-in-evolution (thrombus-in-evolution), begins with slight neurologic deficit and worsens in a day or two. In a completed stroke, neurologic deficits are maximal right at onset.

Signs and symptoms
Clinical features of CVA vary with the artery affected (and, consequently, the portion of the brain it supplies), the severity of damage, and the extent of collateral circulation that develops to help the brain compensate for decreased blood supply.

If the CVA occurs in the left hemisphere, it produces symptoms on the right side; if in the right hemisphere, symptoms are on the left side. However, a CVA that causes cranial nerve damage produces signs of cranial nerve dysfunction on the same side as the hemorrhage.

Symptoms are usually classified according to the artery affected:

• *middle cerebral artery:* aphasia, dysphasia, visual field cuts, and hemiparesis on the affected side (more severe in the face and arm than in the leg)

• *carotid artery:* weakness, paralysis, numbness, sensory changes, and visual disturbances on the affected side; altered level of consciousness (LOC), bruits, headaches, aphasia, and ptosis

• *vertebrobasilar artery:* weakness on the affected side, numbness around the lips and mouth, visual field cuts, diplopia, poor coordination, dysphagia, slurred speech, dizziness, amnesia, and ataxia

• *anterior cerebral artery:* confusion, weakness and numbness (especially in the leg) on the affected side, incontinence, loss of coordination, impaired motor and sensory functions, and personality changes

• *posterior cerebral arteries:* visual field cuts, sensory impairment, dyslexia, coma, and cortical blindness. Usually, paralysis is absent.

Symptoms can also be classified as premonitory, generalized, and focal. Premonitory symptoms, such as drowsiness, dizziness, headache, and mental confusion, are rare. Generalized symptoms, such as headache, vomiting, mental impairment, convulsions, coma, nuchal rigidity, fever, and disorientation, are typical. Focal symptoms, such as sensory and reflex changes, reflect the site of hemorrhage or infarction and may worsen.

Diagnosis
Confirmation of CVA is based on observation of clinical features, a history of risk factors, and the results of diagnostic tests.

• *Computed tomography scan* shows evidence of hemorrhagic stroke immediately but may not show evidence of thrombotic infarction for 48 to 72 hours.

• *Magnetic resonance imaging* may help identify ischemic or infarcted areas and cerebral swelling.

• *Brain scan* shows ischemic areas but may not be positive for up to 2 weeks after the CVA.

• *Lumbar puncture* reveals bloody cerebrospinal fluid in hemorrhagic stroke.

• *Ophthalmoscopy* may show signs of hypertension and atherosclerotic changes in retinal arteries.

• *Angiography* outlines blood vessels and pinpoints occlusion or rupture site.

• *EEG* helps to localize the damaged area.

Other baseline laboratory studies include urinalysis, coagulation studies, complete blood count, serum osmolality, and electrolyte, glucose, triglyceride, creatinine, and blood urea nitrogen levels.

Treatment
Surgery performed to improve cerebral circulation for patients with thrombotic or embolic CVA includes an endarterectomy (the removal of atherosclerotic plaque from the inner arterial wall) or a microvascular bypass (the surgical anastamosis of an extracranial vessel to an intracranial vessel).

Medications useful in treating CVA include:

• ticlopidine, an antiplatelet drug, which may be more effective than aspirin in preventing CVA and reducing the risk of recurrent CVA after therapy has begun

• tissue plasminogen activator used experimentally in clot dissolution

• anticonvulsants, such as phenytoin or phenobarbital, to treat or prevent seizures

• stool softeners, such as dioctyl sodium sulfosuccinate, to avoid straining, which increases intracranial pressure (ICP)

• corticosteroids, such as dexamethasone, to minimize associated cerebral edema

• analgesics, such as codeine, to relieve the headache that typically follows hemorrhagic CVA.

Special considerations

• Maintain a patent airway and oxygenation. Loosen constricting clothes. Watch for ballooning of the cheek with respiration. The side that balloons is the side affected by the stroke.

• If the patient is unconscious, he could aspirate saliva, so keep him in a lateral position to allow secretions to drain naturally or suction secretions as needed. Insert an artificial airway, and start mechanical ventilation or supplemental oxygen, if necessary.

• Check the patient's vital signs and neurologic status and record observations. Watch closely for any significant changes.

• Monitor blood pressure, LOC, pupillary changes, motor function (voluntary and involuntary movements), sensory function, speech, skin color, temperature, signs of increased ICP, and nuchal rigidity or flaccidity.

• Be especially alert for a sudden rise in blood pressure, rapid and bounding pulse, and complaints of headache. These are all signs of impending CVA.

• Watch for signs of pulmonary emboli, such as chest pains, shortness of breath, dusky color, tachycardia, fever, and changed sensorium. If the patient is unresponsive, monitor his blood gas levels often, looking for increased partial pressure of carbon dioxide or decreased partial pressure of oxygen.

• Watch for signs of other complications such as infection.

• Maintain fluid and electrolyte balance. If the patient can take liquids by mouth, offer them as often as fluid limitations permit. Administer I.V.

fluids as needed. Never give too much too fast, because this can increase ICP.

• Offer the urinal or bedpan every 2 hours. If the patient is incontinent, he may need an indwelling urinary catheter; but this should be avoided, if possible, because of the risk of infection.

• Ensure adequate nutrition. Check the patient's gag reflex before offering small oral feedings of semisolid foods. Place the food tray within the patient's visual field. If oral feedings aren't possible, insert a nasogastric tube.

• Manage GI problems. Be alert for signs that the patient is straining during defecation because this increases ICP. Modify diet and administer stool softeners and laxatives as needed. If the patient vomits (usually during the first few days), keep him positioned on his side to prevent aspiration.

• Give careful mouth care. Clean and irrigate the patient's mouth to remove food particles. Care for his dentures as needed.

• Provide meticulous eye care. Remove secretions from the patient's eyes with a cotton ball and sterile normal saline solution. Instill eyedrops if needed. Patch the patient's affected eye if he can't close the lid.

• Position the patient, and align his extremities correctly. Use high-topped sneakers to prevent footdrop and contractures and egg crate, flotation, or pulsating mattresses or sheepskin to prevent pressure ulcers.

• To prevent pneumonia, turn the patient at least every 2 hours. Elevate the affected hand to control dependent edema, and place it in a functional position.

• Assist the patient with exercise. Perform range-of-motion exercises for both the affected and unaffected sides. Teach and encourage the patient to use his unaffected side to exercise his affected side.

• Give medications as needed and watch for adverse effects.

• Establish and maintain communication with the patient. If he is aphasic, set up a simple method of communicating basic needs. Remember to phrase your questions so he'll be able to answer using this system. Repeat yourself quietly and calmly (remember, he isn't deaf!) and use gestures if necessary to help him understand. Even the unresponsive patient can hear, so don't say anything in his presence you wouldn't want him to hear and remember.

• Provide psychological support. Set realistic short-term goals. Involve the patient's family in his care when possible, and explain his deficits and strengths.

• Begin your rehabilitation of the patient with CVA on admission. The amount of teaching you'll have to do depends on the extent of neurologic deficit.

• Establish rapport with the patient. Spend time with him, and provide a means of communication. Simplify your language, asking yes-or-no questions whenever possible. Don't correct his speech or treat him like a child. Remember that building rapport may be difficult because of the mood changes that may result from brain damage or as a reaction to being dependent.

• If necessary, teach the patient to comb his hair, dress, and wash. With the aid of a physical and an occupational therapist, obtain appliances, such as walking frames, hand bars by the toilet, and ramps as needed.

• If speech therapy is indicated, encourage the patient to begin as soon as possible and follow through with the speech pathologist's suggestions.

• To reinforce teaching, involve the patient's family in all aspects of rehabilitation. With their cooperation and support, devise realistic discharge goals, and let them help decide when the patient can return home.

• Before discharge, warn the patient or his family to report any premonitory signs of a CVA, such as severe headache, drowsiness, confusion, and dizziness. Emphasize the importance of regular follow-up visits.

• If aspirin has been prescribed to minimize the risk of embolic stroke, tell the patient to watch for possible GI bleeding related to ulcer formation. Make sure the patient realizes that he can't substitute acetaminophen for aspirin.

• To help patients prevent CVA, stress the need to control diseases such as diabetes or hypertension. Teach all patients (especially those at high risk) the importance of following a low-cholesterol, low-salt diet; watching their weight; increasing activity; avoiding smoking and prolonged bed rest; and minimizing stress.

CERVICAL CANCER

The third most common cancer of the female reproductive system, cervical cancer is classified as either preinvasive or invasive.

Preinvasive carcinoma ranges from minimal cervical dysplasia, in which the lower third of the epithelium contains abnormal cells, to carcinoma in situ, in which the full thickness of epithelium contains abnormally proliferating cells (also known as cervical intraepithelial neoplasia).

Preinvasive cancer is curable 75% to 90% of the time with early detection and proper treatment. If untreated (and depending on the form in which it appears), it may progress to invasive cervical cancer.

In invasive carcinoma, cancer cells penetrate the basement membrane and can spread directly to contiguous pelvic structures or disseminate to distant sites by lymphatic routes. Invasive carcinoma of the uterine cervix is responsible for 8,000 deaths annually in the United States alone.

In almost all cases (95%), the histologic type is squamous cell carcinoma, which varies from well-differentiated cells to highly anaplastic spindle cells. Only 5% are adenocarcinomas. Usually, invasive carcinoma occurs between ages 30 and 50; rarely, under age 20.

Causes

Although the cause is unknown, several predisposing factors have been related to the development of cervical cancer: intercourse at a young age (under age 16), multiple sexual partners, multiple pregnancies, and herpesvirus II and other bacterial or viral venereal infections.

Signs and symptoms

Preinvasive cervical cancer produces no symptoms or other clinically apparent changes. Early invasive cervical cancer causes abnormal vaginal bleeding, persistent vaginal discharge, and postcoital pain and bleeding. In advanced stages, it causes pelvic pain, vaginal leakage of urine and feces from a fistula, anorexia, weight loss, and anemia.

Diagnosis

A cytologic examination (Papanicolaou [Pap] smear) can detect cervical cancer before clinical evidence appears. (Systems of Pap smear classification may vary from hospital to hospital.) Abnormal cervical cytology routinely calls for colposcopy, which can detect the presence and extent of preclinical lesions requiring a biopsy and histologic examination.

Staining with Lugol's solution (strong iodine) or Schiller's solution (iodine, potassium iodide, and purified water) may identify areas for a biopsy when the smear shows abnormal cells but there's no obvious lesion. Although the tests are nonspecific, they do distinguish between normal and abnormal tissues: Normal tissues absorb the iodine and turn brown; abnormal tissues are devoid of glycogen and won't change color.

Additional studies, such as lymphangiography, cystography, and scans, can detect metastasis. (See *Staging cervical cancer.*)

Treatment

Appropriate treatment depends on accurate clinical staging. Preinvasive lesions may be treated with a total excisional biopsy, cryosurgery, laser destruction, conization (and frequent Pap smear follow-up) or, rarely, hysterectomy. Therapy for invasive squamous cell carcinoma may include radical hysterectomy and radiation therapy (internal, external, or both).

Special considerations

• If the patient needs a biopsy, drape and prepare her as for a routine Pap smear and pelvic examination. Have a container of formaldehyde ready to preserve the specimen during transfer to the pathology laboratory. Explain to the patient that she may feel pressure, minor abdominal cramps, or a pinch from the punch forceps. Reassure her that pain will be minimal because the cervix has few nerve endings.

• If the patient is having cryosurgery, drape and prepare her as if for a routine Pap smear and pelvic examination. Explain that the procedure takes approximately 15 minutes, during which time refrigerant will be used to freeze the cervix. Warn the patient that she may experience abdominal cramps, headache, and sweating, but reassure her that she'll feel little, if any, pain.

• If the patient needs laser therapy, drape and prepare her as if for a routine Pap smear and pelvic examina-

STAGING CERVICAL CANCER

Cervical cancer treatment decisions depend on accurate staging. The International Federation of Gynecology and Obstetrics defines cervical cancer stages as follows.

Stage 0 — carcinoma in situ, intraepithelial carcinoma

Stage I — cancer confined to the cervix (extension to the corpus should be disregarded)

Stage IA — preclinical malignant lesions of the cervix (diagnosed only microscopically)

Stage IA1 — minimal microscopically evident stromal invasion

Stage IA2 — lesions detected microscopically, measuring 5 mm or less from the base of the epithelium, either surface or glandular, from which it originates; lesion width shouldn't exceed 7 mm

Stage IB — lesions measuring more than 5 mm deep and 7 mm wide, whether seen clinically or not (preformed space involvement shouldn't alter the staging but should be recorded for future treatment decisions)

Stage II — extension beyond the cervix but not to the pelvic wall; the cancer involves the vagina but hasn't spread to the lower third

Stage IIA — no obvious parametrial involvement

Stage IIB — obvious parametrial involvement

Stage III — extension to the pelvic wall; on rectal examination, no cancer-free space exists between the tumor and the pelvic wall; the tumor involves the lower third of the vagina; this includes all cases with hydronephrosis or nonfunctioning kidney

Stage IIIA — no extension to the pelvic wall

Stage IIIB — extension to the pelvic wall and hydronephrosis, or nonfunctioning kidney, or both

Stage IV — extension beyond the true pelvis or involvement of the bladder or the rectal mucosa

Stage IVA — spread to adjacent organs

Stage IVB — spread to distant organs

---

tion. Explain that the procedure takes approximately 30 minutes and may cause abdominal cramps.

• After an excisional biopsy, cryosurgery, and laser therapy, tell the patient to expect a discharge or spotting for about 1 week after these procedures, and advise her not to douche, use tampons, or engage in sexual intercourse during this time. Tell her to watch for and report signs of infection. Stress the need for a follow-up Pap smear and a pelvic examination within 3 to 4 months after these procedures and periodically thereafter.

• Tell the patient what to expect postoperatively if she'll have a hysterectomy.

• After surgery, monitor vital signs every 4 hours.

• Watch for signs and symptoms of complications, such as bleeding, abdominal distention, severe pain, and breathing difficulties.

• Administer analgesics, prophylactic antibiotics, and S.C. heparin as needed.

• Encourage deep-breathing and coughing exercises.

• Find out if the patient is to have internal or external therapy, or both. Usually, internal radiation therapy is the first procedure.

• Explain the internal radiation procedure, and answer the patient's questions. Internal radiation requires a 2- to 3-day hospital stay, bowel preparation, a povidone-iodine vaginal douche, a clear liquid diet, and nothing by mouth the night before the implantation; it also requires an indwelling urinary catheter.

• Tell the patient that the procedure is performed in the operating room under general anesthesia and that an applicator containing radioactive material (such as radium or cesium) will be implanted.

• Remember that safety precautions—time, distance, and shielding—begin as soon as the radioactive source is in place. Inform the patient that she'll require a private room.

• Encourage the patient to lie flat and limit movement while the implant is in place. If she prefers, elevate the head of the bed slightly.

• Check vital signs every 4 hours; watch for skin reaction, vaginal bleeding, abdominal discomfort, or evidence of dehydration. Make sure the patient can reach everything she needs without stretching or straining.

• Assist the patient in range-of-motion *arm* exercises (leg exercises and other body movements could dislodge the implant). If needed, administer a tranquilizer to help the patient relax and remain still. Organize the time you spend with the patient to minimize your exposure to radiation.

• Inform visitors of safety precautions, and hang a sign listing these precautions on the patient's door.

• Explain that external outpatient radiation therapy, when necessary, continues for 4 to 6 weeks.

• Teach the patient to watch for and report uncomfortable effects. Because radiation therapy may increase susceptibility to infection by lowering the white blood cell count, warn the patient to avoid persons with obvious infections during therapy.

• Teach the patient to use a vaginal dilator to prevent vaginal stenosis and to facilitate vaginal examinations and sexual intercourse.

• Reassure the patient that this disease and its treatment shouldn't radically alter her lifestyle or prohibit sexual intimacy.

CHALAZION

A common eye disorder, a chalazion is a granulomatous inflammation of a meibomian gland in the upper or lower eyelid. This disorder is characterized by localized swelling and usually develops slowly over several weeks.

A chalazion may become large enough to press on the eyeball, producing astigmatism; a large chalazion seldom subsides spontaneously. It's generally benign and chronic and can occur at any age; in some patients, it's apt to recur.

Causes
Obstruction of the meibomian (sebaceous) gland duct causes a chalazion.

Signs and symptoms
A chalazion occurs as a painless, hard lump that usually *points toward* the conjunctival side of the eyelid. Eversion of the lid reveals a red or red-yellow elevated area on the conjunctival surface. (See *Identifying a chalazion.)*

Diagnosis
Visual examination and palpation of the eyelid reveal a small bump or nodule. Persistently recurrent chalazions, especially in an adult, necessitate a biopsy to rule out meibomian cancer.

Treatment

Initial treatment consists of the application of warm compresses to open the lumen of the gland and, occasionally, instillation of sulfonamide eye drops. If such therapy fails, or if the chalazion presses on the eyeball or causes a severe cosmetic problem, steroid injection or incision and curettage under local anesthetic may be necessary.

After such surgery, a pressure eye patch applied for 8 to 24 hours controls bleeding and swelling. After removal of the patch, treatment again consists of warm compresses applied for 10 to 15 minutes, two to four times daily, and antimicrobial eye drops or ointment to prevent secondary infection.

Special considerations

• Teach proper lid hygiene to the patient disposed to chalazions (water and mild baby shampoo applied with a cotton applicator).

• Instruct the patient how to properly apply *warm* compresses: Tell him to take special care to avoid burning the skin, to always use a clean cloth, and to discard used compresses. Also tell him to start applying warm compresses at the first sign of lid irritation to increase the blood supply and keep the lumen open.

CHANCROID

Painful genital ulcers and inguinal adenitis characterize chancroid, or soft chancre. This sexually transmitted disease (STD) occurs worldwide but is particularly common in tropical countries; it affects men more often than women.

Chancroidal lesions may heal spontaneously and usually respond well to treatment in the absence of secondary infections. A high rate of human immunodeficiency virus (HIV) infection has been reported among patients with chancroid.

IDENTIFYING A CHALAZION

A chalazion is a nontender granulomatous inflammation of a meibomian gland on the eyelid.

Causes

Chancroid results from *Haemophilus ducreyi*, a gram-negative streptobacillus, and is transmitted through sexual contact. Poor hygiene may predispose men — especially those who are uncircumcised — to this disease.

Signs and symptoms

After a 3- to 5-day incubation period, a small papule appears at the site of entry, usually the groin or inner thigh. In men, it may appear on the penis; in women, on the vulva, vagina, or cervix. Occasionally, this papule may erupt on the tongue, lip, breast, or navel.

The papule rapidly ulcerates, becoming painful, soft, and malodorous; it bleeds easily and produces pus. It's gray and shallow, with irregular edges, and measures up to 1″ (2.5 cm) in diameter. Within 2 to 3 weeks, inguinal adenitis develops, creating suppurated, inflamed nodes that may rupture into large ulcers or buboes. Headache and malaise occur in 50% of patients. During the healing stage, phimosis may develop.

Diagnosis
Gram stain smears of ulcer exudate or bubo aspirate are 50% reliable; blood agar cultures are 75% reliable. A biopsy confirms the diagnosis but is reserved for resistant cases or cases in which cancer is suspected. Dark-field examination and serologic testing rule out other STDs that cause similar ulcers. Testing for HIV infection should be done at the time of the diagnosis.

Treatment
Drug therapy consists of azithromycin, 1 g by mouth (P.O.) in a single dose; erythromycin, 500 mg P.O. q.i.d. for 7 days; or ceftriaxone, 250 mg I.M. in a single dose. The safety of azithromycin for pregnant or lactating women hasn't been established. Aspiration of fluid-filled nodes helps prevent spreading the infection.

Special considerations
• Practice universal precautions.
• Make sure the patient isn't allergic to any drug before giving the first dose.
• Instruct the patient not to apply lotions, creams, or oils on or near the genitalia or on other lesion sites.
• Tell the patient to abstain from sexual contact until healing is complete (usually about 2 weeks after treatment begins) and to wash the genitalia daily with soap and water. Instruct uncircumcised men to retract the foreskin for thorough cleaning.
• To prevent chancroid, advise patients to avoid sexual contact with infected persons, to use condoms during sexual activity, and to wash the genitalia with soap and water after sexual activity.

CHEST INJURIES, BLUNT

One-fourth of all trauma deaths in the United States result from chest injuries. Many are blunt chest injuries, which include myocardial contusion, and rib and sternal fractures that may be simple, multiple, displaced, or jagged. Such fractures may cause potentially fatal complications, such as hemothorax, pneumothorax, hemorrhagic shock, and diaphragmatic rupture.

Causes
Most blunt chest injuries result from automobile accidents. Other common causes include sports and blast injuries.

Signs and symptoms
Rib fractures produce tenderness, slight edema over the fracture site, and pain that worsens with deep breathing and movement; this painful breathing causes the patient to display shallow, splinted respirations that may lead to hypoventilation.

Sternal fractures, which are usually transverse and located in the middle or upper sternum, produce persistent chest pain, even at rest. If a fractured rib tears the pleura and punctures a lung, it causes pneumothorax, which usually produces severe dyspnea, cyanosis, agitation, extreme pain, and, when air escapes into chest tissue, subcutaneous emphysema.

Effects of multiple fractures
Multiple rib fractures may cause flail chest: a portion of the chest wall "caves" in, which causes a loss of chest

wall integrity and prevents adequate lung inflation. Bruised skin, extreme pain caused by rib fracture and disfigurement, paradoxical chest movements, and rapid, shallow respirations are all signs of flail chest, as are tachycardia, hypotension, respiratory acidosis, and cyanosis.

Flail chest can also cause tension pneumothorax, a condition in which air enters the chest but can't be ejected during exhalation; life-threatening thoracic pressure buildup causes lung collapse and subsequent mediastinal shift. The cardinal symptoms of tension pneumothorax include tracheal deviation (away from the affected side), cyanosis, severe dyspnea, absent breath sounds (on the affected side), agitation, distended jugular veins, and shock.

Hemothorax

When a rib lacerates lung tissue or an intercostal artery, hemothorax occurs, causing blood to collect in the pleural cavity, thereby compressing the lung and limiting respiratory capacity. It can also result from rupture of large or small pulmonary vessels.

Massive hemothorax is the most common cause of shock following chest trauma. Although slight bleeding occurs even with mild pneumothorax, such bleeding resolves very quickly, usually without changing the patient's condition.

Rib fractures may also cause pulmonary contusion (resulting in hemoptysis, hypoxia, dyspnea, and possible obstruction), large myocardial tears (which can be rapidly fatal), and small myocardial tears (which can cause pericardial effusion).

Further complications

Myocardial contusions produce electrocardiogram abnormalities. Laceration or rupture of the aorta is nearly always immediately fatal. Rarely, aortic laceration may develop 24 hours after blunt injury, so patient observation is critical.

Diaphragmatic rupture (usually on the left side) causes severe respiratory distress. Unless treated early, abdominal viscera may herniate through the rupture into the thorax, compromising both circulation and the lungs' vital capacity.

Other complications of blunt chest trauma may include cardiac tamponade, pulmonary artery tears, ventricular rupture, and bronchial, tracheal, or esophageal tears or rupture.

Diagnosis

A history of trauma with dyspnea, chest pain, and other typical clinical features suggest a blunt chest injury. A physical examination and diagnostic tests determine the extent of injury.

• *Percussion* reveals dullness in hemothorax and tympany in tension pneumothorax.

• *Auscultation* may reveal a change in position of the loudest heart sound in tension pneumothorax.

• *Chest X-rays* may confirm rib and sternal fractures, pneumothorax, flail chest, pulmonary contusions, lacerated or ruptured aorta, tension pneumothorax, diaphragmatic rupture, lung compression, or atelectasis with hemothorax.

• *Electrocardiography* may show abnormalities with cardiac damage, including multiple premature ventricular contractions, unexplained tachycardias, atrial fibrillation, bundle-branch heart block (usually right), and ST-segment changes.

• *Serial aspartate aminotransferase, alanine aminotransferase, lactate dehydrogenase, creatine kinase (CK),* and *CK-MB* levels are elevated.

• *Retrograde aortography* and *transesophageal echocardiography* reveal aortic laceration or rupture.

• *Contrast studies* and *liver* and *spleen scans* detect diaphragmatic rupture.

• *Echocardiography, computed tomography scans*, and *cardiac* and *lung scans* show the injury's extent.

Treatment and special considerations

• Blunt chest injuries call for immediate physical assessment, control of bleeding, maintenance of a patent airway, adequate ventilation, and fluid and electrolyte balance.

• Check all pulses and level of consciousness. Also evaluate color and temperature of skin, depth of respiration, use of accessory muscles, and length of inhalation compared with exhalation.

• Check pulse oximetry values for adequate oxygenation.

• Observe tracheal position. Look for distended jugular veins and paradoxical chest motion. Listen to heart and breath sounds carefully; palpate for subcutaneous emphysema (crepitation) or a lack of structural integrity of the ribs.

• Obtain a history of the injury. Unless severe dyspnea is present, ask the patient to locate the pain, and ask if he's having trouble breathing. Obtain an order for laboratory studies (arterial blood gas analysis, cardiac enzyme studies, complete blood count, and typing and crossmatching).

• For simple rib fractures, give mild analgesics, encourage bed rest, and apply heat. Don't strap or tape the chest.

• For more severe fractures, intercostal nerve blocks may be needed. Obtain X-rays before and after the nerve blocks to rule out pneumothorax.

• Intubate the patient with excessive bleeding or hemopneumothorax. Chest tubes may be inserted to treat hemothorax and to assess the need for thoracotomy. To prevent atelectasis, turn the patient frequently and encourage coughing and deep breathing.

• For pneumothorax, the patient may need a chest tube placed anterior to the midaxillary line at the fifth intercostal space to aspirate as much air as possible from the pleural cavity and to reexpand the lungs. When time permits, insert chest tubes attached to water-seal drainage and suction.

• For flail chest, place the patient in a semi-Fowler's position. Reexpansion of the lung is the first definitive care measure. Administer oxygen at a high flow rate under positive pressure. Suction the patient frequently, as completely as possible. Maintain acid-base balance. Observe carefully for signs of tension pneumothorax.

• Start I.V. therapy for the patient with flail chest. Use lactated Ringer's solution or normal saline solution. Beware of both excessive and insufficient fluid resuscitation.

• For hemothorax, treat shock with I.V. infusions of lactated Ringer's solution or normal saline solution. Administer packed red blood cells for blood losses greater than 1,500 ml or circulating blood volume losses exceeding 30%. Autotransfusion is an option. Administer oxygen.

• The patient with hemothorax will also need insertion of chest tubes in the fifth or sixth intercostal space anterior to the midaxillary line to remove blood. Monitor and document vital signs and blood loss. Watch for falling blood pressure, rising pulse rate, and hemorrhage — all require thoracotomy to stop bleeding.

• For pulmonary contusions, give limited amounts of colloids (for example, salt-poor albumin, whole blood, or plasma) to replace volume and maintain oncotic pressure. Give analgesics, diuretics and, if necessary, corticosteroids as needed. Monitor blood gas levels to ensure adequate ventilation; provide oxygen therapy, mechanical ventilation, and chest tube care.

• For suspected cardiac damage, close intensive care or telemetry may detect arrhythmias and prevent cardiogenic shock. Impose bed rest in semi-Fowler's position (unless the patient requires shock position); as needed, administer oxygen, analgesics, and supportive drugs to control heart failure or supraventricular arrhythmia.

• Watch for cardiac tamponade, which calls for pericardiocentesis. Essentially, provide the same care as for a patient who has suffered a myocardial infarction.

• For myocardial rupture, septal perforations, and other cardiac lacerations, immediate surgical repair is mandatory; less severe ventricular wounds require use of a digital or balloon catheter; atrial wounds require a clamp or balloon catheter.

• For the few patients with aortic rupture or laceration who reach the hospital alive, immediate surgery is mandatory, using synthetic grafts or anastomosis to repair the damage. Give large volumes of I.V. fluids (lactated Ringer's or normal saline solution) and whole blood, along with oxygen at very high flow rates; then transport the patient promptly to the operating room.

• For tension pneumothorax, the patient will need insertion of a spinal or 14G to 16G needle into the second intercostal space at the midclavicular line, to release pressure in the chest. Following this, insert a chest tube to normalize pressure and reexpand the lung. Administer oxygen under positive pressure, along with I.V. fluids.

• For a diaphragmatic rupture, insert a nasogastric tube to temporarily decompress the stomach, and prepare the patient for surgical repair.

CHEST WOUNDS, PENETRATING

Depending on their size, penetrating chest wounds may cause varying degrees of damage to bones, soft tissue, blood vessels, and nerves. Mortality and morbidity from a chest wound depend on the size and severity of the wound.

Gunshot wounds are usually more serious than stab wounds, both because they cause more severe lacerations and cause rapid blood loss and because ricochet often damages large areas and multiple organs. With prompt, aggressive treatment, up to 90% of patients with penetrating chest wounds recover.

Causes

Stab wounds from a knife or ice pick are the most common penetrating chest wounds; gunshot wounds are a close second. Wartime explosions or firearms fired at close range are the usual source of large, gaping wounds.

Signs and symptoms

In addition to the obvious chest injuries, penetrating chest wounds can also cause the following:

• A sucking sound occurs as the diaphragm contracts and air enters the chest cavity through the opening in the chest wall.

• Level of consciousness varies, depending on the extent of the injury. If the patient is awake and alert, he may be in severe pain, which will make him splint his respirations, thereby reducing his vital capacity.

• Tachycardia stems from anxiety and blood loss.

• A weak, thready pulse results from massive blood loss and hypovolemic shock.

Penetrating chest wounds may also cause lung lacerations (bleeding and substantial air leakage through the chest tube); arterial lacerations (loss of more than 100 ml of blood/hour through the chest tube); and exsanguination. Pneumothorax (air in the pleural space causing loss of negative intrathoracic pressure and lung collapse), tension pneumothorax (intrapleural air accumulation causing potentially fatal mediastinal shift), and hemothorax can also result.

Other effects may include arrhythmias, cardiac tamponade, mediastinitis, subcutaneous emphysema, esophageal perforation, and bronchopleural fistula. Tracheobronchial, abdominal, or diaphragmatic injuries can also occur.

Diagnosis

An obvious chest wound and a sucking sound during breathing confirm the diagnosis. Consider any lower thoracic chest injury a thoracicoabdominal injury until proven otherwise.

Further tests to provide baseline data include:

• *pulse oximetry* and *arterial blood gas analysis* to assess respiratory status
• *chest X-rays* before and after chest tube placement to evaluate the injury and tube placement; however, in an emergency, don't wait for chest X-ray results before inserting the chest tube
• *complete blood count,* including hemoglobin, hematocrit, and differential (low hemoglobin and hematocrit reflect severe blood loss; in early blood loss, these values may be normal)
• *palpation* and *auscultation* of the chest and abdomen to evaluate damage to adjacent organs and structures.

Treatment and special considerations

Penetrating chest wounds require immediate support of respiration and circulation, prompt surgical repair, and measures to prevent complications.

• Immediately assess airway, breathing, and circulation. Establish a patent airway, support ventilation, and monitor pulses frequently.
• Place an occlusive dressing over the sucking wound. Monitor for signs of tension pneumothorax (tracheal shift, respiratory distress, tachycardia, tachypnea, and diminished or absent breath sounds on the affected side); if tension pneumothorax develops, temporarily remove the occlusive dressing to create a simple pneumothorax.
• Control blood loss (also remember to look *under* the patient to estimate loss), type and crossmatch blood, and replace blood and fluids as necessary.
• Prepare the patient for chest X-rays and placement of chest tubes (using water-seal drainage) to reestablish intrathoracic pressure and to drain blood in hemothorax. A second X-ray will evaluate the position of tubes and their function.
• Emergency surgery may be needed to repair the damage caused by the wound.
• Throughout treatment, monitor central venous pressure and blood pressure to detect hypovolemia, and assess vital signs. Provide analgesics as appropriate. Tetanus and antibiotic prophylaxis may be necessary.
• Reassure the patient, especially if he's been the victim of a violent crime. Report the incident to the police in accordance with local laws. Help contact the patient's family, and offer them reassurance as well.

CHLAMYDIAL INFECTIONS

Urethritis in men and urethritis and cervicitis in women compose a group of infections that are linked to one organism: *Chlamydia trachomatis*. These chlamydial infections are the most common sexually transmitted diseases in the United States, affecting an estimated 4 million Americans each year.

Trachoma inclusion conjunctivitis, a chlamydial infection that occurs rarely in the United States, is a leading cause of blindness in Third World countries. Lymphogranuloma venereum, a rare disease in the United States, is also caused by *C. trachomatis*.

Untreated, chlamydial infections can lead to such complications as acute epididymitis, salpingitis, pelvic inflammatory disease and, eventually, sterility. Some studies show that chlamydial infections in pregnant women are associated with spontaneous abortion and premature delivery. Other studies haven't confirmed these findings.

Causes

Transmission of *C. trachomatis* primarily follows vaginal or rectal intercourse or oral-genital contact with an infected person. Because signs and symptoms of chlamydial infections commonly appear late in the course of the disease, sexual transmission of the organism typically occurs unknowingly.

Children born of mothers who have chlamydial infections may contract associated conjunctivitis, otitis media, and pneumonia during passage through the birth canal.

Signs and symptoms

Both men and women with chlamydial infections may be asymptomatic or may show signs of infection on physical examination. Individual signs and symptoms vary with the specific type of chlamydial infection and are determined by the organism's route of transmission to susceptible tissue.

Clinical features in women

Women who have *cervicitis* may develop cervical erosion, mucopurulent discharge, pelvic pain, and dyspareunia.

Women who have *endometritis* or *salpingitis* may experience signs of pelvic inflammatory disease, such as pain and tenderness of the abdomen, cervix, uterus, and lymph nodes; chills; fever; breakthrough bleeding; bleeding after intercourse; and vaginal discharge. They may also have dysuria.

Women with *urethral syndrome* may experience dysuria, pyuria, and urinary frequency.

Clinical features in men

Men who have *urethritis* may experience dysuria, erythema, tenderness of the urethral meatus, urinary frequency, pruritus, and urethral discharge. In urethritis, such discharge may be copious and purulent or scant and clear or mucoid.

Men with *epididymitis* may experience painful scrotal swelling and urethral discharge.

Men who have *prostatitis* may have lower back pain, urinary frequency, dysuria, nocturia, and painful ejaculation.

In *proctitis*, patients may have diarrhea, tenesmus, pruritus, bloody or mucopurulent discharge, and diffuse or discrete ulceration in the rectosigmoid colon.

TEACHING CHECKLIST

WHAT YOUR PATIENT NEEDS TO KNOW ABOUT CHLAMYDIA

Before discharge, teach the patient with a chlamydial infection to:
• complete drug therapy, even after symptoms subside
• follow meticulous personal hygiene
• avoid touching the discharge

• wash and dry his hands before touching his eyes
• abstain from intercourse until he and his partner are cured
• inform sexual contacts of his infection
• return for follow-up testing.

Diagnosis

The following laboratory tests provide a definitive diagnosis of chlamydial infections:
• A *swab* from the site of infection (urethra, cervix, or rectum) establishes a diagnosis of urethritis, cervicitis, salpingitis, endometritis, or proctitis.
• A *culture* of aspirated material establishes a diagnosis of epididymitis.
• Antigen detection methods, including the *enzyme-linked immunosorbent assay* and the *direct fluorescent antibody test,* are the diagnostic tests of choice for identifying chlamydial infection, although tissue cell cultures are more sensitive and specific.
• Newer *nucleic acid probes* using polymerase chain reactions are also commercially available.

Treatment

The recommended first-line treatment for adults and adolescents who have chlamydial infections is drug therapy with oral doxycycline for 7 days or oral azithromycin in a single dose. (See *What your patient needs to know about chlamydia.*)

For pregnant women with chlamydial infections, erythromycin (stearate base) is the treatment of choice.

Special considerations

• Practice universal precautions when caring for a patient with a chlamydial infection.
• Teach the patient what he needs to know before discharge.
• Make sure that the patient fully understands the dosage requirements of any prescribed medications for this infection.
• If required in your state, report all cases of chlamydial infection to the appropriate local public health authorities who will then conduct follow-up notification of the patient's sexual contacts.
• Suggest that the patient and his sexual partners receive testing for the human immunodeficiency virus.
• Check newborns of infected mothers for signs of chlamydial infection. Obtain appropriate specimens for diagnostic testing.

CHLORIDE IMBALANCE

Hypochloremia and hyperchloremia are, respectively, conditions of deficient or excessive serum levels of the anion chloride. A predominantly extracellular anion, chloride accounts for two-thirds of all serum anions.

Secreted by stomach mucosa as hydrochloric acid, chloride provides an acid medium conducive to digestion and activation of enzymes. It also participates in maintaining acid-base and body water balances, influences the osmolality or tonicity of extracellular fluid, plays a role in the exchange of oxygen and carbon dioxide in red blood cells, and helps activate salivary amylase (which, in turn, activates the digestive process).

Causes

Chloride imbalance can stem from a variety of causes.

Hypochloremia

Insufficient serum chloride levels can result from decreased chloride intake or absorption, as in low dietary sodium intake, sodium deficiency, potassium deficiency, and metabolic alkalosis. Prolonged use of mercurial diuretics and administration of dextrose I.V. without electrolytes can also interfere with chloride absorption.

Excessive chloride loss can result from prolonged diarrhea or diaphoresis, as well as loss of hydrochloric acid in gastric secretions from vomiting, gastric suctioning, or gastric surgery.

Hyperchloremia

Excessive chloride intake or absorption — as in hyperingestion of ammonium chloride, or ureterointestinal anastomosis — can lead to hyperchloremia by allowing reabsorption of chloride by the bowel. Hemoconcentration from dehydration can also lead to excess serum chloride.

Compensatory mechanisms for other metabolic abnormalities can also cause hyperchloemia. These abnormalities include metabolic acidosis, brain stem injury causing neurogenic hyperventilation, and hyperparathyroidism.

Signs and symptoms

Because of the natural affinity of sodium and chloride ions, chloride imbalance frequently produces signs and symptoms also associated with sodium imbalance.

Hypochloremia

Indications of hypochloremia include the characteristic muscular weakness and twitching that mark hyponatremia, because renal chloride loss always accompanies sodium loss, and sodium reabsorption isn't possible without chloride.

However, if chloride depletion results from metabolic alkalosis secondary to loss of gastric secretions, chloride is lost independently from sodium. Typical symptoms include muscle hypertonicity, tetany, and shallow, depressed breathing.

Hyperchloremia

The clinical effects of hyperchloremia typically match those of hypernatremia and resulting extracellular fluid volume excess: agitation, tachycardia, hypertension, pitting edema, and dyspnea. Hyperchloremia associated with metabolic acidosis results from excretion of base bicarbonate by the kidneys and induces deep, rapid breathing; weakness; diminished cognitive ability and, ultimately, coma.

Diagnosis

A serum chloride level that's less than 98 mEq/L confirms hypochloremia; supportive values with metabolic alkalosis include a serum pH greater than 7.45 and a serum carbon dioxide level greater than 32 mEq/L.

A serum chloride level greater than 108 mEq/L confirms hyperchloremia; with metabolic acidosis, serum pH is less than 7.35 and the serum carbon dioxide level is less than 22 mEq/L.

Treatment
In either kind of chloride imbalance, treatment must correct the underlying disorder.

Hypochloremia
Besides correcting the condition that caused excessive chloride loss, treatment can include giving oral replacement such as salty broth. When oral therapy isn't possible or when emergency measures are necessary, treatment may include normal saline solution I.V. (if hypovolemia is present) or chloride-containing drugs, such as ammonium chloride, to increase serum chloride levels, and potassium chloride for metabolic alkalosis.

Hyperchloremia
For severe hyperchloremic acidosis, treatment consists of sodium bicarbonate I.V. to raise serum bicarbonate level and permit renal excretion of the chloride anion, because bicarbonate and chloride compete for combination with sodium. For mild hyperchloremia, lactated Ringer's solution is administered; it converts to bicarbonate in the liver, thus increasing base bicarbonate to correct acidosis.

Special considerations
For hypochloremia:
• Monitor serum chloride levels frequently, particularly during I.V. therapy.
• Watch for signs of hyperchloremia or hypochloremia. Be alert for respiratory difficulty.
• To prevent hypochloremia, monitor laboratory results (serum electrolyte and arterial blood gas levels) and fluid intake and output of patients who are vulnerable to chloride imbalance, particularly those recovering from gastric surgery.
• Watch for excessive or continuous loss of gastric secretions, as well as prolonged infusion of dextrose in water without saline.

For hyperchloremia:
• Check serum electrolyte levels every 3 to 6 hours. If the patient is receiving high doses of sodium bicarbonate, watch for signs of overcorrection (metabolic alkalosis, respiratory depression) or lingering signs of hyperchloremia, which indicate inadequate treatment.
• To prevent hyperchloremia, check laboratory results for elevated serum chloride or potassium imbalance if the patient is receiving I.V. solutions containing sodium chloride, and monitor fluid intake and output.
• Watch for signs of metabolic acidosis. When administering I.V. fluids containing lactated Ringer's solution, monitor flow rate according to the patient's age, physical condition, and bicarbonate level, watching for irregularities.

CHOLELITHIASIS, CHOLECYSTITIS, AND RELATED DISORDERS

Diseases of the gallbladder and biliary tract are common and often painful conditions that usually require surgery and may be life-threatening. They are often associated with deposition of calculi and inflammation. (See *Common sites of calculi formation,* page 196.)

In most cases, gallbladder and bile duct diseases occur during middle age. Between ages 20 and 50, they're six times more common in women, but incidence in men and women becomes equal after age 50. Incidence rises with each succeeding decade.

Causes

The origin and frequency of gallbladder and biliary tract disease vary with the particular disorder.

Cholelithiasis

The presence of stones or calculi (gallstones) in the gallbladder results from changes in bile components. Gallstones are made of cholesterol, calcium bilirubinate, or a mixture of cholesterol and bilirubin pigment. They arise during periods of sluggishness in the gallbladder resulting from pregnancy, oral contraceptives, diabetes mellitus, celiac disease, cirrhosis of the liver, and pancreatitis.

Cholelithiasis is the fifth leading cause of hospitalization among adults, and accounts for 90% of all gallbladder and duct diseases. The prognosis is usually good with treatment unless infection occurs, in which case the prognosis depends on its severity and response to antibiotics.

Choledocholithiasis

One out of every ten patients with gallstones develops choledocholithiasis, or gallstones in the common bile duct (sometimes called common duct stones). This occurs when stones passed out of the gallbladder lodge in the hepatic and common bile ducts and obstruct the flow of bile into the duodenum. The prognosis is good unless infection occurs.

Cholangitis

An infection of the bile duct, cholangitis is often associated with choledocholithiasis and may follow percutaneous transhepatic cholangiography. Predisposing factors may include bacterial or metabolic alteration of bile acids. Widespread inflammation may cause fibrosis and stenosis of the common bile duct. The prognosis for this rare condition is poor without stenting or surgery.

Cholecystitis

This acute or chronic inflammation of the gallbladder is usually associated with a gallstone impacted in the cystic duct, causing painful distention of the gallbladder. Cholecystitis accounts for 10% to 25% of all patients requiring gallbladder surgery.

The acute form is most common during middle age; the chronic form, among elderly people. The prognosis is good with treatment.

Cholesterolosis

Cholesterol polyps or cholesterol crystal deposits in the gallbladder's submucosa may result from bile secretions containing high concentrations of cholesterol and insufficient bile salts. The polyps may be localized or speckle the entire gallbladder. Cholesterolosis, the most common pseudotumor, isn't related to widespread inflammation of the mucosa or lining of the gallbladder. The prognosis is good with surgery.

Biliary cirrhosis

An ascending infection of the biliary system, biliary cirrhosis sometimes follows viral destruction of liver and duct cells, but the primary cause is unknown. This condition usually leads to obstructive jaundice and involves the portal and periportal spaces of the liver. It strikes women ages 40 to 60 nine times more often than men. The prognosis is poor without liver transplantation.

Gallstone ileus

This disorder results from a gallstone lodging at the terminal ileum. Gallstone ileus is more common in elderly people. The prognosis is good with surgery.

COMMON SITES OF CALCULI FORMATION

Stones vary in size; small stones may travel.

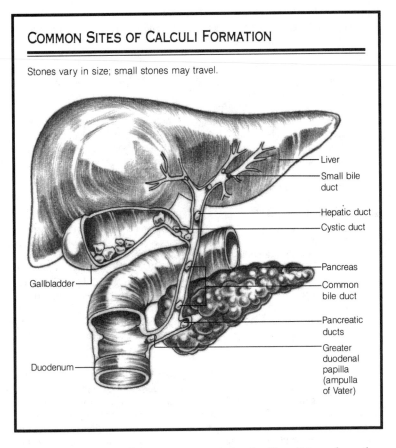

Liver
Small bile duct
Hepatic duct
Cystic duct
Pancreas
Common bile duct
Pancreatic ducts
Greater duodenal papilla (ampulla of Vater)
Gallbladder
Duodenum

Postcholecystectomy syndrome

This syndrome commonly results from residual gallstones or stricture of the common bile duct. It occurs in 1% to 5% of all patients whose gallbladders have been surgically removed and may produce right upper quadrant abdominal pain, biliary colic, fatty food intolerance, dyspepsia, and indigestion. The prognosis is good with selected radiologic procedures, endoscopic procedures, or surgery.

Complications

Each of these disorders produces its own set of complications. Cholelithiasis may lead to any of the disorders associated with gallstone formation: cholangitis, cholecystitis, choledocholithiasis, and gallstone ileus.

Cholecystitis can progress to gallbladder complications, such as empyema, hydrops or mucocele, or gangrene. Gangrene may lead to perforation, resulting in peritonitis, fistula formation, pancreatitis, limy bile, and porcelain gallbladder. Other complications include chronic cholecystitis and cholangitis.

Choledocholithiasis may lead to cholangitis, obstructive jaundice, pancreatitis, and secondary biliary cirrhosis. Cholangitis, especially in the suppurative form, may progress to septic shock and death. Gallstone ileus may cause bowel obstruction, which can lead to intestinal perforation, peritonitis, septicemia, secondary infection, and septic shock.

Signs and symptoms
Although gallbladder disease may produce no symptoms, acute cholelithiasis, acute cholecystitis, choledocholithiasis, and cholesterolosis produce the symptoms of a classic gallbladder attack. Such attacks often follow meals rich in fats or may occur at night, suddenly awakening the patient.

They begin with acute abdominal pain in the right upper quadrant that may radiate to the back, between the shoulders, or to the front of the chest. The pain may be so severe that the patient seeks emergency department care.

Other features may include recurring fat intolerance, biliary colic, belching, flatulence, indigestion, diaphoresis, nausea, vomiting, chills, low-grade fever, jaundice (if a stone obstructs the common bile duct), and clay-colored stools (with choledocholithiasis).

Clinical features of cholangitis include a rise in eosinophils, jaundice, abdominal pain, high fever, and chills. Biliary cirrhosis may produce jaundice, related itching, weakness, fatigue, slight weight loss, and abdominal pain. Gallstone ileus produces signs of small bowel obstruction—nausea, vomiting, abdominal distention, and absent bowel sounds if the bowel is completely obstructed. Its most telling sign is intermittent recurrence of colicky pain over several days.

Diagnosis
Echography and X-rays detect gallstones. Specific procedures include the following:
• *Ultrasonography* reflects stones in the gallbladder with 96% accuracy.

• *Percutaneous transhepatic cholangiography* allows imaging under fluoroscopic control that distinguishes between gallbladder or bile duct disease and cancer of the pancreatic head in patients with jaundice.

• *Endoscopic retrograde cholangiopancreatography* visualizes the biliary tree after insertion of an endoscope down the esophagus into the duodenum, cannulation of the common bile and pancreatic ducts, and injection of contrast medium.

• *Hida scan* of the gallbladder detects obstruction of the cystic duct.

• *Computed tomography scan,* although not used routinely, helps distinguish between obstructive and nonobstructive jaundice.

• *Flat plate of the abdomen* identifies calcified, but not cholesterol, stones with 15% accuracy.

• *Oral cholecystography* shows stones in the gallbladder and biliary duct obstruction.

• *I.V. cholangiography* visualizes the ductal system, although it's rarely used.

Elevated icteric index, total bilirubin, urine bilirubin, and alkaline phosphatase support the diagnosis. White blood cell count is slightly elevated during a cholecystitis attack.

Differential diagnosis is essential because gallbladder disease can mimic other diseases (myocardial infarction, angina, pancreatitis, pancreatic head cancer, pneumonia, peptic ulcer, hiatal hernia, esophagitis, and gastritis). Serum amylase distinguishes gallbladder disease from pancreatitis. With suspected heart disease, serial enzyme tests and an electrocardiogram should precede gallbladder and upper GI diagnostic tests.

Treatment
Surgery, usually elective, is the treatment of choice for gallbladder and bile duct diseases. Surgery may include open or laparoscopic cholecystectomy,

cholecystectomy with operative cholangiography and, possibly, exploration of the common bile duct.

Other treatment includes a low-fat diet to prevent attacks and vitamin K for itching, jaundice, and bleeding tendencies resulting from vitamin K deficiency. Treatment during an acute attack may include insertion of a nasogastric tube and an I.V. line and, possibly, antibiotic administration.

A nonsurgical treatment for choledocholithiasis involves insertion of a flexible catheter, formed around a T tube, through a sinus tract into the common bile duct. Guided by fluoroscopy, the catheter is directed toward the stone. A Dormia basket is threaded through the catheter, opened, twirled to entrap the stone, closed, and withdrawn.

Chenodiol, which dissolves radiolucent stones, provides an alternative for patients who are poor surgical risks or who refuse surgery. However, use of chenodiol is limited by the need for prolonged treatment, the high incidence of adverse effects, and the frequency of stone reformation after treatment ends.

Special considerations
• Before surgery, teach the patient to deep-breathe, cough, expectorate, and perform leg exercises that are necessary after surgery. Also teach splinting, repositioning, and ambulation techniques. Explain the procedures that will be performed before, during, and after surgery to help ease the patient's anxiety and to help ensure his cooperation.
• After surgery, monitor vital signs for indications of bleeding, infection, or atelectasis.
• Evaluate the incision site for bleeding. Serosanguineous and bile drainage is common during the first 24 to 48 hours if the patient has a wound

drain such as a Jackson-Pratt or Penrose drain.
• If, after a choledochostomy, a T-tube drain is placed in the duct and attached to a drainage bag, make sure that the drainage tube has no kinks. Also check that the connecting tubing from the T tube is well secured to the patient to prevent dislodgment.
• Measure and record drainage daily (200 to 300 ml is normal).
• Teach patients who will be discharged with a T tube how to perform dressing changes and routine skin care.
• Monitor intake and output. Allow the patient nothing by mouth for 24 to 48 hours or until bowel sounds return and nausea and vomiting cease (postoperative nausea may indicate a full urinary bladder).
• If the patient doesn't void within 8 hours (or if the amount voided is inadequate based on I.V. fluid intake), percuss over the symphysis pubis for bladder distention (especially in patients receiving anticholinergics). Patients who have had a laparoscopic cholecystectomy may be discharged the same day or within 48 hours after surgery. These patients should have minimal pain, be able to tolerate a regular diet within 24 hours after surgery, and be able to return to normal activity within a few days to a week.
• Encourage deep-breathing and leg exercises every hour. The patient should ambulate after surgery. Provide elastic stockings to support leg muscles and promote venous blood flow in order to prevent stasis and clot formation.
• Evaluate the location, duration, and character of any pain. Administer adequate medication to relieve pain, especially before such activities as deep breathing and ambulation, which increase pain. Abdominal distention resolves spontaneously as bowel function returns.
• At discharge (usually 1 to 2 days after laparoscopy), advise the patient

against heavy lifting or straining for 6 weeks. Urge him to walk daily. Tell him that food restrictions are unnecessary unless he has an intolerance to a specific food or some underlying condition (such as diabetes, atherosclerosis, or obesity) that requires such restriction.

CHRONIC FATIGUE AND IMMUNE DYSFUNCTION SYNDROME

This recently recognized illness goes by several names, including chronic fatigue and immune dysfunction syndrome (CFIDS), chronic fatigue syndrome, chronic Epstein-Barr virus (EBV), myalgic encephalomyelitis, and "Yuppie flu." It's typically marked by debilitating fatigue, neurologic abnormalities, and persistent symptoms that suggest chronic mononucleosis. It commonly occurs in adults under age 45, primarily in women.

Causes
Although the cause of CFIDS is unknown, researchers suspect that it may be found in human herpesvirus-6 or in other herpesviruses, enteroviruses, or retroviruses. Rising levels of antibodies to EBV, once thought to implicate EBV infection as the cause of CFIDS, are now considered a result of this disease.

CFIDS may be associated with a reaction to viral illness that is complicated by dysfunctional immune response and by other factors that may include gender, age, genetic disposition, prior illness, stress, and environment.

Signs and symptoms
The characteristic symptom of CFIDS is prolonged, often overwhelming fatigue that is commonly associated with a varying complex of other symptoms. To aid identification of the disease, the Centers for Disease Control (CDC) uses a "working case definition" to group symptoms and severity. (See *CDC Criteria for Diagnosing CFIDS*, page 200.)

Diagnosis
The cause and nature of CFIDS are still unknown and no single test unequivocally confirms its presence. Therefore, the diagnosis is based on the patient's history and the CDC's criteria. Because the CDC criteria are admittedly a working concept that may not include all forms of this disease and are based on symptoms that can result from other diseases, a diagnosis is difficult and uncertain.

Treatment
No therapy is known to cure CFIDS. Experimental treatments include the antiviral acyclovir and selected immunomodulating agents such as I.V. gamma globulin, ampligen, transfer factor, and others.

Treatment of symptoms may include tricyclic antidepressants (doxepin), histamine$_2$-blocking agents (cimetidine), and antianxiety agents (alprazolam). In some patients, avoidance of environmental irritants and certain foods may help to relieve symptoms.

Special considerations
• Refer the patient to the CFIDS Association for information as well as to local support groups; supportive contact with others who share this disease may benefit the patient.
• If appropriate, suggest psychological counseling.

CDC Criteria for Diagnosing CFIDS

To meet the case definition by the Centers for Disease Control and Prevention (CDC) for chronic fatigue and immune dysfunction syndrome (CFIDS), a patient must fulfill two "major criteria": either 8 of 11 "symptom criteria," or 6 of the "symptom criteria" and 2 of 3 "physical criteria."

Major criteria
• New onset of persistent or relapsing debilitating fatigue in a person without a history of similar symptoms; fatigue doesn't resolve with bed rest and is severe enough to reduce or impair average daily activity by 50% for 6 months.
• Exclusion of other disorders after evaluation through history, physical examination, and laboratory findings.

Symptom criteria
The symptom criteria include the initial development of the main symptom complex over a few hours or days and the following 10 other symptoms:

• profound or prolonged fatigue, especially after exercise levels that would have been easily tolerated before
• low-grade fever
• painful lymph nodes
• muscle weakness
• sleep disturbances (insomnia or hypersomnia)
• headaches of a new type, severity, or pattern
• migratory arthralgia without joint swelling or redness
• photophobia, forgetfulness, irritability, confusion, depression, transient visual scotomata, difficulty thinking, and inability to concentrate.

Physical criteria
These criteria must be recorded on at least two occasions, at least 1 month apart:
• low-grade fever
• nonexudative pharyngitis
• palpable or tender nodes.

Chronic Granulomatous Disease

In this disease, abnormal neutrophil metabolism impairs phagocytosis—one of the body's chief defense mechanisms—resulting in increased susceptibility to low-virulent or nonpathogenic organisms, such as *Staphylococcus epidermidis*, *Escherichia coli*, *Aspergillus*, and *Nocardia*. Phagocytes attracted to sites of infection can engulf these invading organisms but are unable to destroy them. Patients with chronic granulomatous disease (CGD) may develop granulomatous inflammation, which leads to ischemic tissue damage.

Causes
CGD is usually inherited as an X-linked trait, although a variant form—probably autosomal recessive—also exists. The genetic defect may be linked to deficiency of the enzyme NADH, NADPH oxidase, or NADH reductase.

Signs and symptoms

Usually, the patient with CGD displays signs and symptoms by age 2, associated with infections of the skin, lymph nodes, lung, liver, and bone. Skin infection is characterized by small, well-localized areas of tenderness. Seborrheic dermatitis of the scalp and axilla is also common. Lymph node infection typically causes marked lymphadenopathy with draining lymph nodes and hepatosplenomegaly.

Many patients develop liver abscess, which may be recurrent and multiple. Abdominal tenderness, fever, anorexia, and nausea point to abscess formation. Other common infections include osteomyelitis, which causes localized pain and fever; pneumonia; and gingivitis with severe periodontal disease.

Diagnosis

Clinical features of osteomyelitis, pneumonia, liver abscess, or chronic lymphadenopathy in a young child provide the first clues to a diagnosis of CGD.

An important tool for confirming this diagnosis is the nitroblue tetrazolium (NBT) test. A clear yellow dye, NBT is normally reduced by neutrophil metabolism, resulting in a color change from yellow to blue. Quantifying this color change estimates the degree of neutrophil metabolism. Patients with CGD show impaired NBT reduction, indicating abnormal neutrophil metabolism. Another test measures the rate of intracellular killing by neutrophils. In CGD, killing is delayed or absent.

Other laboratory values may support the diagnosis or help monitor disease activity. Osteomyelitis typically causes an elevated white blood cell count and erythrocyte sedimentation rate; bone scans help locate and measure such infections. Recurrent liver or lung infection may eventually cause abnormal function studies. Cell-mediated and humoral immunity are usually normal in CGD, although some patients have hypergammaglobulinemia.

Treatment

Early, aggressive treatment of infection is the chief goal in caring for a patient with CGD. Areas of suspected infection should be biopsied or cultured, with broad-spectrum antibiotics usually started immediately—without waiting for the results of cultures. Confirmed abscesses may be drained or surgically removed.

Many patients with CGD receive a combination of I.V. antibiotics, often extended beyond the usual 10- to 14-day course. However, for fungal infections with *Aspergillus* or *Nocardia,* treatment involves amphotericin B in gradually increasing doses to achieve a maximum cumulative dose.

To help treat life-threatening or antibiotic-resistant infection or to help localize infection, the patient may receive granulocyte transfusions—usually once daily until the crisis has passed. Transfusions shouldn't be given for 6 hours before or after amphotericin B to avoid severe pulmonary edema and possibly respiratory arrest.

Interferon is an experimental but promising treatment in CGD.

Special considerations

• If prophylactic antibiotics are ordered, teach the patient and his family how to administer them and how to recognize adverse reactions. Advise them to promptly report any signs or symptoms of infection. Stress the importance of good nutrition and hygiene, especially meticulous skin and mouth care.

• During hospitalizations, encourage the patient to continue his activities of daily living as much as possible. Try to arrange for a tutor to help the child keep up with his schoolwork.

• Provide meticulous wound care after drainage or removal of an abscess, including irrigation or packing.

• During I.V. drug therapy, monitor vital signs frequently and rotate the I.V. site every 48 to 72 hours.

• During granulocyte transfusions, watch for fever and chills. (These effects can sometimes be prevented by premedication with acetaminophen.)

CHRONIC MUCOCUTANEOUS CANDIDIASIS

This form of candidiasis (moniliasis) usually develops during the first year of life but occasionally may occur as late as the twenties. It affects both males and females.

Chronic mucocutaneous candidiasis is characterized by repeated infection with *Candida albicans* that may result from an inherited defect in the cell-mediated (T cell) immune system. (The humoral immune system, mediated by B cells, is intact and gives a normal antibody response to *C. albicans*.) In some patients, an autoimmune response affecting the endocrine system may induce various endocrinopathies.

Despite chronic candidiasis, these patients rarely die of systemic infection. Instead, they usually die of hepatic or endocrine failure. The prognosis for chronic mucocutaneous candidiasis depends on the severity of the associated endocrinopathy. Patients with associated endocrinopathy rarely live beyond their thirties.

Causes

Although no characteristic immunologic defects have been identified in this infection, many patients are anergic to various antigens or to *Candida* alone. In some patients, anergy may result from deficient migration inhibition factor, a mediator normally produced by lymphocytes.

Signs and symptoms

Chronic candidal infections can affect the skin, mucous membranes, nails, and vagina, usually causing large, circular lesions. These infections rarely produce systemic symptoms, but in late stages they may be associated with recurrent respiratory tract infections.

Other associated conditions include severe viral infections that may precede the onset of endocrinopathy and, sometimes, hepatitis. Involvement of the mouth, nose, and palate may cause speech and eating difficulties.

Signs and symptoms of endocrinopathy are peculiar to the organ involved. Tetany and hypocalcemia are most common and are associated with hypoparathyroidism. Addison's disease, hypothyroidism, diabetes, and pernicious anemia are also connected with chronic mucocutaneous candidiasis. Psychiatric disorders are likely because of disfigurement and multiple endocrine aberrations.

Diagnosis

Laboratory findings usually show a normal circulating T cell count, although it may be decreased. Most patients don't have delayed hypersensitivity skin tests to *Candida*, even during the infectious stage. Migration inhibiting factor that indicates the presence of activated T cells may not respond to *Candida*.

Nonimmunologic abnormalities result from endocrinopathy and may include hypocalcemia, abnormal liver function studies, hyperglycemia, iron deficiency, and abnormal vitamin B_{12} absorption (pernicious anemia). The diagnosis must rule out other immunodeficiency disorders associated with chronic *Candida* infection, especially DiGeorge's syndrome, ataxia-telangiectasia, and severe combined immunodeficiency disease, all of which produce severe immunologic defects.

After a diagnosis, the patient needs evaluation of adrenal, pituitary, thyroid, gonadal, pancreatic, and parathyroid functions, with careful follow-up. The disease is progressive, and most patients eventually develop endocrinopathy.

Treatment

Although treatment aims to control infection, it isn't always successful. Topical antifungal agents are often ineffective against chronic mucocutaneous candidiasis. Miconazole and nystatin are sometimes useful, but ultimately fail to control this infection.

Systemic infections may not be fatal, but they're serious enough to warrant vigorous treatment. Oral ketaconazole and injected thymosin and levamisole have had some positive effect. Oral or intramuscular iron replacement may also be necessary.

Treatment may also include plastic surgery, when possible.

Special considerations

• Teach the patient about the progressive manifestations of the disease and emphasize the importance of seeing an endocrinologist for regular checkups.
• Suggest counseling to help the patient cope with disfigurement.

CHRONIC OBSTRUCTIVE PULMONARY DISEASE

This chronic airway obstruction — also called chronic obstructive lung disease — results from emphysema, chronic bronchitis, asthma, or any combination of these disorders. Usually, more than one of these underlying conditions coexist; most often, bronchitis and emphysema occur together. (See *Understanding chronic obstructive pulmonary disease,* pages 204 to 207.)

The most common chronic lung disease, chronic obstructive pulmonary disease (COPD) affects an estimated 17 million Americans, and its incidence is rising. It affects men more often than women, probably because, until recently, men were more likely to smoke heavily. It doesn't always produce symptoms and causes only minimal disability in many patients. However, COPD tends to worsen with time.

Causes

Predisposing factors include cigarette smoking, recurrent or chronic respiratory infections, air pollution, and allergies. Familial and hereditary factors (for example, deficiency of $alpha_1$-antitrypsin) may also predispose a person to COPD.

Smoking is by far the most important of these factors; it impairs ciliary action and macrophage function, and causes inflammation in airways, increased mucus production, destruction of alveolar septae, and peribronchiolar fibrosis. Early inflammatory changes may reverse if the patient stops smoking before lung destruction is extensive.

Signs and symptoms

The typical patient, a long-term cigarette smoker, has no symptoms until middle age, when his ability to exercise or do strenuous work gradually starts to decline, and he begins to develop a productive cough. While subtle at first, these signs become more pronounced as the patient gets older and the disease progresses.

Eventually the patient develops dyspnea on minimal exertion, frequent respiratory infections, intermittent or

(Text continues on page 206.)

UNDERSTANDING CHRONIC OBSTRUCTIVE PULMONARY DISEASE

DISEASE	CAUSES AND PATHOPHYSIOLOGY	CLINICAL FEATURES
Emphysema • Abnormal irreversible enlargement of air spaces distal to terminal bronchioles due to destruction of alveolar walls, resulting in decreased elastic recoil properties of lungs • Most common cause of death from respiratory disease in the United States	• Cigarette smoking, deficiency of alpha$_1$-antitrypsin • Recurrent inflammation associated with release of proteolytic enzymes from cells in lungs causes bronchiolar and alveolar wall damage and, ultimately, destruction. Loss of lung supporting structure results in decreased elastic recoil and airway collapse on expiration. Destruction of alveolar walls decreases surface area for gas exchange.	• Insidious onset, with dyspnea the predominant symptom • *Other signs and symptoms of long-term disease:* chronic cough, anorexia, weight loss, malaise, barrel chest, use of accessory muscles of respiration, prolonged expiratory period with grunting, pursed-lip breathing and tachypnea, and peripheral cyanosis • *Complications* include recurrent respiratory tract infections, cor pulmonale, and respiratory failure.
Chronic bronchitis • Excessive mucus production with productive cough for at least 3 months a year for 2 successive years • Only a minority of patients with the clinical syndrome of chronic bronchitis develop significant airway obstruction.	• Severity of disease related to amount and duration of smoking; respiratory infection exacerbates symptoms. • Hypertrophy and hyperplasia of bronchial mucous glands, increased goblet cells, damage to cilia, squamous metaplasia of columnar epithelium, and chronic leukocytic and lymphocytic infiltration of bronchial walls; widespread inflammation, distortion, narrowing of airways, and mucus within the airways produce resistance in small airways and cause severe ventilation-perfusion imbalance	• Insidious onset, with productive cough and exertional dyspnea as predominant symptoms • *Other signs and symptoms:* colds associated with increased sputum production and worsening dyspnea that take progressively longer to resolve; copious sputum (gray, white, or yellow); weight gain due to edema; cyanosis; tachypnea; wheezing; prolonged expiratory time, use of accessory muscles of respiration

CONFIRMING DIAGNOSTIC MEASURES

MANAGEMENT

• *Physical examination:* hyperresonance on percussion, decreased breath sounds, expiratory prolongation, quiet heart sounds
• *Chest X-ray:* in advanced disease, flattened diaphragm, reduced vascular markings at lung periphery, overaeration of lungs, vertical heart, enlarged anteroposterior chest diameter, large retrosternal air space
• *Pulmonary function tests:* increased residual volume, total lung capacity, and compliance; decreased vital capacity, diffusing capacity, and expiratory volumes
• *Arterial blood gases (ABGs):* reduced Po_2 with normal Pco_2 until late in disease
• *Electrocardiography (ECG):* tall, symmetrical P waves in leads II, III, and AV_F; vertical QRS axis; signs of right ventricular hypertrophy late in disease
• *Red blood cells:* increased hemoglobin late in disease when persistent severe hypoxia is present

• Bronchodilators, such as beta-adrenergics and theophylline, to reverse bronchospasm and promote mucociliary clearance
• Antibiotics to treat respiratory infection; flu vaccine to prevent influenza; Pneumovax to prevent pneumococcal pneumonia; and mucolytics
• Adequate fluid intake and, in selected patients, chest physiotherapy to mobilize secretions
• O_2 at low-flow settings to treat hypoxia
• Avoidance of smoking and air pollutants
• Aerosolized or systemic corticosteroids

• *Physical examination:* rhonchi and wheezing on auscultation, expiratory prolongation, neck vein distention, pedal edema
• *Chest X-ray:* may show hyperinflation and increased bronchovascular markings
• *Pulmonary function tests:* increased residual volume, decreased vital capacity and forced expiratory volumes, normal static compliance and diffusing capacity
• *Arterial blood gases:* decreased Po_2, normal or increased Pco_2
• *Sputum:* contains evidence of infection
• *ECG:* may show atrial arrhythmias; peaked P waves in leads II, III, and AV_F; and, occasionally, right ventricular hypertrophy

• Antibiotics for infections
• Avoidance of smoking and air pollutants
• Bronchodilators to relieve bronchospasm and facilitate mucociliary clearance
• Adequate fluid intake and chest physiotherapy to mobilize secretions
• Ultrasonic or mechanical nebulizer treatments to loosen secretions and aid in mobilization
• Occasionally, corticosteroids
• Diuretics for edema
• Oxygen for hypoxia

(continued)

Understanding Chronic Obstructive Pulmonary Disease
(continued)

DISEASE	CAUSES AND PATHOPHYSIOLOGY	CLINICAL FEATURES
Asthma • Increased bronchial reactivity to a variety of stimuli, which produces episodic bronchospasm and airway obstruction in conjunction with airway inflammation. • Asthma with onset in adulthood: often without distinct allergies; asthma with onset in childhood: often associated with definite allergens. Status asthmaticus is an acute asthma attack with severe bronchospasm that fails to clear with bronchodilator therapy. • *Prognosis:* More than half of asthmatic children become asymptomatic as adults; more than half of asthmatics with onset after age 15 have persistent disease with occasional severe attacks.	• Possible mechanisms include allergy (family tendency, seasonal occurrence); allergic reaction results in release of mast cell vasoactive and bronchospastic mediators. • Upper airway infection, exercise, anxiety and, rarely, coughing or laughing can precipitate an asthma attack; nocturnal flare-ups are common. • Paroxysmal airway obstruction associated with nasal polyps may be seen in response to aspirin or indomethacin ingestion. • Airway obstruction from spasm of bronchial smooth muscle narrows airways; inflammatory edema of the bronchial wall and inspissation of tenacious mucoid secretions are also important, particularly in status asthmaticus.	• History of intermittent attacks of dyspnea and wheezing • Mild wheezing progresses to severe dyspnea, audible wheezing, chest tightness (a feeling of being unable to breathe), and a cough that produces thick mucus. • *Other signs:* prolonged expiration, intercostal and supraclavicular retraction on inspiration, use of accessory muscles of respiration, flaring nostrils, tachypnea, tachycardia, perspiration, and flushing; patients often have symptoms of eczema and allergic rhinitis (hay fever). • Status asthmaticus, unless treated promptly, can progress to respiratory failure.

continuous hypoxemia, and grossly abnormal pulmonary function studies. In its advanced form, COPD may cause thoracic deformities, overwhelming disability, cor pulmonale, severe respiratory failure, and death.

Treatment

The main goal of treatment is to relieve symptoms and prevent complications. Bronchodilators can help alleviate bronchospasm and enhance mucociliary clearance of secretions. Effective coughing, postural drainage, and chest physiotherapy can help mobilize secretions.

Administration of low concentrations of oxygen helps relieve symptoms; arterial blood gas analysis determines oxygen need and helps avoid carbon dioxide narcosis.

Antibiotics allow treatment of respiratory infections. Pneumococcal vaccination and annual influenza vaccinations are important preventive measures.

CONFIRMING DIAGNOSTIC MEASURES

- *Physical examination:* usually normal between attacks; auscultation shows rhonchi and wheezing throughout lung fields on expiration and, at times, inspiration; absent or diminished breath sounds during severe obstruction. Loud bilateral wheezes may be grossly audible; chest is hyperinflated.
- *Chest X-ray:* hyperinflated lungs with air trapping during attack; normal during remission
- *Sputum:* presence of Curschmann's spirals (casts of airways), Charcot-Leyden crystals, and eosinophils
- *Pulmonary function tests:* during attacks, decreased forced expiratory volumes that improve significantly after inhaled bronchodilator; increased residual volume and, occasionally, total lung capacity; may be normal between attacks
- *ABGs:* decreased Po_2; decreased, normal, or increased Pco_2 (in severe attack)
- *ECG:* sinus tachycardia during an attack; severe attack may produce signs of cor pulmonale (right axis deviation, peaked P wave) that resolve after the attack.
- *Skin tests:* may identify allergens

MANAGEMENT

- Aerosol containing beta-adrenergic agents such as metaproterenol or albuterol; also oral beta-adrenergic agents (terbutaline) and oral methylxanthines (theophylline). Many patients require inhaled, oral, or I.V. corticosteroids.
- *Emergency treatment:* O_2 therapy, corticosteroids, and bronchodilators, such as S.C. epinephrine, I.V. theophylline, and inhaled agents (such as metaproterenol, albuterol, or ipratropium bromide).
- Monitor for deteriorating respiratory status and note sputum characteristics; provide adequate fluid intake and oxygen.
- *Prevention:* Tell the patient to avoid possible allergens and to use antihistamines, decongestants, cromolyn powder by inhalation, and oral or aerosol bronchodilators, as needed. Explain the influence of stress and anxiety on asthma as well as its frequent association with exercise (particularly running), cold air, and nighttime flare-ups.

Special considerations

Most COPD patients receive outpatient treatment, so provide the following comprehensive patient teaching to help them comply with therapy and understand the nature of this chronic, progressive disease.

- If programs in pulmonary rehabilitation are available, encourage the patient to enroll.
- Urge the patient to stop smoking and avoid other respiratory irritants. Suggest that he install an air conditioner with an air filter in his home; it may prove helpful.
- Familiarize the patient with his prescribed bronchodilators.
- Teach the patient and his family how to recognize early signs of infection; warn the patient to avoid contact with persons with respiratory infections.
- Encourage good oral hygiene to help prevent infection.
- If the patient is receiving an antibiotic, stress the need to complete the prescribed course.

• To strengthen the muscles of respiration, teach the patient to take slow, deep breaths and exhale through pursed lips.

• To help mobilize secretions, teach the patient how to cough effectively.

• If the patient with copious secretions has difficulty mobilizing secretions, teach his family how to perform postural drainage and chest physiotherapy.

• If secretions are thick, urge the patient to drink 12 to 15 8-ounce (240-ml) glasses of fluid a day. A home humidifier may be beneficial, particularly in the winter.

• If the patient is to continue oxygen therapy at home, teach him how to use the equipment correctly. Patients with COPD rarely require more than 2 to 3 L/minute to maintain adequate oxygenation. Higher flow rates will further increase the partial pressure of oxygen level, but patients whose ventilatory drive is largely based on hypoxemia will often develop a markedly increased partial pressure of carbon dioxide. In such patients, chemoreceptors in the brain are relatively insensitive to the increase in carbon dioxide.

• Teach the patient and his family that excessive oxygen therapy may eliminate the hypoxic respiratory drive, causing confusion and drowsiness, which are signs of carbon dioxide narcosis.

• Emphasize the importance of a balanced diet. Because the patient may tire easily when eating, suggest frequent, small meals and consider using oxygen, administered by nasal cannula, during meals.

• Help the patient and his family adjust their lifestyles to accommodate the limitations imposed by this debilitating chronic disease. Instruct the patient to allow for daily rest periods and to exercise daily as directed.

• As COPD progresses, encourage the patient to discuss his fears.

• To help prevent COPD, advise all people, especially those with a family history of COPD or those in its early stages, not to smoke.

• Assist in the early detection of COPD by urging persons to have periodic physical examinations, including spirometry and medical evaluation of a chronic cough, and to seek treatment for recurring respiratory infections promptly.

• Set a good example by not smoking.

CIRRHOSIS

This chronic hepatic disease is characterized by diffuse destruction and fibrotic regeneration of hepatic cells. As necrotic tissue yields to fibrosis, cirrhosis alters liver structure and normal vasculature, impairs blood and lymph flow, and ultimately causes hepatic insufficiency. (See *Circulation in portal hypertension*.)

Cirrhosis is twice as common in men as in women and is especially prevalent among malnourished chronic alcoholics over age 50. Mortality is high: Many patients die within 5 years of onset. The prognosis is better in noncirrhotic forms of hepatic fibrosis, which cause minimal hepatic dysfunction and don't destroy liver cells.

Causes
The following clinical types of cirrhosis reflect its diverse etiology:

• *Portal, nutritional,* or *alcoholic cirrhosis* (Laënnec's), the most common type, occurs in 30% to 50% of cirrhotic patients, up to 90% of whom have a history of alcoholism. Liver damage results from malnutrition, especially of dietary protein, and chronic alcohol ingestion. Fibrous tissue forms

Circulation in Portal Hypertension

As portal pressure rises, blood will back up into the spleen and flow through collateral channels to the venous system, bypassing the liver and causing esophageal varices.

Esophagus

Esophageal varices

Relative increase in hepatic artery flow

Portal vein pressure rises from 10 to 20 mm Hg or above

Superior vena cava

Azygos vein

Right atrium

Inferior vena cava

Hepatic vein

Enlarged spleen

Short gastric vein

Left gastric vein

Splenic vein

in portal areas and around central veins.

• *Biliary cirrhosis* (15% to 20% of patients) results from bile duct diseases, which suppress bile flow.

• *Postnecrotic (posthepatitic) cirrhosis* (10% to 30% of patients) stems from various types of hepatitis.

• *Pigment cirrhosis* (5% to 10% of patients) may stem from disorders such as hemochromatosis.

• *Cardiac cirrhosis* (rare) refers to liver damage caused by right heart failure.

• *Idiopathic cirrhosis* (about 10% of patients) has no known cause.

Noncirrhotic fibrosis may result from schistosomiasis or congenital hepatic fibrosis, or may be idiopathic.

Signs and symptoms

Clinical manifestations of cirrhosis and fibrosis are similar for all types, regardless of cause. Early indications are vague but usually include GI symptoms (anorexia, indigestion, nausea, vomiting, constipation, or diarrhea) and dull abdominal ache.

Major and late symptoms develop as a result of hepatic insufficiency and portal hypertension, and include the following:

• *respiratory* — pleural effusion and limited thoracic expansion because of abdominal ascites, interfering with efficient gas exchange and leading to hypoxia

• *central nervous system* — progressive symptoms of hepatic encephalopathy:

lethargy, mental changes, slurred speech, asterixis (flapping tremor), peripheral neuritis, paranoia, hallucinations, extreme obtundation, and coma
• *hematologic* — bleeding tendencies (nosebleeds, easy bruising, bleeding gums), anemia
• *endocrine* — testicular atrophy, menstrual irregularities, gynecomastia, and loss of chest and axillary hair
• *skin* — severe pruritus, extreme dryness, poor tissue turgor, abnormal pigmentation, spider angiomas, palmar erythema and, possibly, jaundice
• *hepatic* — jaundice, hepatomegaly, ascites, edema of the legs, hepatic encephalopathy, and hepatorenal syndrome constitute the other major effects of full-fledged cirrhosis
• *miscellaneous* — musty breath, enlarged superficial abdominal veins, muscle atrophy, pain in the upper right abdominal quadrant that worsens when the patient sits up or leans forward, palpable liver or spleen, and a temperature of 101° to 103° F (38.3° to 39.4° C). Bleeding from esophageal varices results from portal hypertension.

Diagnosis
A liver biopsy, the definitive test for cirrhosis, detects destruction and fibrosis of hepatic tissue. A liver scan shows abnormal thickening and a liver mass.

Cholecystography and cholangiography visualize the gallbladder and the biliary duct system, respectively; splenoportal venography visualizes the portal venous system. Percutaneous transhepatic cholangiography differentiates extrahepatic from intrahepatic obstructive jaundice and discloses hepatic pathology and the presence of gallstones.

The following laboratory findings are characteristic of cirrhosis:
• decreased white blood cell count and decreased levels of hemoglobin and hematocrit, albumin, serum electrolytes (sodium, potassium, chloride, and magnesium), and cholinesterase
• elevated levels of globulin, serum ammonia, total bilirubin, alkaline phosphatase, serum aspartate aminotransferase, serum alanine aminotransferase, and lactate dehydrogenase and increased thymol turbidity
• anemia, neutropenia, and thrombocytopenia, characterized by prolonged prothrombin and partial thromboplastin times
• deficiencies of vitamins A, B_{12}, C, and K; folic acid; and iron
• positive tests for galactose tolerance and urine bilirubin
• fecal urobilinogen levels greater than 280 mg/24 hours
• urine urobilinogen levels greater than 1.16 mg/24 hours.

Treatment
The goals of treatment include removing or alleviating the underlying cause of cirrhosis or fibrosis, preventing further liver damage, and preventing or treating complications.

Dietary measures
The patient may benefit from a high-calorie and moderate- to high-protein diet, but developing hepatic encephalopathy mandates restricted protein intake. In addition, sodium is usually restricted to 200 to 500 mg/day, fluids to 1,000 to 1,500 ml/day.

If the patient's condition continues to deteriorate, he may need tube feedings or hyperalimentation. Other supportive measures include supplemental vitamins — A, B complex, D, and K — to compensate for the liver's inability to store them, and vitamin B_{12}, folic acid, and thiamine for deficiency anemia. Rest, moderate exercise, and avoidance of exposure to infections and toxic agents are essential.

Drug therapy

In cirrhosis, drug therapy requires special caution because the cirrhotic liver can't detoxify harmful substances efficiently. Alcohol is prohibited; sedatives should be avoided or prescribed with great care.

When absolutely necessary, antiemetics, such as trimethobenzamide or benzquinamide, may be given for nausea; vasopressin, for esophageal varices; and diuretics, such as furosemide or spironolactone, for edema. However, diuretics require careful monitoring; fluid and electrolyte imbalance may precipitate hepatic encephalopathy.

Other treatment

Paracentesis and infusions of salt-poor albumin may alleviate ascites. Surgical procedures include ligation of varices, splenectomy, esophagogastric resection, and splenorenal or portacaval anastomosis to relieve portal hypertension. Programs for prevention of cirrhosis usually emphasize avoidance of alcohol.

Special considerations

• Check skin, gums, stools, and emesis regularly for bleeding. Apply pressure to injection sites to prevent bleeding. Warn the patient against taking aspirin, straining during defecation, and blowing his nose or sneezing too vigorously. Suggest using an electric razor and soft toothbrush.
• Observe closely for signs of behavioral or personality changes, especially increasing stupor, lethargy, hallucinations, and neuromuscular dysfunction. Arouse the patient periodically to determine his level of consciousness. Watch for asterixis, a sign of developing hepatic encephalopathy.
• To assess fluid retention, weigh the patient and measure his abdominal girth daily, inspect the ankles and sacrum for dependent edema, and accurately record intake and output. Carefully evaluate the patient before, during, and after paracentesis; this drastic loss of fluid may induce shock.
• To prevent skin breakdown associated with edema and pruritus, avoid using soap when you bathe the patient; instead, use lubricating lotion or moisturizing agents. Handle the patient gently, and turn and reposition him often to keep his skin intact.
• Tell the patient that rest and good nutrition will conserve energy and decrease metabolic demands on the liver. Urge him to eat frequent small meals. Stress the need to avoid infections and abstain from alcohol.
• Refer the patient to Alcoholics Anonymous, if necessary.

CLUBFOOT

The most common congenital disorder of the lower extremities, clubfoot, or talipes, is marked primarily by a deformed talus and shortened Achilles tendon, which give the foot a characteristic clublike appearance. In talipes equinovarus, the foot points downward (equinus) and turns inward (varus), while the front of the foot curls toward the heel (forefoot adduction).

Clubfoot, which has an incidence of approximately 1 per 1,000 live births, usually occurs bilaterally and is twice as common in boys as in girls. It may be associated with other birth defects, such as myelomeningocele, spina bifida, and arthrogryposis. Clubfoot is correctable with prompt treatment.

Causes

A combination of genetic and environmental factors in utero appears to cause clubfoot. Heredity is a definite factor in some cases, although the mechanism of transmission is undetermined. If a child is born with club-foot, his sibling has a 1 in 35 chance of being born with the same anomaly. Children of a parent with clubfoot have 1 chance in 10.

In children without a family history of clubfoot, this anomaly seems linked to arrested development during the ninth and tenth weeks of embryonic life when the feet are formed. Researchers also suspect muscle abnormalities, leading to variations in length and tendon insertions, as possible causes of clubfoot.

Signs and symptoms

Talipes equinovarus varies in severity. Deformity may be so extreme that the toes touch the inside of the ankle, or it may be only vaguely apparent.

In every case, the talus is deformed, the Achilles tendon shortened, and the calcaneus somewhat shortened and flattened. Depending on the degree of the varus deformity, the calf muscles are shortened and underdeveloped, with soft-tissue contractures at the site of the deformity. The foot is tight in its deformed position and resists manual efforts to push it back into normal position.

Clubfoot is painless, except in older, arthritic patients. In older children, clubfoot may be secondary to paralysis, poliomyelitis, or cerebral palsy, in which case treatment must include management of the underlying disease.

Diagnosis

An early diagnosis of clubfoot is usually no problem because the deformity is obvious. In subtle deformity, however, true clubfoot must be distinguished from apparent clubfoot (metatarsus varus or pigeon toe).

Apparent clubfoot results when a fetus maintains a position in utero that gives his feet a clubfoot appearance at birth. This can usually be corrected manually.

Another form of apparent clubfoot is inversion of the feet, resulting from the peroneal type of progressive muscular atrophy and progressive muscular dystrophy. In true clubfoot, X-rays show superimposition of the talus and the calcaneus and a ladderlike appearance of the metatarsals.

Treatment

Appropriate treatment for clubfoot is administered in three stages:
• correcting the deformity
• maintaining the correction until the foot regains normal muscle balance
• observing the foot closely for several years to prevent the deformity from recurring.

In newborns, corrective treatment for true clubfoot should begin *at once*. An infant's foot contains large amounts of cartilage; the muscles, ligaments, and tendons are supple. The ideal time to begin treatment is during the first few days and weeks of life—when the foot is most malleable.

Sequential correction

Clubfoot deformities are usually corrected in sequential order: forefoot adduction first, then varus (or inversion), then equinus (or plantar flexion). Trying to correct all three deformities at once only results in a misshapen, rocker-bottomed foot.

Forefoot adduction is corrected by uncurling the front of the foot away from the heel (forefoot abduction); the varus deformity is corrected by turning the foot so the sole faces outward (eversion); and finally, equinus is corrected by casting the foot with the toes pointing up (dorsiflexion). This last correction may have to be supplemented with a subcutaneous tenotomy of the Achilles tendon and posterior capsulotomy of the ankle joint.

Treatment methods

Several therapeutic methods have been tested and found effective in correcting clubfoot. The first is simple manipulation and casting, whereby the foot is gently manipulated into a partially corrected position, then held there in a cast for several days or weeks. (The skin should be painted with a nonirritating adhesive liquid beforehand to prevent the cast from slipping.)

After the cast is removed, the foot is manipulated into an even better position and casted again. This procedure is repeated as many times as necessary. In some cases, the shape of the cast can be transformed through a series of wedging maneuvers, instead of changing the cast each time.

After correction of clubfoot, proper foot alignment should be maintained through exercise, night splints, and orthopedic shoes. With manipulating and casting, correction usually takes about 3 months. The Denis Browne splint, a device that consists of two padded, metal footplates connected by a flat, horizontal bar, is sometimes used as a follow-up measure to help promote bilateral correction and strengthen the foot muscles.

Resistant clubfoot may require surgery. Older children, for example, with recurrent or neglected clubfoot usually need surgery.

Tenotomy, tendon transfer, stripping of the plantar fascia, and capsulotomy are some of the surgical procedures that may be used. In severe cases, bone surgery (wedge resections, osteotomy, or astragalectomy) may be appropriate. After surgery, a cast is applied to preserve the correction.

Whenever clubfoot is severe enough to require surgery, it's rarely totally correctable. However, surgery can usually ameliorate the deformity.

Special considerations

• Look for any exaggerated attitudes in an infant's feet. Make sure you can recognize the difference between true clubfoot and apparent clubfoot. Don't use excessive force in trying to manipulate a clubfoot. The foot with apparent clubfoot moves easily.

• Stress the importance of prompt treatment to parents. Make sure they understand that clubfoot demands immediate therapy and orthopedic supervision until growth is completed.

• After casting, elevate the child's feet with pillows. Check the toes every 1 to 2 hours for temperature, color, sensation, motion, and capillary refill time; watch for edema. Before a child in a clubfoot cast is discharged, teach parents to recognize circulatory impairment.

• Insert plastic petals over the top edges of a new cast while it's still wet to keep urine from soaking and softening the cast. When the cast is dry, "petal" the edges with adhesive tape to keep out plaster crumbs and prevent skin irritation.

• Perform good skin care under the cast edges every 4 hours. After washing and drying the skin, rub it with alcohol. (Don't use oils or powders; they tend to macerate the skin.)

• Warn parents of an older child not to let the foot part of the cast get soft and thin from wear. If it does, much of the correction may be lost.

• When the wedging method is being used, check circulatory status frequently; it may be impaired because of increased pressure on tissues and blood vessels. The equinus correction especially places considerable strain on ligaments, blood vessels, and tendons.

• After surgery, elevate the child's feet with pillows to decrease swelling and pain. Watch for signs of discomfort or pain. Try to locate the source of pain — it may result from cast pressure, not the incision. If bleeding occurs under the cast, circle the location and mark the time on the cast. Watch for indications that the bleeding is spreading.

• Explain to the older child and his parents that surgery can improve clubfoot with good function, but can't totally correct it; the affected calf muscle will remain slightly underdeveloped.

• Emphasize the need for long-term orthopedic care to maintain correction. Teach the parents the prescribed exercises that their child can do at home.

• Urge the parents to make their child wear corrective shoes as ordered and splints during naps and at night. Make sure they understand that treatment for clubfoot continues during the entire growth period. Correcting this defect permanently takes time and patience.

COAL WORKER'S PNEUMOCONIOSIS

This disease goes by several names, including black lung disease, coal miner's disease, miner's asthma, anthracosis, anthracosilicosis, and coal worker's pneumoconiosis (CWP). This progressive nodular pulmonary disease occurs in two forms.

Simple CWP is characterized by small lung opacities. In complicated CWP, also known as progressive massive fibrosis (PMF), masses of fibrous tissue occasionally develop in the lungs of patients with simple CWP.

The risk of developing CWP depends upon the duration of exposure to coal dust (usually 15 years or longer), intensity of exposure (dust count, particle size), location of the mine, silica content of the coal (anthracite coal has the highest silica content), and the worker's susceptibility. Incidence of CWP is highest among anthracite coal miners in the eastern United States.

The prognosis varies. Simple asymptomatic disease is self-limiting, although progression to complicated CWP is more likely if CWP begins after a relatively short period of exposure. Complicated CWP may be disabling, resulting in severe ventilatory failure and right heart failure secondary to pulmonary hypertension.

Causes

CWP is caused by the inhalation and prolonged retention of respirable coal dust particles (less than 5 microns in diameter).

Simple CWP

This form of CWP results in the formation of macules (accumulations of macrophages laden with coal dust) around the terminal and respiratory bronchioles, surrounded by a halo of dilated alveoli. Macule formation leads to atrophy of supporting tissue, causing permanent dilation of small airways (focal emphysema).

Complicated CWP

Simple CWP may progress to the more complicated form if the disease involves one or both lungs. If this happens, fibrous tissue masses enlarge and coalesce, causing gross distortion of pulmonary structures (destruction of vasculature, alveoli, and airways).

Signs and symptoms

Simple CWP is asymptomatic, especially in nonsmokers. Symptoms appear if PMF develops that include exertional dyspnea and a cough that occasionally produces inky-black sputum when fibrotic changes undergo avascular necrosis and their centers cavitate.

Other clinical features of CWP include increasing dyspnea and a cough that produces milky, gray, clear, or coalflecked sputum. Recurrent bronchial and pulmonary infections produce yellow, green, or thick sputum.

Complications include pulmonary hypertension, right ventricular hypertrophy and cor pulmonale, and pulmonary tuberculosis. In cigarette smokers, chronic bronchitis and emphysema may also complicate the disease.

Diagnosis

The patient history reveals exposure to coal dust. Physical examination shows a barrel chest, hyperresonant lungs with areas of dullness, diminished breath sounds, crackles, rhonchi, and wheezes.

In simple CWP, chest X-rays show small opacities (less than 10 mm in diameter), which may be present in all lung zones but are more prominent in the upper lung zones. In complicated CWP, one or more large opacities (1 to 5 cm in diameter), possibly exhibiting cavitation, are seen.

The results of pulmonary function studies include the following:
• *Vital capacity* is normal in simple CWP, but decreased with PMF.
• *Forced vital capacity* is decreased in complicated disease.
• *Residual volume and total lung capacity* remains normal in simple CWP but is decreased in PMF.
• *Diffusing capacity of the lungs for carbon monoxide* is significantly decreased in complicated CWP as alveolar septae are destroyed and pulmonary capillaries obliterated.

Arterial blood gas studies show the following:
• *Partial pressure of oxygen* is normal in simple CWP, but decreased in PMF.
• *Partial pressure of carbon dioxide* usually remains normal in simple CWP but may decrease because of hyperventilation. It may also increase if the patient is hypoxic and has severe impairment of alveolar ventilation.

Treatment

The goal of treatment is to relieve respiratory symptoms, to manage hypoxia and cor pulmonale, and to avoid respiratory tract irritants and infection. If tuberculosis develops, the patient will need antitubercular therapy.

Respiratory symptoms may be relieved through bronchodilator therapy with theophylline or aminophylline (if bronchospasm is reversible), oral or inhaled sympathomimetic amines (metaproterenol), corticosteroids (oral prednisone or an aerosol form of a corticosteroid), or cromolyn sodium aerosol. Chest physiotherapy techniques, such as controlled coughing and segmental bronchial drainage, combined with chest percussion and vibration help remove secretions.

Other measures include increased fluid intake (at least 3 qt [3 L] daily) and respiratory therapy techniques, such as aerosol therapy, inhaled mucolytics, and intermittent positive pressure breathing (IPPB). Diuretics, digitalis glycosides, and salt restriction may be indicated in cor pulmonale.

In severe cases, oxygen may be administered by cannula or mask (1 to 2 L/minute) if the patient has chronic hypoxia or by mechanical ventilation if arterial oxygen can't be maintained above 40 mm Hg. Respiratory infections require prompt administration of antibiotics.

Special considerations

• Watch for signs of developing tuberculosis.
• Teach the patient to prevent infections by avoiding crowds and persons with respiratory infections and by receiving influenza and pneumococcal vaccines.
• Encourage the patient to stay active to avoid a deterioration in his physical condition, but to pace his activities and practice relaxation techniques.

COCCIDIOIDOMYCOSIS

Also known as valley fever and San Joaquin Valley fever, coccidioidomycosis is caused by the fungus *Coccidioides immitis*. It occurs primarily as a respiratory infection, although generalized dissemination may occur.

The primary pulmonary form is usually self-limiting and rarely fatal. The rare secondary (progressive, disseminated) form produces abscesses throughout the body and carries a mortality of up to 60%, even with treatment. Such dissemination is more common in dark-skinned men, pregnant women, and patients who are receiving immunosuppressives.

Causes

Coccidioidomycosis is endemic to the southwestern United States, especially between the San Joaquin Valley in California and southwestern Texas. It's also found in Mexico, Guatemala, Honduras, Venezuela, Colombia, Argentina, and Paraguay.

It may result from inhalation of *C. immitis* spores found in the soil in these areas or from inhalation of spores from dressings or plaster casts of infected persons. It's most prevalent during warm, dry months.

Because of population distribution and an occupational link (it's common in migrant farm laborers), coccidioidomycosis generally strikes Filipino Americans, Mexican Americans, Native Americans, and blacks. In primary infection, the incubation period is from 1 to 4 weeks.

Signs and symptoms

Chronic pulmonary cavitation can occur in both the primary and the disseminated forms, causing hemoptysis with or without chest pain. Other signs and symptoms vary with the form of the disease.

Primary coccidioidomycosis

Acute or subacute respiratory symptoms (dry cough, pleuritic chest pain, pleural effusion), fever, sore throat, chills, malaise, headache, and an itchy macular rash usually accompany the primary form of the disease. Occasionally, the sole symptom is a fever that persists for weeks. From 3 days to several weeks after onset, some patients, particularly Caucasian women, may develop tender red nodules (erythema nodosum) on their legs, especially the shins, with joint pain in the knees and ankles. Generally, the primary form heals spontaneously within a few weeks.

Disseminiated coccidioidomycosis

In rare cases, coccidioidomycosis spreads to other organs several weeks or months after the primary infection. Disseminated coccidioidomycosis causes fever and abscesses throughout the body, especially in skeletal, central nervous system (CNS), splenic, hepatic, renal, and subcutaneous tissues. Depending on the location of these abscesses, disseminated coccidioidomycosis may cause bone pain and meningitis.

Diagnosis

Typical clinical features and skin and serologic studies confirm the diagnosis. The primary form — and sometimes the disseminated form — produces a positive coccidioidin skin test. In the first week of illness, complement fixation for immunoglobulin G antibodies or, in the first month, positive serum precipitins (immunoglobulins) also establish this diagnosis.

Examination or, more recently, immunodiffusion testing of sputum, pus from lesions, and a tissue biopsy may show *C. immitis* spores. The presence of antibodies in pleural and joint fluid, and a rising serum or body fluid antibody titer indicate dissemination.

Other abnormal laboratory results include an increased white blood cell (WBC) count, eosinophilia, increased erythrocyte sedimentation rate, and a chest X-ray showing bilateral diffuse infiltrates.

In coccidioidal meningitis, examination of cerebrospinal fluid shows the WBC count increased to more than 500/mm^3 (primarily because of mononuclear leukocytes) and increased protein and decreased glucose levels. Ventricular fluid obtained from the brain may contain complement fixation antibodies.

After the diagnosis has been reached, the results of serial skin tests, blood cultures, and serologic testing may document the effectiveness of therapy.

Treatment

Usually, mild primary coccidioidomycosis requires only bed rest and relief of symptoms. Severe primary disease and dissemination, however, also require long-term I.V. infusion or, in CNS dissemination, intrathecal administration of amphotericin B and, possibly, excision or drainage of lesions. Severe pulmonary lesions may require lobectomy. Miconazole and ketoconazole suppress *C. immitis* but don't eradicate it.

Special considerations

• Don't wash off the circle marked on the skin for serial skin tests; this aids in reading test results.
• In mild primary disease, encourage bed rest and adequate fluid intake. Record the amount and color of sputum. Watch for shortness of breath that may point to pleural effusion. In patients with arthralgia, provide analgesics.
• Coccidioidomycosis requires strict secretion precautions if the patient has draining lesions. A "no-touch" dressing technique and careful hand washing are essential.
• In CNS dissemination, monitor the patient carefully for a decreased level of consciousness or a change in mood or affect.
• Before intrathecal administration of amphotericin B, explain the procedure to the patient, and reassure him that he'll receive analgesics before a lumbar puncture.
• If the patient is to receive I.V. amphotericin B, infuse it slowly; rapid infusion may cause circulatory collapse. During infusion, monitor his vital signs. (His temperature may rise but should return to normal within 1 to 2 hours.)
• In patients receiving amphotericin B, watch for decreased urinary output, and monitor laboratory results for elevated blood urea nitrogen and creatinine levels and hypokalemia. Tell patients to immediately report hearing loss, tinnitus, dizziness, and all signs of toxicity. To ease adverse reactions, give antiemetics and antipyretics.

COLD INJURIES

Overexposure to cold air or water causes cold injuries. They occur in two major forms: localized injuries (such as frostbite) and systemic injuries (such as hypothermia). Untreated or improperly treated frostbite can lead to gangrene and may necessitate amputation; severe hypothermia can be fatal.

The risk of serious cold injuries, especially hypothermia, is increased by youth, lack of insulating body fat, wet or inadequate clothing, old age, drug abuse, cardiac disease, smoking, fatigue, hunger and depletion of caloric reserves, and excessive alcohol intake (which draws blood into the capillaries and away from body organs).

Causes

The specific causes of frostbite and hypothermia vary.

Frostbite

Localized cold injuries occur when ice crystals form in the tissues and expand extracellular spaces. With compression of the tissue cell, the cell membrane ruptures, interrupting enzymatic and metabolic activities. Increased capillary permeability accompanies the release of histamine, resulting in aggregation of red blood cells and microvascular occlusion. Frostbite results from prolonged exposure to dry temperatures far below freezing.

Hypothermia

Chemical changes result from hypothermia that slow the functions of most major organ systems, such as decreased renal blood flow and decreased glomerular filtration. Hypothermia results from cold-water near-drowning and prolonged exposure to cold temperatures.

Signs and symptoms

Both frostbite and hypothermia produce distinctive clinical features.

Frostbite

Two types of frostbite can occur: deep or superficial. Superficial frostbite affects skin and subcutaneous tissue, especially of the face, ears, extremities, and other exposed body areas. Although it may go unnoticed at first, upon returning to a warm place, frostbite produces burning, tingling, numbness, swelling, and a mottled, blue-gray skin color.

Deep frostbite extends beyond subcutaneous tissue and usually affects the hands or feet. The skin becomes white until it's thawed; then it turns purplish blue. Deep frostbite also produces pain, skin blisters, tissue necrosis, and gangrene.

Hypothermia

Indications of hypothermia (a core body temperature below 95° F [35° C]) vary with severity.
- *Mild hypothermia* produces a temperature of 89.6° to 95° F (32° to 35° C), severe shivering, slurred speech, and amnesia.
- *Moderate hypothermia* results in a temperature of 86° to 89.6° F (30° to 32° C), unresponsiveness or confusion, muscle rigidity, peripheral cyanosis and, with improper rewarming, signs of shock.
- In *severe hypothermia,* core temperature drops to 77° to 86° F (25° to 30° C), with loss of deep tendon reflexes and ventricular fibrillation. The patient may appear dead, with no palpable pulse or audible heart sounds. His pupils may dilate, and he appears to be in a state of rigor mortis. A temperature drop below 77° F causes cardiopulmonary arrest and death.

Diagnosis

A history of severe and prolonged exposure to cold may make this diagnosis obvious. Nevertheless, hypothermia can be overlooked if outdoor temperatures are above freezing or if the patient is comatose.

Treatment

In a localized cold injury, treatment consists of rewarming the injured part, supportive measures, and sometimes a fasciotomy to increase circulation by lowering edematous tissue pressure. However, if gangrene occurs, amputation may be necessary.

In hypothermia, therapy consists of immediate resuscitative measures, careful monitoring, and gradual rewarming of the body.

Frostbite

• Remove constrictive clothing and jewelry. Slowly rewarm the affected part in tepid water (about 100° to 108° F [37.8° to 42.2° C]). Give the patient warm fluids to drink.

• When the affected part begins to rewarm, the patient will feel pain, so give analgesics. Check for a pulse. If the injury is on the foot, place cotton or gauze sponges between the toes to prevent maceration. (See *Precaution in frostbite.*) Instruct the patient not to walk.

• If the injury has caused an open skin wound, give antibiotics and tetanus prophylaxis.

• If a pulse fails to return, the patient may develop compartment syndrome and need fasciotomy to restore circulation. If gangrene occurs, prepare the patient for amputation.

Hypothermia

• If the patient has no pulse or respiration, begin cardiopulmonary resuscitation (CPR) immediately and, if necessary, continue it for 2 to 3 hours. (*Remember:* Hypothermia helps protect the brain from anoxia, which normally accompanies prolonged cardiopulmonary arrest. Therefore, even after the patient has been unresponsive for a long time, resuscitation may be possible, especially after cold-water near-drownings.) Perform CPR until the patient is adequately rewarmed.

• Move the patient to a warm area, remove wet clothing, and keep him dry. If he's conscious, give warm fluids with high sugar content, such as tea with sugar. If the patient's core temperature is above 89.6° F (32° C), use external warming techniques. Bathe him in water that's 104° F (40° C), cover him with a heating blanket set at 97.9° to 99.9° F (36.6° to 37.7° C), and cautiously apply hot water bottles at 104° F

HAZARD

◪ PRECAUTION IN FROSTBITE

When treating a patient with frostbite, *never* rub the injured area. This aggravates tissue damage. Also, be careful not to rupture any blebs.

---

to groin and axillae, guarding against burns.

• If the patient's core temperature is below 89.6° F (32° C), use internal and external warming methods. Rewarm his body core and surface 1° to 2° F (0.5° to 1.1° C) per hour concurrently. (If you rewarm the surface first, rewarming shock could cause potentially fatal ventricular fibrillation.)

• To warm inhalations, provide oxygen heated to 107.6° to 114.8° F (42° to 46° C). Infuse I.V. solutions that have been warmed to 98.6° F (37° C), and perform nasogastric lavage with normal saline solution that has been warmed to the same temperature.

• The patient may need peritoneal lavage, using normal saline solution (full or half strength) warmed to 104° to 113° F (40° to 45° C); in severe hypothermia, the patient may need heart and lung bypass at controlled temperatures and thoracotomy with a direct cardiac warm-saline bath. Avoid using arterial venous catheters in patients with severe hypothermia to prevent arrhythmias.

Special considerations

• Before discharging the patient with frostbite, tell him about possible long-term effects: increased sensitivity to cold, burning and tingling, and increased sweating. Warn against smoking; this causes vasoconstriction and slows healing.

• During treatment for hypothermia, monitor arterial blood gas levels, intake and output, central venous pressure, temperature, and cardiac and neurologic status every half hour. Monitor laboratory results, such as complete blood count, blood urea nitrogen level, electrolytes, prothrombin time, and partial thromboplastin time.

• If the patient is a child, suspect neglect or abuse; make sure a thorough patient history is performed.

• If the patient developed a cold injury because of inadequate clothes or housing, refer him to a community social service agency.

• To help prevent future cold injuries, tell the patient to wear mittens (not gloves); windproof, water-resistant, many-layered clothing; two pairs of socks (cotton next to the skin, then wool); and a scarf and a hat that cover the ears (to avoid substantial heat loss through the head).

• Advise the patient not to drink alcohol or smoke and to get adequate food and rest before prolonged exposure.

• Caution the patient to find shelter early or increase physical activity if caught in a severe snowstorm.

COLORADO TICK FEVER

A benign infection, colorado tick fever results from the Colorado tick fever virus, an arbovirus, and is transmitted to humans by a hard-shelled wood tick called *Dermacentor andersoni*. The adult tick acquires the virus when it bites infected rodents and remains permanently infective.

Colorado tick fever occurs in the Rocky Mountain region of the United States, mostly in April and May at lower altitudes and in June and July at higher altitudes. Because of occupational or recreational exposure, it's more common in men than in women. Colorado tick fever apparently confers long-lasting immunity against reinfection.

Signs and symptoms

After a 3- to 6-day incubation period, Colorado tick fever begins abruptly with chills; a temperature of 104° F (40° C); severe aching of the back, arms, and legs; lethargy; and headache with eye movement. Photophobia, abdominal pain, nausea, and vomiting may occur. Rare effects include petechial or maculopapular rashes and central nervous system involvement.

After several days, symptoms subside but return within 2 to 3 days and continue for 3 more days before slowly disappearing. Complete recovery usually follows.

Diagnosis

A history of recent exposure to ticks and moderate to severe leukopenia, complement fixation tests, or virus isolation confirm the diagnosis.

Treatment and special considerations

After correct removal of the tick, supportive treatment relieves symptoms, combats secondary infection, and maintains fluid balance.

• Carefully remove the tick by grasping it with forceps or gloved fingers and pulling gently. Be careful not to crush the tick's body. Keep it for identification.

• Thoroughly wash the wound with soap and water. If the tick's head remains embedded, surgical removal is necessary. Give a tetanus-diphtheria booster as needed.

• Be alert for secondary infection.

• Monitor fluid and electrolyte balance, and provide replacement accordingly.

• Reduce fever with antipyretics and tepid sponge baths.

• To prevent tickborne infection, tell the patient to avoid tick bites by wearing protective clothing (long pants tucked into boots) and carefully checking his body and scalp for ticks several times a day whenever in infested areas.

COLORECTAL CANCER

In the United States and Europe, colorectal cancer is the second most common visceral neoplasm. Incidence is equally distributed between men and women.

Colorectal malignant tumors are almost always adenocarcinomas. About half of these are sessile lesions of the rectosigmoid area; the rest are polypoid lesions.

Colorectal cancer tends to progress slowly and remains localized for a long time. Consequently, it's potentially curable in 75% of patients if an early diagnosis allows resection before nodal involvement. With early diagnosis, the overall 5-year survival rate is nearing 50%. (See *Staging colorectal cancer,* page 222.)

Causes

The exact cause of colorectal cancer is unknown, but studies showing concentration in areas of higher economic development suggest a relationship to diet (excess animal fat, particularly beef, and low fiber). Other factors that magnify the risk of developing colorectal cancer include:

• other diseases of the digestive tract
• age (over 40)

• history of ulcerative colitis (the average interval before onset of cancer is 11 to 17 years)

• familial polyposis (cancer almost always develops by age 50).

Signs and symptoms

Manifestations of colorectal cancer result from local obstruction and, in later stages, from direct extension to adjacent organs (bladder, prostate, ureters, vagina, sacrum) and distant metastasis (usually to the liver).

In the early stages, signs and symptoms are typically vague and depend on the anatomical location and function of the bowel segment containing the tumor. Later, they generally include pallor, cachexia, ascites, hepatomegaly, or lymphangiectasis.

Cancer on the right side

On the right side of the colon (which absorbs water and electrolytes), early tumor growth causes no signs of obstruction because the tumor tends to grow along the bowel rather than surround the lumen, and the fecal content in this area is normally liquid. It may, however, cause black, tarry stools; anemia; and abdominal aching, pressure, or dull cramps.

As the disease progresses, the patient develops weakness, fatigue, exertional dyspnea, vertigo and, eventually, diarrhea, obstipation, anorexia, weight loss, vomiting, and other signs and symptoms of intestinal obstruction. In addition, a tumor on the right side may be palpable.

Cancer on the left side

On the left side, a tumor causes signs and symptoms of an obstruction even in early stages because, in this area, stools are of a formed consistency. It commonly causes rectal bleeding (often ascribed to hemorrhoids), intermittent abdominal fullness or cramping, and rectal pressure.

STAGING COLORECTAL CANCER

Named for pathologist Cuthbert Dukes, the Dukes Cancer Classification System assigns tumors to four stages. These stages (with substages) reflect the extent of bowel-mucosa and bowel-wall infiltration, lymph node involvement, and metastasis.

Stage A
Malignant cells are confined to the bowel mucosa, and the lymph nodes contain no cancer cells. Treated promptly, about 80% of these patients remain disease-free 5 years later.

Stage B
Malignant cells extend through the bowel mucosa but remain within the bowel wall. The lymph nodes are normal. In substage B_2, all bowel wall layers and immediately adjacent structures contain malignant cells, but the lymph nodes remain normal. About 50% of patients with substage B_2 survive for 5 or more years.

Stage C
Malignant cells extend into the bowel wall and the lymph nodes. In substage C_2, malignant cells extend through the entire thickness of the bowel wall and into the lymph nodes. The 5-year survival rate for patients with stage C disease is about 25%.

Stage D
Metastasized to distant organs by way of the lymph nodes and mesenteric vessels, malignant cells typically lodge in the lungs and liver. Only 5% of patients with stage D cancer survive 5 or more years.

As the disease progresses, the patient develops obstipation, diarrhea, or "ribbon" or pencil-shaped stools. Typically, he notices that passage of stools or flatus relieves the pain. At this stage, bleeding from the colon becomes obvious, with dark or bright red blood in the feces and mucus in or on the stools.

Rectal tumor signs

With a rectal tumor, the first symptom is a change in bowel habits, often beginning with an urgent need to defecate on arising ("morning diarrhea") or obstipation alternating with diarrhea. Other indications include blood or mucus in stools and a sense of incomplete evacuation.

Late in the disease, pain begins as a feeling of rectal fullness that later becomes a dull, and sometimes constant, ache confined to the rectum or sacral region.

Diagnosis

Only a tumor biopsy can verify colorectal cancer, but the following tests help detect it:

• *Digital examination* can detect almost 15% of colorectal cancers.

• *Hemoccult test* (guaiac) can detect blood in stools.

• *Proctoscopy* or *sigmoidoscopy* can detect up to 66% of colorectal cancers.

• *Colonoscopy* permits visual inspection (and photographs) of the colon up to the ileocecal valve, and gives access for polypectomies and biopsies of suspected lesions.

• *Computed tomography scan* helps to detect areas affected by metastasis.

• *Barium X-ray,* utilizing a dual contrast with air, can locate lesions that are undetectable manually or visually. Barium examination should *follow* endoscopy or excretory urography because the barium sulfate interferes with these tests.

• *Carcinoembryonic antigen,* though not specific or sensitive enough for an early diagnosis, is helpful in monitoring patients before and after treatment to detect metastasis or recurrence.

Treatment

The most effective treatment for colorectal cancer is surgery to remove the malignant tumor and adjacent tissues as well as any lymph nodes that may contain cancer cells. The type of surgery depends on the location of the tumor:

• *Cecum and ascending colon:* A right hemicolectomy (for advanced disease) is performed. It may include resection of the terminal segment of the ileum, cecum, ascending colon, and the right half of the transverse colon with corresponding mesentery.

• *Proximal and middle transverse colon:* A right colectomy is performed that includes the transverse colon and mesentery corresponding to midcolic vessels, or segmental resection of the transverse colon and associated midcolic vessels.

• *Sigmoid colon:* Surgery is usually limited to sigmoid colon and mesentery.

• *Upper rectum:* Anterior or low anterior resection is performed. A newer method, using a stapler, allows for resections much lower than were previously possible.

• *Lower rectum:* Abdominoperineal resection and permanent sigmoid colostomy is performed.

Chemotherapy is indicated for patients with metastasis, residual disease, or a recurrent inoperable tumor. Drugs used in such treatment commonly include fluorouracil with levamisole, leucovorin, methotrexate, or streptozocin. Patients whose tumor has extended to regional lymph nodes may receive fluorouracil and levamisole for 1 year postoperatively.

Radiation therapy induces tumor regression and may be used before or after surgery or combined with chemotherapy, especially fluorouracil.

Special considerations

Before surgery:

• Monitor the patient's diet modifications, laxatives, enemas, and antibiotics — all used to clean the bowel and to decrease abdominal and perineal cavity contamination during surgery.

• If the patient is having a colostomy, teach him and his family about the procedure.

• Emphasize that the stoma will be red, moist, and swollen and that postoperative swelling will eventually subside.

• Show them a diagram of the intestine before and after surgery, stressing how much of the bowel will remain intact. Supplement your teaching with instructional aids. Arrange a postsurgical visit from a recovered ostomate.

• Prepare the patient for postoperative I.V. infusions, a nasogastric tube, and an indwelling urinary catheter.

• Discuss the importance of cooperating during deep-breathing and coughing exercises.

After surgery:

• Explain to the patient's family the importance of their positive reactions to the patient's adjustment. Consult with an enterostomal therapist, if available, to help set up a regimen for the patient.

• Encourage the patient to look at the stoma and participate in its care as soon as possible. Teach good hygiene and skin care. Allow him to shower or bathe as soon as the incision heals.

• If appropriate, instruct the patient with a sigmoid colostomy to do his own irrigation as soon as he can after surgery. Advise him to schedule irrigation for the time of day when he normally evacuated before surgery. Many patients find that irrigating every 1 to 3 days is necessary for regularity.

• If flatus, diarrhea, or constipation occurs, eliminate suspected causative foods from the patient's diet. He may reintroduce them later.

• After several months, many ostomates establish control with irrigation and no longer need to wear a pouch. A stoma cap or gauze sponge placed over the stoma protects it and absorbs mucoid secretions.

• Before achieving such control, the patient can resume physical activities, including sports, but he should avoid injury to the stoma or surrounding abdominal muscles.

• Inform the patient that a structured, gradually progressive exercise program to strengthen abdominal muscles may be instituted under medical supervision.

• Instruct the patient to avoid heavy lifting because herniation or prolapse may occur through weakened muscles in the abdominal wall.

• If appropriate, refer the patient to a home health agency for follow-up care and counseling. Suggest sexual counseling for male patients; most are impotent after an abdominoperineal resection.

• Anyone who's had colorectal cancer is at increased risk for another primary cancer. Instruct the patient to have yearly screening and testing and to maintain a high-fiber diet.

COMMON COLD

This acute, usually afebrile viral infection causes inflammation of the upper respiratory tract. It accounts for more time lost from school or work than any other cause and is the most common infectious disease. Although it's benign and self-limiting, it can lead to secondary bacterial infections.

Causes

The common cold is more prevalent in children than in adults; in adolescent boys than in girls; and in women than in men. In temperate zones, it occurs more often in the colder months; in the tropics, during the rainy season.

About 90% of colds stem from a viral infection of the upper respiratory passages and consequent mucous membrane inflammation; occasionally, colds result from *Mycoplasma*.

Over a hundred viruses can cause the common cold. Major offenders include rhinoviruses, coronaviruses, myxoviruses, adenoviruses, coxsackieviruses, and echoviruses.

Transmission occurs through airborne respiratory droplets, contact with contaminated objects, and hand-to-hand transmission. Children acquire new strains from their schoolmates and pass them on to family members. Fatigue or drafts doesn't increase susceptibility.

Signs and symptoms

After a 1- to 4-day incubation period, the common cold produces pharyngitis, nasal congestion, rhinitis, headache, and burning, watery eyes; there may be fever (in children), chills, myalgia, arthralgia, malaise, lethargy, and a hacking, nonproductive, or nocturnal cough.

As the cold progresses, clinical features develop more fully. After a day, symptoms include a feeling of fullness with a copious nasal discharge that often irritates the nose, adding to discomfort. About 3 days after onset, major signs diminish, but the "stuffed-up" feeling often persists for a week.

Reinfection (with productive cough) is common, but complications (sinusitis, otitis media, pharyngitis, lower respiratory tract infection) are rare. A cold is communicable for 2 to 3 days after the onset of symptoms.

Diagnosis

No explicit diagnostic test exists to isolate the specific organis n responsible for the common cold. Consequently, the diagnosis rests on a cold's typically mild, localized, and afebrile upper respiratory symptoms. Despite infection, white blood cell count and differential are within normal limits.

A diagnosis must rule out allergic rhinitis, measles, rubella, and other disorders that produce similar early symptoms. A fever higher than 100° F (37.8° C), severe malaise, anorexia, tachycardia, exudate on the tonsils or throat, petechiae, and tender lymph glands may point to more serious disorders and require additional diagnostic tests.

Treatment

The primary treatment—aspirin or acetaminophen, fluids, and rest—is purely symptomatic, as the common cold has no cure. Aspirin eases myalgia and headache; fluids help loosen accumulated respiratory secretions and maintain hydration; and rest combats fatigue and weakness. In a child with a fever, acetaminophen is the drug of choice.

Decongestants can relieve congestion. Throat lozenges relieve soreness. Steam encourages expectoration. In infants, saline nose drops and mucus aspiration with a bulb syringe may be beneficial.

Nasal douching, sinus drainage, and antibiotics aren't necessary except in complications or chronic illness. Pure antitussives relieve severe coughs but are contraindicated with productive coughs, when cough suppression is harmful. The role of vitamin C remains controversial.

Currently, no known measure can prevent the common cold. Vitamin

therapy, interferon administration, and ultraviolet irradiation are under investigation.

Special considerations

- Emphasize that antibiotics don't cure the common cold.
- Tell the patient to maintain bed rest during the first few days, use a lubricant on his nostrils to decrease irritation, relieve throat irritation with hard candy or cough drops, increase his fluid intake, and eat light meals.
- Inform the patient that warm baths or heating pads can reduce aches and pains but won't hasten a cure. Suggest hot or cold steam vaporizers. Commercial expectorants are available, but their effectiveness is questionable.
- Advise the patient against overuse of nose drops or sprays; these may cause rebound congestion.
- To help prevent colds, warn the patient to minimize contact with people who have colds.
- To avoid spreading colds, teach the patient to wash his hands often, to cover coughs and sneezes, and to avoid sharing towels and drinking glasses.

COMMON VARIABLE IMMUNODEFICIENCY

Also called acquired hypogammaglobulinemia and agammaglobulinemia with immunoglobulin-bearing B cells, common variable immunodeficiency is characterized by progressive deterioration of B-cell (humoral) immunity. This results in increased susceptibility to infection.

Unlike X-linked hypogammaglobulinemia, this disorder usually causes symptoms after infancy and childhood, between ages 25 and 40. It affects men and women equally and usually doesn't interfere with normal life span or with normal pregnancy and offspring.

Causes
Exactly what causes common variable immunodeficiency isn't known. Most patients have a normal circulating B-cell count but defective synthesis or release of immunoglobulins. Many also exhibit progressive deterioration of T-cell (cell-mediated) immunity, which is revealed by delayed hypersensitivity skin testing.

Signs and symptoms
In common variable immunodeficiency, pyogenic bacterial infections are characteristic but tend to be chronic rather than acute (as in X-linked hypogammaglobulinemia). Recurrent sinopulmonary infections, chronic bacterial conjunctivitis, and malabsorption (often associated with infestation by *Giardia lamblia*) are usually the first clues to immunodeficiency.

Common variable immunodeficiency may be associated with auto-immune diseases, such as systemic lupus erythematosus, rheumatoid arthritis, hemolytic anemia, and pernicious anemia, as well as with cancers, such as leukemia and lymphoma.

Diagnosis
Characteristic diagnostic markers in this disorder include decreased serum immunoglobulin M (IgM), IgA, and IgG detected by immunoelectrophoresis, along with a normal circulating B-cell count. Antigenic stimulation confirms an inability to produce specific antibodies; cell-mediated immunity may be intact or delayed. X-rays usually show signs of chronic lung disease or sinusitis.

Treatment
Patients with common variable immunodeficiency need essentially the same treatment as patients with X-linked hypogammaglobulinemia.

Injection of immune globulin (usually weekly to monthly) helps maintain immune response. Because immune globulin is composed primarily of IgG, the patient may also need fresh frozen plasma infusions to provide IgA and IgM.

Antibiotics are the mainstay for combating infection. Regular X-rays and pulmonary function studies help monitor infection in the lungs; chest physiotherapy may forestall or help clear such infection.

Special considerations
• Because immune globulin injections are very painful, give them deep into a large muscle mass, such as the gluteal or thigh muscles, and massage well. If the dosage is more than 1.5 ml, divide the dose and inject it into more than one site; for frequent injections, rotate the injection sites.
• To help prevent severe infection, teach the patient and his family how to recognize its early signs. Warn them to avoid crowds and persons who have active infections.
• Stress the importance of good nutrition and regular follow-up care.

COMPLEMENT DEFICIENCIES

A series of circulating enzymatic serum proteins with nine functional components make up complement. Components of complement are labeled C1 through C9. The first four complement components are numbered out of sequence (in order of their discovery) — C1, C4, C2, and C3 — but the remaining five are numbered sequentially.

When immunoglobulin G (IgG) or IgM reacts with antigens as part of an immune response, they activate C1, which then combines with C4, initiating the classic complement pathway, or cascade. (An alternative complement pathway involves the direct activation of C3 by the serum protein properdin, bypassing the initial components [C1, C4, C2] of the classic pathway.)

Complement then combines with the antigen-antibody complex and undergoes a sequence of reactions that amplify the immune response against the antigen. This complex process is called complement fixation.

Complement deficiency or dysfunction may increase susceptibility to infection and also seems related to certain autoimmune disorders. Theoretically, any complement component may be deficient or dysfunctional, and many such disorders are under investigation.

Primary complement deficiencies are rare. The most common ones are C2, C4, C6, and C8 deficiencies and C5 familial dysfunction.

More common secondary complement abnormalities have been confirmed in patients with lupus erythematosus, in some with dermatomyositis, in one with scleroderma (and in his family), and in a few with gonococcal and meningococcal infections. The prognosis varies with the abnormality and the severity of associated diseases.

Causes

Primary complement deficiencies are inherited as autosomal recessive traits, except for deficiency of C1 esterase inhibitor, which is autosomal dominant. Secondary deficiencies may follow complement-fixing (complement-consuming) immunologic reactions, such as drug-induced serum sickness, acute streptococcal glomerulonephritis, and acute active systemic lupus erythematosus.

Signs and symptoms

Clinical effects vary with the specific deficiency as follows:
• C2 and C3 deficiencies and C5 familial dysfunction increase susceptibility to bacterial infection (which may involve several body systems simultaneously).
• C2 and C4 deficiencies are also associated with collagen vascular disease, such as lupus erythematosus, and with chronic renal failure.
• C5 dysfunction, a familial defect in infants, causes failure to thrive, diarrhea, and seborrheic dermatitis.
• C1 esterase inhibitor deficiency (hereditary angioedema) may cause periodic swelling in the face, hands, abdomen, or throat, with potentially fatal laryngeal edema.

Diagnosis

Careful interpretation of both clinical features and laboratory results help to make this difficult diagnosis. Total serum complement level (CH50) is low in various complement deficiencies.

In addition, specific assays may be done to confirm deficiency of specific complement components. For example, detection of complement components and IgG by immunofluorescent examination of glomerular tissues in glomerulonephritis strongly suggests complement deficiency.

Treatment

Primary complement deficiencies have no known cure. Associated infection, collagen vascular disease, or renal disease requires prompt, appropriate treatment.

Transfusion of fresh frozen plasma to provide replacement of complement components is controversial, because replacement therapy doesn't cure complement deficiencies and any beneficial effects are transient. Bone marrow transplant may be helpful but can cause a potentially fatal graft-versus-host (GVH) reaction. Anabolic steroids, such as danazol, and antifibrinolytic agents are often used to reduce acute swelling in patients with C1 esterase inhibitor deficiency.

Special considerations

• Teach the patient (or his family, if he's a child) the importance of avoiding infection, how to recognize its early signs and symptoms, and the need for prompt treatment if it occurs.

• After bone marrow transplantation, monitor the patient closely for signs of transfusion reaction and GVH reaction.

• Provide meticulous patient care to help speed recovery and prevent complications. A patient with renal infection, for example, will need careful monitoring of intake and output, tests for serum electrolytes and acid-base balance, and observation for signs of renal failure.

• When caring for a patient with hereditary angioedema, be prepared for emergency management of laryngeal edema; keep airway equipment on hand.

CONCUSSION

By far the most common head injury, concussion results from a blow to the head—a blow hard enough to jostle the brain and make it hit against the skull, causing temporary neural dysfunction, but not hard enough to cause a cerebral contusion. Most concussion victims recover completely within 24 to

48 hours. Repeated concussions, however, exact a cumulative toll on the brain.

Causes

The blow that causes a concussion is usually sudden and forceful—a fall to the ground, a punch to the head, an automobile accident. Also, such a blow sometimes results from child abuse. Whatever the cause, the resulting injury is mild compared to the damage done by cerebral contusions or lacerations.

Signs and symptoms

Concussion may produce a short-term loss of consciousness, vomiting, and both anterograde and retrograde amnesia, in which the patient not only can't recall what happened immediately after the injury but also has difficulty recalling events that led up to the traumatic incident. The presence of anterograde amnesia and the duration of retrograde amnesia reliably correlate with the severity of the injury.

The injury often causes adults to be irritable or lethargic, to behave out of character, and to complain of dizziness, nausea, or severe headache. Some children have no apparent ill effects, but many grow lethargic and somnolent in a few hours. All these signs occur normally with a concussion.

Postconcussion syndrome—characterized by headache, dizziness, vertigo, anxiety, and fatigue—may persist for several weeks after the injury.

Diagnosis

Differentiating between concussion and more serious head injuries requires a thorough history of the trauma and a neurologic examination. Such an examination must evaluate the patient's level of consciousness (LOC), mental status, cranial nerve and motor function, deep tendon reflexes, and orientation to time, place, and person.

If no abnormalities are found, and if severe head injury appears unlikely, the patient should be observed for signs of more severe cerebral trauma. Observation provides a baseline for gauging any deterioration in the patient's condition.

Computed tomography (CT) scans may rule out fractures and more serious injuries; obtain them whenever you suspect severe head injuries. Skull X-rays remain controversial and are, in any case, being supplanted by CT scans.

Treatment and special considerations

• Obtain a thorough history of the trauma from the patient (if he's not suffering from amnesia), his family, eyewitnesses, or ambulance personnel. Ask whether the patient lost consciousness.

• Monitor vital signs and check for additional injuries. Palpate the skull for tenderness or hematomas.

• If the patient has an altered LOC or if a neurologic examination reveals abnormalities, the injury may be more severe than a concussion; in such a case, the patient should undergo a CT scan and a neurosurgeon should be consulted immediately.

• If a neurologic examination reveals no abnormalities, observe the patient in the emergency department. Check his vital signs, LOC, and pupil size every 15 minutes. The patient who is stable after 4 or more hours of observation can be discharged (with a head injury instruction sheet) in the care of a responsible adult.

CONJUNCTIVITIS

Hyperemia of the conjunctiva from infection, allergy, or chemical reactions characterize conjunctivitis. This disorder usually occurs as benign, self-limiting pinkeye; it may also be chronic, possibly indicating degenerative changes or damage from repeated acute attacks. In the Western hemisphere, conjunctivitis is probably the most common eye disorder.

Causes

The most common causative organisms are the following:

• *bacterial: Staphylococcus aureus, Streptococcus pneumoniae, Neisseria gonorrhoeae, Neisseria meningitidis*

• *chlamydial: Chlamydia trachomatis* (inclusion conjunctivitis)

• *viral:* adenovirus types 3, 7, and 8; herpes simplex virus, type 1.

Other causes include allergic reactions to pollen, grass, topical medications, air pollutants, and smoke; occupational irritants (acids and alkalies); rickettsial diseases (Rocky Mountain spotted fever); parasitic diseases caused by *Phthirus pubis, Schistosoma haematobium;* and, rarely, fungal infections.

Vernal conjunctivitis (also called seasonal or warm-weather conjunctivitis) results from allergy to an unidentified allergen. This form of conjunctivitis is bilateral; it usually begins before puberty and persists for about 10 years. It's sometimes associated with other signs and symptoms of allergy commonly related to grass or pollen sensitivity.

An idiopathic form of conjunctivitis may be associated with certain systemic diseases, such as erythema multiforme, chronic follicular conjunctivitis (orphan's conjunctivitis), and thy-

CLINICAL EFFECTS OF CONJUNCTIVITIS

Allergy, infection, or physical or chemical trauma can cause an inflammation of the conjunctiva, which produces redness, pain, swelling, lacrimation, and possible discharge.

roid disease. Conjunctivitis may be secondary to pneumococcal dacryocystitis or canaliculitis from candidal infection.

Signs and symptoms

Conjunctivitis commonly produces hyperemia of the conjunctiva, sometimes accompanied by discharge, tearing, pain, and, with corneal involvement, photophobia. (See *Clinical effects of conjunctivitis.*) It generally doesn't affect vision. Conjunctivitis usually begins in one eye and rapidly spreads to the other by contamination of towels, washcloths, or the patient's own hand.

Acute bacterial form

In acute bacterial conjunctivitis (pinkeye), the infection usually lasts only 2 weeks. The patient typically complains of itching, burning, and the sensation of a foreign body in his eye. The eyelids show a crust of sticky, mucopurulent discharge. If the disorder stems from *N. gonorrhoeae*, however, the patient exhibits a profuse, purulent discharge.

Viral form

Viral conjunctivitis produces copious tearing with minimal exudate, and enlargement of the preauricular lymph node. Some viruses follow a chronic course and produce severe disabling disease; others last 2 to 3 weeks.

Diagnosis

Physical examination reveals injection of the bulbar conjunctival vessels. In children, possible systemic symptoms include sore throat or fever.

Monocytes are predominant in stained smears of conjunctival scrapings if conjunctivitis is caused by a virus. Polymorphonuclear cells (neutrophils) predominate if conjunctivitis stems from bacteria; eosinophils, if it's allergy-related. Culture and sensitivity tests identify the causative bacterial organism and indicate appropriate antibiotic therapy.

Treatment

The cause of conjunctivitis dictates the treatment. Bacterial conjunctivitis requires topical application of the appropriate antibiotic or sulfonamide.

Although viral conjunctivitis resists treatment, a sulfonamide or broad-spectrum antibiotic eye drops may prevent secondary infection.

Herpes simplex infection generally responds to treatment with trifluridine drops or vidarabine ointment or oral acyclovir, but the infection may persist for 2 to 3 weeks. Treatment of vernal (allergic) conjunctivitis includes administration of corticosteroid drops followed by cromolyn sodium, cold compresses to relieve itching and, occasionally, oral antihistamines.

Instillation of a one-time dose of tetracycline or erythromycin into the eyes of newborns prevents gonococcal conjunctivitis.

Special considerations

• Teach proper hand-washing technique because some forms of conjunctivitis are highly contagious. Stress the risk of spreading infection to family members by sharing washcloths, towels, and pillows. Warn against rubbing the infected eye, which can spread the infection to the other eye and to other persons.

• Apply warm compresses and therapeutic ointment or drops. Don't irrigate the eye; this will only spread infection. Have the patient wash his hands before he uses the medication, and use clean washcloths or towels frequently so he doesn't infect his other eye.

• Teach the patient to instill eyedrops and ointments correctly — without touching the bottle tip to his eye or lashes.

• Stress the importance of safety glasses for the patient who works near chemical irritants.

• Notify public health authorities if cultures show *N. gonorrhoeae.*

CONVERSION DISORDER

This disorder allows a patient to resolve a psychological conflict through the loss of a specific physical function — for example, by paralysis, blindness, or inability to swallow.

Unlike factitious disorders or malingering, conversion disorder results in an involuntary loss of physical function. (For more information, see *Factitious disorders,* page 232.) However, laboratory tests and diagnostic procedures fail to disclose an organic cause.

Conversion disorder can occur in either sex at any age. An uncommon disorder, it usually begins in adolescence or early adulthood. The conversion symptom itself isn't life-threatening and usually has a short duration.

Causes

The patient suddenly develops the conversion symptom soon after experiencing a traumatic conflict that he believes he can't handle. Two theories may explain why this occurs.

According to the first, the patient achieves a "primary gain" when the symptom keeps a psychological conflict out of conscious awareness. For example, a person may experience blindness after witnessing a violent crime.

The second theory suggests that the patient achieves "secondary gain" from the symptom by avoiding a traumatic activity. For example, a soldier may develop a "paralyzed" hand that prevents him from entering into combat.

Signs and symptoms

The history of a patient with conversion disorder may reveal the sudden onset of a single, debilitating sign or symptom that prevents normal function of the affected body part, such as

FACTITIOUS DISORDERS

Marked by the irrational, repetitive simulation of a physical or mental illness for the purpose of obtaining medical treatment, factitious disorders are severe psychopathologic conditions. The symptoms are intentionally produced and can be either physical or psychological. These disorders are more common in men than in women.

Factitious disorder with physical symptoms

Also called Munchausen syndrome, this is the most common factitious disorder. The patient convincingly presents with intentionally feigned symptoms. These symptoms may be fabricated (acute abdominal pain with no underlying disease), self-inflicted (deliberately infecting an open wound), an exacerbation or exaggeration of a preexisting disorder (taking penicillin despite a known allergy), or a combination of all the above.

The history of a patient with Munchausen syndrome may include:
• multiple admissions to various hospitals, typically across a wide geographic area
• extensive knowledge of medical terminology
• pathologic lying
• evidence of previous treatment such as surgery
• shifting complaints and signs and symptoms

• eagerness to undergo hazardous and painful procedures
• discharge against medical advice to avoid detection
• poor interpersonal relationships
• refusal of psychiatric examination
• psychoactive substance or analgesic abuse.

Factitious disorder with psychological symptoms

Causing severely impaired function, this disorder is characterized by intentional feigning of symptoms suggesting a mental disorder. However, the symptoms represent how the patient views the mental disorder and seldom coincide with any of the diagnostic categories documented in the *Diagnostic and Statistical Manual of Mental Disorders*, 4th edition.

This disorder almost always coexists with a severe personality disorder. Most patients have a history of psychoactive substance use, often in an attempt to elicit the desired symptoms.

paralysis of a leg. The patient may describe a very psychologically stressful event that recently preceded the symptom. Oddly, the patient doesn't display the affect and concern that such a severe symptom usually elicits.

Assessment findings obtained during a physical examination are inconsistent with the primary symptom. For instance, tendon reflexes may be normal in a "paralyzed" part of the body, loss of function fails to follow anatomic patterns of innervation, or pupillary responses and evoked poten-

tials are normal in a patient who complains of blindness.

Diagnosis

A thorough physical evaluation must rule out any physical cause, especially diseases that typically produce vague physical symptoms (such as multiple sclerosis or systemic lupus erythematosus). The *Diagnostic and Statistical Manual of Mental Disorders*, 4th edition, describes symptoms characteristic of patients with this disorder. (See *Diagnosing conversion disorder.*)

DIAGNOSING CONVERSION DISORDER

The diagnosis of conversion disorder is based on the following criteria put forth in the *Diagnostic and Statistical Manual of Mental Disorders*, 4th edition:
• The person has one or more symptoms or deficits affecting voluntary motor or sensory function that suggest a neurologic or other general medical condition.
• The person exhibits psychological factors judged to be associated with the symptom or deficit because conflicts or other stressors preceded the symptom's or deficit's manifestation.
• The person's symptom or deficit isn't intentionally produced or feigned.

• The person's symptom or deficit can't, after appropriate investigation, be fully explained by a general medical condition, by the direct effects of a substance, or as a culturally sanctioned behavior or experience.
• The person's symptom or deficit warrants medical evaluation, causes clinically significant distress, or impairs social, occupational, or other important areas of functioning.
• The person's symptom or deficit isn't limited to pain or sexual dysfunction, doesn't occur exclusively during the course of somatization disorder, and isn't better accounted for by another mental disorder.

Treatment
Psychotherapy, family therapy, relaxation therapy, behavioral therapy, or hypnosis may be used alone or in combination (two or more).

Special considerations
• Help the patient maintain integrity of the affected system. Regularly exercise paralyzed limbs to prevent muscle wasting and contractures.
• Frequently change the bedridden patient's position to prevent pressure ulcers from forming.
• Ensure adequate nutrition, even if the patient is complaining of GI distress.
• Provide a supportive environment, and encourage the patient to discuss the stressful event that provoked the conversion disorder.
• Don't force the patient to talk, but convey a caring attitude to help him share his feelings.
• Don't insist that the patient use the affected system. This will only anger him and prevent the two of you from forming a therapeutic relationship.

• Add your support to the recommendation for psychiatric care.
• Include the patient's family in all care. They may be contributing to the patient's stress, and they are essential to help him regain normal functioning.

COR PULMONALE

The World Health Organization defines chronic cor pulmonale as "hypertrophy of the right ventricle resulting from diseases affecting the function and/or the structure of the lungs, except when these pulmonary alterations are the result of diseases that primarily affect the left side of the heart or of congenital heart disease."

Invariably, cor pulmonale follows some disorder of the lungs, pulmonary vessels, chest wall, or respiratory control center. For instance, chronic obstructive pulmonary disease (COPD) produces pulmonary hypertension, which leads to right ventricular hypertrophy and failure. Because cor pulmonale generally occurs late during the course of COPD and other irreversible diseases, the prognosis is generally poor.

Causes

Approximately 85% of patients with cor pulmonale have COPD, and 25% of patients with COPD eventually develop cor pulmonale.

Other respiratory disorders that produce cor pulmonale include:
- obstructive lung diseases—for example, bronchiectasis and cystic fibrosis
- restrictive lung diseases—for example, pneumoconiosis, interstitial pneumonitis, scleroderma, and sarcoidosis
- loss of lung tissue after extensive lung surgery
- pulmonary vascular diseases such as recurrent thromboembolism, primary pulmonary hypertension, schistosomiasis, and pulmonary vasculitis
- respiratory insufficiency without pulmonary disease, as seen in chest wall disorders such as kyphoscoliosis, neuromuscular incompetence resulting from muscular dystrophy and amyotrophic lateral sclerosis, polymyositis, and spinal cord lesions above C6
- obesity hypoventilation syndrome (pickwickian syndrome) and upper airway obstruction
- living at high altitudes (chronic mountain sickness).

Pathophysiology

Pulmonary capillary destruction and pulmonary vasoconstriction (usually secondary to hypoxia) reduce the cross-sectional area of the pulmonary vascular bed. This increases pulmonary vascular resistance and causes pulmonary hypertension.

To compensate for the extra work needed to force blood through the lungs, the right ventricle dilates and hypertrophies. In response to low oxygen content, the bone marrow produces more red blood cells (RBCs), causing erythrocytosis. When the hematocrit exceeds 55%, blood viscosity increases, which further aggravates pulmonary hypertension and increases the hemodynamic load on the right ventricle. Right ventricular failure is the result.

Incidence

Cor pulmonale accounts for about 25% of all types of heart failure. It's most common in areas of the world where the incidence of cigarette smoking and COPD is high.

Cor pulmonale affects middle-aged to elderly men more often than women, but its incidence in women is increasing. In children, cor pulmonale may be a complication of cystic fibrosis, hemosiderosis, upper airway obstruction, scleroderma, extensive bronchiectasis, neurologic diseases affecting respiratory muscles, or abnormalities of the respiratory control center.

Signs and symptoms

As long as the heart can compensate for the increased pulmonary vascular resistance, clinical features reflect the underlying disorder and occur mostly in the respiratory system. They include chronic productive cough, exertional dyspnea, wheezing respirations, fatigue, and weakness.

Progression of cor pulmonale is associated with dyspnea (even at rest) that worsens on exertion, tachypnea, orthopnea, edema, weakness, and right upper quadrant discomfort. Chest examination reveals findings characteristic of the underlying lung disease.

Signs of cor pulmonale and right ventricular failure include dependent edema; distended neck veins; enlarged, tender liver; prominent parasternal or epigastric cardiac impulse; hepatojugular reflux; and tachycardia.

Decreased cardiac output may cause a weak pulse and hypotension.

Thoracic assessment

Chest examination yields various findings, depending on the underlying cause of cor pulmonale. In COPD, auscultation reveals wheezing, rhonchi, and diminished breath sounds. When the disease is secondary to upper airway obstruction or damage to central nervous system respiratory centers, chest findings may be normal except for a right ventricular lift, gallop rhythm, and loud pulmonic component of S_2.

Tricuspid insufficiency produces a pansystolic murmur heard at the lower left sternal border; its intensity increases on inspiration, distinguishing it from a murmur caused by mitral valve disease. A right ventricular early murmur that increases on inspiration can be heard at the left sternal border or over the epigastrium. A systolic pulmonic ejection click may also be heard.

Drowsiness and alterations in consciousness may occur.

Diagnosis

Pulmonary artery pressure measurements show increased right ventricular and pulmonary artery pressures as a result of increased pulmonary vascular resistance. Right ventricular systolic and pulmonary artery systolic pressures will exceed 30 mm Hg. Pulmonary artery diastolic pressure will exceed 15 mm Hg.

• *Echocardiography* or *angiography* indicates right ventricular enlargement, and echocardiography can estimate pulmonary artery pressure.

• *Chest X-ray* shows large central pulmonary arteries and suggests right ventricular enlargement by rightward enlargement of cardiac silhouette on an anterior chest film.

• *Arterial blood gas (ABG) analysis* shows decreased partial pressure of arterial oxygen (PaO_2) — often less than 70 mm Hg and usually no more than 90 mm Hg on room air.

• *Electrocardiography* frequently shows arrhythmias, such as premature atrial and ventricular contractions and atrial fibrillation during severe hypoxia; it may also show right bundle-branch heart block, right axis deviation, prominent P waves and an inverted T wave in right precordial leads, and right ventricular hypertrophy.

• *Pulmonary function tests* show results consistent with the underlying pulmonary disease.

• *Hematocrit* is often greater than 50%.

Treatment

The goals of treatment include reducing hypoxemia, increasing the patient's exercise tolerance, and, when possible, correcting the underlying condition. In addition to bed rest, treatment may include administration of:

• *digitalis glycosides* (digoxin)

• *antibiotics* when respiratory infection is present (a culture and sensitivity of a sputum specimen aids in the selection of antibiotics)

• *potent pulmonary artery vasodilators* (such as diazoxide, nitroprusside, hydralazine, angiotensin converting enzyme inhibitors, calcium channel blockers, or prostaglandins) in primary pulmonary hypertension

• *oxygen* by mask or cannula in concentrations ranging from 24% to 40%, depending on PaO_2, as necessary; in acute cases, therapy may also include mechanical ventilation; patients with underlying COPD generally shouldn't receive high concentrations of oxygen because of possible subsequent respiratory depression

• *low-salt diet, restricted fluid intake,* and *diuretics* such as furosemide to reduce edema

• *phlebotomy* to reduce the RBC count

• *anticoagulation* with small doses of heparin to reduce the risk of thromboembolism.

Depending on the underlying cause, some variations in treatment may be necessary. For example, a tracheotomy may be necessary if the patient has an upper airway obstruction, and steroids may be used in patients with a vasculitis autoimmune phenomenon or acute exacerbations of COPD.

Special considerations
• The patient will need a diet carefully planned in consultation with the staff dietitian. Because the patient may lack energy and tire easily when eating, provide small, frequent feedings rather than three heavy meals.
• Prevent fluid retention by limiting the patient's fluid intake to 1,000 to 2,000 ml/day and providing a low-sodium diet.
• Monitor serum potassium levels closely if the patient is receiving diuretics. Low serum potassium levels can potentiate the risk of arrhythmias associated with digitalis glycosides.
• Watch the patient for signs of digitalis toxicity, such as complaints of anorexia, nausea, vomiting, and yellow halos around visual images; monitor for cardiac arrhythmias.
• Teach the patient to check his radial pulse before taking digoxin or any digitalis glycoside and to report any changes in pulse rate.
• Reposition bedridden patients often to prevent atelectasis.
• Provide meticulous respiratory care, including oxygen therapy and, for COPD patients, pursed-lip breathing exercises.
• Periodically measure ABG levels and watch for signs of respiratory failure, such as a change in pulse rate; deep, labored respirations; and increased fatigue produced by exertion.

Before discharge:
• Make sure the patient understands the importance of maintaining a low-salt diet, weighing himself daily, and watching for and immediately reporting edema. Teach him to detect edema by pressing the skin over his shins with one finger, holding it for a second or two, then checking for a finger impression.
• Instruct the patient to allow himself frequent rest periods and to do his breathing exercises regularly.
• If the patient needs suctioning or supplemental oxygen therapy at home, refer him to a social service agency that can help him obtain the necessary equipment, and, as necessary, arrange for follow-up examinations.
• Because pulmonary infection often exacerbates COPD and cor pulmonale, instruct the patient to watch for and immediately report early signs of infection, such as increased sputum production, a change in sputum color, increased coughing or wheezing, chest pain, fever, and tightness in the chest.
• Tell the patient to avoid crowds and persons known to have pulmonary infections, especially during the flu season.
• Warn the patient to avoid nonprescribed medications, such as sedatives, that may depress the ventilatory drive.

CORNEAL ABRASION

Often caused by a foreign body, a corneal abrasion is a scratch on the surface epithelium of the cornea. An abrasion or foreign body in the eye is the most common eye injury. With treatment, the prognosis is usually good.

Causes

A corneal abrasion usually results from a foreign body, such as a cinder or a piece of dust, dirt, or grit, that becomes embedded under the eyelid. Even if the foreign body is washed out by tears, it may still injure the cornea.

Small pieces of metal that get in the eyes of workers who don't wear protective glasses quickly form a rust ring on the cornea and cause corneal abrasion. Such abrasions also commonly occur in the eyes of persons who fall asleep wearing hard contact lenses.

A corneal scratch produced by a fingernail, a piece of paper, or other organic substance may cause a persistent lesion. The epithelium doesn't always heal properly, and a recurrent corneal erosion may develop, with delayed effects more severe than the original injury.

Signs and symptoms

Typically, corneal abrasions produce redness, increased tearing, a sensation of "something in the eye" and, because the cornea is richly endowed with nerve endings from the trigeminal nerve (cranial nerve V), pain disproportionate to the size of the injury. A corneal abrasion may affect visual acuity, depending on the size and location of the injury.

Diagnosis

A history of eye trauma or prolonged wearing of contact lenses, as well as typical symptoms, suggest corneal abrasion. Staining the cornea with fluorescein stain confirms the diagnosis: The injured area appears green when examined with a flashlight. Slit-lamp examination discloses the depth of the abrasion.

Examining the eye with a flashlight may reveal a foreign body on the cornea; the eyelid must be everted to check for a foreign body embedded under the lid.

Before beginning treatment, a test to determine visual acuity provides a medical baseline and a legal safeguard.

Treatment

The first steps in treatment include examining the eye and checking visual acuity. If the foreign object is visible, the eye can be irrigated with normal saline solution.

Removal of a deeply embedded foreign body is done with a foreign body spud, using a topical anesthetic. A rust ring on the cornea can be removed with an ophthalmic burr, after applying a topical anesthetic. When only partial removal is possible, re-epithelialization lifts the ring again to the surface and allows complete removal the following day.

Treatment also includes instillation of broad-spectrum antibiotic eyedrops in the affected eye every 3 to 4 hours. Initial application of a pressure patch prevents further corneal irritation when the patient blinks.

Special considerations

• Tell the patient with an eyepatch to leave the patch in place for 24 to 48 hours. Warn that wearing a patch alters depth perception, so advise caution in everyday activities, such as climbing stairs or stepping off a curb.

• Reassure the patient that the corneal epithelium usually heals in 24 to 48 hours.

• Stress the importance of instilling prescribed antibiotic eyedrops because an untreated corneal infection can lead to ulceration and permanent loss of vision. Teach the patient the proper way to instill eye medications.

• Emphasize the importance of safety glasses to protect workers' eyes from flying fragments. Also review instructions for wearing and caring for contact lenses, to prevent further trauma.

CORNEAL ULCERS

A major cause of blindness worldwide, ulcers produce corneal scarring or perforation. They occur in the central or marginal areas of the cornea, vary in shape and size, and may be singular or multiple. Marginal ulcers are the most common form. Prompt treatment (within hours of onset) can prevent visual impairment.

Causes

Corneal ulcers generally result from protozoan, bacterial, viral, or fungal infections. Common bacterial sources include *Staphylococcus aureus, Pseudomonas aeruginosa, Streptococcus viridans, Streptococcus (Diplococcus) pneumoniae,* and *Moraxella liquefaciens;* viral sources, herpes simplex type 1, variola, vaccinia, and varicella-zoster viruses; and common fungal sources, *Candida, Fusarium,* and *Cephalosporium.*

Other causes include trauma, exposure, reactions to bacterial infections, toxins, and allergens. Tuberculoprotein causes a classic phlyctenular keratoconjunctivitis; vitamin A deficiency results in xerophthalmia; and fifth cranial nerve lesions, in neurotropic ulcers.

Signs and symptoms

Typically, corneal ulceration begins with pain (aggravated by blinking) and photophobia, followed by increased tearing. Eventually, central corneal ulceration produces pronounced visual blurring. The eye may appear infected. If a bacterial ulcer is present, purulent discharge is possible.

Diagnosis

A history—of trauma or use of contact lenses—and flashlight examination that reveals an irregular corneal surface suggest corneal ulcer. Exudate may be present on the cornea, and a hypopyon (accumulation of white cells or pus in the anterior chamber) may produce cloudiness or color change.

Fluorescein dye, instilled in the conjunctival sac, stains the outline of the ulcer and confirms the diagnosis. Culture and sensitivity testing of corneal scrapings may identify the causative bacteria or fungus and indicate appropriate antibiotic or antifungal therapy.

Treatment

Prompt treatment is essential for all forms of corneal ulcer to prevent complications and permanent visual impairment. Treatment aims to eliminate the underlying cause of the ulcer and to relieve pain.

Until culture results identify the causative organism, treatment consists of systemic and topical broad-spectrum antibiotics. Once the causative agent is identified, specific treatments vary.

• P. aeruginosa *infection* is treated with polymyxin B and gentamicin, administered topically and by subconjunctival injection, or I.V. carbenicillin and tobramycin. Because this type of corneal ulcer spreads so rapidly, it can cause corneal perforation and loss of the eye within 48 hours. Immediate treatment and isolation of hospitalized patients are required.

Treatment of a corneal ulcer should never include an eye patch because patching creates the dark, warm, moist environment ideal for bacterial growth.

• *Herpes simplex type 1 virus* is treated with hourly topical applications of idoxuridine or vidarabine. Corneal ulcers resulting from a viral infection often recur. In this case, trifluridine becomes the treatment of choice.

• *Varicella-zoster virus* calls for treatment with topical sulfonamide ointment applied three to four times daily to prevent secondary infection.

• *Fungi* are treated with topical instillation of natamycin for *Fusarium, Cephalosporium,* and *Candida.*

• *Hypovitaminosis A* requires correction of dietary deficiency or GI malabsorption of vitamin A.

• *Neurotropic ulcers* or *exposure keratitis* is treated with frequent instillation of artificial tears or lubricating ointments and use of a plastic bubble eye shield.

Special considerations

• Lesions caused by varicella-zoster virus are unilateral, following the pathway of the fifth cranial nerve, and are typically quite painful. Give analgesics as needed. Associated anterior uveitis requires cycloplegic eye drops.

• Watch for signs of secondary glaucoma (transient vision loss and halos around lights).

• Keep the room darkened and orient the patient as necessary.

CORNS AND CALLUSES

Usually located on areas of repeated trauma (most often the feet), corns and calluses are acquired skin conditions marked by hyperkeratosis of the stratum corneum. The prognosis is good with proper foot care.

Causes and incidence

A corn is a hyperkeratotic area that usually results from external pressure such as that from ill-fitting shoes. Less commonly, it results from internal pressure such as that caused by a protruding underlying bone (from arthritis, for example).

A callus is an area of thickened skin, generally found on the foot or hand, produced by external pressure or fric-

tion. Persons whose activities produce repeated trauma (for example, manual laborers or guitarists) commonly develop calluses.

The severity of a corn or callus depends on the degree and duration of trauma.

Signs and symptoms

Both corns and calluses cause pain through pressure on underlying tissue by localized thickened skin.

Corns

Containing a central keratinous core, corns are smaller and more clearly defined than calluses and are usually more painful. The pain they cause may be dull and constant or sharp when pressure is applied.

Soft corns are caused by the pressure of a bony prominence. They appear as whitish thickenings and are commonly found between the toes, most often in the fourth interdigital web. Hard corns are sharply delineated and conical and appear most frequently over the dorsolateral aspect of the fifth toe.

Calluses

Often quite large, calluses have indefinite borders. They usually produce dull pain on pressure, rather than constant pain. Although calluses commonly appear over plantar warts, they're distinguished from these warts by normal skin markings.

Diagnosis

Careful physical examination of the affected area and a patient history revealing chronic trauma lead to a diagnosis.

Treatment

Surgical debridement may be performed to remove the nucleus of a corn, usually under a local anesthetic.

In intermittent debridement, keratolytics — usually 40% salicylic acid plasters — are applied to affected areas. Injections of corticosteroids beneath the corn may be necessary to relieve pain.

However, the simplest and best treatment is essentially preventive — avoidance of trauma. Corns and calluses disappear after the source of trauma has been removed. Metatarsal pads may redistribute the weight-bearing areas of the foot; corn pads may prevent painful pressure.

Patients with persistent corns or calluses require referral to a podiatrist or dermatologist; those with corns or calluses caused by a bony malformation, as in arthritis, require orthopedic consultation.

Special considerations
• Teach the patient how to apply salicylic acid plasters. Make sure the plaster is large enough to cover the affected area. Place the sticky side down on the foot, then cover the plaster with adhesive tape.
• Plasters are usually taken off after an overnight application but may be left in place for as long as 7 days. After removing the plaster, instruct the patient to soak the area in water and abrade the soft, macerated skin with a towel or pumice stone. Show him how to reapply the plaster, and tell him to repeat the entire procedure until he has removed all the hyperkeratotic skin.
• Warn the patient against removing corns or calluses with a sharp instrument, such as a razor blade.
• Advise the patient to wear properly fitted shoes. Suggest the use of metatarsal or corn pads to relieve pressure. Refer him to a podiatrist, dermatologist, or orthopedist, if necessary.
• Assure the patient that good foot care can correct this condition.

CORONARY ARTERY DISEASE

The dominant effect of coronary artery disease (CAD) is the loss of oxygen and nutrients to myocardial tissue because of diminished coronary blood flow. This disease is near epidemic in the Western world.

CAD occurs more often in men than in women, in whites, and in middle-aged and elderly people. In the past, this disorder rarely affected women who were premenopausal; but that's no longer the case, perhaps because many women now take oral contraceptives, smoke cigarettes, and are employed in stressful jobs that used to be held exclusively by men.

Causes
Atherosclerosis is the usual cause of CAD. In this form of arteriosclerosis, fatty, fibrous plaques narrow the lumen of the coronary arteries, reduce the volume of blood that can flow through them, and lead to myocardial ischemia. Plaque formation also predisposes to thrombosis, which can provoke myocardial infarction (MI).

Atherosclerosis usually develops in high-flow, high-pressure arteries, such as those in the heart, brain, kidneys, and aorta, especially at bifurcation points. It has been linked to many risk factors: family history, hypertension, obesity, smoking, diabetes mellitus, stress, a sedentary lifestyle, and high serum cholesterol and triglyceride levels.

Uncommon causes of reduced coronary artery blood flow include dissecting aneurysms, infectious vasculitis, syphilis, and congenital defects in the coronary vascular system. Coronary artery spasms may also impede blood flow. (See *Coronary artery spasm,* page 242.)

Signs and symptoms

The classic symptom of CAD is angina, the direct result of inadequate flow of oxygen to the myocardium. It's usually described as a burning, squeezing, or tight feeling in the substernal or precordial chest that may radiate to the left arm, neck, jaw, or shoulder blade.

Typically, the patient clenches his fist over his chest or rubs his left arm when describing the pain, which may be accompanied by nausea, vomiting, fainting, sweating, and cool extremities. Anginal episodes most often follow physical exertion but may also follow emotional excitement, exposure to cold, or a large meal.

Angina has three major forms:
• *Stable* angina causes pain that's predictable in frequency and duration and can be relieved with nitrates and rest.
• *Unstable* angina causes pain that increases in frequency and duration. It is more easily induced.
• *Prinzmetal's* angina causes unpredictable coronary artery spasm.

Severe and prolonged anginal pain generally suggests MI, with potentially fatal arrhythmias and mechanical failure.

Diagnosis

The patient history—including the frequency and duration of angina and the presence of associated risk factors—is crucial in evaluating CAD. Additional diagnostic measures include the following:
• *Electrocardiography (ECG)* during angina shows ischemia and, possibly, arrhythmias such as premature ventricular contractions. The ECG is apt to be normal when the patient is pain-free. Arrhythmias may occur without MI, secondary to ischemia.
• *Treadmill* or *bicycle exercise test* may provoke chest pain and ECG signs of myocardial ischemia.
• *Coronary angiography* reveals coronary artery stenosis or obstruction, possible collateral circulation, and the arteries' condition beyond the narrowing.
• *Myocardial perfusion imaging* with thallium-201 or cardiolite during treadmill exercise detects ischemic areas of the myocardium, visualized as "cold spots."

Treatment

The goal of treatment in patients with angina is to either reduce myocardial oxygen demand or increase oxygen supply. Therapy consists primarily of nitrates, such as nitroglycerin (given sublingually, orally, transdermally, or topically in ointment form), isosorbide dinitrate (given sublingually or orally), beta-adrenergic blockers (given orally), or calcium channel blockers (given orally). Obstructive lesions may necessitate coronary artery bypass surgery and the use of vein grafts.

Angioplasty may be performed during cardiac catheterization to compress fatty deposits and relieve occlusion in patients with no calcification and partial occlusion. (See *Relieving occlusions with angioplasty,* page 243.) A certain risk is associated with this procedure, but its morbidity is lower than that for surgery. Laser angioplasty, a newer procedure, corrects occlusion by melting fatty deposits.

Prevention

Because CAD is so widespread, prevention is of incalculable importance. Dietary restrictions aimed at reducing intake of calories (in obesity) and of salt, fats, and cholesterol serve to minimize the risk, especially when supplemented with regular exercise. Absten-

CORONARY ARTERY SPASM

A spontaneous, sustained contraction of one or more coronary arteries causes ischemia and dysfunction of the heart muscle in coronary artery spasm. This disorder also causes Prinzmetal's angina and even myocardial infarction in patients with unoccluded coronary arteries.

Cause

Although the cause of coronary artery spasm is unknown, possible contributing factors include:
• intimal hemorrhage into the medial layer of the blood vessel
• hyperventilation
• elevated catecholamine levels
• fatty buildup in the lumen
• cocaine use.

Signs and symptoms

Angina is the major symptom of coronary artery spasm. But unlike classic angina, this pain often occurs spontaneously and may not be related to physical exertion or emotional stress; it's also more severe, usually lasts longer, and may be cyclic, frequently recurring every day at the same time.

These ischemic episodes may cause arrhythmias, altered heart rate, lower blood pressure and, occasionally, fainting from diminished cardiac output. Spasm in the left coronary artery may result in mitral insufficiency, producing a loud systolic murmur and, possibly, pulmonary edema, with dyspnea, crackles, hemoptysis, or sudden death.

Diagnosis and treatment

Coronary angiography and electrocardiography (ECG) allow a diagnosis. The patient may receive calcium channel blockers (verapamil, nifedipine, or diltiazem) to reduce coronary artery spasm and vascular resistance as well as nitrates (nitroglycerin or isosorbide dinitrate) to relieve chest pain.

Special considerations

• When caring for a patient with coronary artery spasm, explain all necessary procedures and teach him how to take his medications safely.
• For calcium antagonist therapy, monitor blood pressure, pulse rate, and ECG patterns to detect arrhythmias.
• For nifedipine and verapamil therapy, monitor digoxin levels and check for signs of digitalis toxicity. Because nifedipine may cause peripheral and periorbital edema, watch for fluid retention.
• Because coronary artery spasm is sometimes associated with atherosclerotic disease, advise the patient to stop smoking, avoid overeating, use alcohol sparingly, and maintain a balance between exercise and rest.

tion from smoking and reduction of stress are also beneficial.

Other preventive actions include control of hypertension (with sympathetic blocking agents, such as methyldopa and propranolol, or diuretics, such as hydrochlorothiazide), control of elevated serum cholesterol or triglyceride levels (with antilipemics such as clofibrate), and measures to minimize platelet aggregation and the danger of blood clots (with aspirin or sulfinpyrazone).

Special considerations

• During anginal episodes, monitor blood pressure and heart rate. Take an ECG during anginal episodes and be-

RELIEVING OCCLUSIONS WITH ANGIOPLASTY

For a patient with an occluded coronary artery, percutaneous transluminal coronary angioplasty can open the artery without opening the chest — an important advantage over bypass surgery.

First, coronary angiography must confirm the presence and location of the arterial occlusion. Then, a guide catheter is threaded through the patient's femoral artery into the coronary artery under fluoroscopic guidance, as shown on the right.

When angiography shows the guide catheter positioned at the occlusion site, a smaller double-lumen balloon catheter is carefully inserted through the guide catheter and the balloon directed through the occlusion (lower left). A marked pressure gradient will be obvious.

The balloon is alternately inflated and deflated until an angiogram verifies successful arterial dilation (lower right) and the pressure gradient has decreased.

Guide catheter

Balloon catheter at occlusion in coronary artery

Plaque

Deflated balloon

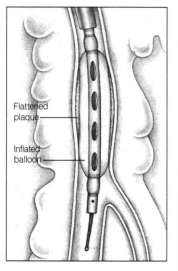

Flattened plaque

Inflated balloon

fore administering nitroglycerin or other nitrates. Record the duration of pain, amount of medication required to relieve it, and accompanying symptoms.

• Keep nitroglycerin available for immediate use. Instruct the patient to call immediately whenever he feels chest, arm, or neck pain.

• Before cardiac catheterization, explain the procedure to the patient. Make sure he knows why it's necessary, understands the risks, and realizes that it may indicate a need for surgery.

• After catheterization, review the expected course of treatment with the patient and family. Monitor the catheter site for bleeding. Also, check for distal pulses. To counter the diuretic effect of the dye, make sure the patient drinks plenty of fluids. Assess potassium levels.

• If the patient is scheduled for surgery, explain the procedure to the patient and family. Give them a tour of the intensive care unit, and introduce them to the staff.

• After surgery, monitor blood pressure, intake and output, breath sounds, chest tube drainage, and ECG, watching for signs of ischemia and arrhythmias. Also, observe for and treat chest pain and possible dye reactions. Give vigorous chest physiotherapy and guide the patient in coughing and deepbreathing exercises.

• Before discharge, stress the need to follow the prescribed drug regimen (antihypertensives, nitrates, antilipemics, for example), exercise program, and diet. Encourage regular, moderate exercise. Refer the patient to a self-help program to stop smoking.

CROHN'S DISEASE

Also know as regional enteritis and granulomatous colitis, Crohn's disease is an inflammation of any part of the GI tract (usually the terminal ileum). It can extend through all layers of the intestinal wall and may also involve regional lymph nodes and the mesentery.

Crohn's disease is most prevalent in adults ages 20 to 40. It's two to three times more common in people of Jewish ancestry and least common in blacks.

Causes

Although the exact cause of Crohn's disease is unknown, possible causes include allergies and other immune disorders and infection. However, no infecting organism has been isolated.

Several factors also implicate a genetic cause: Crohn's disease sometimes occurs in monozygotic twins, and up to 20% of patients with Crohn's disease have one or more affected relatives. However, no simple pattern of mendelian inheritance has been identified.

Whatever the cause of Crohn's disease, lacteal blockage in the intestinal wall leads to edema and, eventually, to inflammation, ulceration, stenosis, and possibly the development of abscesses and fistulas.

Signs and symptoms

Clinical effects vary according to the location and extent of the lesion, and at first, they may be mild and nonspecific.

Acute disease

Acute inflammatory signs and symptoms mimic appendicitis and include steady, colicky, pain in the right lower quadrant; cramping; tenderness; flatulence; nausea; fever; and diarrhea. Bleeding may occur and, although usually mild, may be massive. Bloody stools may also occur.

Chronic disease

Chronic symptoms, which are more typical of the disease, are more persistent and less severe; they include diarrhea (four to six stools a day) with pain in the right lower abdominal quadrant, steatorrhea, marked weight loss and, rarely, clubbing of fingers. The patient may complain of weakness and fatigue.

Complications

Crohn's disease may lead to intestinal obstruction, fistula formation between the small bowel and the bladder, perianal and perirectal abscesses and fistulas, intra-abdominal abscesses, and perforation.

Diagnosis

Laboratory findings often indicate increased white blood cell count and erythrocyte sedimentation rate, hypokalemia, hypocalcemia, hypomagnesemia, and decreased hemoglobin. A barium enema showing the string sign (segments of stricture separated by normal bowel) supports this diagnosis.

Sigmoidoscopy and colonoscopy may show patchy areas of inflammation, thus helping to rule out ulcerative colitis. However, a definitive diagnosis is possible only after a biopsy.

Treatment

No cure for Crohn's disease exists; treatment is symptomatic. In debilitated patients, therapy includes I.V. hyperalimentation to maintain nutrition while resting the bowel.

Drug therapy may include anti-inflammatory corticosteroids, immunosuppressive agents, such as azathioprine, and antibacterial agents, such as

sulfasalazine. Metronidazole has proven to be effective in some patients. Opium tincture and diphenoxylate may help combat diarrhea but are contraindicated in patients with significant intestinal obstruction.

Effective treatment requires important changes in lifestyle: physical rest, restricted fiber diet (no fruit or vegetables), and elimination of dairy products for lactose intolerance.

Surgery may be necessary to correct bowel perforation, massive hemorrhage, fistulas, or acute intestinal obstruction. Colectomy with ileostomy is often necessary in patients with extensive disease of the large intestine and rectum.

Special considerations

• Record fluid intake and output (including the amount of stools), and weigh the patient daily. Watch for dehydration and maintain fluid and electrolyte balance.

• Be alert for signs of intestinal bleeding (bloody stools); check stools daily for occult blood.

• If the patient is receiving steroids, watch for adverse reactions such as GI bleeding. Remember that steroids can mask signs of infection.

• Check hemoglobin and hematocrit regularly. Give iron supplements and blood transfusions as needed.

• Give analgesics as needed.

• Provide good patient hygiene and meticulous mouth care if the patient is restricted to nothing by mouth.

• After each bowel movement, give good skin care. Always keep a clean, covered bedpan within the patient's reach. Ventilate the room to eliminate odors.

• Observe the patient for fever and pain or pneumaturia, which may signal bladder fistula. Abdominal pain and distention and fever may indicate intestinal obstruction. Watch for stools from the vagina and an enterovaginal fistula.

• Before ileostomy, arrange for a visit by an enterostomal therapist.

• After surgery, frequently check the patient's I.V. and nasogastric tube for proper functioning. Monitor vital signs and fluid intake and output. Watch for wound infection.

• Provide meticulous stoma care, and teach it to the patient and family.

• Realize that ileostomy changes the patient's body image, so offer reassurance and emotional support.

• Stress the need for a severely restricted diet and bed rest, which may be trying, particularly for the young patient.

• Encourage the patient to try to reduce tension. If stress is clearly an aggravating factor, refer him for counseling.

CROUP

This severe inflammation and obstruction of the upper airway can occur as acute laryngotracheobronchitis (most common), laryngitis, and acute spasmodic laryngitis; it must always be distinguished from epiglottitis.

Croup is a childhood disease affecting boys more often than girls (typically between ages 3 months and 3 years) that usually occurs during the winter. Up to 15% of patients have a strong family history of croup. Recovery is usually complete.

Causes
Croup usually results from a viral infection. Parainfluenza viruses cause two-thirds of such infections; adenoviruses, respiratory syncytial virus (RSV), influenza and measles viruses, and bacteria (pertussis and diphtheria) account for the rest.

Signs and symptoms
The onset of croup usually follows an upper respiratory tract infection. Clinical features include inspiratory stridor, hoarse or muffled vocal sounds, varying degrees of laryngeal obstruction and respiratory distress, and a characteristic sharp, barklike cough. These symptoms may last only a few hours or persist for a day or two.

As croup progresses, it causes inflammatory edema and, possibly, spasm, which can obstruct the upper airway and severely compromise ventilation. Each form of croup has additional characteristics.

Laryngotracheobronchitis
The symptoms of this form of croup seem to worsen at night. Inflammation causes edema of the bronchi and bronchioles and increasingly difficult expiration, which frightens the child. Other characteristic features include fever, diffusely decreased breath sounds, expiratory rhonchi, and scattered crackles.

Laryngitis
Resulting from vocal cord edema, laryngitis is usually mild and produces no respiratory distress except in infants. Early indications include a sore throat and cough that, rarely, may progress to marked hoarseness, suprasternal and intercostal retractions, inspiratory stridor, dyspnea, diminished breath sounds, and restlessness. In later stages, severe dyspnea and exhaustion may result.

Acute spasmodic laryngitis
This form of croup affects children between ages 1 and 3, particularly those with allergies and a family history of croup. It typically begins with mild to moderate hoarseness and nasal discharge, followed by the characteristic cough and noisy inspiration (which often awaken the child at night), la-

bored breathing with retractions, rapid pulse, and clammy skin.

The child understandably becomes anxious, which may lead to increasing dyspnea and transient cyanosis. These severe symptoms diminish after several hours but reappear in a milder form on the next night or two.

Diagnosis
When bacterial infection is the cause, throat cultures may identify organisms and their sensitivity to antibiotics as well as rule out diphtheria. A neck X-ray may show areas of upper airway narrowing and edema in subglottic folds; laryngoscopy may reveal inflammation and obstruction in epiglottal and laryngeal areas.

In evaluating the patient, consider foreign body obstruction (a common cause of croupy cough in young children) as well as masses and cysts.

Treatment
For most children with croup, home care with rest, cool humidification during sleep, and antipyretics, such as acetaminophen, relieve symptoms. However, respiratory distress that interferes with oral hydration requires hospitalization and parenteral fluid replacement to prevent dehydration.

If bacterial infection is the cause, antibiotic therapy is necessary. Oxygen therapy may also be required.

Special considerations
• Monitor and support respiration, and control fever. Because croup is so frightening to the child and his family, also provide support and reassurance.
• Carefully monitor cough and breath sounds, hoarseness, severity of retractions, inspiratory stridor, cyanosis, respiratory rate and character (especially prolonged and labored respirations), restlessness, fever, and cardiac rate.

• Keep the child as quiet as possible, but avoid sedation, which can depress respiration.
• If the patient is an infant, position him in an infant seat or prop him up with a pillow.
• Place an older child in Fowler's position. If an older child requires a cool mist tent to help him breathe, explain why it's needed.
• Isolate patients suspected of having RSV and parainfluenza infections, if possible. Wash your hands carefully before leaving the room to avoid transmission to other children, particularly infants. Instruct parents and others involved in the care of these children to take similar precautions.
• Control fever with sponge baths and antipyretics. Keep a hypothermia blanket on hand for temperatures above 102° F (38.9° C). Watch for seizures in infants and young children with high fevers. Give I.V. antibiotics as necessary.
• Relieve sore throat with soothing, water-based ices such as fruit sherbet and popsicles. Avoid thicker, milk-based fluids if the child is producing heavy mucus or has great difficulty in swallowing.
• Apply petroleum jelly or another ointment around the nose and lips to soothe irritation from nasal discharge and mouth breathing.
• Maintain a calm, quiet environment and offer reassurance. Explain all procedures and answer any questions.
• When croup doesn't require hospitalization, provide thorough patient and family teaching for effective home care. Suggest the use of a cool mist humidifier (vaporizer).
• To relieve croupy spells, tell parents to carry the child into the bathroom, shut the door, and turn on the hot water. Breathing in warm, moist air quickly eases an acute spell of croup.
• Warn parents that ear infections and pneumonia are complications of croup,

which may appear about 5 days after recovery. Stress the importance of reporting earache, productive cough, high fever, or increased shortness of breath immediately.

CRYPTOCOCCOSIS

The fungus *Cryptococcus neoformans* causes this disease, also called torulosis and European blastomycosis. Cryptococcosis usually begins as an asymptomatic pulmonary infection but disseminates to extrapulmonary sites, usually to the central nervous system (CNS), but also to the skin, bones, prostate gland, liver, or kidneys.

Cryptoscoccosis is most prevalent in men, usually those between ages 30 and 60, and is rare in children. It's especially likely to develop in immuno-compromised patients, such as those with Hodgkin's disease, sarcoidosis, leukemia, or lymphoma and those who are receiving immunosuppressive agents. Currently, patients with acquired immunodeficiency syndrome (AIDS) are by far the most commonly affected group.

With appropriate treatment, the prognosis in pulmonary cryptococcosis is good. CNS infection, however, can be fatal, but treatment dramatically reduces mortality.

Causes
Transmission is through inhalation of *C. neoformans* in particles of dust contaminated by pigeon feces that harbor this organism. Therefore, cryptococcosis is primarily an urban infection.

Signs and symptoms
Typically, pulmonary cryptococcosis is asymptomatic. Onset of CNS involvement is gradual (cryptococcal meningitis), and causes progressively severe frontal and temporal headache, diplopia, blurred vision, dizziness, ataxia, aphasia, vomiting, tinnitus, memory changes, inappropriate behavior, irritability, psychotic symptoms, convulsions, and fever.

If untreated, symptoms progress to coma and death, usually a result of cerebral edema or hydrocephalus. Complications include optic atrophy, ataxia, hydrocephalus, deafness, paralysis, chronic brain syndrome, and personality changes.

Skin involvement produces red facial papules and other skin abscesses, with or without ulcerations; bone involvement produces painful osseous lesions of the long bones, skull, spine, and joints.

Diagnosis
A routine chest X-ray showing a pulmonary lesion may point to pulmonary cryptococcosis. However, this infection usually escapes diagnosis until it disseminates.

A firm diagnosis requires identification of *C. neoformans* by culture of sputum, urine, prostatic secretions, bone marrow aspirate or biopsy, or pleural biopsy; and, in CNS infection, by an India ink preparation of cerebrospinal fluid (CSF) and culture. Blood cultures are positive only in severe infection.

Supportive values include an increased antigen titer in serum and CSF in disseminated infection; increased CSF pressure, protein, and white blood cell count in CNS infection; and moderately decreased CSF glucose in about half of these patients. The diagnosis must rule out cancer and tuberculosis.

Treatment
The patient with pulmonary cryptococcosis will require close medical observation for a year after diagnosis. Treatment is unnecessary unless ex-

trapulmonary lesions develop or pulmonary lesions progress.

Treatment of disseminated infection calls for I.V. amphotericin B or fluconazole. Patients with AIDS will also need long-term therapy, usually with oral fluconazole.

Special considerations
• Cryptococcosis doesn't require isolation.
• Check the patient's vital functions, and note any changes in mental status, orientation, pupillary response, and motor function.
• Watch for headache, vomiting, and nuchal rigidity.
• Before giving I.V. amphotericin B, check for phlebitis. Infuse slowly and dilute—rapid infusion may cause circulatory collapse.
• Before therapy, draw blood for a serum electrolyte analysis to determine baseline renal status.
• During drug therapy, watch for decreased urine output, elevated blood urea nitrogen and creatinine levels, and hypokalemia.
• Monitor results of complete blood count, urinalysis, magnesium and potassium levels, and hepatic function tests. Ask the patient to report hearing loss, tinnitus, or dizziness.
• Give analgesics, antihistamines, and antiemetics for fever, chills, nausea, and vomiting.
• Provide psychological support to help the patient cope with long-term hospitalization.

CUSHING'S SYNDROME

A cluster of clinical abnormalities characterize Cushing's syndrome. These abnormalities result from excessive levels of adrenocortical hormones (particularly cortisol) or related corticosteroids and, to a lesser extent, androgens and aldosterone. Its unmistakable signs include rapidly developing adiposity of the face (moon face), neck, and trunk and purple striae on the skin.

Cushing's syndrome is most common in women. The prognosis depends on the underlying cause; it's poor in untreated persons and in those with untreatable ectopic corticotropin-producing carcinoma.

Causes
In approximately 70% of patients, Cushing's syndrome results from excess production of corticotropin and consequent hyperplasia of the adrenal cortex. Overproduction of corticotropin may stem from pituitary hypersecretion (Cushing's disease), a corticotropin-producing tumor in another organ (particularly bronchogenic or pancreatic carcinoma), or excessive administration of exogenous glucocorticoids.

In the remaining 30% of patients, Cushing's syndrome results from a cortisol-secreting adrenal tumor that's usually benign. In infants, the usual cause of Cushing's syndrome is adrenal carcinoma.

Signs and symptoms
Like other endocrine disorders, Cushing's syndrome induces changes in multiple body systems, depending on the adrenocortical hormone involved. Specific clinical effects vary with the system affected.
• *Endocrine and metabolic systems:* diabetes mellitus, with decreased glucose tolerance, fasting hyperglycemia, and glucosuria
• *Musculoskeletal system:* muscle weakness resulting from hypokalemia or loss of muscle mass from increased catabolism, pathologic fractures from decreased bone mineral, and skeletal growth retardation in children

- *Skin:* purplish striae; fat pads above the clavicles, over the upper back (buffalo hump), on the face (moon face), and throughout the trunk, with slender arms and legs; little or no scar formation; poor wound healing; acne and hirsutism in women
- *GI system:* peptic ulcer, resulting from increased gastric secretions and pepsin production, and decreased gastric mucus
- *Central nervous system (CNS):* irritability and emotional lability, ranging from euphoric behavior to depression or psychosis; insomnia
- *Cardiovascular system:* hypertension resulting from sodium and water retention; left ventricular hypertrophy; capillary weakness from protein loss, which leads to bleeding, petechiae, and ecchymosis
- *Immunologic system:* increased susceptibility to infection because of decreased lymphocyte production and suppressed antibody formation, decreased resistance to stress; suppressed inflammatory response may mask even a severe infection
- *Renal and urologic systems:* sodium and secondary fluid retention, increased potassium excretion, inhibited secretion of antidiuretic hormone, ureteral calculi from increased bone demineralization with hypercalciuria
- *Reproductive system:* increased androgen production, with clitoral hypertrophy, mild virilism, and amenorrhea or oligomenorrhea in women; sexual dysfunction also occurs.

Diagnosis

Initially, the diagnosis of Cushing's syndrome requires determination of plasma steroid levels. In persons with normal hormone balance, plasma cortisol levels are higher in the morning and decrease gradually through the day (diurnal variation). In patients with Cushing's syndrome, cortisol levels don't fluctuate and typically remain consistently elevated; a 24-hour urine sample demonstrates elevated free cortisol levels.

Suppression test

A low-dose dexamethasone suppression test confirms the diagnosis of Cushing's syndrome. A high-dose dexamethasone suppression test can determine if Cushing's syndrome results from pituitary dysfunction (Cushing's disease).

In this test, dexamethasone suppresses plasma cortisol levels, and urinary 17-hydroxycorticosteroids (17-OHCS) and 17-ketogenic steroids fall to 50% or less of basal levels. Failure to suppress these levels indicates that the syndrome results from an adrenal tumor or a nonendocrine, corticotropin-secreting tumor. This test can produce false-positive results.

Stimulation test

In a stimulation test, administration of metyrapone, which blocks cortisol production by the adrenal glands, tests the ability of the pituitary gland and the hypothalamus to detect and correct low levels of plasma cortisol by increasing corticotropin production. The patient with Cushing's disease reacts to this stimulus by secreting an excess of plasma corticotropin as measured by levels of urinary 17-OHCS.

If the patient has an adrenal or a nonendocrine corticotropin-secreting tumor, the pituitary gland—which is suppressed by the high cortisol levels—can't respond normally, so steroid levels remain stable or fall.

Other tests

Ultrasonography, a computed tomography (CT) scan, or angiography localizes adrenal tumors; a CT scan and magnetic resonance imaging of the head identify pituitary tumors.

Treatment

Radiation, drug therapy, and surgery are among the treatments used to restore hormone balance and reverse Cushing's syndrome. For example, pituitary-dependent Cushing's syndrome with adrenal hyperplasia and severe cushingoid symptoms—such as psychosis, poorly controlled diabetes mellitus, osteoporosis, and severe pathologic fractures—may require hypophysectomy or pituitary irradiation. If the patient fails to respond, bilateral adrenalectomy may be performed.

Nonendocrine corticotropin-producing tumors require excision of the tumor. Drug therapy follows (for example, with mitotane, metyrapone, or aminoglutethimide) to decrease cortisol levels if symptoms persist.

Aminoglutethimide and ketoconazole decrease cortisol levels and have been beneficial for many cushingoid patients. Aminoglutethimide alone, or in combination with metyrapone, may also be useful in metastatic adrenal carcinoma.

Before surgery, the patient with cushingoid symptoms should have special management to control hypertension, edema, diabetes, and cardiovascular manifestations and to prevent infection. Glucocorticoid administration on the morning of surgery can help prevent acute adrenal insufficiency during surgery.

Cortisol therapy is essential during and after surgery to help the patient tolerate the physiologic stress imposed by removal of the pituitary or adrenals. If normal cortisol production resumes, steroid therapy may be gradually tapered and eventually discontinued. However, bilateral adrenalectomy or total hypophysectomy mandates lifelong steroid replacement therapy to correct hormonal deficiencies. (See *Dealing with lifelong treatment,* page 252.)

Special considerations

• Frequently monitor vital signs, especially blood pressure. Carefully observe the hypertensive patient who also has cardiac disease.

• Check laboratory reports for hypernatremia, hypokalemia, hyperglycemia, and glycosuria.

• Because the cushingoid patient is likely to retain sodium and water, check for edema, and monitor daily weight and intake and output carefully.

• To minimize weight gain, edema, and hypertension, ask the dietary department to provide a diet that's high in protein and potassium but low in calories, carbohydrates, and sodium.

• Watch for infection—a particular problem in Cushing's syndrome.

• If the patient has osteoporosis and is bedridden, perform passive range-of-motion exercises carefully because of the severe risk for pathologic fractures.

• *Remember:* Cushing's syndrome produces emotional lability. Record incidents that upset the patient, and try to prevent such situations from occurring, if possible. Help him get the physical and mental rest he needs—by sedation, if necessary.

• Offer support to the emotionally labile patient throughout the difficult testing period.

After surgery:

• Watch carefully for wound drainage or temperature elevation. Use strict aseptic technique in changing the patient's dressings.

• Administer analgesics and replacement steroids as necessary.

• Monitor urinary output and check vital signs carefully, watching for signs of shock (decreased blood pressure, increased pulse rate, pallor, and cold, clammy skin).

• If shock develops, give vasopressors and increase the rate of I.V. fluids. Because mitotane, aminoglutethimide, and metyrapone decrease mental alertness and produce physical weakness, assess neurologic and behavioral status, and warn the patient of adverse CNS effects.

• Watch for severe nausea, vomiting, and diarrhea.

• Check laboratory reports for hypoglycemia from removal of the source of cortisol, a hormone that maintains blood glucose levels.

• Check for abdominal distention and return of bowel sounds following adrenalectomy.

• Check regularly for signs of adrenal hypofunction — orthostatic hypotension, apathy, weakness, fatigue — indicators that steroid replacement is inadequate.

• In the patient undergoing pituitary surgery, be alert for signs of increased intracranial pressure (confusion, agitation, changes in level of consciousness, nausea, and vomiting). Also watch for hypopituitarism.

CUTANEOUS LARVA MIGRANS

Also called creeping eruption, cutaneous larva migrans is a skin reaction to infestation by nematodes (hookworms or roundworms) that usually infect dogs and cats. This parasitic infection most often affects persons who come in contact with infected soil or sand, such as children and farmers. Eruptions associated with cutaneous larva migrans clear completely with treatment.

Causes
Under favorable conditions — warmth, moisture, sandy soil — hookworm or roundworm ova present in feces of affected animals (such as dogs and cats) hatch into larvae, which can then burrow into human skin on contact. After penetrating its host, the larva becomes trapped under the skin, unable to reach the intestines to complete its normal life cycle.

Then the parasite begins to move around, producing the peculiar, tunnel-like lesions that are alternately meandering and linear, reflecting the nematode's persistent and unsuccessful attempts to escape its host.

Signs and symptoms

A transient rash or, possibly, a small vesicle appears at the point of penetration, usually on an exposed area that has come in contact with the ground, such as the feet, legs, or buttocks. The incubation period may be weeks or months, or the parasite may be active almost as soon as it enters the skin.

As the parasite migrates, it etches a noticeable thin, raised, red line on the skin, which may become vesicular and encrusted. Pruritus quickly develops, often with crusting and secondary infection following excoriation.

The larva's apparently random path can cover from 1 mm to 1 cm a day. Penetration of more than one larva may involve a much larger area of the skin, marking it with many tracks.

Diagnosis

Characteristic migratory lesions strongly suggest cutaneous larva migrans. A thorough patient history usually reveals contact with warm, moist soil within the past several months.

Treatment

Cutaneous larva migrans infections may require oral administration of 50 mg/kg thiabendazole for 2 or 3 days. Topical thiabendazole may also be effective.

Special considerations

• Reassure the patient that larva migrans lesions usually clear 1 to 2 weeks after treatment, especially if he is sensitive about his appearance. Stress the importance of adhering to the treatment regimen exactly as ordered.

• Have the patient's nails cut short to prevent skin breaks and secondary bacterial infection from scratching. Apply cool, moist compresses to alleviate itching.

• Tell the patient receiving systemic thiabendazole treatment to watch for and report adverse reactions, including nausea, vomiting, abdominal pain, and dizziness.

• Encourage the patient to verbalize feelings about the infestation, including embarrassment, fear of rejection by others, and body image disturbance.

• Instruct the patient and his family in good hand-washing technique, and stress the importance of preventing the spread of the infection among family members.

• To prevent cutaneous larva migrans, teach patients about the existence of these parasites, sanitation of beaches and sandboxes, and proper pet care.

CYSTIC FIBROSIS

Sometimes called mucoviscidosis, cystic fibrosis is a generalized dysfunction of the exocrine glands that affects multiple organ systems. Transmitted as an autosomal recessive trait, it's the most common fatal genetic disease of white children.

Cystic fibrosis is a chronic disease. About 50% of affected children die by age 16; of the rest, some survive to age 30 or beyond, depending on the patient's genotype.

Incidence of cystic fibrosis is highest (1 in 2,000 live births) in people of northern European ancestry and lowest in blacks (1 in 17,000 live births), Native Americans, and people of Asian ancestry. The disease occurs equally in both sexes.

Causes

The recently identified gene responsible for cystic fibrosis encodes a protein that involves chloride transport across epithelial membranes.

The immediate causes of symptoms are increased viscosity of bronchial, pancreatic, and other mucous gland secretions and consequent obstruction of glandular ducts. Cystic fibrosis accounts for almost all cases of pancreatic enzyme deficiency in children.

Signs and symptoms

The clinical effects of cystic fibrosis may become apparent soon after birth or may take years to develop. They include major aberrations in sweat gland, respiratory, and GI functions.

Sweat gland dysfunction

In cystic fibrosis, sweat gland dysfunction is the most consistent abnormality. Increased concentrations of sodium and chloride in the sweat lead to hyponatremia and hypochloremia and can eventually induce fatal shock and arrhythmias, especially in hot weather.

Respiratory symptoms

Such symptoms reflect obstructive changes in the lungs: wheezy respirations; a dry, nonproductive, paroxysmal cough; dyspnea; and tachypnea. These changes stem from thick, tenacious secretions in the bronchioles and alveoli and eventually lead to severe atelectasis and emphysema.

Children with cystic fibrosis display a barrel chest, cyanosis, and clubbing of the fingers and toes. They suffer recurring bronchitis and pneumonia and associated nasal polyps and sinusitis. Death typically results from pneumonia, emphysema, or atelectasis.

GI symptoms

The GI effects of cystic fibrosis occur mainly in the intestines, pancreas, and liver. One early symptom is meconium ileus; the newborn with cystic fibrosis doesn't excrete meconium, a dark green mucilaginous material found in the intestine at birth. He develops symptoms of intestinal obstruction, such as abdominal distention, vomiting, constipation, dehydration, and electrolyte imbalance.

Eventually, obstruction of the pancreatic ducts and resulting deficiency of trypsin, amylase, and lipase prevent the conversion and absorption of fat and protein in the intestinal tract. The undigested food is then excreted in frequent, bulky, foul-smelling, and pale stools with a high fat content.

This malabsorption induces poor weight gain, poor growth, ravenous appetite, distended abdomen, thin extremities, and sallow skin with poor turgor. The inability to absorb fats produces deficiency of fat-soluble vitamins (A, D, E, and K), leading to clotting problems, retarded bone growth, and delayed sexual development. Males may experience azoospermia and sterility; females may experience secondary amenorrhea but can reproduce.

A common complication in infants and children is rectal prolapse. This stems from malnutrition and wasting of perirectal supporting tissues.

In the pancreas, fibrotic tissue, multiple cysts, thick mucus and, eventually, fat replace the acini (small, saclike swellings normally found in this gland). This results in signs of pancreatic insufficiency: insufficient insulin production, abnormal glucose tolerance, and glycosuria.

About 15% of patients are pancreatic sufficient, having adequate pancreatic exocrine function for normal digestion. These patients have a better prognosis.

Biliary obstruction and fibrosis may prolong neonatal jaundice. In some patients, cirrhosis and portal hypertension may lead to esophageal varices, episodes of hematemesis and, occasionally, hepatomegaly.

Diagnosis

The Cystic Fibrosis Foundation sets the following standards for a definitive diagnosis:

• *Two sweat tests* using a pilocarpine solution (a sweat inducer) are clearly positive; the patient also has either an obstructive pulmonary disease, confirmed pancreatic insufficiency or failure to thrive, or a family history of cystic fibrosis.

• *Chest X-rays* indicate early signs of obstructive lung disease.

• *Stool specimen analysis* indicates the absence of trypsin, suggesting pancreatic insufficiency.

The following test results may support the diagnosis:

• *Deoxyribonucleic acid testing* can now locate the presence of the Delta F 508 deletion (found in about 70% of cystic fibrosis patients, although the disease can cause more than 100 other mutations). This test can also be used for carrier detection and a prenatal diagnosis in families with a previously affected child.

• *Pulmonary function tests* reveal decreased vital capacity, elevated residual volume from air entrapments, and decreased forced expiratory volume in 1 second. This test is used if pulmonary exacerbation already exists.

• *Liver enzyme test* may reveal hepatic insufficiency.

• *Sputum culture* reveals organisms that cystic fibrosis patients typically and chronically colonize, such as *Staphylococcus* and *Pseudomonas*.

• *Serum albumin levels* help assess nutritional status.

• *Electrolyte analysis* assesses dehydration and glucose levels.

Treatment

The aim of treatment is to help the child lead as normal a life as possible. Specific treatment depends on the organ systems involved.

• To combat sweat electrolyte losses, treatment includes generous salting of foods and, during hot weather, administration of sodium supplements.

• To offset pancreatic enzyme deficiencies, treatment includes oral pancreatic enzymes with meals and snacks. The child's diet should be low in fat but high in protein and calories, and it should include supplements of watermiscible, fat-soluble vitamins (A, D, E, and K).

• Management of pulmonary dysfunction includes chest physiotherapy, postural drainage, and breathing exercises several times daily to aid removal of secretions from lungs. Antihistamines are contraindicated; they have a drying effect on mucous membranes, making expectoration of mucus difficult or impossible.

Aerosol therapy includes intermittent nebulizer treatments before postural drainage, to loosen secretions. Dornase alfa, a genetically engineered pulmonary enzyme given by aerosol nebulizer, helps thin airway mucus, improving lung function and reducing the risk of pulmonary infection.

A patient with pulmonary infection will need mucopurulent secretions loosened and removed, using an intermittent nebulizer and postural drainage to relieve obstruction. Use of a mist tent is controversial because mist particles may become trapped in the esophagus and stomach and never even reach the lungs. Broad-spectrum antimicrobials help combat infection. Oxygen therapy is used as needed.

Recently, some patients have undergone lung transplants to reduce the effects of the disease. Also, clinical trials of aerosol gene therapy show promise in reducing pulmonary symptoms.

Special considerations
• Suggest the use of air conditioners and humidifiers to help decrease vulnerability to respiratory infections.
• Throughout this illness, teach the patient and his family about the disease and its treatment.
• Provide emotional support, and refer the patient and his family for genetic counseling and to the Cystic Fibrosis Foundation.

CYSTINURIA

An autosomal recessive disorder, cystinuria is an inborn error of amino acid transport in the kidneys and intestine that allows excessive urinary excretion of cystine and other dibasic amino acids and results in recurrent cystine renal calculi. It's the most common defect of amino acid transport.

Cystinuria is inherited as an autosomal recessive defect and occurs in approximately 1 in 15,000 live births. It's more prevalent in persons of short stature; the reason for this is unknown. Although this disorder affects both sexes, it's more severe in males. With proper treatment, the prognosis is good.

Causes
Impaired renal tubular reabsorption of dibasic amino acids (cystine, lysine, arginine, and ornithine) results in excessive amino acid concentration and excretion in the urine. When cystine concentration exceeds its solubility, it precipitates and forms crystals, precursors of cystine calculi. Excessive excretion of the other three amino acids produces no ill effects.

Signs and symptoms
The clinical effects of cystinuria result from cystine or mixed cystine calculi. These develop most frequently between ages 10 and 30.

Typically, such calculi may cause dull flank pain from renal parenchymal and capsular distention. They also cause nausea, vomiting, abdominal distention from acute renal colic (the result of smooth-muscle spasm and hyperperistalsis), hematuria, and tenderness in the costovertebral angle or over the kidneys.

Renal calculi may also cause urinary tract obstruction, with resultant secondary infection (chills; fever; burning, itching, or pain on urination; frequency; and foul-smelling urine). With prolonged ureteral obstruction, marked hydronephrosis and a visible or palpable flank mass may result.

Diagnosis
Typical clinical features and a positive family history of renal disease or kidney stones suggest cystinuria, but the following laboratory data confirm it:
• *Chemical analysis of calculi* shows cystine crystals, with a variable amount of calcium. Pure cystine stones are radiolucent on X-rays, but most contain some calcium. These stones are light yellow or brownish-yellow, and granular; they may be large.
• *Blood studies* may show an elevated serum white blood cell count, especially with a urinary tract infection, and elevated clearance of cystine, lysine, arginine, and ornithine.
• *Urinalysis* with amino acid chromatography indicates aminoaciduria, consisting of cystine, lysine, arginine, and ornithine. Urine pH is usually less than 5.
• *Microscopic examination of urine* shows hexagonal, flat cystine crystals. When glacial acetic acid is added to chilled urine, cystine crystals resemble benzene rings.

• *Cyanide-nitroprusside test* is positive. In cystinuria, a urine specimen made alkaline by adding ammonia turns magenta when nitroprusside is added to it.

Confirming tests also include excretory urography to determine renal function, and kidney-ureter-bladder X-rays to determine the size and location of calculi.

Treatment
No effective treatment exists to decrease cystine excretion. Increasing fluid intake to maintain a minimum 24-hour urine volume of 3,000 ml and reduce urine cystine concentration is the primary means of dissolving excess cystine and preventing cystine stones.

Sodium bicarbonate and an alkaline-ash diet (high in vegetables and fruit, low in protein) alkalinize urine, increasing cystine solubility. However, this therapy may provide a favorable environment for formation of calcium phosphate stones. Penicillamine can also increase cystine solubility but should be used with caution because of its toxic side effects and high incidence of allergic reaction.

Treatment may also include surgical removal of calculi, when necessary, and appropriate measures to prevent and treat urinary tract infection.

Special considerations
• Explain to the patient the importance of complying with his treatment regimen.
• Emphasize the need to maintain increased, evenly spaced fluid intake, even through the night.
• Teach the patient how to recognize signs and symptoms of renal calculi and urinary tract infection, and tell him to report them immediately.
• Teach the patient to check urine pH and record the results.
• Carefully monitor sodium bicarbonate administration because metabolic alkalosis may develop. Arterial bicarbonate level can be estimated by subtracting 2 from the serum carbon dioxide level.
• Explain to the patient receiving penicillamine that it may cause an allergic or serum sickness–type reaction. Other adverse reactions may include severe proteinuria, neutropenia, tinnitus, and taste impairment.

CYTOMEGALOVIRUS INFECTION

Also called generalized salivary gland disease and cytomegalic inclusion disease, cytomegalovirus (CMV) infection is caused by the cytomegalovirus, which is a deoxyribonucleic acid, ether-sensitive virus belonging to the herpes family. The disease occurs worldwide and is transmitted by human contact.

About four out of five people over age 35 have been infected with cytomegalovirus, usually during childhood or early adulthood. In most of these people, the disease is so mild that it's overlooked. However, CMV infection during pregnancy can be hazardous to the fetus, possibly leading to stillbirth, brain damage, and other birth defects or to severe neonatal illness.

Causes
Cytomegalovirus has been found in the saliva, urine, semen, breast milk, feces, blood, and vaginal and cervical secretions of infected persons. Transmission usually happens through contact with these infected secretions, which harbor the virus for months or even years.

The virus may be transmitted by sexual contact and can travel across the placenta of a pregnant woman, causing a congenital infection. Immunosuppressed patients, especially those who have received transplanted organs, run a 90% chance of contracting CMV infection. Recipients of blood transfusions from donors with positive CMV antibodies are at some risk.

Signs and symptoms

Cytomegalovirus probably spreads through the body in lymphocytes or mononuclear cells to the lungs, liver, GI tract, eyes, and central nervous system, where it often produces inflammatory reactions.

Most patients with CMV infection have mild, nonspecific complaints, or none at all, even though antibody titers indicate infection. In these patients, the disease usually runs a self-limiting course.

Immunodeficient patients, such as those with aquired immunodeficiency syndrome (AIDS), and those receiving immunosuppressives may develop pneumonia or other secondary infections. AIDS patients may also develop disseminated CMV infection, which may cause chorioretinitis (resulting in blindness), colitis, or encephalitis.

Infected infants ages 3 to 6 months usually appear asymptomatic but may develop hepatic dysfunction, hepatosplenomegaly, spider angiomas, pneumonitis, and lymphadenopathy.

Congenital CMV infection is seldom apparent at birth, though the infant's urine contains CMV. About 1% of all newborns have CMV.

The virus can cause brain damage that may not show up for months after birth. Occasionally, it produces a rapidly fatal neonatal illness characterized by jaundice, petechial rash, hepatosplenomegaly, thrombocytopenia, hemolytic anemia, microcephaly, psychomotor retardation, mental deficiency, and hearing loss.

In some adults, CMV may cause cytomegalovirus mononucleosis, with 3 weeks or more of irregular, high fever.

Other findings may include a normal or elevated white blood cell (WBC) count, lymphocytosis, and increased atypical lymphocytes.

Diagnosis

Although virus isolation in urine is the most sensitive laboratory method, a diagnosis can also rest on virus isolation from saliva, throat, cervix, WBC, and biopsy specimens.

Other laboratory tests support the diagnosis, including complement fixation studies, hemagglutination inhibition antibody tests, and, for congenital infections, indirect immunofluorescent tests for CMV immunoglobulin M antibody.

Treatment

Because CMV infection is usually self-limiting, treatment aims to relieve symptoms and prevent complications. In the immunosuppressed patient, however, CMV is treated with acyclovir, ganciclovir, and foscarnet.

Special considerations

• Provide parents of children with severe congenital CMV infection with counseling to help them cope with the possibility of brain damage or death.

• To help prevent CMV infection, warn immunosuppressed patients and pregnant women to avoid exposure to confirmed or suspected CMV infection. Tell pregnant patients that maternal CMV infection can cause serious fetal abnormalities.

• Urge patients with CMV infection — especially young children — to wash their hands thoroughly to prevent spreading it.

• Observe universal precautions when handling body secretions.

Dacryocystitis

A common infection of the lacrimal sac, dacryocystitis results from an obstruction (dacryostenosis) of the nasolacrimal duct, occurring most often in women over age 40. In infants, it results from congenital atresia of the nasolacrimal duct. Dacryocystitis can be acute or chronic.

Causes
The most common infecting organism in acute dacryocystitis is *Staphylococcus aureus* or, occasionally, beta-hemolytic streptococci. In chronic dacryocystitis, *Streptococcus pneumoniae* or sometimes a fungus, such as *Actinomyces* or *Candida albicans,* is the causative organism.

In infants, atresia of the nasolacrimal ducts results from failure of canalization or, in the first few months of life, from blockage when the membrane that separates the lower part of the nasolacrimal duct and the inferior nasal meatus fails to open spontaneously before tear secretion. It may also result from obstruction of the duct by gross abnormalities of the nasal bones.

Signs and symptoms
The hallmark of both acute and chronic dacryocystitis is constant tearing. Other symptoms of the acute form include inflammation and tenderness over the nasolacrimal sac; pressure over this area may produce purulent discharge from the punctum. In the chronic form, a mucoid discharge may be expressed from the tear sac.

Diagnosis
Clinical features and a physical examination suggest dacryocystitis.

Culture of the discharged material demonstrates *S. aureus* and, occasionally, beta-hemolytic streptococci in acute dacryocystitis and *S. pneumoniae* or *C. albicans* in the chronic form. The white blood cell count may be elevated in the acute form; in the chronic form, it's generally normal.

X-ray after injection of a radiopaque medium (dacryocystography) locates the atresia.

Treatment
Therapy for acute dacryocystitis consists of warm compresses, topical and systemic antibiotic therapy and, occasionally, incision and drainage. Chronic dacryocystitis may eventually require dacryocystorhinostomy.

Treatment for nasolacrimal duct obstruction in an infant consists of careful massage of the area over the lacrimal sac four times a day for 6 to 9 months. If this fails to open the duct, dilation of the punctum and probing of the duct are necessary. Postoperative management requires a pressure patch over this area of the eye.

Special considerations
• Check the patient history for possible allergy to antibiotics before giving them. Emphasize the importance of precise compliance with the prescribed antibiotic regimen.

• Tell the adult patient what to expect after surgery: He'll have ice compresses over the surgical site and will have bruising and swelling.
• Monitor blood loss by counting dressings used to collect the blood.
• Apply ice compresses postoperatively. A small adhesive bandage may be placed over the suture line to protect it from damage.

DELUSIONAL DISORDERS

According to the *Diagnostic and Statistical Manual of Mental Disorders*, 4th edition *(DSM-IV)*, delusional disorders are marked by false beliefs with a plausible basis in reality. Formerly referred to as paranoid disorders, delusional disorders involve erotomanic, grandiose, jealous, somatic, or persecutory themes. Some patients experience several types of delusions, whereas others experience unspecified delusions with no dominant theme.

Delusional disorders commonly begin in middle or late adulthood, usually between ages 40 and 55, but they can occur at a younger age. These uncommon illnesses affect less than 1% of the population; the incidence is about equal in men and women.

Typically chronic, these disorders often interfere with social and marital relationships but seldom impair intellectual or occupational functioning significantly.

Causes
Delusional disorders of later life strongly suggest a hereditary predisposition. At least one study has linked the development of delusional disorders to inferiority feelings in the family.

Some researchers suggest that delusional disorders are the product of specific early childhood experiences with an authoritarian family structure. Others hold that anyone with a sensitive personality is particularly vulnerable to developing a delusional disorder.

Certain medical conditions — head injury, chronic alcoholism, and deafness — and aging are known to increase the risks of delusional disorders. Predisposing factors linked to aging include isolation, lack of stimulating interpersonal relationships, physical illness, and impaired hearing and vision.

Severe stress (such as a move to a foreign country) may also precipitate a delusional disorder.

Signs and symptoms
Aside from behavior related to his delusions, the psychiatric history of a delusional patient may be unremarkable. This helps distinguish it from disorders that result in behavior more dissociated from reality, such as paranoid schizophrenia. (For more information, see *Delusional disorder or paranoid schizophrenia?*)

The delusional patient is likely to report problems with social and marital relationships, including depression or sexual dysfunction. He may describe a life marked by social isolation or hostility. He may deny feeling lonely, relentlessly criticizing or placing unreasonable demands on others.

Gathering accurate information from a delusional patient may prove difficult. He may deny his feelings, disregard the circumstances that lead to his hospitalization, and refuse treatment.

However, his responses and behavior during the assessment interview provide clues that can help to identify his disorder. Family members may confirm observations — for example, by reporting that the patient is chronically jealous or suspicious.

Assessment clue: Communication

The patient's ability to communicate can be another indicator. He may be evasive or reluctant to answer questions. Or he may be overly talkative, explaining events in great detail and emphasizing what he has achieved, prominent people he knows, or places he has traveled.

The patient may make statements that at first seem logical but later prove irrelevant. Some of his answers may be contradictory, jumbled, or irrational.

A delusional patient may make expressions of denial, projection, and rationalization. Once delusions become firmly entrenched, the patient will no longer seek to justify his beliefs. However, if he's still struggling to maintain his delusional defenses, he may make statements that reveal his condition, such as "People at work won't talk to me because I'm smarter than they are."

Accusatory statements are also characteristic of the delusional patient. Pervasive delusional themes (for example, grandiose or persecutory) may become apparent.

The patient may also display nonverbal cues, such as excessive vigilance or obvious apprehension on entering the room. During questions, he may listen intently, reacting defensively to imagined slights or insults. He may sit at the edge of his seat or fold his arms as if to shield himself. If he carries papers or money, he may clutch them firmly.

Diagnosis

The DSM-IV describes a characteristic set of behaviors that mark the patient with delusional disorder. (See *Diagnosing delusional disorder,* page 262.)

DELUSIONAL DISORDER OR PARANOID SCHIZOPHRENIA?

To distinguish between these two disorders, consider the following characteristics.

Delusional disorder

In a delusional disorder, the patient's delusions reflect reality and are arranged into a coherent system. They're based on misinterpretations of, or elaborations on, reality.

The patient doesn't experience hallucinations, and his affect and behavior are normal.

Paranoid schizophrenia

In paranoid schizophrenia, the patient's delusions are scattered, illogical, and incoherently arranged with no relation to reality.

The patient may have hallucinations, his affect is inappropriate and inconsistent, and his behavior is bizarre.

In addition, blood and urine tests, psychological tests, and neurologic evaluation can rule out organic causes of the delusions, such as amphetamine-induced psychoses and Alzheimer's disease. Endocrine function tests rule out hyperadrenalism, pernicious anemia, and thyroid disorders such as "myxedema madness."

Treatment

Effective treatment of delusional disorders, consisting of a combination of drug therapy and psychotherapy, must correct the behavior and mood disturbances that result from the patient's mistaken belief system. Treatment also may include mobilizing a support system for the isolated elderly patient.

DIAGNOSING DELUSIONAL DISORDER

In an individual with a suspected delusional disorder, psychiatric examination confirms the diagnosis. The examiner bases the diagnosis on the following criteria set forth in the *Diagnostic and Statistical Manual of Mental Disorders*, 4th edition:

• Nonbizzare delusions of at least 1 month's duration are present, involving real-life situations, such as being followed, poisoned, infected, loved at a distance, or deceived by one's spouse or lover.

• The patient's symptoms have never met the criteria known as characteristic symptoms of schizophrenia. However, tactile and olfactory hallucinations may be present if they are related to a delusional theme.

• Apart from being affected by the delusion or its ramifications, the patient isn't markedly impaired functionally nor is his behavior obviously odd or bizarre.

• If mood disturbances have occurred concurrently with delusions, their total duration has been brief relative to the duration of the delusional disturbance.

• The disturbance doesn't result from the direct physiologic effects of a substance or a general medical condition.

Antipsychotic drug therapy

Drug treatment with antipsychotic agents is similar to that used in schizophrenic disorders. Antipsychotics appear to work by blocking postsynaptic dopamine receptors. These drugs reduce the incidence of psychotic symptoms, such as hallucinations and delusions, and relieve anxiety and agitation.

Other psychiatric drugs, such as antidepressants and anxiolytics, may be prescribed to control associated symptoms.

High-potency antipsychotics include fluphenazine, haloperidol, thiothixene, and trifluoperazine. Loxapine, molindone, and perphenazine are intermediate in potency, and chlorpromazine and thioridazine are low-potency agents.

Haloperidol decanoate, fluphenazine decanoate, and fluphenazine enanthate are depot formulations that are implanted I.M. They release the drug gradually over a 30-day period, improving compliance.

Clozapine, which differs chemically from other antipsychotic drugs, may be prescribed for severely ill patients who fail to respond to standard treatment. This agent effectively controls a wider range of psychotic symptoms without the usual adverse effects.

However, clozapine can cause drowsiness, sedation, excessive salivation, tachycardia, dizziness, and seizures as well as agranulocytosis, a potentially fatal blood disorder characterized by a low white blood cell count and pronounced neutropenia.

Routine blood monitoring is essential to detect the estimated 1% to 2% of all patients taking clozapine who develop agranulocytosis. If caught in the early stages, this disorder is reversible.

Special considerations

• In dealing with the delusional patient, be direct, straightforward, and dependable. Whenever possible, elicit his feedback. Move slowly, in a matter-of-fact manner, and respond without anger or defensiveness to his hostile remarks.

• Respect the patient's privacy and space needs. Don't touch him unnecessarily.

• Take steps to reduce social isolation, if the patient allows. Gradually increase social contacts after he has become comfortable with the staff.

• Watch for refusal of medication or food, resulting from the patient's irrational fear of poisoning.

• Monitor the patient carefully for adverse effects of antipsychotic drugs: drug-induced parkinsonism, acute dystonia, akathisia, tardive dyskinesia, and malignant neuroleptic syndrome.

• If the patient is taking clozapine, stress the importance of returning weekly to the hospital or an outpatient setting to have his blood monitored.

• Involve the family in treatment. Teach them how to recognize signs of an impending relapse — tension, nervousness, insomnia, decreased concentration ability, and apathy — and suggest ways to manage them.

DEPERSONALIZATION DISORDER

Persistent or recurrent episodes of detachment characterize depersonalization disorder. During these episodes, self-awareness is temporarily altered or lost; the patient often perceives this alteration in consciousness as a barrier between himself and the outside world.

The patient's sense of depersonalization may be restricted to a single body part, such as a limb, or it may encompass the whole self. Although he seldom loses touch with reality completely, the episodes of depersonalization may cause him severe distress.

Depersonalization disorder usually has a sudden onset in adolescence or early in adult life. It follows a chronic course, with periodic exacerbations and remissions, and resolves gradually.

Causes

Depersonalization disorder typically stems from severe stress, including war experiences, accidents, and natural disasters.

Signs and symptoms

The patient with depersonalization disorder may complain of feeling detached from his entire being and body, as if he were watching himself from a distance or living in a dream. He also may report sensory anesthesia, a loss of self-control, difficulty speaking, and feelings of derealization and losing touch with reality.

Common findings during the assessment interview include symptoms of depression, obsessive rumination, somatic concerns, anxiety, fear of going insane, a disturbed sense of time, and a prolonged recall time, as well as physical complaints such as dizziness.

Diagnosis

The *Diagnostic and Statistical Manual of Mental Disorders*, 4th edition, describes a set of symptoms characteristic of patients with this condition. (See *Diagnosing depersonalization disorder,* page 264.)

Treatment

Psychotherapy aims to establish a trusting, therapeutic relationship in which the patient recognizes the traumatic event that triggered the disorder and the anxiety it evoked. The therapist subsequently teaches the patient to use reality-based coping strategies, rather than to detach himself from the situation.

DIAGNOSING DEPERSONALIZATION DISORDER

The depersonalization disorder diagnosis is made when the patient's symptoms match the following criteria from the *Diagnostic and Statistical Manual of Mental Disorders*, 4th edition:

• The patient has persistent or recurrent experiences of feeling detached from his mind or body (as if the person were an outside observer) or feeling like an automaton (as if the person were in a dream).

• During the depersonalization experience, reality testing remains intact.

• The depersonalization causes clinically significant distress or impairment in social, occupational, or other important areas of functioning.

• The depersonalization experience doesn't occur exclusively during the course of another mental disorder, such as schizophrenia, panic disorder, acute stress disorder, or another dissociative disorder and doesn't result from the direct physiologic effects of a substance or a general medical condition.

Special considerations

• When providing care in this disorder, assist the patient in using reality-based coping strategies under stress, rather than those strategies that distort reality.

• Help the patient who has depersonalization disorder recognize and deal with anxiety-producing experiences.

• Establish a therapeutic, nonjudgmental relationship with the patient.

DEPRESSION, MAJOR

Also known as unipolar disorder, major depression is a syndrome of persistently sad, dysphoric mood accompanied by disturbances in sleep and appetite, lethargy, and an inability to experience pleasure (anhedonia). Major depression occurs in up to 17% of adults, affecting all racial, ethnic, and socioeconomic groups. It affects both sexes but is more common in women.

About half of all depressed patients experience a single episode and recover completely; the rest have at least one recurrence. Major depression can profoundly alter social, family, and occupational functioning.

However, suicide is the most serious complication of major depression, resulting when the patient's feelings of worthlessness, guilt, and hopelessness are so overwhelming that he no longer considers life worth living. Nearly twice as many women as men attempt suicide, but men are far more likely to succeed.

Causes

The multiple causes of depression are not completely understood. Current research suggests possible genetic, familial, biochemical, physical, psychological, and social causes.

Psychological factors

Such causes may include feelings of helplessness and vulnerability, anger, hopelessness and pessimism, and low self-esteem; they may be related to abnormal character and behavior patterns and troubled personal relationships.

In many patients, the history identifies a specific personal loss or severe stressor that probably interacts with the person's predisposition to provoke major depression.

Medical conditions

Depression may be secondary to a specific medical condition — for example, metabolic disturbances, such as hypoxia and hypercalcemia; endocrine disorders, such as diabetes and Cushing's disease; neurologic diseases, such as Parkinson's and Alzheimer's disease; and cancer, especially of the pancreas.

Other medical conditions that may underlie depression include viral and bacterial infections, such as influenza and pneumonia; cardiovascular disorders such as congestive heart failure; pulmonary disorders such as chronic obstructive lung disease; musculoskeletal disorders such as degenerative arthritis; GI disorders such as irritable bowel syndrome; genitourinary problems such as incontinence; collagen vascular diseases such as lupus; and anemias.

Drugs

Drugs prescribed for medical and psychiatric conditions, as well as many commonly abused substances, can also cause depression. Examples include antihypertensives, psychotropics, narcotic and nonnarcotic analgesics, antiparkinsonian drugs, numerous cardiovascular medications, oral antidiabetics, antimicrobials, steroids, chemotherapeutic agents, cimetidine, and alcohol.

Signs and symptoms

The primary features of major depression are a predominantly sad mood and a loss of interest or pleasure in daily activities. Symptoms tend to be more severe than those caused by dysthymic disorder, which is a milder, chronic form of depression. (See *Dysthymic disorder: A chronic affective disorder.*)

The depressive patient may complain of feeling "down in the dumps," express doubts about his self-worth or ability to cope, or simply appear un-

---

DYSTHYMIC DISORDER: A CHRONIC AFFECTIVE DISORDER

This disorder is characterized by a chronic dysphoric mood (irritable mood in children), persisting at least 2 years in adults and 1 year in children and adolescents.

Signs and symptoms

During periods of depression, the patient also may experience poor appetite or overeating, insomnia or hypersomnia, low energy or fatigue, low self-esteem, poor concentration or difficulty making decisions, and feelings of hopelessness.

Diagnosis

Dysthymic disorder is confirmed when the patient exhibits at least two of the symptoms listed above nearly every day, with intervening normal moods lasting no more than 2 months during a 2-year period.

The disorder typically begins in childhood, adolescence, or early adulthood and causes only mild social or occupational impairment. In adults, it's more common in women; in children and adolescents, it's equally common in both sexes.

---

happy and apathetic. He also may report feeling angry or anxious.

Other common signs include difficulty concentrating or thinking clearly, distractibility, and indecisiveness. Take special note if the patient reveals suicidal thoughts, a preoccupation with death, or previous suicide attempts.

The psychosocial history may reveal life problems or losses that can account for the depression. Alternatively, the patient's medical history may implicate a physical disorder or the use

DIAGNOSING MAJOR DEPRESSION

A patient is diagnosed with major depression when he fulfills the following criteria for a single major depressive episode from the *DSM-IV:*

• At least five of the following symptoms must have been present during the same 2-week period and must represent a change from previous functioning; one of these symptoms must be either depressed mood or loss of interest in previously pleasurable activities:

— depressed mood (irritable mood in children and adolescents) most of the day, nearly every day, as indicated by either subjective account or observation by others

— markedly diminished interest or pleasure in all, or almost all, activities most of the day, nearly every day

— significant weight loss or weight gain when not dieting or decrease or increase in appetite nearly every day (in children, consider failure to make expected weight gains)

— insomnia or hypersomnia nearly every day

— psychomotor agitation or retardation nearly every day

— fatigue or loss of energy nearly every day

— feelings of worthlessness or excessive or inappropriate guilt nearly every day

— diminished ability to think or concentrate, or indecisiveness, nearly every day

— recurrent thoughts of death, recurrent suicidal ideation without a specific plan, a suicide attempt, or a specific plan for committing suicide.

• The symptoms do not meet criteria for a mixed episode.

• The symptoms cause clinically significant distress or impairment in social, occupational, or other important areas of functioning.

• The symptoms are not due to the direct physiologic effects of a substance or a general medical condition.

• The symptoms are not better accounted for by bereavement, the symptoms persist for longer than 2 months, or the symptoms are characterized by marked functional impairment, morbid preoccupation with worthlessness, suicidal ideation, psychotic symptoms, or psychomotor retardation.

of prescription, nonprescription, or illegal drugs that can cause depression.

The patient may report an increase or a decrease in appetite, sleep disturbances (for example, insomnia or early awakening), a lack of interest in sexual activity, constipation, or diarrhea. Other signs that you may note during a physical examination include agitation (such as hand wringing or restlessness) and reduced psychomotor activity (for example, slowed speech).

Diagnosis

The *Diagnostic and Statistical Manual of Mental Disorders,* 4th edition, describes specific characteristics of patients with this condition. (See *Diagnosing major depression.*)

The diagnosis of major depression is supported by psychological tests, such as the Beck Depression Inventory, which may help determine the onset, severity, duration, and progression of depressive symptoms.

A toxicology screening may suggest drug-induced depression.

Treatment

Depression is difficult to treat, especially in children, adolescents, elderly patients, and those with a history of chronic disease. The primary treatment methods are drug therapy, electroconvulsive therapy (ECT), and psychotherapy.

Drug therapy

In depression, drug therapy includes tricyclic antidepressants (TCAs) such as amitriptyline, serotonin reuptake inhibitors such as fluoxetine, and monoamine oxidase (MAO) inhibitors such as isocarboxazid, maprotiline, and trazodone.

• The most widely used class of antidepressant drugs, TCAs prevent the reuptake of norepinephrine or serotonin (or both) into the presynaptic nerve endings, resulting in increased synaptic concentrations of these neurotransmitters. They also cause a gradual loss in the number of beta-adrenergic receptors.

• Selective serotonin reuptake inhibitors, including fluoxetine, paroxetine, and sertraline, are increasingly becoming the drugs of choice. They are effective and produce fewer adverse effects than the TCAs; however, they're associated with sleep and GI problems and alterations in sexual desire and function.

• MAO inhibitors block the enzymatic degradation of norepinephrine and serotonin. These agents often are prescribed for patients with atypical depression (for example, depression marked by an increased appetite and need for sleep, rather than anorexia and insomnia) and for some patients who fail to respond to TCAs.

MAO inhibitors are associated with a high risk of toxicity; patients treated with one of these drugs must be able to comply with the necessary dietary restrictions. Conservative doses of an MAO inhibitor may be combined with a TCA for patients refractory to either drug alone.

Maprotiline is a potent blocker of norepinephrine uptake, whereas trazodone is a selective serotonin uptake blocker. The mechanism of action of bupropion is unknown.

ECT

When a depressed patient is incapacitated, suicidal, or psychotically depressed, or when antidepressants are contraindicated or ineffective, ECT often is the treatment of choice. Six to 12 treatments usually are needed, although improvement often is evident after only a few treatments. Researchers hypothesize that ECT affects the same receptor sites as antidepressants.

Psychotherapy

Short-term psychotherapy also is effective in treating major depression. Many psychiatrists believe that the best results are achieved with a combination of individual, family, or group psychotherapy and medication.

After resolution of the acute episode, patients with a history of recurrent depression may be maintained on low doses of antidepressants as a preventive measure.

Special considerations

• Share your observations of the patient's behavior with him. For instance, you might say, "You're sitting all by yourself, looking very sad. Is that how you feel?" Because the patient may think and react sluggishly, speak slowly and allow ample time for him to respond.

• Avoid feigned cheerfulness. However, don't hesitate to laugh with the patient and point out the value of humor.

• Show the patient that he's important by listening attentively and respectfully, preventing interruptions, and avoiding judgmental responses.

• Provide a structured routine, including noncompetitive activities, to build the patient's self-confidence and encourage interaction with others. Urge him to join group activities and to socialize.

• Inform the patient that he can help ease depression by expressing his feelings, participating in pleasurable activities, and improving grooming and hygiene.

• Ask the patient if he thinks of death or suicide. Such thoughts signal an immediate need for consultation and assessment. Failure to detect suicidal thoughts early may encourage the patient to attempt suicide. The risk of suicide increases as the depression lifts.

• While tending to the patient's psychological needs, don't forget his physical needs. If he's too depressed to take care of himself, help him with personal hygiene. Encourage him to eat, or feed him if necessary. If he's constipated, add high-fiber foods to his diet; offer small, frequent meals; and encourage physical activity and fluid intake. Offer warm milk or back rubs at bedtime to improve sleep.

• If the patient is taking an antidepressant, monitor him for evidence of seizures. Some antidepressants significantly lower the seizure threshold.

• Recognize that antidepressants may take several weeks to produce an effect.

• Teach the patient about depression. Emphasize that effective methods are available to relieve his symptoms. Help him to recognize distorted perceptions that may contribute to his depression. Once the patient learns to recognize depressive thought patterns, he can consciously begin to substitute self-affirming thoughts.

• Instruct the patient about prescribed medications. Stress the need for compliance and review adverse effects. For drugs that produce strong anticholinergic effects, such as amitriptyline and amoxapine, suggest sugarless gum or hard candy to relieve dry mouth.

• Many antidepressants are sedating (for example, amitriptyline and trazodone); warn the patient taking one of these drugs to avoid activities that require alertness, including driving and operating mechanical equipment, until the central nervous system (CNS) effects of the drug are known.

• Caution the patient taking a TCA to avoid drinking alcoholic beverages or taking other CNS depressants during therapy.

• If the patient is taking an MAO inhibitor, emphasize that he must avoid foods that contain tyramine, caffeine, or tryptophan. The ingestion of tyramine can cause a hypertensive crisis. Examples of foods that contain these substances are cheese, sour cream, pickled herring, liver, canned figs, raisins, bananas, avocados, chocolate, soy sauce, fava beans, yeast extracts, meat tenderizers, coffee, colas, and beer, chianti, and sherry.

DERMATITIS

An inflammation of the skin, dermatitis occurs in several forms: atopic (discussed here), seborrheic, nummular, contact, chronic, localized neurodermatitis, exfoliative, and stasis. (See *Types of dermatitis,* pages 270 to 273.)

Atopic dermatitis (atopic or infantile eczema, neurodermatitis constitutionalis, Besnier's prurigo) is a chronic inflammatory response often associated with other atopic diseases, such as bronchial asthma and allergic rhinitis. It usually develops in infants and toddlers between ages 1 month and 1 year, commonly in those with strong family histories of atopic disease. These children often acquire other atopic disorders as they grow older.

Typically, this form of dermatitis flares and subsides repeatedly before finally resolving during adolescence. However, it can persist into adulthood. Atopic dermatitis affects about 9 out of every 1,000 persons.

Causes

The cause of atopic dermatitis is unknown, but there is a genetic predisposition exacerbated by factors such as food allergies, infections, irritating chemicals, temperature and humidity, and emotions. Approximately 10% of childhood cases are caused by allergy to certain foods, particularly eggs, peanuts, milk, and wheat.

Atopic dermatitis tends to flare up in response to extremes in temperature and humidity. Other causes of flare-ups are sweating and psychological stress.

An important secondary cause of atopic dermatitis is irritation, which seems to change the epidermal structure, allowing immunoglobulin E (IgE) activity to increase. Consequently, chronic skin irritation usually continues even after exposure to the allergen has ended or after the irritation has been systemically controlled.

Signs and symptoms

Atopic skin lesions generally begin as erythematous areas on excessively dry skin. In children, such lesions typically appear on the forehead, cheeks, and extensor surfaces of the arms and legs; in adults, at flexion points (antecubital fossa, popliteal area, and neck).

During flare-ups, pruritus and scratching cause edema, crusting, and scaling. Eventually, chronic atopic lesions lead to multiple areas of dry, scaly skin, with white dermatographia, blanching, and lichenification.

Common secondary conditions associated with atopic dermatitis include viral, fungal, or bacterial infections and ocular disorders.

Because of intense pruritus, the upper eyelid is commonly hyperpigmented and swollen, and a double fold occurs under the lower lid (Morgan's, Dennie's, or Mongolian fold). Atopic cataracts are unusual but may develop between ages 20 and 40.

Kaposi's varicelliform eruption, a potentially fatal generalized viral infection, may develop if the patient comes in contact with a person who's infected with herpes simplex.

Diagnosis

A family history of allergy and chronic inflammation suggests atopic dermatitis.

Typical distribution of skin lesions rules out other inflammatory skin lesions, such as diaper rash (lesions confined to the diapered area), seborrheic dermatitis (no pigmentation changes, or lichenification occurs in chronic lesions), and chronic contact dermatitis (lesions affect hands and forearms, sparing antecubital and popliteal areas). Serum IgE levels are often elevated.

Treatment

Effective treatment of atopic lesions consists of eliminating allergens and avoiding irritants, extreme temperature changes, and other precipitating factors. Local and systemic measures relieve itching and inflammation.

Topical application of a corticosteroid ointment, especially after bathing, often alleviates inflammation. Between steroid doses, application of a moisturizing cream can help retain moisture. Systemic corticosteroid therapy should be used only during extreme exacerbations.

Weak tar preparations and ultraviolet B light therapy are used to increase the thickness of the stratum corneum. Antibiotics are appropriate if a bacterial agent has been cultured.

(Text continues on page 272.)

TYPES OF DERMATITIS

TYPE	CAUSES	SIGNS AND SYMPTOMS
Seborrheic dermatitis An acute or subacute skin disease that affects the scalp, face, and occasionally other areas and is characterized by lesions covered with yellow or brownish gray scales	• Unknown; stress and neurologic conditions may be predisposing factors; may be related to the yeast *Pityrosporum ovale*	• Eruptions in areas with many sebaceous glands (usually scalp, face, and trunk) and in skin folds • Itching, redness, and inflammation of affected areas; lesions may appear greasy; fissures may occur • Indistinct, occasionally yellowish, scaly patches from excess stratum corneum (Dandruff may be a mild seborrheic dermatitis.)
Nummular dermatitis Chronic form of dermatitis characterized by inflammation of coin-shaped, vesicular, crusted scales and, possibly, pruritic lesions	• Possibly precipitated by stress, skin dryness, irritants, or scratching	• Round, nummular (coin-shaped) lesions, usually on arms and legs, with distinct borders of crusts and scales • Possible oozing and severe itching • Summertime remissions common, with wintertime recurrence
Contact dermatitis Often sharply demarcated inflammation and irritation of the skin resulting from contact with concentrated substances to which the skin is sensitive, such as perfumes, soaps, or chemicals	• Mild irritants: chronic exposure to detergents or solvents • Strong irritants: damage on contact with acids or alkalis • Allergens: sensitization after repeated exposure	• Mild irritants and allergens: erythema and small vesicles that ooze, scale, and itch • Strong irritants: blisters and ulcerations • Classic allergic response: clearly defined lesions, with straight lines following points of contact • Severe allergic reaction: marked edema of affected areas
Chronic dermatitis Characterized by inflammatory eruptions of the hands and feet	• Usually unknown but may result from progressive contact dermatitis • Secondary factors: trauma, infections, redistribution of normal flora, photosensitivity, and food sensitivity, which may perpetuate this condition	• Thick, lichenified, single or multiple lesions on any part of the body (often on the hands) • Inflammation and scaling • Recurrence following long remissions

DIAGNOSIS	TREATMENT AND INTERVENTIONS
• Patient history and physical findings, especially distribution of lesions in sebaceous gland areas, confirm seborrheic dermatitis. • Diagnosis must rule out psoriasis.	• Removal of scales with frequent washing and shampooing with selenium sulfide suspension (most effective), zinc pyrithione, or tar and salicylic acid shampoo • Application of fluorinated corticosteroids to nonhairy areas
• Physical findings and patient history confirm nummular dermatitis; a middle-aged or older patient may have a history of atopic dermatitis. • Diagnosis must rule out fungal infections, atopic or contact dermatitis, and psoriasis.	• Elimination of known irritants • Measures to relieve dry skin: increased humidification, limited frequency of baths and use of bland soap and bath oils, and application of emollients • Application of wet dressings in acute phase • Topical corticosteroids (occlusive dressings or intralesional injections) for persistent lesions • Tar preparations and antihistamines to control itching • Antibiotics for secondary infection • Same as for atopic dermatitis
• Patient history, patch testing to identify allergens, and shape and distribution of lesions suggest contact dermatitis.	• Elimination of known allergens and decreased exposure to irritants; wearing protective clothing, such as gloves; and washing immediately after contact with irritants or allergens • Topical anti-inflammatory agents (including corticosteroids), systemic corticosteroids for edema and bullae, antihistamines, and local applications of Burow's solution (for blisters) • Possible sensitization to topical medications • Same as for atopic dermatitis
• No characteristic pattern or course; diagnosis relies on detailed patient history and physical findings.	• Same as for contact dermatitis • Antibiotics for secondary infection • Avoidance of excessive hand washing and drying and of accumulation of soaps and detergents under rings • Use of emollients with topical corticosteroids

(continued)

TYPES OF DERMATITIS *(continued)*

TYPE	CAUSES	SIGNS AND SYMPTOMS
Localized neurodermatitis (lichen simplex chronicus, essential pruritus) Superficial inflammation of the skin characterized by itching and papular eruptions that appear on thickened, hyperpigmented skin	• Chronic scratching or rubbing of a primary lesion or insect bite, or other skin irritation	• Intense, sometimes continual scratching • Thick, sharp-bordered, possibly dry, scaly lesions with raised papules • Usually affects easily reached areas, such as ankles, lower legs, anogenital area, back of neck, and ears
Exfoliative dermatitis Severe, chronic skin inflammation characterized by redness and widespread erythema and scaling	• Preexisting skin lesions usually progressing to exfoliative stage, such as in contact dermatitis, drug reaction, lymphoma, or leukemia	• Generalized dermatitis, with acute loss of stratum corneum, and erythema and scaling • Sensation of tight skin • Hair loss • Possible fever, sensitivity to cold, shivering, gynecomastia, and lymphadenopathy
Stasis dermatitis Condition usually caused by impaired circulation and characterized by eczema of the legs with edema, hyperpigmentation, and persistent inflammation	• Secondary to peripheral vascular diseases affecting legs, such as recurrent thrombophlebitis and resultant chronic venous insufficiency	• Varicosities and edema common, but obvious vascular insufficiency not always present • Usually affects the lower leg, just above internal malleolus, or sites of trauma or irritation • Early signs: dusky red deposits of hemosiderin in skin, with itching and dimpling of subcutaneous tissue. Later signs: edema, redness, and scaling of large area of legs • Possible fissures, crusts, and ulcers

Special considerations
• Warn that drowsiness is possible with the use of antihistamines to relieve daytime itching. If nocturnal itching interferes with sleep, suggest methods for inducing natural sleep, such as drinking a glass of warm milk, to prevent overuse of sedatives. Antihistamines may also be useful.

• Help the patient set up an individual schedule and plan for daily skin care.
• Instruct the patient to bathe in plain water. (He may have to limit bathing, according to the severity of the lesions.) Tell him to bathe with a special nonfatty soap and tepid water (96° F [35.6°C]) but to avoid using any soap when lesions are acutely inflamed.

DIAGNOSIS	TREATMENT AND INTERVENTIONS
• Physical findings confirm diagnosis.	• Scratching must stop; then lesions will disappear in about 2 weeks. • Fixed dressing or Unna's boot to cover affected area • Topical corticosteroids under occlusion or by intralesional injection • Antihistamines and open wet dressings • Emollients • Patient informed about underlying cause.
• Diagnosis requires identification of the underlying cause.	• Hospitalization, with protective isolation and hygienic measures to prevent secondary bacterial infection • Open wet dressings, with colloidal baths • Bland lotions over topical corticosteroids • Maintenance of constant environmental temperature to prevent chilling or overheating • Careful monitoring of renal and cardiac status • Systemic antibiotics and steroids • Same as for atopic dermatitis
• Diagnosis requires positive history of venous insufficiency and physical findings, such as varicosities.	• Measures to prevent venous stasis: avoidance of prolonged sitting or standing, use of support stockings, and weight reduction in obesity • Corrective surgery for underlying cause • After ulcer develops, encourage rest periods, with legs elevated; open wet dressings; Unna's boot (zinc gelatin dressing provides continuous pressure to affected areas); and antibiotics for secondary infection after wound culture.

• Advise the patient to shampoo frequently and apply corticosteroid solution to the scalp afterward, to keep fingernails short to limit excoriation and secondary infections caused by scratching, and to lubricate his skin after a tub bath.

• To help clear lichenified skin, apply occlusive dressings (such as plastic film) intermittently as necessary.
• Inform the patient that irritants, such as detergents and wool, and emotional stress exacerbate atopic dermatitis.
• Be careful not to show any anxiety or revulsion when touching the lesions during treatment. Help the patient ac-

cept his altered body image, and encourage him to verbalize his feelings. Remember, coping with disfigurement is extremely difficult, especially for children and adolescents.

• Arrange for counseling, if necessary, to help the patient deal with this distressing condition more effectively.

DERMATOPHYTOSIS

Also called tinea, dermatophytosis is a disease that can affect the scalp (tinea capitis), body (tinea corporis), nails (tinea unguium), feet (tinea pedis), groin (tinea cruris), and bearded skin (tinea barbae).

Tinea infections are quite prevalent in the United States and are usually more common in males than in females. With effective treatment, the cure rate is very high, although about 20% of infected persons develop chronic conditions.

Causes
Tinea infections (except for tinea versicolor) result from dermatophytes (fungi) of the genera *Trichophyton, Microsporum,* and *Epidermophyton.*

Transmission can occur directly (through contact with infected lesions) or indirectly (through contact with contaminated articles, such as shoes, towels, or shower stalls).

Signs and symptoms
Lesions vary in appearance and duration with the type of infection:

• *Tinea capitis,* which mainly affects children, is characterized by small, spreading papules on the scalp, causing patchy hair loss with scaling. These papules may progress to inflamed, pus-filled lesions (kerions).

• *Tinea corporis* produces flat lesions on the skin at any site except the scalp,

bearded skin, or feet. These lesions may be dry and scaly or moist and crusty; as they enlarge, their centers heal, causing the classic ring-shaped appearance.

• *Tinea unguium* (onychomycosis) infection typically starts at the tip of one or more toenails (fingernail infection is less common) and produces gradual thickening, discoloration, and crumbling of the nail, with accumulation of subungual debris. Eventually, the nail may be destroyed completely.

• *Tinea pedis* causes scaling and blisters between the toes. Severe infection may result in inflammation, with severe itching and pain on walking. A dry, squamous inflammation may affect the entire sole.

• *Tinea cruris* (jock itch) produces red, raised, sharply defined, itchy lesions in the groin that may extend to the buttocks, inner thighs, and the external genitalia. Warm weather and tight clothing encourage fungus growth.

• *Tinea barbae* is an uncommon infection that affects the bearded facial area of men.

Diagnosis
Microscopic examination of lesion scrapings prepared in potassium hydroxide solution usually confirms tinea infection. Other diagnostic procedures include Wood's light examination (which is useful in only about 5% of cases of tinea capitis) and culture of the infecting organism.

Treatment
Tinea infections usually respond to topical agents such as imidazole cream or to oral griseofulvin, which is especially effective in tinea infections of the skin, hair, and nails.

However, topical therapy is ineffective for tinea capitis; oral griseofulvin for 1 to 3 months is the treatment of choice. Also, griseofulvin is contraindicated in the patient with porphyria, and it may necessitate an increase in dosage during anticoagulant (warfarin) therapy.

In addition to imidazole, other antifungals include naftifine, ciclopirox, terbinafine, haloprogin, and tolnaftate. Topical treatments should continue for 2 weeks after lesions resolve.

Supportive measures include open wet dressings, removal of scabs and scales, and application of keratolytics, such as salicylic acid, to soften and remove hyperkeratotic lesions of the heels or soles.

Special considerations

• For all tinea infections, apply topical agents, watch for sensitivity reactions and secondary bacterial infections, and provide patient teaching.

• Monitor liver function of patients on griseofulvin.

• For tinea capitis, discontinue oral griseofulvin if the patient's condition worsens. Use good hand-washing technique, and teach the patient to do the same. To prevent spreading infection to others, advise him to wash his towels, bedclothes, and combs frequently in hot water and to avoid sharing them. Suggest that family members be checked for tinea capitis.

• For tinea corporis, use abdominal pads between skin folds for the patient with excessive abdominal girth; change pads frequently. Check the patient daily for excoriated, newly denuded areas of skin. If the involved area is moist, apply open wet dressings two or three times daily to decrease inflammation and help remove scales.

• For tinea unguium, keep the patient's nails short and straight. Gently remove debris under the nails with an emery board. Prepare the patient for prolonged therapy and possible adverse effects of griseofulvin, such as headache, nausea, vomiting, and photosensitivity.

• For tinea pedis, encourage the patient to expose his feet to air whenever possible and to wear sandals or leather shoes and clean cotton socks. Instruct the patient to wash his feet twice daily and, after drying them thoroughly, to apply the antifungal cream followed by antifungal powder to absorb perspiration and prevent excoriation.

• For tinea cruris, instruct the patient to dry the affected area thoroughly after bathing and to evenly apply antifungal powder after applying the topical antifungal agent. Advise him to wear loose-fitting clothing, which should be changed frequently and washed in hot water.

• For tinea barbae, suggest that the patient let his beard grow. (Whiskers should be trimmed with scissors, not a razor.) If the patient insists that he must shave, advise him to use an electric razor instead of a blade.

DIABETES INSIPIDUS

A disorder of water metabolism, diabetes insipidus (pituitary diabetes insipidus) results from a deficiency of circulating vasopressin (also called antidiuretic hormone). It's characterized by excessive fluid intake and hypotonic polyuria.

The disorder may start in childhood or early adulthood (median age of onset is 21) and is more common in men than in women. Incidence is slightly higher today than in the past.

In uncomplicated diabetes insipidus, the prognosis is good with adequate water replacement, and patients usually lead normal lives.

Causes

Diabetes insipidus results from intracranial neoplastic or metastatic lesions, hypophysectomy or other neurosurgery, a skull fracture, or head trauma that damages the neurohypophyseal structures.

It can also result from infection, granulomatous disease, and vascular lesions; it may be idiopathic and, rarely, familial. (*Note:* Pituitary diabetes insipidus shouldn't be confused with nephrogenic diabetes insipidus, a rare congenital disturbance of water metabolism that results from renal tubular resistance to vasopressin.)

Normally, the hypothalamus synthesizes vasopressin. The posterior pituitary gland (or neurohypophysis) stores vasopressin and releases it into general circulation, where it causes the kidneys to reabsorb water by making the distal tubules and collecting duct cells water-permeable.

In diabetes insipidus, the absence of vasopressin allows the filtered water to be excreted in the urine instead of being reabsorbed.

Signs and symptoms

The patient's history typically shows an abrupt onset of extreme polyuria (usually 4 to 16 L/day of dilute urine, but sometimes as much as 30 L/day). As a result, the patient is extremely thirsty and drinks great quantities of water to compensate for the body's water loss.

This disorder may also result in nocturia. In severe cases, it may lead to extreme fatigue from inadequate rest caused by frequent voiding and excessive thirst.

Other characteristic features of diabetes insipidus include signs and symptoms of dehydration (poor tissue turgor, dry mucous membranes, constipation, muscle weakness, dizziness, and hypotension). These symptoms usually begin abruptly, commonly appearing within 1 to 2 days after a basal skull fracture, a cerebrovascular accident, or surgery.

Relieving cerebral edema or increased intracranial pressure may cause all of these symptoms to subside just as rapidly as they began.

Diagnosis

Urinalysis reveals almost colorless urine of low osmolality (50 to 200 mOsm/kg, less than that of plasma) and low specific gravity (less than 1.005). However, a diagnosis requires the water deprivation test to provide evidence of vasopressin deficiency, resulting in the kidneys' inability to concentrate urine.

Water deprivation test

In this test, after baseline vital signs, weight, and urine and plasma osmolalities are obtained, the patient is deprived of fluids and observed to make sure he doesn't drink anything surreptitiously. Hourly measurements then record the total volume of urine output, body weight, urine osmolality or specific gravity, and plasma osmolality. Throughout the test, blood pressure and pulse rate must be monitored for signs of orthostatic hypotension.

Fluid deprivation continues until the patient loses 3% of his body weight (indicating severe dehydration). When urine osmolality stops increasing in three consecutive hourly specimens, the patient receives 5 units of aqueous vasopressin S.C.

Hourly measurements of urine volume and specific gravity continue after S.C. injection of aqueous vasopressin. Patients with pituitary diabetes insipidus respond to exogenous vasopressin with decreased urine output and increased specific gravity. Patients with nephrogenic diabetes insipidus show no response to vasopressin.

Treatment

Until the cause of diabetes insipidus can be identified and eliminated, administration of various forms of vasopressin or of a vasopressin stimulant can control fluid balance and prevent dehydration.

Vasopressin injection
This aqueous preparation is administered S.C. or I.M. several times a day because it's effective for only 2 to 6 hours. This form of the drug is used in acute disease and as a diagnostic agent.

Desmopressin acetate
This drug can be given by nasal spray that's absorbed through the mucous membranes or by S.C. or I.V. injection. Desmopressin acetate is effective for 8 to 20 hours, depending on the dosage.

Special considerations
• Record fluid intake and output carefully. Maintain fluid intake that's adequate to prevent severe dehydration.
• Watch for signs of hypovolemic shock, and monitor blood pressure and heart and respiratory rates regularly, especially during the water deprivation test. Check the patient's weight daily.
• If the patient is dizzy or has muscle weakness, institute safety precautions, including keeping the side rails up. Assist him with walking.
• Monitor urine specific gravity between doses. Watch for a decrease in specific gravity accompanied by increasing urine output, indicating the recurrence of polyuria and necessitating administration of the next dose of medication or a dosage increase.
• If constipation develops, add more high-fiber foods and fruit juices to the patient's diet. If necessary, give the patient a mild laxative, such as milk of magnesia.
• Provide meticulous skin and mouth care; apply petroleum jelly, as needed, to cracked or sore lips.
• Urge the patient to verbalize his feelings. Offer encouragement and a realistic assessment of his situation.

• Help the patient identify strengths that he can use in developing coping strategies.
• Before discharge, teach the patient how to monitor intake and output.
• Instruct the patient to administer desmopressin by nasal spray only after the onset of polyuria — not before — to prevent excess fluid retention and water intoxication.
• Tell the patient to report weight gain, which may mean that his medication dosage is too high. Recurrence of polyuria, as reflected on the intake and output sheet, indicates that the dosage is too low.
• Advise the patient to wear a medical identification bracelet and to carry his medication with him at all times.
• Teach the parents of a child with diabetes insipidus about normal growth and development. Discuss how their child may differ from others at his developmental stage.
• Encourage the parents to help identify the child's strengths and to use them in developing coping strategies.
• Refer patients with diabetes insipidus and their families for counseling, if necessary.

DIABETES MELLITUS

A chronic disease of absolute or relative insulin deficiency or resistance, diabetes mellitus is characterized by disturbances in carbohydrate, protein, and fat metabolism.

This condition occurs in two forms: *Type I, insulin-dependent diabetes mellitus,* and the more prevalent *Type II, non-insulin-dependent diabetes mellitus.*

Type I usually occurs before age 30 (although it may occur at any age); the patient is usually thin and requires exogenous insulin and dietary management to achieve control. Conversely, Type II usually occurs in obese adults after age 40 and is most often treated with diet and exercise (possibly in combination with antidiabetic drugs), although treatment may include insulin therapy.

Diabetes mellitus affects an estimated 5% of the population of the United States (10 to 12 million people), about half of whom are undiagnosed. Incidence is equal in men and women and rises with age.

A leading cause of death by disease in the United States, this syndrome contributes to about 50% of myocardial infarctions and about 75% of cerebrovascular accidents, as well as to renal failure and peripheral vascular disease. It's also the leading cause of new blindness.

Causes

The effects of diabetes mellitus result from insulin deficiency. Insulin transports glucose into the cell for use as energy and storage as glycogen. It also stimulates protein synthesis and free fatty acid storage in the fat deposits. Insulin deficiency compromises the body tissues' access to essential nutrients for fuel and storage.

The etiology of both Type I and Type II diabetes remains unknown. Genetic factors may play a part in development of all types; autoimmune disease and viral infections may be risk factors in Type I.

Other risk factors include the following:

• Obesity contributes to the resistance to endogenous insulin.

• Physiologic or emotional stress can cause prolonged elevation of stress hormone levels (cortisol, epinephrine, glucagon, and growth hormone). This raises blood glucose levels, which, in turn, places increased demands on the pancreas.

• Pregnancy causes weight gain and increases levels of estrogen and placental hormones, which antagonize insulin.

• Some medications can antagonize the effects of insulin, including thiazide diuretics, adrenal corticosteroids, and oral contraceptives.

Signs and symptoms

Diabetes may begin dramatically with ketoacidosis in Type I or insidiously. Its most common symptom is fatigue, from energy deficiency and a catabolic state.

Insulin deficiency causes hyperglycemia, which pulls fluid from body tissues, causing osmotic diuresis, polyuria, dehydration, polydipsia, dry mucous membranes, and poor skin turgor. In ketoacidosis and hyperglycemic hyperosmolar nonketotic coma, dehydration may cause hypovolemia and shock. Wasting of glucose in the urine usually produces weight loss and hunger in Type I diabetes, even if the patient eats voraciously.

Long-term effects

In diabetes, long-term effects may include retinopathy, nephropathy, atherosclerosis, and peripheral and autonomic neuropathy.

Peripheral neuropathy usually affects the hands and feet and may cause numbness or pain. Autonomic neuropathy may manifest itself in several ways, including gastroparesis (leading to delayed gastric emptying and a feeling of nausea and fullness after meals), nocturnal diarrhea, impotence, and postural hypotension.

Because hyperglycemia impairs the patient's resistance to infection, diabetes may result in skin and urinary tract infections and vaginitis. Glucose content of the epidermis and urine encourages bacterial growth.

Diagnosis

In nonpregnant adults, one of the following findings confirms diabetes mellitus:

• typical symptoms of uncontrolled diabetes and a random blood glucose level equal to or above 200 mg/dl

• a fasting plasma glucose level equal to or greater than 140 mg/dl on at least two occasions

• if the fasting glucose test is normal, a blood glucose level above 200 mg/dl at 2 hours and on at least one other occasion during the glucose tolerance test.

An ophthalmologic examination may show diabetic retinopathy. Other diagnostic and monitoring tests include urinalysis for acetone and blood testing for glycosylated hemoglobin (hemoglobin A), which reflects recent glucose cortisol.

Treatment

Effective treatment for both types of diabetes normalizes blood glucose and decreases complications.

Type I diabetes

In insulin-dependent diabetes mellitus, treatment includes insulin replacement, diet, and exercise. Current forms of insulin replacement include single-dose, mixed-dose, split-mixed dose, and multiple-dose regimens. The multiple-dose regimens may use an insulin pump.

Insulin may be rapid-acting (Regular), intermediate-acting (NPH), long-acting (Ultralente), or a combination of rapid-acting and intermediate-acting (Mixtard); it may be standard or purified, and it may be derived from beef, pork, or human sources. Purified human insulin is used commonly today.

Pancreas transplantation is experimental and requires chronic immunosuppression.

Type II diabetes

Non-insulin-dependent diabetes mellitus may require oral antidiabetic drugs to stimulate endogenous insulin production, increase insulin sensitivity at the cellular level, and suppress hepatic gluconeogenesis.

Both types

Treatment of both types of diabetes requires a strict diet planned to meet nutritional needs, to control blood glucose levels, and to reach and maintain appropriate body weight.

For the obese patient with Type II diabetes, weight reduction is a goal. In Type I, the calorie allotment may be high, depending on growth stage and activity level. For success, the diet must be followed consistently and meals eaten at regular times.

Complications

Treatment of long-term diabetic complications may include transplantation or dialysis for renal failure, photocoagulation for retinopathy, and vascular surgery for large-vessel disease. Meticulous blood glucose control is essential.

The Diabetes Control and Complications Trial has proved that intensive drug therapy that focuses on keeping glucose at near-normal levels for 5 years or more reduces both the onset and progression of retinopathy (up to 63%), nephropathy (by up to 54%), and neuropathy (by up to 60%).

Special considerations

• Stress that compliance with the prescribed program is essential. Emphasize the effect of blood glucose control on long-term health. (See *What your patient needs to know about diabetes mellitus,* page 280.)

• Watch for acute complications of diabetic therapy, especially hypoglycemia (vagueness, slow cerebration, dizziness, weakness, pallor, tachycar-

---

WHAT YOUR PATIENT NEEDS TO KNOW ABOUT DIABETES MELLITUS

The patient with diabetes mellitus will need careful teaching. Tailor your instruction to the patient's needs, abilities, and developmental stage. Make sure you teach your patient to:
• follow dietary guidelines closely
• understand the purpose and goals of treatment
• correctly administer his medications

• recognize and report adverse reactions to medication
• maintain an exercise program
• follow procedures to monitor his condition
• maintain meticulous hygiene
• watch for and immediately report symptoms of hypoglycemia and hyperglycemia.

---

dia, diaphoresis, seizures, and coma). Immediately give carbohydrates in the form of fruit juice, hard candy, honey or, if the patient is unconscious, glucagon or dextrose I.V.

• Be alert for signs of ketoacidosis (acetone breath, dehydration, weak and rapid pulse, Kussmaul's respirations) and hyperosmolar coma (polyuria, thirst, neurologic abnormalities, stupor). These hyperglycemic crises require I.V. fluids, insulin and, usually, potassium replacement.

• Monitor diabetic control by testing urine for acetone and obtaining blood glucose levels.

• Watch for diabetic effects on the cardiovascular system, such as cerebrovascular, coronary artery, and peripheral vascular impairment, and on the peripheral and autonomic nervous systems.

• Treat all injuries, cuts, and blisters (particularly on the legs or feet) meticulously.

• Be alert for signs of urinary tract infection and renal disease.

• Urge regular ophthalmologic examinations to detect diabetic retinopathy.

• Assess for signs of diabetic neuropathy (numbness or pain in the hands and feet, footdrop, neurogenic bladder). Stress the need for personal safety precautions; explain that decreased sensation can mask injuries. Minimize complications by maintaining strict blood glucose control.

• Teach the patient to care for his feet by washing them daily, drying carefully between toes, and inspecting for corns, calluses, redness, swelling, bruises, and breaks in the skin. Urge him to report any changes. Advise him to wear nonconstricting shoes and to avoid walking barefoot.

• Teach the patient how to manage his diabetes when he has a minor illness, such as a cold, flu, or upset stomach.

• To delay the clinical onset of diabetes, teach persons at high risk to avoid risk factors. Advise genetic counseling for young adult diabetics who are planning families.

• For further information, consult the Juvenile Diabetes Foundation, the American Diabetes Association, and the American Association of Diabetes Educators.

DIABETIC COMPLICATIONS DURING PREGNANCY

Pregnancy places special demands on carbohydrate metabolism and causes the insulin requirement to increase, even in a healthy woman. Consequently, pregnancy may lead to a prediabetic state, to the conversion of an asymptomatic subclinical diabetic state to a clinical one (gestational diabetes occurs in about 1% to 2% of all pregnancies), or to complications in a previously stable diabetic state.

Prevalence of diabetes mellitus increases with age. Maternal and fetal prognoses can be equivalent to those in nondiabetic women if maternal blood glucose is well controlled and ketosis and other complications are prevented. Infant morbidity and mortality depend on recognizing and successfully controlling hypoglycemia, which may develop within hours after delivery.

Causes

In diabetes mellitus, glucose is inadequately used either because insulin isn't synthesized (as in Type I, insulin-dependent diabetes) or because tissues are resistant to the hormonal action of endogenous insulin (as in Type II, non-insulin-dependent diabetes).

Protective mechanisms

During pregnancy, the fetus relies on maternal glucose as a primary fuel source. Pregnancy triggers protective mechanisms that have anti-insulin effects: increased hormone production (placental lactogen, estrogen, and progesterone), which antagonizes the effects of insulin; degradation of insulin by the placenta; and prolonged elevation of stress hormones (cortisol, epinephrine, and glucagon), which raise blood glucose levels.

In a normal pregnancy, an increase in anti-insulin factors is counterbalanced by an increase in insulin production to maintain normal blood glucose levels. However, women who are prediabetic or diabetic can't produce sufficient insulin to overcome the insulin antagonist mechanisms of pregnancy, or their tissues are insulin-resistant.

As insulin requirements rise toward term, the patient who is prediabetic may develop gestational diabetes, necessitating dietary management and, possibly, exogenous insulin to achieve glycemic control. The insulin-dependent patient may need increased insulin dosage.

Signs and symptoms

Indications for diagnostic screening for maternal diabetes mellitus during pregnancy include obesity, excessive weight gain, excessive hunger or thirst, polyuria, recurrent monilial infections, glycosuria, previous delivery of a large infant, polyhydramnios, maternal hypertension, and a family history of diabetes.

Uncontrolled diabetes in a pregnant woman can cause stillbirth, fetal anomalies, premature delivery, and birth of an infant who is large or small for gestational age. Such infants are predisposed to severe episodes of hypoglycemia shortly after birth. These infants may also develop hypocalcemia, hyperbilirubinemia, and respiratory distress syndrome.

Diagnosis

The prevalence of gestational diabetes makes careful screening for hyperglycemia appropriate in all pregnancies in each trimester. Abnormal fasting or postprandial blood glucose levels and clinical signs and history suggest diabetes in patients not previously diabetic. A 3-hour glucose tolerance test confirms diabetes mellitus when two or more values are above normal.

Diagnosis of fetal status

Procedures to assess fetal status include stress and nonstress tests, ultrasonography to determine fetal age and growth, measurement of urinary or serum estriols and of phosphatidylglycerol, and determination of the lecithin-sphingomyelin ratio from amniotic fluid to predict pulmonary maturity.

Treatment

Both the newly diagnosed and the established diabetic need dietary management and insulin administration to maintain blood glucose levels within acceptable limits. Most women with overt diabetes mellitus require hospitalization at the beginning of pregnancy to assess physical status, to check for cardiac and renal disease, and to regulate diabetes.

For pregnant patients with diabetes, therapy includes:

• bimonthly visits to the obstetrician and the internist during the first 6 months of pregnancy; weekly visits may be necessary during the third trimester

• maintenance of blood glucose levels at or below 100 mg/dl during the third trimester

• frequent monitoring for glycosuria and ketonuria (Ketosis presents a grave threat to the fetal central nervous system.)

• weight control (Gain shouldn't exceed 3 to 3½ lb [1.36 to 1.59 kg]/month during the last 6 months of pregnancy.)

• a high-protein diet of 2 g/day/kg of body weight (a minimum of 80 g/day during the second half of pregnancy), a daily calorie intake of 30 to 40 calories/kg of body weight, a daily carbohydrate intake of 200 g, and enough fat to provide 36% of total calories (However, vigorous calorie restriction can cause starvation ketosis.)

• exogenous insulin if diet doesn't control blood glucose levels. Oral antidiabetic agents are contraindicated during pregnancy, because they may cause fetal hypoglycemia and congenital anomalies.

Delivery

Generally, the optimal time for delivery is between 37 and 39 weeks' gestation. The insulin-dependent diabetic requires hospitalization before delivery because bed rest promotes uteroplacental circulation and myometrial tone. In addition, hospitalization permits frequent monitoring of blood glucose levels and prompt intervention if complications develop.

Depending on fetal status and maternal history, labor may be induced or a cesarean section performed. During labor and delivery, the patient with diabetes should receive a continuous I.V. infusion of dextrose with regular insulin in water. Maternal and fetal status must be monitored closely throughout labor.

The patient may benefit from half her prepregnancy dosage of insulin before a cesarean delivery. Her insulin requirement will fall markedly after delivery.

Special considerations

• Be alert for changes in insulin requirements from one trimester to the next and immediately postpartum.

• Teach the newly diagnosed patient about diabetes, including dietary management, insulin administration, home monitoring of blood glucose or urine testing for glucose and ketones, and skin and foot care. Instruct her to report ketonuria immediately.

• Evaluate the diabetic patient's knowledge about this disease, and provide supplementary patient teaching as she requires. Inform the patient that frequent monitoring and adjustment of insulin dosage are necessary throughout the course of her pregnancy.

• Give reassurance that strict compliance to prescribed therapy should ensure a favorable outcome.

• Refer the patient to an appropriate social service agency if financial assistance is necessary because of prolonged hospitalization.

• Encourage medical counseling regarding the prognosis of future pregnancies.

DiGeorge's Syndrome

Also called congenital thymic hypoplasia or aplasia, DiGeorge's syndrome is a disorder known typically by the partial or total absence of cell-mediated immunity that results from a deficiency of T lymphocytes. It characteristically produces life-threatening hypocalcemia that may be associated with cardiovascular and facial anomalies.

Patients rarely live beyond age 2 without fetal thymic transplant; however, the prognosis improves when fetal thymic transplant, correction of hypocalcemia, and repair of cardiac anomalies are possible.

Causes

DiGeorge's syndrome is probably caused by abnormal fetal development of the third and fourth pharyngeal pouches (12th week of gestation) that interferes with the formation of the thymus. As a result, the thymus is completely absent or partially absent and abnormally located, causing deficient cell-mediated immunity.

This syndrome has been associated with maternal alcoholism and resultant fetal alcohol syndrome.

Signs and symptoms

Visible indications are usually obvious at birth or shortly thereafter. An infant with DiGeorge's syndrome may have low-set ears, notched ear pinnae, a fish-shaped mouth, an undersized jaw, and abnormally wide-set eyes (hypertelorism) with antimongoloid eyelid formation (downward slant).

Cardiovascular abnormalities include great blood vessel anomalies (these may also develop soon after birth) and tetralogy of Fallot.

The thymus may be absent, or underdeveloped and abnormally located. An infant with thymic hypoplasia (rather than aplasia) may experience a spontaneous return of cell-mediated immunity but can develop severe T-cell deficiencies later in life, allowing exaggerated susceptibility to viral, fungal, or bacterial infections, which may be overwhelming.

Typically, hypoparathyroidism, usually associated with DiGeorge's syndrome, causes tetany, hyperphosphoremia, and hypocalcemia. Hypocalcemia develops early and is both life-threatening and unusually resistant to treatment. It can lead to seizures, central nervous system damage, and early congestive heart failure.

Diagnosis

Unless the infant shows typical facial anomalies — normally the first clues to the disorder — an immediate diagnosis is difficult.

A definitive diagnosis depends on successful treatment of hypocalcemia and other life-threatening birth defects during the first few weeks of life. Such a diagnosis rests on proof of decreased or absent T lymphocytes (sheep cell test, lymphopenia) and of an absent thymus (chest X-ray).

Immunoglobulin assays are useless, because antibodies present are usually from maternal circulation. Additional tests showing low serum calcium, elevated serum phosphorus, and missing parathyroid hormone confirm hypoparathyroidism.

Treatment

Life-threatening hypocalcemia must be treated immediately, but it's unusually resistant and requires aggressive treatment; for example, with a rapid I.V. infusion of 10% solution of calcium gluconate.

After hypocalcemia is under control, fetal thymic transplant may restore normal cell-mediated immunity. Cardiac anomalies require surgical repair when possible.

Special considerations

• During I.V. infusion of 10% solution of calcium gluconate, monitor heart rate and watch carefully to avoid infiltration.
• Give calcium supplements with vitamin D (or parathyroid hormone) to ensure effective calcium utilization.
• Provide a low-phosphorus diet.
• Take precautions to protect the patient from infection.
• Teach the mother of an infant with DiGeorge's syndrome to watch for signs of infection and have it treated immediately, to keep the infant away from crowds or any other potential sources of infection, and to provide good hygiene and adequate nutrition and hydration.

DISLOCATIONS AND SUBLUXATIONS

In a dislocation, joint bones are displaced so that their articulating surfaces totally lose contact. Subluxations partially displace the articulating surfaces.

Dislocations and subluxations occur at the joints of the shoulders, elbows, wrists, digits, hips, knees, ankles, and feet; the injury may accompany fractures of these joints or result in deposition of fracture fragments between joint surfaces. Prompt reduction can limit the resulting damage to soft tissue, nerves, and blood vessels.

Causes

A dislocation or subluxation may be congenital (as in congenital dislocation of the hip), or it may follow trauma or disease of surrounding joint tissues (for example, Paget's disease).

Signs and symptoms

Dislocation and subluxations produce deformity around the joint, change the length of the involved extremity, impair joint mobility, and cause point tenderness.

When the injury results from trauma, it's extremely painful and often accompanies joint surface fractures. Even in the absence of concomitant fracture, the displaced bone may damage surrounding muscles, ligaments, nerves, and blood vessels, and may cause bone necrosis, especially if reduction is delayed.

Diagnosis

Patient history, X-rays, and clinical examination rule out or confirm fracture.

Treatment

Immediate reduction (before tissue edema and muscle spasm make reduction difficult) can prevent additional tissue damage and vascular impairment.

Closed reduction consists of manual traction under general anesthesia (or local anesthesia and sedatives). During such reduction, morphine I.V. controls pain; midazolam I.V. controls muscle spasm and facilitates muscle stretching during traction.

Some injuries require open reduction under regional block or general anesthesia. Such surgery may include wire fixation of the joint, skeletal traction, and ligament repair.

After reduction, a splint, cast, or traction immobilizes the joint. Generally, immobilizing the digits for 2 weeks, hips for 6 to 8 weeks, and other dislocated joints for 3 to 6 weeks allows surrounding ligaments to heal.

Special considerations

• Until reduction immobilizes the dislocated joint, don't attempt manipulation. Apply ice to ease pain and edema. Splint the extremity "as it lies," even if the angle is awkward.

• Watch for pallor, pain, loss of pulses, paralysis, and paresthesia—signs of severe vascular compromise. If this occurs, an immediate orthopedic examination (and possibly immediate reduction) is necessary.

• When a patient receives narcotics or benzodiazepines I.V., he may develop respiratory depression or arrest. Keep an airway and a hand-held resuscitation bag in the room, and monitor respirations and pulse rate closely.

• To avoid injury from a dressing that's too tight, instruct the patient to report numbness, pain, cyanosis, or coldness of the extremity below the cast or splint.

• To avoid skin damage, watch for signs of pressure injury (pressure, pain, or soreness) both inside and outside the dressing.

• After removal of the cast or splint, inform the patient that he may gradually return to normal joint activity.

• A dislocated hip needs immediate reduction. At discharge, stress the need for follow-up visits to detect aseptic femoral head necrosis from vascular damage.

DISSEMINATED INTRAVASCULAR COAGULATION

Also called consumption coagulopathy and defibrination syndrome, disseminated intravascular coagulation (DIC) occurs as a complication of diseases and conditions that accelerate clotting. This causes small blood vessel occlusion, organ necrosis, depletion of circulating clotting factors and platelets, and activation of the fibrinolytic system—which, in turn, can provoke severe hemorrhage.

Clotting in the microcirculation usually affects the kidneys and extremities but may occur in the brain, lungs, pituitary and adrenal glands, and GI mucosa. Other conditions, such as vitamin K deficiency, hepatic disease, and anticoagulant therapy, may cause a similar hemorrhage.

DIC is generally an acute condition but may be chronic in cancer patients. The prognosis depends on early detection and treatment, the severity of the hemorrhage, and treatment of the underlying disease or condition.

Causes

DIC may result from:

• *infection,* including gram-negative or gram-positive septicemia; viral, fungal, or rickettsial infection; and protozoal infection (falciparum malaria)

• *obstetric complications,* such as abruptio placentae, amniotic fluid embolism, and retained dead fetus

• *neoplastic disease,* including acute leukemia and metastatic carcinoma

• *disorders that produce necrosis,* such as extensive burns and trauma, brain tissue destruction, transplant rejection, and hepatic necrosis.

Other causes include heatstroke, shock, poisonous snakebite, cirrhosis, fat embolism, incompatible blood transfusion, cardiac arrest, surgery necessitating cardiopulmonary bypass, giant hemangioma, severe venous thrombosis, and purpura fulminans.

It's not clear why such disorders lead to DIC; nor is it certain that they lead to it through a common mechanism. In many patients, the triggering mechanisms may be the entrance of foreign protein into the circulation and vascular endothelial injury.

Results of accelerated clotting

Regardless of how DIC begins, the typical accelerated clotting results in generalized activation of prothrombin and a consequent excess of thrombin. Excess thrombin converts fibrinogen to fibrin, producing fibrin clots in the microcirculation.

This process consumes exorbitant amounts of coagulation factors (especially fibrinogen, prothrombin, platelets, and factor V and factor VIII), causing hypofibrinogenemia, hypoprothrombinemia, thrombocytopenia, and deficiencies in factor V and factor VIII. Circulating thrombin activates the fibrinolytic system, which lyses fibrin clots into fibrin degradation products.

The hemorrhage that occurs may largely be the result of the anticoagulant activity of fibrin degradation products as well as depletion of plasma coagulation factors.

Signs and symptoms

The most significant clinical feature of DIC is abnormal bleeding, *without* an accompanying history of a serious hemorrhagic disorder.

Principal signs of such bleeding include cutaneous oozing, petechiae, ecchymoses, and hematomas caused by bleeding into the skin. Bleeding from sites of surgical or invasive procedures (such as incisions or I.V. sites) and from the GI tract are equally significant indications, as are acrocyanosis and signs of acute tubular necrosis.

Related symptoms and other possible effects include nausea, vomiting, dyspnea, oliguria, convulsions, coma, shock, failure of major organ systems, and severe muscle, back, and abdominal pain.

Diagnosis

Abnormal bleeding in the absence of a known hematologic disorder suggests DIC. Initial laboratory findings supporting a tentative diagnosis of DIC include:

• *prolonged prothrombin time:* greater than 15 seconds

• *prolonged partial thromboplastin time:* greater than 60 to 80 seconds

• *decreased fibrinogen levels:* less than 150 mg/dl

• *decreased fibrinogen levels:* less than 150 mg/dl

• *decreased platelets:* less than 100,000/μl

• *increased fibrin degradation products:* often greater than 100 μg/ml.

Other supportive data include positive fibrin monomers, diminished levels of factors V and VIII, fragmentation of red blood cells (RBCs), and decreased hemoglobin (less than 10 g/dl). Assessment of renal status demonstrates a reduction in urinary output (less than 30 ml/hour) and elevated blood urea nitrogen (greater than 25 mg/dl) and serum creatinine (greater than 1.3 mg/dl) levels.

Final confirmation of the diagnosis may be difficult because many of these test results also occur in other disorders (primary fibrinolysis, for example). Additional diagnostic measures determine the underlying disorder.

Treatment
Successful management of DIC necessitates prompt recognition and adequate treatment of the underlying disorder. Treatment may be supportive (when the underlying disorder is self-limiting, for example) or highly specific.

If the patient isn't actively bleeding, supportive care alone may reverse DIC. However, active bleeding may require heparin I.V. and administration of blood, fresh-frozen plasma, platelets, or packed RBCs to support hemostasis.

Special considerations
• To prevent clots from dislodging and causing fresh bleeding, don't scrub bleeding areas. Use pressure, cold compresses, and topical hemostatic agents to control bleeding.
• Protect the patient from injury. Enforce complete bed rest during bleeding episodes. If the patient is very agitated, pad the side rails.
• Check all I.V. and venipuncture sites frequently for bleeding. Apply pressure to injection sites for at least 10 minutes. Alert other personnel to the patient's tendency to hemorrhage.
• Monitor intake and output hourly in acute DIC, especially when administering blood products.
• Watch for transfusion reactions and signs of fluid overload. To measure the amount of blood lost, weigh dressings and linen and record drainage. Weigh the patient daily, particularly in renal involvement.
• Watch for bleeding from the gastrointestinal and genitourinary tracts. If you suspect intra-abdominal bleeding,

measure the patient's abdominal girth at least every 4 hours, and monitor closely for signs of shock.
• Monitor the results of serial blood studies (particularly hematocrit, hemoglobin, and coagulation times).
• Explain all diagnostic tests and procedures. Allow time for questions.
• Inform the family of the patient's progress. Prepare them for his appearance (I.V. lines, nasogastric tubes, bruises, dried blood). Provide emotional support for the patient and family. As needed, enlist the aid of a social worker, chaplain, and other members of the health care team in providing such support.

DISSOCIATIVE AMNESIA

The essential feature of dissociative amnesia is a sudden inability to recall important personal information that cannot be explained by ordinary forgetfulness. The patient typically is unable to recall all events that occurred during a specific time period, but other types of recall disturbance also are possible.

This disorder commonly occurs during war and natural disasters. Although it's more common in adolescents and young adult women, it's also seen in young men after combat experience. The amnesic event typically ends abruptly, and recovery is complete, with rare recurrences.

Causes
Dissociative amnesia follows severe psychosocial stress, often involving a threat of physical injury or death. Amnesia also may occur after thinking about or engaging in unacceptable behavior such as an extramarital affair.

DIAGNOSING DISSOCIATIVE AMNESIA

A diagnosis of dissociative amnesia is made when the patient's symptoms meet the following criteria put forth in the *Diagnostic and Statistical Manual of Mental Disorders,* 4th edition:
• The predominant disturbance is at least one episode of inability to recall important personal information, usually of a traumatic or stressful nature, that is too extensive to be explained by ordinary forgetfulness.
• The disturbance is not due to dissociative identity disorder, dissociative fugue, posttraumatic stress disorder, acute stress disorder, or somatization disorder and is not due to the direct physiologic effects of a substance or a neurologic or other general medical condition.
• The symptoms cause clinically significant distress or impairment in social, occupational, or other important areas of functioning.

Signs and symptoms
During the assessment interview, the amnesic patient may appear perplexed and disoriented, wandering aimlessly. He won't be able to remember the event that precipitated the episode and probably won't recognize his inability to recall information.

After the episode has ended, the patient usually is unaware that he's suffered what is known as a recall disturbance.

Diagnosis
The *Diagnostic and Statistical Manual of Mental Disorders,* 4th edition, describes symptoms characteristic of patients with this condition. (See *Diagnosing dissociative amnesia.*)

Treatment
Psychotherapy aims to help the patient recognize the traumatic event that triggered the amnesia and the anxiety it produced. A trusting, therapeutic relationship is essential to achieving this goal. The therapist subsequently attempts to teach the patient reality-based coping strategies.

Special considerations
• When providing care in this disorder, teach the patient effective coping strategies to use in stressful situations, rather than those strategies that distort reality.
• Help the patient with dissociative amnesia recognize and deal with anxiety-producing experiences.
• Establish a therapeutic, nonjudgmental relationship with the patient.

DISSOCIATIVE FUGUE

The patient suffering from dissociative fugue wanders or travels while mentally blocking out a traumatic event. During the fugue state, he usually assumes a different personality and later can't recall what happened.

The degree of impairment varies, depending on the duration of the fugue and the nature of the personality state it invokes. Dissociative fugue may be related to dissociative identity disorder, narcissistic personality disorder, and sleepwalking.

The age of onset varies. Although the fugue state usually is brief (hours to days), it can last for many months and carry the patient far from home. The prognosis is good for complete recovery, and recurrences are rare.

Causes

Dissociative fugue typically follows an extremely stressful event, such as combat experience, a natural disaster, a violent or abusive confrontation, or personal rejection. Heavy alcohol use may constitute a predisposing factor.

Signs and symptoms

Psychiatric examination of the patient with dissociative fugue may reveal that he has assumed a new, more uninhibited identity. If the new personality is still evolving, he may avoid social contact. On the other hand, he may have traveled to a distant location, set up a new residence, and developed a well-integrated network of social relationships that don't suggest any mental alteration.

The psychosocial history of such a patient may include episodes of violent behavior. After recovery, he typically can't remember these and other events that took place during the fugue state.

Diagnosis

The *Diagnostic and Statistical Manual of Mental Disorders,* 4th edition, lists characteristic findings in patients with this condition. (See *Diagnosing dissociative fugue.*)

Treatment

Psychotherapy aims to help the patient recognize the traumatic event that triggered the fugue state and develop reality-based strategies for coping with anxiety. A trusting, therapeutic relationship is essential for successful therapy.

Special considerations

• When providing care in this disorder, teach the patient effective coping strategies to use in stressful situations, rather than strategies that distort reality.

DIAGNOSING DISSOCIATIVE FUGUE

The diagnosis of dissociative fugue is made when the patient's symptoms match the following criteria put forth in the *Diagnostic and Statistical Manual of Mental Disorders,* 4th edition:

• The predominant disturbance is sudden, unexpected travel away from home or the patient's customary place of work, with an inability to recall the past.

• The person experiences confusion about personal identity or assumption of a new partial or complete identity.

• The disturbance isn't due to dissociative identity disorder, physiologic effects of a substance, or a general medical condition.

• The symptoms cause clinically significant distress or impairment in social, occupational, or other important areas of functioning.

• Help the patient with dissociative fugue recognize and deal with anxiety-producing experiences.

• Establish a therapeutic, nonjudgmental relationship with the patient.

DISSOCIATIVE IDENTITY DISORDER

A complex disturbance of identity and memory, dissociative identity disorder (formerly referred to as multiple personality disorder) is characterized by the existence of two or more distinct, fully integrated personalities in the same person.

DIAGNOSING DISSOCIATIVE IDENTITY DISORDER

The diagnosis of dissociative identity disorder is based on fulfillment of the following criteria established in the *Diagnostic and Statistical Manual of Mental Disorders,* 4th edition:

• Two or more distinct personalities or personality states (each with its own relatively enduring pattern of perceiving, relating to, and thinking about the environment and self) are present.
• At least two of these personalities or personality states recurrently take full control of the person's behavior.
• The person can't recall important personal information that's too extensive to be explained by ordinary forgetfulness.
• The disturbance isn't due to the direct physiologic effects of a substance or a general medical condition.

The personalities alternate in dominance. Each comprises unique memories, behavior patterns, and social relationships; rigid and flamboyant personalities often are combined. Usually, one personality is unaware of the existence of the others.

Dissociative identity disorder usually begins in childhood, but patients seldom seek treatment until much later in life. The disorder is three to nine times more common in women than in men.

Causes
The cause isn't known. The patient typically has experienced abuse, often sexual, or another form of emotional trauma in childhood. A child may evolve multiple personalities to dissociate herself from the traumatic situation. The dissociated contents become linked with one of many possible shaping influences for personality organization.

Signs and symptoms
The patient may seek treatment for a concurrent psychiatric disorder present in one of the personalities. She may have a history of unsuccessful psychiatric treatment, or she may report periods of amnesia and disturbances in time perception. Family members may describe incidents that the patient can't recall as well as alterations in facial presentation, voice, and behavior.

The transition from one personality to another often is triggered by stress or idiosyncratically meaningful social or environmental cues. Although usually sudden, the transition can occur over hours or days. Hypnosis and amobarbital may facilitate transition.

Diagnosis
The *Diagnostic and Statistical Manual of Mental Disorders,* 4th edition, describes characteristic findings of patients with this condition. (See *Diagnosing dissociative identity disorder.*)

Treatment
Psychotherapy is essential to uniting the personalities and preventing the personality from splitting again. Treatment is usually intensive and prolonged, with success linked to the strength of the patient-therapist relationship with each of the personalities. All of the personalities require equal respect and concern.

Special considerations
• Establish an empathetic relationship with each emerging personality.
• Monitor the patient's actions for evidence of self-directed violence or violence directed at others.

• Recognize even small gains.
• Stress the importance of continuing psychotherapy. Point out that the therapy can be prolonged, with alternating successes and failures, and that one or more of the personalities may resist treatment.

DIVERTICULAR DISEASE

In this disorder, bulging pouches (diverticula) in the GI wall push the mucosal lining through the surrounding muscle. The most common site for diverticula is in the sigmoid colon, but they may develop anywhere, from the proximal end of the pharynx to the anus.

Other typical sites are the duodenum, near the pancreatic border or the ampulla of Vater, and the jejunum. Diverticular disease of the stomach is rare and is often a precursor of peptic or neoplastic disease. Diverticular disease of the ileum (Meckel's diverticulum) is the most common congenital anomaly of the GI tract.

Diverticular disease has two clinical forms. In *diverticulosis,* diverticula are present but don't cause symptoms. In *diverticulitis,* diverticula are inflamed and may cause potentially fatal obstruction, infection, or hemorrhage.

Causes
Diverticular disease is most prevalent in men over age 40. Diverticula probably result from high intraluminal pressure on areas of weakness in the GI wall, where blood vessels enter.

Diet may also be a contributing factor because lack of roughage reduces fecal residue, narrows the bowel lumen, and leads to higher intra-abdominal pressure during defecation.

The fact that diverticulosis is most prevalent in Western industrialized nations, where processing removes much of the roughage from foods, supports this theory. Diverticulosis is less common in nations where the diet contains more natural bulk and fiber.

In diverticulitis, retained undigested food mixed with bacteria accumulates in the diverticular sac, forming a hard mass (fecalith). This substance cuts off the blood supply to the thin walls of the sac, making them more susceptible to attack by colonic bacteria.

Inflammation follows, possibly leading to perforation, abscess, peritonitis, obstruction, or hemorrhage. Occasionally, the inflamed colon segment may produce a fistula by adhering to the bladder or other organs.

Signs and symptoms
The two forms of diverticular disease produce different clinical effects.

Diverticulosis
Although diverticulosis usually produces no symptoms, it may cause recurrent left lower quadrant pain. Such pain, often accompanied by alternating constipation and diarrhea, is relieved by defecation or the passage of flatus. Symptoms resemble irritable bowel syndrome and suggest that both disorders may coexist.

In older patients, a rare complication of diverticulosis (without diverticulitis) is hemorrhage from colonic diverticula, usually in the right colon. Such hemorrhage is usually mild to moderate and easily controlled but may occasionally be massive and life-threatening.

Diverticulitis
Mild diverticulitis produces moderate left lower abdominal pain, mild nausea, gas, irregular bowel habits, low-grade fever, and leukocytosis.

In severe diverticulitis, the diverticula can rupture and produce abscesses or peritonitis. Rupture occurs in up to

20% of such patients; its symptoms include abdominal rigidity and left lower quadrant pain.

Peritonitis follows release of fecal material from the rupture site and causes signs of sepsis and shock (high fever, chills, hypotension). Rupture of diverticulum near a vessel may cause microscopic or massive hemorrhage, depending on the vessel's size.

Chronic diverticulitis may cause fibrosis and adhesions that narrow the bowel's lumen and lead to bowel obstruction. Signs and symptoms of incomplete obstruction include constipation, ribbonlike stools, intermittent diarrhea, and abdominal distention. Increasing obstruction causes abdominal rigidity and pain, diminishing or absent bowel sounds, nausea, and vomiting.

Diagnosis

Diverticular disease frequently produces no symptoms and is often found incidental to an upper GI barium X-ray series. An upper GI series confirms or rules out diverticulosis of the esophagus and upper bowel.

A barium enema confirms or rules out diverticulosis of the lower bowel. Barium-filled diverticula can be single, multiple, or clustered like grapes and may have a wide or narrow mouth. Barium outlines, but doesn't fill, diverticula blocked by impacted feces. In patients with acute diverticulitis, a barium enema may rupture the bowel, so this procedure requires caution.

If irritable bowel syndrome accompanies diverticular disease, X-rays may reveal colonic spasm.

A biopsy rules out cancer; however, a colonoscopic biopsy isn't recommended during acute diverticular disease because of the strenuous bowel preparation it requires. Blood studies may show an elevated erythrocyte sedimentation rate in diverticulitis, especially if the diverticula are infected.

Treatment

The two forms of the disease call for different treatment regimens.

Diverticulosis

Asymptomatic diverticulosis generally doesn't require treatment. Intestinal diverticulosis with pain, mild GI distress, constipation, or difficult defecation may respond to a liquid or bland diet, stool softeners, and occasional doses of mineral oil. These measures relieve symptoms, minimize irritation, and lessen the risk of progression to diverticulitis.

After pain subsides, patients also benefit from a high-residue diet and bulk medication such as psyllium.

Diverticulitis

Treatment of mild diverticulitis without signs of perforation aims to prevent constipation and combat infection. It may include bed rest, a liquid diet, stool softeners, a broad-spectrum antibiotic, meperidine to control pain and relax smooth muscle, and an antispasmodic such as propantheline to control muscle spasms.

Diverticulitis that doesn't respond to medical treatment requires a colon resection to remove the involved segment. Perforation, peritonitis, obstruction, or a fistula that accompanies diverticulitis may require a temporary colostomy to drain abscesses and rest the colon, followed by later anastomosis.

Patients who hemorrhage need blood replacement and careful monitoring of fluid and electrolyte balance. Such bleeding usually stops spontaneously.

If bleeding continues, angiography may be performed to guide catheter placement for infusing vasopressin into the bleeding vessel.

Special considerations

If the patient has diverticulosis:

• Explain what diverticula are and how they form.

• Make sure the patient understands the importance of dietary roughage and the harmful effects of constipation and straining during defecation. Encourage increased intake of foods high in undigestible fiber, including fresh fruits and vegetables, whole grain bread, and wheat or bran cereals. Warn that a high-fiber diet may temporarily cause flatulence and discomfort.

• Advise the patient to relieve constipation with stool softeners or bulk-forming cathartics. But caution against taking bulk-forming cathartics without plenty of water; if swallowed dry, they may absorb enough moisture in the mouth and throat to swell and obstruct the esophagus or trachea.

• If the patient with diverticulosis is hospitalized, administer medication as needed; observe his stools carefully for frequency, color, and consistency; and keep accurate pulse and temperature charts because they may signal developing inflammation or complications.

If the patient has diverticulitis:

• In mild disease, administer medications, explain diagnostic tests and preparations for such tests, observe stools carefully, and maintain accurate records of temperature, pulse, respirations, and intake and output.

• If diverticular bleeding occurs, the patient may require angiography and catheter placement for vasopressin infusion. If so, inspect the insertion site frequently for bleeding, check pedal pulses often, and keep the patient from flexing his legs at the groin.

• Watch for vasopressin-induced fluid retention (apprehension, abdominal cramps, convulsions, oliguria, and anuria) and severe hyponatremia (hypotension; rapid, thready pulse; cold, clammy skin; and cyanosis).

After surgery to resect the colon:

• Watch for signs of infection.

• Provide meticulous wound care because perforation may already have infected the area.

• Check drain sites frequently for signs of infection (purulent drainage, foul odor) or fecal drainage.

• Change dressings as necessary.

• Encourage coughing and deep breathing to prevent atelectasis.

• Watch for signs of postoperative bleeding (hypotension, decreased hemoglobin and hematocrit).

• Record intake and output accurately.

• Keep the nasogastric tube patent.

• As needed, teach ostomy care.

• Arrange for a visit by an enterostomal therapist.

DRUG ABUSE AND DEPENDENCE

The National Institute on Drug Abuse defines this condition as the use of a legal or an illegal drug that causes physical, mental, emotional, or social harm. Examples of abused drugs include narcotics, stimulants, depressants, antianxiety agents, and hallucinogens.

Chronic drug abuse, especially I.V. use, can lead to life-threatening complications, such as cardiac and respiratory arrest, intracranial hemorrhage, acquired immunodeficiency syndrome, tetanus, subacute infective endocarditis, hepatitis, vasculitis, septicemia, thrombophlebitis, pulmonary emboli, gangrene, malnutrition and GI disturbances, respiratory infections, musculoskeletal dysfunction, trauma, depression, increased risk of suicide, and psychosis. Materials used to "cut" street drugs also can cause toxic or allergic reactions.

Drug abuse can occur at any age. Experimentation with drugs commonly begins in adolescence or even earlier. Drug abuse often leads to addiction, which may involve physical or psychological dependence or both. The most dangerous form of abuse occurs when users mix several drugs simultaneously—including alcohol.

Causes

Drug abuse commonly results from a combination of low self-esteem, peer pressure, inadequate coping skills, and curiosity.

Most people who are predisposed to drug abuse have few mental or emotional resources against stress, an overdependence on others, and a low tolerance for frustration. Taking the drug gives them pleasure by relieving tension, abolishing loneliness, allowing them to achieve a temporarily peaceful or euphoric state, or simply relieving boredom.

Drug dependence may follow experimentation with drugs in response to peer pressure. It also may follow the use of drugs to relieve physical pain, but this is uncommon.

Signs and symptoms

Indications of acute intoxication vary, depending on the drug.

The drug user seldom seeks treatment specifically for his drug problem. Instead, he may seek emergency treatment for drug-related injuries or complications, such as a motor vehicle accident, burns from freebasing, an overdose, physical deterioration from illness or malnutrition, or symptoms of withdrawal.

Friends, family members, or law enforcement officials may bring the patient to the hospital because of respiratory depression, unconsciousness, acute injury, or a psychiatric crisis.

Physical examination

Examine the patient for signs and symptoms of drug use or drug-related complications as well as for clues to the type of drug ingested. For example, fever can result from stimulant or hallucinogen intoxication, from withdrawal, or from infection from I.V. drug use.

Inspect the eyes for lacrimation from opiate withdrawal, nystagmus from central nervous system (CNS) depressants or phencyclidine intoxication, and drooping eyelids from opiate or CNS depressant use. Constricted pupils occur with opiate use or withdrawal; dilated pupils, with the use of hallucinogens or amphetamines.

Examine the nose for rhinorrhea from opiate withdrawal and the oral and nasal mucosa for signs of drug-induced irritation. Drug sniffing can result in inflammation, atrophy, or perforation of the nasal mucosa. Dental conditions commonly result from the poor oral hygiene associated with chronic drug use. Also inspect under the tongue for evidence of I.V. drug injection.

Inspect the skin. Sweating, a common sign of intoxication with opiates or CNS stimulants, also accompanies most drug withdrawal syndromes. Drug use sometimes induces a sensation of bugs crawling on the skin, known as formication; as a result, the patient's skin may be excoriated from scratching.

Needle marks or tracks are an obvious sign of I.V. drug abuse. Keep in mind that the patient may attempt to conceal or disguise injection sites with tattoos or by selecting an inconspicuous site, such as under the nails.

In addition, self-injection can sometimes cause cellulitis or abscesses, especially in patients who also are chronic alcoholics. Puffy hands can be a late sign of thrombophlebitis or of fascial infection from self-injection on the hands or arms.

Auscultation may disclose bilateral crackles and rhonchi caused by smoking and inhaling drugs or by opiate overdose. Other cardiopulmonary signs of overdose include pulmonary edema, respiratory depression, aspiration pneumonia, and hypotension.

CNS stimulants and some hallucinogens may precipitate refractory acute-onset hypertension or cardiac arrhythmias. Withdrawal from opiates or depressants also can provoke arrhythmias and, occasionally, hypotension.

During opiate withdrawal, the patient may report abdominal pain, nausea, or vomiting. Opiate abusers also commonly complain of hemorrhoids, a consequence of the constipating effects of these drugs. Palpation of an enlarged liver, with or without tenderness, may indicate hepatitis.

Neurologic symptoms of drug abuse include tremors, hyperreflexia, hyporeflexia, and seizures. Abrupt withdrawal may precipitate signs of CNS depression (ranging from lethargy to coma), hallucinations, or signs of overstimulation, including euphoria and violent behavior.

Medical history

Carefully review the patient's medical history. Suspect drug abuse if he reports a painful injury or chronic illness but refuses a diagnostic workup. In his attempt to obtain drugs, the dependent patient may feign illnesses, such as migraine headaches, myocardial infarction, and renal colic; claim an allergy to over-the-counter analgesics; or even request a specific medication.

Also be alert for a previous history of overdose or a high tolerance for potentially addictive drugs. I.V. drug users may have a history of hepatitis or human immunodeficiency virus (HIV) infection from sharing dirty needles.

Female drug users may report a history of amenorrhea.

A patient who abuses drugs may give you a fictitious name and address, be reluctant to discuss previous hospitalizations, or seek treatment at a medical facility across town rather than in his own neighborhood. If possible, interview family members to verify his responses.

If the patient admits to drug use, try to determine the extent to which this behavior interferes with his normal functioning. Note whether he expresses a desire to overcome his dependence on drugs.

If possible, obtain a drug history consisting of substances ingested, amount, frequency, and last dose. Expect incomplete or inaccurate responses. Drug-induced amnesia, a depressed level of consciousness, or ignorance may distort the patient's recollection of the facts; he also may deliberately fabricate answers to avoid arrest or to conceal a suicide attempt.

The hospitalized drug abuser is likely to be uncooperative, disruptive, or even violent. He may experience mood swings, anxiety, impaired memory, sleep disturbances, flashbacks, slurred speech, depression, and thought disorders.

Some patients resort to plays on sympathy, bribery, or threats to obtain drugs. They may also try to manipulate caregivers by pitting one against another.

Diagnosis

The *Diagnostic and Statistical Manual of Mental Disorders,* 4th edition, gives characteristic findings for patients with drug dependence. (See *Diagnosing substance dependence and related disorders,* page 296.)

Various tests can confirm drug use, determine the amount and type of drug taken, and reveal complications. For example, a serum or urine drug screen

DIAGNOSING SUBSTANCE DEPENDENCE AND RELATED DISORDERS

The *Diagnostic and Statistical Manual of Mental Disorders*, 4th edition, identifies the following diagnostic criteria for substance dependence, abuse, intoxication, and withdrawal.

Substance dependence

A maladaptive pattern of substance use leading to clinically significant impairment or distress, as manifested by three or more of the following, occurring at any time in the same 12-month period:

• Tolerance, as defined by either of the following: the need for increased amounts of the substance to achieve intoxication or desired effect, or a markedly diminished effect with continued use of the same amount of the substance

• Withdrawal, as manifested by either of the following: the characteristic withdrawal syndrome for the substance or the same, or similar, substance is taken to relieve or avoid withdrawal symptoms

• The person often takes the substance in larger amounts or over a longer period than was intended.

• The person experiences a persistent desire or unsuccessful efforts to cut down or control substance use.

• The person spends much time obtaining or using the substance or recovering from its effects.

• The person abandons or reduces social, occupational, or recreational activities due to substance use.

• The person continues using the substance despite knowing he has a physical or psychological problem that's likely to have been caused or exacerbated by the substance.

Substance abuse

A maladaptive pattern of substance use leading to clinically significant impairment or distress, as manifested by one or more of the following, occurring within a 12-month period:

• recurrent substance use resulting in a failure to fulfill major role obligations at work, school, or home

• recurrent substance use in physically hazardous situations

• recurrent substance-related legal problems

• continued substance use despite having social or interpersonal problems caused or exacerbated by the effects of the substance.

The symptoms have never met the criteria for substance dependence for this class of substance.

Substance intoxication

• The development of a reversible substance-specific syndrome resulting from recent ingestion of, or exposure to, a substance.

• Clinically significant maladaptive behavioral or psychological changes resulting from the effect of the substance on the central nervous system and developing during or shortly after use of the substance.

• Symptoms aren't caused by a general medical condition and aren't better accounted for by another mental disorder.

Substance withdrawal

• A substance-specific syndrome develops from the cessation or reduction of heavy and prolonged substance use.

• The substance-specific syndrome causes clinically significant distress or impairment in social, occupational, or other areas of functioning.

• The symptoms aren't caused by a general medical condition and aren't better accounted for by another mental disorder.

can detect recently ingested substances.

Characteristic findings in other tests include elevated serum globulin levels, hypoglycemia, leukocytosis, liver function abnormalities, positive Venereal Disease Research Laboratory test results, positive rapid plasma reagin test results because of elevated protein fractions, elevated mean corpuscular hemoglobin levels, elevated uric acid levels, and reduced blood urea nitrogen levels.

Treatment
The patient may first need treatment for drug intoxication, followed by long-term therapy to combat drug dependence.

Drug intoxication
The patient with acute drug intoxication should receive symptomatic treatment based on the drug ingested. Measures include fluid replacement therapy and nutritional and vitamin supplements, if indicated, and detoxification with the same drug or a pharmacologically similar drug. (Exceptions include cocaine, hallucinogens, and marijuana, which aren't used for detoxification.)

Medications include sedatives to induce sleep; anticholinergics and antidiarrheal agents to relieve GI distress; antianxiety drugs for severe agitation, especially in cocaine abusers; and symptomatic treatment of complications.

Depending on the dosage and time elapsed before admission, additional treatments may include gastric lavage, induced emesis, activated charcoal, forced diuresis and, possibly, hemoperfusion or hemodialysis.

Drug dependence
Treatment of drug dependence commonly involves a triad of care: detoxification, short- and long-term rehabilitation, and aftercare. The latter means a lifetime of abstinence, usually aided by participation in Narcotics Anonymous or a similar self-help group.

Detoxification, the controlled and gradual withdrawal of an abused drug, is achieved through substitution of a drug with similar action. Such gradual replacement of the abused drug controls the effects of withdrawal, thereby reducing the patient's discomfort and associated risks.

Depending on which drug the patient has abused, detoxification may be managed on an inpatient or outpatient basis. For example, withdrawal from depressants can produce hazardous adverse reactions, such as generalized tonic-clonic seizures, status epilepticus, and hypotension.

The severity of these reactions determines whether the patient can be safely treated as an outpatient or requires hospitalization. Withdrawal from depressants usually doesn't require detoxification.

Opioid withdrawal causes severe physical discomfort and can even be life-threatening. To minimize these effects, chronic opioid abusers commonly are detoxified with methadone.

To ease withdrawal from opioids, depressants, and other drugs, useful nonchemical measures may include psychotherapy, exercise, relaxation techniques, and nutritional support. Sedatives and tranquilizers may be administered temporarily to help the patient cope with insomnia, anxiety, and depression.

After withdrawal, the patient needs to participate in a rehabilitation program to prevent a recurrence of drug abuse. Rehabilitation programs are available for both inpatients and outpatients; they usually last a month or longer and may include individual, group, and family psychotherapy. During and after rehabilitation, participation in a drug-oriented self-help group may be beneficial. The largest such group is Narcotics Anonymous.

Special considerations
During an acute episode:
• Continuously monitor the patient's vital signs, and observe for complications of overdose and withdrawal, such as cardiopulmonary arrest, seizures, and aspiration.
• Based on standard hospital policy, institute appropriate measures to prevent suicide attempts.
• Give medications as needed to decrease withdrawal symptoms; monitor and record their effectiveness.
• Maintain a quiet, safe environment during withdrawal from any drug, because excessive noise may agitate the patient.
• Remove harmful objects from the patient's room, and use restraints only if you suspect that he might harm himself or others. Institute seizure precautions.
After an acute episode:
• Learn to control your reactions to the patient's undesirable behaviors—commonly, psychological dependency, manipulation, anger, frustration, and alienation.
• Set limits for dealing with demanding, manipulative behavior.
• Promote adequate nutrition and monitor the patient's nutritional intake.
• Administer medications carefully to prevent hoarding by the patient. Check the patient's mouth to ensure that he has swallowed the medication. Closely monitor visitors who might supply the patient with drugs.
• Refer the patient for detoxification and rehabilitation as appropriate. Give him a list of available resources.
• Encourage family members to seek help whether or not the abuser seeks it. You can suggest private therapy or community mental health clinics.

If the patient refuses to participate in a rehabilitation program:
• Teach him how to minimize the risk of drug-related complications. Review measures for preventing HIV infection and hepatitis. Stress that these infections are readily transmitted by sharing needles with other drug users and by unprotected sexual intercourse.
• Advise the patient to use a new needle for every injection or to clean needles with a solution of chlorine bleach and water.
• Emphasize the importance of using a condom during intercourse to prevent disease transmission and pregnancy. If necessary, teach the female drug abuser about other methods of birth control. Explain the devastating effects of drugs on the developing fetus.

DYSMENORRHEA

The most common gynecologic complaint, dysmenorrhea—painful menstruation—is a leading cause of absenteeism from school (affecting 10% of high school girls each month) and work (causing an estimated 140 million work hours lost annually).

Dysmenorrhea can occur as a primary disorder or secondary to an underlying disease. Because dysmenorrhea almost always follows an ovulatory cycle, both the primary and secondary forms are rare during the anovulatory cycles of menses. After age 20, dysmenorrhea is generally secondary.

Primary dysmenorrhea is self-limiting, so the prognosis is generally good. The prognosis for secondary dysmenorrhea depends on the underlying disorder.

Causes

Although primary dysmenorrhea is unrelated to any identifiable cause, possible contributing factors include hormonal imbalances and psychogenic factors. The pain of dysmenorrhea probably results from increased prostaglandin secretion, which intensifies normal uterine contractions.

Dysmenorrhea may also be secondary to such gynecologic disorders as endometriosis, cervical stenosis, uterine leiomyomas, uterine malposition, pelvic inflammatory disease, pelvic tumors, or adenomyosis.

Signs and symptoms

Dysmenorrhea produces sharp, intermittent, cramping, lower abdominal pain, which usually radiates to the back, thighs, groin, and vulva. Such pain starts with or immediately before menstrual flow and peaks within 24 hours.

Dysmenorrhea may also be associated with signs and symptoms of premenstrual syndrome (urinary frequency, nausea, vomiting, diarrhea, headache, chills, abdominal bloating, painful breasts, depression, and irritability).

Diagnosis

Pelvic examination and a detailed patient history may help suggest the cause of dysmenorrhea.

Primary dysmenorrhea is diagnosed when secondary causes are ruled out. Appropriate tests (such as laparoscopy, dilation and curettage, and X-rays) are used to diagnose underlying disorders in secondary dysmenorrhea.

Treatment

Initial treatment aims to relieve pain. Pain-relief measures may include the following:

• *Analgesics,* such as aspirin, relieve mild to moderate pain (most effective taken 24 to 48 hours before the onset of menses). Aspirin is especially effective because it also inhibits prostaglandin synthesis.

• *Narcotics* help lessen severe pain (infrequently used).

• *Prostaglandin inhibitors* (such as ibuprofen) relieve pain by decreasing the severity of uterine contractions.

• *Heat* applied locally to the lower abdomen may relieve discomfort in mature women but isn't recommended in young adolescents, because appendicitis may mimic dysmenorrhea.

Primary dysmenorrhea

Administration of sex steroids is an alternative to treatment with antiprostaglandins or analgesics in primary dysmenorrhea. In such therapy, oral contraceptives relieve pain by suppressing ovulation. However, patients who are attempting pregnancy should rely on antiprostaglandin therapy to relieve symptoms of primary dysmenorrhea.

Because persistently severe dysmenorrhea may have a psychogenic cause, psychological evaluation and appropriate counseling may be helpful.

Secondary dysmenorrhea

Treatment of secondary dysmenorrhea may include surgical treatment of underlying disorders, such as endometriosis or uterine leiomyomas. However, surgical treatment is used only after conservative therapy fails.

Special considerations

• Obtain a history focusing on gynecologic complaints, including symptoms of pelvic disease such as excessive bleeding, changes in bleeding pattern, vaginal discharge, and dyspareunia.

• Explain normal female anatomy and physiology to the patient, as well as the nature of dysmenorrhea. Provide the adolescent patient with information on pregnancy and contraception.

• Tell the patient to record her menstrual symptoms and to seek medical care if her symptoms persist.

DYSPAREUNIA

Defined as genital pain associated with intercourse, dyspareunia may be mild or it may be severe enough to affect enjoyment of intercourse. It's commonly associated with physical problems; less commonly, with a psychological disorder. The prognosis is good if the underlying disorder can be treated successfully.

Causes

Physical causes of dyspareunia include an intact hymen; deformities or lesions of the introitus or vagina; retroversion of the uterus; genital, rectal, or pelvic scar tissue; acute or chronic infections of the genitourinary tract; and disorders of the surrounding viscera (including residual effects of pelvic inflammatory disease or disease of the adnexal and broad ligaments).

Other possible physical causes are endometriosis, benign and malignant growths and tumors, insufficient lubrication, radiation to the area, and allergic reactions to diaphragms, condoms, or other contraceptives.

Psychological causes include fear of pain or of injury during intercourse, recollection of a painful experience, guilt feelings about sex, fear of pregnancy or of injury to the fetus during pregnancy, anxiety caused by a new sexual partner or technique, and fatigue.

Signs and symptoms

Dyspareunia produces mild aches to severe pain before, during, or after intercourse. It also may be associated with vaginal itching or burning.

Diagnosis

Physical examination and laboratory tests help determine the underlying disorder. The diagnosis also depends on a sexual history and the answers to such questions as: When does the pain occur? Does it occur with certain positions or techniques or at certain times during the sexual response cycle? Where does the pain occur? What is its quality, frequency, and duration? What relieves or aggravates it?

When the disorder causes marked distress or interpersonal difficulty, it may fulfill the criteria for a *Diagnostic and Statistical Manual of Mental Disorders,* 4th edition, diagnosis.

Treatment

Among the treatments for physical causes are creams and water-soluble gels for inadequate lubrication, appropriate medications for infections, excision of hymenal scars, and gentle stretching of painful scars at the vaginal opening. The patient may be advised to change her coital position to reduce pain on deep penetration.

Methods for treating psychologically based dyspareunia vary with the patient. Sensate focus exercises deemphasize intercourse and teach foreplay techniques. Education about methods of contraception can reduce fear of pregnancy; education about sexual activity during pregnancy can relieve fear of harming the fetus.

Special considerations

• Provide instruction concerning anatomy and physiology of the reproductive system, contraception, and the human sexual response cycle.
• Provide information on drugs that may affect the patient sexually and on lubricating gels and creams.

EAR CANAL TUMORS, BENIGN

Tumors that are benign may develop anywhere in the ear canal. Common types include keloids, osteomas, and sebaceous cysts. These tumors rarely become malignant, and, with proper treatment, the prognosis is excellent.

Causes

The causes, incidence, and characteristics of benign ear canal tumors vary. (See *Causes and characteristics of benign ear tumors,* page 302.)

Signs and symptoms

A benign ear tumor is usually asymptomatic, unless it becomes infected, in which case pain, fever, or inflammation may result. (Pain is often a sign of cancer.) If the tumor grows large enough to obstruct the ear canal by itself or through accumulated cerumen and debris, it may cause hearing loss and the sensation of pressure.

Diagnosis

Clinical features and the patient history suggest a benign tumor of the ear canal; otoscopy confirms it. A biopsy rules out cancer.

Treatment

Generally, a benign tumor requires surgical excision if it obstructs the ear canal, is cosmetically undesirable, or becomes malignant.

Treatment of keloids may include surgery followed by repeated injections of long-acting steroids into the suture line. Excision must be complete, but even this may not prevent recurrence.

Surgical excision of an osteoma consists of elevating the skin from the surface of the bony growth and shaving the osteoma with a mechanical burr or drill.

Before surgery, a sebaceous cyst requires preliminary treatment with antibiotics, to reduce inflammation. To prevent recurrence, excision must be complete, including the sac or capsule of the cyst.

Special considerations

• Because patients usually don't require hospitalization, they need emotional support and appropriate patient teaching so they'll follow their therapeutic plan properly at home.

• Thoroughly explain diagnostic procedures and treatment to the patient and his family. Reassure them and answer any questions they may have.

• After surgery, instruct the patient in good aural hygiene. Until his ear is completely healed, advise him not to insert anything in his ear or allow water to get in it. Suggest that he cover his ears with a cap when showering.

• Teach the patient how to recognize signs of infection, such as pain, fever, localized redness, and swelling. If he detects any of these signs, instruct him to report them immediately.

CAUSES AND CHARACTERISTICS OF BENIGN EAR TUMORS

TUMOR	CAUSES AND INCIDENCE	CHARACTERISTICS
Keloid	• Surgery or trauma such as ear-piercing • Most common in blacks	• Hypertrophy and fibrosis of scar tissue • Commonly recurs
Osteoma	• Idiopathic growth • Predisposing factor such as swimming in cold water • Three times more common in males than in females • Seldom occurs before adolescence	• Bony outgrowth from wall of external auditory meatus • Usually bilateral and multiple (exostoses) • May be circumscribed or diffuse, nondisplaceable, nontender
Sebaceous cyst	• Obstruction of a sebaceous gland	• Painless, circumscribed, round mass of variable size filled with oily, fatty, glandular secretions • May occur on external ear and outer third of external auditory canal

EARDRUM PERFORATION

Perforation of the eardrum is a rupture of the tympanic membrane. Such injury may cause otitis media and hearing loss.

Causes

The usual cause of perforated eardrum is trauma: the deliberate or accidental insertion of sharp objects (cotton swabs, bobby pins) or sudden excessive changes in pressure (explosion, a blow to the head, flying, or diving). The injury may also result from untreated otitis media and, in children, from acute otitis media.

Signs and symptoms

Sudden onset of severe earache and bleeding from the ear are the first signs of a perforated eardrum. Other symptoms include hearing loss, tinnitus, and vertigo. Purulent otorrhea within 24 to 48 hours of injury signals infection.

Diagnosis

Severe earache and bleeding from the ear with a history of trauma strongly suggest a perforated eardrum; direct visualization of the perforated tympanic membrane with an otoscope confirms it. Additional diagnostic measures include audiometric testing and a check of voluntary facial movements to rule out facial nerve damage.

Treatment

In bleeding from the ear, use a sterile, cotton-tipped applicator to absorb the blood, and check for purulent drainage or evidence of cerebrospinal fluid leakage. A culture of the specimen may be ordered. *Irrigation of the ear is absolutely contraindicated.*

Apply a sterile dressing over the outer ear, and refer the patient to an ear specialist. A large perforation with uncontrolled bleeding may require immediate surgery to approximate the ruptured edges. Treatment may include a mild analgesic, a sedative to decrease anxiety, and an oral antibiotic.

Special considerations
• Find out the cause of the injury, and report suspected child abuse.
• Before discharge, tell the patient not to blow his nose or get water in his ear canal until the perforation heals.

LIFE-THREATENING DISORDER

ELECTRIC SHOCK

When an electric current passes through the body, the damage it does depends on the intensity of the current (amperes, milliamperes, or microamperes), the resistance of the tissues it passes through, the kind of current (AC, DC, or mixed), and the frequency and duration of current flow.

Electric shock may cause ventricular fibrillation, respiratory paralysis, burns, and death. The prognosis depends on the site and extent of damage, the patient's state of health, and the speed and adequacy of treatment. In the United States, about 1,000 people die of electric shock each year.

Causes
Electric shock usually follows accidental contact with exposed parts of electrical appliances or wiring, but it may also result from lightning or the flash of electric arcs from high-voltage power lines or machines.

The increased use of electrical medical devices in the hospital, many of which are connected directly to the patient, has raised serious concern for electrical safety and has led to the development of electrical safety standards. But even well-designed equipment with reliable safety features can cause electric shock if mishandled. (See *Preventing electric shock,* page 304.)

Electric current can cause injury in three ways: true electrical injury as the current passes through the body, arc or flash burns from current that doesn't pass through the body, and thermal surface burns caused by associated heat and flames.

Signs and symptoms
Severe electric shock usually causes muscle contraction, followed by unconsciousness and loss of reflex control, sometimes with respiratory paralysis (by way of prolonged contraction of respiratory muscles, or a direct effect on the respiratory nerve center).

After momentary shock, hyperventilation may follow initial muscle contraction. Passage of even the smallest electric current — if it passes through the heart — may induce ventricular fibrillation or another arrhythmia that progresses to fibrillation or myocardial infarction.

Electric shock from a high-frequency current (which generates more heat in tissues than a low-frequency current) usually causes burns and local tissue coagulation and necrosis. Low-frequency currents can also cause serious burns if the contact with the current is concentrated in a small area (for example, when a toddler bites into an electrical cord).

Contusions, fractures, and other injuries can result from violent muscle contractions or falls during the shock; later, the patient may develop renal shutdown. Residual hearing impairment, cataracts, and vision loss may persist after severe electric shock.

PREVENTING ELECTRIC SHOCK

To protect your patient from electric shock:
• Check for cuts, cracks, or frayed insulation on electric cords, call buttons (also check for warm call buttons), and electric devices attached to the bed. Keep these away from hot or wet surfaces and sharp corners.
• Don't set glasses of water, damp towels, or other wet items on electrical equipment. Wipe up accidental spills before they leak into equipment. Avoid using extension cords because they may circumvent the ground. If they're absolutely necessary, don't place them under carpeting or in areas where they'll be walked on.
• Report faulty equipment promptly to maintenance personnel. If a machine sparks, smokes, seems unusually hot, or gives you or your patient a slight shock, unplug it immediately if doing so won't endanger the patient's life.
• Check inspection labels, and report equipment overdue for inspection.
• Be especially careful when using electrical equipment near patients

with pacemakers or direct cardiac lines because a cardiac catheter or pacemaker can create a direct, low-resistance path to the heart; even a small shock may cause ventricular fibrillation.
• Make sure ground connections on electrical equipment are intact. Line cord plugs should have three prongs; the prongs should be straight and firmly fixed. Check that prongs fit wall outlets properly, and that outlets aren't loose or broken. Don't use adapters on plugs.
• Remember: Dry, calloused, unbroken skin offers more resistance to electric current than mucous membrane, an open wound, or thin, moist skin.
• Make sure defibrillator paddles are free of dry, caked gel before applying fresh gel because poor electrical contact can cause burns. Also, don't apply too much gel. If the gel runs over the edge of the paddle and touches your hand, you'll receive some of the defibrillator shock, while the patient loses some of the energy in the discharge.

Diagnosis
Usually, the cause of electrical injuries is either obvious or suspected. However, an accurate history can define the voltage and the length of contact.

Treatment
Immediate emergency treatment includes carefully separating the victim from the current source, quick assessment of vital functions, and emergency measures, such as cardiopulmonary resuscitation (CPR) and defibrillation.

To separate the victim from the current source, immediately turn it off or

unplug it. If this isn't possible, pull the victim free with a nonconductive device, such as a loop of dry cloth or rubber, a dry rope, or a leather belt.

Emergency measures
Then begin emergency treatment as follows:
• Quickly assess vital functions. If you don't detect a pulse or breathing, start CPR at once. Continue until vital signs return or emergency help arrives with a defibrillator and other life-support equipment. Then monitor the patient's

cardiac rhythm continuously and obtain a 12-lead electrocardiogram.

• Because internal tissue destruction may be much greater than indicated by skin damage, give lactated Ringer's solution I.V. to maintain a urine output of 50 to 100 ml/hour. Insert an indwelling urinary catheter, and send the first specimen to the laboratory.

• Measure intake and output hourly and watch for tea- or port wine–colored urine, which occurs when coagulation necrosis and tissue ischemia liberate myoglobin and hemoglobin. These proteins can precipitate in the renal tubules, causing tubular necrosis and renal shutdown. To prevent this, give mannitol and furosemide.

• Administer sodium bicarbonate to counteract acidosis caused by widespread tissue destruction and anaerobic metabolism.

Special considerations

• Assess the patient's neurologic status frequently because central nervous system damage may result from ischemia or demyelination.

• Watch for sensorimotor deficits because a spinal cord injury may follow cord ischemia or a compression fracture.

• Check for neurovascular damage in the extremities by assessing peripheral pulses and capillary refill and by asking about numbness, tingling, or pain. Elevate any injured extremities.

• Apply a temporary sterile dressing and admit the patient for surgical debridement and observation as needed. Frequent debridement and use of topical and systemic antibiotics can help reduce the risk of infection.

• Prepare the patient for grafting or, if his injuries are extreme, for amputation.

• Protect patients from electric shock in the hospital.

• Tell patients how to avoid electrical hazards at home and at work. Advise parents of small children to put safety guards on all electrical outlets and keep children away from electrical devices. Warn all patients not to use electrical appliances while showering or wet.

• Also warn patients *never* to touch electrical appliances while touching faucets or cold water pipes in the kitchen because these pipes often provide the ground for all circuits in the house.

LIFE-THREATENING DISORDER

ENCEPHALITIS

A severe inflammation of the brain, encephalitis is usually caused by a mosquito-borne or, in some areas, a tickborne virus. However, transmission by means other than arthropod bites may occur through ingestion of infected goat's milk and accidental injection or inhalation of the virus. Eastern equine encephalitis may produce permanent neurologic damage and is often fatal.

In encephalitis, intense lymphocytic infiltration of brain tissues and the leptomeninges causes cerebral edema, degeneration of the brain's ganglion cells, and diffuse nerve cell destruction.

Causes

Encephalitis generally results from infection with arboviruses specific to rural areas. However, in urban areas, it's most frequently caused by enteroviruses (coxsackievirus, poliovirus, and echovirus).

Other causes include herpesvirus, mumps virus, human immunodeficiency virus, adenoviruses, and demyelinating diseases following measles, varicella, rubella, or vaccination.

Between World War I and the Depression, a type of encephalitis known as lethargic encephalitis, von Economo's disease, or sleeping sickness occurred with some regularity. The causative virus was never clearly identified, and the disease is rare today. Even so, the term *sleeping sickness* persists and is often mistakenly used to describe other types of encephalitis as well.

Signs and symptoms

All viral forms of encephalitis have similar clinical features, although certain differences do occur.

Usually, the acute illness begins with sudden onset of fever, headache, and vomiting, and progresses to include signs and symptoms of meningeal irritation (stiff neck and back) and neuronal damage (drowsiness, coma, paralysis, convulsions, ataxia, organic psychoses). After the acute phase of the illness, coma may persist for days or weeks.

The severity of arbovirus encephalitis may range from subclinical to rapidly fatal necrotizing disease. Herpes encephalitis also produces signs and symptoms that vary from subclinical to acute and often fatal fulminating disease. Associated effects include disturbances of taste or smell.

Diagnosis

During an encephalitis epidemic, diagnosis is easily based on clinical findings and patient history. However, sporadic cases are difficult to distinguish from other febrile illnesses, such as gastroenteritis or meningitis. When possible, identification of the virus in cerebrospinal fluid (CSF) or blood confirms this diagnosis.

The common viruses that also cause herpes, measles, and mumps are easier to identify than arboviruses. Arboviruses and herpesviruses can be isolated by inoculating young mice with a specimen taken from the patient. In herpes encephalitis, serologic studies may show rising titers of complement-fixing antibodies.

In all forms of encephalitis, CSF pressure is elevated, and despite inflammation, the fluid is often clear. White blood cell and protein levels in CSF are slightly elevated, but the glucose level remains normal. An EEG reveals abnormalities. Occasionally, a computed tomography scan may be ordered to rule out cerebral hematoma.

Treatment

The antiviral agent acyclovir is effective only against herpes encephalitis. Treatment of all other forms of encephalitis is entirely supportive.

Drug therapy includes phenytoin or another anticonvulsant, usually given I.V.; glucocorticoids to reduce cerebral inflammation and edema; furosemide or mannitol to reduce cerebral swelling; sedatives for restlessness; and aspirin or acetaminophen to relieve headache and reduce fever.

Other supportive measures include adequate fluid and electrolyte intake to prevent dehydration and antibiotics for an associated infection such as pneumonia. Isolation is unnecessary.

Special considerations

During the acute phase of the illness:
• Assess neurologic function often. Observe the patient's level of consciousness and check for signs of increased intracranial pressure (ICP), such as increasing restlessness, plucking at the bedcovers, vomiting, seizures, and changes in pupil size, motor function, and vital signs.
• Also watch for cranial nerve involvement (ptosis, strabismus, diplopia), abnormal sleep patterns, and behavior changes.
• Maintain adequate fluid intake to prevent dehydration, but avoid fluid overload, which may increase cerebral

edema. Measure and record intake and output accurately.

• Give acyclovir by slow I.V. infusion only. The patient must be well hydrated and the infusion given over 1 hour to avoid kidney damage. Watch for adverse effects, such as nausea, diarrhea, pruritus, and rash, and adverse effects of other drugs. Check the infusion site often to avoid infiltration and phlebitis.

• Carefully position the patient to prevent joint stiffness and neck pain, and turn him often. Assist with range-of-motion exercises.

• Maintain adequate nutrition. It may be necessary to give the patient small, frequent meals or to supplement these meals with nasogastric tube or parenteral feedings.

• To prevent constipation and minimize the risk of increased ICP resulting from straining during defecation, give a mild laxative or stool softener.

• Provide good mouth care.

• Maintain a quiet environment. Darkening the room may decrease photophobia and headache. If the patient naps during the day and is restless at night, plan daytime activities to minimize napping and promote sleep at night.

• Provide emotional support and reassurance, since the patient is apt to be frightened by the illness and frequent diagnostic tests.

• If the patient is delirious or confused, attempt to reorient him often. Providing a calendar or a clock in the patient's room may be helpful.

• Reassure the patient and his family that behavior changes caused by encephalitis usually disappear. If a neurologic deficit is severe and appears permanent, refer the patient to a rehabilitation program as soon as the acute phase has passed.

ENDOCARDITIS

Also called infective endocarditis and bacterial endocarditis, endocarditis is an infection of the endocardium, heart valves, or cardiac prosthesis, resulting from bacterial or fungal invasion. This invasion produces vegetative growths on the heart valves, endocardial lining of a heart chamber, or the endothelium of a blood vessel that may embolize to the spleen, kidneys, central nervous system, and lungs.

In endocarditis, fibrin and platelets aggregate on the valve tissue and engulf circulating bacteria or fungi that flourish and produce friable verrucous vegetations. Such vegetations may cover the valve surfaces, causing ulceration and necrosis; they may also extend to the chordae tendineae, leading to their rupture and subsequent valvular insufficiency.

Untreated endocarditis is usually fatal, but with proper treatment, about 70% of patients recover. The prognosis is worst when endocarditis causes severe valvular damage, leading to insufficiency and heart failure, or when it involves a prosthetic valve.

Causes

Most cases of endocarditis occur in I.V. drug abusers, patients with prosthetic heart valves, and those with mitral valve prolapse (especially males with a systolic murmur). These conditions have surpassed rheumatic heart disease as the leading risk factor.

Other predisposing conditions include coarctation of the aorta; tetralogy of Fallot; subaortic and valvular aortic stenosis; ventricular septal defects; pulmonary stenosis; Marfan's syndrome; degenerative heart disease, especially calcific aortic stenosis; and, rarely, syphilitic aortic valve. There are, however, some patients with endocarditis who have no underlying heart disease.

Infecting organisms

Organisms that cause infection differ among these groups. In patients with native valve endocarditis who aren't I.V. drug abusers, causative organisms usually include — in order of frequency — streptococci (especially *S. viridans*), staphylococci, or enterococci.

Although many other bacteria occasionally cause the disorder, fungal causes are rare in this group. The mitral valve is involved most commonly, followed by the aortic valve.

In patients who are I.V. drug abusers, *Staphylococcus aureus* is the most common infecting organism. Less frequently, streptococci, enterococci, gram-negative bacilli, or fungi cause the disorder. The tricuspid valve is involved most commonly, followed by the aortic and then the mitral valve.

In patients with prosthetic valve endocarditis, "early" cases (those that develop within 60 days of valve insertion) are usually due to staphylococcal infection. However, gram-negative aerobic organisms, fungi, streptococci, enterococci, or diphtheroids may also cause the disorder.

The course is often fulminant and is associated with a high mortality rate. "Late" cases (occurring after 60 days) present similarly to native valve endocarditis.

Signs and symptoms

Early clinical features of endocarditis are usually nonspecific and include malaise, weakness, fatigue, weight loss, anorexia, arthralgia, night sweats, chills, valvular insufficiency and, in 90% of patients, an intermittent fever that may recur for weeks. A more acute

onset is associated with highly pathogenic organisms such as *S. aureus*.

Endocarditis often causes a loud, regurgitant murmur typical of the underlying heart lesion. A suddenly changing murmur or the discovery of a new murmur in the presence of fever is a classic physical sign of endocarditis.

In about 30% of patients, embolization from vegetating lesions or diseased valvular tissue may produce typical features of splenic, renal, cerebral, or pulmonary infarction or of peripheral vascular occlusion:

- *splenic infarction:* pain in the left upper quadrant, radiating to the left shoulder; abdominal rigidity
- *renal infarction:* hematuria, pyuria, flank pain, decreased urine output
- *cerebral infarction:* hemiparesis, aphasia, or other neurologic deficits
- *pulmonary infarction* (most common in right-sided endocarditis, which commonly occurs among I.V. drug abusers and after cardiac surgery): cough, pleuritic pain, pleural friction rub, dyspnea, hemoptysis
- *peripheral vascular occlusion:* numbness and tingling in an arm, leg, finger, or toe or signs of impending peripheral gangrene.

Other signs may include splenomegaly; petechiae of the skin (especially common on the upper anterior trunk) and the buccal, pharyngeal, or conjunctival mucosa; and splinter hemorrhages under the nails. Rarely, endocarditis produces Osler's nodes (tender, raised, subcutaneous lesions on the fingers or toes), Roth's spots (hemorrhagic areas with white centers on the retina), and Janeway lesions (purplish macules on the palms or soles).

Diagnosis

Three or more blood cultures in a 24- to 48-hour period identify the causative organism in up to 90% of patients. The remaining 10% may have negative blood cultures, possibly suggesting fungal infection or infections that are difficult to diagnose, such as *Haemophilus parainfluenzae*. Other abnormal but nonspecific laboratory test results include:

• normal or elevated white blood cell count

• abnormal histiocytes (macrophages)

• elevated erythrocyte sedimentation rate

• normocytic, normochromic anemia (in 70% to 90% of endocarditis cases)

• positive serum rheumatoid factor (in about half of all patients with endocarditis after the disease is present for 3 to 6 weeks).

Echocardiography may identify valvular damage; electrocardiography may show atrial fibrillation and other arrhythmias that accompany valvular disease.

Treatment

The goal of treatment is to eradicate the infecting organism. Antimicrobial therapy should start promptly and continue over 4 to 6 weeks. Selection of an antibiotic is based on identification of the infecting organism and on sensitivity studies. While awaiting results, or if blood cultures are negative, empiric antimicrobial therapy is based on the likely infecting organism.

Supportive treatment includes bed rest, aspirin for fever and aches, and sufficient fluid intake. Severe valvular damage, especially aortic or mitral insufficiency, may require corrective surgery if refractory heart failure develops or in cases requiring that an infected prosthetic valve be replaced.

Special considerations

• Before giving antibiotics, obtain a patient history of allergies. Administer antibiotics on time to maintain consistent antibiotic blood levels.

• Observe for signs of infiltration or inflammation at the venipuncture site, possible complications of long-term I.V. drug administration. To reduce the risk of these complications, rotate venous access sites.

• Watch for signs of embolization (hematuria, pleuritic chest pain, left upper quadrant pain, or paresis), a common occurrence during the first 3 months of treatment. Tell the patient to watch for and report these signs, which may indicate impending peripheral vascular occlusion or splenic, renal, cerebral, or pulmonary infarction.

• Monitor the patient's renal status (blood urea nitrogen levels, creatinine clearance, and urine output) to check for signs of renal emboli or evidence of drug toxicity.

• Observe for signs of heart failure, such as dyspnea, tachypnea, tachycardia, crackles, neck vein distention, edema, and weight gain.

• Provide reassurance by teaching the patient and family about this disease and the need for prolonged treatment. Tell them to watch closely for fever, anorexia, and other signs of relapse about 2 weeks after treatment stops. Suggest quiet diversionary activities to prevent excessive physical exertion.

• Make sure susceptible patients understand the need for prophylactic antibiotics before, during, and after dental work, childbirth, and genitourinary, GI, or gynecologic procedures.

• Teach patients how to recognize symptoms of endocarditis, and tell them to notify the doctor immediately if such symptoms occur.

ENDOMETRIOSIS

A diagnosis of endometriosis denotes the presence of endometrial tissue outside the lining of the uterine cavity.

Such ectopic tissue is generally confined to the pelvic area, most commonly around the ovaries, uterovesical peritoneum, uterosacral ligaments, and cul-de-sac, but it can appear anywhere in the body.

This ectopic endometrial tissue responds to normal stimulation in the same way that the endometrium does. During menstruation, the ectopic tissue bleeds, which causes inflammation of the surrounding tissues. This inflammation causes fibrosis, leading to adhesions that produce pain and infertility.

Active endometriosis usually occurs between ages 30 and 40, especially in women who postpone childbearing; it's uncommon before age 20. Severe symptoms of endometriosis may have an abrupt onset or may develop over many years. This disorder usually becomes progressively severe during the menstrual years; after menopause, it tends to subside.

Causes
The mechanisms by which endometriosis causes symptoms, including infertility, are unknown. The main theories to explain this disorder are:
• transtubal regurgitation of endometrial cells and implantation at ectopic sites
• coelomic metaplasia (repeated inflammation may induce metaplasia of mesothelial cells to the endometrial epithelium)
• lymphatic or hematogenous spread to explain extraperitoneal disease.

Signs and symptoms
The classic symptom of endometriosis is acquired dysmenorrhea, which may produce constant pain in the lower abdomen and in the vagina, posterior pelvis, and back. This pain usually begins from 5 to 7 days before menses reaches its peak and lasts for 2 to 3 days.

It differs from primary dysmenorrheal pain, which is more cramplike and concentrated in the abdominal midline. However, the severity of pain doesn't necessarily indicate the extent of the disease.

Other clinical features depend on the location of the ectopic tissue:
• *ovaries* and *oviducts:* infertility and profuse menses
• *ovaries* or *cul-de-sac:* deep-thrust dyspareunia
• *bladder:* suprapubic pain, dysuria, hematuria
• *rectovaginal septum* and *colon:* painful defecation, rectal bleeding with menses, pain in the coccyx or sacrum
• *small bowel* and *appendix:* nausea and vomiting, which worsen before menses, and abdominal cramps
• *cervix, vagina,* and *perineum:* bleeding from endometrial deposits in these areas during menses.

The primary complication of endometriosis is infertility.

Diagnosis
A pelvic examination suggests endometriosis. Palpation may detect multiple tender nodules on uterosacral ligaments or in the rectovaginal septum in one-third of patients. These nodules enlarge and become more tender during menses.

Palpation may also uncover ovarian enlargement in the presence of endometrial cysts on the ovaries or thickened, nodular adnexa (as in pelvic inflammatory disease). Laparoscopy must confirm the diagnosis and determine the stage of the disease before treatment is initiated.

Treatment
How endometriosis is treated varies according to the stage of the disease and the patient's age and desire to have children. Conservative therapy for young women who want to have children includes androgens, such as dan-

azol, which produce a temporary remission in Stages I and II.

Progestins and oral contraceptives also relieve symptoms. Gonadotropin-releasing hormone agonists, by inducing a pseudomenopause and, thus, a "medical oophorectomy," have shown a remission of disease and are commonly used.

When ovarian masses are present (stages III and IV), surgery must rule out cancer. Conservative surgery is possible, but the treatment of choice for women who don't want to bear children and for those with extensive disease (stages III and IV) is a total abdominal hysterectomy with bilateral salpingo-oophorectomy.

Special considerations
• Minor gynecologic procedures are contraindicated immediately before and during menstruation.
• Advise adolescents to use sanitary napkins instead of tampons; this can help prevent retrograde flow in girls with a narrow vagina or small introitus.
• Because infertility is a possible complication, advise the patient who wants children not to postpone childbearing.
• Recommend an annual pelvic examination and Papanicolaou test to all patients.

ENTEROBIASIS

Also called pinworm, seatworm, or threadworm infection or oxyuriasis, enterobiasis is a benign intestinal disease caused by the nematode *Enterobius vermicularis*. Found worldwide, it's common even in temperate regions with good sanitation. It's the most prevalent helminthic infection in the United States.

TEACHING CHECKLIST

☑ PREVENTING ENTEROBIASIS

• To help prevent enterobiasis, tell parents to bathe children daily (showers are preferable to tub baths) and to change underwear and bed linens daily.
• Educate children in proper personal hygiene, and stress the need for handwashing after defecation and before handling food. Discourage nail biting. If the child can't stop, suggest that he wear gloves until the infection clears.
• If the patient with enterobiasis receives pyrantel, tell him and his family that this drug colors stools bright red and may cause vomiting. (The vomitus will also be red.)

Causes
Adult pinworms live in the intestine; female worms migrate to the perianal region to deposit their ova. *Direct transmission* occurs when the patient's hands transfer infective eggs from the anus to the mouth. *Indirect transmission* occurs when he comes in contact with contaminated articles, such as linens and clothing.

Enterobiasis infection and reinfection occur most often in children between ages 5 and 14 and in certain institutionalized groups because of poor hygiene and frequent hand-to-mouth activity. Crowded living conditions often lead to its spread to other family members. (See *Preventing enterobiasis.*)

Signs and symptoms
Asymptomatic enterobiasis is often overlooked. However, intense perianal pruritus may occur, especially at night, when the female worm crawls out of the anus to deposit ova. Pruritus dis-

turbs sleep and causes irritability, scratching, skin irritation, and sometimes, vaginitis. Rarely, complications include appendicitis, salpingitis, and pelvic granuloma.

Diagnosis
A history of pruritus ani suggests enterobiasis; identification of *Enterobius* ova recovered from the perianal area with a cellophane tape swab confirms it. In this test, cellophane tape is placed sticky side out on the base end of a test tube, and the tube is rolled around the perianal region. The tape is then examined under a microscope.

This test should be done before the patient bathes and defecates in the morning. A stool specimen is generally ova- and wormfree, because these worms deposit the ova outside the intestine and die after migration to the anus.

Treatment
Drug therapy with pyrantel, piperazine, or mebendazole destroys these parasites. Effective eradication requires simultaneous treatment of family members and, in institutions, other patients.

Special considerations
• Before giving piperazine, obtain a history of seizure disorders. Piperazine may aggravate these disorders and is contraindicated in a patient with such a history.
• The tablet form of pyrantel is coated with aspirin and shouldn't be given to aspirin-sensitive patients.
• Report *all* outbreaks of enterobiasis to school authorities.
• Teach the patient and his family about adverse drug effects and proper hygiene.

EPICONDYLITIS

Also known as tennis elbow and epitrochlear bursitis, epicondylitis is inflammation of the forearm extensor supinator tendon fibers at their common attachment to the lateral humeral epicondyle, which produces acute or subacute pain.

Causes
Epicondylitis probably begins as a partial tear and is common among tennis players or people whose activities require a forceful grasp, wrist extension against resistance, or frequent rotation of the forearm. Untreated epicondylitis may become disabling.

Signs and symptoms
The patient's initial symptom is elbow pain that gradually worsens and often radiates to the forearm and back of the hand whenever he grasps an object or twists his elbow.

Other associated signs and symptoms include tenderness over the involved lateral or medial epicondyle or over the head of the radius, and a weak grasp. In rare instances, epicondylitis may cause local heat, swelling, or restricted range of motion (ROM).

Diagnosis
Because X-rays are almost always negative, diagnosis typically depends on clinical signs and symptoms and a patient history of playing tennis or engaging in similar activities. The pain can be reproduced by wrist extension and supination with lateral involvement, or by flexion and pronation with medial epicondyle involvement.

Treatment

The aim of treatment is to relieve pain, usually by local injection of corticosteroid and a local anesthetic and by systemic anti-inflammatory therapy with aspirin or indomethacin.

Supportive measures

Supportive treatment includes an immobilizing splint from the distal forearm to the elbow, which generally relieves pain in 2 to 3 weeks; heat therapy, such as warm compresses, short wave diathermy, and ultrasound (alone or in combination with diathermy); and physical therapy, such as manipulation and massage to detach the tendon from the chronically inflamed periosteum.

A "tennis elbow strap" has helped many patients. This strap, which is wrapped snugly around the forearm approximately 1″ (2.5 cm) below the epicondyle, helps relieve the strain on affected forearm muscles and tendons.

If these measures prove ineffective, surgical release of the tendon at the epicondyle may be necessary.

Special considerations

• Assess the patient's level of pain, ROM, and sensory function. Monitor heat therapy to prevent burns.

• Advise the patient to take anti-inflammatory drugs with food to avoid GI irritation.

• Instruct the patient to rest the elbow until inflammation subsides.

• Remove the support daily, and gently move the arm to prevent stiffness and contracture.

• Instruct the patient to follow the prescribed exercise program. For example, he may stretch his arm and flex his wrist to the maximum, then press the back of his hand against a wall until he can feel a pull in his forearm, and hold this position for 1 minute.

• Advise the patient to warm up for 15 to 20 minutes before beginning any sports activity.

• Urge the patient to wear an elastic support or splint during any activity that stresses the forearm or elbow.

EPIDIDYMITIS

This infection of the epididymis, the testicle's cordlike excretory duct, is one of the most common infections of the male reproductive tract. It usually affects adults and is rare before puberty. Epididymitis may spread to the testicle itself, causing orchitis; bilateral epididymitis may cause sterility.

Causes

Epididymitis usually results from pyogenic organisms, such as staphylococci, *Escherichia coli,* and streptococci. Generally, such organisms result from established urinary tract infection or prostatitis and reach the epididymis through the lumen of the vas deferens.

Rarely, epididymitis is secondary to a distant infection, such as pharyngitis or tuberculosis, that spreads through the lymphatics or, less commonly, the bloodstream.

Other causes include trauma, gonorrhea, syphilis, or a chlamydial infection. Trauma may reactivate a dormant infection or initiate a new one. Epididymitis is a complication of prostatectomy and may also result from chemical irritation by extravasation of urine through the vas deferens.

Signs and symptoms

The key symptoms are pain, extreme tenderness, and swelling in the groin and scrotum. Other clinical effects include high fever, malaise, and a characteristic waddle — an attempt to protect the groin and scrotum during walking. An acute hydrocele may also occur as a reaction to the inflammatory process.

Diagnosis

Clinical features suggest epididymitis, but the actual diagnosis is made with the aid of the following laboratory tests:

• *Urinalysis* shows an increased white blood cell (WBC) count, indicating infection.

• *Urine culture and sensitivity tests* may identify the causative organism.

• *Serum WBC count* of more than 10,000/µl indicates infection.

• *Scrotal ultrasonography* may help differentiate acute epididymitis from other conditions, such as testicular torsion, which is a surgical emergency.

Treatment

The goal of treatment is to reduce pain and swelling and combat infection. Therapy must begin immediately, particularly in the patient with bilateral epididymitis because sterility is always a threat.

During the acute phase

Treatment consists of bed rest, scrotal elevation with towel rolls or adhesive strapping, broad-spectrum antibiotics, and analgesics.

An ice bag applied to the area may reduce swelling and relieve pain. (Heat is contraindicated because it may damage germinal cells, which are viable only at or below normal body temperature.) When pain and swelling subside and allow walking, an athletic supporter may prevent pain. Occasionally, corticosteroids may be prescribed to help counteract inflammation, but their use is controversial.

Prevention

In the older patient undergoing open prostatectomy, bilateral vasectomy may be necessary to prevent epididymitis as a postoperative complication; however, antibiotic therapy alone may prevent it. When epididymitis is refractory to antibiotic therapy, epididymectomy under local anesthetic is necessary.

Special considerations

• Watch closely for abscess formation (a localized, hot, red, tender area) and for extension of the infection into the testes. Closely monitor temperature, and ensure adequate fluid intake.

• Since the patient is usually very uncomfortable, administer analgesics as necessary. During bed rest, check often for proper scrotum elevation.

• Before discharge, emphasize the importance of completing the prescribed antibiotic therapy, even after symptoms subside.

• If the patient faces the possibility of sterility, suggest supportive counseling, as necessary.

LIFE-THREATENING DISORDER

EPIGLOTTITIS

Acute epiglottitis is an inflammation of the epiglottis that tends to cause airway obstruction. It typically strikes children between ages 2 and 8. A critical emergency, epiglottitis can prove fatal in 8% to 12% of victims unless it's recognized and treated promptly.

Causes

Epiglottitis usually results from infection with the bacterium *Haemophilus influenzae* type B; occasionally, it results from pneumococci and group A streptococci.

Signs and symptoms

Sometimes preceded by an upper respiratory infection, epiglottitis may rapidly progress to complete upper airway obstruction within 2 to 5 hours.

Laryngeal obstruction results from inflammation and edema of the epiglottis. Accompanying symptoms include high fever, stridor, sore throat, dysphagia, irritability, restlessness, and drooling.

To relieve severe respiratory distress, the child with epiglottitis may hyperextend his neck, sit up, and lean forward with his mouth open, tongue protruding, and nostrils flaring as he tries to breathe. He may develop inspiratory retractions and rhonchi.

Diagnosis
In acute epiglottitis, throat examination reveals a large, edematous, bright red epiglottis. Such examination should follow lateral neck X-rays and, generally, should *not* be performed if the suspected obstruction is large.

Special equipment (a laryngoscope and endotracheal [ET] tubes) should be available because a tongue depressor can cause sudden complete airway obstruction. Trained personnel (such as an anesthesiologist) should be on hand during throat examination to secure an emergency airway.

Treatment
A child with acute epiglottitis and airway obstruction requires emergency hospitalization; he may need emergency ET intubation or a tracheotomy and should be monitored in an intensive care unit. Respiratory distress that interferes with swallowing necessitates parenteral fluid administration to prevent dehydration.

A patient with acute epiglottitis should always receive a 10-day course of parenteral antibiotics — usually a second- or third-generation cephalosporin (if the child is allergic to penicillin, a quinolone or sulfa drug may be substituted). Oxygen therapy and arterial blood gas (ABG) monitoring may be desirable.

Special considerations
• Keep the following equipment available in case of sudden, complete airway obstruction: a tracheotomy tray, ET tubes, a hand-held resuscitation bag, oxygen equipment, and a laryngoscope with blades of various sizes. Monitor ABG levels for hypoxia and hypercapnia.
• Watch for increasing restlessness, rising heart rate, fever, dyspnea, and retractions, which may indicate a need for emergency tracheotomy.
• After tracheotomy, anticipate the patient's needs because he won't be able to cry or call out, and provide emotional support. Reassure the patient and his family that the tracheotomy is a short-term intervention (usually from 4 to 7 days).
• Monitor the patient for rising temperature and pulse rate and hypotension — signs of secondary infection.

EPILEPSY

Seizure disorder, or epilepsy, is a condition of the brain characterized by a susceptibility to recurrent seizures (paroxysmal events associated with abnormal electrical discharges of neurons in the brain). Epilepsy is believed to affect 1% to 2% of the population. The prognosis is good if the patient with epilepsy adheres strictly to his prescribed treatment.

Causes
In about half of all epilepsy cases, the cause is unknown. However, some possible causes include:
• birth trauma (inadequate oxygen supply to the brain, blood incompatibility, or hemorrhage)
• perinatal infection

- anoxia
- infectious diseases (meningitis, encephalitis, or brain abscess)
- ingestion of toxins (mercury, lead, or carbon monoxide)
- tumors of the brain
- inherited disorders or degenerative disease, such as phenylketonuria or tuberous sclerosis
- head injury or trauma
- metabolic disorders, such as hypoglycemia or hypoparathyroidism
- cerebrovascular accident (hemorrhage, thrombosis, or embolism).

Signs and symptoms
The hallmarks of epilepsy are recurring seizures, which can be classified as partial or generalized (some patients may be affected by more than one type).

Partial seizures
Arising from a localized area of the brain, partial seizures cause specific symptoms. In some patients, partial seizure activity may spread to the entire brain, causing a generalized seizure. Partial seizures include jacksonian and complex partial seizures (psychomotor or temporal lobe).

A *jacksonian seizure* begins as a localized motor seizure characterized by a spread of abnormal activity to adjacent areas of the brain. It typically produces a stiffening or jerking in one extremity, accompanied by a tingling sensation in the same area.

For example, it may start in the thumb and spread to the entire hand and arm. The patient seldom loses consciousness. A jacksonian seizure may progress to a generalized tonic-clonic seizure.

A simple partial sensory type involves perceptual distortion, which can include hallucinations. The symptoms of a *complex partial seizure* vary but usually include purposeless behavior. This seizure may begin with an aura, a sensation the patient feels immediately before a seizure.

An aura represents the beginning of abnormal electrical discharges within a focal area of the brain and may include a pungent smell, GI distress (nausea or indigestion), a rising or sinking feeling in the stomach, a dreamy feeling, an unusual taste, or a visual disturbance.

Overt signs of a complex partial seizure include a glassy stare, picking at one's clothes, aimless wandering, lip-smacking or chewing motions, and unintelligible speech. Mental confusion may last several minutes after the seizure; as a result, an observer may mistakenly suspect intoxication with alcohol or drugs, or psychosis.

Generalized seizures
As the term suggests, generalized seizures cause a generalized electrical abnormality within the brain and include several distinct types:
- *Absence seizures* occur most often in children, although they may affect adults as well. They usually begin with a brief change in level of consciousness, indicated by blinking or rolling of the eyes, a blank stare, and slight mouth movements. The patient retains his posture and continues preseizure activity without difficulty. Typically, each seizure lasts from 1 to 10 seconds. If not properly treated, seizures can recur as often as 100 times a day. An absence seizure may progress to a generalized tonic-clonic seizure.
- *Myoclonic (bilateral massive epileptic myoclonus) seizures* are characterized by brief, involuntary muscular jerks of the body or extremities, which may occur in a rhythmic fashion.
- *Generalized tonic-clonic seizures* typically begin with a loud cry, precipitated by air rushing from the lungs through the vocal cords. The patient then falls to the ground, losing consciousness. The body stiffens (tonic

phase), then alternates between episodes of muscular spasm and relaxation (clonic phase). Tongue-biting, incontinence, labored breathing, apnea, and subsequent cyanosis may also occur.

The seizure stops in 2 to 5 minutes, when abnormal electrical conduction of the neurons is completed. The patient then regains consciousness but is somewhat confused and may have difficulty talking. If he can talk, he may complain of drowsiness, fatigue, headache, muscle soreness, and arm or leg weakness. He may fall into deep sleep following the seizure.

• *Akinetic seizures* are characterized by a general loss of postural tone and a temporary loss of consciousness. They occur in young children and are sometimes called "drop attacks" because they cause the child to fall.

• *Status epilepticus* is a continuous seizure state that can occur in all seizure types. The most life-threatening example is generalized tonic-clonic status epilepticus, a continuous generalized tonic-clonic seizure without intervening return of consciousness.

Status epilepticus is accompanied by respiratory distress. It can result from abrupt withdrawal of antiepileptic medications, hypoxic encephalopathy, acute head trauma, metabolic encephalopathy, or septicemia secondary to encephalitis or meningitis.

Diagnosis

Clinically, the diagnosis of epilepsy is based on the occurrence of one or more seizures and proof or the assumption that the condition which led to them is still present.

Diagnostic information is obtained from the patient's history and description of seizure activity and from family history, physical and neurologic examinations, and computed tomography scan or magnetic resonance imaging. These scans offer density readings of the brain and may indicate abnormalities in internal structures.

Confirming evidence

Paroxysmal abnormalities on the EEG confirm the diagnosis by providing evidence of the continuing tendency to have seizures. However, a negative EEG doesn't rule out epilepsy because the paroxysmal abnormalities occur intermittently. Other tests may include serum glucose and calcium studies, skull X-rays, lumbar puncture, brain scan, and cerebral angiography.

Treatment

Generally, treatment of epilepsy consists of drug therapy specific to the type of seizure. The most commonly prescribed drugs include phenytoin, carbamazepine, phenobarbital, or primidone administered individually for generalized tonic-clonic seizures and complex partial seizures.

Valproic acid, clonazepam, and ethosuximide are commonly prescribed for absence seizures. Gabapentin and felbamate are newer anticonvulsant drugs.

A patient taking anticonvulsant medications requires monitoring for signs of toxicity: nystagmus, ataxia, lethargy, dizziness, drowsiness, slurred speech, irritability, nausea, and vomiting.

If drug therapy fails, treatment may include surgical removal of a demonstrated focal lesion to attempt to stop seizures. Emergency treatment of status epilepticus usually consists of diazepam (or lorazepam), phenytoin, or phenobarbital; dextrose 50% I.V. (when seizures are secondary to hypoglycemia); and thiamine I.V. (in chronic alcoholism or withdrawal).

Special considerations

• Encourage the patient and family to express their feelings about the patient's condition. Answer their ques-

☑️ ## FIRST AID FOR SEIZURES

Generalized tonic-clonic seizures may necessitate first aid. Use this checklist when teaching the patient's family how to give such aid correctly:

• Don't restrain the patient during a seizure. Instead, help him to a lying position, loosen any tight clothing, and place something flat and soft, such as a pillow, jacket, or hand, under his head. Clear the area of hard objects.

• If the patient's teeth are clenched, don't force anything into his mouth. This could lacerate his mouth and lips or displace teeth, causing respiratory distress.

• If the patient's mouth is open, protect his tongue by placing a soft object (such as folded cloth) between his teeth.

• Turn his head to provide an open airway.

• After the seizure subsides, reassure him that he's all right, orient him to time and place, and inform him that he's had a seizure.

• If the patient has a complex partial seizure, don't restrain him. Clear the area of any hard objects, and protect him from injury by gently calling his name and directing him away from the source of danger. Afterwards, reassure him and tell him that he's just had a seizure.

scribed medication regimen and that most patients maintain a normal lifestyle.

• Teach the family how to give first aid in case a seizure occurs. (See *First aid for seizures.*)

• Because drug therapy is the treatment of choice for most persons with epilepsy, information about the medications is invaluable.

• Stress the need for compliance with the prescribed drug schedule. Assure the patient that anticonvulsant drugs are safe *when taken as prescribed.*

• Reinforce dosage instructions, and find methods to help the patient remember to take medications. Caution him to monitor the amount of medication left so he doesn't run out of it.

• Warn against possible adverse reactions—drowsiness, lethargy, hyperactivity, confusion, visual and sleep disturbances—all of which indicate the need for dosage adjustment. Phenytoin therapy may lead to hyperplasia of the gums, which may be relieved by conscientious oral hygiene. Instruct the patient to report adverse effects immediately.

• Warn the patient against drinking alcoholic beverages.

• When administering phenytoin I.V., use a large vein and monitor vital signs frequently. Avoid I.M. administration and mixing with dextrose solutions.

• Emphasize the importance of having antiepileptic drug blood levels checked at regular intervals, even if the seizures are under control.

• Know which social agencies in your community can help epileptic patients. Refer the patient to the Epilepsy Foundation of America for general information and to the state motor vehicle department for information about a driver's license.

tions, and help them cope by dispelling some of the myths about epilepsy; for example, that it's contagious. Assure them that epilepsy is controllable for most patients who follow a pre-

EPISTAXIS

Nosebleed, or epistaxis, may either be a primary disorder or occur secondary to another condition. Such bleeding in children generally originates in the anterior nasal septum and tends to be mild. In adults, such bleeding is most likely to originate in the posterior septum and can be severe. Epistaxis is twice as common in children as in adults.

Causes
Epistaxis usually follows trauma from external or internal causes: a blow to the nose, nose picking, or insertion of a foreign body. Less commonly, it follows polyps; acute or chronic infections, such as sinusitis or rhinitis, which cause congestion and eventual bleeding of the capillary blood vessels; or inhalation of chemicals that irritate the nasal mucosa.

Predisposing factors
Such factors include anticoagulant therapy, hypertension, chronic use of aspirin, high altitudes and dry climates, sclerotic vessel disease, Hodgkin's disease, neoplastic disorders, scurvy, vitamin K deficiency, rheumatic fever, blood dyscrasias (hemophilia, purpura, leukemia, and anemias), and hemorrhagic telangiectasia.

Signs and symptoms
Blood oozing from the nostrils usually originates in the anterior nose and is bright red. Blood from the back of the throat originates in the posterior area and may be dark or bright red (often mistaken for hemoptysis due to expectoration).

Epistaxis is generally unilateral, except when due to dyscrasia or severe trauma. In severe epistaxis, blood may seep behind the nasal septum; it may also appear in the middle ear and in the corners of the eyes.

Associated effects
Clinical effects depend on the severity of bleeding. Moderate blood loss may produce light-headedness, dizziness, and slight respiratory difficulty; severe hemorrhage causes hypotension, rapid and bounding pulse, dyspnea, and pallor. Bleeding is considered severe if it persists longer than 10 minutes after pressure is applied. If severe, blood loss can be as great as 1 L/hour in adults.

Diagnosis
Although simple observation confirms epistaxis, inspection with a bright light and nasal speculum is necessary to locate the site of bleeding.

Relevant laboratory values include:
• gradual reduction in hemoglobin and hematocrit (often inaccurate immediately following epistaxis, due to hemoconcentration)
• decreased platelet count in a patient with blood dyscrasia
• prothrombin time and partial thromboplastin time showing a coagulation time twice the control because of a bleeding disorder or anticoagulant therapy.

Diagnosis must rule out underlying systemic causes of epistaxis, especially disseminated intravascular coagulation and rheumatic fever. Bruises or concomitant bleeding elsewhere probably indicates a hematologic disorder.

Treatment
Different treatment measures are used for anterior and posterior bleeding. Drug therapy, transfusions, and surgery may also be necessary.

Local measures
For anterior bleeding, treatment consists of application of a cotton ball saturated with epinephrine to the bleed-

INSERTION OF AN ANTERIOR-POSTERIOR NASAL PACK

The first step in the insertion of an anterior-posterior nasal pack is the insertion of catheters in the nostrils. After drawing the catheters through the mouth, a suture from the pack is tied to each, which positions the pack in place as the catheters are drawn back through the nostrils.

While the sutures are held tightly, packing is inserted into the anterior nose.

The sutures are then secured around a dental roll; the middle suture extends from the mouth and is tied to the cheek.

ing site and external pressure, followed by cauterization with electrocautery or silver nitrate stick. If these measures don't control the bleeding, petrolatum gauze nasal packing may be needed. (See *Insertion of an anterior-posterior nasal pack.*)

For posterior bleeding, treatment includes gauze packing inserted through the nose or postnasal packing inserted through the mouth, depending on the bleeding site. (Gauze packing generally remains in place for 24 to 48 hours; postnasal packing, 3 to 5 days.) An alternate method, the nasal balloon catheter, also controls bleeding effectively.

Other measures
Antibiotics may be appropriate if packing must remain in place for longer than 24 hours. If local measures fail to control bleeding, additional treatment may include supplemental vitamin K and, for severe bleeding, blood transfusions and surgical ligation or embolization of a bleeding artery.

Special considerations
To control epistaxis:
• Sit the patient upright.
• Compress the soft portion of the nostrils against the septum continuously for 5 to 10 minutes. Apply an ice collar or cold, wet compresses to the nose. Bleeding should stop after 10 minutes.
• Administer oxygen as needed.
• Monitor vital signs and skin color; record blood loss.
• Tell the patient to breathe through his mouth and not to swallow blood, talk, or blow his nose.
• Monitor oxygen saturation levels.
• Keep vasoconstrictors, such as phenylephrine, handy.

• Reassure the patient and family that epistaxis usually looks worse than it is.

To prevent a recurrence of epistaxis:
• Instruct the patient not to pick his nose or insert foreign objects in it and to avoid bending or lifting. Emphasize the need for follow-up examinations and periodic blood studies after an episode of epistaxis. Advise the patient to get prompt treatment for nasal infection or irritation.
• Suggest humidifiers for people who live in dry climates or at high elevations or whose homes are heated with circulating hot air.
• Instruct the patient to sneeze with his mouth open.

ERECTILE DISORDER

Also called impotence, erectile disorder refers to a male's inability to attain or maintain penile erection sufficient to complete intercourse. The patient with primary impotence has never achieved a sufficient erection; secondary impotence, which is more common and less serious than the primary form, implies that, despite present inability, the patient has succeeded in completing intercourse in the past.

Transient periods of impotence are not considered dysfunctional and probably occur in half of adult males. Erectile disorder affects all age-groups but increases in frequency with age. The prognosis depends on the severity and duration of impotence and the underlying cause.

Causes
Psychogenic factors are responsible for approximately 50% to 60% of erectile disorder; organic factors, for the rest.

In some patients, psychogenic and organic factors coexist, making isolation of the primary cause difficult.

Psychogenic causes

These causes may be intrapersonal, reflecting personal sexual anxieties, or interpersonal, reflecting a disturbed sexual relationship.

• Intrapersonal factors generally involve guilt, fear, depression, or feelings of inadequacy resulting from previous traumatic sexual experience, rejection by parents or peers, exaggerated religious orthodoxy, abnormal mother-son intimacy, or homosexual experiences.

• Interpersonal factors may stem from differences in sexual preferences between partners, lack of communication, insufficient knowledge of sexual function, or nonsexual personal conflicts. Situational impotence, a temporary condition, may develop in response to stress.

Organic causes

These causes may include chronic diseases, such as cardiopulmonary disease, diabetes, multiple sclerosis, or renal failure; spinal cord trauma; complications of surgery; drug- or alcohol-induced dysfunction; and, rarely, genital anomalies or central nervous system defects.

Signs and symptoms

Secondary erectile disorder is classified as follows:

• *Partial:* The patient is unable to achieve a full erection.

• *Intermittent:* The patient is sometimes potent with the same partner.

• *Selective:* The patient is potent only with certain females.

Some patients lose erectile function suddenly; others lose it gradually. If the cause isn't organic, erection may still be achieved through masturbation.

Patients with psychogenic impotence may appear anxious, with sweating and palpitations, or may lose interest in sexual activity. Patients with psychogenic or drug-induced impotence may suffer extreme depression, which may cause the impotence or result from it.

Diagnosis

A detailed sexual history helps distinguish between organic and psychogenic factors and between primary and secondary impotence.

Questions should include: Does the patient have intermittent, selective, nocturnal, or early-morning erections? Can he achieve erections through other sexual activity? When did his dysfunction begin, and what was his life situation at that time? Did erectile problems occur suddenly or gradually? Is he taking large quantities of prescription or nonprescription drugs?

The diagnosis must rule out chronic disease, such as diabetes and other vascular, neurologic, or urogenital problems.

When the disorder causes marked distress or interpersonal difficulty, it may fulfill the diagnostic criteria for sexual disorders listed in the *Diagnostic and Statistical Manual of Mental Disorders,* 4th edition.

Treatment

Sex therapy, which should include both partners, may effectively cure psychogenic impotence. The course and content of such therapy depend on the specific cause of the dysfunction and the nature of the male-female relationship.

Usually, therapy includes the concept of sensate focus, which restricts the couple's sexual activity and encourages them to become more attuned to the physical sensations of touching. Sex therapy also includes improving verbal communication skills, eliminating unreasonable guilt, and reevaluating attitudes toward sex and sexual roles.

Treatment of organic impotence focuses on reversing the cause, if possible. If not, psychological counseling may help the couple deal realistically with their situation and explore alternatives for sexual expression. Certain patients suffering from organic impotence may benefit from surgically inserted inflatable or noninflatable penile implants.

Special considerations

• When you identify a patient with impotence or with a condition that may cause impotence, help him feel comfortable about discussing his sexuality. Assess his sexual health during your initial history. When appropriate, refer him for further evaluation or treatment.

• After penile implant surgery, instruct the patient to avoid intercourse until the incision heals, usually in 6 weeks.

To help prevent impotence:

• Promote establishment of responsible health and sex education programs at primary, secondary, and college levels.

• Provide information about resuming sexual activity as part of discharge instructions for any patient with a condition that requires modification of daily activities. Such patients include those with cardiac disease, diabetes, hypertension, or chronic obstructive pulmonary disease as well as all postoperative patients.

E. COLI AND OTHER ENTEROBACTERIACEAE INFECTIONS

Enterobacteriaceae — a group of mostly aerobic, gram-negative bacilli — cause local and systemic infections, including an invasive diarrhea resembling shigella and, more often, a noninvasive toxin-mediated diarrhea resembling cholera.

Escherichia coli and other Enterobacteriaceae cause most nosocomial infections. Noninvasive, enterotoxin-producing *E. coli* infections may be a major cause of diarrheal illness in children in the United States.

The prognosis in mild to moderate infection is good. But severe infection requires immediate fluid and electrolyte replacement to avoid fatal dehydration, especially among children, in whom mortality may be quite high.

Causes

Although some strains of *E. coli* exist as part of the normal GI flora, infection usually results from certain nonindigenous strains. For example:

• Noninvasive diarrhea results from two toxins produced by strains called enterotoxic or enteropathogenic *E. coli*. These toxins interact with intestinal juices and promote excessive loss of chloride and water.

• In the invasive form, *E. coli* directly invades the intestinal mucosa without producing enterotoxins, thereby causing local irritation, inflammation, and diarrhea. Normal strains can cause infection in immunocompromised patients.

Transmission can occur directly from an infected person or indirectly by ingestion of contaminated food or water or contact with contaminated utensils. Incubation takes 12 to 72 hours.

Incidence

The incidence of *E. coli* infection is highest among travelers returning from other countries, particularly Mexico, Southeast Asia, and South America. *E. coli* infection also induces other diseases, especially in people whose resistance is low. A new strain, *E. coli 0157:H7*, has been reported. It's associated with undercooked hamburger.

Signs and symptoms

Effects of noninvasive diarrhea depend on the causative toxin but may include the abrupt onset of watery diarrhea with cramping abdominal pain and, in severe illness, acidosis. Invasive infection produces chills, abdominal cramps, and diarrheal stools containing blood and pus.

Infantile diarrhea from an *E. coli* infection is usually noninvasive; it begins with loose, watery stools that change from yellow to green and contain little mucus or blood. Vomiting, listlessness, irritability, and anorexia often precede diarrhea. This condition can progress to fever, severe dehydration, acidosis, and shock. Bloody diarrhea may occur from an *E. coli 0157:H7* infection.

Diagnosis

Because certain strains of *E. coli* normally reside in the GI tract, culturing is of little value; a working diagnosis depends on clinical observation alone.

A firm diagnosis requires sophisticated identification procedures, such as bioassays, that are expensive, time-consuming, and, consequently, not widely available. The diagnosis must rule out salmonellosis and shigellosis, other common infections that produce similar signs and symptoms.

Treatment

Effective treatment consists of isolation, correction of fluid and electrolyte imbalance, and, in an infant, I.V. antibiotics based on the organism's drug sensitivity. For cramping and diarrhea, bismuth subsalicylate may be given.

Special considerations

• Keep accurate intake and output records. Measure stool volume and note the presence of blood and pus. Replace fluids and electrolytes as needed, monitoring for decreased serum sodium and chloride levels and signs of gram-negative shock. Watch for signs of dehydration, such as poor skin turgor and dry mouth.

• For infants, provide isolation, give nothing by mouth, administer antibiotics, and maintain body warmth.

To prevent spread of this infection:

• Screen all hospital personnel and visitors for diarrhea, and prevent them from making direct patient contact during epidemics. Report cases to local public health authorities.

• Use proper handwashing technique. Teach personnel, patients, and their families to do the same.

• Use enteric precautions: private room, gown and gloves while handling feces, and handwashing before entering and after leaving the patient's room.

• To prevent accumulation of these water-loving organisms, discard suction bottles, irrigating fluid, and open bottles of saline solution every 24 hours. Be sure to change I.V. tubing according to hospital policy and empty the ventilator water reservoirs before refilling them with sterile water. Remember to use suction catheters only once.

• Advise travelers to foreign countries to avoid unbottled water and uncooked vegetables.

ESOPHAGEAL CANCER

Nearly always fatal, esophageal cancer usually develops in men over age 60. This disease occurs worldwide, but incidence varies geographically. It's most common in Japan, China, the Middle East, and parts of South Africa.

Causes

The cause of esophageal cancer is unknown, but predisposing factors include chronic irritation caused by heavy smoking and excessive use of alcohol, stasis-induced inflammation, and nutritional deficiency. Esophageal tumors are usually fungating and infiltrating. Most arise in squamous cell epithelium; a few are adenocarcinomas; fewer still are melanomas and sarcomas.

Esophageal cancer has a 5-year survival rate below 10% and regional metastasis occurs early via submucosal lymphatics. Metastasis produces such serious complications as tracheoesophageal fistulas, mediastinitis, and aortic perforation. Common sites of distant metastasis include the liver and lungs. (See *Staging esophageal cancer.*)

Signs and symptoms

Dysphagia and weight loss are the most common presenting symptoms. Dysphagia is mild and intermittent at first, but it soon becomes constant. Pain, hoarseness, coughing, and esophageal obstruction follow. Cachexia usually develops.

Diagnosis

X-rays of the esophagus, with barium swallow and motility studies, reveal structural and filling defects and reduced peristalsis. Endoscopic examination of the esophagus, punch and

STAGING ESOPHAGEAL CANCER

The TNM (tumor, node, metastasis) staging system accepted by the American Joint Committee on Cancer classifies esophageal cancer as follows.

Primary tumor
TX — primary tumor can't be assessed
T0 — no evidence of primary tumor
Tis — carcinoma in situ
T1 — tumor invades lamina propria or submucosa
T2 — tumor invades muscularis propria
T3 — tumor invades adventitia
T4 — tumor invades adjacent structures

Regional lymph nodes
NX — regional lymph nodes can't be assessed
N0 — no regional lymph node metastasis
N1 — regional lymph node metastasis

Distant metastasis
MX — distant metastasis can't be assessed
M0 — no known distant metastasis
M1 — distant metastasis

Staging categories
Esophageal cancer progresses from mild to severe as follows:
Stage 0 — Tis, N0, M0
Stage I — T1, N0, M0
Stage IIA — T2, N0, M0; T3, N0, M0
Stage IIB — T1, N1, M0; T2, N1, M0
Stage III — T3, N1, M0; T4, any N, M0
Stage IV — any T, any N, M1

brush biopsies, and exfoliative cytologic tests confirm esophageal tumors.

Treatment

Whenever possible, treatment includes resection to maintain a passageway for food. This may require such radical surgery as esophagogastrectomy with jejunal or colonic bypass grafts. Palliative surgery may include a feeding gastrostomy. Other therapies may consist of radiation, chemotherapy with cisplatin, or the insertion of prosthetic tubes to bridge the tumor and alleviate dysphagia.

Treatment complications

Complications of treatment may be severe. Surgery may precipitate an anastomotic leak, a fistula, pneumonia, and empyema. Rarely, radiation may cause esophageal perforation, pneumonitis and pulmonary fibrosis, or myelitis of the spinal cord. Prosthetic tubes may dislodge and perforate the mediastinum or erode the tumor.

Special considerations

• Before surgery, answer the patient's questions and let him know what to expect after surgery, such as gastrostomy tubes, closed chest drainage, and nasogastric suctioning.
• After surgery, monitor vital signs and watch for unexpected changes. If surgery included an esophageal anastomosis, keep the patient flat on his back to avoid tension on the suture line.
• Promote adequate nutrition and assess the patient's nutritional and hydration status to determine the need for supplementary parenteral feedings.
• Prevent aspiration of food by placing the patient in Fowler's position for meals and allowing plenty of time to eat. Provide high-calorie, high-protein, pureed food as needed. Because the patient will probably regurgitate some food, clean his mouth carefully

after each meal. Keep mouthwash handy.
• If the patient has a gastrostomy tube, give food slowly, using gravity to adjust the flow rate. The prescribed amount usually ranges from 200 to 500 ml. Offer him something to chew before each feeding to promote gastric secretions and a semblance of normal eating.
• Instruct the family in gastrostomy tube care (checking tube patency before each feeding, providing skin care around the tube, and keeping the patient upright during and after feedings).
• Provide emotional support for the patient and family; refer them to appropriate organizations such as the American Cancer Society.

ESOPHAGEAL DIVERTICULA

Hollow outpouchings of one or more layers of the esophageal wall, esophageal diverticula occur in three main areas: just above the upper esophageal sphincter (Zenker's, or pulsion, diverticulum, the most common type), near the midpoint of the esophagus (traction), and just above the lower esophageal sphincter (epiphrenic).

Generally, esophageal diverticula occur later in life—although they can affect infants and children—and are three times more common in men than in women. Epiphrenic diverticula usually occur in middle-aged men; Zenker's, in men over age 60.

Causes

Esophageal diverticula are due either to primary muscular abnormalities that may be congenital or to inflammatory processes adjacent to the esophagus.

Zenker's diverticulum

When the pouch results from increased intraesophageal pressure, Zenker's diverticulum occurs. It's caused by developmental muscular weakness of the posterior pharynx above the border of the cricopharyngeal muscle. The pressure of swallowing aggravates this weakness, as does contraction of the pharynx before relaxation of the sphincter.

Traction diverticulum

When the pouch is pulled out by adjacent inflamed tissue or lymph nodes, a midesophageal (traction) diverticulum occurs. It's a response to scarring and pulling on esophageal walls by an external inflammatory process such as tuberculosis. Some authorities classify all diverticula as traction diverticula.

Epiphrenic diverticulum

This rare condition is generally right-sided and usually accompanies an esophageal motor disturbance, such as esophageal spasm or achalasia. It's thought to be caused by traction and pulsation.

Signs and symptoms

Both midesophageal and epiphrenic diverticula with an associated motor disturbance (achalasia or spasm) seldom produce symptoms but may cause dysphagia and heartburn. However, Zenker's diverticulum produces distinctly staged symptoms: initially, throat irritation and, later, dysphagia and near-complete obstruction.

In early stages, regurgitation occurs soon after eating; in later stages, regurgitation after eating is delayed and may even occur during sleep, leading to food aspiration and pulmonary infection. Other symptoms include noise when liquids are swallowed, chronic cough, hoarseness, a bad taste in the mouth or foul breath, and, rarely, bleeding.

Diagnosis

X-rays taken following a barium swallow usually confirm the diagnosis by showing characteristic outpouching. Esophagoscopy can rule out another lesion; however, the procedure risks rupturing the diverticulum by passing the scope into it rather than into the lumen of the esophagus, a special danger with Zenker's diverticulum.

Treatment

The treatment depends on the type of diverticulum. For example:

• Treatment of Zenker's diverticulum is usually palliative; it includes a bland diet, thorough chewing, and drinking water after eating to flush out the sac. However, severe symptoms or a large diverticulum necessitates surgery to remove the sac or facilitate drainage. An esophagomyotomy may be necessary to prevent recurrence.

• A midesophageal diverticulum seldom requires therapy except when esophagitis aggravates the risk of rupture. Then, treatment includes antacids and an antireflux regimen: keeping the head elevated, maintaining an upright position for 2 hours after eating, eating small meals, controlling chronic coughing, and avoiding constrictive clothing.

• Epiphrenic diverticulum requires treatment of accompanying motor disorders, such as achalasia, by repeated dilations of the esophagus; of acute spasm by anticholinergic administration and diverticulum excision; and of dysphagia or severe pain by surgical excision or suspending the diverticulum to promote drainage.

• Depending on the patient's nutritional status, treatment may also include insertion of a nasogastric tube (passed carefully to prevent perforation) and tube feedings to prepare for the stress of surgery.

ADVICE FOR PATIENTS WITH CORROSIVE ESOPHAGITIS

• Because the adult who has ingested a corrosive agent has usually done so with suicidal intent, encourage and assist him and his family to seek psychological counseling.
• Provide emotional support for parents whose child has ingested a chemical. They'll be distraught and may feel guilty about the accident.
• After the emergency and without emphasizing blame, teach appropriate preventive measures, such as locking accessible cabinets and keeping all corrosive agents out of a child's reach.

Special considerations

• Carefully observe and document symptoms.
• Regularly assess nutritional status (weight, caloric intake, appearance).
• If the patient has dysphagia, record well-tolerated foods and what circumstances ease swallowing. Provide a pureed diet, with vitamin or protein supplements, and encourage thorough chewing.
• If the patient regurgitates food and mucus, protect against aspiration by positioning him carefully with his head elevated or turned to one side. To prevent aspiration, tell the patient to empty any visible outpouching in the neck by massage or postural drainage before retiring.
• Teach the patient about this disorder. Explain treatment instructions and diagnostic procedures.

ESOPHAGITIS, CORROSIVE

Inflammation and damage to the esophagus after ingestion of a caustic chemical is called corrosive esophagitis. Similar to a burn, this injury may be temporary or may lead to permanent stricture (narrowing or stenosis) of the esophagus that's correctable only through surgery.

Severe injury can quickly lead to esophageal perforation, mediastinitis, and death from infection, shock, and massive hemorrhage (due to aortic perforation).

Causes

The most common chemical injury to the esophagus follows the ingestion of lye or other strong alkalies; less often, the ingestion of strong acids. The type and amount of chemical ingested determine the severity and location of the damage.

In children, household chemical ingestion is accidental; in adults, it's usually a suicide attempt or gesture. (See *Advice for patients with corrosive esophagitis.*) The chemical may damage only the mucosa or submucosa, or may damage all layers of the esophagus.

Esophageal tissue damage occurs in three phases: the acute phase, edema and inflammation; the latent phase, ulceration, exudation, and tissue sloughing; and the chronic phase, diffuse scarring.

Signs and symptoms

Effects vary from none at all to intense pain in the mouth and anterior chest, marked salivation, inability to swallow, and tachypnea. Bloody vomitus containing pieces of esophageal tissue signals severe damage. Signs of esophageal perforation and mediastinitis, especially crepitation, indicate destruction of the entire esophagus. Inability to speak suggests laryngeal damage.

The acute phase subsides in 3 to 4 days, enabling the patient to eat again. Fever suggests secondary infection. Symptoms of dysphagia return if stricture develops, usually within weeks; rarely, stricture is delayed and develops several years after the injury.

Diagnosis

A history of chemical ingestion and physical examination revealing oropharynhgeal burns (including white membranes and edema of the soft palate and uvula) usually confirm the diagnosis. The type and amount of the chemical ingested must be identified; this may sometimes be done by examining empty containers of the ingested material or by calling the poison control center.

Two procedures are helpful in evaluating the severity of the injury:
• *Endoscopy* (in the first 24 hours after ingestion) delineates the extent and location of the esophageal injury and assesses the depth of the burn. This procedure may also be performed a week after ingestion to assess stricture development.
• *Barium swallow* (1 week after ingestion and every 3 weeks thereafter) may identify segmental spasm or fistula but doesn't always show mucosal injury.

Treatment

Conservative treatment may be effective; or the patient may need bougienage or surgery.

Conservative treatment

The usual treatment for corrosive esophagitis and stricture includes monitoring the victim's condition; administering corticosteroids, such as prednisone and hydrocortisone, to control inflammation and inhibit fibrosis; administering a broad-spectrum antibiotic, such as ampicillin, to protect the corticosteroid-immunosuppressed patient against infection by his own mouth flora; and performing endoscopy early.

Bougienage

This procedure involves passing a slender, flexible, cylindrical instrument called a bougie into the esophagus to dilate it and minimize stricture. Some doctors begin bougienage immediately and continue it regularly to maintain a patent lumen and prevent stricture; others delay it for a week to avoid the risk of esophageal perforation.

Surgery

Immediate surgery may be necessary for esophageal perforation; it may also be done later to correct stricture untreatable with bougienage. Corrective surgery may involve transplanting a piece of the colon to the damaged esophagus. However, even after surgery, stricture may recur at the site of the anastomosis.

Supportive treatment

Other treatment includes I.V. therapy to replace fluids or total parenteral nutrition while the patient can't swallow, gradually progressing to clear liquids and a soft diet.

Special considerations

If you're the first health-care professional to see the person who has ingested a corrosive chemical, the quality of your emergency care will be critical. Follow these important guidelines:

• *Don't induce vomiting or lavage* because this will expose the esophagus and oropharynx to injury a second time.
• *Don't perform gastric lavage* because the corrosive chemical may cause further damage to the mucous membrane of the GI lining.
• Provide vigorous support of vital functions as needed, such as oxygen, mechanical ventilation, I.V. fluids, and treatment for shock, depending on the severity of the injury.
• Carefully observe and record intake and output.
• Before X-rays and endoscopy, explain the procedure to the patient to lessen anxiety during the tests and to obtain his cooperation.
• Help patients and families prevent future incidents of corrosive esophagitis.

EXOPHTHALMOS

Proptosis or exophthalmos is the unilateral or bilateral bulging or protrusion of the eyeballs or their apparent forward displacement (with lid retraction). The prognosis depends on the underlying cause.

Causes
Exophthalmos commonly results from ophthalmic Graves' disease, in which the eyeballs are displaced forward and the lids retract. Unilateral exophthalmos may also result from trauma (such as fracture of the ethmoid bone, which allows air from the sinus to enter the orbital tissue, displacing soft tissue and the eyeball).

Exophthalmos may also stem from hemorrhage, varicosities, thrombosis, and edema, all of which similarly displace one or both eyeballs.

Other systemic and ocular causes include:
• *infection:* orbital cellulitis, panophthalmitis, and infection of the lacrimal gland or orbital tissues
• *tumors and neoplastic diseases:* especially in children—rhabdomyosarcomas, leukemia, gliomas of the optic nerve, dermoid cysts, teratomas, metastatic neuroblastomas, and lymphoma; in adults—lacrimal gland tumors, mucoceles, cavernous hemangioma, meningiomas, metastatic carcinomas, and lymphoma
• *parasitic cysts:* in surrounding tissue
• *pseudoexophthalmos paralysis of extraocular muscles:* relaxation of eyeball retractors, congenital macrophthalmia, and high myopia.

Signs and symptoms
The obvious sign is a bulging eyeball, commonly with diplopia, if extraocular muscle edema causes misalignment. A rim of the sclera may be visible around the limbus, and the patient may blink infrequently.

Other symptoms depend on the cause: pain may accompany traumatic exophthalmos; a tumor may produce conjunctival hyperemia or chemosis; retraction of the upper lid predisposes to exposure keratitis.

If exophthalmos is associated with cavernous sinus thrombosis, the patient may exhibit paresis of the muscles supplied by cranial nerves III, IV, and VI; limited ocular movement; and a septic-type (high) fever.

Diagnosis
Exophthalmos is usually obvious on physical examination; exophthalmometer readings confirm the diagnosis by showing the degree of anterior projection and asymmetry between the eyes (normal bar readings range from 12 to 20 mm). The following diagnostic measures identify the cause:

• *Computed tomography scan* detects lesions in the optic nerve, orbit, or ocular muscle within the orbit.

• *Culture* of discharge determines the infecting organism; sensitivity testing indicates appropriate antibiotic therapy.

• *Biopsy* of orbital tissue may be necessary if initial treatment fails.

Treatment

Effective treatment varies with the cause. For example:

• Eye trauma may require cold compresses for the first 24 hours, followed by warm compresses, and prophylactic antibiotic therapy. After edema subsides, surgery may sometimes be necessary.

• Eye infection requires treatment with broad-spectrum antibiotics during the 24 hours preceding positive identification of the organism, followed by specific antibiotics.

• A patient with exophthalmos resulting from an orbital tumor may initially benefit from antibiotic or corticosteroid therapy. Eventually, surgical exploration of the orbit and excision of the tumor, enucleation, or exenteration may be necessary. When primary orbital tumors, such as rhabdomyosarcoma, can't be fully excised as encapsulated lesions, radiation and chemotherapy may be used.

• Treatment of Graves' disease may include antithyroid drug therapy or partial or total thyroidectomy to control hyperthyroidism; initial high doses of systemic corticosteroids, such as prednisone, for optic neuropathy; and, if lid retraction is severe, protective lubricants.

Surgery may include lateral tarsorrhaphy (suturing the lateral sections of the eyelids together) to correct lid retraction or orbital decompression (removal of the superior and lateral orbital walls) if vision is threatened.

Special considerations

• Administer medication.

• Record the patient's response to therapy.

• Apply cold and warm compresses for fractures or other trauma.

• Provide postoperative care.

• Explain tests and procedures and give emotional support.

• Protect the exposed cornea with lubricants and patching when appropriate.

EXTRAOCULAR MOTOR NERVE PALSIES

Dysfunctions of the third, fourth, and sixth cranial nerves are called extraocular motor nerve palsies. Each of these nerves innervates specific muscles, as follows:

• The oculomotor (third cranial) nerve innervates the inferior, medial, and superior rectus muscles; the inferior oblique extraocular muscles; the pupilloconstrictor muscles; and the levator palpebrae muscles.

• The trochlear (fourth cranial) nerve innervates the superior oblique muscles.

• The abducens (sixth cranial) nerve innervates the lateral rectus muscles.

The superior oblique muscles control downward rotation, intorsion, and abduction of the eye. Complete dysfunction of the third cranial nerve is called total oculomotor ophthalmoplegia and may be associated with other central nervous system abnormalities.

Causes

The most common causes of extraocular motor nerve palsies are diabetic neuropathy and pressure from an aneurysm or brain tumor. Other causes of these disorders vary, depending on the cranial nerve involved:

• *Third-nerve (oculomotor) palsy* (acute ophthalmoplegia) also results from brain stem ischemia or other cerebrovascular disorders, poisoning (lead, carbon monoxide, botulism), alcohol abuse, infections (measles, encephalitis), trauma to the extraocular muscles, myasthenia gravis, or tumors in the cavernous sinus area.

• *Fourth-nerve (trochlear) palsy* also results from closed-head trauma (blowout fracture) or sinus surgery.

• *Sixth-nerve (abducens) palsy* also results from increased intracranial pressure, brain abscess, meningitis, arterial brain occlusion, infections of the petrous bone (rare), lateral sinus thrombosis, myasthenia gravis, and thyrotropic exophthalmos.

Signs and symptoms

The most characteristic clinical effect of extraocular motor nerve palsies is diplopia of recent onset, which varies in different visual fields, depending on the muscles affected:

• Typically, the patient with third-nerve palsy exhibits ptosis, exotropia (in which the eye looks outward), pupil dilation, and unresponsiveness to light; the eye is unable to move and cannot accommodate.

• The patient with fourth-nerve palsy displays diplopia and an inability to rotate the eye downward or upward. Such a patient develops ocular torticollis (wryneck) from repeatedly tilting his head to the affected side to compensate for vertical diplopia.

• Sixth-nerve palsy causes one eye to turn; the eye cannot abduct beyond the midline. To compensate for diplopia, the patient turns his head to the unaffected side and develops torticollis.

Diagnosis

A complete neuro-ophthalmologic examination and a thorough patient history are needed to diagnose these palsies. Differential diagnosis of third-, fourth-, or sixth-nerve palsy depends on the specific motor defect exhibited by the patient.

For all extraocular motor nerve palsies, skull X-rays and computed tomography scans rule out tumors. The patient is also evaluated for an aneurysm or diabetes. If sixth-nerve palsy results from infection, culture and sensitivity tests identify the causative organism and determine specific antibiotic therapy.

Treatment

Identification of the underlying cause is essential because treatment of extraocular motor nerve palsies varies accordingly. Neurosurgery is necessary if the cause is a brain tumor or an aneurysm. For infection, massive doses of antibiotics I.V. may be appropriate.

Special considerations

• After treatment of the primary condition, the patient may need to perform exercises that stretch the neck muscles to correct acquired torticollis.

• Other treatment and care measures are aimed at relieving signs and symptoms.

FALLOPIAN TUBE CANCER

Primary fallopian tube cancer is extremely rare, accounting for fewer than 0.5% of all gynecologic cancers. It usually occurs in postmenopausal women in their 50s and 60s but occasionally is found in younger women. Because this disease is generally well advanced before diagnosis (up to 30% of such cancers are bilateral with extratubal spread), the prognosis is poor.

Causes

The causes of fallopian tube cancer aren't clear, but this disease appears to be linked with nulliparity. In fact, over half the women with this disease have never had children.

Signs and symptoms

Generally, early-stage fallopian tube cancer produces no symptoms. Late-stage disease is characterized by an enlarged abdomen with a palpable mass, amber-colored vaginal discharge, and excessive bleeding during menstruation.

Other symptoms include abdominal cramps, frequent urination, bladder pressure, persistent constipation, weight loss, and unilateral colicky pain produced by hydrops tubae profluens. (This last symptom occurs when the abdominal end of the fallopian tube closes, causing the tube to become greatly distended until its accumulated secretions suddenly overflow into the uterus.)

Metastasis develops by local extension or by lymphatic spread to the abdominal organs or to the pelvic, aortic, and inguinal lymph nodes. Extra-abdominal metastasis is rare.

Diagnosis

Unexplained postmenopausal bleeding and an abnormal Papanicolaou test (suspicious or positive in up to 50% of all cases) suggest this diagnosis, but laparotomy is usually necessary to confirm fallopian tube cancer. When such cancer involves both the ovary and fallopian tube, the primary site is very difficult to identify.

The preoperative workup includes:
• *ultrasound or plain film* of the abdomen to help delineate tumor mass
• *excretory urography* to assess renal function and to show urinary tract anomalies and ureteral obstruction
• *chest X-ray* to rule out metastasis
• *barium enema* to rule out intestinal obstruction
• *routine blood studies*
• *electrocardiogram.*

Treatment

Fallopian tube cancer is treated with total abdominal hysterectomy, bilateral salpingo-oophorectomy, or omentectomy; chemotherapy with progestogens, fluorouracil, melphalan, cyclophosphamide, and cisplatin; and external radiation for 5 to 6 weeks.

All patients should receive some form of adjunctive therapy (radiation or chemotherapy), even when surgery has removed all evidence of the disease.

Special considerations
Before surgery:
• Explain diagnostic and treatment procedures and the need for preoperative studies. Tell the patient what to expect: fasting from the evening before surgery; an enema to clear her bowel; insertion of an indwelling urinary catheter attached to a drainage bag; abdominal and, possibly, pelvic preparation; placement of an I.V. line; and, possibly, a sedative.
• Describe the tubes and dressings the patient can expect to have in place when she returns from surgery. Teach her deep breathing and coughing techniques to prepare for postoperative exercises.

After surgery:
• Check vital signs every 4 hours. Watch for fever, tachycardia, and hypotension.
• Monitor I.V. fluids.
• Change dressings regularly, and check for excessive drainage and bleeding and signs of infection.
• Provide antiembolism stockings.
• Encourage regular deep breathing and coughing.
• If necessary, institute incentive spirometry.
• Turn the patient often, and help her reposition herself, using pillows for support.
• Auscultate for bowel sounds. When the patient's bowel function returns, ask the dietitian to provide a clear liquid diet; then, when tolerated, a regular diet.
• Encourage the patient to walk within 24 hours after surgery. Reassure her that she won't harm herself or cause wound dehiscence by sitting up or walking.
• Provide psychological support. Encourage the patient to express anxieties and fears. If she seems worried

about the effect of surgery on her sexual activity, reassure her that this surgery won't inhibit sexual intimacy.
• Before radiation therapy begins, explain that the area to be irradiated will be marked with ink to precisely locate the treatment field. Explain that radiation may cause a skin reaction, bladder irritation, myelosuppression, and other systemic reactions.
• During and after treatment, watch for and treat side effects of radiation and chemotherapy.
• Before discharge, to minimize adverse effects during outpatient radiation and chemotherapy, advise the patient to maintain a high-carbohydrate, high-protein, low-fat, low-bulk diet to maintain caloric intake but reduce bulk. Suggest that she eat several small meals a day instead of three large ones.
• Include the patient's husband or other close relatives in patient care and teaching as much as possible.
• To help detect fallopian tube and other gynecologic cancers early, stress the importance of a regular pelvic examination to *all* patients. Tell them to contact a doctor promptly about any gynecologic symptom.

FATTY LIVER

Steatosis, or fatty liver, a common disorder, is the accumulation of triglycerides and other fats in liver cells. In severe fatty liver, fat constitutes as much as 40% of the liver's weight (as opposed to 5% in a normal liver) and the liver's weight may increase from 3.3 lb (1.5 kg) to as much as 11 lb (4.9 kg).

Minimal fatty changes are temporary and asymptomatic; severe or persistent changes may cause liver dysfunction. Fatty liver is usually reversible by simply eliminating the cause.

(See *Reversing fatty liver.*) However, this disorder may result in recurrent infection or sudden death from fat emboli in the lungs.

Causes

The most common cause of fatty liver in the United States and in Europe is chronic alcoholism, with the severity of hepatic disease directly related to the amount of alcohol consumed.

Other causes include malnutrition (especially protein deficiency), obesity, diabetes mellitus, jejunoileal bypass surgery, Cushing's syndrome, Reye's syndrome, pregnancy, large doses of hepatotoxins — such as I.V. tetracycline — carbon tetrachloride intoxication, prolonged I.V. hyperalimentation, and DDT poisoning.

Whatever the cause, fatty infiltration of the liver probably results from mobilization of fatty acids from adipose tissues or altered fat metabolism.

Signs and symptoms

Clinical features of fatty liver vary with the degree of lipid infiltration, and many patients are asymptomatic. The most typical sign is a large, tender liver (hepatomegaly). Common symptoms include upper right quadrant pain (with massive or rapid infiltration), ascites, edema, jaundice, and fever (all with hepatic necrosis or biliary stasis).

Nausea, vomiting, and anorexia are less common. Splenomegaly usually accompanies cirrhosis. Rarer changes are spider angiomas, varices, transient gynecomastia, and menstrual disorders.

Diagnosis

Typical clinical features — especially in patients with chronic alcoholism, malnutrition, poorly controlled diabetes mellitus, or obesity — suggest fatty liver. *A liver biopsy* confirms excessive fat in the liver. The following liver function tests support this diagnosis:

TEACHING CHECKLIST

☑️ **REVERSING FATTY LIVER**

- Suggest counseling for alcoholics. Provide emotional support for their families as well.
- Teach diabetic patients and their families about proper care, such as the purpose of insulin injections, diet, and exercise. Refer them to public health nurses or to group classes, as necessary, to promote compliance with the treatment plan. Emphasize the need for long-term medical supervision, and urge diabetic patients to report any changes in their health immediately.
- Instruct obese patients and their families about proper diet. Warn against fad diets because they may be nutritionally inadequate.
- Recommend medical supervision for patients more than 20% overweight.
- Encourage the patient to attend a group diet and exercise program and, if necessary, suggest behavior modification programs to correct eating habits.
- Advise patients receiving hepatotoxins and those who risk occupational exposure to DDT to watch for and immediately report signs of toxicity.
- Inform all patients that fatty liver is reversible *only* if they strictly follow the therapeutic program; otherwise, they risk permanent liver damage.

- *albumin* — somewhat low
- *globulin* — usually elevated
- *cholesterol* — usually elevated
- *total bilirubin* — elevated
- *alkaline phosphatase* — elevated
- *transaminase* — usually low (less than 300 units)
- *prothrombin time* — possibly prolonged.

Other findings may include anemia, leukocytosis, an elevated white blood cell count, albuminuria, hyperglycemia or hypoglycemia, and deficiencies of iron, folic acid, and vitamin B_{12}.

Treatment

The treatment for fatty liver is essentially supportive and consists of correcting the underlying condition or eliminating its cause. For instance, when fatty liver results from I.V. hyperalimentation, decreasing the rate of carbohydrate infusion may correct the disease.

In alcoholic fatty liver, abstinence from alcohol and a proper diet can begin to correct liver changes within 4 to 8 weeks. Such correction requires comprehensive patient teaching.

Special considerations

• Assess for malnutrition, especially protein deficiency, in those with chronic illness. Suggest an adequate diet.

• If your patient is obese, be sure to follow up on his progress in losing weight. Provide positive reinforcement for any weight loss.

• Do comprehensive patient teaching, especially for obese, alchoholic, and diabetic patients.

FOLIC ACID DEFICIENCY ANEMIA

A common, slowly progressive, megaloblastic anemia, folic acid deficiency anemia occurs most often in infants, adolescents, pregnant and lactating females, alcoholics, the elderly, and in persons with malignant or intestinal diseases.

Causes

Folic acid deficiency anemia may result from:

• *alcohol abuse* (may suppress metabolic effects of folate).

• *poor diet* (common in alcoholics, elderly persons living alone, and infants, especially those with infections or diarrhea).

• *impaired absorption* (due to intestinal dysfunction from disorders such as celiac disease, tropical sprue, regional jejunitis, or bowel resection).

• *bacteria* competing for available folic acid.

• *excessive cooking,* which can destroy a high percentage of folic acids in foods.

• *limited storage capacity* in infants.

• *prolonged drug therapy* (anticonvulsants, estrogens).

• *increased folic acid requirement* during pregnancy; during rapid growth in infancy (common because of a recent increase in the survival of premature infants); during childhood and adolescence (because of general use of folate-poor cow's milk); and in patients with neoplastic diseases and some skin diseases (chronic exfoliative dermatitis).

Signs and symptoms

Folic acid deficiency anemia gradually produces clinical features characteristic of other megaloblastic anemias, without the neurologic manifestations: progressive fatigue, shortness of breath, palpitations, weakness, glossitis, nausea, anorexia, headache, fainting, irritability, forgetfulness, pallor, and slight jaundice.

Folic acid deficiency anemia doesn't cause neurologic impairment unless it's associated with vitamin B_{12} deficiency, as in pernicious anemia.

Diagnosis

The Schilling test and a therapeutic trial of vitamin B_{12} injections distinguish between folic acid deficiency anemia and pernicious anemia. Significant findings include macrocytosis, a decreased reticulocyte count, abnormal platelets, and a serum folate level less than 4 mg/ml.

Treatment

Folic acid supplements and the elimination of contributing causes are the primary treatments. Folic acid supplements may be given orally (usually 1 to 5 mg/day) or parenterally (to patients who are severely ill, have malabsorption, or are unable to take oral medication). Many patients respond favorably to a well-balanced diet.

If the patient has combined B_{12} and folate deficiencies, folic acid replenishment alone may aggravate neurologic dysfunction.

Special considerations

• Teach the patient to meet daily folic acid requirements by including a food from each food group in every meal.
• If the patient has a severe deficiency, explain that diet only reinforces folic acid supplementation and isn't therapeutic by itself.
• Urge compliance with the prescribed course of therapy. Advise the patient not to stop taking the supplements when he begins to feel better.
• If the patient has glossitis, emphasize the importance of good oral hygiene. Suggest regular use of mild or diluted mouthwash and a soft toothbrush.
• Watch fluid and electrolyte balance, particularly in the patient who has severe diarrhea and is receiving parenteral fluid replacement therapy.
• Because anemia causes severe fatigue, schedule regular rest periods until the patient is able to resume normal activity.
• To prevent folic acid deficiency anemia, emphasize the importance of a well-balanced diet high in folic acid. Identify alcoholics with poor dietary habits, and try to arrange for appropriate counseling.
• Tell mothers who aren't breast-feeding to use commercially prepared formulas.

FOLLICULITIS, FURUNCULOSIS, AND CARBUNCULOSIS

A bacterial infection of the hair follicle, folliculitis causes the formation of a pustule. The infection can be superficial (follicular impetigo or Bockhart's impetigo) or deep (sycosis barbae).

Folliculitis may also lead to the development of furuncles (furunculosis), commonly known as boils, or carbuncles (carbunculosis). The prognosis depends on the severity of the infection and on the patient's physical condition and ability to resist infection.

Causes

The most common cause of folliculitis, furunculosis, or carbunculosis is coagulase-positive *Staphylococcus aureus*. Predisposing factors include an infected wound, poor hygiene, debilitation, diabetes, occlusive cosmetics, tight clothes, friction, exposure to chemicals, and the treatment of skin lesions with tar or with occlusive therapy using steroids.

Furunculosis often follows folliculitis exacerbated by irritation, pressure, friction, or perspiration. Carbunculosis follows persistent *S. aureus* infection and furunculosis.

Signs and symptoms

Folliculitis, furunculosis, and carbunculosis have different signs and symptoms. For example:

- Folliculitis pustules usually appear on the scalp, arms, and legs in children; on the face of bearded men (sycosis barbae); and on the eyelids (styes). Deep folliculitis may be painful.
- Furunculosis — hard, painful nodules that commonly develop on the neck, face, axillae, and buttocks — may follow folliculitis. For several days, these nodules enlarge and then rupture, discharging pus and necrotic material. After the nodules rupture, pain subsides, but erythema and edema may persist for days or weeks.
- Carbunculosis is marked by extremely painful, deep abscesses that drain through multiple openings onto the skin surface, usually around several hair follicles. Fever and malaise may accompany these lesions.

Diagnosis

The obvious skin lesion confirms folliculitis, furunculosis, or carbunculosis. Wound culture shows *S. aureus.* In carbunculosis, patient history reveals preexistent furunculosis. A complete blood count may show an elevated white blood cell count (leukocytosis).

Treatment

Appropriate treatment includes the following:
- Folliculitis is treated by cleaning the infected area thoroughly with soap and water; applying warm, wet compresses to promote vasodilation and drainage from the lesions; applying topical antibiotics, such as mupirocin ointment; and, in extensive infection, administering systemic antibiotics (erythromycin or dicloxacillin).
- Furunculosis may also require incision and drainage of ripe lesions after application of warm, wet compresses, and topical antibiotics after drainage.
- Carbunculosis requires systemic antibiotic therapy.

Special considerations

- Care for folliculitis, furunculosis, and carbunculosis is basically supportive and emphasizes teaching the patient scrupulous personal and family hygiene measures. Taking the necessary precautions to prevent spreading infection is also an important part of care.
- Caution the patient never to squeeze a boil, since this may cause it to rupture into the surrounding area.
- To avoid spreading bacteria to family members, urge the patient not to share towels and washcloths. Tell him that these items should be laundered in hot water before being reused. The patient should change his clothes and bedsheets daily, and these also should be washed in hot water. Encourage the patient to change dressings frequently and to discard them promptly in paper bags.
- Advise the patient with recurrent furunculosis to have a physical examination because an underlying disease, such as diabetes, may be present.

GALACTOSEMIA

Any disorder of galactose metabolism is called galactosemia. It produces symptoms ranging from cataracts and liver damage to mental retardation and occurs in two forms: *classic galactosemia* and *galactokinase-deficiency galactosemia.* Although a galactose-free diet relieves most symptoms, galactosemia-induced mental impairment is irreversible; some residual vision impairment may also persist.

Causes
Both forms of galactosemia are inherited as autosomal recessive defects and occur in about 1 in 60,000 births in the United States.

Up to 1.25% of the population is heterozygous for the classic galactosemia gene. Classic galactosemia results from a defect in the enzyme galactose-1-phosphate uridyl transferase.

The rarer form of this disorder, galactokinase-deficiency galactosemia stems from a deficiency of the enzyme galactokinase.

In both forms of galactosemia, the inability to normally metabolize the sugar galactose (which is mainly formed by digestion of the disaccharide lactose that's present in milk) causes galactose accumulation.

Signs and symptoms
In children who are homozygous for the classic galactosemia gene, signs are evident at birth or begin within a few days after milk ingestion, and include failure to thrive, vomiting, and diarrhea.

Other clinical effects include liver damage (which causes jaundice, hepatomegaly, cirrhosis, ascites), splenomegaly, galactosuria, proteinuria, and aminoaciduria. Cataracts may also be present at birth or develop later. Pseudotumor cerebri may occur.

Continued ingestion of galactose or lactose-containing foods may cause mental retardation, malnourishment, progressive hepatic failure, and death—from the still unknown process of galactose metabolites accumulating in body tissues.

Although treatment may prevent mental impairment, galactosemia can produce a short attention span, difficulty with spatial and mathematical relationships, and apathetic, withdrawn behavior. Cataracts may be the only sign of galactokinase deficiency, resulting from the accumulation of galactitol, a metabolic by-product of galactose, in the lens.

Diagnosis
Deficiency of the enzyme galactose-1-phosphate uridyl transferase in red blood cells (RBCs) confirms classic galactosemia; decreased RBC levels of galactokinase confirm galactokinase deficiency. Other related laboratory results include increased galactose levels in blood (the normal value in children is less than 20 mg/dl) and urine.

Galactose measurements in blood and urine must be interpreted carefully, because some children who consume large amounts of milk have elevated plasma galactose concentrations and galactosuria but are not galactosemic. Also, neonates excrete galactose in their urine for about a week after birth; premature infants, even longer. Other test results include:

• *liver biopsy:* typical acinar formation
• *liver enzymes (AST, ALT):* elevated
• *urinalysis:* albumin in urine
• *ophthalmoscopy:* punctate lesions in the fetal lens nucleus (with treatment, cataracts regress)
• *amniocentesis:* prenatal diagnosis of galactosemia (recommended for heterozygous and homozygous parents).

Treatment
Elimination of galactose and lactose from the diet causes most effects to subside. The infant gains weight; liver anomalies, nausea, vomiting, galactosemia, proteinuria, and aminoaciduria disappear; and cataracts regress.

To eliminate galactose and lactose from an infant's diet, replace cow's milk formula or breast milk with a meat-base or soybean formula. As the child grows, a balanced, galactose-free diet must be maintained.

A pregnant woman who is heterozygous or homozygous for galactosemia should also follow a galactose-restricted diet. Such a diet supports normal growth and development and may delay symptoms of galactosemia in the neonate.

Special considerations
• Teach the parents about dietary restrictions and stress the importance of compliance. Warn them to read medication labels carefully and avoid giving their child any drugs that contain lactose fillers.

• If the child has a learning disability, help his parents secure educational assistance.
• Refer those parents who want to have other children for genetic counseling. In some states, screening of all neonates for galactosemia is required by law.

GALLBLADDER AND BILE DUCT CANCERS

Cancer of the gallbladder is rare, constituting fewer than 1% of all cancer cases. It's usually found coincidentally in patients with cholecystitis; 1 in 400 cholecystectomies reveals cancer.

This disease is most prevalent in females over age 60. It's rapidly progressive and usually fatal; patients seldom live a year after diagnosis. The poor prognosis is due to late diagnosis; gallbladder cancer usually isn't diagnosed until after cholecystectomy, when it's typically in an advanced, metastatic stage.

Extrahepatic bile duct cancer is the cause of approximately 3% of all cancer deaths in the United States. It occurs in both males and females (incidence is slightly higher in males) between ages 60 and 70. The usual site is at the bifurcation in the common duct.

Cancer at the distal end of the common duct is often confused with pancreatic cancer. Characteristically, metastatis occurs in local lymph nodes, the liver, the lungs, and the peritoneum.

Causes
Many consider gallbladder cancer a complication of gallstones. However, this inference rests on circumstantial evidence from postmortem examina-

tions: 60% to 90% of all gallbladder cancer patients also have gallstones; but postmortem data from patients with gallstones show gallbladder cancer in only 0.5%.

Adenocarcinoma accounts for 85% to 95% of all cases of gallbladder cancer; squamous cell, 5% to 15%. Mixed-tissue types are rare.

Lymph node metastasis is present in 25% to 70% of patients at diagnosis. Direct extension to the liver is common (in 46% to 89%); direct extension to both the cystic and the common bile ducts, stomach, colon, duodenum, and jejunum also occurs, and produces obstructions. Metastasis also occurs through the portal or hepatic veins to the peritoneum, ovaries, and lower lung lobes.

The cause of extrahepatic bile duct cancer isn't known; however, statistics reveal an unexplained increased incidence of this cancer in patients with ulcerative colitis. This association may be due to a common cause — perhaps an immune mechanism, or chronic use of certain drugs by the colitis patient.

Signs and symptoms

Clinically, gallbladder cancer is almost indistinguishable from cholecystitis: pain in the epigastrium or right upper quadrant, weight loss, anorexia, nausea, vomiting, and jaundice. However, chronic, progressively severe pain in an afebrile patient suggests cancer. In patients with simple gallstones, pain is sporadic.

Another telling clue to cancer is a palpable gallbladder (in the right upper quadrant) with obstructive jaundice. Some patients may also have hepatosplenomegaly.

Signs of bile duct cancer

Progressive profound jaundice is commonly the first sign of obstruction due to extrahepatic bile duct cancer. The jaundice is usually accompanied by chronic pain in the epigastrium or the right upper quadrant, radiating to the back. Other common symptoms, if associated with active cholecystitis, include pruritus, skin excoriations, anorexia, weight loss, chills, and fever.

Diagnosis

No test or procedure is, in itself, diagnostic of gallbladder cancer. However, the following laboratory tests support this diagnosis when they suggest hepatic dysfunction and extrahepatic biliary obstruction:

• *baseline studies* (complete blood count, routine urinalysis, electrolyte studies, enzymes)

• *liver function tests* (typically reveal elevated serum bilirubin, urine bile and bilirubin, and urobilinogen levels in more than 50% of patients as well as consistently elevated serum alkaline phosphatase levels)

• *occult blood in stools* (linked to the associated anemia)

• *cholecystography* (may show stones or calcification)

• *cholangiography* (may locate the site of common duct obstruction)

• *magnetic resonance imaging* (detects tumors).

The following tests help compile data that confirm extrahepatic bile duct cancer:

• *liver function studies* (indicate biliary obstruction: elevated levels of bilirubin [5 to 30 mg/dl], alkaline phosphatase, and blood cholesterol as well as prolonged prothrombin time)

• *endoscopic retrograde cannulization of the pancreas* (identifies the tumor site and allows access for obtaining a biopsy specimen).

Treatment

Surgical treatment of gallbladder cancer is essentially palliative and includes various procedures, such as cholecystectomy, common bile duct exploration, T-tube drainage, and wedge excision of hepatic tissue.

If the cancer invades gallbladder musculature, the survival rate is less than 5%, even with massive resection. Although some cases of long-term survival (4 to 5 years) have been reported, few patients survive longer than 6 months after surgery for gallbladder cancer.

Surgery is normally indicated to relieve the obstruction and jaundice that result from extrahepatic bile duct cancer. The type of procedure used to relieve obstruction depends on the site of the cancer. Such procedures may include cholecystoduodenostomy or T-tube drainage of the common duct.

Other palliative measures for both kinds of cancers include radiation, radiation implants (mostly used for local and incisional recurrences), and chemotherapy (with combinations of fluorouracil, doxorubicin, and lomustine). All of these treatment measures have limited effects.

Special considerations

After biliary resection:
• Monitor vital signs.
• Use strict aseptic technique when caring for the incision and the surrounding area.
• Place the patient in low Fowler's position.
• Prevent respiratory problems by encouraging deep breathing and coughing. The high incision makes the patient want to take shallow breaths; taking analgesics and splinting his abdomen with a pillow or an abdominal binder may make breathing easier.
• Monitor bowel sounds and bowel movements. Observe the patient's tolerance of his diet.
• Provide pain-control measures.
• Check intake and output carefully. Watch for electrolyte imbalance; monitor I.V. solutions to avoid overloading the cardiovascular system.

• Monitor the nasogastric tube, which will be in place for 24 to 72 hours postoperatively to relieve distention, and the T tube. Record amount and color of drainage each shift. Secure the T tube to minimize tension on it and prevent its being pulled out.
• Help the patient and his family cope with their initial fears and reactions to the diagnosis by offering information and support.
• Before discharge, teach the patient how to manage the biliary catheter.
• Advise the patient of the adverse effects of both chemotherapy and radiation therapy, and monitor him for these effects.

LIFE-THREATENING DISORDER

GAS GANGRENE

Local infection with the anaerobic, spore-forming, gram-positive rod *Clostridium perfringens* (or another clostridial species) causes gas gangrene. It occurs in devitalized tissues and results from compromised arterial circulation following trauma or surgery.

This rare infection carries a high mortality unless therapy begins immediately. However, with prompt treatment, 80% of patients with gas gangrene of the extremities survive; the prognosis is poorer for gas gangrene in other sites, such as the abdominal wall or the bowel. The usual incubation period is 1 to 4 days but can vary from 3 hours to 6 weeks or longer.

Causes

C. perfringens is a normal inhabitant of the GI and female genital tracts; it's also prevalent in soil. The organism is typically transmitted during trauma or surgery. Because *C. perfringens* is anaerobic, gas gangrene is most often found in deep wounds, especially those in which tissue necrosis further reduces oxygen supply.

When *C. perfringens* invades soft tissues, it produces thrombosis of regional blood vessels, tissue necrosis, and localized edema. Such necrosis releases both carbon dioxide and hydrogen subcutaneously, producing interstitial gas bubbles. Gas gangrene occurs most commonly in the extremities and in abdominal wounds; less frequently, in the uterus. (See *Growth cycle of* Clostridium perfringens *in a closed wound.*)

Signs and symptoms

True gas gangrene produces myositis and another form of this disease, involving only soft tissue, called anaerobic cellulitis. Most signs of infection develop within 72 hours of trauma or surgery. The hallmark of gas gangrene is crepitation, a result of carbon dioxide and hydrogen accumulation as a metabolic by-product in necrotic tissues.

Local symptoms

Other typical indications are severe localized pain, swelling, and discoloration (often dusky brown or reddish), with formation of bullae and necrosis within 36 hours from onset of symptoms. Soon the skin over the wound may rupture, revealing dark red or black necrotic muscle, a foul-smelling watery or frothy discharge, intravascular hemolysis, thrombosis of blood vessels, and evidence of infection spread.

Toxemia and hypovolemia

In addition to these local symptoms, gas gangrene produces early signs of toxemia and hypovolemia (tachycardia, tachypnea, and hypotension) and a moderate fever that usually doesn't exceed 101° F (38.3° C). Although pale,

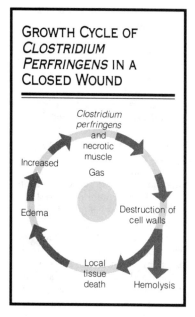

GROWTH CYCLE OF *CLOSTRIDIUM PERFRINGENS* IN A CLOSED WOUND

Clostridium perfringens and necrotic muscle

Gas

Increased

Destruction of cell walls

Edema

Local tissue death

Hemolysis

prostrate, and motionless, most patients remain alert and oriented and are extremely apprehensive.

Usually death occurs suddenly, often during surgery for removal of necrotic tissue. Less often, death is preceded by delirium and coma, sometimes accompanied by vomiting, profuse diarrhea, and circulatory collapse.

Diagnosis

A history of recent surgery or a deep puncture wound and the rapid onset of pain and crepitation around the wound suggest this diagnosis. It's confirmed by anaerobic cultures of wound drainage showing *C. perfringens;* a Gram stain of wound drainage showing large, gram-positive, rod-shaped bacteria; X-rays showing gas in tissues; and blood studies showing leukocytosis and, later, hemolysis.

The diagnosis must rule out synergistic gangrene and necrotizing fasciitis; unlike gas gangrene, both of these disorders anesthetize the skin around the wound.

Treatment
Effective treatment includes careful observation for signs of myositis and cellulitis and *immediate treatment* if these signs appear, and *immediate* wide surgical excision of all affected tissues and necrotic muscle in myositis.

Note: Delayed or inadequate surgical excision is a *fatal* mistake.

Treatment also includes I.V. administration of high-dose penicillin and, after adequate debridement, hyperbaric oxygenation, if available.

In addition, for 1 to 3 hours every 6 to 8 hours, the patient is placed in a hyperbaric chamber and is exposed to pressures designed to increase oxygen tension and prevent multiplication of the anaerobic clostridia. Surgery may be done within the hyperbaric chamber if the chamber is large enough.

Special considerations
Before diagnosis:
• Look for signs of ischemia (cool skin; pallor or cyanosis; sudden, severe pain; sudden edema; and loss of pulses in involved limb).

After diagnosis:
• Throughout this illness, provide adequate fluid replacement, and assess pulmonary and cardiac functions often. Maintain airway and ventilation.
• To prevent skin breakdown and further infection, give good skin care. After surgery, provide meticulous wound care.
• Before penicillin administration, obtain a patient history of allergies; afterward, watch closely for signs of hypersensitivity.
• Provide psychological support. This is critical because these patients can remain alert until death, knowing that death is imminent and unavoidable.
• Deodorize the room to control foul odor from the wound. Prepare the patient emotionally for a large wound after surgical excision, and refer him for physical rehabilitation as necessary.
• Institute wound precautions. Dispose of drainage material properly (double-bag dressings in plastic bags for incineration), and wear sterile gloves when changing dressings. No special cleaning measures are required after the patient is discharged.
• Take measures to prevent gas gangrene. Routinely take precautions to render all wound sites unsuitable for growth of clostridia by attempting to keep granulation tissue viable; adequate debridement is imperative to reduce anaerobic growth conditions.
• Be alert for devitalized tissues.
• Position the patient to facilitate drainage, and eliminate all dead spaces in closed wounds.

GASTRIC CANCER

Common throughout the world, gastric cancer affects all races. However, unexplained geographic and cultural differences in incidence occur; for example, mortality is high in Japan, Iceland, Chile, and Austria. In the United States, incidence has decreased 50% during the past 25 years, and the death rate from gastric cancer is one-third that of 30 years ago.

The decrease in gastric cancer incidence in the United States has been attributed, without proof, to the balanced American diet and to refrigeration, which reduces nitrate-producing bacteria in food.

Incidence is higher in males over age 40. The prognosis depends on the stage of the disease at the time of diagnosis; however, overall, the 5-year survival rate is approximately 15%.

SITES OF GASTRIC CANCER

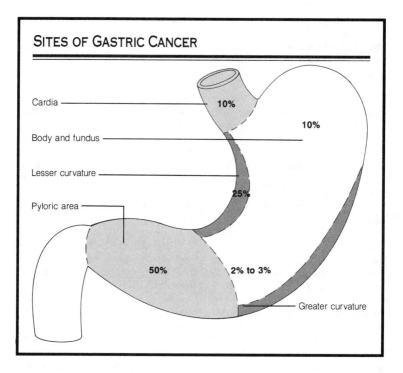

Cardia — **10%**

10%

Body and fundus —

Lesser curvature —

25%

Pyloric area —

50%   **2% to 3%**

Greater curvature

Causes

The cause of gastric cancer is unknown. This cancer is often associated with gastritis with gastric atrophy, which is now thought to be a result of gastric cancer rather than a precursor state. Predisposing factors include environmental influences, such as smoking and high alcohol intake.

Genetic factors have also been implicated because this disease occurs more frequently among people with type A blood than among those with type O; similarly it occurs more frequently in people with a family history of such cancer.

Dietary factors also seem related, including types of food preparation, physical properties of some foods, and certain methods of food preservation (especially smoking, pickling, or salting).

Classification

According to gross appearance, gastric cancer can be classified as polypoid, ulcerating, ulcerating and infiltrating, or diffuse. The parts of the stomach affected by gastric cancer, listed in order of decreasing frequency, are the pylorus and antrum, the lesser curvature, the cardia, the body of the stomach, and the greater curvature. (See *Sites of gastric cancer.*)

Metastasis

Gastric cancer metastasizes rapidly to the regional lymph nodes, omentum, liver, and lungs by the following routes: walls of the stomach, duodenum, and esophagus; lymphatic system; adjacent organs; bloodstream; and peritoneal cavity.

Signs and symptoms

Early clues to gastric cancer are chronic dyspepsia and epigastric discomfort, followed in later stages by weight loss, anorexia, a feeling of fullness after eating, anemia, and fatigue. If the cancer is in the cardia, the first symptom may be dysphagia and, later, vomiting (typically coffee-ground vomitus). Affected patients may also have blood in their stools.

The course of gastric cancer may be insidious or fulminating. Unfortunately, the patient typically treats himself with antacids until the symptoms of advanced stages appear.

Diagnosis

The diagnosis depends primarily on reinvestigations of any persistent or recurring GI changes and complaints. To rule out other conditions producing similar symptoms, a diagnostic evaluation must include the testing of blood, stools, and stomach fluid specimens.

Diagnosis of gastric cancer often requires these studies:
• *Barium X-rays of the GI tract, with fluoroscopy* show changes (a tumor or filling defect in the outline of the stomach, loss of flexibility and distensibility, and abnormal gastric mucosa with or without ulceration).
• *Gastroscopy with fiber-optic endoscopy* helps rule out other diffuse gastric mucosal abnormalities by allowing direct visualization and gastroscopic biopsy to evaluate gastric mucosal lesions.
• *Photography with fiber-optic endoscopy* provides a permanent record of gastric lesions that can later be used to determine the progress of the disease and the effect of treatment.

The following studies may rule out metastasis to specific organs: computed tomography scans, chest X-rays, liver and bone scans, and a liver biopsy. (See *Staging gastric cancer.*)

Treatment

Surgery is often the treatment of choice. Excision of the lesion with appropriate margins is possible in over one-third of patients. Even in patients whose disease isn't considered surgically curable, resection offers palliation and improves potential benefits from chemotherapy and radiation.

Types of surgery

The nature and extent of the lesion determine what kind of surgery is most appropriate. Common surgical procedures include subtotal gastric resection (subtotal gastrectomy) and total gastric resection (total gastrectomy).

When cancer involves the pylorus and antrum, gastric resection removes the lower stomach and duodenum (gastrojejunostomy or Billroth II). If metastasis has occurred, the omentum and spleen may also have to be removed.

If gastric cancer has spread to the liver, peritoneum, or lymph glands, palliative surgery may include gastrostomy, jejunostomy, or a gastric or partial gastric resection. Such surgery may temporarily relieve vomiting, nausea, pain, and dysphagia, while allowing enteral nutrition to continue.

Other treatments

Chemotherapy for GI cancers may help to control symptoms and prolong survival. Adenocarcinoma of the stomach has responded to several agents, including fluorouracil, carmustine, doxorubicin, cisplatin, methotrexate, and mitomycin.

Antiemetics can control nausea, which increases as the cancer advances. In the more advanced stages, sedatives and tranquilizers may be necessary to control overwhelming anxiety. Narcotics are often necessary to relieve severe and unremitting pain.

Radiation has been particularly useful when combined with chemotherapy

STAGING GASTRIC CANCER

Both the prognosis and treatment of gastric cancer depend on its type and stage. Using the TNM (tumor, node, metastasis) system, the American Joint Committee on Cancer describes the following stages of gastric cancer.

Primary tumor
TX — primary tumor can't be assessed
T0 — no evidence of primary tumor
Tis — carcinoma in situ: intraepithelial tumor doesn't penetrate the lamina propria
T1 — tumor penetrates the lamina propria or submucosa
T2 — tumor penetrates the muscularis propria or subserosa
T3 — tumor penetrates the serosa (visceral peritoneum) without invading adjacent structures
T4 — tumor invades adjacent structures

Regional lymph nodes
NX — regional lymph nodes can't be assessed
N0 — no evidence of regional lymph node metastasis

N1 — involvement of perigastric lymph nodes within 3 cm of the edge of the primary tumor
N2 — involvement of the perigastric lymph nodes more than 3 cm from the edge of the primary tumor, or in lymph nodes along the left gastric, common hepatic, splenic, or celiac arteries

Distant metastasis
MX — distant metastasis can't be assessed
M0 — no evidence of distant metastasis
M1 — distant metastasis

Staging categories
Gastric cancer stages progress from mild to severe as follows:
Stage 0 — Tis, N0, M0
Stage IA — T1, N0, M0
Stage IB — T1, N1, M0; T2, N0, M0
Stage II — T1, N2, M0; T3, N0, M0
Stage IIIA — T2, N2, M0; T3, N1, M0; T4, N0, M0
Stage IIIB — T3, N2, M0; T4, N1, M0
Stage IV — T4, N2, M0; any T, any N, M1

---

in patients who have unresectable or partially resectable disease. It should be given on an empty stomach, and shouldn't be used preoperatively, since it may damage viscera and impede healing.

Treatment with antispasmodics and antacids may help relieve GI distress.

Special considerations
• Before surgery, prepare the patient for its effects and for postsurgical procedures, such as insertion of a nasogastric (NG) tube for drainage and I.V. lines.

• Reassure the patient who's having a partial gastric resection that he may eventually be able to eat normally.

• Prepare the patient who's having a total gastrectomy for slow recovery and only partial return to a normal diet.

• Include the family in all phases of the patient's care.

• Emphasize the importance of changing position every 2 hours and of deep breathing.

• After surgery, provide meticulous supportive care to promote recovery and prevent complications.

• After any type of gastrectomy, pulmonary complications may result and oxygen may be needed. Regularly assist the patient with turning, coughing, and deep breathing. Turning the patient hourly and administering analgesic narcotics may prevent pulmonary problems. Incentive spirometry may also be needed for complete lung expansion. Proper positioning is important as well: semi-Fowler's position facilitates breathing and drainage.

• After gastrectomy, little (if any) drainage comes from the NG tube because no secretions form after stomach removal. Without a stomach for storage, many patients experience dumping syndrome. Intrinsic factor is absent from gastric secretions, leading to malabsorption of vitamin B_{12}.

• To prevent vitamin B_{12} deficiency, the patient must take a replacement vitamin for the rest of his life as well as an iron supplement.

• During radiation treatment, encourage the patient to eat high-calorie, well-balanced meals. Offer fluids, such as ginger ale, to minimize such radiation side effects as nausea and vomiting.

• Patients who experience poor digestion and absorption after gastrectomy need a special diet: frequent feedings of small amounts of clear liquids, increasing to small, frequent feedings of bland food.

• After total gastrectomy, patients must eat small meals for the rest of their lives. (Some patients need pancreatin and sodium bicarbonate after meals to prevent or control steatorrhea and dyspepsia.)

• Wound dehiscence and delayed healing, stemming from decreased protein, anemia, and avitaminosis, may occur. Preoperative vitamin and protein replacement can prevent such complications.

• Observe the wound regularly for redness, swelling, failure to heal, or warmth. Parenteral administration of vitamin C may improve wound healing.

• Vitamin deficiency may result from obstruction, diarrhea, or an inadequate diet. Ascorbic acid, thiamine, riboflavin, nicotinic acid, and vitamin K supplements may be beneficial.

• Good nutrition promotes weight gain, strength, independence, a positive outlook, and tolerance for surgery, radiation therapy, or chemotherapy. Aside from meeting caloric needs, nutrition must provide adequate protein, fluid, and potassium intake to facilitate glycogen and protein synthesis.

• Anabolic agents, such as methandrostenolone, may induce nitrogen retention. Steroids, antidepressants, wine, or brandy may boost the appetite.

When all treatments have failed:

• Concentrate on keeping the patient comfortable and free of pain, and provide as much psychological support as possible.

• If the patient is going home, discuss continuing care needs with the caregiver or refer the patient to an appropriate home health care agency.

• Encourage the patient and the caregivers to express their feelings and concerns. Answer their questions honestly with tact and sensitivity.

GASTRITIS

An inflammation of the gastric mucosa, gastritis may be acute or chronic and can occur at any age. *Acute gastritis* produces mucosal reddening, edema, hemorrhage, and erosion. *Chronic gastritis* is common among elderly people and people with pernicious anemia. It's often present as chronic atrophic gastritis, in which all stomach mucosal layers are inflamed, with reduced numbers of chief and parietal cells.

Causes

Acute and chronic gastritis have different causes.

Acute gastritis

Acute gastritis has numerous causes including:

• chronic ingestion of irritating foods, such as hot peppers (or an allergic reaction to them), or alcohol

• drugs such as aspirin and other nonsteroidal anti-inflammatory agents (in large doses), cytotoxic agents, caffeine, corticosteroids, antimetabolites, phenylbutazone, and indomethacin

• ingestion of poisons, especially DDT, ammonia, mercury, carbon tetrachloride, and corrosive substances

• endotoxins released from infecting bacteria, such as staphylococci, *Escherichia coli,* or salmonella.

Acute gastritis also may develop in acute illnesses, especially when the patient has had major traumatic injuries; burns; severe infection; hepatic, renal, or respiratory failure; or major surgery.

Chronic gastritis

Chronic gastritis may be associated with peptic ulcer disease or gastrostomy, both of which cause chronic reflux of pancreatic secretions, bile, and bile acids from the duodenum into the stomach.

Recurring exposure to irritating substances, such as drugs, alcohol, cigarette smoke, or environmental agents, also may lead to chronic gastritis. Chronic gastritis may occur with pernicious anemia, renal disease, or diabetes mellitus.

Bacterial infection with *Helicobacter pylori* is a common cause of nonerosive chronic gastritis.

Signs and symptoms

After exposure to the offending substance, the patient with acute gastritis typically reports a rapid onset of symptoms, such as epigastric discomfort, indigestion, cramping, anorexia, nausea, vomiting, and hematemesis. The symptoms last from a few hours to a few days.

The patient with chronic gastritis may describe similar symptoms or may have only mild epigastric discomfort. Or his complaints may be vague, such as an intolerance for spicy or fatty foods or slight pain relieved by eating. The patient with chronic atrophic gastritis may be asymptomatic.

Diagnosis

The following tests are used to diagnose gastritis:

• Laboratory analyses can detect occult blood in vomitus or stools (or both) if the patient has gastric bleeding.

• Hemoglobin level and hematocrit are decreased if the patient has developed anemia from bleeding.

• Gastroscopy (with a biopsy) confirms gastritis when done before lesions heal (usually within 24 hours). This test is contraindicated after ingestion of a corrosive agent.

Treatment

To eliminate the cause of gastritis, bacterial gastritis is treated with antibiotics and ingested poisons are neutralized with the appropriate antidote.

Histamine$_2$-receptor antagonists, such as cimetidine, may block gastric secretions. Antacids may be used as buffers.

For critically ill patients, antacids administered hourly, with or without histamine antagonists, may reduce the frequency of gastritis attacks. Some patients also require analgesics. Until healing occurs, oxygen needs, blood volume, and fluid and electrolyte balance must be monitored.

When gastritis causes massive bleeding, treatment includes blood replacement; iced saline lavage, possibly with norepinephrine; angiography with vasopressin infused in normal saline solution; and, sometimes, surgery.

Vagotomy and pyloroplasty have achieved limited success when conservative treatments fail. Rarely, partial or total gastrectomy may be required.

Simply avoiding aspirin and spicy foods may relieve chronic gastritis. If symptoms develop or persist, antacids may be taken. If pernicious anemia is the cause, vitamin B_{12} may be administered parenterally. A combination of bismuth and an antibiotic, such as amoxicillin, may relieve *H. pylori* infection, but eradication is difficult.

Special considerations
• For vomiting, give antiemetics and, as needed, I.V. fluids. Monitor fluid intake and output and electrolyte levels.
• Monitor the patient for recurrent symptoms as food is reintroduced; provide a bland diet.
• Offer smaller, more frequent meals to reduce irritating gastric secretions. Eliminate foods that cause gastric upset.
• Administer antacids and other prescribed medications.
• If pain or nausea interferes with the patient's appetite, give analgesics or antiemetics 1 hour before meals.
• Tell the patient to avoid alcohol, caffeine, and irritating foods, such as spicy or highly seasoned foods.
• If the patient smokes, refer him to a smoking-cessation program.
• Urge the patient to seek immediate attention for recurring symptoms, such as hematemesis, nausea, or vomiting.
• Urge the patient to take prophylactic medications as prescribed. To reduce gastric irritation, advise the patient to take steroids with milk, food, or antacids. Instruct him to take antacids between meals and at bedtime and to avoid aspirin-containing compounds.

GASTROENTERITIS

Also called intestinal flu, traveler's diarrhea, viral enteritis, and food poisoning, gastroenteritis is a self-limiting disorder characterized by diarrhea, nausea, vomiting, and abdominal cramping. It occurs in persons of all ages and is a major cause of morbidity and mortality in underdeveloped nations.

In the United States, gastroenteritis ranks second to the common cold as a cause of lost work time and fifth as the cause of death among young children. It also can be life-threatening in elderly and debilitated people.

Causes
Gastroenteritis has many possible causes, including the following:
• bacteria (responsible for acute food poisoning): *Staphylococcus aureus, Salmonella, Shigella, Clostridium botulinum, Escherichia coli, Clostridium perfringens*
• amoebae: especially *Entamoeba histolytica*
• parasites: *Ascaris, Enterobius,* and *Trichinella spiralis*
• viruses (may be responsible for traveler's diarrhea): adeno-, echo-, or coxsackieviruses
• ingestion of toxins: plants or toadstools
• drug reactions: antibiotics
• enzyme deficiencies
• food allergens.

The bowel reacts to any of these enterotoxins with hypermotility, producing severe diarrhea and secondary depletion of intracellular fluid.

Signs and symptoms
Clinical manifestations vary depending on the pathologic organism and on the level of GI tract involved. How-

ever, gastroenteritis in adults is usually a self-limiting, nonfatal disease producing diarrhea, abdominal discomfort (ranging from cramping to pain), nausea, and vomiting. Other possible symptoms include fever, malaise, and borborygmi.

In children and elderly and debilitated people, gastroenteritis produces the same symptoms, but these patients' inability to tolerate electrolyte and fluid losses leads to a higher mortality.

Diagnosis
Patient history can aid diagnosis of gastroenteritis. A stool culture (by direct rectal swab) or blood culture identifies causative bacteria or parasites.

Treatment
Usually supportive, treatment consists of bed rest, nutritional support, and increased fluid intake.

When gastroenteritis is severe or affects a young child or an elderly or debilitated person, hospitalization may be needed. Treatment may also require specific antimicrobials, I.V. fluid and electrolyte replacement, bismuth-containing compounds such as Pepto-Bismol, and antiemetics (oral, I.M., or rectal suppositories), such as prochlorperazine or trimethobenzamide.

Special considerations
• Administer medications; correlate dosages, routes, and times appropriately with the patient's meals and activities (for example, give antiemetics 30 to 60 minutes before meals).
• If the patient can eat, replace lost fluids and electrolytes with broth, ginger ale, and lemonade as tolerated. Vary his diet to make it more enjoyable, and allow some choice of foods. Warn the patient to avoid milk and milk products, which may provoke recurrence.

• Record intake and output carefully. Watch for signs of dehydration, such as dry skin and mucous membranes, fever, and sunken eyes.
• Wash your hands thoroughly after giving care to avoid spreading infection.
• To ease anal irritation, provide warm sitz baths or apply witch hazel compresses.
• If food poisoning is probable, contact public health authorities so they can interview patients and food handlers, and take samples of the suspected contaminated food.
• Teach good hygiene to prevent recurrence. Instruct patients to thoroughly cook foods, especially pork; to refrigerate perishable foods, such as milk, mayonnaise, potato salad, and cream-filled pastry; and to always wash their hands with warm water and soap before handling food, especially after using the bathroom.
• Teach patients to clean utensils thoroughly, to avoid drinking water or eating raw fruit or vegetables when visiting a foreign country, and to eliminate flies and roaches in their home.

GASTROESOPHAGEAL REFLUX

The backflow of gastric or duodenal contents, or both, into the esophagus and past the lower esophageal sphincter (LES), without associated belching or vomiting, is called gastroesophageal reflux. Reflux may or may not cause symptoms or pathologic changes. Persistent reflux may cause reflux esophagitis (inflammation of the esophageal mucosa). The prognosis varies with the underlying cause.

☑ COPING WITH
REFLUX

• Teach the patient what causes reflux, how to avoid reflux with an antireflux regimen (medication, diet, and positional therapy), and what symptoms to watch for and report.
• Instruct the patient to avoid any circumstance that increases intraabdominal pressure (such as bending, coughing, vigorous exercise, tight clothing, constipation, and obesity) or any substance that reduces sphincter control (cigarettes, alcohol, fatty foods, and certain drugs).
• Advise the patient to sit upright, particularly after meals, and to eat small, frequent meals. Tell him to avoid highly seasoned food, acidic juices, alcoholic drinks, bedtime snacks, and foods high in fat or carbohydrates, which reduce LES pressure. He should eat meals at least 2 to 3 hours before lying down.
• Tell the patient to take antacids, as ordered (usually 1 hour and 3 hours after meals and at bedtime).

Causes

The function of the LES — a high-pressure area in the lower esophagus, just above the stomach — is to prevent gastric contents from backing up into the esophagus. Normally, the LES creates pressure, closing the lower end of the esophagus, but relaxes after each swallow to allow food into the stomach.

Reflux occurs when LES pressure is deficient or when pressure within the stomach exceeds LES pressure.

Studies have shown that a person with symptomatic reflux can't swallow often enough to create sufficient peristaltic amplitude to clear gastric acid from the lower esophagus. This results in prolonged periods of acidity in the esophagus when reflux occurs.

Predisposing factors include:
• pyloric surgery (alteration or removal of the pylorus), which allows reflux of bile or pancreatic juice.
• long-term nasogastric (NG) intubation (more than 4 or 5 days).
• any agent that lowers LES pressure, such as food, alcohol, cigarettes, anticholinergics (atropine, belladonna, propantheline), and other drugs (morphine, diazepam, and meperidine).
• hiatal hernia (especially in children).
• any condition or position that increases intra-abdominal pressure.

Signs and symptoms

Gastroesophageal reflux doesn't always cause symptoms, and in patients showing clinical effects, physiologic reflux isn't always confirmable. The most common feature of gastroesophageal reflux is heartburn, which may become more severe with vigorous exercise, bending, or lying down, and may be relieved by antacids or sitting upright. (See *Coping with reflux.*)

The pain of esophageal spasm resulting from reflux esophagitis tends to be chronic and may mimic angina pectoris, radiating to the neck, jaws, and arms. Other symptoms include odynophagia, which may be followed by a dull substernal ache from severe, long-term reflux; dysphagia from esophageal spasm, stricture, or esophagitis; and bleeding (bright red or dark brown).

Rarely, nocturnal regurgitation wakens the patient with coughing, choking, and a mouthful of saliva. Reflux may be associated with hiatal hernia. Direct hiatal hernia becomes clinically significant *only* when reflux is confirmed.

Pulmonary symptoms result from reflux of gastric contents into the throat and subsequent aspiration and include chronic pulmonary disease or nocturnal wheezing, bronchitis, asthma, morning hoarseness, and cough.

In children, other signs consist of failure to thrive and forceful vomiting from esophageal irritation. Such vomiting sometimes causes aspiration pneumonia.

Diagnosis

After a careful history and physical examination, tests to confirm gastroesophageal reflux include barium swallow fluoroscopy, esophageal pH probe, and esophagoscopy. In children, barium esophagography under fluoroscopic control can show reflux. Recurrent reflux after age 6 weeks is abnormal.

An acid perfusion (Bernstein) test can show that reflux is the cause of symptoms. Finally, endoscopy and a biopsy allow visualization and confirmation of any pathologic changes in the mucosa.

Treatment

Effective management relieves symptoms by reducing intra-abdominal pressure and reflux through gravity, neutralizing gastric contents, strengthening the LES with drug therapy, and in severe cases, performing surgery.

Positional therapy

To reduce intra-abdominal pressure and reflux, the patient should sleep in a reverse Trendelenburg position (with the head of the bed elevated) and should avoid lying down after meals and late-night snacks. In uncomplicated cases, positional therapy is especially useful in infants and children.

Antacids

Antacids given 1 hour and 3 hours after meals and at bedtime are effective for intermittent reflux. Hourly administration is necessary for intensive therapy. A nondiarrheal, nonmagnesium antacid (aluminum carbonate, aluminum hydroxide) may be preferred, depending on the patient's bowel status.

Drug therapy

Bethanechol, a drug to increase LES pressure, stimulates smooth-muscle contraction and decreases esophageal acidity after meals (proven with pH probe). Metoclopramide and cimetidine have also been used with beneficial results.

If possible, NG intubation should not be continued for more than 4 or 5 days because the tube interferes with sphincter integrity and itself allows reflux, especially when the patient lies flat.

Surgery

Surgical intervention may be necessary to control severe and refractory symptoms, such as pulmonary aspiration, hemorrhage, obstruction, severe pain, perforation, incompetent LES, or associated hiatal hernia.

Surgical procedures that create an artificial closure at the gastroesophageal junction include the Belsey Mark IV operation (which invaginates the esophagus into the stomach) and the Hill or Nissen procedures (which create a gastric wraparound with or without fixation). Also, vagotomy or pyloroplasty may be combined with an antireflux regimen to modify gastric contents.

Special considerations

• Teach the patient correct preparation for diagnostic testing. For example, he should not eat for 6 to 8 hours before having a barium X-ray or endoscopy.

• After surgery using a thoracic approach, carefully watch and record chest tube drainage and respiratory status. If needed, give chest physiotherapy and oxygen. Place the patient

with an NG tube in semi-Fowler's position to help prevent reflux. Offer reassurance and emotional support.
• Teach the patient how to avoid and treat reflux.

GAUCHER'S DISEASE

The most common form of lipidosis, Gaucher's disease causes an abnormal accumulation of glucocerebrosides in reticuloendothelial cells. It occurs in three forms: type 1 (adult); type 2 (infantile); and type 3 (juvenile). Type 2 can prove fatal within 9 months of onset, usually from pulmonary involvement.

Causes
Gaucher's disease results from an autosomal recessive inheritance, which causes decreased activity of the enzyme glucocerebrosidase. Type 1 is 30 times more prevalent in people of Eastern European Jewish ancestry. Types 2 and 3 are less common.

Signs and symptoms
Key signs of all types of Gaucher's disease are hepatosplenomegaly and bone lesions.

Type 1
In type 1, bone lesions lead to thinning of cortices, pathologic fractures, collapsed hip joints, and, eventually, vertebral compression. Severe episodic pain may develop in the legs, arms, and back but usually not until adolescence. (The adult form of Gaucher's disease is generally diagnosed while the patient is in his teens; the word "adult" is used loosely here.)

Other clinical effects of type 1 are fever, abdominal distention (from hypotonicity of the large bowel), respiratory problems (pneumonia or, rarely, cor pulmonale), easy bruising and bleeding, anemia, and, rarely, pancytopenia. Older patients may develop a yellow pallor and brown-yellow pigmentation on the face and legs.

Type 2
In type 2, motor dysfunction and spasticity occur at ages 6 to 7 months. Other signs of the infantile form of Gaucher's disease include abdominal distention, strabismus, muscular hypertonicity, retroflexion of the head, neck rigidity, dysphagia, laryngeal stridor, hyperreflexia, seizures, respiratory distress, and easy bruising and bleeding.

Type 3
Clinical effects of type 3 after infancy include seizures, hypertonicity, strabismus, poor coordination and mental ability and, possibly, easy bruising and bleeding.

Diagnosis
Bone marrow aspiration showing Gaucher's cells and direct assay of glucocerebrosidase activity, which can be performed on venous blood, confirm this diagnosis. Supportive laboratory results include an increased serum acid phosphatase level, decreased platelet count and serum iron level and, in type 3, an abnormal EEG after infancy.

Treatment
Supportive treatment consists of vitamins, supplemental iron or liver extract to prevent anemia caused by iron deficiency and to alleviate other hematologic problems, blood transfusions for anemia, splenectomy for thrombocytopenia, and strong analgesics for bone pain. Enzyme replacement therapy is still experimental but looks promising.

Special considerations

• If the patient is confined to bed, prevent pathologic fractures by turning him carefully. If he's ambulatory, see that he's assisted when getting out of bed or walking.

• Observe the patient closely for changes in pulmonary status.

• Explain all diagnostic tests and procedures to the patient and his family. Help the patient accept the limitations imposed by this disorder.

• Recommend genetic counseling for parents who want to have another child.

GENITAL HERPES

An acute inflammatory disease of the genitalia, genital herpes' prognosis varies, depending on the patient's age, the strength of his immune defenses, and the infection site. Primary genital herpes usually is self-limiting but may cause painful local or systemic disease.

In neonates and immunocompromised patients, such as those with acquired immunodeficiency syndrome, genital herpes is commonly severe, resulting in complications and high mortality.

Causes

Genital herpes usually is caused by infection with herpes simplex virus type 2, but some studies report increasing incidence of infection with herpes simplex virus type 1. This disease typically is transmitted through sexual intercourse, orogenital sexual activity, kissing, and hand-to-body contact.

Pregnant women may transmit the infection to neonates during vaginal delivery. Such transmitted infection may be localized (for instance, in the eyes) or disseminated and may be associated with central nervous system involvement.

Signs and symptoms

After a 3- to 7-day incubation period, fluid-filled vesicles appear, usually on the cervix (the primary infection site) and possibly on the labia, perianal skin, vulva, or vagina of the female and on the glans penis, foreskin, or penile shaft of the male. Extragenital lesions may appear on the mouth or anus.

In both males and females, the vesicles, usually painless at first, will rupture and develop into extensive, shallow, painful ulcers, with redness, marked edema, tender inguinal lymph nodes, and the characteristic yellow oozing centers.

Other features

Initial mucocutaneous infection also may cause fever, malaise, dysuria and, in females, leukorrhea. Rare complications — generally from extragenital lesions — include herpetic keratitis, which may lead to blindness, and potentially fatal herpetic encephalitis.

Diagnosis

In genital herpes, the diagnosis is based on the physical examination and patient history. Helpful (but nondiagnostic) measures include laboratory data showing increased antibody titers, smears of genital lesions showing atypical cells, and cytologic preparations (Tzanck test) that reveal giant cells.

The diagnosis can be confirmed by demonstration of the herpes simplex virus in vesicular fluid, using tissue culture techniques, or by antigen tests that identify specific antigens.

Treatment

Acyclovir has proved to be an effective treatment for genital herpes. I.V. administration may be required for patients who are hospitalized with severe genital herpes or for those who are immunocompromised and have a potentially life-threatening herpes infection.

Oral acyclovir may be prescribed for patients with first-time infections or recurrent outbreaks. Daily prophylaxis with acyclovir reduces the frequency of recurrences by at least 50%.

Special considerations

- Practice universal precautions.
- Encourage the patient to get adequate rest and nutrition and to keep the lesions dry.
- Advise the patient to avoid sexual intercourse during the active stage of this disease (while lesions are present) and to use condoms during all sexual exposures. Urge him to have his sexual partners seek medical examination.
- Advise the female patient to have a Papanicolaou test every 6 months.
- Explain to the infected pregnant patient the risk to her newborn child from vaginal delivery. Urge her to consider a cesarean delivery.
- Refer patients to the Herpes Resource Center, an American Social Health Association group, for support.

GENITAL WARTS

Also called venereal warts and condylomata acuminata, genital warts consist of papillomas with fibrous tissue overgrowth from the dermis and thickened epithelial coverings. They're uncommon before puberty or after menopause. Certain types of human papillomavirus (HPV) infections have been strongly associated with genital dysplasia and, over a period of years, with cervical neoplasia.

Causes

Infection with one of the more than 60 known strains of HPV causes condylomata acuminata. Genital warts are transmitted through sexual contact. They grow rapidly in the presence of heavy perspiration, poor hygiene, or pregnancy and often accompany other genital infections.

Signs and symptoms

After a 1- to 6-month incubation period (usually 2 months), genital warts develop on moist surfaces: in males, on the subpreputial sac, within the urethral meatus and, less commonly, on the penile shaft; in females, on the vulva and on vaginal and cervical walls.

In both sexes, papillomas spread to the perineum and the perianal area. These painless warts start as tiny red or pink swellings that grow (sometimes to 4″ [10 cm]) and become pedunculated. Typically, multiple swellings give them a cauliflower-like appearance. If infected, these warts become malodorous.

Most patients report no symptoms; a few complain of itching or pain.

Diagnosis

A dark-field examination of scrapings from wart cells shows marked vascularization of epidermal cells, which helps to differentiate genital warts from condylomata lata associated with second-stage syphilis. Applying 5% acetic acid (white vinegar) to the warts turns them white.

Treatment

The initial goal of treatment is to eradicate associated genital infections. Warts often resolve spontaneously. Topical drug therapy (10% to 25% podophyllum in tincture of benzoin, trichloroacetic acid, or bichloroacetic acid) removes small warts. (Podophyllum is contraindicated in pregnancy.)

Warts that are larger than 1″ (2.5 cm) are generally removed by carbon dioxide laser treatment, cryosurgery, or electrocautery. Treatment aims to remove exophytic warts and to ameliorate signs and symptoms. No therapy has proved effective in eradicating HPV. Relapse is common.

Special considerations

• Use universal precautions.

• Tell the patient to wash off the podophyllum with soap and water 4 to 6 hours after applying it. Recommend that he abstain from sexual intercourse or use a condom until healing is complete.

• Encourage the patient's sexual partners to be examined for HPV, human immunodeficiency virus, and other sexually transmitted diseases.

• Encourage annual Papanicolaou tests for women.

GIARDIASIS

Also known as *Giardia* enteritis and lambliasis, giardiasis is an infection of the small bowel caused by the symmetrical flagellate protozoan *Giardia lamblia*. A mild infection may not produce intestinal symptoms. In untreated giardiasis, symptoms wax and wane; with treatment, recovery is complete.

Causes

G. lamblia has two stages: the cystic stage and the trophozoite stage. Ingestion of *G. lamblia* cysts in fecally contaminated water or the fecal-oral transfer of cysts by an infected person results in giardiasis.

When cysts enter the small bowel, they become trophozoites and attach themselves with their sucking disks to the bowel's epithelial surface. Follow-

ing this, the trophozoites encyst again, travel down the colon, and are excreted. Unformed feces that pass quickly through the intestine may contain trophozoites as well as cysts.

Incidence

Giardiasis occurs worldwide but is most common in developing countries and other areas where sanitation and hygiene are poor. In the United States, giardiasis is most common in travelers who've recently returned from endemic areas and in campers who drink unpurified water from contaminated streams.

Probably because of frequent hand-to-mouth activity, children are more likely to become infected with *G. lamblia* than adults. In addition, hypogammaglobulinemia also appears to predispose persons to this disorder. Giardiasis doesn't confer immunity, so reinfections may occur. (See *Preventing and treating giardiasis,* page 358.)

Signs and symptoms

Attachment of *G. lamblia* to the intestinal lumen causes superficial mucosal invasion and destruction, inflammation, and irritation. All of these destructive effects decrease food transit time through the small intestine and result in malabsorption.

Such malabsorption results in chronic GI complaints—such as abdominal cramps—and pale, loose, greasy, malodorous, and frequent stools (from 2 to 10 daily) with concurrent nausea. Stools may contain mucus but not pus or blood. Chronic giardiasis may produce fatigue and weight loss in addition to these typical signs and symptoms.

Diagnosis

Suspect giardiasis when travelers to endemic areas or campers who may have drunk unpurified water develop symptoms.

☑ PREVENTING AND TREATING GIARDIASIS

• To keep from spreading giardiasis, teach good personal hygiene, particularly proper hand-washing technique.

• Warn travelers to endemic areas not to drink water or eat uncooked and unpeeled fruits or vegetables. (They may have been rinsed in contaminated water.) Prophylactic drug therapy isn't recommended. Advise campers to purify all stream water before drinking it.

• Inform the patient receiving metronidazole of the expected adverse effects of this drug: commonly headache, anorexia, and nausea; less commonly, vomiting, diarrhea, and abdominal cramps.

• Before administering metronidazole to a female patient with giardiasis, ask if she's pregnant — metronidazole is contraindicated during pregnancy.

• Warn patients against drinking alcoholic beverages while taking metronidazole because they may provoke a disulfiram-like reaction.

• When talking to family members and other suspected contacts, emphasize the importance of stool examination for *G. lamblia* cysts.

Actual diagnosis requires laboratory examination of a fresh stool specimen for cysts or examination of duodenal aspirate for trophozoites. A barium X-ray of the small bowel may show mucosal edema and barium segmentation. Diagnosis must also rule out other causes of diarrhea and malabsorption.

Treatment

Giardiasis responds readily to a 10-day course of metronidazole or a 7-day course of quinacrine and oral furazolidone. Severe diarrhea may require parenteral fluid replacement to prevent dehydration if oral fluid intake is inadequate.

Special considerations

• If hospitalization is required, apply enteric precautions. The patient will require a private room if he's a child or an incontinent adult.

• When caring for such a patient, pay strict attention to hand washing, particularly after handling feces. Quickly dispose of fecal material. (Normal sewage systems can remove and process infected feces adequately.)

• Report epidemic situations to the public health authorities.

• Teach patients about possible drug reactions and about how to avoid spreading or contracting giardiasis.

GLAUCOMA

A group of disorders characterized by an abnormally high intraocular pressure, glaucoma can damage the optic nerve. If untreated, it can lead to gradual vision loss and, ultimately, blindness.

Glaucoma occurs in several forms: chronic open-angle (primary), acute angle-closure, congenital (inherited as an autosomal recessive trait), and secondary to other causes.

Glaucoma affects 2% of the U.S. population over age 40 and accounts for 12% of all cases of new blindness in the U.S. Its incidence is highest among blacks. The prognosis is good with early treatment.

Causes

The cause of glaucoma varies according to the type of disorder:

• *Chronic open-angle glaucoma* results from overproduction of aqueous humor or obstructed outflow of aqueous humor through the trabecular meshwork or the canal of Schlemm. This form of glaucoma frequently runs in families and affects 90% of all patients with glaucoma.

• *Acute angle-closure (narrow-angle) glaucoma* results from obstructed outflow of aqueous humor due to anatomically narrow angles between the anterior iris and the posterior corneal surface, shallow anterior chambers, a thickened iris that causes angle closure on pupil dilation, or a bulging iris that presses on the trabeculae, closing the angle (peripheral anterior synechiae).

• *Secondary glaucoma* can result from uveitis, trauma, or drugs (such as steroids.) Neovascularization in the angle can result from vein occlusion or diabetes.

Signs and symptoms

Clinical features vary with the form of glaucoma.

Chronic open-angle glaucoma

Usually bilateral, chronic open-angle glaucoma has an insidious onset and a slowly progressive course. Symptoms appear late in the disease and include mild aching in the eyes, loss of peripheral vision, seeing halos around lights, and reduced visual acuity (especially at night) that's uncorrectable with glasses.

Acute angle-closure glaucoma

An ophthalmic emergency, acute angle-closure glaucoma typically has a rapid onset. Symptoms may include unilateral inflammation and pain, pressure over the eye, moderate pupil dilation that's nonreactive to light, a cloudy cornea, blurring and decreased visual acuity, photophobia, and seeing halos around lights.

Increased intraocular pressure (IOP) may induce nausea and vomiting, which may cause glaucoma to be misinterpreted as GI distress. Unless treated promptly, this acute form of glaucoma produces blindness in 3 to 5 days.

Diagnosis

Loss of peripheral vision and disk changes confirm that glaucoma is present. Relevant diagnostic tests include the following:

• *Tonometry* (using an applanation, Schiøtz, or air-puff tonometer) measures IOP and provides a baseline for reference.

Normal IOP ranges between 8 and 21 mm Hg. However, patients who fall in this normal range can develop signs and symptoms of glaucoma. Furthermore, patients who have abnormally high pressure may have no clinical effects.

Fingertip tension is another way to measure IOP. On gentle palpation of closed eyelids, one eye feels harder than the other in acute closed-angle glaucoma.

• *Slit-lamp examination* provides a look at the anterior structures of the eye, including the cornea, iris, and lens.

• *Gonioscopy,* by determining the angle of the anterior chamber of the eye, allows differentiation between chronic open-angle glaucoma and acute angle-closure glaucoma. The angle is normal in chronic open-angle glaucoma. However, in older patients partial closure of the angle may also occur, so two forms of glaucoma may coexist.

• *Ophthalmoscopy* provides a look at the fundus, where cupping and atrophy of the optic disk are visible in chronic open-angle glaucoma. These

CUPPING OF THE OPTIC DISK

Ophthalmoscopy and slit-lamp examination show cupping of the optic disk, which is characteristic of chronic glaucoma.

changes appear later in chronic closed-angle glaucoma, if the disease is not brought under control. (For more information, see *Cupping of the optic disk.*) A pale disk appears in acute closed-angle glaucoma.

• *Perimetry or visual field tests* help evaluate the extent of chronic open-angle deterioration by determining peripheral vision loss.

• *Fundus photography* can monitor the disk for any changes.

Treatment

Drug therapy is the treatment of choice for chronic open-angle glaucoma. If this fails, argon laser trabeculoplasty (ALT) or trabeculectomy is performed. Acute angle-closure glaucoma is treated with drugs, laser iridotomy, or surgical peripheral iridectomy.

Drug therapy for open-angle glaucoma

For chronic open-angle glaucoma, treatment initially decreases aqueous humor production through beta blockers, such as timolol (contraindicated for asthmatic patients or those with bradycardia) or betaxolol, a beta$_1$-blocker; epinephrine to lower IOP; or diuretics such as acetazolamide.

Drug treatment also includes miotic eyedrops, such as pilocarpine, to facilitate the outflow of aqueous humor. Patients who are unresponsive to drug therapy may be candidates for an iridectomy, a surgical filtering procedure that creates an opening for aqueous outflow.

Argon laser trabeculoplasty

In ALT, an argon laser beam is focused on the trabecular meshwork of an open angle. This produces a thermal burn that changes the surface of the meshwork and increases the outflow of aqueous humor.

Trabeculectomy

In trabeculectomy, a flap of sclera is dissected free to expose the trabecular meshwork. Then this discrete tissue block is removed and a peripheral iridectomy is performed. This produces an opening for aqueous outflow under the conjunctiva, creating a filtering bleb.

Angle-closure glaucoma treatment

This condition is an ocular emergency requiring immediate treatment to lower the high IOP. If pressure doesn't decrease with drug therapy, laser iridotomy or surgical peripheral iridectomy must be performed promptly to save the patient's vision.

Iridectomy relieves pressure by excising part of the iris to reestablish aqueous humor outflow. A prophylactic iridectomy is performed a few days later on the other eye to prevent an acute episode of glaucoma in the normal eye.

Preoperative drug therapy lowers IOP with acetazolamide, pilocarpine (which constricts the pupil, forcing the iris away from the trabeculae, allowing fluid to escape), and I.V. mannitol (20%) or oral glycerin (50%) to force fluid from the eye by making the blood hypertonic. Severe pain may necessitate narcotic analgesics.

Special considerations

• Stress the importance of meticulous compliance with prescribed drug therapy to prevent disk changes, loss of vision, and an increase in IOP.
• For the patient with acute angle-closure glaucoma, give medications and prepare him physically and psychologically for laser iridotomy or surgery.
• Postoperative care after peripheral iridectomy includes cycloplegic eyedrops to relax the ciliary muscle and to decrease inflammation, thus preventing adhesions. Cycloplegics must be used only in the affected eye. The use of these drops in the normal eye may precipitate an attack of acute angle-closure glaucoma in this eye, threatening the patient's residual vision.
• Encourage ambulation immediately after surgery.
• Following surgical filtering, postoperative care includes dilation and topical steroids to rest the pupil.
• Stress the importance of glaucoma screening for early detection and prevention. All people over age 35, especially those with a family history of glaucoma, should have an annual tonometric examination.

LIFE-THREATENING DISORDER

GLOMERULONEPHRITIS, ACUTE POSTSTREPTOCOCCAL

Also called acute glomerulonephritis, acute poststreptococcal glomerulonephritis (APSGN) is a relatively common bilateral inflammation of the glomeruli. It follows a streptococcal infection of the respiratory tract or, less often, a skin infection, such as impetigo.

APSGN is most common in boys ages 3 to 7 but can occur at any age. Up to 95% of children and up to 70% of adults with APSGN recover fully; the rest may progress to chronic renal failure within months.

Causes

APSGN results from the entrapment and collection of antigen-antibody (which is produced as an immunologic mechanism in response to streptococcus) in the glomerular capillary membranes, inducing inflammatory damage and impeding glomerular function.

Sometimes, the immune complement further damages the glomerular membrane. The damaged and inflamed glomerulus loses the ability to be selectively permeable, and allows red blood cells (RBCs) and proteins to filter through as the glomerular filtration rate falls. Uremic poisoning may result.

Signs and symptoms
APSGN begins within 1 to 3 weeks after untreated pharyngitis. Symptoms are mild to moderate edema, oliguria (less than 400 ml/24 hours), proteinuria, azotemia, hematuria, and fatigue.

Mild to severe hypertension may result from either sodium or water retention (due to decreased glomerular filtration rate) or inappropriate renin release. Congestive heart failure from hypervolemia leads to pulmonary edema.

Diagnosis
A detailed patient history, assessment of clinical symptoms, and laboratory tests are needed to diagnose this disease. The following tests support the diagnosis:
• *Urinalysis* typically reveals proteinuria and hematuria. RBCs, white blood cells, and mixed cell casts are common in urinary sediment.
• *Blood tests* show elevated serum creatinine levels, a low creatinine clearance, and impaired glomerular filtration.
• *Elevated antistreptolysin-O titers* (in 80% of patients), *elevated streptozyme and anti-DNase B titers, and low serum complement levels* verify recent streptococcal infection.
• *Throat culture* may also show group A beta-hemolytic streptococci.
• *Renal ultrasound* may show a normal or slightly enlarged kidney.

• *Renal biopsy* may confirm the diagnosis in a patient with APSGN or assess renal tissue status.

Treatment
The goals of treatment are relief of symptoms and prevention of complications. Vigorous supportive care includes bed rest, fluid and dietary sodium restrictions, and correction of electrolyte imbalances (possibly with dialysis, although this is rarely necessary).

Therapy may include diuretics, such as metolazone or furosemide, to reduce extracellular fluid overload, and an antihypertensive such as hydralazine. The use of antibiotics to prevent secondary infection or transmission to others is controversial.

Special considerations
• APSGN usually resolves within 2 weeks, so patient care is primarily supportive.
• Check vital signs and electrolyte values. Monitor intake and output and daily weight. Assess renal function daily through serum creatinine and blood urea nitrogen levels and urine creatinine clearance. Watch for signs of acute renal failure (oliguria, azotemia, and acidosis).
• Consult the dietitian to provide a diet high in calories and low in protein, sodium, potassium, and fluids.
• Protect the debilitated patient against secondary infection by providing good nutrition, using good hygienic technique, and preventing contact with infected persons.
• Bed rest is necessary during the acute phase. Allow the patient to gradually resume normal activities as symptoms subside.
• Provide emotional support for the patient and family. If the patient's on dialysis, explain the procedure fully.
• Advise the patient with a history of chronic upper respiratory tract infec-

tions to immediately report signs of infection (fever, sore throat).

• Tell the patient that follow-up examinations are necessary to detect chronic renal failure. Stress the need for regular blood pressure, urinary protein, and renal function assessments during the convalescent months to detect recurrence. After APSGN, gross hematuria may recur during nonspecific viral infections; abnormal urinary findings may persist for years.

• Encourage pregnant women with a history of APSGN to have frequent medical evaluations because pregnancy further stresses the kidneys and increases the risk of chronic renal failure.

GLOMERULONEPHRITIS, CHRONIC

A slowly progressive disease, chronic glomerulonephritis is characterized by inflammation of the glomeruli, which results in sclerosis, scarring, and eventual renal failure.

This condition usually remains subclinical until the progressive phase begins, marked by proteinuria, cylindruria (presence of granular tube casts), and hematuria. By the time it produces symptoms, chronic glomerulonephritis is usually irreversible.

Causes
Common causes of chronic glomerulonephritis include primary renal disorders, such as membranoproliferative glomerulonephritis, membranous glomerulopathy, focal glomerulosclerosis, rapidly progressive glomerulonephritis, and, less often, poststreptococcal glomerulonephritis.

Systemic disorders that may cause chronic glomerulonephritis include lupus erythematosus, Goodpasture's syndrome, or hemolytic-uremic syndrome.

Signs and symptoms
Chronic glomerulonephritis usually develops insidiously and asymptomatically, often over many years. At any time, however, it may suddenly become progressive, producing nephrotic syndrome, hypertension, proteinuria, and hematuria.

Late stages
In late stages of progressive chronic glomerulonephritis, it may accelerate to uremic symptoms, such as azotemia, nausea, vomiting, pruritus, dyspnea, malaise, and fatigability. Mild to severe edema and anemia may accompany these symptoms.

Severe hypertension may cause cardiac hypertrophy, leading to congestive heart failure (CHF), and may accelerate the development of advanced renal failure, eventually necessitating dialysis or transplantation.

Diagnosis
Patient history and physical assessment seldom suggest glomerulonephritis. Suspicion develops from:

• *urinalysis,* which reveals proteinuria, hematuria, cylindruria, and red blood cell casts

• *rising blood urea nitrogen and serum creatinine levels,* which indicate advanced renal insufficiency

• *X-ray or ultrasonography,* which shows smaller kidneys

• *kidney biopsy,* which identifies underlying disease and provides data needed to guide therapy.

Treatment
Effective treatment, essentially nonspecific and symptomatic, aims to control hypertension with antihyper-

tensives and a sodium-restricted diet, to correct fluid and electrolyte imbalances through restrictions and replacement, to reduce edema with diuretics such as furosemide, and to prevent CHF.

Treatment may also include antibiotics (for symptomatic urinary tract infections), dialysis, or transplantation.

Special considerations
• Patient care is primarily supportive, focusing on continual observation and sound patient teaching.
• Accurately monitor vital signs, intake and output, and daily weight to evaluate fluid retention. Observe for signs of fluid, electrolyte, and acid-base imbalances.
• Ask the dietitian to plan low-sodium, high-calorie meals with adequate protein.
• Administer medications and provide good skin care (because of pruritus and edema) and oral hygiene. Instruct the patient to continue taking prescribed antihypertensives as scheduled, even if he's feeling better, and to report any adverse effects.
• Advise the patient to take diuretics in the morning so he won't have to disrupt his sleep to void, and teach him how to assess ankle edema.
• Warn the patient to report signs of infection, particularly urinary tract infection, and to avoid contact with people who have infections. Urge follow-up examinations to assess renal function.
• Help the patient adjust to this illness by encouraging him to express his feelings. Explain all necessary procedures beforehand, and answer the patient's questions about them.

GLYCOGEN STORAGE DISEASES

Consisting of at least eight distinct errors of metabolism, all inherited, glycogen storage diseases alter the synthesis or degradation of glycogen, the form in which glucose is stored in the body.

Normally, muscle and liver cells store glycogen. Muscle glycogen is used in muscle contraction; liver glycogen can be converted into free glucose, which can then diffuse out of the liver cells to increase blood glucose levels.

Glycogen storage diseases manifest as dysfunctions of the liver, the heart, or the musculoskeletal system. Symptoms vary from mild and easily controlled hypoglycemia to severe organ involvement that may lead to cardiac and respiratory failure.

Causes
Almost all glycogen storage diseases (types I through V and type VII) are transmitted as autosomal recessive traits. The mode of transmission of type VI is unknown; type VIII may be an X-linked trait.

The most common glycogen storage disease is type I—von Gierke's, or hepatorenal glycogen storage disease—which results from a deficiency of the liver enzyme glucose-6-phosphatase. This enzyme converts glucose-6-phosphate into free glucose and is necessary for the release of stored glycogen and glucose into the bloodstream to relieve hypoglycemia.

Infants may die of acidosis before age 2; if they survive past this age, with proper treatment, they may grow normally and live to adulthood, with only minimal hepatomegaly. However, there's a danger of adenomatous liver nodules, which may be premalignant.

Signs and symptoms

Primary clinical features of the liver glycogen storage diseases (types I, III, IV, VI, and VIII) are hepatomegaly and rapid onset of hypoglycemia and ketosis when food is withheld. Symptoms of the muscle glycogen storage diseases (types II, V, and VII) include poor muscle tone; type II may result in death from heart failure.

In addition, type I may produce the following symptoms:
• *infants:* acidosis, hyperlipidemia, GI bleeding, coma
• *children:* low resistance to infection and, without proper treatment, short stature
• *adolescents:* gouty arthritis and nephropathy; chronic tophaceous gout; bleeding (especially epistaxis); small superficial vessels visible in skin, due to impaired platelet function; and fat deposits in cheeks, buttocks, and subcutaneous tissues.

Other symptoms include poor muscle tone; enlarged kidneys; xanthomas over extensor surfaces of arms and legs; steatorrhea; multiple, bilateral, yellow lesions in fundi; and osteoporosis, probably secondary to negative calcium balance. Proper treatment of glycogen storage disease should prevent all of these effects.

Diagnosis

Liver and muscle biopsies are the key tests in diagnosing type I glycogen storage disease:
• *Liver biopsy* confirms the diagnosis by showing normal glycogen synthetase and phosphorylase enzyme activities but reduced or absent glucose-6-phosphatase activity. Glycogen structure is normal, but amounts are elevated.
• *Laboratory studies* of plasma demonstrate low glucose levels but high levels of free fatty acids, triglycerides, cholesterol, and uric acid. Serum analysis reveals high pyruvic acid levels and high lactic acid levels. Diagnoses can be made prenatally for types II, III, and IV.
• *Injection of glucagon or epinephrine* increases pyruvic and lactic acid levels but doesn't increase blood glucose levels. The glucose tolerance test curve typically shows depletional hypoglycemia and reduced insulin output. An intrauterine diagnosis is possible.

Treatment

For type I, the aims of treatment are to maintain glucose homeostasis and prevent secondary consequences of hypoglycemia through frequent feedings and a constant nocturnal nasogastric (NG) drip with an enteral nutrition formula or dextrose. Treatment includes a low-fat diet, with normal amounts of protein and calories; carbohydrates should contain glucose or glucose polymers only.

Therapy for type III includes frequent feedings and a high-protein diet. Type IV requires a high-protein, high-calorie diet; bed rest; diuretics; sodium restriction; and paracentesis, if necessary, to relieve ascites.

Types V and VII require no treatment except avoidance of strenuous exercise. No treatment is necessary for types VI and VIII, and no effective treatment exists for type II.

Special considerations

When managing type I disease:
• Advise the patient or parents to include carbohydrate foods containing mainly starch in his diet and to sweeten foods with glucose only.
• Before discharge, teach the patient or a family member how to pass an NG tube, use a pump with alarm capacity, monitor blood glucose levels with glucose reagent strips, and recognize symptoms of hypoglycemia.

• Watch for signs of infection (fever, chills, myalgia) and of hepatic encephalopathy (mental confusion, stupor, asterixis, coma) due to increased blood ammonia levels.

When managing other types:

• *Type II:* Explain test procedures, such as electromyography and electroencephalography, thoroughly.

• *Type III:* Instruct the patient to eat a high-protein diet (eggs, nuts, fish, meat, poultry, and cheese).

• *Type IV:* Watch for signs of hepatic failure (nausea, vomiting, irregular bowel function, clay-colored stools, right upper quadrant pain, jaundice, dehydration, electrolyte imbalance, edema, and changes in mental status, progressing to coma).

When caring for patients with type II, III, or IV glycogen storage disease, offer the parents reassurance and emotional support. Recommend and arrange for genetic counseling, if appropriate.

• *Types V through VIII:* Care for these patients is minimal. Explain the disorder to the patient and his family, and help them accept the limitations imposed by his particular type of glycogen storage disease.

GOITER

Nontoxic or simple goiter — thyroid gland enlargement not caused by inflammation or a neoplasm — is commonly classified as endemic or sporadic.

Endemic goiter usually results from inadequate dietary intake of iodine associated with such factors as iodine-depleted soil or malnutrition. *Sporadic goiter* follows ingestion of certain drugs or foods.

Simple goiter affects more females than males, especially during adolescence, pregnancy, and menopause, when the demand on the body for thyroid hormone increases. Sporadic goiter affects no particular population segment. With appropriate treatment, the prognosis is good for either type of goiter.

Causes

Simple goiter occurs when the thyroid gland can't secrete enough thyroid hormone to meet metabolic requirements. As a result, the thyroid gland enlarges to compensate for inadequate hormone synthesis. Such compensation usually overcomes mild to moderate hormonal impairment.

Because thyroid-stimulating hormone (TSH) levels are generally within normal limits in patients with simple goiter, goitrogenicity probably results from impaired intrathyroidal hormone synthesis and depletion of glandular iodine, which increases the thyroid gland's sensitivity to TSH. However, increased levels of TSH may be transient and therefore missed.

Endemic goiter

Endemic goiter usually results from inadequate dietary intake of iodine, which leads to inadequate secretion of thyroid hormone. The use of iodized salt prevents this deficiency.

Sporadic goiter

Sporadic goiter commonly results from the ingestion of large amounts of goitrogenic foods or the use of goitrogenic drugs.

Goitrogenic foods contain agents that decrease thyroxine (T_4) production. Such foods include rutabagas, cabbage, soybeans, peanuts, peaches, peas, strawberries, spinach, and radishes.

Goitrogenic drugs include propylthiouracil, iodides, phenylbutazone, para-aminosalicylic acid, cobalt, and lithium. In a pregnant woman, such

---

---

substances may cross the placenta and affect the fetus.

Both types
Inherited defects may be responsible for insufficient T_4 synthesis or impaired iodine metabolism. Because families tend to congregate in a single geographic area, this familial factor may contribute to the incidence of both endemic and sporadic goiters.

Signs and symptoms
Thyroid enlargement may range from a mildly enlarged gland to a massive, multinodular goiter. Because simple goiter doesn't alter the patient's metabolic state, clinical features arise solely from enlargement of the thyroid gland.

The patient may complain of respiratory distress and dysphagia from compression of the trachea and esophagus, and swelling and distention of the neck.

In addition, large goiters may obstruct venous return, produce venous engorgement and in rare cases, induce development of collateral venous circulation in the chest. Such obstruction may cause dizziness or syncope (Pemberton's sign) when the patient raises her arms above her head.

Diagnosis
An accurate diagnosis of simple goiter requires a thorough patient history and physical examination to rule out disorders with similar clinical effects, such as Graves' disease, Hashimoto's thyroiditis, and thyroid carcinoma. A detailed patient history also may reveal goitrogenic medications or foods or endemic influence.

The results of diagnostic laboratory tests include the following:
• *TSH:* high or normal
• *Serum T_4 concentrations:* low-normal or normal
• *Iodine 131 uptake:* normal or increased (50% of the dose at 24 hours).

Treatment
The goal of treatment is to reduce thyroid hyperplasia. The following measures are used:
• Exogenous thyroid hormone replacement with levothyroxine is the treatment of choice; it inhibits TSH secretion and allows the gland to rest. (See *Patient instructions in goiter.*)
• Small doses of iodine (Lugol's or potassium iodide solution) commonly relieve goiter that's due to iodine deficiency. Sporadic goiter requires avoidance of known goitrogenic drugs and foods.

• A large goiter that's unresponsive to treatment may require subtotal thyroidectomy.

Special considerations
• Measure the patient's neck circumference daily to check for progressive thyroid gland enlargement. Also check for the development of hard nodules in the gland, which may indicate carcinoma.
• Monitor the patient taking goitrogenic drugs for signs of sporadic goiter.
• Teach the patient about iodized salt, medications, and the symptoms of thyrotoxicosis.

GONORRHEA

A common venereal disease, gonorrhea is an infection of the genitourinary tract (especially the urethra and cervix) and, occasionally, the rectum, pharynx, and eyes. Untreated gonorrhea can spread through the blood to the joints, tendons, meninges, and endocardium; in females, it can also lead to chronic pelvic inflammatory disease (PID) and sterility.

After adequate treatment, the prognosis in both males and females is excellent, although reinfection is common. Gonorrhea is especially prevalent among young people and people with multiple partners, particularly between ages 19 and 25.

Causes
Transmission of *Neisseria gonorrhoeae,* the organism that causes gonorrhea, almost exclusively follows sexual contact with an infected person. Children born of infected mothers can contract gonococcal ophthalmia neonatorum during passage through the birth canal. Children and adults with gonorrhea can contract gonococcal conjunctivitis by touching their eyes with contaminated hands.

Signs and symptoms
Although many infected males may be asymptomatic, after a 3- to 6-day incubation period, some develop symptoms of urethritis, including dysuria and purulent urethral discharge, with redness and swelling at the site of infection. Most infected females remain asymptomatic but may develop inflammation and a greenish-yellow discharge from the cervix—the most common gonorrheal symptoms in females.

Other clinical features vary according to the site involved:
• *urethra:* dysuria, urinary frequency and incontinence, purulent discharge, itching, red and edematous meatus
• *vulva:* occasional itching, burning, and pain due to exudate from an adjacent infected area. Vulval symptoms tend to be more severe before puberty or after menopause.
• *vagina* (most common site in children over age 1): engorgement, redness, swelling, and profuse purulent discharge
• *pelvis:* severe pelvic and lower abdominal pain, muscular rigidity, tenderness, and abdominal distention. As the infection spreads, nausea, vomiting, fever, and tachycardia may develop in patients with salpingitis or PID.
• *liver:* right upper quadrant pain in patients with perihepatitis.

Other possible symptoms include pharyngitis, tonsillitis, and rectal burning, itching, and bloody mucopurulent discharge.

Gonococcal septicemia
Gonococcal septicemia is more common in females than in males. Its characteristic signs include tender papillary skin lesions on the hands and feet;

these lesions may be pustular, hemorrhagic, or necrotic.

Gonococcal septicemia may also produce migratory polyarthralgia, and polyarthritis and tenosynovitis of the wrists, fingers, knees, or ankles. Untreated septic arthritis leads to progressive joint destruction.

Eye involvement

Signs of gonococcal ophthalmia neonatorum include lid edema, bilateral conjunctival infection, and abundant purulent discharge 2 to 3 days after birth. Adult conjunctivitis, most common in men, causes unilateral conjunctival redness and swelling. Untreated gonococcal conjunctivitis can progress to corneal ulceration and blindness.

Diagnosis

A culture from the site of infection (urethra, cervix, rectum, or pharynx), grown on a Thayer-Martin or Transgrow medium, usually establishes the diagnosis by isolating the organism. A Gram stain showing gram-negative diplococci supports the diagnosis and may be sufficient to confirm gonorrhea in males.

Confirmation of gonococcal arthritis requires identification of gramnegative diplococci on smears made from joint fluid and skin lesions. Complement fixation and immunofluorescent assays of serum reveal antibody titers four times the normal rate. Culture of conjunctival scrapings confirms gonococcal conjunctivitis.

Treatment

For adults and adolescents, the recommended treatment for uncomplicated gonorrhea caused by susceptible non-penicillinase-producing *N. gonorrhoeae* is a single 125-mg dose of ceftriaxone I.M.; for presumptive treatment of concurrent *Chlamydia tra-*

chomatis infection, 100 mg doxycycline P.O. twice daily for 7 days.

A single dose of ceftriaxone and erythromycin for 7 days is recommended for pregnant patients and those allergic to penicillin.

The recommended initial regimen for disseminated gonococcal infection in adults and adolescents is 1 g ceftriaxone I.M. or I.V. every 24 hours, or for patients allergic to beta-lactam drugs, 2 g spectinomycin I.M. every 12 hours.

All regimens should be continued for 24 to 48 hours after improvement begins; then therapy may be switched to one of the following regimens to complete a full week of antimicrobial therapy: 400 mg cefixime P.O. twice daily, or 500 mg ciprofloxacin P.O. twice daily. Ciprofloxacin is contraindicated for children, adolescents under age 18, and pregnant or lactating women.

Treatment of gonococcal conjunctivitis requires a single 1-g dose of ceftriaxone I.M. and lavage of the infected eye with saline solution once.

Routine instillation of 1% silver nitrate or erythromycin drops into neonates' eyes has greatly reduced the incidence of gonococcal ophthalmia neonatorum.

Special considerations

• Before treatment, establish whether the patient has any drug sensitivities, and watch closely for adverse drug reactions during therapy.
• Warn the patient that until cultures prove negative, he's still infectious and can transmit gonococcal infection.
• Practice universal precautions.
• In the patient with gonococcal arthritis, apply moist heat to ease pain in affected joints.
• Urge the patient to inform sexual contacts of his infection so that they can seek treatment, even if cultures are negative. Advise them to avoid sexual

intercourse until treatment is complete.

• Report all cases of gonorrhea to local public health authorities for follow-up on sexual contacts. Examine and test all people exposed to gonorrhea as well as newborn infants of infected mothers.

• Routinely instill two drops of 1% silver nitrate or erythromycin in the eyes of all neonates immediately after birth. Check newborn infants of infected mothers for any signs of infection. Take specimens for culture from the infant's eyes, pharynx, and rectum.

• To prevent gonorrhea, tell patients to avoid anyone even *suspected* of being infected, to use condoms during intercourse, to wash their genitalia with soap and water before and after intercourse, and to avoid sharing washcloths or douche equipment.

• Report all cases of gonorrhea in children to child abuse authorities.

GOODPASTURE'S SYNDROME

In Goodpasture's syndrome, hemoptysis and rapidly progressive glomerulonephritis follow the deposition of antibodies against the alveolar and glomerular basement membranes. This syndrome may occur at any age but is most common in men between ages 20 and 30. The prognosis improves with aggressive immunosuppressive and antibiotic therapy and with dialysis or kidney transplantation.

Causes

The cause of Goodpasture's syndrome is unknown. Although some cases have been associated with exposure to hydrocarbons or type 2 influenza, many have no precipitating events. The high incidence of the human leukocyte antigen HLA-DRw2 in these patients suggests a genetic predisposition.

Abnormal production and deposition of antibodies against the glomerular basement membrane (GBM) and the alveolar basement membrane (ABM) activates the complement (C) and inflammatory responses, resulting in glomerular and alveolar tissue damage.

Signs and symptoms

Goodpasture's syndrome may initially cause malaise, fatigue, and pallor associated with severe iron deficiency anemia. Pulmonary findings range from slight dyspnea and cough with blood-tinged sputum to hemoptysis and frank pulmonary hemorrhage. Subclinical pulmonary bleeding may precede overt hemorrhage and renal disease by months or years.

Usually, renal findings are more subtle, although some patients note hematuria and peripheral edema.

Diagnosis

Confirmation of Goodpasture's syndrome requires measurement of circulating anti-GBM antibody by radioimmunoassay and linear staining of GBM and ABM by immunofluorescence. The following test results support the diagnosis:

• *Immunofluorescence of ABM* shows linear deposition of immunoglobulin, as well as C3 and fibrinogen.

• *Immunofluorescence of GBM* also shows linear deposition of immunoglobulin combined with detection of circulating anti-GBM antibodies. This finding distinguishes Goodpasture's from other pulmonary-renal syndromes, such as Wegener's granulomatosis, polyarteritis, and systemic lupus erythematosus.

• *Lung biopsy* shows interstitial and intra-alveolar hemorrhage with hemosiderin-laden macrophages.

• *Chest X-ray* reveals pulmonary infiltrates in a diffuse, nodular pattern.

• *Renal biopsy* frequently shows focal necrotic lesions and cellular crescents.

• *Serum creatinine and blood urea nitrogen (BUN) levels* typically increase to two to three times the normal rate.

• *Urinalysis* may reveal red blood cells and cellular casts, which typify glomerular inflammation. Granular casts and proteinuria may also be observed.

Treatment
The aim of treatment is to remove antibody by plasmapheresis and to suppress antibody production with immunosuppressive drugs. Patients with renal failure may benefit from dialysis or transplantation. Aggressive ultrafiltration helps relieve pulmonary edema that may aggravate pulmonary hemorrhage. High-dose I.V. steroids also help control pulmonary hemorrhage.

Special considerations
• Promote adequate oxygenation by elevating the head of the bed and administering humidified oxygen. Encourage the patient to conserve his energy.

• Assess respirations and breath sounds regularly; note sputum quantity and quality.

• Monitor vital signs, arterial blood gas levels, hematocrit, and coagulation studies.

• Transfuse blood and administer steroids as needed. Observe closely for drug adverse effects.

• Assess renal function by monitoring symptoms, intake and output, daily weight, creatinine clearance, and BUN and creatinine levels.

• Teach the patient and his family what signs and symptoms to expect and how to relieve them. Carefully describe other treatment measures such as dialysis.

GOUT

Gouty arthritis, or gout, is a metabolic disease marked by urate deposits in the joints, which cause painfully arthritic joints. It can strike any joint but favors those in the feet and legs. *Primary gout* usually occurs in men older than age 30 and in postmenopausal women. *Secondary gout* occurs in older people.

Gout follows an intermittent course and often leaves patients totally free of symptoms for years between attacks. Gout can lead to chronic disability or incapacitation and, rarely, severe hypertension and progressive renal disease. The prognosis is good with treatment.

Causes
Although the exact cause of primary gout remains unknown, it seems linked to a genetic defect in purine metabolism, which causes overproduction of uric acid (hyperuricemia), retention of uric acid, or both.

In secondary gout, which develops during the course of another disease (such as obesity, diabetes mellitus, hypertension, sickle cell anemia, and renal disease), hyperuricemia results from the breakdown of nucleic acid.

Secondary gout can also follow drug therapy, especially use of hydrochlorothiazide or pyrazinamide, which interferes with urate excretion. Increased concentration of uric acid leads to urate deposits, called tophi, in joints or tissues, causing local necrosis or fibrosis.

Pseudogout
Another condition — pseudogout — results when calcium pyrophosphate crystals collect in the periarticular joint structures. (See *Pseudogout,* page 372.)

PSEUDOGOUT

Also called calcium pyrophosphate disease, pseudogout results when calcium pyrophosphate crystals collect in periarticular joint structures. Without treatment, it leads to permanent joint damage in about half of the patients it affects, most of whom are elderly.

Signs and symptoms

Like gout, pseudogout causes abrupt joint pain and swelling — most commonly affecting the knee, wrist, ankle, and other peripheral joints. These recurrent, self-limiting attacks may be triggered by stress, trauma, surgery, severe dieting, thiazide therapy, and alcohol abuse. Associated symptoms are similar to those of rheumatoid arthritis.

Diagnosis and treatment

In pseudogout, the diagnosis depends on joint aspirations and a synovial biopsy to detect calcium pyrophosphate crystals. X-rays reveal calcific densities in the fibrocartilage and linear markings along bone ends. Blood tests may detect an underlying endocrine or metabolic disorder.

Effective treatment of pseudogout may include joint aspiration to relieve fluid pressure; instillation of steroids; administration of analgesics, phenylbutazone, salicylates, or other nonsteroidal anti-inflammatories; and, if appropriate, treatment of the underlying endocrine or metabolic disorder.

Signs and symptoms

Gout develops in four stages: asymptomatic, acute, intercritical, and chronic.

Asymptomatic stage

In asymptomatic gout, serum urate levels rise but produce no symptoms.

Acute stage

As the disease progresses, it may cause hypertension or nephrolithiasis, with severe back pain. The first acute attack strikes suddenly and peaks quickly. Although it generally involves only one or a few joints, this initial attack is extremely painful. Affected joints appear hot, tender, inflamed, dusky-red, or cyanotic.

The metatarsophalangeal joint of the great toe usually becomes inflamed first (podagra), then the instep, ankle, heel, knee, or wrist joints. Sometimes a low-grade fever is present. Mild acute attacks often subside quickly but tend to recur at irregular intervals. Severe attacks may persist for days or weeks.

Intercritical stage

Symptom-free intervals between gout attacks are called intercritical periods. Most patients have a second attack within 6 months to 2 years, but in some the second attack is delayed for 5 to 10 years. Delayed attacks are more common in those who are untreated and tend to be longer and more severe than initial attacks.

Such attacks are also polyarticular, invariably affecting joints in the feet and legs, and are sometimes accompanied by fever. A migratory attack sequentially strikes various joints and the Achilles tendon, and is associated with either subdeltoid or olecranon bursitis.

Chronic stage

Eventually, chronic polyarticular gout sets in. This final, unremitting stage of the disease (chronic or tophaceous gout) is marked by persistent painful polyarthritis with large, subcutaneous tophi in cartilage, synovial membranes, tendons, and soft tissue.

Tophi form in fingers, hands, knees, feet, ulnar sides of the forearms, helix of the ear, Achilles tendons and, rarely, in internal organs, such as the kidneys and myocardium.

The skin over the tophus may ulcerate and release a chalky, white exudate or pus. Chronic inflammation and tophaceous deposits precipitate secondary joint degeneration, with eventual erosions, deformity, and disability. Kidney involvement, with associated tubular damage, leads to chronic renal dysfunction. Hypertension and albuminuria occur in some patients; urolithiasis is common.

Diagnosis

The presence of monosodium urate monohydrate crystals in synovial fluid taken from an inflamed joint or tophous establishes the diagnosis. Aspiration of synovial fluid (arthrocentesis) or of tophaceous material reveals needlelike intracellular crystals of sodium urate.

Although hyperuricemia isn't specifically diagnostic of gout, serum uric acid is above normal. Urinary uric acid is usually higher in secondary gout than in primary gout.

Initially, X-ray examinations are normal. However, in chronic gout, X-rays show damage of the articular cartilage and subchondral bone. Outward displacement of the overhanging margin from the bone contour characterizes gout.

Treatment

Correct management seeks to terminate an acute attack, reduce hyperuricemia, and prevent recurrence, complications, and the formation of renal calculi.

Acute gout

Treatment for the patient with acute gout consists of bed rest; immobilization and protection of the inflamed, painful joints; and local application of heat or cold.

Analgesics, such as acetaminophen, relieve the pain associated with mild attacks, but acute inflammation requires concomitant treatment with colchicine (oral or I.V.) every hour for 8 hours until the pain subsides or until nausea, vomiting, cramping, or diarrhea develops.

Phenylbutazone or indomethacin in therapeutic doses may be used instead but is less specific. Resistant inflammation may require corticosteroids or corticotropin (I.V. drip or I.M.), or joint aspiration and an intra-articular corticosteroid injection.

Chronic gout

Treatment of chronic gout consists of the following:

• A continuing maintenance dosage of allopurinol is often given to suppress uric acid formation or control uric acid levels, preventing further attacks. However, this powerful drug should be used cautiously in patients with renal failure.

• Colchicine prevents recurrent acute attacks until uric acid returns to its normal level, but it doesn't affect the acid level. Uricosuric agents — probenecid and sulfinpyrazone — promote uric acid excretion and inhibit accumulation of uric acid, but their value is limited in patients with renal impairment. These medications should not be given to patients with urinary calculi.

• Other therapeutic measures include a few dietary restrictions, primarily the avoidance of alcohol and purine-rich foods. Obese patients should try to lose weight because obesity puts additional stress on painful joints.

• In some cases, surgery may be necessary to improve joint function or correct deformities. Tophi must be excised and drained if they become infected or ulcerated. They can also be excised to prevent ulceration, improve the patient's appearance, or make it easier for him to wear shoes or gloves.

Special considerations
• Encourage bed rest, but use a bed cradle to keep bedcovers off extremely sensitive, inflamed joints.
• Give pain medication, as needed, especially during acute attacks. Apply hot or cold packs to inflamed joints. Administer anti-inflammatory medication and other drugs, and watch for adverse effects. Be alert for GI disturbances with colchicine.
• Urge the patient to drink plenty of fluids (up to 2 L/day) to prevent formation of renal calculi.
• When forcing fluids, record intake and output accurately. Be sure to monitor serum uric acid levels regularly. Alkalinize urine with sodium bicarbonate or another agent as needed.
• Watch for acute gout attacks 24 to 96 hours after surgery. Even minor surgery can precipitate an attack. Before and after surgery, administer colchicine to help prevent gout attacks as needed.
• Make sure the patient understands the importance of having serum uric acid levels checked periodically. Tell him to avoid high-purine foods, such as anchovies, liver, sardines, kidneys, sweetbreads, lentils, and alcoholic beverages — especially beer and wine — which raise the urate level.
• Explain the principles of a gradual weight reduction diet to obese patients. Such a diet features foods containing moderate amounts of protein and very little fat.
• Advise the patient receiving allopurinol, probenecid, and other drugs to report any adverse effects immediately. (These may include drowsiness, dizziness, nausea, vomiting, urinary frequency, and dermatitis.)
• Warn the patient taking probenecid

or sulfinpyrazone to avoid aspirin and other salicylates. Their combined effect causes urate retention.
• Inform the patient that long-term colchicine therapy is essential during the first 3 to 6 months of treatment with uricosuric drugs or allopurinol.

GRANULOCYTOPENIA AND LYMPHOCYTOPENIA

In *granulocytopenia (agranulocytosis),* a marked reduction in the number of circulating granulocytes occurs. Although this implies that all the granulocytes (neutrophils, basophils, eosinophils) are reduced, granulocytopenia usually refers to decreased neutrophils.

This disorder, which can occur at any age, is associated with infections and ulcerative lesions of the throat, GI tract, other mucous membranes, and skin. Its severest form is known as agranulocytosis.

Lymphocytopenia (lymphopenia), a rare disorder, is a deficiency of circulating lymphocytes (leukocytes produced mainly in lymph nodes).

In both granulocytopenia and lymphocytopenia, the total white blood cell (WBC) count may reach dangerously low levels, leaving the body unprotected against infection. The prognosis in both disorders depends on the underlying cause and whether or not it can be treated. Untreated, severe granulocytopenia can be fatal in 3 to 6 days.

Causes
Granulocytopenia and lymphocytopenia have several causes.

Granulocytopenia

Granulocytopenia may result from decreased production of granulocytes in bone marrow, increased peripheral destruction of granulocytes, or greater utilization of granulocytes.

Decreased production of granulocytes in bone marrow generally stems from radiation or drug therapy; it's a common adverse effect of antimetabolites and alkylating agents and may occur in the patient who's hypersensitive to phenothiazines, sulfonamides (and some sulfonamide derivatives such as chlorothiazide), antibiotics, or antiarrhythmic drugs.

Drug-induced granulocytopenia usually develops slowly and typically correlates with the dosage and duration of therapy. Production of granulocytes also decreases in such conditions as aplastic anemia and bone marrow cancers and in some hereditary disorders, such as infantile genetic agranulocytosis.

The growing loss of peripheral granulocytes is due to increased splenic sequestration, diseases that destroy peripheral blood cells (viral and bacterial infections), and drugs that act as haptens (carrying antigens that attack blood cells and causing acute idiosyncratic or non-dose-related drug reactions).

Infections such as infectious mononucleosis may result in granulocytopenia because of increased utilization of granulocytes.

Lymphocytopenia

Similarly, lymphocytopenia may result from the decreased production, increased destruction, or loss of lymphocytes. Decreased production of lymphocytes may occur secondary to a genetic or a thymic abnormality or to immunodeficiency disorders, such as ataxia-telangiectasia or thymic dysplasia. Increased destruction of lymphocytes may occur secondary to radiation or chemotherapy (with alkylating agents).

Loss of lymphocytes may follow postsurgical thoracic duct drainage, intestinal lymphangiectasia, or impaired intestinal lymphatic drainage (as in Whipple's disease). Lymphocyte depletion can also result from elevated plasma corticoid levels (due to stress, corticotropin or steroid treatment, or congestive heart failure).

Other associated disorders include Hodgkin's disease, leukemia, aplastic anemia, sarcoidosis, myasthenia gravis, lupus erythematosus, protein-calorie malnutrition, renal failure, terminal cancer, tuberculosis and, in infants, severe combined immunodeficiency disease (SCID).

Signs and symptoms

Patients with granulocytopenia typically experience slowly progressive fatigue and weakness, followed by the sudden onset of signs of overwhelming infection (fever, chills, tachycardia, anxiety, headache, and extreme prostration); ulcers in the mouth or colon; pharyngeal ulceration, possibly with associated necrosis; pneumonia; and septicemia, possibly leading to mild shock.

If granulocytopenia is caused by an idiosyncratic drug reaction, signs of infection develop abruptly, without slowly progressive fatigue and weakness.

Patients with lymphocytopenia may exhibit enlarged lymph nodes, spleen, and tonsils and signs of an associated disease.

Diagnosis

Granulocytopenia is diagnosed by a thorough patient history to check for precipitating factors. Physical examination for clinical effects of underlying disorders is also essential. The following test results confirm the diagnosis:

• Complete blood count (CBC) reveals a marked reduction in neutrophils (less than 500/µl leads to severe bacterial infections) and a WBC count lower than 2,000/µl, with few observable granulocytes.

• Examination of bone marrow generally shows a scarcity of granulocytic precursor cells beyond the most immature forms, but this finding may vary, depending on the cause.

• A lymphocyte count less than 1,500/µl in adults or less than 3,000/µl in children indicates lymphocytopenia. Identifying the cause by evaluation of the patient's clinical status, bone marrow and lymph node biopsies, or other appropriate diagnostic tests helps establish the diagnosis.

Treatment

Effective management of granulocytopenia must identify and eliminate the cause and control infection until the bone marrow can generate more leukocytes. This often means that drug or radiation therapy must be stopped and antibiotic treatment begun immediately, even while awaiting test results. Treatment may also include antifungal preparations.

Administration of granulocyte- or granulocyte-macrophage colony-stimulating factor is a newer treatment used to stimulate bone marrow production of neutrophils. Spontaneous restoration of leukocyte production in bone marrow generally occurs within 1 to 3 weeks.

Treatment of lymphocytopenia includes eliminating the cause and managing any underlying disorders. For infants with SCID, therapy may include bone marrow transplantation.

Special considerations

• Monitor vital signs frequently. Obtain cultures from blood, throat, urine, and sputum. Give antibiotics as scheduled.

• Explain the necessity of protective isolation (preferably with laminar air flow) to the patient and family.

• Teach proper hand-washing technique and how to correctly use gowns and masks. Prevent patient contact with staff members or visitors with respiratory tract infections.

• Maintain adequate nutrition and hydration, since malnutrition aggravates immunosuppression. Make sure the patient with mouth ulcerations receives a high-calorie liquid diet (for example, high-protein milk shakes). Offer a straw to make drinking less painful.

• Provide warm saline water gargles and rinses, analgesics, and anesthetic lozenges because good oral hygiene promotes patient comfort and facilitates the healing process.

• Ensure adequate rest, which is essential to the mobilization of the body's defenses against infection. Provide good skin and perineal care.

• Monitor CBC and differential, blood culture results, serum electrolyte levels, intake and output, and daily weight.

• To help detect granulocytopenia and lymphocytopenia in the early, most treatable stages, monitor the WBC count of any patient receiving radiation or chemotherapy. After the patient has developed bone marrow depression, he must zealously avoid exposure to infection.

• Advise the patient with known or suspected sensitivity to a drug that may lead to granulocytopenia or lymphocytopenia to alert medical personnel to this sensitivity in the future.

GUILLAIN-BARRÉ SYNDROME

Also known as infectious polyneuritis, Landry-Guillain-Barré syndrome, and acute idiopathic polyneuritis, Guillain-Barré syndrome is an acute, rapidly progressive and potentially fatal form of polyneuritis that causes muscle weakness and mild distal sensory loss.

This syndrome can occur at any age but is most common between ages 30 and 50; it affects both sexes equally. Recovery is spontaneous and complete in about 95% of patients, although mild motor or reflex deficits in the feet and legs may persist. The prognosis is best when symptoms clear between 15 and 20 days after onset.

Causes

The precise cause of Guillain-Barré syndrome is unknown, but it may be a cell-mediated immune response with an attack on peripheral nerves in response to a virus. The major pathologic effect is segmental demyelination of the peripheral nerves.

Since this syndrome causes inflammation and degenerative changes in both the posterior (sensory) and anterior (motor) nerve roots, signs of sensory and motor losses occur simultaneously.

Precipitating factors

About 50% of patients with Guillain-Barré syndrome have a recent history of minor febrile illness, usually an upper respiratory tract infection or, less often, gastroenteritis. When infection precedes the onset of Guillain-Barré syndrome, signs of infection subside before neurologic features appear.

Other possible precipitating factors include surgery, rabies or swine influenza vaccination, viral illness, Hodgkin's or some other malignant disease, and systemic lupus erythematosus.

Signs and symptoms

Muscle weakness, the major neurologic sign, usually appears in the legs first (ascending type), then extends to the arms and facial nerves in 24 to 72 hours. Sometimes, muscle weakness develops in the arms first (descending type), or in the arms and legs simultaneously. In milder forms of this disease, muscle weakness may affect only the cranial nerves or may not occur at all.

Paresthesia, another common neurologic sign, sometimes precedes muscle weakness but tends to vanish quickly. However, some patients with this disorder never develop this symptom.

Other clinical features may include facial diplegia (possibly with ophthalmoplegia [ocular paralysis]), dysphagia or dysarthria, and, less often, weakness of the muscles supplied by cranial nerve XI (spinal accessory).

Muscle weakness develops so quickly that muscle atrophy doesn't occur, but hypotonia and areflexia do. Stiffness and pain in the form of a severe "charley horse" often occur.

Three-phase course

The clinical course of Guillain-Barré syndrome is divided into three phases:

• The *initial phase* begins when the first definitive symptom develops; it ends 1 to 3 weeks later, when no further deterioration is noted.

• The *plateau phase* lasts several days to 2 weeks.

• The *recovery phase* is believed to coincide with remyelination and axonal process regrowth. This phase extends over a period of 4 to 6 months; patients with severe disease may take up to 2 years to recover, and recovery may not be complete.

Complications

Significant complications of Guillain-Barré syndrome include mechanical ventilatory failure, aspiration, pneumonia, sepsis, joint contractures, and deep vein thrombosis. Unexplained autonomic nervous system involvement may cause sinus tachycardia or bradycardia, hypertension, postural hypotension, or loss of bladder and bowel sphincter control.

Diagnosis

A history of preceding febrile illness (usually a respiratory tract infection) and typical clinical features suggest Guillain-Barré syndrome.

Several days after onset of signs and symptoms, the cerebrospinal fluid (CSF) protein level begins to rise, peaking in 4 to 6 weeks, probably as a result of widespread inflammatory disease of the nerve roots. The CSF's white blood cell count remains normal, but in severe disease CSF pressure may rise above normal.

Probably because of predisposing infection, the complete blood count shows leukocytosis with the presence of immature forms early in the illness, but blood studies soon return to normal. Electromyography may show repeated firing of the same motor unit, instead of widespread sectional stimulation.

Nerve conduction velocities are slowed soon after paralysis develops. The diagnosis must rule out similar diseases such as acute poliomyelitis.

Treatment

Primarily supportive, treatment consists of endotracheal intubation or tracheotomy if the patient has difficulty clearing secretions.

A trial dose of prednisone may be tried if the course of the disease is relentlessly progressive. If prednisone produces no noticeable improvement after 7 days, the drug is discontinued.

Plasmapheresis is useful during the initial phase but offers no benefit if begun 2 weeks after onset.

Special considerations

• Watch for ascending sensory loss, which precedes motor loss. Also, monitor vital signs and level of consciousness.

• Assess and treat respiratory dysfunction. If respiratory muscles are weak, take serial vital capacity recordings. Use a respirometer with a mouthpiece or a face mask for bedside testing.

• Obtain arterial blood gas measurements. Because neuromuscular disease results in primary hypoventilation with hypoxemia and hypercapnia, watch for a partial pressure of oxygen (PaO_2) below 70 mm Hg, which signals respiratory failure. Be alert for signs of a rising partial pressure of carbon dioxide (confusion, tachypnea).

• Auscultate for breath sounds, turn and reposition the patient regularly, and encourage coughing and deep breathing.

• Begin respiratory support at the first sign of dyspnea (in adults, a vital capacity less than 800 ml; in children, less than 12 ml/kg of body weight) or a decreasing PaO_2.

• If respiratory failure becomes imminent, establish an emergency airway with an endotracheal tube.

• Give meticulous skin care to prevent skin breakdown and contractures.

• Establish a strict turning schedule; inspect the skin (especially sacrum, heels, and ankles) for breakdown, and reposition the patient every 2 hours.

• After each position change, stimulate circulation by carefully massaging pressure points. Also, use foam, gel, or alternating pressure pads at points of contact.

• Perform passive range-of-motion exercises within the patient's pain limits, perhaps using a Hubbard tank. (Although this disease doesn't produce pain, exercising little-used muscles will.) Remember that the proximal muscle group of the thighs, shoulders, and trunk will be the most tender and will cause the most pain on passive movement and turning.

• When the patient's condition stabilizes, change to gentle stretching and active assistance exercises.

• To prevent aspiration, test the gag reflex, and elevate the head of the bed before giving the patient anything to eat. If the gag reflex is absent, give nasogastric feedings until this reflex returns.

• As the patient regains strength and can tolerate a vertical position, be alert for postural hypotension. Monitor blood pressure and pulse during tilting periods and, if necessary, apply toe-to-groin elastic bandages or an abdominal binder to prevent postural hypotension.

• Inspect the patient's legs regularly for signs of thrombophlebitis (localized pain, tenderness, erythema, edema, positive Homans' sign), a common complication of Guillain-Barré syndrome.

• To prevent thrombophlebitis, apply antiembolism stockings and give prophylactic anticoagulants as needed.

• If the patient has facial paralysis, give eye and mouth care every 4 hours.

• Protect the corneas with isotonic eyedrops and conical eye shields.

• Encourage adequate fluid intake (2,000 ml/day), unless contraindicated.

• Watch for urine retention. Measure and record intake and output every 8 hours, and offer the bedpan every 3 to 4 hours.

• If urine retention develops, begin intermittent catheterization as needed. Because the abdominal muscles are weak, the patient may need manual pressure on the bladder (Credé's method) before he can urinate.

• To prevent and relieve constipation, offer prune juice and a high-bulk diet. If necessary, give daily or alternate-day suppositories (glycerin or bisacodyl), or Fleet enemas.

• Before discharge, prepare a home care plan. Teach the patient how to transfer from bed to wheelchair and from wheelchair to toilet or to tub and how to walk short distances with a walker or a cane.

• Teach the family how to help the patient eat, compensating for facial weakness, and how to help him avoid skin breakdown. Stress the need for a regular bowel and bladder routine.

• Refer the patient for physical therapy as needed.

HAEMOPHILUS INFLUENZAE INFECTION

A small, gram-negative, pleomorphic aerobic bacillus, *Haemophilus influenzae* causes diseases in many organ systems but most frequently attacks the respiratory system. In exudates, this organism predominantly resembles a coccobacillus.

H. influenzae is a common cause of epiglottitis, laryngotracheobronchitis, pneumonia, bronchiolitis, otitis media, and meningitis. Less often, it causes bacterial endocarditis, conjunctivitis, facial cellulitis, septic arthritis, and osteomyelitis.

H. influenzae pneumonia is an increasingly common nosocomial infection. It infects about half of all children before age 1 and virtually all children by age 3, although a new vaccine given at ages 2, 4, and 6 months has reduced this number.

Signs and symptoms

H. influenzae provokes a characteristic tissue response — acute suppurative inflammation.

When *H. influenzae* infects the larynx, the trachea, and the bronchial tree, it leads to mucosal edema and thick exudate; when it invades the lungs, it leads to bronchopneumonia.

In the pharynx, *H. influenzae* usually produces no remarkable changes, except when it causes epiglottitis, which generally affects both the laryngeal and pharyngeal surfaces.

The pharyngeal mucosa may be reddened, rarely with soft yellow exudate. More commonly, however, it appears normal or shows only slight diffuse redness, even while severe pain makes swallowing difficult or impossible. These infections typically cause high fever and generalized malaise.

Diagnosis

Isolation of the organism, usually with a blood culture, confirms *H. influenzae* infection. Other laboratory findings include:

- polymorphonuclear leukocytosis (15,000 to 30,000/µl)
- leukopenia (2,000 to 3,000/µl) in young children with severe infection
- *H. influenzae* bacteremia, found frequently in patients with meningitis.

Treatment

H. influenzae infections usually respond to a 2-week course of ampicillin (resistant strains are becoming more common), cephalosporins, or chloramphenicol.

Special considerations

- Maintain adequate respiratory function through proper positioning, humidification (croup tent) in children, and suctioning as needed.
- Monitor the rate and type of respirations.
- Watch for signs of cyanosis and dyspnea, which necessitate intubation or a tracheotomy.
- For home treatment, suggest that the patient use a room humidifier or

breathe moist air from a shower or bath as necessary.

• Check the patient's history for drug allergies before giving antibiotics.

• Monitor the complete blood count for signs of bone marrow depression when therapy includes chloramphenicol.

• Monitor intake (including I.V. infusions) and output. Watch for signs of dehydration, such as decreased skin turgor, parched lips, concentrated urine, decreased urine output, and increased pulse.

• Organize your physical care measures beforehand, and do them quickly so as not to disrupt the patient's rest.

• Take preventive measures, such as giving the *H. influenzae* vaccine to children ages 2 (or younger) to 6, maintaining respiratory isolation, using proper hand-washing technique, properly disposing of respiratory secretions, placing soiled tissues in a plastic bag, and decontaminating all equipment.

Hallux Valgus

A lateral deviation of the great toe at the metatarsophalangeal joint, hallux valgus occurs with medial enlargement of the first metatarsal head and bunion formation (bursa and callus formation at the bony prominence).

Causes

Hallux valgus may be congenital or familial but is more often acquired from degenerative arthritis or prolonged pressure on the foot, especially from narrow-toed, high-heeled shoes that compress the forefoot. Consequently, hallux valgus is more common in women.

In congenital hallux valgus, abnormal bony alignment (increased space between the first and second metatarsal [metatarsus primus varus]) causes bunion formation. In acquired hallux valgus, bony alignment is normal at the outset of the disorder.

Signs and symptoms

Hallux valgus characteristically begins as a tender bunion covered by deformed, hard, erythematous skin and palpable bursa, often distended with fluid. The first indication of hallux valgus may be pain over the bunion from shoe pressure. Pain can also stem from traumatic arthritis, bursitis, or abnormal stresses on the foot, since hallux valgus changes the body's weight-bearing pattern.

In an advanced stage, a flat, splayed forefoot may occur, with severely curled toes (hammer toes) and formation of a small bunion on the fifth metatarsal.

Diagnosis

A red, tender bunion makes hallux valgus obvious. X-rays confirm the diagnosis by showing medial deviation of the first metatarsal and lateral deviation of the great toe.

Treatment

In the very early stages of acquired hallux valgus, good foot care and proper shoes may eliminate the need for further treatment. Other useful measures for early management include felt pads to protect the bunion, foam pads or other devices to separate the first and second toes at night, and a supportive pad and exercises to strengthen the metatarsal arch.

Early treatment is vital in patients predisposed to foot problems, such as those with rheumatoid arthritis or diabetes mellitus.

Bunionectomy

If the disease progresses to severe deformity with disabling pain, bunionectomy is necessary. After surgery, the toe is immobilized in its corrected position one of two ways: with a soft compression dressing (which may cover the entire foot or just the great toe and the second toe, which serves as a splint) or with a short cast (such as a light slipper spica cast).

The patient may need crutches or controlled weight-bearing. Depending on the extent of surgery, some patients walk on their heels a few days after surgery; others must wait 4 to 6 weeks to bear weight on the affected foot. Supportive treatment may include physical therapy, such as warm compresses, soaks, and exercises, and analgesics to relieve pain and stiffness.

Special considerations

• Before bunionectomy, obtain a patient history and assess the neurovascular status of the foot (temperature, color, sensation, blanching sign). If necessary, teach the patient how to walk with crutches.

After bunionectomy:

• Apply ice to reduce swelling. Increase negative venous pressure and reduce edema by supporting the foot with pillows, elevating the foot of the bed, or putting the bed in a Trendelenburg position.

• Record the neurovascular status of the toes, including the patient's ability to move the toes (dressing may inhibit movement), every hour for the first 24 hours, then every 4 hours. Watch for any change in neurovascular status.

• Prepare the patient for walking by having him dangle his foot over the side of the bed for a short time before he gets up, allowing a gradual increase in venous pressure.

• If crutches are needed, supervise the patient in using them, and make sure this skill is mastered before discharge. The patient should have a proper cast shoe or boot to protect the cast or dressing.

• Before discharge, instruct the patient to limit activities, to rest frequently with feet elevated, to elevate his feet whenever he feels pain or has edema, and to wear wide-toed shoes and sandals after the dressings are removed.

• Teach proper foot care, such as cleanliness, massages, and cutting toenails straight across to prevent ingrown nails and infection.

• Suggest exercises to do at home to strengthen foot muscles, such as standing at the edge of a step on the heel, then raising and inverting the top of the foot.

• Stress the importance of follow-up care and prompt medical attention for painful bunions, corns, and calluses.

LIFE-THREATENING DISORDER

HANTAVIRUS PULMONARY SYNDROME

Mainly occurring in the southwestern United States, but not confined to that area, hantavirus pulmonary syndrome is a new viral disease first reported in May 1993. The syndrome, which rapidly progresses from flulike symptoms to respiratory failure and, possibly, death, is known for its high mortality.

The hantavirus strain that causes disease in Asia and Europe — mainly hemorrhagic fever and renal disease — is distinctly different from the one currently described in North America.

Causes

A member of the Bunyaviridae family, the genus *Hantavirus* (first isolated in 1977) is responsible for hantavirus pulmonary syndrome. Disease transmission is associated with exposure to infected rodents, the primary reservoir for this virus.

Data suggest that the deer mouse is the main source, but piñon mice, brush mice, and western chipmunks in close proximity to humans in rural areas are also sources.

Infected rodents manifest no apparent illness but shed the virus in feces, urine, and saliva. Human infection may occur from inhalation, ingestion (of contaminated food or water, for example), contact with rodent excrement, or rodent bites. Transmission from person to person or by mosquitos, fleas, or other arthropods hasn't been reported.

Hantavirus infections have been documented in people whose activities are associated with rodent contact, such as farming, hiking or camping in rodent-infested areas, and occupying rodent-infested dwellings.

Signs and symptoms

Noncardiogenic pulmonary edema distinguishes the syndrome. Common chief complaints include myalgia, fever, headache, nausea and vomiting, and cough. Respiratory distress typically follows the onset of a cough. Fever, hypoxia and, in some patients, serious hypotension typify the hospital course.

Other signs and symptoms include a rising respiratory rate (28 breaths/minute or more) and an increased heart rate (120 beats/minute or more).

Diagnosis

Despite ongoing efforts to identify clinical and laboratory features that distinguish hantavirus pulmonary syndrome from other infections with similar features, diagnosis currently is based on clinical suspicion along with a process of elimination developed by the Centers for Disease Control and Prevention (CDC) with the Council of State and Territorial Epidemiologists. (See *Screening for hantavirus pulmonary syndrome,* page 384.)

Note: The CDC and state health departments can perform definitive testing for hantavirus exposure and antibody formation.

Laboratory tests usually reveal an elevated white blood cell count with a predominance of neutrophils, myeloid precursors, and atypical lymphocytes; elevated hematocrit; decreased platelet count; elevated partial thromboplastin time; and a normal fibrinogen level.

Usually, laboratory findings demonstrate only minimal abnormalities in renal function, with serum creatinine levels no higher than 2.5 mg/dl.

Chest X-rays eventually show bilateral diffuse infiltrates in almost all patients (findings consistent with adult respiratory distress syndrome).

Treatment

Primarily supportive, treatment consists of maintaining adequate oxygenation, monitoring vital signs, and intervening to stabilize the patient's heart rate and blood pressure.

Drug therapy includes administering vasopressors, such as dopamine or epinephrine, for hypotension. Fluid volume replacement may also be ordered (with precautions not to overhydrate the patient).

Clinical trials with ribavirin are currently underway.

Special considerations

• Assess the patient's respiratory status and arterial blood gas values often.
• Monitor the patient's serum electrolyte levels and correct imbalances as appropriate.
• Maintain a patent airway by suctioning. Ensure adequate humidification, and check ventilator settings frequently.
• In patients with hypoxemia, assess neurologic status frequently along with heart rate and blood pressure.
• Administer drug therapy and monitor the patient's response.

SCREENING FOR HANTAVIRUS PULMONARY SYNDROME

The Centers for Disease Control and Prevention (CDC) has developed a screening procedure to track cases of hantavirus pulmonary syndrome. The screening criteria identify potential and actual cases.

Potential cases
For a diagnosis of possible hantavirus pulmonary syndrome, a patient must have one of the following:
• a febrile illness (temperature equal to or above 101° F [38.3° C]) occurring in a previously healthy person and characterized by unexplained adult respiratory distress syndrome
• bilateral interstitial pulmonary infiltrates that develop within 1 week of hospitalization with respiratory compromise that requires supplemental oxygen
• an unexplained respiratory illness resulting in death and autopsy findings demonstrating noncardiogenic pulmonary edema without an identifiable specific cause of death.

Exclusions
Of the patients who meet the criteria for having potential hantavirus pulmonary syndrome, the CDC excludes those who have any of the following:
• a predisposing underlying medical condition (for example, severe underlying pulmonary disease, solid tumors or hematologic cancers, congenital or acquired immunodeficiency disorders, or medical conditions—such as rheumatoid arthritis or organ transplantation—requiring immunosuppressive drug therapy [for example, steroids or cytotoxic chemotherapy])
• an acute illness that provides a likely explanation for the respiratory illness (for example, a recent major trauma, burn, or surgery; recent seizures or a history of aspiration; bacterial sepsis; another respiratory disorder such as respiratory syncytial virus in young children; influenza; or legionella pneumonia).

Confirmed cases
Cases of confirmed hantavirus pulmonary syndrome must include the following:
• at least one serum or tissue specimen available for laboratory testing for evidence of hantavirus infection
• in a patient with a compatible clinical illness, serologic evidence (presence of hantavirus-specific immunoglobulin M [IgM] or rising titers of IgG), polymerase chain reaction for hantavirus ribonucleic acid, or positive immunohistochemistry for the hantavirus antigen.

• Provide I.V. fluid therapy based on results of hemodynamic monitoring.
• Provide emotional support for the patient and his family.
• Report cases of hantavirus pulmonary syndrome to your state health department.
• Provide prevention guidelines. (Until more is known about hantavirus pulmonary syndrome, preventive measures currently focus on rodent control.)

HEADACHE

The most common patient complaint, headache usually occurs as a symptom of an underlying disorder. Ninety percent of all headaches are vascular, muscle contraction, or a combination; 10% are due to underlying intracranial, systemic, or psychological disorders.

Migraine headaches, probably the most intensively studied, are throbbing, vascular headaches that usually begin to appear in childhood or adolescence and recur throughout adulthood. Affecting up to 10% of Americans, they're more common in females and have a strong familial incidence.

Causes

Most chronic headaches result from tension – muscle contraction – which may be caused by emotional stress, fatigue, menstruation, or environmental stimuli (noise, crowds, bright lights).

Other possible causes include glaucoma; inflammation of the eyes or mucosa of the nasal or paranasal sinuses; diseases of the scalp, teeth, extracranial arteries, or external or middle ear; and muscle spasms of the face, neck, or shoulders.

In addition, headaches may be caused by vasodilators (nitrates, alcohol, histamine), systemic disease, hypoxia, hypertension, head trauma and tumor, intracranial bleeding, abscess, or aneurysm.

Migraine headaches

The cause of migraine headache is unknown, but these headaches are associated with constriction and dilation of intracranial and extracranial arteries. Certain biochemical abnormalities are thought to occur during a migraine attack. These include local leakage of a vasodilator polypeptide called neurokinin through the dilated arteries and a decrease in the plasma level of serotonin.

Headache pain

Pain may emanate from the pain-sensitive structures of the skin, scalp, muscles, arteries, veins; cranial nerves V, VII, IX, and X; and cervical nerves 1, 2, and 3. Intracranial mechanisms of headache include traction or displacement of arteries, venous sinuses, or venous tributaries, and inflammation or direct pressure on the cranial nerves with afferent pain fibers.

Signs and symptoms

Migraine headaches and muscle contraction headaches have different signs and symptoms.

Migraine headaches

Initially, migraine headache usually produces unilateral, pulsating pain, which later becomes more generalized. The headache is often preceded by a scintillating scotoma, hemianopsia, unilateral paresthesia, or speech disorders. The patient may experience irritability, anorexia, nausea, vomiting, and photophobia. (See *Clinical features of migraine headaches,* page 386.)

Muscle contraction headaches

These headaches produce a dull, persistent ache, tender spots on the head and neck, and a feeling of tightness around the head, with a characteristic "hatband" distribution. The pain is often severe and unrelenting.

If caused by intracranial bleeding, these headaches may result in neurologic deficits, such as paresthesia and muscle weakness; narcotics fail to relieve pain in these cases. If caused by a tumor, pain is most severe when the patient awakens.

Diagnosis

An accurate diagnosis requires a history of recurrent headaches and physical examination of the head and neck. Such examination includes percussion, auscultation for bruits, inspection for signs of infection, and palpation for defects, crepitus, or tender spots (especially after trauma).

A firm diagnosis also requires a complete neurologic examination, assessment for other systemic diseases –

CLINICAL FEATURES OF MIGRAINE HEADACHES

TYPE	SIGNS AND SYMPTOMS
Common migraine *(most prevalent, 85%)* Usually occurs on weekends and holidays	• Prodromal symptoms (fatigue, nausea and vomiting, and fluid imbalance) precede headache by about a day. • Sensitivity to light and noise (most prominent feature) • Headache pain (unilateral or bilateral, aching or throbbing) lasts longer than in classic migraine.
Classic migraine *(incidence 10%)* Usually occurs in compulsive personalities and within families	• Prodromal symptoms include visual disturbances, such as zigzag lines and bright lights (most common); sensory disturbances (tingling of face, lips, and hands); or motor disturbances (staggering gait). • Recurrent and periodic headaches
Hemiplegic and ophthalmoplegic migraine *(rare)* Usually occurs in young adults	• Severe, unilateral pain; extraocular muscle palsies (involving third cranial nerve) and ptosis • With repeated headaches, possible permanent third cranial nerve injury • In hemiplegic migraine, neurologic deficits (hemiparesis, hemiplegia) may persist after headache subsides.
Basilar artery migraine Occurs in young women before their menstrual periods	• Prodromal symptoms usually include partial vision loss followed by vertigo, ataxia, dysarthria, tinnitus and, sometimes, tingling of fingers and toes, lasting from several minutes to almost an hour. • Headache pain, severe occipital throbbing, vomiting

such as hypertension—and a psychosocial evaluation (when such factors are suspected.)

Diagnostic tests include skull X-rays (including cervical spine and sinuses), an EEG, computed tomography and brain scans, and lumbar puncture.

Treatment

Depending on the type of headache, analgesics—ranging from aspirin to codeine or meperidine—may provide symptomatic relief. A tranquilizer, such as diazepam, may help during acute attacks.

Other measures include identification and elimination of causative factors and, possibly, psychotherapy for headaches caused by emotional stress.

Chronic tension headaches may also require muscle relaxants.

Migraine treatment

For migraine headache, ergotamine alone or with caffeine may be an effective treatment. These drugs and others, such as metoclopramide or naproxen, work best when taken early in the course of an attack. If nausea and vomiting make oral administration impossible, these drugs may be given as rectal suppositories.

Sumatriptan is considered by many clinicians to be the drug of choice for acute migraine attacks or cluster headaches. Drugs that can help prevent migraine headache include propranolol, atenolol, clonidine, and amitriptyline.

Special considerations

• Headaches rarely require hospitalization unless caused by a serious disorder. If that's the case, direct your care to the primary problem.

• Obtain a complete patient history: the duration and location of the headache; the time of day it usually begins; the nature of the pain; the headache's concurrence with other symptoms such as blurred vision; and precipitating factors, such as tension, menstruation, loud noises, menopause, alcohol use, use of medications such as oral contraceptives, or prolonged fasting.

• Using the history as a guide, help the patient avoid precipitating factors.

• Advise the patient to lie down in a dark, quiet room during an attack and to place ice packs on his forehead or a cold cloth over his eyes.

• Instruct the patient to take the prescribed medication at the onset of migraine symptoms, to prevent dehydration by drinking plenty of fluids after nausea and vomiting subside, and to use other headache relief measures.

• Bear in mind that the patient with migraine usually needs to be hospitalized only if nausea and vomiting are severe enough to induce dehydration and possibly shock.

HEARING LOSS

Loss of hearing results from a mechanical or nervous impediment to the transmission of sound waves. Hearing loss is classified into three major forms:

• *Conductive loss* is the interrupted passage of sound from the external ear to the junction of the stapes and oval window.

• *Sensorineural loss* is impaired cochlear or acoustic (eighth cranial) nerve dysfunction, causing failure of transmission of sound impulses within the inner ear or brain.

• *Mixed loss* is a combination of conductive and sensorineural hearing loss.

Hearing loss may be partial or complete and is calculated from the American Medical Association formula: Hearing is 1.5% impaired for every decibel (dB) that the pure tone average exceeds 25 dB.

Causes

Hearing loss may be congenital, or it may be caused by drugs or illness, loud noise, or aging.

Congenital hearing loss

Hearing loss may be transmitted as a dominant, autosomal dominant, autosomal recessive, or sex-linked recessive trait. In neonates, it may also result from trauma, toxicity, or infection during pregnancy or delivery.

Predisposing factors include a family history of hearing loss or known hereditary disorders (otosclerosis, for example), maternal exposure to rubella or syphilis during pregnancy, use of ototoxic drugs during pregnancy, prolonged fetal anoxia during delivery, and congenital abnormalities of the ears, nose, or throat.

Premature or low-birth-weight infants are most likely to have structural or functional hearing impairments; those with serum bilirubin levels greater than 20 mg/dl also risk hearing impairment from the toxic effect of high serum bilirubin levels on the brain.

In addition, trauma during delivery may cause intracranial hemorrhage and damage the cochlea or acoustic nerve.

Sudden deafness

Sudden hearing loss may occur in a person with no prior hearing impairment. This condition is considered a medical emergency because prompt treatment may restore full hearing. Its causes and predisposing factors may include:

• acute infections, especially mumps (the most common cause of unilateral sensorineural hearing loss in children), and other bacterial and viral infections, such as rubella, rubeola, influenza, herpes zoster, and infectious mononucleosis; and mycoplasma infections

• metabolic disorders (diabetes mellitus, hypothyroidism, hyperlipoproteinemia)

• vascular disorders, such as hypertension and arteriosclerosis

• head trauma or brain tumors

• ototoxic drugs (tobramycin, streptomycin, quinine, gentamicin, furosemide, ethacrynic acid)

• neurologic disorders (multiple sclerosis, neurosyphilis)

• blood dyscrasias (leukemia and hypercoagulation).

Noise-induced hearing loss
Hearing loss caused by loud noise may be transient or permanent, may follow prolonged exposure to loud noise (85 to 90 dB) or brief exposure to extremely loud noise (more than 90 dB). Such hearing loss is common in workers subjected to constant industrial noise and in military personnel, hunters, and rock musicians.

Presbycusis
An otologic effect of aging, presbycusis results from a loss of hair cells in the organ of Corti. This disorder causes sensorineural hearing loss, usually of high-frequency tones.

Signs and symptoms
The four types of hearing loss have different signs and symptoms:

• Although congenital hearing loss may produce no obvious signs of hearing impairment at birth, a deficient response to auditory stimuli generally becomes apparent within 2 to 3 days

of birth. As the child grows older, hearing loss impairs speech development.

• Sudden deafness may be conductive, sensorineural, or mixed, depending on etiology. Associated clinical features depend on the underlying cause.

• Noise-induced hearing loss causes sensorineural damage, the extent of which depends on the duration and intensity of the noise. Initially, the patient loses perception of certain frequencies (around 4,000 Hz) but, with continued exposure, eventually loses perception of all frequencies.

• Presbycusis usually produces tinnitus and the inability to understand the spoken word.

Diagnosis
Patient, family, and occupational histories and a complete audiologic examination usually provide ample evidence of hearing loss and suggest possible causes or predisposing factors. The Weber and Rinne tests and other specialized audiologic tests differentiate between conductive and sensorineural hearing loss.

Treatment
Measures for treating each type of hearing loss vary.

Congenital hearing loss
After identifying the underlying cause, therapy for congenital hearing loss refractory to surgery consists of developing the patient's ability to communicate through sign language, speech reading, or other effective means.

Measures to prevent congenital hearing loss include aggressively immunizing children against rubella to reduce the risk of maternal exposure during pregnancy; educating pregnant women about the dangers of exposure to drugs, chemicals, or infection; and careful monitoring of the fetus during labor and delivery to prevent fetal anoxia.

Sudden deafness

Treatment of sudden deafness requires prompt identification of the underlying cause. Prevention requires educating patients and health care professionals about the many causes of sudden deafness and the ways to recognize and treat them.

Noise-induced hearing loss

In persons with noise-induced hearing loss, overnight rest usually restores normal hearing in those who have been exposed to noise levels greater than 90 dB for several hours; but not in those who have been exposed to such noise repeatedly. As hearing deteriorates, treatment must include speech and hearing rehabilitation, since hearing aids are rarely helpful.

Prevention of noise-induced hearing loss requires public recognition of the dangers of noise exposure and insistence on the use, as mandated by law, of protective devices, such as earplugs, during occupational exposure to noise.

Presbycusis

Patients with presbycusis usually require a hearing aid.

Special considerations

• When speaking to a patient with hearing loss who can read lips, stand directly in front of him, with the light on your face, and speak slowly and distinctly. Approach the patient within his visual range, and elicit his attention by raising your arm or waving; touching him may be unnecessarily startling.
• Make other staff members and hospital personnel aware of the patient's handicap and his established method of communication.
• Carefully explain all diagnostic tests

and hospital procedures in a way the patient understands.
• Make sure the patient with a hearing loss is in an area where he can observe unit activities and persons approaching because such a patient depends totally on visual clues.
• When addressing an older patient, speak slowly and distinctly in a low tone; avoid shouting.
• Provide emotional support and encouragement to the patient learning to use a hearing aid. Teach him how the aid works and how to maintain it.
• Refer children with suspected hearing loss to an audiologist or otolaryngologist for further evaluation.
• To help prevent hearing loss, watch for signs of hearing impairment in patients receiving ototoxic drugs. Emphasize the danger of excessive exposure to noise; stress the danger of exposure to drugs, chemicals, and infection (especially rubella) to pregnant women; and encourage the use of protective devices in a noisy environment.

LIFE-THREATENING DISORDER

HEART FAILURE

A syndrome characterized by myocardial dysfunction, heart failure leads to impaired pump performance (reduced cardiac output) or to frank heart failure and abnormal circulatory congestion. Congestion of systemic venous circulation may result in peripheral edema or hepatomegaly; congestion of pulmonary circulation may cause pulmonary edema, an acute, life-threatening emergency.

Pump failure usually occurs in a damaged left ventricle (left-sided heart failure) but may occur in the right ventricle (right-sided heart failure) either as a primary disorder or secondary to left-sided heart failure. Sometimes, left- and right-sided heart failure develop simultaneously.

Although heart failure may be acute (as a direct result of myocardial infarction), it's generally a chronic disorder associated with retention of sodium and water by the kidneys. Advances in diagnostic and therapeutic techniques have greatly improved the outlook for patients with heart failure, but the prognosis still depends on the underlying cause and its response to treatment.

Causes

Heart failure may result from a primary abnormality of the heart muscle — such as an infarction — inadequate myocardial perfusion due to coronary artery disease, or cardiomyopathy. Other causes include:

• mechanical disturbances in ventricular filling during diastole when there's too little blood for the ventricle to pump, as in mitral stenosis secondary to rheumatic heart disease or constrictive pericarditis and atrial fibrillation

• systolic hemodynamic disturbances, such as excessive cardiac workload due to volume overloading or pressure overload, that limit the heart's pumping ability.

These disturbances can result from mitral or aortic insufficiency, which causes volume overloading, and aortic stenosis or systemic hypertension, which results in increased resistance to ventricular emptying.

Reduced cardiac output triggers three compensatory mechanisms: ventricular dilation, hypertrophy, and increased sympathetic activity. These mechanisms improve cardiac output at the expense of increased ventricular work.

Cardiac dilation

In cardiac dilation, an increase in end-diastolic ventricular volume (preload) causes increased stroke work and stroke volume during contraction, stretching cardiac muscle fibers beyond optimum limits and producing pulmonary congestion and pulmonary hypertension, which in turn lead to right ventricular failure.

Ventricular hypertrophy

In ventricular hypertrophy, an increase in muscle mass or diameter of the left ventricle allows the heart to pump against increased resistance (impedance) to the outflow of blood.

An increase in ventricular diastolic pressure necessary to fill the enlarged ventricle may compromise diastolic coronary blood flow, limiting the oxygen supply to the ventricle and causing ischemia and impaired myocardial contractility.

Increased sympathetic activity

As a response to decreased cardiac output and blood pressure, increased sympathetic activity occurs by enhancing peripheral vascular resistance, contractility, heart rate, and venous return.

Signs of increased sympathetic activity, such as cool extremities and clamminess, may indicate impending heart failure. Increased sympathetic activity also restricts blood flow to the kidneys, which respond by reducing the glomerular filtration rate and increasing tubular reabsorption of sodium and water, in turn expanding the circulating blood volume. This renal mechanism, if unchecked, can aggravate congestion and produce overt edema.

Chronic heart failure may worsen as a result of respiratory tract infections, pulmonary embolism, stress, increased sodium or water intake, or failure to comply with the prescribed treatment regimen.

Signs and symptoms

Left-sided heart failure primarily produces pulmonary signs and symptoms; right-sided heart failure, primarily systemic signs and symptoms. However, heart failure often affects both sides of the heart.

Left-sided heart failure

Clinical signs of left-sided heart failure include dyspnea, orthopnea, crackles, possibly wheezing, hypoxia, respiratory acidosis, cough, cyanosis or pallor, palpitations, arrhythmias, elevated blood pressure, and pulsus alternans.

Right-sided heart failure

Clinical signs of right-sided heart failure include dependent peripheral edema, hepatomegaly, splenomegaly, jugular vein distention, ascites, slow weight gain, arrhythmias, hepatojugular reflex, abdominal distention, nausea, vomiting, anorexia, weakness, fatigue, dizziness, and syncope.

Complications

These typically include pulmonary edema, venostasis with a predisposition to thromboembolism (associated primarily with prolonged bed rest), cerebral insufficiency, and renal insufficiency with severe electrolyte imbalance. (See *Pulmonary edema: How to intervene,* pages 392 and 393.)

Diagnosis

The following tests are used to diagnose heart failure:

• *Electrocardiography* reflects heart strain, enlargement, or ischemia. It may also reveal atrial enlargement, tachycardia, and extrasystole.

• *Chest X-ray* shows increased pulmonary vascular markings, interstitial edema, or pleural effusion and cardiomegaly.

• *Pulmonary artery monitoring* typically demonstrates elevated pulmonary artery and pulmonary artery wedge pressures, left ventricular end-diastolic pressure in left-sided heart failure, and elevated right atrial pressure or central venous pressure in right-sided heart failure.

Treatment

The aim of therapy is to improve pump function by reversing the compensatory mechanisms producing the symptoms. Heart failure can be controlled quickly by treatment consisting of:

• diuresis to reduce total blood volume and circulatory congestion

• prolonged bed rest

• digoxin to strengthen myocardial contractility

• vasodilators to increase cardiac output by reducing the impedance to ventricular outflow (afterload)

• antiembolism stockings to prevent venostasis and thromboembolus formation.

Special considerations

During the acute phase:

• Place the patient in Fowler's position and give him supplemental oxygen to help him breathe more easily.

• Weigh the patient daily and check for peripheral edema. Carefully monitor his I.V. intake and urine output, vital signs, and mental status. Auscultate the heart for abnormal sounds (S_3 gallop) and the lungs for crackles or rhonchi.

• Frequently monitor levels of blood urea nitrogen and serum creatinine, potassium, sodium, chloride, and magnesium.

• The patient should have continuous cardiac monitoring during acute and advanced stages to identify and treat arrhythmias promptly.

• To prevent deep vein thrombosis due to vascular congestion, assist the patient with range-of-motion exercises. Enforce bed rest and apply antiembolism stockings. Check regularly for calf pain and tenderness.

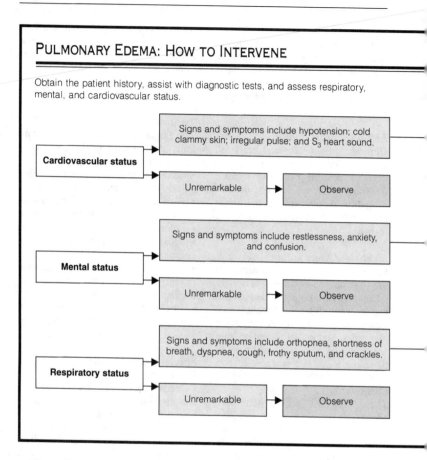

PULMONARY EDEMA: HOW TO INTERVENE

Obtain the patient history, assist with diagnostic tests, and assess respiratory, mental, and cardiovascular status.

Cardiovascular status
- Signs and symptoms include hypotension; cold clammy skin; irregular pulse; and S₃ heart sound.
- Unremarkable → Observe

Mental status
- Signs and symptoms include restlessness, anxiety, and confusion.
- Unremarkable → Observe

Respiratory status
- Signs and symptoms include orthopnea, shortness of breath, dyspnea, cough, frothy sputum, and crackles.
- Unremarkable → Observe

• Allow adequate rest periods.
  Before discharge:
• Advise the patient to avoid foods high in sodium, such as canned or commercially prepared foods and dairy products, to curb fluid overload.
• Explain to the patient that the potassium he loses through diuretic therapy must be replaced by taking a prescribed potassium supplement and eating high-potassium foods, such as bananas, apricots, and orange juice.
• Stress the need for regular checkups.
• Stress the importance of taking digoxin exactly as prescribed. Tell the patient to watch for and immediately report signs of toxicity, such as anorexia, vomiting, and yellow vision.
• Tell the patient to promptly report any unusual pulse irregularities or a pulse rate less than 60 beats/minute. He should also report dizziness, blurred vision, shortness of breath, persistent dry cough, palpitations, increased fatigue, paroxysmal nocturnal dyspnea, swollen ankles, decreased urine output, or rapid weight gain (3 to 5 lb [1.35 to 2.25 kg] in a week).

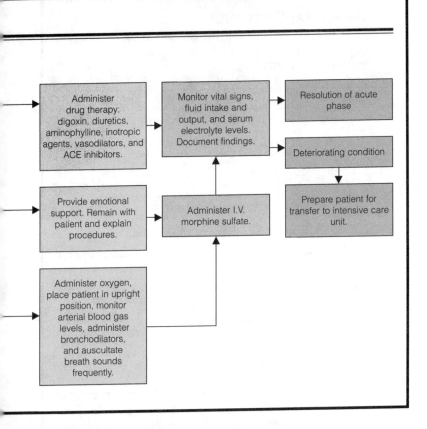

HEAT SYNDROME

Resulting from environmental or internal conditions that increase heat production or impair heat dissipation, heat syndromes fall into three categories: heat cramps, heat exhaustion, and heatstroke. (See *Managing heat syndrome,* page 394.)

Causes

Normally, humans adjust to excessive temperatures by complex cardiovascular and neurologic changes, which are coordinated by the hypothalamus. Heat loss offsets heat production to regulate the body temperature. It does this by evaporation (sweating) or vasodilation, which cools the body's surface by radiation, conduction, and convection.

However, heat production increases with exercise, infection, and drugs such as amphetamines.

Heat loss decreases with high temperatures or humidity, lack of acclimatization, excess clothing, obesity, dehydration, cardiovascular disease,

MANAGING HEAT SYNDROME

TYPE AND PREDISPOSING FACTORS	SIGNS AND SYMPTOMS	MANAGEMENT
HEAT CRAMPS		
• Commonly affect young adults • Strenuous activity without training or acclimatization • Normal to high temperature or high humidity	• Muscle twitching and spasms, weakness, severe muscle cramps • Nausea • Normal temperature or slight fever • Normal central nervous system findings • Diaphoresis	• Hospitalization usually unnecessary. • To replace fluid and electrolytes, give salt tablets and balanced electrolyte drink. • Loosen patient's clothing, and have him lie down in a cool place. Massage his muscles. If muscle cramps are severe, start an I.V. infusion with normal saline solution.
HEAT EXHAUSTION		
• Commonly affects young people • Physical activity without acclimatization • Decreased heat dissipation • High temperature and humidity	• Muscle cramps (infrequent) • Nausea and vomiting • Decreased blood pressure • Thready, rapid pulse • Cool, pallid skin • Headache, mental confusion, syncope, giddiness • Oliguria, thirst • No fever	• Hospitalization usually unnecessary. • *Immediately* give salt tablets and balanced electrolyte drink. • Loosen patient's clothing, and put him in a shock position in a cool place. Massage his muscles. If cramps are severe, start an I.V. infusion. • If needed, give oxygen.
HEATSTROKE		
• Exertional heatstroke commonly affects young, healthy people who are involved in strenuous activity. • Classical heatstroke commonly affects elderly, inactive people who have cardiovascular disease or who take drugs that influence temperature regulation. • High temperature and humidity without any wind	• Hypertension followed by hypotension • Atrial or ventricular tachycardia • Hot, dry, red skin, which later turns gray; no diaphoresis • Confusion, progressing to seizures and loss of consciousness • Temperature higher than 104° F (40° C) • Dilated pupils • Slow, deep respirations; then Cheyne-Stokes respirations	• Initiate ABCs (airway, breathing, and circulation) of life support. • To lower patient's body temperature, cool rapidly with ice packs on arterial pressure points and hypothermia blankets. • To replace fluids and electrolytes, start an I.V. infusion. • Hospitalization needed. • Insert nasogastric tube to prevent aspiration. • Give diazepam to control seizures; chlorpromazine I.V. to reduce shivering; or mannitol to maintain urine output. • Monitor temperature, intake, output, and cardiac status. Give dobutamine to correct cardiogenic shock. (Vasoconstrictors are contraindicated.)

sweat gland dysfunction, and drugs, such as phenothiazines and anticholinergics.

So when heat loss mechanisms fail to offset heat production, the body retains heat and may develop heat syndrome.

Special considerations

• Heat illnesses are easily preventable, so it's important to educate the public about the various factors that cause them. This information is especially vital for athletes, laborers, and soldiers in field training.

• Advise your patients to avoid heat syndrome by taking the following precautions in hot weather: wear loose-fitting, lightweight clothing; rest frequently; avoid hot places; and drink adequate fluids.

• Advise patients who are obese, elderly, or taking drugs that impair heat regulation to avoid overheating.

• Tell patients who've had heat cramps or heat exhaustion to exercise gradually and to increase their salt and water intake.

• Warn patients with heatstroke that residual hypersensitivity to high temperatures may persist for several months.

HEMOPHILIA

A hereditary bleeding disorder, hemophilia results from the deficiency of specific clotting factors. *Hemophilia A* (classic hemophilia), which affects over 80% of all hemophiliacs, results from a deficiency of factor VIII; *hemophilia B* (Christmas disease), which affects 15% of hemophiliacs, from a deficiency of factor IX. However, recent evidence suggests that hemophilia is believed to result from nonfunctioning factors VIII and IX, rather than from their deficiency.

The severity and prognosis of bleeding disorders vary with the degree of deficiency and the site of bleeding. The overall prognosis is best in mild hemophilia, which doesn't cause spontaneous bleeding and joint deformities.

Advances in treatment have greatly improved the prognosis, and many hemophiliacs live normal life spans. Surgical procedures can be done safely at special treatment centers for hemophiliacs under the guidance of a hematologist.

Causes

Hemophilia A and B are inherited as X-linked recessive traits. This means that female carriers have a 50% chance of transmitting the gene to each daughter, who would then be a carrier, and a 50% chance of transmitting the gene to each son, who would be born with hemophilia.

Incidence

Hemophilia is the most common X-linked genetic disease, occurring in approximately 1.25 in 10,000 live male births. Hemophilia A is five times more common than hemophilia B. Hemophilia causes abnormal bleeding because of a specific clotting factor malfunction. After a person with hemophilia forms a platelet plug at a bleeding site, clotting factor deficiency impairs capacity to form a stable fibrin clot.

Signs and symptoms

Hemophilia produces abnormal bleeding, which may be mild, moderate, or severe, depending on the degree of factor deficiency.

Mild hemophilia

The mild form of hemophilia frequently goes undiagnosed until adulthood, because the patient with a mild deficiency doesn't bleed spontaneously or after minor trauma but has prolonged bleeding if challenged by major trauma or surgery. Postoperative bleeding continues as a slow ooze or ceases and starts again up to 8 days after surgery.

Moderate and severe hemophilia

Severe hemophilia causes spontaneous bleeding. The first sign of severe hemophilia is commonly excessive bleeding after circumcision. Later, spontaneous bleeding or severe bleeding after minor trauma may produce large subcutaneous and deep intramuscular hematomas. (See *Managing hemophilia.*)

Bleeding into joints and muscles causes pain, swelling, extreme tenderness, and possibly permanent deformity. Bleeding near peripheral nerves may cause peripheral neuropathies, pain, paresthesia, and muscle atrophy.

If bleeding impairs blood flow through a major vessel, it can cause ischemia and gangrene. Pharyngeal, lingual, intracardial, intracerebral, and intracranial bleeding may all lead to shock and death.

Moderate hemophilia causes symptoms similar to severe hemophilia but produces only occasional spontaneous bleeding episodes.

Diagnosis

A history of prolonged bleeding after trauma or surgery (including dental extractions) or of episodes of spontaneous bleeding into muscles or joints usually indicates some defect in the hemostatic mechanism.

Specific coagulation factor assays can diagnose the type and severity of hemophilia. A positive family history can also help diagnose hemophilia, but 20% of all cases have no family history.

Characteristic findings in hemophilia A include:

- factor VIII assay 0% to 30% of normal
- prolonged activated partial thromboplastin time (PTT)
- normal platelet count and function, bleeding time, and prothrombin time.

Characteristics of hemophilia B include:

- deficient factor IX assay
- baseline coagulation results similar to hemophilia A, with normal factor VIII.

In hemophilia A or B, the degree of factor deficiency determines severity:

- mild hemophilia—factor levels 5% to 40% of normal
- moderate hemophilia—factor levels 1% to 5% of normal
- severe hemophilia—factor levels less than 1% of normal.

Treatment

Hemophilia is not curable, but treatment can prevent crippling deformities and prolong life expectancy. Correct treatment quickly stops bleeding by increasing plasma levels of deficient clotting factors to help prevent disabling deformities that result from repeated bleeding into muscles and joints. Treatment varies according to the type of hemophilia:

- In hemophilia A, cryoprecipitated antihemophilic factor (AHF), lyophilized AHF, or both, given in doses large enough to raise clotting factor levels above 25% of normal, can permit normal hemostasis. Before surgery, AHF is administered to raise clotting factors to hemostatic levels. Levels are then kept within a normal range until the wound has completely healed.
- In hemophilia B, administration of factor IX concentrate during bleeding episodes increases factor IX levels.

A person with hemophilia who undergoes surgery needs careful management by a hematologist with expertise in hemophilia care. The patient will

☑ Managing Hemophilia

Teach parents how to care for their child with hemophilia as follows.

Risk for injury and bleeding

• Instruct parents to notify the doctor immediately after even a minor injury, but especially after an injury to the head, neck, or abdomen. Such injuries may require special blood factor replacement. Also, they should check with the doctor before allowing dental extractions or any other surgery.

• Stress the importance of regular, careful toothbrushing to prevent the need for dental surgery. The child should use a soft toothbrush.

• Teach parents to be alert for signs of severe internal bleeding, such as severe pain or swelling in a joint or muscle; stiffness; decreased joint movement; severe abdominal pain; blood in the urine; black, tarry stools; and severe headache.

Risk for other disorders

• Because the child receives blood components, he's at risk for hepatitis. Early signs—headache, fever, decreased appetite, nausea, vomiting, abdominal tenderness, and pain over the liver—may appear 3 weeks to 6 months after treatment with blood components.

• Discuss the increased risk for human immunodeficiency virus (HIV) infection if the child received a blood product before routine screening of blood products for HIV began. Tell his parents to ask the doctor about periodic testing for HIV.

Precautions and treatment

• Urge parents to make sure their child wears a medical identification bracelet at all times.

• *Warn parents never to give their child aspirin.* It can increase the tendency to bleed. Advise them to give acetaminophen instead.

• Instruct parents to protect their child from injury, but to avoid unnecessary restrictions that impair his development. For example, they can sew padded patches into the knees and elbows of a toddler's clothing to protect these joints during falls. They must forbid an older child to play contact sports such as football but can encourage swimming or playing golf.

• Teach parents to apply cold compresses or ice bags to an injured area and to elevate it or to apply light pressure to a bleeding site. To prevent recurrence of bleeding, advise parents to restrict their child's activity for 48 hours after his bleeding is under control.

• If parents have been trained to give blood factor components at home to avoid hospitalization, make sure they know venipuncture and infusion techniques and don't delay treatment during bleeding episodes.

• Instruct parents to keep blood factor concentrate and infusion equipment on hand, even on vacation.

• Emphasize the importance of having the child keep routine appointments at the local hemophilia center.

Importance of genetic screening

• Daughters should have genetic screening and testing to determine if they're hemophilia carriers. Affected males should have counseling as well. If they mate with a noncarrier, all of their daughters will be carriers; if they mate with a carrier, each male or female child has a 25% chance of being affected.

• For more information, refer parents to the National Hemophilia Foundation.

require deficient factor replacement before and after surgery. Such replacement may be necessary even for minor surgery such as a dental extraction.

In addition, epsilon-aminocaproic acid is frequently used for oral bleeding to inhibit the active fibrinolytic system present in the oral mucosa. Preventive treatment teaches the patient how to avoid trauma, manage minor bleeding, and recognize bleeding that requires immediate medical intervention. Genetic counseling helps those who are carriers understand how this disease is transmitted.

Special considerations

During bleeding episodes:
• Give deficient clotting factor or plasma as needed. The body uses up AHF in 48 to 72 hours, so repeat infusions, as needed, until bleeding stops.
• Apply cold compresses or ice bags and raise the injured part.
• To prevent recurrence of bleeding, restrict activity for 48 hours after bleeding is under control.
• Control pain with an analgesic, such as acetaminophen, propoxyphene, codeine, or meperidine, as needed. Avoid I.M. injections because of possible hematoma formation at the injection site. Aspirin and aspirin-containing medications are contraindicated because they decrease platelet adherence and may increase the bleeding.

If the patient has bled into a joint:
• Immediately elevate the joint.
• To restore joint mobility, begin range-of-motion exercises at least 48 hours after the bleeding is controlled. Tell the patient to avoid weight bearing until bleeding stops and swelling subsides.

After bleeding episodes and surgery:
• Watch closely for signs of further bleeding, such as increased pain and swelling, fever, or symptoms of shock.
• Closely monitor PTT.

• Teach parents special precautions to prevent bleeding episodes, signs of internal bleeding, and how to administer emergency first aid.
• Refer new patients to a hemophilia treatment center for evaluation. The center will devise a treatment plan for the patient's primary doctor and serve as a resource for everyone involved in the patient's care.
• People who have been exposed to the human immunodeficiency virus through contaminated blood products need special support.
• Refer the patient and family for genetic counseling.

HEMORRHOIDS

Varicosities or hemorrhoids may occur in the superior or inferior hemorrhoidal venous plexus. Dilation and enlargement of the superior plexus produce internal hemorrhoids; dilation and enlargement of the inferior plexus produce external hemorrhoids, which may protrude from the rectum. Hemorrhoids occur in both sexes. Incidence is generally highest between ages 20 and 50.

Causes

Hemorrhoids probably result from increased intravenous pressure in the hemorrhoidhal plexus. Predisposing factors include occupations that require prolonged standing or sitting; straining due to constipation, diarrhea, coughing, sneezing, or vomiting; and heart failure.

Other factors include hepatic disease, such as cirrhosis, amebic abscesses or hepatitis; alcoholism; anorectal infections; loss of muscle tone due to old age, rectal surgery, or episiotomy; anal intercourse; and pregnancy.

Signs and symptoms

Hemorrhoids are classified as *first-degree, second-degree,* or *third-degree,* depending on their severity. Signs and symptoms vary accordingly:

• Although first-degree hemorrhoids may produce no symptoms, they characteristically cause painless, intermittent bleeding during defecation. Bright-red blood appears in stools or on toilet paper because of injury of the fragile mucosa covering the hemorrhoid. First-degree hemorrhoids may itch from poor anal hygiene.

• When second-degree hemorrhoids prolapse, they're usually painless and spontaneously return to the anal canal following defecation.

• Third-degree hemorrhoids cause constant discomfort and prolapse in response to any increase in intra-abdominal pressure. They must be manually reduced. Thrombosis of external hemorrhoids produces sudden rectal pain and a subcutaneous, large, firm lump that the patient can feel.

If hemorrhoids cause severe or recurrent bleeding, they may lead to secondary anemia with significant pallor, fatigue, and weakness. However, such systemic complications are rare.

Diagnosis

Physical examination confirms external hemorrhoids. Proctoscopy confirms internal hemorrhoids and rules out rectal polyps.

Treatment

Effective treatment depends on the type and severity of the hemorrhoid and on the patient's overall condition.

Nonsurgical treatments

Generally, treatment includes measures to ease pain, combat swelling and congestion, and regulate bowel habits. Patients can relieve constipation by increasing the amount of raw vegetables,

fruit, and whole grain cereal in the diet or by using stool softeners.

Venous congestion can be prevented by avoiding prolonged sitting on the toilet; local swelling and pain can be decreased with local anesthetic agents (lotions, creams, or suppositories), astringents, or cold compresses, followed by warm sitz baths or thermal packs. Rarely, the patient with chronic, profuse bleeding may require blood transfusion.

Other nonsurgical treatments are injection of a sclerosing solution to produce scar tissue that decreases prolapse, manual reduction, and hemorrhoid ligation or laser ablation.

Hemorrhoidectomy

The most effective treatment, hemorrhoidectomy is necessary for patients with severe bleeding, intolerable pain and pruritus, and large prolapse. This procedure is contraindicated in patients with blood dyscrasias (acute leukemia, aplastic anemia, or hemophilia) or gastric cancer and during the first trimester of pregnancy.

Special considerations

• To prepare the patient for hemorrhoidectomy, administer an enema (usually 2 to 4 hours before surgery), and record the results. Shave the perianal area, and clean the anus and surrounding skin.

• Postoperatively, check for signs of prolonged rectal bleeding, administer adequate analgesics, and provide sitz baths.

• As soon as the patient can resume oral feedings, administer a bulk medication, such as psyllium, about 1 hour after the evening meal to ensure a daily bowel movement.

• Warn against using a stool softener soon after hemorrhoidectomy because firm stools act as a natural dilator to prevent anal stricture from the scar tissue. (Some patients may need re-

peated digital dilation to prevent such narrowing.)
• Keep the wound site clean to prevent infection and irritation.
• Before discharge, stress the importance of regular bowel habits and good anal hygiene.
• Warn against too-vigorous wiping with washcloths and using harsh soaps.
• Encourage the use of medicated astringent pads and white toilet paper (the fixative in colored paper can irritate the skin).

HEMOTHORAX

In hemothorax, blood from damaged intercostal, pleural, mediastinal, and (infrequently) lung parenchymal vessels enters the pleural cavity. Depending on the amount of bleeding and the underlying cause, hemothorax may be associated with varying degrees of lung collapse and mediastinal shift. Pneumothorax — air in the pleural cavity — often accompanies hemothorax.

Causes
Hemothorax usually results from blunt or penetrating chest trauma; in fact, about 25% of patients with such trauma have hemothorax. Less often, it results from thoracic surgery, pulmonary infarction, neoplasm, dissecting thoracic aneurysm, or anticoagulant therapy.

Signs and symptoms
The patient with hemothorax may experience chest pain, tachypnea, and mild to severe dyspnea, depending on the amount of blood in the pleural cavity and associated pathology. If respiratory failure results, the patient may appear anxious, restless, possibly stuporous, and cyanotic; marked blood loss produces hypotension and shock.

The affected side of the chest expands and stiffens, while the unaffected side rises and falls with the patient's gasping respirations.

Diagnosis
The following clinical test results, along with a history of trauma, strongly suggest hemothorax:
• *Percussion* reveals dullness and, on auscultation, decreased to absent breath sounds over the affected side.
• *Thoracentesis* yields blood or serosanguineous fluid.
• *Chest X-rays* show pleural fluid with or without mediastinal shift.
• *Arterial blood gas (ABG) analysis* may document respiratory failure.
• *Hemoglobin* may be decreased, depending on blood loss.

Treatment
Effective treatment stabilizes the patient's condition, stops the bleeding, evacuates blood from the pleural space, and re-expands the underlying lung. Mild hemothorax usually clears rapidly in 10 to 14 days, requiring only observation for further bleeding.

In severe hemothorax, thoracentesis serves not only as a diagnostic tool, but also as a method of removing fluid from the pleural cavity.

After the diagnosis is confirmed, a chest tube is inserted into the sixth intercostal space at the posterior axillary line. Suction may be used; a large-bore tube is used to prevent clot blockage. If the chest tube doesn't improve the patient's condition, he may need a thoracotomy to evacuate blood and clots and to control bleeding.

Special considerations
• Give oxygen by face mask or nasal cannula.
• Give I.V. fluids and blood transfusions (monitored by a central venous pressure line), as needed, to treat shock. Monitor ABG levels often.

• Explain all procedures to the patient to allay his fears. Assist with thoracentesis. Warn the patient not to cough during this procedure.

• Observe chest tube drainage carefully, and record the volume drained at least every hour. Milk the chest tube every hour to keep it open and free of clots. If the tube is warm and full of blood, and the bloody fluid level in the water-seal bottle is rising rapidly, the patient may need immediate surgery.

• Watch the patient closely for pallor and gasping respirations. Monitor his vital signs diligently. Falling blood pressure and rising pulse and respiratory rates may indicate shock or massive bleeding.

HEPATIC ENCEPHALOPATHY

Also known as hepatic coma, hepatic encephalopathy is a neurologic syndrome that develops as a complication of chronic liver disease. Most common in patients with cirrhosis, this syndrome is caused primarily by ammonia intoxication of the brain. It may be acute and self-limiting, or chronic and progressive.

Treatment requires correction of the precipitating cause and reduction of blood ammonia levels. In advanced stages, the prognosis is extremely poor despite vigorous treatment.

Causes
Hepatic encephalopathy follows rising blood ammonia levels. Several factors cause these levels to rise.

Improper shunting of blood
Normally, the ammonia produced by protein breakdown in the bowel is metabolized to urea in the liver. When portal blood shunts past the liver, ammonia directly enters the systemic circulation and is carried to the brain.

Such shunting may result from the collateral venous circulation that develops in portal hypertension or from surgically created portal-systemic shunts. Cirrhosis further compounds this problem because impaired hepatocellular function prevents conversion of ammonia that reaches the liver.

Other factors
Other factors that predispose rising ammonia levels include excessive protein intake, sepsis, excessive accumulation of nitrogenous body wastes (from constipation or GI hemorrhage), and bacterial action on protein and urea to form ammonia.

Certain other factors heighten the brain's sensitivity to ammonia intoxication: fluid and electrolyte imbalances (especially metabolic alkalosis), hypoxia, azotemia, impaired glucose metabolism, infection, and administration of sedatives, narcotics, and general anesthetics.

Signs and symptoms
Clinical manifestations of hepatic encephalopathy vary (depending on the severity of neurologic involvement) and develop in four stages:

• *prodromal stage*: often overlooked because early symptoms, such as slight personality changes (disorientation, forgetfulness, slurred speech) and a slight tremor, are subtle

• *impending stage*: tremor progressing to asterixis (liver flap, flapping tremor), the hallmark of hepatic encephalopathy. Asterixis is characterized by quick, irregular extensions and flexions of the wrists and fingers when the wrists are held out straight and the hands flexed upward. Lethargy, aberrant behavior, and apraxia also occur.

• *stuporous stage*: hyperventilation; patient is stuporous but noisy and abusive when aroused

• *comatose stage*: hyperactive reflexes, a positive Babinski's sign, fetor hepaticus (musty, sweet odor to the breath), and coma.

Diagnosis

Clinical features, a positive history of liver disease, and elevated serum ammonia levels in venous and arterial samples confirm hepatic encephalopathy. Other supportive test results include an EEG that slows as the disease progresses, an elevated bilirubin level, and prolonged prothrombin time.

Treatment

Effective treatment stops the progression of encephalopathy by reducing blood ammonia levels. Such treatment eliminates ammonia-producing substances from the GI tract by:

• administration of neomycin to suppress bacterial flora (preventing them from converting amino acids into ammonia)

• sorbitol-induced catharsis to produce osmotic diarrhea

• continuous aspiration of blood from the stomach

• reduction of dietary protein intake

• administration of lactulose to reduce the blood ammonia levels.

Neomycin

Neomycin is usually given in a dose of 3 to 4 g daily P.O. or by retention enema. Although neomycin is nonabsorbable at the recommended dosage, an amount that exceeds 4 g daily may produce irreversible hearing loss and nephrotoxicity.

Lactulose

Lactulose traps ammonia in the bowel and promotes its excretion. It's effective because bacterial enzymes change lactulose to lactic acid, thereby rendering the colon too acidic for bacterial growth. At the same time, the resulting increase in free hydrogen ions prevents diffusion of ammonia through the mucosa; lactulose promotes conversion of systemically absorbable ammonia to ammonium, which is poorly absorbed and can be excreted.

The usual dosage of lactulose syrup is 30 to 45 ml P.O. three or four times daily. For acute hepatic coma, 300 ml diluted with 700 ml of water may be administered by retention enema. Lactulose therapy requires careful monitoring of fluid and electrolyte balance.

Other treatments

Treatment may also include potassium supplements (80 to 120 mEq/day P.O. or I.V.) to correct alkalosis (from increased ammonia levels), especially if the patient is taking diuretics. Sometimes, hemodialysis can temporarily clear toxic blood. Exchange transfusions may provide dramatic but temporary improvement; however, they require a large amount of blood.

Salt-poor albumin may be used to maintain fluid and electrolyte balance, replace depleted albumin levels, and restore plasma.

Special considerations

• Frequently assess and record the patient's level of consciousness. Continually orient him to place and time. Remember to keep a daily record of the patient's handwriting to monitor the progression of neurologic involvement.

• Monitor intake, output, and fluid and electrolyte balance. Check daily weight and measure abdominal girth. Watch for, and immediately report, signs of anemia (decreased hemoglobin), infection, alkalosis (increased serum bicarbonate levels), and GI bleeding (melena, hematemesis).

• Give prescribed drugs and watch for adverse effects.

• Ask the dietitian to provide the specified low-protein diet, with carbohydrates supplying most of the calories. Provide good mouth care.

• Promote rest, comfort, and a quiet atmosphere. Discourage strenuous exercise.

• Use restraints, if necessary, but avoid sedatives. Protect the comatose patient's eyes from corneal injury by using artificial tears or eye patches.

• Provide emotional support for the patient's family in the terminal stage of encephalopathy.

HEPATITIS, NONVIRAL

Classified as toxic or drug-induced (idiosyncratic) hepatitis, nonviral hepatitis is an inflammation of the liver. Most patients recover from this illness, although a few develop fulminating hepatitis or cirrhosis.

Causes

Nonviral hepatitis usually results from exposure to certain chemicals or drugs.

Toxic hepatitis

Various hepatotoxins—carbon tetrachloride, acetaminophen, trichloroethylene, poisonous mushrooms, vinyl chloride—can cause the toxic form of this disease. Following exposure to these agents, liver damage usually occurs within 24 to 48 hours, depending on the size of the dose. Alcohol, anoxia, and preexisting liver disease exacerbate the toxic effects of some of these agents.

Drug-induced hepatitis

Idiosyncratic hepatitis may stem from a hypersensitivity reaction unique to the affected individual, unlike toxic hepatitis, which appears to affect all

people indiscriminately. Among the drugs that may cause this type of hepatitis are niacin, halothane, sulfonamides, isoniazid, methyldopa, and phenothiazines (cholestasis-induced hepatitis).

In hypersensitive people, symptoms of hepatic dysfunction may appear at any time during or after exposure to these drugs but usually emerge after 2 to 5 weeks of therapy. Not all adverse drug reactions are toxic. Oral contraceptives, for example, may impair liver function and produce jaundice without causing necrosis, fatty infiltration of liver cells, or hypersensitivity.

Signs and symptoms

Clinical features of toxic and drug-induced hepatitis vary with the severity of the liver damage and the causative agent. In most patients, symptoms resemble those of viral hepatitis: anorexia, nausea, vomiting, jaundice, dark urine, hepatomegaly, possible abdominal pain (with acute onset and massive necrosis), and clay-colored stools or pruritus with the cholestatic form of hepatitis.

Carbon tetrachloride poisoning also produces headache, dizziness, drowsiness, and vasomotor collapse; halothane-related hepatitis produces fever, moderate leukocytosis, and eosinophilia; chlorpromazine produces a rash, abrupt fever, arthralgias, lymphadenopathy, and epigastric or right upper quadrant pain.

Diagnosis

Diagnostic findings include elevations in serum aspartate aminotransferase and alanine aminotransferase, both total and direct bilirubin (with cholestasis), alkaline phosphatase, white blood cell (WBC) count, and eosinophil count (possible in the drug-induced type).

A liver biopsy may help identify the underlying pathology, especially infiltration with WBCs and eosinophils. Liver function tests have limited value in distinguishing between nonviral and viral hepatitis.

Treatment

Effective treatment must remove the causative agent by lavage, catharsis, or hyperventilation, depending on the route of exposure. Acetylcysteine may serve as an antidote for toxic hepatitis caused by acetaminophen poisoning but doesn't prevent drug-induced hepatitis caused by other substances.

Corticosteroids may be ordered for patients with the drug-induced type. Thioctic acid, an investigational drug, may be successful with mushroom poisoning.

Special considerations

To prevent this disease, teach the patient the proper use of drugs and the proper handling of cleaning agents and solvents.

HEPATITIS, VIRAL

A fairly common systemic disease, viral hepatitis is marked by hepatic cell destruction, necrosis, and autolysis, leading to anorexia, jaundice, and hepatomegaly. In most patients, hepatic cells eventually regenerate with little or no residual damage. However, old age and serious underlying disorders make complications more likely. The prognosis is poor if edema and hepatic encephalopathy develop.

There are five types of hepatitis:
• *Type A* (infectious or short-incubation hepatitis) is rising among homosexuals and in people with immunosuppression related to human immunodeficiency virus (HIV) infection.

• *Type B* (serum or long-incubation hepatitis) also is increasing among HIV-positive individuals. Routine screening of donor blood for the hepatitis B surface antigen (HBsAg) has decreased the incidence of posttransfusion cases, but transmission by needles shared by drug abusers remains a major problem.
• *Type C* accounts for about 20% of all viral hepatitis cases and for most posttransfusion cases.
• *Type D* (delta hepatitis) is responsible for about 50% of all cases of fulminant hepatitis, which has a high mortality. Developing in 1% of patients, fulminant hepatitis causes unremitting liver failure with encephalopathy. It progresses to coma and commonly leads to death within 2 weeks.

In the United States, type D is confined to people who are frequently exposed to blood and blood products, such as I.V. drug users and hemophiliacs.
• *Type E* (formerly grouped with type C under the name non-A, non-B hepatitis) occurs primarily in people who've recently returned from an endemic area (such as India, Africa, Asia, or Central America); it's more common in young adults and more severe in pregnant women.

Causes

The five major forms of viral hepatitis result from infection with the causative viruses: A, B, C, D, or E.

Type A hepatitis

Hepatitis A is highly contagious and is usually transmitted by the fecal-oral route. However, it may also be transmitted parenterally. Hepatitis A usually results from ingestion of contaminated food, milk, or water. Outbreaks of this type are often traced to ingestion of seafood from polluted water.

Type B hepatitis

Once thought to be transmitted only by the direct exchange of contaminated blood, hepatitis B is now known to be transmitted also by contact with human secretions and feces. As a result, nurses, doctors, laboratory technicians, and dentists are frequently exposed to type B hepatitis, often as a result of wearing defective gloves.

Transmission also occurs during intimate sexual contact and through perinatal transmission.

Type C hepatitis

Although hepatitis C viruses have been isolated, only a small percentage of patients have tested positive for them — perhaps reflecting the test's poor specificity. Usually, this type of hepatitis is transmitted through transfused blood from asymptomatic donors.

Type D hepatitis

Hepatitis D is found only in patients with an acute or chronic episode of hepatitis B and requires the presence of HBsAg. The type D virus depends on the double-shelled type B virus to replicate. For this reason, type D infection can't outlast a type B infection.

Type E hepatitis

Hepatitis E is transmitted enterically, much like type A. Because this virus is inconsistently shed in feces, detection is difficult.

Signs and symptoms

Assessment findings are similar for the different types of hepatitis. Typically, signs and symptoms progress in three stages — the prodromal (preicteric), clinical (icteric), and recovery (posticteric).

Prodromal stage

In this stage, the patient typically complains of easy fatigue and anorexia (possibly with mild weight loss), generalized malaise, depression, headache, weakness, arthralgia, myalgia, photophobia, and nausea with vomiting. He also may describe changes in his senses of taste and smell.

Assessment of vital signs may reveal a fever of 100° to 102° F (37.8° to 38.9° C). As the prodromal stage draws to a close, usually 1 to 5 days before the onset of the clinical jaundice stage, inspection of urine and stool specimens may reveal dark-colored urine and clay-colored stools.

Clinical stage

If the patient has progressed to the clinical jaundice stage, he may report pruritus, abdominal pain or tenderness, and indigestion. Early in this stage, he may complain of anorexia; later, his appetite may return. Inspection of the sclerae, mucous membranes, and skin may reveal jaundice, which can last for 1 to 2 weeks.

Jaundice indicates that the damaged liver is unable to remove bilirubin from the blood; however, its presence doesn't indicate the severity of the disease. Occasionally, hepatitis occurs without jaundice.

During the clinical jaundice stage, inspection of the skin may detect rashes, erythematous patches, or urticaria, especially if the patient has hepatitis B or C. Palpation may disclose abdominal tenderness in the right upper quadrant, an enlarged and tender liver and, in some cases, splenomegaly and cervical adenopathy.

Recovery stage

During the recovery stage, most of the patient's symptoms decrease or subside. On palpation, a decrease in liver enlargement may be noted. The recovery phase commonly lasts from 2 to 12 weeks, although sometimes this phase lasts longer in patients with hepatitis B, C, or E.

☑ PREVENTING A RECURRENCE OF HEPATITIS

- Before discharge, emphasize the importance of having regular medical checkups for at least 1 year. The patient will have an increased risk of developing hepatoma.
- Warn the patient against using any alcohol or nonprescription drugs for 1 year.
- Teach the patient to recognize the signs of a recurrence.

Diagnosis

In suspected viral hepatitis, a hepatitis profile is routinely performed. This study identifies antibodies specific to the causative virus, establishing the type of hepatitis as follows:

- *Type A:* Detection of an antibody to hepatitis A confirms the diagnosis.
- *Type B:* The presence of HBsAg and hepatitis B antibodies confirms the diagnosis.
- *Type C:* The diagnosis depends on serologic testing for the specific antibody 1 or more months after the onset of acute hepatitis. Until then, the diagnosis is established primarily by obtaining negative test results for hepatitis A, B, and D.
- *Type D:* The detection of intrahepatic delta antigens or immunoglobulin M (IgM) antidelta antigens in acute disease (or IgM and IgG in chronic disease) establishes the diagnosis.
- *Type E:* Detection of hepatitis E antigens supports the diagnosis; however, the diagnosis may also be determined by ruling out hepatitis C.

Additional findings from liver function studies support the diagnosis:

- *Serum aspartate aminotransferase* and *serum alanine aminotransferase levels* are increased in the prodromal stage of acute viral hepatitis.
- *Serum alkaline phosphatase levels* are slightly increased.
- *Serum bilirubin levels* are elevated. Levels may continue to be high late in the disease, especially in severe cases.
- *Prothrombin time* is prolonged (more than 3 seconds longer than normal indicates severe liver damage).
- *White blood cell counts* commonly reveal transient neutropenia and lymphopenia followed by lymphocytosis.
- *Liver biopsy* is performed if chronic hepatitis is suspected. (It's performed for acute hepatitis only if the diagnosis is questionable.)

Treatment

No specific drug therapy has been developed for hepatitis, with the exception of hepatitis C, which has been treated somewhat successfully with interferon alfa. Instead, the patient is advised to rest in the early stages of the illness and to combat anorexia by eating small, high-calorie, high-protein meals.

Protein intake should be reduced if signs of precoma—lethargy, confusion, and mental changes—develop. Large meals are usually better tolerated in the morning because many patients experience nausea late in the day.

In acute viral hepatitis, hospitalization usually is required only for patients with severe symptoms or complications. Parenteral nutrition may be required if the patient experiences persistent vomiting and is unable to maintain oral intake.

Antiemetics (trimethobenzamide or benzquinamide) may be given a half hour before meals to relieve nausea and prevent vomiting; phenothiazines have a cholestatic effect and should be avoided. For severe pruritus, the resin cholestyramine may be given.

Special considerations
• Use enteric precautions when caring for patients with type A or E hepatitis. Practice universal precautions for all patients.
• Inform visitors about isolation precautions.
• Provide rest periods throughout the day. Schedule treatments and tests so that the patient can rest between bouts of activity.
• Because inactivity may make the patient anxious, include diversional activities as part of his care. Gradually add activities to his schedule as he begins to recover.
• Encourage the patient to eat. Don't overload his meal tray or overmedicate him because this will diminish his appetite.
• Force fluids (at least 4,000 ml/day). Encourage the anorectic patient to drink fruit juices. Also offer chipped ice and effervescent soft drinks to maintain hydration without inducing vomiting.
• Administer supplemental vitamins and commercial feedings. If symptoms are severe and the patient can't tolerate oral intake, provide I.V. therapy and parenteral nutrition.
• Record the patient's weight daily, and keep intake and output records. Observe stools for color, consistency, and amount, and record the frequency of bowel movements.
• Watch for signs of fluid shift, such as weight gain and orthostasis.

• Watch for signs of hepatic coma, dehydration, pneumonia, vascular problems, and pressure ulcers.
• In fulminant hepatitis, maintain electrolyte balance and a patent airway, prevent infections, and control bleeding. Correct hypoglycemia and any other complications while awaiting liver regeneration and repair.
• Before the patient is discharged, discuss restrictions and how to prevent a recurrence of hepatitis. (See *Preventing a recurrence of hepatitis.*)

HERNIATED DISK

Also called a ruptured or slipped disk or a herniated nucleus pulposus, a herniated disk occurs when all or part of the nucleus pulposus — the soft, gelatinous, central portion of an intervertebral disk (nucleus pulposus) — is forced through the disk's weakened or torn outer ring (anulus fibrosus).

When this happens, the extruded disk may impinge on spinal nerve roots as they exit from the spinal canal or on the spinal cord itself, resulting in back pain and other signs of nerve root irritation. Herniated disks usually occur in adults (mostly men) under age 45.

Causes
Herniated disks may result from severe trauma or strain or may be related to intervertebral joint degeneration. In older patients, whose disks have begun to degenerate, minor trauma may cause herniation. About 90% of herniated disks occur in the lumbar and lumbosacral regions, 8% occur in the cervical area, and 1% to 2% in the thoracic area.

Patients with a congenitally small lumbar spinal canal or with osteophyte formation along the vertebrae may be more susceptible to nerve root compression with a herniated disk and more likely to have neurologic symptoms.

Signs and symptoms

The overriding symptom of lumbar herniated disk is severe, low back pain, which radiates to the buttocks, legs, and feet, usually unilaterally. When herniation follows trauma, the pain may begin suddenly, subside in a few days, then recur at shorter intervals and with progressive intensity.

Sciatic pain follows, beginning as a dull pain in the buttocks. Valsalva's maneuver, coughing, sneezing, or bending intensifies the pain, which is often accompanied by muscle spasms. A herniated disk may also cause sensory and motor loss in the area innervated by the compressed spinal nerve root and, in later stages, weakness and atrophy of leg muscles.

Diagnosis

Obtaining a careful patient history is vital because the mechanisms that intensify disk pain are diagnostically significant. The following test results support the diagnosis:

• *The straight-leg-raising test* and its variants are perhaps the best tests for diagnosing a herniated disk. For this test, the patient lies in a supine position while the examiner places one hand on the patient's ilium, to stabilize the pelvis, and the other hand under the ankle, then slowly raises the patient's leg. The test is positive only if the patient complains of posterior leg (sciatic) pain, not back pain.

• In *LeSegue's test,* the patient lies flat while the thigh and knee are flexed to a 90-degree angle. Resistance and pain, as well as loss of ankle or knee-jerk reflex, indicate spinal root compression.

• *X-rays of the spine* are essential to rule out other abnormalities but may not diagnose a herniated disk because a marked disk prolapse can be present despite a normal X-ray.

• *Peripheral vascular status check* — including posterior tibial and dorsalis pedis pulses, and the skin temperature of extremities — helps rule out ischemic disease, another cause of leg pain or numbness.

• Aside from the physical examination and X-rays, *myelography, a computed tomography scan,* and *magnetic resonance imaging* provide the most specific diagnostic information, showing spinal canal compression by herniated disk material.

Treatment

Treatment measures are initially conservative and consist of several weeks of bed rest (possibly with pelvic traction), heat applications, an exercise program, and medication. If neurologic impairment progresses rapidly, surgery may be necessary.

Drug therapy

Aspirin reduces inflammation and edema at the site of injury; rarely, corticosteroids, such as dexamethasone, may be prescribed for the same purpose. Muscle relaxants, especially diazepam or methocarbamol, also may be beneficial.

Surgery

A herniated disk that fails to respond to conservative treatment may necessitate surgery. The most common procedure, laminectomy, involves excision of a portion of the lamina and removal of the protruding disk (nucleus pulposus).

If laminectomy doesn't alleviate pain and disability, a spinal fusion may be necessary to overcome segmental instability. Laminectomy and spinal fusion are sometimes performed concurrently to stabilize the spine.

Other treatments

Chemonucleolysis — injection of the enzyme chymopapain into the herniated disk to dissolve nucleus polposus — is a possible alternative to laminectomy. Microdiskectomy can also be used to remove fragments of nucleus polposus.

Special considerations

• Herniated disk requires supportive care, careful patient teaching, and strong emotional support to help the patient cope with the discomfort and frustration of chronic low back pain.

• If the patient requires myelography, reinforce the need for this test, and tell the patient to expect some pain. Assure him that he'll receive a sedative before the test, if needed, to keep him as calm and comfortable as possible.

• Before myelography, question the patient carefully about allergies to iodides, iodine-containing substances, or seafood, since such allergies may indicate sensitivity to the test's radiopaque dye.

• After myelography, urge the patient to remain in bed with his head elevated (especially if metrizamide was used) and to drink plenty of fluids. Monitor intake and output. Watch for seizures and an allergic reaction.

• During conservative treatment, watch for any deterioration in neurologic status (especially during the first 24 hours after admission), which may indicate an urgent need for surgery.

• Apply antiembolism stockings, as prescribed, and encourage the patient to move his legs, as allowed. Provide high-topped sneakers to prevent footdrop. Work closely with the physical therapy department to ensure a consistent regimen of leg- and back-strengthening exercises.

• Give plenty of fluids to prevent renal stasis.

• Remind the patient to cough, deep-breathe, and use blow bottles or an incentive spirometer to prevent pulmonary complications.

• Provide good skin care.

• Assess for bowel function. Use a fracture bedpan for the patient on complete bed rest.

• After laminectomy, microdiskectomy, or spinal fusion, enforce bed rest. If a blood drainage system (Hemovac) is in use, check the tubing frequently for kinks and a secure vacuum. Empty the Hemovac at the end of each shift, and record the amount and color of drainage.

• Report colorless moisture on dressings (possible cerebrospinal fluid leakage) or excessive drainage immediately. Observe the neurovascular status of the legs (color, motion, temperature, sensation).

• Monitor vital signs, and check for bowel sounds and abdominal distention. Use the logrolling technique to turn the patient.

• Administer analgesics, especially 30 minutes before initial attempts at sitting or walking. Help the patient during his first attempt to walk. Provide a straight-backed chair for limited sitting.

• Teach the patient who has undergone spinal fusion how to wear a brace. Assist with straight-leg-raising and toe-pointing exercises as necessary.

• Before discharge, teach proper body mechanics — bending at the knees and hips (never at the waist), standing straight, carrying objects close to the body.

• Advise the patient to lie down when tired and to sleep on his side (never on his abdomen) on an extra-firm mattress or a bed board. Urge him to maintain proper weight to prevent lordosis caused by obesity.

• Before chemonucleolysis, ask the patient about allergies to meat tenderizers (chymopapain is a similar substance). Such an allergy contraindicates the use of this enzyme, which can produce severe anaphylaxis in a sensitive patient. Enforce bed rest. Administer analgesics and apply heat as needed. Urge the patient to cough and deep-breathe. Assist with special exercises, and tell the patient to continue these exercises after discharge.

• Tell the patient who must receive a muscle relaxant of possible adverse effects, especially drowsiness. Warn him to avoid activities that require alertness until he has built up a tolerance to the drug's sedative effects.

• Provide emotional support. Try to cheer the patient during periods of frustration and depression. Assure him of his progress, and offer encouragement.

HERPANGINA

An acute infection, herpangina is generally caused by group A coxsackieviruses (usually types 1 through 10, 16, and 23). It's less commonly caused by group B coxsackieviruses and echoviruses. The disease characteristically produces vesicular lesions on the mucous membranes of the soft palate, tonsillar pillars, and throat.

Causes

Because fecal-oral transfer is the main mode of transmission, herpangina usually affects children under age 10 (except neonates, because of maternal antibodies). It occurs slightly more often in late summer and fall and can be sporadic, endemic, or epidemic. Herpangina generally subsides in 4 to 7 days.

Signs and symptoms

After a 2- to 9-day incubation period, herpangina begins abruptly with a sore throat, pain on swallowing, headache, a temperature of 100° to 104° F (37.8°

to 40° C) that persists for 1 to 4 days and may cause seizures, anorexia, vomiting, malaise, diarrhea, and pain in the stomach, back of the neck, legs, and arms.

After this, up to 12 grayish white papulovesicles appear on the soft palate and, less frequently, on the tonsils, uvula, tongue, and larynx. These lesions grow from 1 to 2 mm in diameter to large, punched-out ulcers surrounded by small, inflamed margins.

Diagnosis

Characteristic oral lesions suggest this diagnosis; isolation of the virus from mouth washings or feces, and elevated specific antibody titer confirm it. Other routine test results are normal except for slight leukocytosis.

A diagnosis requires distinguishing the mouth lesions in herpangina from those in streptococcal tonsillitis (no ulcers; lesions confined to tonsils).

Treatment and special considerations

• Effective treatment for herpangina is entirely symptomatic, emphasizing measures to reduce fever and prevent seizures and possible dehydration. Herpangina doesn't require isolation or hospitalization but does require careful hand washing and sanitary disposal of excretions.

• Teach parents to give adequate fluids, enforce bed rest, and administer tepid sponge baths and antipyretics.

HERPES SIMPLEX

A recurrent viral infection, herpes simplex is caused by *Herpesvirus hominis (HVH)*, a widespread infectious agent. Herpes type I, which is transmitted by oral and respiratory secretions, affects the skin and mucous membranes and commonly produces cold sores and fever blisters.

Herpes type II primarily affects the genital area and is transmitted by sexual contact. However, cross-infection may result from orogenital sex.

Causes

About 85% of all HVH infections are subclinical. The others produce localized lesions and systemic reactions. After the first infection, a patient is a carrier susceptible to recurrent infections, which may be provoked by fever, menses, stress, heat, and cold. However, in recurrent infections, the patient usually has no constitutional signs and symptoms.

Incidence

Primary HVH is the leading cause of childhood gingivostomatitis in children ages 1 to 3. It causes the most common nonepidemic encephalitis and is the second most common viral infection in pregnant women. It can pass to the fetus transplacentally and, in early pregnancy, may cause spontaneous abortion or premature birth.

Herpes is equally common in males and females. It occurs worldwide and is most prevalent among children in lower socioeconomic groups who live in crowded environments. Saliva, feces, urine, skin lesions, and purulent eye exudate are potential sources of infection.

Signs and symptoms

In neonates, HVH symptoms usually appear a week or two after birth. They range from localized skin lesions to a disseminated infection of such organs as the liver, lungs, or brain. Common complications include seizures, mental retardation, blindness, chorioretinitis, deafness, microcephaly, diabetes insipidus, and spasticity. Up to 90% of infants with disseminated disease will die.

Primary infection in childhood may be generalized or localized.

Generalized infection

After an incubation period of from 2 to 12 days, onset of generalized infection begins with fever, pharyngitis, erythema, and edema. After brief prodromal tingling and itching, typical primary lesions erupt as vesicles on an erythematous base, eventually rupturing and leaving a painful ulcer, followed by a yellowish crust. Healing begins 7 to 10 days after onset and is complete in 3 weeks.

Vesicles may form on any part of the oral mucosa, especially the tongue, gingiva, and cheeks. In generalized infection, vesicles occur with submaxillary lymphadenopathy, increased salivation, halitosis, anorexia, and fever of up to 105° F (40.6° C). Herpetic stomatitis may lead to severe dehydration in children.

A generalized infection usually runs its course in 4 to 10 days. In this form, virus reactivation causes cold sores— single or grouped vesicles in and around the mouth.

Localized infection

Genital herpes usually affects adolescents and young adults. Typically painful, the initial attack produces fluid-filled vesicles that ulcerate and heal in 1 to 3 weeks. Fever, regional lymphadenopathy, and dysuria may also occur.

Usually, herpetic keratoconjunctivitis is unilateral and causes only local symptoms: conjunctivitis, regional adenopathy, blepharitis, and vesicles on the lid. Other ocular symptoms may be excessive lacrimation, edema, chemosis, photophobia, and purulent exudate.

☑ TREATING AND PREVENTING HERPES SIMPLEX

• Teach the patient with genital herpes to use warm compresses or take sitz baths several times a day. Tell him to use a drying agent, such as povidone-iodine solution, to increase his fluid intake, and to avoid all sexual contact during the active stage.

• Recommend that pregnant women with *Herpesvirus hominis* infection have weekly viral cultures of the cervix and external genitalia starting at 32 weeks' gestation.

• Instruct patients with herpetic whitlow not to share towels or utensils with uninfected people. Educate staff members and other susceptible people about the risk of contracting the disease.

• Tell patients with cold sores not to kiss infants or people with eczema. (Those with genital herpes pose no risk to infants if their hygiene is meticulous.)

Other signs and symptoms

Both types of HVH can cause acute sporadic encephalitis with an altered level of consciousness, personality changes, and seizures. Other effects may include smell and taste hallucinations and neurologic abnormalities such as aphasia.

Herpetic whitlow, an HVH finger infection, commonly affects health care workers. First the finger tingles and then it becomes red, swollen, and painful. Vesicles with a red halo erupt and may ulcerate or coalesce. Other effects may include satellite vesicles, fever, chills, malaise, and a red streak up the arm.

Diagnosis

Typical lesions may suggest HVH infection. However, confirmation requires isolation of the virus from local lesions and a histologic biopsy. A rise in antibodies and moderate leukocytosis may support the diagnosis.

Treatment

Symptomatic and supportive therapy is essential. Generalized primary infection usually requires an analgesic-antipyretic to reduce fever and relieve pain. Anesthetic mouthwashes, such as viscous lidocaine, may reduce the pain of gingivostomatitis, enabling the patient to eat and preventing dehydration. Drying agents, such as calamine lotion, make labial lesions less painful.

Refer patients with eye infections to an ophthalmologist. Topical corticosteroids are contraindicated in active infection, but idoxuridine, trifluridine, and vidarabine are effective.

A 5% acyclovir ointment may bring relief to patients with genital herpes or to immunosuppressed patients with HVH skin infections. Acyclovir I.V. helps treat more severe infections. (See *Treating and preventing herpes simplex.*)

Special considerations

• Abstain from direct patient care if you have herpetic whitlow.

• Patients with central nervous system infection alone need no isolation.

• Teach patients how to care for themselves during an outbreak of HVH and how to avoid infecting others.

HERPES ZOSTER

Also called shingles, herpes zoster is an acute unilateral and segmental inflammation of the dorsal root ganglia caused by infection with the herpesvirus varicella-zoster (V-Z), which also causes chickenpox. This infection usually occurs in adults. It produces localized vesicular skin lesions confined to a dermatome, and severe neuralgic pain in peripheral areas innervated by the nerves arising in the inflamed root ganglia.

The prognosis is good unless the infection spreads to the brain. Eventually, most patients recover completely, except for possible scarring and, in corneal damage, visual impairment. Occasionally, neuralgia may persist for months or years.

Herpes zoster is found primarily in adults, especially those past age 50. It seldom recurs.

Causes

Herpes zoster results from reactivation of varicella virus that has lain dormant in the cerebral ganglia (extramedullary ganglia of the cranial nerves) or the ganglia of posterior nerve roots since a previous episode of chickenpox.

Exactly how or why this reactivation occurs isn't clear. Some believe that the virus multiplies as it's reactivated and that it's neutralized by antibodies remaining from the initial infection. But if effective antibodies aren't present, the virus continues to multiply in the ganglia, destroy the host neuron, and spread down the sensory nerves to the skin.

Signs and symptoms

Herpes zoster usually runs a typical course with classic signs and symptoms. However, serious complications sometimes occur.

Onset of disease

Herpes zoster begins with fever and malaise. Within 2 to 4 days, severe deep pain, pruritus, and paresthesia or hyperesthesia develop, usually on the trunk and occasionally on the arms and legs in a dermatomal distribution. Pain may be continuous or intermittent and usually lasts from 1 to 4 weeks.

Skin lesions

Up to 2 weeks after the first symptoms, small red nodular skin lesions erupt on the painful areas. (These lesions commonly spread unilaterally around the thorax or vertically over the arms or legs.) Sometimes nodules don't appear at all, but when they do, they quickly become vesicles filled with clear fluid or pus.

About 10 days after they appear, the vesicles dry and form scabs. (See *Skin lesions in herpes zoster,* page 414.) When they rupture, such lesions often become infected and, in severe cases, may lead to the enlargement of regional lymph nodes; they may even become gangrenous. Intense pain may occur before the rash appears and after the scabs form.

Nerve involvement

Occasionally, herpes zoster involves the cranial nerves, especially the trigeminal and geniculate ganglia or the oculomotor nerve. Geniculate zoster may cause vesicle formation in the external auditory canal, ipsilateral facial palsy, hearing loss, dizziness, and loss of taste.

Trigeminal ganglion involvement causes eye pain and, possibly, corneal and scleral damage and impaired vision. Rarely, oculomotor involvement causes conjunctivitis, extraocular

SKIN LESIONS IN HERPES ZOSTER

Characteristic skin lesions in herpes zoster are fluid-filled vesicles that dry and form scabs after about 10 days.

weakness, ptosis, and paralytic mydriasis.

Rare complications

In rare cases, herpes zoster leads to generalized central nervous system infection, muscle atrophy, motor paralysis (usually transient), acute transverse myelitis, and ascending myelitis. More often, generalized infection causes acute retention of urine and unilateral paralysis of the diaphragm. In postherpetic neuralgia, a complication most common in elderly patients, intractable neuralgic pain may persist for years. Scars may be permanent.

Diagnosis

A positive diagnosis of herpes zoster usually isn't possible until the characteristic skin lesions develop. Before then, the pain may mimic that of appendicitis, pleurisy, or other conditions. Diagnostic test results include:
• *Examination of vesicular fluid and infected tissue* shows eosinophilic intranuclear inclusions and varicella virus.
• *Lumbar puncture* shows increased pressure; examination of cerebrospinal fluid shows increased protein levels and, possibly, pleocytosis.
• *Staining antibodies from vesicular fluid and identification under fluorescent light* differentiates herpes zoster from localized herpes simplex.

Treatment

No specific treatment exists. The primary goal of supportive treatment is to relieve itching and neuralgic pain with calamine lotion or another antipruritic; aspirin, possibly with codeine or another analgesic; and, occasionally, collodion or tincture of benzoin applied to unbroken lesions.

If bacteria have infected ruptured vesicles, treatment usually includes an appropriate systemic antibiotic.

Trigeminal zoster with corneal involvement calls for instillation of idoxuridine ointment or another antiviral agent.

To help a patient cope with the intractable pain of postherpetic neuralgia, administer a systemic corticosteroid—such as cortisone or, possibly, corticotropin—to reduce inflammation, tranquilizers, sedatives, or tricyclic antidepressants with phenothiazines.

Acyclovir seems to stop progression of the rash and prevent visceral complications. In immunocompromised patients—both children and adults—acyclovir therapy may be administered I.V. The drug appears to prevent disseminated, life-threatening disease in some patients.

Special considerations

• Keep the patient comfortable, maintain meticulous hygiene, and prevent infection. During the acute phase, encourage him to get adequate rest and give supportive care to promote proper healing of lesions.

• Apply calamine lotion liberally to the lesions. If lesions are severe and widespread, apply a wet dressing.

• Instruct the patient to avoid scratching the lesions.

• If vesicles rupture, apply a cold compress.

• To decrease the pain of oral lesions, tell the patient to use a soft toothbrush, eat a soft diet, and use saline mouthwash.

• To minimize neuralgic pain, never withhold or delay administration of analgesics. Give them exactly on schedule, because the pain of herpes zoster can be severe. In postherpetic neuralgia, avoid narcotic analgesics because of the danger of addiction.

• Repeatedly reassure the patient that herpetic pain will eventually subside. Provide the patient with diversionary activity to take his mind off the pain and pruritus.

HIATAL HERNIA

Hiatus or hiatal hernia is a defect in the diaphragm that permits a portion of the stomach to pass through the diaphragmatic opening into the chest. Three types of hiatal hernia can occur: *sliding hernia, paraesophageal ("rolling") hernia,* or *mixed hernia,* which includes features of both. (See *Two types of hiatal hernia,* page 416.)

In a sliding hernia, both the stomach and the gastroesophageal junction slip up into the chest, so the gastroesophageal junction is above the diaphragmatic hiatus. In paraesophageal hernia, a part of the greater curvature of the stomach rolls through the diaphragmatic defect. Treatment can prevent such complications as strangulation of the herniated intrathoracic portion of the stomach.

Causes

Usually, hiatal hernia results from muscle weakening that's common with aging and may be secondary to esophageal cancer, kyphoscoliosis, trauma, or certain surgical procedures. It may also result from certain diaphragmatic malformations that may cause congenital weakness.

In hiatal hernia, the muscular collar around the esophageal and diaphragmatic junction loosens, permitting the lower portion of the esophagus and the stomach to rise into the chest when intra-abdominal pressure increases (possibly causing gastroesophageal reflux). Such increased intra-abdominal pressure may result from ascites, pregnancy, obesity, constrictive clothing, bending, straining, coughing, Valsalva's maneuver, or extreme physical exertion.

Incidence

A sliding hernia is three to ten times more common than paraesophageal and mixed hernias combined. The incidence of hiatal hernia is higher in women than in men (especially the paraesophageal type) and increases with age.

Signs and symptoms

Typically, a paraesophageal hernia produces no symptoms; it's usually an incidental finding on barium swallow. Since this type of hernia leaves the closing mechanism of the cardiac sphincter unchanged, it rarely causes acid reflux and reflux esophagitis.

Symptoms result from displacement or stretching of the stomach and may include a feeling of fullness in the chest

Two Types of Hiatal Hernia

Normal stomach

Esophagus

Diaphragm

Cardia

Stomach

Duodenum

Sliding hiatal hernia

Esophagus

Pleura

Sac

Diaphragm

Cardia

Stomach

Duodenum

Paraesophageal or rolling hernia

Esophagus

Pleura

Diaphragm

Sac

Stomach

Duodenum

or pain resembling angina pectoris. Even if it produces no symptoms, this type of hernia needs surgical treatment because of the high risk of strangulation.

A sliding hernia without an incompetent sphincter produces no reflux or symptoms and, consequently, doesn't require treatment. When a sliding hernia does cause symptoms, they are typical of gastric reflux (resulting from the incompetent lower esophageal sphincter), and may include the following:

• *Pyrosis* (heartburn) occurs from 1 to 4 hours after eating and is aggravated by reclining, belching, and increased intra-abdominal pressure. It may be accompanied by regurgitation or vomiting.

• *Retrosternal or substernal chest pain* results from reflux of gastric contents, distention of the stomach, and spasm or altered motor activity. Chest pain occurs most often after meals or at bedtime and is aggravated by reclining, belching, and increased intra-abdominal pressure.

Other common symptoms reflect possible complications:

• *Dysphagia* occurs when the hernia produces esophagitis, esophageal ulceration, or stricture, especially with ingestion of very hot or cold foods, alcoholic beverages, or a large amount of food.

• *Bleeding* may be mild or massive, frank or occult; the source may be esophagitis or erosions of the gastric pouch.

• *Severe pain and shock* result from incarceration, in which a large portion of the stomach is caught above the diaphragm. (This usually occurs with paraesophageal hernia.) Incarceration may lead to the perforation of a gastric ulcer as well as strangulation and gangrene of the herniated portion of the stomach. It requires immediate surgery.

Diagnosis

Hiatal hernia is diagnosed based on typical clinical features and on the results of the following laboratory studies and procedures:

• *Chest X-ray* occasionally shows an air shadow behind the heart with a large hernia and infiltrates in the lower lobes if the patient has aspirated.

• In a *barium study,* the hernia may appear as an outpouching containing barium at the lower end of the esophagus. (Small hernias are difficult to recognize.) This study also shows diaphragmatic abnormalities.

• *Endoscopy and biopsy* differentiate between hiatal hernia, varices, and other small gastroesophageal lesions; identify the mucosal junction and the edge of the diaphragm indenting the esophagus; and can rule out malignant tumors that otherwise might be difficult to detect.

• *Esophageal motility studies* assess the presence of esophageal motor abnormalities before surgical repair of the hernia.

• *pH studies* assess for reflux of gastric contents.

• *Acid perfusion (Bernstein) test* indicates that heartburn results from esophageal reflux when perfusion of hydrogen chloride through the nasogastric (NG) tube provokes this symptom.

The following laboratory tests may indicate GI bleeding as a complication of hiatal hernia:

• *Complete blood count* may show hypochromic microcytic anemia when bleeding from esophageal ulceration occurs.

• *Stool guaiac test* may be positive.

• *Analysis of gastric contents* may reveal blood.

Treatment

The primary goals of treatment are to relieve symptoms by minimizing or correcting the incompetent cardia and to manage and prevent complications. Medical therapy is used first, because symptoms usually respond to it and because hiatal hernia tends to recur after surgery.

Medical therapy

Such therapy attempts to modify or reduce reflux by changing the quantity or quality of refluxed gastric contents, by strengthening the lower esophageal sphincter muscle pharmacologically, or by decreasing the amount of reflux through gravity.

Specific measures include restricting any activity that increases intra-abdominal pressure (coughing, straining, bending), giving antiemetics and cough suppressants, avoiding constrictive clothing, modifying diet, giving stool softeners or laxatives to prevent straining during defecation, and discouraging smoking because it stimulates gastric acid production.

Modifying the diet means eating small, frequent, bland meals at least 2 hours before lying down (no bedtime snacks); eating slowly; and avoiding spicy foods, fruit juices, alcoholic beverages, and coffee. Antacids also modify the fluid refluxed into the esophagus and are probably the best treatment for intermittent reflux.

Intensive antacid therapy may call for hourly administration; however, the choice of antacid should take into consideration the patient's bowel function. Cimetidine also modifies the fluid refluxed into the esophagus.

To reduce the amount of reflux, the overweight patient should lose weight to decrease intra-abdominal pressure. Elevating the head of the bed about 6″ (15 cm) reduces gastric reflux by gravity.

Drug therapy to strengthen cardiac sphincter tone may include a cholinergic agent such as bethanecol. Metoclopramide has also been used to stimulate smooth-muscle contraction, increase cardiac sphincter tone, and decrease reflux after eating.

Surgery

Failure to control symptoms medically, or the onset of such complications as stricture, bleeding, pulmonary aspiration, strangulation, or incarceration, requires surgical repair.

Surgery creates an artificial closing mechanism at the gastroesophageal junction to strengthen the lower esophageal sphincter's barrier function. An abdominal or a thoracic approach may be used, or the hernia may be repaired by laparoscopic surgery, which allows for less dependence on an NG tube and a shorter hospital stay.

Special considerations

• To enhance compliance with treatment, teach the patient about this disorder. Explain treatments, diagnostic tests, and significant symptoms.
• Prepare the patient for diagnostic tests as needed. After endoscopy, watch for signs of perforation (falling blood pressure, rapid pulse, shock, sudden pain).
• If surgery is scheduled, reinforce patient teaching about the procedure and any preoperative and postoperative considerations. Tell the patient he probably won't be allowed to eat or drink and will have an NG tube in place, with low suction, for 2 to 3 days postoperatively. Don't manipulate the tube.
• After surgery, carefully record intake and output, including NG tube and wound drainage.
• While the NG tube is in place, provide meticulous mouth and nose care. Give ice chips to moisten oral mucous membranes.
• If a thoracic approach was used, the patient will have chest tubes in place. Carefully observe chest tube drainage and respiratory status, and perform pulmonary physiotherapy.

• Before discharge, tell the patient what foods he can eat, and recommend small, frequent meals. Warn against activities that cause increased intraabdominal pressure, and advise a slow return to normal functions (within 6 to 8 weeks).

HIRSCHSPRUNG'S DISEASE

A congenital disorder of the large intestine, Hirschsprung's disease is also called congenital megacolon and congenital aganglionic megacolon. It's characterized by the absence or marked reduction of parasympathetic ganglion cells in the colorectal wall.

This disorder impairs intestinal motility and causes severe, intractable constipation. Without prompt treatment, an infant with colonic obstruction may die within 24 hours from enterocolitis that leads to severe diarrhea and hypovolemic shock. With prompt treatment, the prognosis is good.

Causes

In Hirschsprung's disease, the aganglionic bowel segment contracts without the reciprocal relaxation needed to propel feces forward. In 90% of patients, this aganglionic segment is in the rectosigmoid area, but it occasionally extends to the entire colon and parts of the small intestine.

Incidence

Hirschsprung's disease is believed to be a familial, congenital defect; it occurs in 1 in 2,000 to 1 in 5,000 live births. It's up to seven times more common in males than in females (although the aganglionic segment is usually shorter in males than in females) and is more prevalent in whites. Total aganglionosis affects both sexes equally. Females with Hirschsprung's disease are at higher risk for having affected children.

This disease often coexists with other congenital anomalies, particularly trisomy 21 and anomalies of the urinary tract such as megaloureter.

Signs and symptoms
Clinical effects usually appear shortly after birth, but mild symptoms may not be recognized until later in childhood or during adolescence (usually) or adulthood (rarely).

In infants
The neonate with Hirschsprung's disease commonly fails to pass meconium within 24 to 48 hours, shows signs of obstruction (bile-stained or fecal vomiting, abdominal distention), irritability, feeding difficulties (poor sucking, refusal to take feedings), failure to thrive, dehydration (pallor, loss of skin turgor, dry mucous membranes, sunken eyes), and overflow diarrhea.

The infant may also exhibit abdominal distention that causes rapid breathing and grunting. Rectal examination reveals a rectum empty of stools and, when the examining finger is withdrawn, an explosive gush of malodorous gas and liquid stools. Such examination may temporarily relieve GI symptoms.

In infants, the main cause of death is enterocolitis, caused by fecal stagnation that leads to bacterial overgrowth, production of bacterial toxins, intestinal irritation, profuse diarrhea, hypovolemic shock, and perforation.

In older children
The older child has intractable constipation (usually requiring laxatives and enemas), abdominal distention, and easily palpated fecal masses. In severe cases, failure to grow is characterized

by wasted extremities and loss of subcutaneous tissue, with a large protuberant abdomen.

In adults
Adult megacolon, although rare, usually affects men. The patient has abdominal distention, rectal bleeding (rare), and a history of chronic intermittent constipation. He's generally in poor physical condition.

Diagnosis
Diagnostic test results for Hirschsprung's disease include the following:
• *Rectal biopsy* provides a definitive diagnosis by showing the absence of ganglion cells. Suction aspiration using a small tube inserted into the rectum may be performed initially. If the findings of suction aspiration are inconclusive, diagnosis requires a full-thickness surgical biopsy under general anesthesia.
• *Barium enema* in older infants shows a narrowed segment of distal colon with a sawtooth appearance and a funnel-shaped segment above it that confirms the diagnosis and assesses the extent of intestinal involvement.

Significantly, infants with Hirschsprung's disease retain barium longer than the usual 12 to 24 hours, so delayed films are often helpful when other characteristic signs are absent.
• *Rectal manometry* detects failure of the internal anal sphincter to relax and contract, and *upright plain films of the abdomen* show marked colonic distention.

Treatment
Surgical treatment involves pulling the normal ganglionic segment through to the anus. However, such corrective surgery is usually delayed until the infant is at least 10 months old and better able to withstand it.

Management of an infant until the time of surgery consists of daily colonic lavage to empty the bowel. If total obstruction is present in the newborn, a temporary colostomy or ileostomy is necessary to decompress the colon. A preliminary bowel prep with an antibiotic, such as neomycin or nystatin, is necessary before surgery.

The surgical technique used is based on the three main corrective procedures: the Duhamel, Soave, or Swenson pull-through procedure.

Special considerations
Before emergency decompression surgery:
• Maintain fluid and electrolyte balance, and prevent shock. Provide adequate nutrition, and hydrate with I.V. fluids as needed. Transfusions may be necessary to correct shock or dehydration. Relieve respiratory distress by keeping the patient in an upright position. (Place an infant in an infant seat.)

After colostomy or ileostomy:
• Place the infant in a heated incubator, with the temperature set at 98° to 99° F (36.6° to 37.2° C), or in a radiant warmer. Monitor vital signs, watching for sepsis and enterocolitis (an increased respiratory rate with abdominal distention).
• Carefully monitor and record fluid intake and output (including drainage from ileostomy or colostomy) and electrolytes. Ileostomy is especially likely to cause excessive electrolyte loss.
• Measure and record nasogastric (NG) drainage, and replace fluids and electrolytes. Check stools carefully for excess water — a sign of fluid loss.
• Check urine for specific gravity, glucose (hyperalimentation may lead to osmotic diuresis), and blood.
• To prevent aspiration pneumonia and skin breakdown, turn and reposition the patient often. Also, suction the nasopharynx frequently.

• Keep the area around the stoma clean and dry, and cover it with dressings or a colostomy or ileostomy appliance to absorb drainage. Use aseptic technique until the wound heals.
• Watch for prolapse, discoloration, or excessive bleeding. (Slight bleeding is common.) To prevent excoriation, use a powder such as karaya gum or a protective stoma disk.
• Oral feeding can begin when bowel sounds return. An infant may tolerate predigested formulas best.
• Teach parents to recognize the signs of fluid loss and dehydration (decreased urine output, sunken eyes, poor skin turgor) and of enterocolitis (sudden marked abdominal distention, vomiting, diarrhea, fever, lethargy).
• Before discharge, if possible, make sure the parents consult with an enterostomal therapist for valuable tips on ostomy care.

Before corrective surgery:
• At least once a day, colonic lavage with normal saline solution is necessary to evacuate the colon, since ordinary enemas and laxatives won't clean it adequately. Keep accurate records of how much lavage solution is instilled. Repeat lavage until the return solution is completely free of fecal particles.
• Administer antibiotics for bowel preparation.

After corrective surgery:
• Keep the wound clean and dry, and check for significant inflammation (some inflammation is normal). Don't use a rectal thermometer or suppository until the wound has healed. After 3 to 4 days, the infant will have a first bowel movement consisting of liquid stools, which will probably create discomfort. Record the number of stools.
• Check urine for blood, especially in a boy; extensive surgical manipulation may cause bladder trauma.
• Watch for signs of possible anastomic leaks (the sudden development of abdominal distention unrelieved by

gastric aspiration, temperature spike, extreme irritability), which may lead to pelvic abscess.

• Begin oral feedings when active bowel sounds begin and NG drainage decreases. As an additional check, clamp the NG tube for brief, intermittent periods. If abdominal distention develops, the patient isn't ready to begin oral feedings. Begin oral feedings with clear fluids, increasing bulk as tolerated.

• Instruct the parents to watch for foods that increase the number of stools and to avoid offering these foods.

• Reassure the parents that their child will probably gain sphincter control and be able to eat a normal diet. But warn them that complete continence may take several years to develop and constipation may recur at times.

• Because an infant with Hirschsprung's disease needs surgery and hospitalization so early in life, parents have difficulty establishing an emotional bond with their child. To promote bonding, encourage them to participate in their child's care as much as possible.

HIRSUTISM

A distressing disorder usually found in women and children, hirsutism is the excessive growth of body hair, typically in an adult male distribution pattern.

This condition commonly occurs spontaneously but may also develop as a secondary disorder of various underlying diseases. It must always be distinguished from hypertrichosis. The prognosis varies with the cause and the effectiveness of treatment.

Causes

Idiopathic hirsutism probably stems from a hereditary trait, because the patient usually has a family history of the disorder.

Causes of secondary hirsutism include endocrine abnormalities related to pituitary dysfunction (acromegaly, precocious puberty), adrenal dysfunction (Cushing's disease, congenital adrenal hyperplasia, or Cushing's syndrome), and ovarian lesions (such as polycystic ovary syndrome); and iatrogenic factors (such as the use of minoxidil, androgen steroids, or testosterone).

Signs and symptoms

Hirsutism typically produces enlarged hair follicles as well as enlargement and hyperpigmentation of the hairs themselves. Excessive facial hair growth is the complaint for which most patients seek medical help. The pattern of hirsutism varies widely, depending on the patient's race and age. An elderly woman, for example, commonly shows increased hair growth on the chin and upper lip.

In secondary hirsutism, signs of masculinization may appear—deepening of the voice, increased muscle mass, increased size of genitalia, menstrual irregularity, and decreased breast size.

Diagnosis

A family history of hirsutism, the absence of menstrual abnormalities or signs of masculinization, and a normal pelvic examination strongly suggest idiopathic hirsutism. Tests for secondary hirsutism depend on associated symptoms that suggest an underlying disorder.

Treatment

At the patient's request, treatment of idiopathic hirsutism consists of eliminating excess hair by scissors, shaving, depilatory creams, or removal of the entire hair shaft with tweezers or wax. Bleaching with hydrogen peroxide may also be satisfactory.

Electrolysis, a slow and expensive process, can destroy hair bulbs permanently, but it works best when only a few hairs need to be removed. (A history of keloid formation contraindicates this procedure.) Hirsutism due to elevated androgen levels may require a low dose of dexamethasone, oral contraceptives, or antiandrogens. These drugs vary in effectiveness.

Treatment of secondary hirsutism varies depending on the nature of the underlying disorder.

Special considerations
• Care for patients with idiopathic hirsutism focuses on emotional support and patient teaching; care for patients with secondary hirsutism depends on how the underlying disease is treated.
• Provide emotional support by being sensitive to the patient's feelings about her appearance.
• Watch for signs of contact dermatitis in patients being treated with depilatory creams, especially the elderly ones. Also watch for infection of hair follicles after hair removal with tweezers or wax.
• Suggest consulting a cosmetologist about makeup or bleaching agents.

HISTOPLASMOSIS

Also called Ohio Valley disease, Central Mississippi Valley disease, Appalachian Mountain disease, and Darling's disease, histoplasmosis is a fungal infection caused by *Histoplasma capsulatum*.

In the United States, it occurs in three forms: *primary acute histoplasmosis, progressive disseminated histoplasmosis* (acute disseminated or chronic disseminated disease), and *chronic pulmonary (cavitary) histoplasmosis,* which produces cavitations in the lung similar to those in pulmonary tuberculosis.

A fourth form, *African histoplasmosis,* occurs only in Africa and is caused by the fungus *Histoplasma capsulatum* var. *duboisii.*

The prognosis varies with each form. The primary acute disease is benign; the progressive disseminated disease is fatal in approximately 90% of patients; and without proper chemotherapy, chronic pulmonary histoplasmosis is fatal in 50% of patients within 5 years.

Causes
H. capsulatum is found in the feces of birds and bats or in soil contaminated by their feces, such as that near roosts, chicken coops, barns, caves, or underneath bridges. Transmission is through inhalation of *H. capsulatum* or *H. duboisii* spores or through the invasion of spores after minor skin trauma.

The incubation period is 5 to 18 days, although chronic pulmonary histoplasmosis may progress slowly for many years.

Incidence
Histoplasmosis occurs worldwide, especially in the temperate areas of Asia, Africa, Europe, and North and South America. In the United States, it's most prevalent in the central and eastern states, especially in the Mississippi and Ohio River valleys.

Probably because of occupational exposure, histoplasmosis is more common in adult males. Fatal disseminated disease, however, is more common in infants and elderly men.

Signs and symptoms

Symptoms vary with each form of this disease, as follows:

• Primary acute histoplasmosis may be asymptomatic or may cause symptoms of a mild respiratory illness similar to a severe cold or influenza. Typical symptoms may include fever, malaise, headache, myalgia, anorexia, cough, and chest pain.

• Progressive disseminated histoplasmosis causes hepatosplenomegaly, general lymphadenopathy, anorexia, weight loss, fever, and possibly ulceration of the tongue, palate, epiglottis, and larynx, with resulting pain, hoarseness, and dysphagia. It may also cause endocarditis, meningitis, pericarditis, and adrenal insufficiency.

• Chronic pulmonary histoplasmosis mimics pulmonary tuberculosis and causes a productive cough, dyspnea, and occasional hemoptysis. Eventually, it produces weight loss, extreme weakness, breathlessness, and cyanosis.

• African histoplasmosis produces cutaneous nodules, papules, and ulcers; lymphadenopathy; lesions of the skull and long bones; and visceral involvement without pulmonary lesions.

Diagnosis

A history of exposure to contaminated soil in an endemic area, miliary calcification in the lung or spleen, and a positive histoplasmin skin test indicate exposure to histoplasmosis. Rising complement fixation and agglutination titers (more than 1:32) strongly suggest histoplasmosis.

The diagnosis of histoplasmosis requires morphologic examination of a tissue biopsy and culture of *H. capsulatum* from sputum in acute primary and chronic pulmonary histoplasmosis; and from bone marrow, lymph nodes, blood, and infection sites in disseminated histoplasmosis. However, cultures take several weeks to grow these organisms.

A faster diagnosis is possible with stained biopsies using Gomori's stains (methenamine silver) or periodic acid-Schiff reaction. Findings must rule out tuberculosis and other diseases that produce similar symptoms.

The diagnosis of histoplasmosis caused by *H. duboisii* necessitates examination of a tissue biopsy and culture of the affected site.

Treatment

Histoplasmosis treatment consists of antifungal therapy, surgery, and supportive care, as follows:

• Antifungal therapy is most important. Except for asymptomatic primary acute histoplasmosis (which resolves spontaneously) and the African form, histoplasmosis requires high-dose or long-term (10-week) therapy with amphotericin B or fluconazole. For a patient who also has acquired immunodeficiency syndrome, lifelong therapy with fluconazole is indicated.

• Supportive care usually includes oxygen for respiratory distress, glucocorticoids for adrenal insufficiency, and parenteral fluids for dysphagia due to oral or laryngeal ulcerations.

• Histoplasmosis doesn't require the patient to be isolated.

Special considerations

• Give drugs and teach patients about possible adverse effects. Since amphotericin B may cause chills, fever, nausea, and vomiting, give appropriate antipyretics and antiemetics.

• Patients with chronic pulmonary or disseminated histoplasmosis also need psychological support because of long-term hospitalization.

• As needed, refer the patient to a social worker or occupational therapist. Help parents of children with this disease arrange for a visiting teacher.

STAGING HODGKIN'S DISEASE

Treatment of Hodgkin's disease depends on the stage it has reached—that is, the number, location, and degree of involved lymph nodes. The Ann Arbor Classification System, adopted in 1971, divides Hodgkin's disease into four stages, which are then subdivided into categories.

Category A includes patients with undefined signs and symptoms, and category B includes patients who experience such defined signs as recent unexplained weight loss, fever, and night sweats.

Stage I
Hodgkin's disease appears in a single lymph node region (I) or a single extralymphatic organ (IE).

• To help prevent histoplasmosis, teach persons in endemic areas to watch for early signs of this infection and to seek treatment promptly. Instruct persons who risk occupational exposure to contaminated soil to wear face masks.

HODGKIN'S DISEASE

A neoplastic disease, Hodgkin's disease is characterized by painless, progressive enlargement of lymph nodes, spleen, and other lymphoid tissue resulting from proliferation of lymphocytes, histiocytes, eosinophils, and Reed-Sternberg giant cells. The latter cells are its special histologic feature.

Untreated, Hodgkin's disease follows a variable but relentlessly progressive and ultimately fatal course. However, recent advances in therapy make Hodgkin's disease potentially curable, even in advanced stages, and appropriate treatment yields a 5-year survival rate of approximately 90%.

Causes
The cause of Hodgkin's disease is unknown. This disease is most common in young adults and occurs more often in males than in females. It occurs in all races but is slightly more common in whites. Incidence peaks in two age-groups: ages 15 to 38 and after age 50—except in Japan, where it occurs exclusively among people over age 50.

Signs and symptoms
Symptoms vary, depending on the stage of the disease.

Early signs
The first sign of Hodgkin's disease is usually a painless swelling of one of the cervical lymph nodes (but sometimes the axillary, mediastinal, or inguinal lymph nodes), occasionally in a

Stage II
The disease appears in two or more nodes on the same side of the diaphragm (II) and in an extralymphatic organ (IIE).

Stage III
Hodgkin's disease spreads to both sides of the diaphragm (III) and perhaps to an extralymphatic organ (IIIE), the spleen (IIIS), or both (IIIES).

Stage IV
The disease disseminates, involving one or more extralymphatic organs or tissues, with or without associated lymph node involvement.

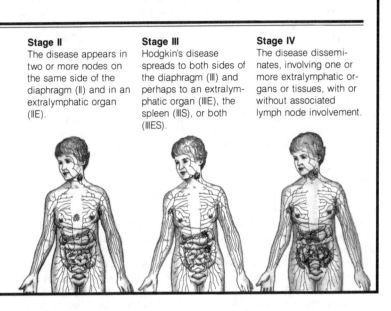

patient who has a history of recent upper respiratory infection.

In older patients, the first symptoms may be nonspecific—persistent fever, night sweats, fatigue, weight loss, and malaise. Rarely, if the mediastinum is initially involved, Hodgkin's may produce respiratory symptoms.

Another early and characteristic indication of Hodgkin's disease is pruritus, which, while mild at first, becomes acute as the disease progresses. Other symptoms depend on the degree and location of systemic involvement.

Lymph nodes may enlarge rapidly, producing pain and obstruction, or enlarge slowly and painlessly for months or years. It's not unusual to see the lymph nodes "wax and wane," but they usually don't return to normal.

Late signs
Sooner or later, most patients develop systemic manifestations, including enlargement of retroperitoneal nodes and nodular infiltrations of the spleen, the liver, and bones. At this late stage, other symptoms include edema of the face and neck, progressive anemia, possible jaundice, nerve pain, and increased susceptibility to infection.

Diagnosis
Diagnostic measures for confirming Hodgkin's disease include a thorough medical history and a complete physical examination, followed by a lymph node biopsy checking for abnormal histiocyte proliferation of Reed-Sternberg cells and nodular fibrosis and necrosis.

Other appropriate diagnostic tests include bone marrow, liver, mediastinal, lymph node, and spleen biopsies and a routine chest X-ray, an abdominal computed tomography scan, a lung scan, a bone scan, and lymphangiography to detect lymph node or organ involvement. Laparoscopy and a lymph node biopsy are performed to complete staging.

Hematologic tests show mild to severe normocytic anemia; normochromic anemia (in 50% of patients); and an elevated, normal, or reduced white blood cell count and differential showing any combination of neutrophilia, lymphocytopenia, monocytosis, and eosinophilia. An elevated serum alkaline phosphatase level indicates liver or bone involvement.

The same diagnostic tests are also used for staging. A staging laparotomy is necessary for patients under age 55 or without obvious stage III or stage IV disease, lymphocyte predominance subtype histology, or medical contraindications. Diagnosis must also rule out other disorders that also enlarge the lymph nodes. (See *Staging Hodgkin's disease,* pages 424 and 425.)

Treatment
Appropriate therapy (chemotherapy, radiation, or both, depending on the stage of the disease) is based on a careful physical examination with accurate histologic interpretation and proper clinical staging. Correct and timely treatment allows longer survival and even induces an apparent cure in many patients.

Chemotherapy and radiation therapy
Radiation therapy is used alone for stage I and stage II, and in combination with chemotherapy for stage III. Chemotherapy is used for stage IV, sometimes inducing a complete remission. The well-known MOPP protocol (mechlorethamine, vincristine [Oncovin], procarbazine, and prednisone) was the first to provide significant cures in patients with generalized Hodgkin's.

Another useful combination is ABVD (doxorubicin [Adriamycin], bleomycin, vinblastine, and dacarbazine). Treatment with these drugs may require concomitant antiemetics, sedatives, or antidiarrheals to combat GI adverse effects.

Other treatments
New treatments include high-dose chemotherapeutic agents with autologous bone marrow transplantation or autologous peripheral blood stem cell transfusions. Biotherapy alone hasn't proven effective.

Special considerations
Because many patients with Hodgkin's disease receive radiation or chemotherapy as outpatients, tell the patient to observe the following precautions:
• Watch for and promptly report adverse effects of radiation and chemotherapy (particularly anorexia, nausea, vomiting, diarrhea, fever, and bleeding).
• Minimize adverse effects of radiation therapy by maintaining good nutrition (aided by eating small, frequent meals of his favorite foods), drinking plenty of fluids, pacing his activities to counteract therapy-induced fatigue, and keeping the skin in radiated areas dry.
• Control pain and bleeding of stomatitis by using a soft toothbrush, cotton swab, or anesthetic mouthwash such as viscous lidocaine; by applying petroleum jelly to the patient's lips; and by avoiding astringent mouthwashes.
• If a female patient is of childbearing age, advise her to delay pregnancy until prolonged remission, because radiation and chemotherapy can cause genetic mutations and spontaneous abortions.
• Because the patient with Hodgkin's disease has usually been healthy up until this point, he's likely to be especially distressed. Provide emotional support and offer appropriate reassur-

ance. Ease the patient's anxiety by sharing your optimism about his prognosis.

• Make sure the patient and his family know that the local chapter of the American Cancer Society is available for information, financial assistance, and supportive counseling.

HOOKWORM DISEASE

Also known as uncinariasis, hookworm disease is an infection of the upper intestine caused by *Ancylostoma duodenale* (found in the eastern hemisphere) or *Necator americanus* (in the western hemisphere). Sandy soil, high humidity, a warm climate, and failure to wear shoes all favor its transmission.

In the United States, hookworm disease is most common in the southeast. Although this disease can cause cardiopulmonary complications, it's rarely fatal, except in debilitated persons or infants under age 1.

Causes
Both forms of hookworm disease are transmitted to humans through direct skin penetration (usually in the foot) by hookworm larvae in soil contaminated with feces containing hookworm ova. These ova develop into infectious larvae in 1 to 3 days.

Larvae travel through the lymphatics to the pulmonary capillaries, where they penetrate alveoli and move up the bronchial tree to the trachea and epiglottis. There they are swallowed and enter the GI tract. When they reach the small intestine, they mature, attach to the jejunal mucosa, and suck blood, oxygen, and glucose from the intestinal wall.

These mature worms then deposit ova, which are excreted in stools,

starting the cycle anew. Hookworm larvae mature in approximately 5 to 6 weeks.

Signs and symptoms
Most cases of hookworm disease produce few symptoms and may be overlooked until worms are passed in stools. The earliest signs and symptoms include irritation, pruritus, and edema at the site of entry, which are sometimes accompanied by secondary bacterial infection with pustule formation.

When the larvae reach the lungs, they may cause pneumonitis and hemorrhage with fever, sore throat, crackles, and cough. Finally, intestinal infection may cause fatigue, nausea, weight loss, dizziness, melena, and uncontrolled diarrhea.

In severe and chronic infection, anemia from blood loss may lead to cardiomegaly (a result of increased oxygen demands), heart failure, and generalized massive edema.

Diagnosis
Identification of hookworm ova in stools confirms the diagnosis. Anemia suggests severe chronic infection. In infected patients, blood studies show:

• hemoglobin level of 5 to 9 g (in severe cases)
• leukocyte count as high as 47,000/μl
• eosinophil count of 500 to 700/μl.

Treatment
The usual treatment for hookworm infection includes administering mebendazole or pyrantel and providing an iron-rich diet or iron supplements to prevent or correct anemia.

Special considerations
• Obtain a complete history, with special attention to travel or residency in endemic areas. Note the sequence and onset of symptoms. Interview the family and other close contacts to see if

they too have any symptoms.

• Carefully assess the patient, noting signs of entry, lymphedema, and respiratory status.

If the patient has confirmed hookworm infestation:

• Segregate the incontinent patient.

• Wash your hands thoroughly after every patient contact.

• For severe anemia, administer oxygen at a low to moderate flow rate. Make sure the oxygen is humidified, because the patient may already have upper airway irritation from the parasites.

• Encourage coughing and deep breathing to stimulate removal of blood or secretions from involved lung areas and to prevent secondary infection.

• Allow frequent rest periods because the patient may tire easily.

• If anemia causes immobility, reposition the patient often to prevent skin breakdown.

• Closely monitor intake and output. Note the quantity and frequency of diarrheal stools. Dispose of feces promptly, and wear gloves when doing so.

• To help assess nutritional status, weigh the patient daily.

• To combat malnutrition, emphasize the importance of good nutrition, with particular attention to foods high in iron and protein. If the patient receives iron supplements, explain that they will darken stools.

• Administer anthelmintics on an empty stomach, but without a purgative.

• To help prevent reinfection, educate the patient in proper hand-washing technique and sanitary disposal of feces. Tell him to wear shoes in endemic areas.

HUNTINGTON'S DISEASE

Also called Huntington's chorea, hereditary chorea, chronic progressive chorea, and adult chorea, Huntington's disease is a hereditary disease in which degeneration in the cerebral cortex and basal ganglia causes chronic progressive chorea and mental deterioration, ending in dementia.

Huntington's disease usually strikes persons between ages 25 and 55 (the average age is 35); however, 2% of cases occur in children, and 5%, as late as age 60. Death usually results 10 to 15 years after onset, from suicide, congestive heart failure, or pneumonia.

Causes

The cause of Huntington's disease is unknown. Because this disease is transmitted as an autosomal dominant trait, either sex can transmit and inherit it. Each child of a parent with this disease has a 50% chance of inheriting it; however, the child who doesn't inherit it can't pass it on to his own children.

Because of hereditary transmission, Huntington's disease is prevalent in areas where affected families have lived for several generations. A study is being made of children in families with Huntington's disease in order to develop ways of identifying this disease before the onset of symptoms.

Signs and symptoms

Onset is insidious. The patient eventually becomes totally dependent—emotionally and physically—through loss of musculoskeletal control.

Choreic movements

Gradually, he develops progressively severe choreic movements. Such movements are rapid, often violent, and purposeless. Initially, they are unilateral and more prominent in the face and arms than in the legs, progressing from mild fidgeting to grimacing, tongue smacking, dysarthria (indistinct speech), athetoid movements (especially of the hands) related to emotional state, and torticollis.

Dementia

Ultimately, the patient with Huntington's disease develops dementia, although the dementia doesn't always progress at the same rate as the chorea. Dementia can be mild at first but eventually severely disrupts the personality.

Such personality changes include obstinacy, carelessness, untidiness, moodiness, apathy, inappropriate behavior, loss of memory and concentration, and sometimes paranoia.

Diagnosis

Huntington's disease can be detected by positron emission tomography and deoxyribonucleic acid analysis. The diagnosis is based on a characteristic clinical history: progressive chorea and dementia, onset of the disorder in early middle age (ages 35 to 40), and confirmation of a genetic link.

A computed tomography scan and magnetic resonance imaging demonstrate brain atrophy. Molecular genetics may detect the gene for Huntington's disease in people at risk while they're still asymptomatic.

Treatment

Because Huntington's disease has no known cure, treatment is supportive, protective, and aimed at relieving symptoms. Tranquilizers as well as chlorpromazine, haloperidol, or imipramine help control choreic movements, but they can't stop mental deterioration. They also alleviate discomfort and depression, making the patient easier to manage. However, tranquilizers increase patient rigidity.

To control choreic movements without rigidity, choline may be prescribed. Institutionalization is often necessary because of mental deterioration.

Special considerations

• Provide physical support by attending to the patient's basic needs, such as hygiene, skin care, bowel and bladder care, and nutrition. Increase this support as mental and physical deterioration make him increasingly immobile.

• Offer emotional support to the patient and family. Teach them about the disease, and listen to their concerns and special problems. Keep in mind the patient's dysarthria, and allow him extra time to express himself, thereby decreasing frustration. Teach the family to participate in the patient's care.

• Stay alert for possible suicide attempts. Control the patient's environment to protect him from suicide or other self-inflicted injury. Pad the side rails of the bed, but avoid restraints, which may cause the patient to injure himself with violent, uncontrolled movements.

• If the patient has difficulty walking, provide a walker to help him maintain his balance.

• Make sure affected families receive genetic counseling. All affected family members should realize that each of their offspring has a 50% chance of inheriting this disease.

• Refer people at risk who desire genetic testing to specialized centers where psychosocial support is available.

• Refer the patient and family to appropriate community organizations.

• For more information about this degenerative disease, refer the patient and family to the Huntington's Disease Association.

HYDROCEPHALUS

An excessive accumulation of cerebrospinal fluid (CSF) within the ventricular spaces of the brain, hydrocephalus occurs most often in neonates. But it can also occur in adults as a result of injury or disease. In infants, hydrocephalus enlarges the head; and in both infants and adults, the resulting compression can damage brain tissue.

With early detection and surgical intervention, the prognosis improves but remains guarded. Even after surgery, such complications as mental retardation, impaired motor function, and vision loss can persist. Without surgery, the prognosis is poor: Mortality may result from increased intracranial pressure (ICP) in people of all ages; infants may also die prematurely of infection and malnutrition.

Causes
Hydrocephalus may result from an obstruction in CSF flow (noncommunicating hydrocephalus) or from faulty absorption of CSF (communicating hydrocephalus).

Noncommunicating hydrocephalus
In this type of hydrocephalus, the obstruction occurs most frequently between the third and fourth ventricles, at the aqueduct of Sylvius, but it can also occur at the outlets of the fourth ventricle (foramina of Luschka and Magendie) or, rarely, at the foramen of Monro.

This obstruction may result from faulty fetal development, infection (syphilis, granulomatous diseases,

meningitis), a tumor, a cerebral aneurysm, or a blood clot (after intracranial hemorrhage).

Communicating hydrocephalus
In this type of hydrocephalus, faulty absorption of CSF may result from surgery to repair a myelomeningocele, adhesions between meninges at the base of the brain, or meningeal hemorrhage. Rarely, a tumor in the choroid plexus causes overproduction of CSF, producing hydrocephalus.

Signs and symptoms
In infants, the unmistakable sign of hydrocephalus is enlargement of the head clearly disproportionate to the infant's growth. Other characteristic changes include distended scalp veins; thin, fragile-looking, and shiny scalp skin; and underdeveloped neck muscles. (See *Characteristics of hydrocephalus.*)

In severe hydrocephalus, the roof of the orbit is depressed, the eyes are displaced downward, and the sclera are prominent. A high-pitched, shrill cry; abnormal muscle tone in the legs; irritability; anorexia; and projectile vomiting often occur.

In adults and older children, indicators of hydrocephalus include a decreased level of consciousness (LOC), ataxia, incontinence, and impaired intellect.

Diagnosis
In infants, abnormally large head size for the patient's age strongly suggests hydrocephalus. Skull X-rays show thinning of the skull with separation of sutures and widening of fontanels.

Other diagnostic tests for hydrocephalus, including angiography, computed tomography scan, and magnetic resonance imaging, can differentiate between hydrocephalus and intracranial lesions and can also demonstrate the Arnold-Chiari deformity, which may occur in an infant with hydrocephalus.

Treatment

Surgical correction is the only treatment for hydrocephalus. Usually, such surgery consists of insertion of a ventriculoperitoneal shunt, which transports excess fluid from the lateral ventricle into the peritoneal cavity.

A less common procedure is insertion of a ventriculoatrial shunt, which drains fluid from the brain's lateral ventricle into the right atrium of the heart, where the fluid makes its way into the venous circulation.

Complications of surgery include shunt infection, septicemia (after ventriculoatrial shunt), adhesions and paralytic ileus, migration, peritonitis, and intestinal perforation (with peritoneal shunt).

Special considerations

On initial assessment:
• Obtain a complete history from the patient or the family. Note the patient's general behavior, especially irritability, apathy, or decreased LOC.
• Perform a neurologic assessment. Examine the eyes: pupils should be equal and reactive to light. In adults and older children, evaluate movements and motor strength in extremities. (Watch especially for ataxia.)
• Ask the patient if he has headaches, and watch for projectile vomiting; both are signs of increased ICP. Also watch for seizures and note changes in vital signs.

Before surgery to insert a shunt:
• Encourage maternal-infant bonding when possible. When caring for the infant yourself, hold him on your lap for feeding; stroke and cuddle him, and speak soothingly.
• Check fontanels for tension or fullness, and measure and record head circumference. On the patient's chart, draw a picture showing where to mea-

CHARACTERISTICS OF HYDROCEPHALUS

In infants, changes characteristic of hydrocephalus include marked enlargement of the head; distended scalp veins; thin, shiny, and fragile-looking scalp skin; and underdeveloped neck muscles.

sure the head so that other staff members measure it in the same place, or mark the forehead with ink.
• To prevent postfeeding aspiration and hypostatic pneumonia, place the infant on his side and reposition him every 2 hours, or prop him up in an infant seat.
• To prevent skin breakdown, make sure his earlobe is flat, and place a sheepskin or rubber foam under his head.
• When turning the infant, move his head, neck, and shoulders with his body to reduce strain on his neck.
• Feed the infant slowly. To lessen the strain from the weight of the infant's head on your arm while holding him during feeding, place his head, neck, and shoulders on a pillow.

After surgery:
• Place the infant on the side opposite the operative site, with his head level with his body.

• Check temperature, pulse rate, blood pressure, and LOC. Also check the fontanels for fullness daily. Watch for vomiting, which may be an early sign of increased ICP and shunt malfunction.
• Watch for signs of infection, especially meningitis: fever, stiff neck, irritability, or tense fontanelles. Also watch for redness, swelling, or other signs of local infection over the shunt tract. Check the dressing often for drainage.
• Listen for bowel sounds after ventriculoperitoneal shunt.
• Check the infant's growth and development periodically, and help the parents set goals consistent with ability and potential.
• Help the parents focus on their child's strengths, not his weaknesses. Discuss special education programs, and emphasize the infant's need for sensory stimulation appropriate for his age.
• Teach the parents to watch for signs of shunt malfunction, infection, and paralytic ileus. Tell them that shunt insertion requires periodic surgery to lengthen the shunt as the child grows older, to correct malfunctioning, or to treat infection.

HYDRONEPHROSIS

An abnormal dilation of the renal pelvis and the calyces of one or both kidneys, hydronephrosis is caused by an obstruction of urine flow in the genitourinary tract. Although partial obstruction and hydronephrosis may not produce symptoms initially, the pressure built up behind the area of obstruction eventually results in symptomatic renal dysfunction.

Causes
Almost any type of obstructive uropathy can result in hydronephrosis. The most common causes are benign prostatic hypertrophy, urethral strictures, and calculi; less common causes include strictures or stenosis of the ureter or bladder outlet, congenital abnormalities, abdominal tumors, blood clots, and neurogenic bladder.

Sites of obstruction
If obstruction is in the urethra or bladder, hydronephrosis is usually bilateral; if obstruction is in a ureter, it's usually unilateral. Obstructions distal to the bladder cause the bladder to dilate and act as a buffer zone, delaying hydronephrosis. Total obstruction of urine flow with dilation of the collecting system ultimately causes complete cortical atrophy and cessation of glomerular filtration.

Signs and symptoms
Clinical features of hydronephrosis vary with the cause of the obstruction. In some patients, hydronephrosis produces no symptoms or only mild pain and slightly decreased urinary flow; in others, it may produce severe, colicky renal pain or dull flank pain that may radiate to the groin, and gross urinary abnormalities, such as hematuria, pyuria, dysuria, alternating oliguria and polyuria, or complete anuria.

Other symptoms of hydronephrosis include nausea, vomiting, abdominal fullness, pain on urination, dribbling, or hesitancy. Unilateral obstruction may cause pain on only one side, usually in the flank area.

Complications
The most common complication of an obstructed kidney is infection (pyelonephritis) due to stasis that exacerbates renal damage and may create a life-threatening crisis. Paralytic ileus

frequently accompanies acute obstructive uropathy.

Diagnosis

While the patient's clinical features may suggest hydronephrosis, excretory urography, retrograde pyelography, renal ultrasound, and renal function studies are necessary to confirm it.

Treatment

The goals of treatment are to preserve renal function and prevent infection through surgical removal of the obstruction, such as dilation for stricture of the urethra or prostatectomy for benign prostatic hypertrophy.

If renal function has already been affected, therapy may include a diet low in protein, sodium, and potassium. This diet is designed to stop the progression of renal failure before surgery.

Inoperable obstructions may require decompression and drainage of the kidney using a nephrostomy tube placed temporarily or permanently in the renal pelvis. Concurrent infection requires appropriate antibiotic therapy.

Special considerations

• Explain hydronephrosis as well as the purpose of excretory urography and other diagnostic procedures. Find out if the patient is allergic to the dye used in excretory urography.
• Administer medication for pain, as needed.
• Postoperatively, closely monitor intake and output, vital signs, and fluid and electrolyte status. Watch for a rising pulse rate and cold, clammy skin, which indicate possible impending hemorrhage and shock. Monitor renal function studies daily.
• If a nephrostomy tube has been inserted, check it frequently for bleeding and patency. Irrigate the tube, but don't clamp it.

• If the patient is to be discharged with a nephrostomy tube in place, teach him how to care for it properly.
• To prevent progression of hydronephrosis to irreversible renal disease, urge older men (especially those with family histories of benign prostatic hyperplasia or prostatitis) to have routine medical checkups. Teach them to recognize and report symptoms of hydronephrosis (colicky pain, hematuria) or urinary tract infection.

HYPERHIDROSIS

The excessive secretion of sweat from the eccrine glands, hyperhydrosis usually occurs in the axillae (typically after puberty) and on the palms and soles (often starting during infancy or childhood).

Causes

Possible causes of hyperhidrosis include the following:
• Genetic factors may contribute to the development of hyperhidrosis, and in susceptible individuals, emotional stress appears to be the most common cause. Increased central nervous system (CNS) impulses may provoke excessive release of acetylcholine, producing a heightened sweat response.
• Exercise and a hot climate can cause profuse sweating in these patients.
• Certain drugs, such as antipyretics, emetics, meperidine, and anticholinesterase, have been known to increase sweating.
• In addition, hyperhidrosis often occurs as a clinical manifestation of an underlying disorder. Infections and chronic diseases, such as tuberculosis, malaria, or lymphoma, may cause excessive nighttime sweating. Diabetic patients often demonstrate hyperhidrosis during a hypoglycemic crisis.

• Other predisposing conditions include pheochromocytomas; cardiovascular disorders, such as shock or heart failure; CNS disturbances (most often lesions of the hypothalamus); withdrawal from drugs or alcohol; menopause; and Graves' disease.

Signs and symptoms

Axillary hyperhidrosis frequently produces such extreme sweating that patients often ruin their clothes in 1 day and develop contact dermatitis from clothing dyes; similarly, hyperhidrosis of the soles can easily damage a pair of shoes.

Profuse sweating from both the soles and palms hinders the patient's ability to work and interact socially. Patients with this condition often report increased emotional strain.

Diagnosis

Clinical observations and the patient history confirm hyperhidrosis.

Treatment

The treatment of choice is application of 20% aluminum chloride in absolute ethanol. (Most antiperspirants contain a 5% solution.) Formaldehyde may also be used but may lead to allergic contact sensitization.

Glutaraldehyde produces less contact sensitivity than formaldehyde but stains the skin; it's used more often on the feet than on the hands, as a soak or applied directly several times a week and then weekly as needed. Therapy sometimes includes anticholinergics, except in patients with glaucoma or benign prostatic hyperplasia.

Severe hyperhidrosis that's unresponsive to conservative therapy may require local axillary removal of sweat glands or, as a last resort, a cervicothoracic or lumbar sympathectomy.

Special considerations

• Provide support and reassurance since hyperhidrosis may be socially embarrassing.
• Tell the patient to apply aluminum chloride in absolute ethanol nightly to dry axillae, soles, or palms. The area should be covered with plastic wrap for 6 to 8 hours, preferably overnight, then washed with soap and water. Repeat this procedure for several nights, until profuse daytime sweating subsides. Frequency of treatments can then be reduced.
• Advise the patient with hyperhidrosis of the soles to wear leather sandals and white or colorfast cotton socks.

HYPERLIPOPROTEINEMIA

About one in five people with elevated plasma lipid and lipoprotein levels has hyperlipoproteinemia, an inherited disorder marked by increased plasma concentrations of one or more lipoproteins. Hyperlipoproteinemia may also occur secondary to other conditions, such as diabetes, pancreatitis, hypothyroidism, or renal disease.

This disorder affects lipid transport in serum and produces varied clinical changes, from relatively mild symptoms that can be corrected by dietary management to potentially fatal pancreatitis.

Hyperlipoproteinemia occurs as five distinct metabolic disorders. Types I and III are transmitted as autosomal recessive traits; types II, IV, and V are transmitted as autosomal dominant traits.

Causes

Each type of hyperlipoproteinemia has distinct causes and incidence. (See *Types of hyperlipoproteinemia.*)

Types of Hyperlipoproteinemia

TYPE	CAUSES AND INCIDENCE	DIAGNOSTIC FINDINGS
I (Frederickson's hyperlipoproteinemia, fat-induced hyperlipemia, idiopathic familial)	• Deficient or abnormal lipoprotein lipase, resulting in decreased or absent postheparin lipolytic activity • Relatively rare • Present at birth	• Chylomicrons (very-low-density lipoprotein [VLDL], low-density lipoprotein [LDL], and high-density lipoprotein) in plasma 14 hours or more after last meal • Highly elevated serum chylomicron and triglyceride levels; slightly elevated serum cholesterol level • Lower serum lipoprotein lipase level • Leukocytosis
II (Familial hyperbetalipoproteinemia, essential familial hypercholesterolemia)	• Deficient cell surface receptor that regulates LDL degradation and cholesterol synthesis, resulting in increased levels of plasma LDL over joints and pressure points • Onset between ages 10 and 30	• Increased plasma concentrations of LDL • Increased serum LDL and cholesterol levels • Amniocentesis shows increased LDL levels.
III (Familial broad-beta disease, xanthoma tuberosum)	• Unknown underlying defect results in deficient conversion of triglyceride-rich VLDL to LDL. • Uncommon; usually occurs after age 20 but can occur earlier in men	• Abnormal serum beta-lipoprotein • Elevated cholesterol and triglyceride levels • Slightly elevated glucose tolerance • Hyperuricemia
IV (Endogenous hypertriglyceridemia, hyperbetalipoproteinemia)	• Usually occurs secondary to obesity, alcoholism, diabetes, or emotional disorders • Relatively common, especially in middle-aged men	• Elevated VLDL levels • Abnormal levels of triglycerides in plasma; variable increase in serum • Normal or slightly elevated serum cholesterol level • Mildly abnormal glucose tolerance • Family history • Early coronary artery disease
V (Mixed hypertriglyceridemia, mixed hyperlipidemia)	• Defective triglyceride clearance causes pancreatitis; usually secondary to another disorder, such as obesity or nephrosis • Uncommon; onset usually occurs in late adolescence or early adulthood.	• Chylomicrons in plasma • Elevated plasma VLDL levels • Elevated serum cholesterol and triglyceride levels

Signs and symptoms

Clinical features of hyperlipoprotein-emia vary according to the type of disorder:

• *Type I:* recurrent attacks of severe abdominal pain similar to pancreatitis, usually preceded by fat intake; abdominal spasm, rigidity, or rebound tenderness; hepatosplenomegaly, with liver or spleen tenderness; papular or eruptive xanthomas (pinkish yellow cutaneous deposits of fat) over pressure points and extensor surfaces; lipemia retinalis (reddish white retinal vessels); malaise; anorexia; and fever

• *Type II:* tendinous xanthomas (firm masses) on the Achilles tendons and tendons of the hands and feet, tuberous xanthomas, xanthelasma, juvenile corneal arcus (opaque ring surrounding the corneal periphery), accelerated atherosclerosis and premature coronary artery disease, and recurrent polyarthritis and tenosynovitis

• *Type III:* peripheral vascular disease manifested by claudication or tuboeruptive xanthomas (soft, inflamed, pedunculated lesions) over the elbows and knees; palmar xanthomas on the hands, particularly fingertips; premature atherosclerosis

• *Type IV:* predisposition to atherosclerosis and early coronary artery disease, exacerbated by excessive calorie intake, obesity, diabetes, and hypertension

• *Type V:* abdominal pain (most common), pancreatitis, peripheral neuropathy, eruptive xanthomas on extensor surfaces of the arms and legs, lipemia retinalis, and hepatosplenomegaly.

Diagnosis

Diagnostic findings vary among the five types of hyperlipoproteinemia. (See *Types of hyperlipoproteinemia,* page 435.)

Treatment

The first goal is to identify and treat any underlying problem such as diabetes. If no underlying problem exists, the primary treatment for types II, III, and IV is dietary management, especially restriction of cholesterol intake. Drug therapy (cholestyramine, clofibrate, or niacin) may also be used to lower the plasma triglyceride or cholesterol level when diet alone is ineffective.

Type I

In type I hyperlipoproteinemia, treatment requires long-term weight reduction, with fat intake restricted to less than 20 g/day. A 20- to 40-g/day medium-chain triglyceride diet may be ordered to supplement calorie intake. The patient should also avoid alcoholic beverages to decrease plasma triglycerides. The prognosis is good with treatment; without treatment, death can result from pancreatitis.

Type II

For type II, dietary management to restore normal lipid levels and decrease the risk of atherosclerosis includes restriction of cholesterol intake to less than 300 mg/day for adults and less than 150 mg/day for children; triglyceride levels must be restricted to less than 100 mg/day for children and adults. The diet should also be high in polyunsaturated fats.

In familial hypercholesterolemia, nicotinic acid with a bile acid usually normalizes low-density lipoprotein levels. For severely affected children, portacaval shunt is a last resort to reduce plasma cholesterol levels.

The prognosis remains poor regardless of treatment; in homozygotes, myocardial infarction usually causes death before age 30.

Type III

For type III, dietary management includes restriction of cholesterol intake to less than 300 mg/day; carbohydrates must also be restricted, while polyunsaturated fats are increased. Clofibrate and niacin help lower blood lipid levels. Weight reduction is helpful. With strict adherence to prescribed diet, the prognosis is good.

Type IV

For type IV, weight reduction may normalize blood lipid levels without additional treatment. Long-term dietary management includes restricted cholesterol intake, increased polyunsaturated fats, and avoidance of alcoholic beverages. Clofibrate and niacin may lower plasma lipid levels.

The prognosis remains uncertain, however, because of predisposition to premature coronary artery disease.

Type V

The most effective treatment for type V is weight reduction and long-term maintenance of a low-fat diet. Alcoholic beverages must be avoided. Niacin, clofibrate, gemfibrozil, and a 20- to 40-g/day medium-chain triglyceride diet may prove helpful.

The prognosis is uncertain because of the risk of pancreatitis. Increased fat intake may cause recurrent bouts of illness, possibly leading to pseudocyst formation, hemorrhage, and death.

Special considerations

• Care for hyperlipoproteinemia emphasizes careful monitoring for adverse reactions to drugs and teaching the importance of long-term dietary management.

• Administer cholestyramine before meals or before bedtime. This drug must not be given with other medications. Watch for adverse reactions, such as nausea, vomiting, constipation, steatorrhea, rashes, and hyperchloremic acidosis. Also watch for malabsorption of other medications and fat-soluble vitamins.

• Give clofibrate as prescribed. Watch for adverse reactions, such as cholelithiasis, cardiac dysrhythmias, intermittent claudication, thromboembolism, nausea, weight gain (from fluid retention), and myositis.

• *Don't* administer niacin to patients with active peptic ulcers or hepatic disease. Use with caution in patients with diabetes. In other patients, watch for adverse reactions, such as flushing, pruritus, hyperpigmentation, and exacerbation of inactive peptic ulcers.

• Urge the patient to adhere to his diet (usually 1,000 to 1,500 calories/day), to avoid excess sugar and alcoholic beverages, to minimize intake of saturated fats (higher in meats, coconut oil), and to increase intake of polyunsaturated fats (vegetable oils).

• Instruct the patient, for the 2 weeks preceding serum cholesterol and serum triglyceride tests, to maintain a steady weight and to adhere strictly to the prescribed diet. He should also fast for 12 hours preceding the test.

• Instruct women with elevated serum lipid levels to avoid oral contraceptives or drugs that contain estrogen.

HYPERPARATHYROIDISM

Characterized by overactivity of one or more of the four parathyroid glands, hyperparathyroidism results in excessive secretion of parathyroid hormone (PTH). Such hypersecretion of PTH promotes bone resorption and leads to hypercalcemia and hypophosphatemia. (See *Bone resorption in primary hyperparathyroidism,* page 438.)

In turn, increased renal and GI absorption of calcium occurs.

BONE RESORPTION IN PRIMARY HYPERPARATHYROIDISM

Erosion of middle phalanx

Demineralization of phalangeal tuft

Primary hyperparathyroidism usually occurs between ages 30 and 50 but can also occur in children and elderly people. It affects women two to three times more frequently than men.

Causes

Hyperparathyroidism may be primary or secondary:

• In primary hyperparathyroidism, one or more of the parathyroid glands enlarges, increasing PTH secretion and elevating serum calcium levels. The most common cause is a single adenoma. Other causes include a genetic disorder or multiple endocrine neoplasia.

• In secondary hyperparathyroidism, excessive compensatory production of PTH stems from a hypocalcemia-producing abnormality outside the parathyroid gland, which causes a resistance to the metabolic action of PTH. Some hypocalcemia-producing abnormalities are rickets, vitamin D deficiency, chronic renal failure, or osteomalacia due to phenytoin or laxative abuse.

Signs and symptoms

Clinical effects of primary hyperparathyroidism result from hypercalcemia and are typically present in several body systems:

• *Renal:* nephrocalcinosis due to elevated levels of calcium and possibly recurring nephrolithiasis, which may lead to renal insufficiency. Renal manifestations, including polyuria, are the most common effects of hyperparathyroidism.

• *Skeletal and articular:* chronic low back pain and easy fracturing due to bone degeneration; bone tenderness; chondrocalcinosis; occasionally severe osteopenia, especially on the vertebrae; erosions of the juxta-articular surface; subchondrial fractures; traumatic synovitis; and pseudogout

• *GI:* pancreatitis, causing constant, severe epigastric pain radiating to the back; peptic ulcers, causing abdominal pain, anorexia, nausea, and vomiting

• *Neuromuscular:* marked muscle weakness and atrophy, particularly in the legs

• *Central nervous system:* psychomotor and personality disturbances, depression, overt psychosis, stupor, and, possibly, coma

• *Other:* skin necrosis, cataracts, calcium microthrombi to lungs and pancreas, polyuria, anemia, and subcutaneous calcification.

Similarly, in secondary hyperparathyroidism, decreased serum calcium levels may produce the same features of calcium imbalance, with skeletal deformities of the long bones (rickets, for example), as well as symptoms of the underlying disease.

Diagnosis

Findings differ in primary and secondary disease.

Primary disease

In primary disease, a high concentration of serum PTH on radioimmunoassay with accompanying hypercalcemia confirms the diagnosis. In addition, X-rays show diffuse demineralization of bones, bone cysts, outer cortical bone absorption, and subperiosteal erosion of the phalanges and distal clavicles.

Microscopic examination of the bone with such tests as X-ray spectrophotometry typically demonstrates increased bone turnover. Laboratory tests reveal elevated urine and serum calcium, chloride, and alkaline phosphatase levels and decreased serum phosphorus levels.

Hyperparathyroidism may also raise uric acid and creatinine levels and increase basal acid secretion and serum immunoreactive gastrin. Increased serum amylase levels may indicate acute pancreatitis.

Secondary disease

Laboratory findings in secondary hyperparathyroidism show normal or slightly decreased serum calcium levels and variable serum phosphorus levels, especially when hyperparathyroidism is due to rickets, osteomalacia, or renal disease. The patient history may reveal familial renal disease, seizure disorders, or drug ingestion.

Other laboratory values and physical examination findings identify the cause of secondary hyperparathyroidism.

Treatment

Effective treatment varies, depending on the cause of the disease.

Primary disease

Treatment for primary hyperparathyroidism may include surgery to remove the adenoma or, depending on the extent of hyperplasia, all but half of one gland (the remaining part of the gland is necessary to maintain normal PTH levels). Such surgery may relieve bone pain within 3 days. However, renal damage may be irreversible.

Preoperatively—or if surgery isn't feasible or necessary—other treatments can decrease calcium levels. These include forcing fluids; limiting dietary intake of calcium; and promoting sodium and calcium excretion through forced diuresis using normal saline solution (up to 6 L in life-threatening circumstances), furosemide, or ethacrynic acid.

Other treatments include administering oral sodium or potassium phosphate, S.C. calcitonin, I.V. mithramycin, or I.V. biphosphonates.

Therapy for potential postoperative magnesium and phosphate deficiencies includes I.V. administration of magnesium and phosphate, or sodium phosphate solution given by mouth or retention enema. In addition, during the first 4 or 5 days after surgery, when serum calcium falls to low normal levels, supplemental calcium may be necessary; vitamin D or calcitriol may also be used to raise the serum calcium level.

Secondary disease

Treatment of secondary hyperparathyroidism must correct the underlying cause of parathyroid hypertrophy. It consists of vitamin D therapy or, in the patient with renal disease, administration of an oral calcium preparation for hyperphosphatemia.

In the patient with renal failure, dialysis is necessary to lower calcium levels and may have to continue for the remainder of the patient's life.

In the patient with chronic secondary hyperparathyroidism, the enlarged glands may not revert to normal size and function even after calcium levels have been controlled.

Special considerations

• Care emphasizes prevention of complications from the underlying disease and its treatment.

• Obtain pretreatment baseline serum potassium, calcium, phosphate, and magnesium levels because these values may change abruptly during treatment.

• During hydration to reduce serum calcium level, record intake and output accurately. Strain the urine to check for calculi. Provide at least 3 L of fluid a day, including cranberry or prune juice to increase urine acidity and help prevent calculus formation.

• Obtain blood and urine samples to measure sodium, potassium, and magnesium levels, especially for the patient taking furosemide.

• Auscultate for breath sounds often. Listen for signs of pulmonary edema in the patient receiving large amounts of saline solution I.V., especially if he has pulmonary or cardiac disease.

• Monitor the patient on digitalis glycosides carefully because elevated calcium levels can rapidly produce toxic effects.

• Because the patient is predisposed to pathologic fractures, take safety precautions to minimize the risk of injury. Assist him with walking, keep the bed at its lowest position, and raise the side rails. Lift the immobilized patient carefully to minimize bone stress.

• Schedule care to allow the patient with muscle weakness as much rest as possible.

• Watch for signs of peptic ulcer and administer antacids as appropriate.

After parathyroidectomy:

• Check frequently for respiratory distress, and keep a tracheotomy tray at bedside. Watch for postoperative complications, such as laryngeal nerve damage, or, rarely, hemorrhage. Monitor intake and output carefully.

• Check for swelling at the operative site. Place the patient in semi-Fowler's position, and support his head and neck with sandbags to decrease edema, which may cause pressure on the trachea.

• Watch for signs of mild tetany, such as complaints of tingling in the hands and around the mouth. These symptoms should subside quickly but may be prodromal signs of tetany, so keep calcium gluconate I.V. available for emergency administration. Watch for increased neuromuscular irritability and other signs of severe tetany.

• Ambulate the patient as soon as possible postoperatively, even though he may find this uncomfortable, because pressure on bones speeds up bone recalcification.

• Check laboratory results for low serum calcium and magnesium levels.

• Monitor the patient's mental status and watch for listlessness. In the patient with persistent hypercalcemia, check for muscle weakness and psychiatric symptoms.

• Before discharge, advise the patient of the possible adverse effects of drug therapy. Emphasize the need for periodic follow-up through laboratory blood tests. If hyperparathyroidism wasn't corrected surgically, warn the patient to avoid calcium-containing antacids and thiazide diuretics.

HYPERSPLENISM

A syndrome marked by exaggerated splenic activity and possible splenomegaly, hypersplenism results in peripheral blood cell deficiency as the spleen traps and destroys peripheral blood cells.

Causes

Hypersplenism may be idiopathic (primary) or secondary to an extrasplenic disorder, such as chronic malaria, polycythemia vera, or rheumatoid arthritis. In hypersplenism, the spleen's normal filtering and phagocytic functions accelerate indiscriminately, automatically removing antibody-coated, aging, and abnormal cells, even though some cells may be functionally normal.

The spleen may also temporarily sequester normal platelets and red blood cells (RBCs), withholding them from circulation. In this manner, the enlarged spleen may trap as much as 90% of the body's platelets and up to 45% of its RBC mass.

Signs and symptoms

Most patients with hypersplenism develop anemia, leukopenia, or thrombocytopenia, often with splenomegaly. They may contract bacterial infections frequently, bruise easily, hemorrhage spontaneously from the mucous membranes and GI or genitourinary tract, and suffer ulcerations of the mouth, legs, and feet. They commonly develop fever, weakness, and palpitations.

Patients with secondary hypersplenism may have other clinical abnormalities, depending on the underlying disease.

Diagnosis

Splenomegaly and evidence of abnormal splenic destruction or sequestration of RBCs or platelets is necessary to diagnose hypersplenism.

• The most definitive test measures the accumulation of erythrocytes in the spleen and liver after I.V. infusion of chromium-labeled RBCs or platelets. A high spleen-to-liver ratio of radioactivity indicates splenic destruction or sequestration.

• Complete blood count shows a decreased hemoglobin level (as low as 4 g/dl), white blood cell count (less than 4,000/µl), platelet count (less than 125,000/µl), and reticulocyte count.

• Splenic biopsy, scan, and angiography may be useful; a biopsy is hazardous, however, and should be avoided, if possible.

Treatment

Splenectomy is indicated only in transfusion-dependent patients who are refractory to medical therapy. Splenectomy rarely cures the patient but it does correct the effects of cytopenia.

Postoperative complications may include infection and thromboembolic disease. Occasionally, splenectomy may result in accelerated blood cell destruction in the bone marrow and liver. Secondary hypersplenism necessitates treatment of the underlying disease.

Special considerations

• If splenectomy is scheduled, administer preoperative transfusions of blood or blood products (fresh frozen plasma, platelets) to replace deficient blood elements. Symptoms or complications of any underlying disorder should be treated also.

• Postoperatively, monitor vital signs.

• Check for any excessive drainage or apparent bleeding.

• Watch for infection, thromboembolism, and abdominal distention.

• Keep the nasogastric tube patent; listen for bowel sounds.

• Instruct the patient to perform deep-breathing exercises, and encourage early ambulation to prevent respiratory complications and venous stasis.

HYPERTENSION

An intermittent or sustained elevation in diastolic or systolic blood pressure, hypertension occurs as two major types: essential (idiopathic) hypertension, the most common, and secondary hypertension, which results from renal disease or another identifiable cause. Malignant hypertension is a severe, fulminant form of hypertension common to both types.

Hypertension is a major cause of cerebrovascular accident, cardiac disease, and renal failure. The prognosis is good if this disorder is detected early and if treatment begins before complications develop. Severely elevated blood pressure (hypertensive crisis) may be fatal.

Causes

Hypertension affects 15% to 20% of adults in the United States. If untreated, it carries a high mortality.

Risk factors

Family history, race (most common in blacks), stress, obesity, a high intake of saturated fats or sodium, use of tobacco, sedentary lifestyle, and aging are risk factors for essential hypertension.

Secondary hypertension may result from renal vascular disease; pheochromocytoma; primary hyperaldosteronism; Cushing's syndrome; thyroid, pituitary, or parathyroid dysfunction; coarctation of the aorta; pregnancy; neurologic disorders; and use of oral contraceptives or other drugs, such as cocaine, epoetin alfa (erythropoietin), and cyclosporine.

Blood pressure regulators

Cardiac output and peripheral vascular resistance determine blood pressure. Increased blood volume, cardiac rate, and stroke volume as well as arteriolar vasoconstriction can raise blood pressure. The link to sustained hypertension, however, is unclear. Hypertension may also result from the failure of the following intrinsic regulatory mechanisms:

• Renal hypoperfusion causes the release of renin, which is converted by angiotensinogen, a liver enzyme, to angiotensin I. Angiotensin I is converted to angiotensin II, a powerful vasoconstrictor. The resulting vasoconstriction increases afterload.

Angiotensin II stimulates adrenal secretion of aldosterone, which increases sodium reabsorption. Hypertonic-stimulated release of antidiuretic hormone from the pituitary gland follows, increasing water reabsorption, plasma volume, cardiac output, and blood pressure.

• Autoregulation changes the diameter of an artery to maintain perfusion despite fluctuations in systemic blood pressure. The intrinsic mechanisms that are responsible include stress relaxation (vessels gradually dilate when blood pressure rises to reduce peripheral resistance) and capillary fluid shift (plasma moves between vessels and extravascular spaces to maintain intravascular volume).

• When the blood pressure drops, baroreceptors in the aortic arch and carotid sinuses decrease their inhibition of the medulla's vasomotor center, which increases sympathetic stimulation of the heart by norepinephrine. This, in turn, increases cardiac output by strengthening the contractile force, increasing the heart rate, and augmenting peripheral resistance by vasoconstriction.

Stress can also stimulate the sympathetic nervous system to increase cardiac output and peripheral vascular resistance.

Signs and symptoms

Hypertension usually doesn't produce clinical effects until vascular changes in the heart, brain, or kidneys occur. Highly elevated blood pressure damages the intima of small vessels, resulting in fibrin accumulation in the vessels, development of local edema and, possibly, intravascular clotting.

Symptoms produced by this process depend on the location of the damaged vessels:

• brain: cerebrovascular accident
• retina: blindness
• heart: myocardial infarction (MI)

• kidneys: proteinuria, edema and, eventually, renal failure.

Hypertension increases the heart's workload, causing left ventricular hypertrophy and, later, left ventricular failure, left- and right-sided heart failure, and pulmonary edema.

Diagnosis

Serial blood pressure measurements that are greater than 140/90 mm Hg in people under age 50 or greater than 150/95 mm Hg in those over age 50 confirm hypertension. Auscultation may reveal bruits over the abdominal aorta and the carotid, renal, and femoral arteries; ophthalmoscopy reveals arteriovenous nicking and, in hypertensive encephalopathy, papilledema.

The patient history and the following additional tests may show predisposing factors and help identify an underlying cause such as renal disease:

• *Urinalysis:* The presence of protein, red blood cells, and white blood cells may indicate glomerulonephritis.

• *Excretory urography:* Renal atrophy indicates chronic renal disease; one kidney that's more than ⅝″ (1.5 cm) shorter than the other suggests unilateral renal disease.

• *Serum potassium:* Levels less than 3.5 mEq/L may indicate adrenal dysfunction (primary hyperaldosteronism).

• *Blood urea nitrogen (BUN) and serum creatinine levels:* A BUN level that's normal or elevated to more than 20 mg/dl and a serum creatinine level that's normal or elevated to more than 1.5 mg/dl suggest renal disease.

Other tests help detect cardiovascular damage and other complications:

• *Electrocardiography* may show left ventricular hypertrophy or ischemia.

• *Chest X-ray* may show cardiomegaly.

• *Echocardiography* may show left ventricular hypertrophy.

Treatment

Secondary hypertension treatment focuses on correcting the underlying cause and controlling hypertensive effects.

The National Institutes of Health recommend the following stepped-care approach for treating primary hypertension:

• *Step 1:* Help the patient initiate necessary lifestyle modifications, including weight reduction, moderation of alcohol intake, regular physical exercise, reduction of sodium intake, and smoking cessation.

• *Step 2:* If the patient fails to achieve the desired blood pressure or make significant progress, continue lifestyle modifications and begin drug therapy. Preferred drugs include diuretics or beta blockers. These drugs have proved effective in reducing cardiovascular morbidity and mortality.

If diuretics or beta blockers are ineffective or unacceptable, the doctor may prescribe angiotensin-converting enzyme inhibitors, calcium antagonists, alpha$_1$-receptor blockers, or alpha-beta blockers. These drugs, while effective in reducing blood pressure, have yet to prove effective in reducing morbidity and mortality.

• *Step 3:* If the patient fails to achieve the desired blood pressure or make significant progress, increase the drug dosage, substitute a drug in the same class, or add a drug from a different class.

• *Step 4:* If the patient fails to achieve the desired blood pressure or make significant progress, add a second or third agent or a diuretic (if one isn't already prescribed). Second or third agents may include direct-acting vasodilators, alpha$_1$-antagonists, and peripherally acting adrenergic neuron antagonists.

Hypertensive emergencies

Examples of hypertensive emergencies include hypertensive encephalopathy, intracranial hemorrhage, acute left ventricular failure with pulmonary edema, and dissecting aortic aneurysm. Hypertensive emergencies are also associated with eclampsia or severe pregnancy-related hypertension, unstable angina, and acute MI.

Typically, hypertensive emergencies require parenteral administration of a vasodilator or an adrenergic inhibitor or oral administration of a selected drug, such as nifedipine, captopril, clonidine, or labetalol, to rapidly reduce blood pressure.

Hypertension without accompanying symptoms or target-organ disease rarely requires emergency drug therapy.

Special considerations

• To encourage compliance with antihypertensive therapy, suggest that the patient establish a daily routine for taking his medication. Warn that uncontrolled hypertension may cause stroke and heart attack.
• Tell the patient to report adverse reactions to drugs.
• Advise the patient to avoid high-sodium antacids and over-the-counter cold and sinus medications, which contain harmful vasoconstrictors.
• Encourage a change in the patient's dietary habits. Help the obese patient plan a weight-reduction diet; tell him to avoid high-sodium foods (pickles, potato chips, canned soups, cold cuts) and table salt.
• Help the patient examine and modify his lifestyle (for example, by reducing stress and exercising regularly).

If a patient is hospitalized with hypertension:
• Find out if he was taking his prescribed medication. If he wasn't, ask why. If the patient can't afford the medication, refer him to an appropriate social service agency.
• Tell the patient and his family to keep a record of drugs used in the past, noting especially which ones were or were not effective. Suggest recording this information on a card so that the patient can show it to his doctor.

When routine blood pressure screening reveals elevated pressure:
• Make sure the cuff size is appropriate for the patient's upper arm circumference.
• Take the pressure in both arms in lying, sitting, and standing positions.
• Ask the patient if he smoked, drank a beverage containing caffeine, or was emotionally upset before the test.
• Advise the patient to return for blood pressure testing at frequent and regular intervals.

To help identify hypertension and prevent untreated hypertension:
• Participate in public education programs dealing with hypertension and ways to reduce risk factors.
• Encourage public participation in blood pressure screening programs. Routinely screen all patients, especially those at risk (blacks and persons with family histories of hypertension, stroke, or heart attack).

LIFE-THREATENING DISORDER

HYPERTENSION, PREGNANCY-INDUCED

Toxemia of pregnancy, or pregnancy-induced hypertension, usually develops late in the second trimester or in the third trimester. *Preeclampsia,* the nonconvulsive form of toxemia, develops in about 7% of pregnancies. It may be mild or severe, and the incidence is significantly higher in low socioeconomic groups.

Eclampsia is the convulsive form of toxemia. About 5% of females with preeclampsia develop eclampsia; of these, about 15% die from toxemia itself or its complications. Fetal mortality is high because of the increased incidence of premature delivery.

Causes

The cause of pregnancy-induced hypertension is unknown, but it appears to be related to inadequate prenatal care (especially poor nutrition), parity (more prevalent in primigravidas), multiple pregnancies, preexisting diabetes mellitus, or hypertension.

Age is also a factor. Adolescents and primaparas over age 35 are at higher risk for preeclampsia. Other theories postulate a long list of potential toxic sources, such as autolysis of placental infarcts, autointoxication, uremia, maternal sensitization to total proteins, and pyelonephritis.

Signs and symptoms

• Mild preeclampsia generally produces the following signs: hypertension, proteinuria, generalized edema, and a sudden weight gain of more than 3 lb (1.36 kg) a week during the second trimester or more than 1 lb (0.45 kg) a week during the third trimester.
• Severe preeclampsia is marked by increased hypertension and proteinuria, eventually leading to the development of oliguria. Hemolysis, elevated liver enzyme levels, and a low platelet count (the HELLP syndrome) is often severe.

Other symptoms that may indicate worsening preeclampsia include blurred vision due to retinal arteriolar spasms, epigastric pain or heartburn, irritability, emotional tension, and severe frontal headache.
• In eclampsia, all the clinical manifestations of preeclampsia are magni-

fied and are associated with seizures and possibly coma, premature labor, stillbirth, renal failure, and hepatic damage.

Diagnosis

The following findings suggest mild preeclampsia:
• *elevated blood pressure readings:* 140 mm Hg systolic, or a rise of 30 mm Hg or more above the patient's normal systolic pressure, measured on two occasions, 6 hours apart; 90 mm Hg diastolic, or a rise of 15 mm Hg or more above the patient's normal diastolic pressure, measured on two occasions, 6 hours apart
• *proteinuria:* more than 500 mg/24 hours.

These findings suggest severe preeclampsia:
• *much higher blood pressure readings:* 160/110 mm Hg or higher on two occasions, 6 hours apart, while on bed rest
• *increased proteinuria:* 5 g or more/24 hours
• *oliguria:* urine output less than or equal to 400 ml/24 hours
• *deep tendon reflexes:* possibly hyperactive as central nervous system (CNS) irritability increases.

Typical clinical features — especially seizures — with typical findings for severe preeclampsia strongly suggest eclampsia. An ophthalmoscopic examination may reveal vascular spasm, papilledema, retinal edema or detachment, and arteriovenous nicking or hemorrhage.

Real-time ultrasonography and stress and nonstress tests evaluate fetal well-being. In the stress test, oxytocin stimulates contractions; fetal heart tones are then monitored electronically.

In the nonstress test, fetal heart tones are monitored electronically during periods of fetal activity, without oxytocin stimulation. Electronic monitoring reveals stable or increased fetal heart tones during periods of fetal activity.

Treatment

Adequate nutrition, good prenatal care, and control of preexisting hypertension during pregnancy decrease the incidence and severity of preeclampsia. Early recognition and prompt treatment of preeclampsia can prevent progression to eclampsia.

Therapy for preeclampsia is designed to halt the disorder's progress — specifically, the early effects of eclampsia, such as convulsions, residual hypertension, and renal shutdown — and to ensure fetal survival. Some doctors advocate the prompt induction of labor, especially if the patient is near term; others follow a more conservative approach.

Conservative measures

Therapy may include sedatives, such as phenobarbital, along with complete bed rest, to relieve anxiety, reduce hypertension, and evaluate response to therapy. If renal function remains adequate, a high-protein, low-sodium, low-carbohydrate diet with increased fluid intake is recommended.

If blood pressure fails to respond to bed rest and sedation and persistently rises above 160/100 mm Hg, or if CNS irritability increases, magnesium sulfate may produce general sedation, promote diuresis, reduce blood pressure, and prevent seizures.

Cesarean section

If these measures fail to improve the patient's condition, or if fetal life is endangered (as determined by stress or nonstress tests), cesarean section or oxytocin induction may be required to terminate the pregnancy.

Treatment for seizures

Emergency treatment of eclamptic seizures consists of immediate administration of diazepam I.V., followed by magnesium sulfate (I.V. drip), oxygen administration, and electronic fetal monitoring. After the patient's condition stabilizes, a cesarean section may be performed.

Special considerations

• Monitor regularly for changes in blood pressure, pulse rate, respiration, fetal heart tones, vision, level of consciousness, and deep tendon reflexes and for headache unrelieved by medication. Assess these signs before administering medications. Absence of patellar reflexes may indicate magnesium sulfate toxicity.

• Assess fluid balance by measuring intake and output and by checking daily weight.

• Observe for signs of fetal distress by closely monitoring the results of stress and nonstress tests.

• Instruct the patient to lie in a left lateral position to increase venous return, cardiac output, and renal blood flow.

• Keep emergency resuscitative equipment and drugs (including diazepam and magnesium sulfate) available in case of seizures and cardiac or respiratory arrest. Also keep calcium gluconate at the bedside, since it counteracts the toxic effects of magnesium sulfate.

• To protect the patient from injury, maintain seizure precautions. Don't leave an unstable patient unattended.

• Give emergency treatment to the patient having seizures. Provide a quiet, darkened room until the patient's condition stabilizes, and enforce absolute bed rest. Carefully monitor administration of magnesium sulfate; give oxygen. Don't administer anything by mouth. Insert an indwelling urinary catheter for accurate measurement of intake and output.

• Provide emotional support for the patient and family.

• If the patient's condition necessitates premature delivery, point out that infants of mothers with toxemia are usually small for gestational age but sometimes fare better than other premature babies of the same weight, possibly because they've developed adaptive responses to stress in utero.

HYPERTHYROIDISM

Also called Graves' disease, Basedow's disease, and thyrotoxicosis, hyperthyroidism is a metabolic imbalance that results from thyroid hormone overproduction. The most common form of hyperthyroidism is Graves' disease, which increases thyroxine production, enlarges the thyroid gland (goiter), and causes multiple system changes. (See *Other forms of hyperthyroidism,* page 448.)

Incidence of Graves' disease is highest between ages 30 and 40, especially in people with family histories of thyroid abnormalities; only 5% of hyperthyroid patients are younger than age 15.

With treatment, most patients can lead normal lives. However, thyroid storm — an acute exacerbation of hyperthyroidism — is a medical emergency that may lead to life-threatening cardiac, hepatic, or renal failure.

Causes

Hyperthyroidism may result from both genetic and immunologic factors. For example:

• An increased incidence of this disorder in monozygotic twins points to an inherited factor, probably an autosomal recessive gene.

• This disease occasionally coexists with abnormal iodine metabolism and other endocrine abnormalities, such as diabetes mellitus, thyroiditis, and hyperparathyroidism.

• Hyperthyroidism is also associated with the production of autoantibodies (thyroid-stimulating immunoglobulin and thyroid-stimulating hormone [TSH]–binding inhibitory immunoglobulin), possibly because of a defect in suppressor–T-lymphocyte function that allows formation of autoantibodies.

• In latent hyperthyroidism, excessive dietary intake of iodine and, possibly, stress can precipitate clinical hyperthyroidism.

• In a person with inadequately treated hyperthyroidism, stress — including surgery, infection, toxemia of pregnancy, and diabetic ketoacidosis — can precipitate thyroid storm.

Signs and symptoms

The classic features of Graves' disease are an enlarged thyroid (goiter), nervousness, heat intolerance, weight loss despite increased appetite, sweating, diarrhea, tremor, and palpitations. Exophthalmos is considered most characteristic but is absent in many patients with hyperthyroidism.

Many other symptoms are common because hyperthyroidism profoundly affects virtually every body system:

• *Central nervous system:* difficulty in concentrating because increased thyroxine secretion accelerates cerebral function; excitability or nervousness due to increased basal metabolic rate; fine tremor, shaky handwriting, and clumsiness from increased activity in the spinal cord area that controls muscle tone; emotional instability and mood swings, ranging from occasional outbursts to overt psychosis

• *Skin, hair, and nails:* smooth, warm, flushed skin (patient sleeps with minimal covers and little clothing); fine,

OTHER FORMS OF HYPERTHYROIDISM

Varied forms of hyperthyroidism may include the following.

Toxic adenoma
This small, benign nodule in the thyroid gland that secretes thyroid hormone is the second most common cause of hyperthyroidism. The cause of toxic adenoma is unknown; incidence is highest in elderly people. Clinical effects are essentially similar to those of Graves' disease, except that toxic adenoma doesn't induce ophthalmopathy, pretibial myxedema, or acropachy.

Presence of adenoma is confirmed by iodine 131 (^{131}I) uptake and a thyroid scan, which show a single hyperfunctioning nodule suppressing the rest of the gland. Treatment includes ^{131}I therapy, or surgery to remove adenoma after antithyroid drugs achieve a euthyroid state.

Thyrotoxicosis factitia
This form of hyperthyroidism results from a chronic ingestion of thyroid hormone for thyrotropin suppression in patients with thyroid carcinoma, or from thyroid hormone abuse by persons who are trying to lose weight.

Functioning metastatic thyroid carcinoma
This rare disease causes excess production of thyroid hormone.

TSH-secreting pituitary tumor
A pituitary tumor that secretes thyroid-stimulating hormone (TSH) causes overproduction of thyroid hormone.

Subacute thyroiditis
This is a virus-induced granulomatous inflammation of the thyroid, producing transient hyperthyroidism associated with fever, pain, pharyngitis, and tenderness in the thyroid gland.

Silent thyroiditis
Self-limiting, silent thyroiditis is a transient form of hyperthyroidism, with histologic thyroiditis but no inflammatory symptoms.

soft hair; premature graying and increased hair loss in both sexes; friable nails and onycholysis (distal nail separated from the bed); pretibial myxedema (dermopathy), producing thickened skin; and accentuated hair follicles, raised red patches of skin that are itchy and sometimes painful, with occasional nodule formation. Microscopic examination shows increased mucin deposits.
• *Cardiovascular system:* tachycardia; full, bounding pulse; wide pulse pressure; cardiomegaly; increased cardiac output and blood volume; visible point of maximal impulse; paroxysmal supraventricular tachycardia and atrial fibrillation (especially in elderly people); and, occasionally, a systolic murmur at the left sternal border
• *Respiratory system:* dyspnea on exertion and at rest, possibly from cardiac decompensation and increased cellular oxygen utilization
• *GI system:* possible anorexia; nausea and vomiting due to increased GI motility and peristalsis; increased defecation; soft stools or, with severe disease, diarrhea; and liver enlargement
• *Musculoskeletal system:* weakness, fatigue, and muscle atrophy; rare coexistence with myasthenia gravis; possibly generalized or localized paralysis associated with hypokalemia; and oc-

casional acropachy (soft-tissue swelling, accompanied by underlying bone changes where new bone formation occurs)

• *Reproductive system:* in females, oligomenorrhea or amenorrhea, decreased fertility, higher incidence of spontaneous abortions; in males, gynecomastia due to increased estrogen levels; in both sexes, diminished libido

• *Eyes:* exophthalmos (produced by the combined effects of accumulation of mucopolysaccharides and fluids in the retroorbital tissues that force the eyeball outward, and of lid retraction that produces the characteristic staring gaze); occasional inflammation of conjunctivae, corneas, or eye muscles; diplopia; and increased tearing.

When hyperthyroidism escalates to thyroid storm, these symptoms can be accompanied by extreme irritability, hypertension, tachycardia, vomiting, temperature up to 106° F (41.1° C), delirium, and coma.

Diagnosis

The diagnosis of hyperthyroidism usually is straightforward and depends on a careful clinical history and physical examination, a high index of suspicion, and routine hormone determinations. The following tests confirm the disorder:

• *Radioimmunoassay* shows increased serum thyroxine (T_4) and triiodothyronine (T_3) concentrations.

• *Thyroid scan* reveals increased uptake of radioactive iodine 131 (^{131}I). This test is contraindicated if the patient is pregnant.

• *TSH* levels are decreased.

• *Thyroid-releasing hormone (TRH) stimulation test* indicates hyperthyroidism if the TSH level fails to rise within 30 minutes after the administration of TRH.

• *Ultrasonography* confirms subclinical ophthalmopathy.

Treatment

A number of approaches are utilized for the treatment of hyperthyroidism. The primary forms of therapy include antithyroid drugs, ^{131}I, and surgery. Appropriate treatment depends on the size of the goiter, the causes, the patient's age and parity, and how long surgery will be delayed (if the patient is an appropriate candidate for surgery).

Antithyroid therapy

Therapy with antithyroid drugs is used for children, young adults, pregnant women, and patients who refuse surgery or ^{131}I treatment. Treatment options include the following:

• Thyroid hormone antagonists include propylthiouracil and methimazole, which block thyroid hormone synthesis. Although hypermetabolic symptoms subside within 4 to 8 weeks after such therapy begins, the patient must continue the medication for 6 months to 2 years, depending on the clinical circumstances.

• Propranolol may be given concomitantly to manage tachycardia and other peripheral effects of excessive hypersympathetic activity.

• During pregnancy, antithyroid medication should be kept at the minimum dosage required to keep maternal thyroid function within the high-normal range until delivery and to minimize the risk of fetal hypothyroidism.

Most infants of hyperthyroid mothers are born with mild and transient hyperthyroidism. Neonatal hyperthyroidism may even necessitate treatment with antithyroid medications and propranolol for 2 to 3 months.

Because hyperthyroidism is sometimes exacerbated in the puerperal period, continuous control of maternal thyroid function is essential. Approximately 3 to 6 months postpartum, antithyroid drug administration can be gradually tapered and thyroid function reassessed.

The mother receiving low-dose antithyroid treatment may breast-feed as long as the infant's thyroid function is checked periodically. Small amounts of the drug can be found in breast milk.

^{131}I

Another major form of therapy for hyperthyroidism is a single oral dose of ^{131}I — the treatment of choice for patients not planning to have children. (Patients of reproductive age must give informed consent for this treatment, since small amounts of ^{131}I concentrate in the gonads.)

During treatment with ^{131}I, the thyroid gland picks up the radioactive element as it would regular iodine. Subsequently, the radioactivity destroys some of the cells that normally concentrate iodine and produce T_4, thus decreasing thyroid hormone production and normalizing thyroid size and function.

In most patients, hypermetabolic symptoms diminish from 6 to 8 weeks after such treatment. However, some patients may require a second dose.

Surgery

Subtotal (partial) thyroidectomy, which decreases the thyroid gland's capacity for hormone production, is indicated for patients with a large goiter whose hyperthyroidism has repeatedly relapsed after drug therapy or patients who refuse or aren't candidates for ^{131}I treatment.

Preoperatively, the patient may receive iodides (Lugol's solution or saturated solution of potassium iodide), antithyroid drugs, or high doses of propranolol, to help prevent thyroid storm. If euthyroidism isn't achieved, surgery should be delayed and propranolol administered to decrease the systemic effects (cardiac arrhythmias) caused by hyperthyroidism.

After ablative treatment with ^{131}I or surgery, patients require regular medical supervision for the rest of their lives because they usually develop hypothyroidism, sometimes as long as several years after treatment.

Treatment for hyperthyroid ophthalmopathy

Therapy includes local application of topical medications but may require high doses of corticosteroids. A patient with severe exophthalmos that causes pressure on the optic nerve may require external-beam radiation therapy or surgical decompression to lessen pressure on the orbital contents.

Treatment for thyroid storm

This includes administration of an antithyroid drug, I.V. propranolol to block sympathetic effects, a corticosteroid to inhibit the conversion of T_4 to T_3 and to replace depleted cortisol levels, and an iodide to block release of thyroid hormone.

Supportive measures include administration of nutrients, vitamins, fluids, and sedatives.

Special considerations

• Patients with hyperthyroidism require vigilant care to prevent acute exacerbations and complications.
• Record vital signs and weight.
• Monitor serum electrolytes, and check periodically for hyperglycemia and glycosuria.
• Carefully monitor cardiac function if the patient is elderly or has coronary artery disease. If the heart rate is more than 100 beats/minute, check blood pressure and pulse rate often.
• Check the patient's level of consciousness and urine output.
• If the patient is pregnant, tell her to watch closely during the first trimester for signs of spontaneous abortion (spotting, occasional mild cramps) and report such signs immediately.

• Encourage bed rest, and keep the patient's room cool, quiet, and dark. The patient with dyspnea will be most comfortable sitting upright or in high Fowler's position.

• Remember, extreme nervousness may produce bizarre behavior. Reassure the patient and his family that such behavior will probably subside with treatment. Provide sedatives, as necessary, and encourage the patient to verbalize his feelings about changes in body image.

• To promote weight gain, provide a balanced diet, with six meals a day. If the patient has edema, suggest a low-sodium diet.

• If iodide is part of the treatment, mix it with milk, juice, or water to prevent GI distress, and administer it through a straw to prevent tooth discoloration.

• Watch for signs of thyroid storm (tachycardia, hyperkinesis, fever, vomiting, hypertension).

• Check intake and output carefully to ensure adequate hydration and fluid balance.

• Closely monitor blood pressure, cardiac rate and rhythm, and temperature. If the patient has a high fever, reduce it with appropriate hypothermic measures. Maintain an I.V. line and give drugs as needed.

• If the patient has exophthalmos or another ophthalmopathy, suggest sunglasses or eyepatches to protect his eyes from light. Moisten the conjunctivae often with isotonic eyedrops. Warn the patient with severe lid retraction to avoid sudden physical movements that might cause the lid to slip behind the eyeball. Instruct him to report signs of decreased visual acuity.

• Avoid excessive palpation of the thyroid to avoid precipitating thyroid storm.

After thyroidectomy:

• Check often for respiratory distress, and keep a tracheotomy tray at bedside.

• Watch for evidence of hemorrhage into the neck, such as a tight dressing with no blood on it. Change dressings and perform wound care; check the *back* of the dressing for drainage. Keep the patient in semi-Fowler's position, and support his head and neck with sandbags to ease tension on the incision.

• Check for dysphagia or hoarseness from possible laryngeal nerve injury.

• Watch for signs of hypoparathyroidism (tetany, numbness), a complication that results from accidental removal of the parathyroid glands during surgery.

• Stress the importance of regular medical follow-up after discharge because hypothyroidism may develop from 2 to 4 weeks postoperatively.

Drug therapy and ^{131}I therapy require careful monitoring and comprehensive patient teaching, as follows:

• After ^{131}I therapy, tell the patient not to expectorate or cough freely because his saliva is radioactive for 24 hours. Stress the need for repeated measurement of serum thyroxine levels.

• If the patient is taking propylthiouracil and methimazole, monitor the complete blood count periodically to detect leukopenia, thrombocytopenia, and agranulocytosis. Instruct him to take these medications with meals to minimize GI distress, and to avoid over-the-counter cough preparations because many contain iodine.

• Tell him to report signs of hypersensitivity—fever, enlarged cervical lymph nodes, sore throat, mouth sores, and other signs of blood dyscrasias and any rash or skin eruptions.

• Watch the patient taking propranolol for signs of hypotension (dizziness, decreased urine output). Tell him to rise slowly after sitting or lying down to prevent orthostatic hypotension.

• Instruct the patient receiving antithyroid drugs or ^{131}I therapy to report any symptoms of hypothyroidism.

DIAGNOSING HYPOCHONDRIASIS

A diagnosis of hypochondriasis is made when the patient's symptoms meet the following criteria from the *Diagnostic and Statistical Manual of Mental Disorders*, 4th edition:
• Preoccupation with the fear of having or the belief that one has a serious disease based on the person's misinterpretation of bodily symptoms.
• The preoccupation persists despite appropriate medical evaluation and reassurance.
• The fear of having or the belief that one has a serious disease is not of delusional intensity (as in delusional disorder, somatic type) and is not restricted to a circumscribed concern about appearance (as in body dysmorphic disorder).
• The preoccupation causes clinically significant distress or impairment in social, occupational, or other important areas of functioning.
• The disturbance has persisted for at least 6 months.
• The preoccupation is not better accounted for by generalized anxiety disorder, obsessive-compulsive disorder, panic disorder, a major depressive episode, separation anxiety, or another somatoform disorder.

HYPOCHONDRIASIS

The dominant feature of hypochondriasis is an unrealistic misinterpretation of the severity and significance of physical signs or sensations as abnormal. This leads to preoccupation with fear of having a serious disease, which persists despite medical reassurance to the contrary.

Hypochondriasis causes severe social and occupational impairment. It doesn't result from other mental disorders, such as schizophrenia, mood disorder, or somatization disorder.

Hypochondriasis appears to be equally common in men and women. It can begin at any age, but onset most frequently occurs between ages 20 and 30. The course of the disorder usually is chronic, although the severity of symptoms may vary.

Causes
Hypochondriasis is not linked to any specific cause. However, this disorder frequently develops in people who have experienced an organic disease or in their relatives. It allows the patient to assume a dependent sick role to ensure that his needs are met. Such a patient is unaware of these unmet needs and does not consciously cause his symptoms. Stress increases the risk of developing hypochondriasis.

Signs and symptoms
The dominant feature of hypochondriasis is the misinterpretation of symptoms — usually multiple complaints that involve a single organ system — as signs of serious illness. As the medical evaluation proceeds, complaints may shift and change.

Symptoms can range from specific to general, vague complaints and often are associated with a preoccupation with normal body functions.

The hypochondriacal patient will relate a chronic history of waxing and waning symptoms. Commonly, he will have undergone multiple evaluations for similar symptoms or complaints of serious illness. His past contacts with health care professionals make him quite knowledgeable about illness, diagnosis, and treatment.

Diagnosis

For characteristic findings in patients with this condition, see *Diagnosing hypochondriasis.*

Treatment

The goal of treatment is to help the patient continue to lead a productive life despite distressing symptoms and fears. After medical evaluation is complete, the patient should be told clearly that he doesn't have a serious disease but that continued medical follow-up will help monitor his symptoms. Providing a diagnosis won't make hypochondriasis disappear, but it may ease the patient's anxiety.

Regular outpatient follow-up can help the patient deal with his symptoms and is necessary to detect organic illness. (Up to 30% of these patients develop an organic disease.) Because the patient can be demanding and irritating, consistent follow-up may be difficult.

Most patients don't acknowledge any psychological influence on their symptoms and resist psychiatric treatment.

Special considerations

• Provide a supportive relationship that lets the patient feel cared for and understood. The patient with hypochondriasis feels real pain and distress, so don't deny his symptoms or challenge his behavior.

• Firmly state that medical test results were negative. Instead of reinforcing his symptoms, encourage him to discuss his other problems, and urge his family to do the same.

• Recognize that the patient will never be symptom-free, and don't become angry when he won't give up his disease. Such anger can drive him to yet another unnecessary medical evaluation.

• Help the patient and family find new ways to deal with stress other than development of physical symptoms.

HYPOGLYCEMIA

An abnormally low glucose level in the bloodstream, hypoglycemia occurs when glucose burns up too rapidly, when the glucose release rate falls behind tissue demands, or when excessive insulin enters the bloodstream.

Hypoglycemia is classified as reactive or fasting. *Reactive hypoglycemia* results from the reaction to the disposition of meals or the administration of excessive insulin. *Fasting hypoglycemia* causes discomfort during long periods of abstinence from food — for example, in the early morning hours before breakfast.

Although hypoglycemia is a specific endocrine imbalance, its symptoms are often vague and depend on how quickly the patient's glucose levels drop. If not corrected, severe hypoglycemia may result in coma, irreversible brain damage, and death.

Causes

The two forms of hypoglycemia have different causes and occur in different types of patients.

Reactive hypoglycemia

Several forms of reactive hypoglycemia occur. In a diabetic patient, it may result from administration of too much insulin or — less commonly — too much oral hypoglycemia medication. In a mildly diabetic patient (or one in the early stages of diabetes mellitus), reactive hypoglycemia may result from delayed and excessive insulin production after carbohydrate ingestion.

Similarly, a nondiabetic patient may suffer reactive hypoglycemia from a sharp increase in insulin output after a meal. Sometimes called *postprandial hypoglycemia,* this type of reactive hypoglycemia usually disappears when the patient eats something sweet.

In some patients, reactive hypoglycemia may have no known cause (idiopathic reactive) or may result from hyperalimentation due to gastric dumping syndrome or from impaired glucose tolerance.

Fasting hypoglycemia

This type of hypoglycemia usually results from an excess of insulin or insulin-like substance or from a decrease in counterregulatory hormones. It can be *exogenous,* resulting from such external factors as alcohol or drug ingestion, or *endogenous,* resulting from organic problems.

Endogenous hypoglycemia may result from tumors or liver disease. Insulinomas, small islet cell tumors in the pancreas, secrete excessive amounts of insulin, which inhibits hepatic glucose production. They're generally benign (in 90% of patients).

Extrapancreatic tumors, though uncommon, can also cause hypoglycemia by increasing glucose utilization and inhibiting glucose output. Such tumors occur primarily in the mesenchyma, liver, adrenal cortex, GI system, and lymphatic system. They may be benign or malignant.

Among nonendocrine causes of fasting hypoglycemia are severe liver diseases, including hepatitis, cancer, cirrhosis, and liver congestion associated with congestive heart failure. All of these conditions reduce the uptake and release of glycogen from the liver.

Some endocrine causes include destruction of pancreatic islet cells; adrenocortical insufficiency, which contributes to hypoglycemia by reducing the production of cortisol and cortisone needed for gluconeogenesis; and pituitary insufficiency, which reduces corticotropin and growth hormone levels.

Causes in infants and children

Hypoglycemia is at least as common in neonates and children as it is in adults. Usually, infants develop hypoglycemia because of an increased number of cells per unit of body weight and because of increased demands on stored liver glycogen to support respirations, thermoregulation, and muscular activity.

In full-term neonates, hypoglycemia may occur 24 to 72 hours after birth and is usually transient. In infants who are premature or small for gestational age, onset of hypoglycemia is much more rapid — it can occur as soon as 6 hours after birth — due to their small, immature livers, which produce much less glycogen.

Maternal disorders that can produce hypoglycemia in infants within 24 hours after birth include diabetes mellitus, toxemia, erythroblastosis, and glycogen storage disease.

Signs and symptoms

Reactive hypoglycemia causes fatigue and malaise, nervousness, irritability, trembling, tension, headache, hunger, cold sweats, and rapid heart rate. These same clinical effects usually characterize fasting hypoglycemia.

In addition, fasting hypoglycemia may also cause central nervous system (CNS) disturbances; for example, blurry or double vision, confusion, motor weakness, hemiplegia, seizures, or coma.

In infants and children, signs and symptoms of hypoglycemia are vague. A newborn's refusal to feed may be the primary clue to underlying hypoglycemia. Associated CNS effects include tremors, twitching, weak or high-pitched cry, sweating, limpness, seizures, and coma.

Diagnosis

Reagent or glucose reagent strips provide quick screening methods for determining blood glucose level. A color change that corresponds to less than 45 mg/dl indicates the need for a venous blood sample.

Laboratory testing confirms the diagnosis by showing decreased blood glucose values. The following values indicate hypoglycemia:
• *full-term infants:* less than 30 mg/dl before a feeding; less than 40 mg/dl after a feeding
• *preterm infants:* less than 20 mg/dl before a feeding; less than 30 mg/dl after a feeding
• *children and adults:* less than 40 mg/dl before a meal; less than 50 mg/dl after a meal.

In addition, a 5-hour glucose tolerance test may be administered to provoke reactive hypoglycemia. Following a 12-hour fast, laboratory testing to detect plasma insulin and plasma glucose levels may identify fasting hypoglycemia.

Treatment

Reactive hypoglycemia and fasting hypoglycemia require different treatments.

Reactive hypoglycemia

Effective treatment of reactive hypoglycemia requires dietary modification to help delay glucose absorption and gastric emptying. Usually, this includes small, frequent meals; ingestion of complex carbohydrates, fiber, and fat; and avoidance of simple sugars, alcohol, and fruit drinks.

The patient may also receive anticholinergic drugs to slow gastric emptying and intestinal motility and to inhibit vagal stimulation of insulin release.

Fasting hypoglycemia

In fasting hypoglycemia, surgery and drug therapy are usually required. In patients with insulinoma, removal of the tumor is the treatment of choice. Drug therapy may include nondiuretic thiazides, such as diazoxide, to inhibit insulin secretion; streptozocin; and hormones, such as glucocorticoids and long-acting glycogen.

In neonates

Therapy for neonates who have hypoglycemia or who are at risk of developing it includes preventive measures. A hypertonic solution of 10% dextrose, calculated at 5 to 10 ml/kg of body weight administered I.V. over 10 minutes and followed by 4 to 8 mg/kg/minute for maintainence, should correct a severe hypoglycemic state in newborns.

To reduce the chance of hypoglycemia in high-risk infants, they should receive feedings—either breast milk or a solution of 5% to 10% glucose and water—as soon after birth as possible.

Special considerations

• Watch for signs of hypoglycemia (such as poor feeding) in high-risk infants.
• Monitor infusion of hypertonic glucose in the newborn to avoid hyperglycemia, circulatory overload, and cellular dehydration. Terminate glucose solutions gradually, to prevent hypoglycemia caused by hyperinsulinemia.
• Explain the purpose and procedure for any diagnostic tests. Collect blood samples at the appropriate times.
• Monitor the effects of drug therapy, and watch for the development of any adverse effects.
• Teach the patient which foods to include in his diet (complex carbohydrates, fiber, fat) and which foods to avoid (simple sugars, alcohol). Refer

the patient and family for dietary counseling as appropriate.

HYPOGONADISM

A condition resulting from decreased androgen production in males, hypogonadism may impair spermatogenesis (causing infertility) and inhibit the development of normal secondary sex characteristics. The clinical effects of androgen deficiency depend on age at onset.

Causes

Hypogonadism may be primary or secondary; each type has different causes.

Primary hypogonadism

This type results directly from interstitial (Leydig's cell) cellular or seminiferous tubular damage due to faulty development or mechanical damage. This causes increased secretion of gonadotropins by the pituitary in an attempt to increase the testicular functional state and is therefore termed hypergonadotropic hypogonadism.

It includes the following: Klinefelter's syndrome, Reifenstein's syndrome, male Turner's syndrome, Sertoli-cell–only syndrome, anorchism, orchitis, and sequelae of irradiation.

Secondary hypogonadism

This type results from faulty interaction within the hypothalamic-pituitary axis resulting in failure to secrete normal levels of gonadotropins, and is therefore termed hypogonadotropic hypogonadism.

It includes the following: hypopituitarism, isolated follicle-stimulating hormone deficiency, isolated luteinizing hormone deficiency, Kallmann's syndrome, and Prader-Willi syndrome.

Depending on the patient's age at onset, hypogonadism may cause eunuchism (complete gonadal failure) or eunuchoidism (partial failure).

Signs and symptoms

Although symptoms vary, depending on the specific cause of hypogonadism, some characteristic findings may include delayed closure of hepiphyses and immature bone age; delayed puberty; infantile penis and small, soft testes; below-average muscle development and strength; fine, sparse facial hair; scant or absent axillary, pubic, and body hair; and a high-pitched, effeminate voice.

In an adult, hypogonadism diminishes sex drive and potency and causes regression of secondary sex characteristics.

Diagnosis

An accurate diagnosis necessitates a detailed patient history, physical examination, and hormonal studies. Serum and urinary gonadotropin levels increase in primary, or hypergonadotropic, hypogonadism but decrease in secondary, or hypogonadotropic, hypogonadism.

Other relevant hormonal studies include assessment of neuroendocrine functions, such as thyrotropin, adrenocorticotropin, growth hormone, and vasopressin levels. Chromosomal analysis may determine the specific causative syndrome. A testicular biopsy and semen analysis determine sperm production, identify impaired spermatogenesis, and assess low levels of testosterone.

Treatment

Depending on the underlying cause, treatment may consist of hormonal replacement, especially with testosterone, methyltestosterone, or human chorionic gonadotropin (HCG) for primary hypogonadism, and with HCG for secondary hypogonadism.

Fertility can't be restored after permanent testicular damage. However, eunuchism that results from hypothalamic-pituitary lesions can be corrected when administration of gonadotropins stimulates normal testicular function.

Special considerations

• Because patients with hypogonadism tend to have multiple associated physical problems, your care should be tailored to meet their specific needs.

• When caring for an adolescent boy with hypogonadism, make every possible effort to promote his self-confidence. If he feels sensitive about his underdeveloped body, provide access to a private bathroom.

• Explain hypogonadism to the boy's parents. Encourage them to express their concerns about their son's delayed development. Reassure them and the patient that effective treatment is available.

• Make sure the parents and the patient understand hormonal replacement therapy fully, including expected adverse reactions, such as acne and water retention.

HYPOPARATHYROIDISM

A deficiency of parathyroid hormone (PTH), hypoparathyroidism is caused by disease, injury, or congenital malfunction of the parathyroid glands. Since the parathyroid glands primarily regulate calcium balance, hypoparathyroidism causes hypocalcemia, producing neuromuscular symptoms ranging from paresthesia to tetany.

The clinical effects of hypoparathyroidism are usually correctable with replacement therapy. However, some complications of long-term hypocalcemia, such as cataracts and basal ganglion calcifications, are irreversible.

Causes

Hypoparathyroidism may be acute or chronic and is classified as idiopathic or acquired, as follows:

• Idiopathic hypoparathyroidism may result from an autoimmune genetic disorder or the congenital absence of the parathyroid glands.

• Acquired hypoparathyroidism often results from accidental removal of or injury to one or more parathyroid glands during thyroidectomy or other neck surgery or, rarely, from massive thyroid irradiation. It may also result from ischemic infarction of the parathyroids during surgery, or from hemochromatosis, sarcoidosis, amyloidosis, tuberculosis, neoplasms, or trauma.

• Acquired, reversible hypoparathyroidism may result from hypomagnesemia-induced impairment of hormone synthesis, from suppression of normal gland function due to hypercalcemia, or from delayed maturation of parathyroid function.

PTH is not regulated by the pituitary or hypothalamus. It normally maintains blood calcium levels by increasing bone resorption and GI absorption of calcium. It also maintains an inverse relationship between serum calcium and phosphate levels by inhibiting phosphate reabsorption in the renal tubules.

Abnormal PTH production disrupts this balance. Incidence of the idiopathic and reversible forms is highest in children; that of the irreversible acquired form, in older patients who have undergone surgery for hyperthyroidism or other head and neck conditions.

Signs and symptoms

Although mild hypoparathyroidism may be asymptomatic, it usually produces hypocalcemia and high serum phosphate levels that affect the central nervous system (CNS) as well as other body systems.

Chronic hypoparathyroidism

In the chronic form, the disease typically causes neuromuscular irritability, increased deep tendon reflexes, Chvostek's sign (hyperirritability of the facial nerve, producing a characteristic spasm when it's tapped), dysphagia, organic brain syndrome, psychosis, mental deficiency in children, and tetany.

Chronic tetany is usually unilateral; it may cause difficulty in walking and a tendency to fall. It can lead to laryngospasm, stridor, and, eventually, cyanosis, and seizures.

Acute hypoparathyroidism

More severe than chronic tetany, acute (overt) tetany begins with a tingling in the fingertips, around the mouth, and, occasionally, in the feet. This tingling spreads and becomes more severe, producing muscle tension and spasms and consequent adduction of the thumbs, wrists, and elbows. Pain varies with the degree of muscle tension but rarely affects the face, legs, and feet.

Like chronic tetany, acute tetany may cause laryngospasm, stridor, cyanosis, and seizures.

These CNS abnormalities tend to be exaggerated during hyperventilation, pregnancy, infection, withdrawal of thyroid hormone, and administration of diuretics and before menstruation.

Other clinical effects include abdominal pain; dry, lusterless hair; spontaneous hair loss; brittle fingernails that develop ridges or fall out; dry, scaly skin; cataracts; and weakened tooth enamel, which causes teeth to stain, crack, and decay easily.

Hypocalcemia may induce cardiac arrhythmias and may eventually lead to congestive heart failure.

Diagnosis

The following test results confirm the diagnosis of hypoparathyroidism:

• *radioimmunoassay for parathyroid hormone:* decreased PTH concentration
• *serum calcium:* decreased level
• *serum phosphorus:* increased level
• *Electrocardiogram (ECG):* prolonged QT and ST intervals due to hypocalcemia.

The following test helps provoke clinical evidence of hypoparathyroidism: Inflating a blood pressure cuff on the upper arm to between diastolic and systolic blood pressure and maintaining this inflation for 3 minutes elicits Trousseau's sign (carpal spasm).

Treatment

Because calcium absorption from the small intestine requires the presence of vitamin D, treatment includes vitamin D and calcium supplements. Such therapy is usually lifelong, except for the reversible form of the disease.

If the patient can't tolerate the pure form of vitamin D, alternatives include dihydrotachysterol, if hepatic and renal function are adequate, and calcitriol, if they are severely compromised.

Acute, life-threatening tetany requires immediate I.V. administration of 10% calcium gluconate to raise serum calcium levels. The patient who's awake and able to cooperate can help raise serum calcium levels by breathing into a paper bag and then inhaling his own carbon dioxide; this produces hypoventilation and mild respiratory acidosis.

Sedatives and anticonvulsants may control spasms until calcium levels rise. Chronic tetany requires maintenance therapy with oral calcium and vitamin

D supplements. (See *Discharge instructions in hypoparathyroidism.*)

Special considerations

• While awaiting the diagnosis of hypoparathyroidism in a patient with a history of tetany, maintain a patent I.V. line and keep calcium I.V. available. Because the patient is vulnerable to convulsions, maintain seizure precautions.

• Keep a tracheotomy tray and endotracheal tube at bedside because laryngospasm may result from hypocalcemia.

• For the patient with tetany, administer 10% calcium gluconate slow I.V. (1 mg/minute), and maintain a patent airway. Such a patient may also require intubation, and sedation with diazepam I.V.

• Monitor vital signs often after administration of diazepam I.V. to make certain blood pressure and heart rate return to normal.

• When caring for the patient with chronic disease, particularly a child, stay alert for minor muscle twitching (especially in the hands) and for signs of laryngospasm (respiratory stridor or dysphagia) because these effects may signal onset of tetany.

• Because the patient with chronic disease has prolonged QT intervals on an

ECG, watch for heart block and signs of decreasing cardiac output.

• Closely monitor the patient receiving both digitalis glycosides and calcium because calcium potentiates the effect of digitalis glycosides. Stay alert for signs of digitalis toxicity (arrhythmias, nausea, fatigue, visual changes).

• Do careful patient teaching.

Idiopathic Thrombocytopenic Purpura

Idiopathic thrombocytopenic purpura (ITP), thrombocytopenia that results from immunologic platelet destruction, may be acute (postviral thrombocytopenia) or chronic (Werlhof's disease, purpura hemorrhagica, essential thrombocytopenia, autoimmune thrombocytopenia). Acute ITP usually affects children between ages 2 and 6; chronic ITP mainly affects adults under age 50, especially women between ages 20 and 40.

The prognosis for acute ITP is excellent; nearly four out of five patients recover without treatment. The prognosis for chronic ITP is good; remissions lasting weeks or years are common, especially among women.

Causes

ITP may be an autoimmune disorder, since antibodies that reduce the life span of platelets have been found in nearly all patients. The spleen probably helps to remove platelets modified by the antibody. Acute ITP usually follows a viral infection, such as rubella or chickenpox, and can follow immunization with a live virus vaccine. Chronic ITP rarely follows infection and is often linked to immunologic disorders, such as systemic lupus erythematosus. It's also linked to drug reactions.

Signs and symptoms

Clinical features of ITP common to all forms of thrombocytopenia include petechiae, ecchymoses, and mucosal bleeding from the mouth, nose, or GI tract. Generally, hemorrhage is a rare physical finding. Purpuric lesions may occur in vital organs, such as the lungs, kidneys, or brain, and may prove fatal.

In acute ITP, which commonly occurs in children, onset is usually sudden and without warning, causing easy bruising, epistaxis, and bleeding gums. Onset of chronic ITP is insidious.

Diagnosis

Platelet count less than 20,000/µl and prolonged bleeding time suggest ITP. Platelet size and morphologic appearance may be abnormal; anemia may be present if bleeding has occurred.

As in thrombocytopenia, bone marrow studies show an abundance of megakaryocytes and a shortened circulating platelet survival time (hours or days). Occasionally, platelet antibodies may be found in vitro, but this diagnosis is usually inferred from platelet survival data and the absence of an underlying disease.

Treatment

Acute ITP may be allowed to run its course without intervention or may be treated with glucorticoids or immune globulin. For chronic ITP, corticosteroids may be the initial treatment of choice. Patients who fail to respond within 1 or 4 months or who need high steroid dosage are candidates for splenectomy, which may be successful in 85%. Alternative treatments include immunosuppression, high-dose I.V. gamma globulin, and immunoabsorption apheresis using staphylococcal protein-A columns.

Before splenectomy, the patient may require blood, blood components, and vitamin K to correct anemia and coagulation defects. After splenectomy, he may need blood and component replacement and platelet concentrate. Normally, platelets increase spontaneously after splenectomy.

Special considerations

• Patient care for ITP is essentially the same as for other types of thrombocytopenia, with emphasis on teaching the patient to observe for petechiae, ecchymoses, and other signs of recurrence.

• Monitor patients receiving immunosuppressives for signs of bone marrow depression, infection, mucositis, GI ulcers, and severe diarrhea or vomiting.

• Tell the patient to avoid aspirin and ibuprofen.

IgA DEFICIENCY, SELECTIVE

Selective deficiency of immunoglobulin A (IgA), also known as Janeway Type 3 dysgammaglobulinemia, is the most common immunoglobulin deficiency, appearing in as many as 1 in 800 persons. IgA—the major immunoglobulin in human saliva, nasal and bronchial fluids, and intestinal secretions—guards against bacterial and viral reinfections. Consequently, IgA deficiency leads to chronic sinopulmonary infections, GI diseases, and other disorders.

The prognosis is good for patients who receive correct treatment, especially if they're free of associated disorders. Such patients have been known to survive to age 70.

Causes

IgA deficiency seems to be linked to autosomal dominant or recessive inheritance. The presence of normal numbers of peripheral blood lymphocytes carrying IgA receptors and of normal amounts of other immunoglobulins suggests that B cells may not be secreting IgA. In an occasional patient, suppressor T cells appear to inhibit IgA.

IgA deficiency also seems related to autoimmune disorders because many patients with rheumatoid arthritis or systemic lupus erythematosus (SLE) are also IgA deficient. Some drugs, such as anticonvulsants, may cause transient IgA deficiency.

Signs and symptoms

Some IgA-deficient patients have no symptoms, possibly because they have extra amounts of low-molecular-weight IgM, which takes over IgA function and helps maintain immunologic defenses. Among patients who do develop symptoms, chronic sinopulmonary infection is most common.

Other effects are respiratory allergy, often triggered by infection; GI tract diseases, such as celiac disease, ulcerative colitis, and regional enteritis; autoimmune diseases, such as rheumatoid arthritis, SLE, immunohemolytic anemia, and chronic hepatitis; and malignant tumors, such as squamous cell carcinoma of the lungs, reticulum cell sarcoma, and thymoma.

The age of onset varies. Some IgA-deficient children with recurrent respiratory disease and middle-ear inflammation may begin to synthesize

IgA spontaneously as recurrent infections subside and their condition improves.

Diagnosis
Immunologic analyses of IgA-deficient patients show serum IgA levels below 5 mg/dl. While IgA is usually absent from secretions in IgA-deficient patients, levels may be normal in rare cases. The IgE level is normal, while the IgM level may be normal or elevated in serum and secretions. Normally absent low-molecular-weight IgM may be present.

Tests may also indicate autoantibodies and antibodies against IgG (rheumatoid factor), IgM, and bovine milk. Cell-mediated immunity and secretory piece (the glycopeptide that transports IgA) are usually normal, and most circulating B cells appear normal.

Treatment
Selective IgA deficiency has no known cure. Treatment aims to control symptoms of associated diseases, such as respiratory and GI infections. *Don't* give an IgA-deficient patient immune globulin because sensitization may lead to anaphylaxis during future administration of blood products.

Special considerations
• If transfusion with blood products is necessary, minimize the risk of adverse reaction by using washed red blood cells or avoid the reaction completely by crossmatching the patient's blood with that of an IgA-deficient donor.
• Because this is a lifelong disorder, teach the patient to prevent infection, to recognize its early signs, and to seek treatment promptly.

IMPETIGO

A contagious, superficial skin infection, impetigo (also known as impetigo contagiosa) occurs in nonbullous and bullous forms. This vesiculopustular eruptive disorder spreads most easily among infants, young children, and elderly people.

Predisposing factors such as poor hygiene, anemia, malnutrition, and a warm climate favor outbreaks of this infection, most of which occur during the late summer and early fall. Impetigo can complicate chickenpox, eczema, or other skin conditions marked by open lesions.

Causes
Coagulase-positive *Staphylococcus aureus* and, less commonly, group A beta-hemolytic streptococci usually produce nonbullous impetigo; *S. aureus* (especially of phage type 71) generally causes bullous impetigo.

Signs and symptoms
Common nonbullous impetigo typically begins with a small red macule that turns into a vesicle, becoming pustular with a honey-colored crust within hours. When the vesicle breaks, a thick yellow crust forms from the exudate. Autoinoculation may cause satellite lesions. Other features include pruritus, burning, and regional lymphadenopathy.

A rare but serious complication of streptococcal impetigo is glomerulonephritis. Infants and young children may develop aural impetigo or otitis externa; the lesions usually clear without treatment in 2 to 3 weeks, unless an underlying disorder, such as eczema, is present.

In *bullous impetigo,* a thin-walled vesicle opens, and a thin, clear crust forms from the exudate. The lesion consists of a central clearing, circumscribed by an outer rim — much like a ringworm lesion — and commonly appears on the face or other exposed areas. Both forms usually produce painless itching; they may appear simultaneously and be clinically indistinguishable.

Diagnosis

Characteristic lesions suggest impetigo (see *Viewing impetigo vesicles*). Microscopic visualization of the causative organism in a Gram stain of vesicle fluid usually confirms *S. aureus* infection and justifies antibiotic therapy.

Culture and sensitivity testing of fluid or denuded skin may indicate the most appropriate antibiotic, but therapy shouldn't be delayed for laboratory results, which can take 3 days. The white blood cell count may be elevated if an infection is present.

Treatment

Generally, treatment consists of the administration of systemic antibiotics (usually a pencillinase-resistant penicillin, cephalosporin, or erythromycin) for 10 days. A topical antibiotic, such as mupirocin ointment, may be used for minor infections.

Therapy also includes removal of the exudate by washing the lesions two or three times a day with soap and water or, for stubborn crusts, warm soaks or compresses of normal saline or a diluted soap solution.

Special considerations

• Urge the patient not to scratch because this spreads impetigo. Advise parents to cut the child's fingernails.
• Give medications as necessary; remember to check for penicillin allergy. Stress the need to continue prescribed medications for 7 to 10 days, even after the lesions have healed.

VIEWING IMPETIGO VESICLES

In impetigo, when the vesicles break, crust forms from the exudate. This infection is especially contagious among young children.

• Teach the patient or his family how to care for impetiginous lesions. To prevent further spread of this highly contagious infection, encourage frequent bathing using a bactericidal soap.
• Tell the patient not to share towels, washcloths, or bed linens with family members. Emphasize the importance of following proper hand-washing technique.
• Check family members for impetigo. If this infection is present in a schoolchild, notify his school.

INACTIVE COLON

Also known as lazy colon, colonic stasis, and atonic constipation, inactive colon is a state of chronic constipation that, if untreated, may lead to fecal impaction. It's common in elderly persons and invalids because of their inactivity and is often relieved with diet and exercise.

Causes

Inactive colon usually results from some deficiency in the three elements necessary for normal bowel activity: dietary bulk, fluid intake, and exercise. Other possible causes can include habitual disregard of the impulse to defecate, emotional conflicts, chronic use of laxatives, or prolonged dependence on enemas, which dull rectal sensitivity to the presence of feces.

Signs and symptoms

The primary symptom of inactive colon is chronic constipation. The patient often strains to produce dry, hard stools accompanied by mild abdominal discomfort. Straining can aggravate other rectal conditions such as hemorrhoids.

Diagnosis

A patient history of dry, hard stools and infrequent bowel movements suggests inactive colon. A digital rectal examination reveals stools in the lower portion of the rectum and a palpable colon. Proctoscopy may show an unusually small colon lumen, prominent veins, and an abnormal amount of mucus. Diagnostic tests to rule out other causes include an upper GI series, barium enema, and examination of stools for occult blood from neoplasms.

Treatment

Effective treatment varies with the patient's age and condition. A higher bulk diet, sufficient exercise, and increased fluid intake often relieve constipation. (See *Breaking the constipation habit.*)

Treatment for severe constipation may include bulk-forming laxatives, such as psyllium, or well-lubricated glycerin suppositories; for fecal impaction, manual removal of feces is necessary. Administration of an oil-

retention enema usually precedes feces removal; an enema is also necessary afterward. For lasting relief of constipation, the patient with inactive colon must modify his bowel habits.

Special considerations

• Autosuggestion, relaxation, and use of a small footstool to promote thigh flexion while sitting on the toilet may be helpful. To help the patient relax, suggest that he bring pleasant reading material.

• Tell the patient to respond promptly to the urge to defecate. If he worries about constipation, assure him that a 2- to 3-day interval between bowel movements can be normal.

• Advise the patient to take bulk-forming laxatives, such as psyllium, with at least 8 oz (240 ml) of liquid. Juices, soft drinks, or other pleasant-tasting liquids help mask this drug's grittiness.

If the patient with inactive colon is hospitalized:

• Assist the elderly patient with inactive colon to a bedside commode for a bowel movement, since using a bedpan causes additional strain.

Caution: If the patient has a history of arteriosclerosis, congestive heart failure, or hypertension, constipation and straining may induce a "bathroom coronary" or a cerebrovascular accident.

• If the patient must use a bedpan, have him sit in Fowler's position, or on the pan at the side of his bed, to facilitate elimination.

• Occasional digital rectal stimulation or abdominal massage near the sigmoid area may help stimulate a bowel movement.

• If the patient requires enemas, avoid using a sodium biphosphate enema too often. Its hypertonic solution can absorb as much as 10% of the colon's sodium content or draw intestinal fluids into the colon, causing dehydration.

TEACHING CHECKLIST

BREAKING THE CONSTIPATION HABIT

Patient education can often help break the constipation habit. Advise the patient to follow these guidelines:
• Drink at least eight to ten glasses (at least 2 qt [2 L]) of liquid every day because fluids help keep the intestinal contents in a semisolid state for easier passage. This is particularly important for an older patient.
• Stimulate the bowel with a drink of hot coffee, warm lemonade, iced liquids — plain or with lemon — or prune juice before breakfast or in the evening.
• Add fiber to the diet with foods such as whole-grain cereals (rolled oats, bran, shredded wheat, brown rice, whole-wheat bread, oatmeal) to contribute bulk and induce peristalsis. However, too much bran can create an irritable bowel, so check labels on foods for fiber content (low fiber — 0.3 to 1 g; moderate fiber — 1.1 to 2 g; high fiber — 2.1 to 4.2 g).
• Increase the bulk content of the diet

slowly to prevent flatulence, which is sometimes a transient effect of a high-bulk diet. Include fresh fruits, with skins, in the diet for additional bulk. Also include raw and coarse vegetables (broccoli, Brussels sprouts, cabbage, cauliflower, cucumbers, lettuce, and turnips).
• Consume fat-containing foods, such as bacon, butter, cream, and oil, in moderation; they will help to soften intestinal contents but sometimes cause diarrhea.
• Avoid highly refined foods, such as white rice, cream of wheat, farina, white bread, pie or cake, macaroni, spaghetti, noodles, candy, cookies, and ice cream.
• Rest at least 6 hours every night.
• Incorporate moderate exercise, such as walking, into the daily routine.
• Avoid overuse of laxatives, and maintain a regular time for bowel movements (usually after breakfast).

Also, don't use other types of enemas frequently.

INCLUSION CONJUNCTIVITIS

A fairly common disease, inclusion conjunctivitis (also called inclusion blennorrhea) is an acute ocular inflammation resulting from infection by *Chlamydia trachomatis.* Although inclusion conjunctivitis occasionally becomes chronic, the prognosis is generally good.

Causes
C. trachomatis is an obligate intracellular organism of the lymphogranuloma venereum serotype group. It usually infects the urethra in males and the cervix in females and is transmitted during sexual activity.

Because contaminated cervical secretions infect the eyes of the neonate during birth, inclusion conjunctivitis is an important cause of ophthalmia neonatorum. Rarely, inclusion conjunctivitis results from autoinfection, by hand-to-eye transfer of the virus from the genitourinary tract.

Signs and symptoms

Inclusion conjunctivitis develops 5 to 10 days after contamination (it takes longer to develop than gonococcal ophthalmia). In a neonate, the lower eyelids redden and a thick, purulent discharge develops. In children and adults, follicles appear inside the lower eyelids; such follicles don't form in infants because the lymphoid tissue isn't yet well developed. Children and adults also develop preauricular lymphadenopathy and, as a complication, otitis media.

Inclusion conjunctivitis may persist for weeks or months, possibly with superficial corneal involvement. In neonates, pseudomembranes may form, which can lead to conjunctival scarring.

Diagnosis

Clinical features and a history of sexual contact with an infected individual suggest inclusion conjunctivitis. Examination of Giemsa-stained conjunctival scraping reveals cytoplasmic inclusion bodies in conjunctival epithelial cells, many polymorphonuclear leukocytes, and a negative culture for bacteria.

Treatment

Treatment consists of eyedrops of 1% tetracycline in oil, erythromycin ophthalmic ointment, or sulfonamide eyedrops 5 or 6 times daily for 2 weeks for infants, and oral tetracycline or erythromycin for 3 weeks for adults. In severe disease, adults may require concomitant systemic sulfonamide therapy.

Prophylactic tetracycline or erythromycin ointment is applied once, 1 hour after delivery.

Special considerations

• Keep the patient's eyes as clean as possible using aseptic technique. Clean the eyes from the inner to the outer canthus. Apply warm soaks as needed. Record the amount and color of drainage.

• Remind the patient not to rub his eyes, which can irritate them.

• If the patient's eyes are sensitive to light, keep the room dark or suggest that he wear dark glasses.

• To prevent further spread of inclusion conjunctivitis, wash your hands thoroughly before and after administering eye medications.

• Suggest a pelvic examination for the mother of an infected neonate or for any adult with inclusion conjunctivitis.

• Obtain a history of recent sexual contacts, so they can be examined for inclusion conjunctivitis.

INFERTILITY, FEMALE

Infertility affects approximately 10% to 15% of all couples in the United States. About 40% to 50% of all infertility is attributed to the female. (See also "Male Infertility," pages 469 and 470.) Following extensive investigation and treatment, approximately 50% of these infertile couples achieve pregnancy. Of the 50% who don't, 10% have no pathologic basis for infertility; the prognosis in this group becomes extremely poor if pregnancy isn't achieved after 3 years.

Causes

The causes of female infertility may be functional, anatomic, or psychological.

Functional causes

Complex hormonal interactions determine the normal function of the female reproductive tract and require an intact hypothalamic-pituitary-ovarian axis, a system that stimulates and regulates the production of hormones necessary for normal sexual development and function.

Any defect or malfunction of this system axis can cause infertility, due to insufficient gonadotropin secretions (both luteinizing hormone and follicle-stimulating hormone). The ovary controls, and is controlled by, the hypothalamus through a system of negative and positive feedback mediated by estrogen production. Insufficient gonadotropin levels may result from infections, tumors, or neurologic disease of the hypothalamus or pituitary gland. Hypothyroidism also impairs fertility.

Anatomic causes
The anatomic causes of female infertility include the following:
• *Ovarian factors* related to anovulation and oligoovulation (infrequent ovulation) are a major cause of infertility. Presumptive signs of ovulation include regular menses, cyclic changes reflected in basal body temperature readings, postovulatory progesterone levels, and endometrial changes due to the presence of progesterone. Absence of presumptive signs suggests anovulation.

Ovarian failure, in which no ova are produced by the ovaries, may result from ovarian dysgenesis or premature menopause. Amenorrhea is often associated with ovarian failure. Oligoovulation may be due to a mild hormonal imbalance in gonadotropin production and regulation and may be caused by polycystic disease of the ovary or abnormalities in the adrenal or thyroid gland that adversely affect hypothalamic-pituitary functioning.
• *Uterine abnormalities* may include a congenitally absent uterus, bicornuate or double uterus, leiomyomas, or Asherman's syndrome, in which the ante-

rior and posterior uterine walls adhere because of scar tissue formation.
• *Tubal and peritoneal factors* are due to faulty tubal transport mechanisms and unfavorable environmental influences affecting the sperm, ova, or recently fertilized ovum. Tubal loss or impairment may occur secondary to ectopic pregnancy.

Frequently, tubal and peritoneal factors result from anatomic abnormalities: bilateral occlusion of the tubes due to salpingitis (resulting from gonorrhea, tuberculosis, or puerperal sepsis), peritubal adhesions (resulting from endometriosis, pelvic inflammatory disease, use of an intrauterine device for contraception, diverticulosis, or childhood rupture of the appendix), and uterotubal obstruction due to tubal spasm.
• *Cervical factors* may include a malfunctioning cervix that produces deficient or excessively viscous mucus and is impervious to sperm, preventing entry into the uterus. In cervical infection, viscous mucus may contain spermicidal macrophages. The possible existence of cervical antibodies that immobilize sperm is also under investigation.

Psychological problems
Such problems probably account for relatively few cases of infertility. Occasionally, ovulation may stop because of stress, which results in failure of the body to release luteinizing hormone. Marital discord may affect the frequency of intercourse. More often, however, psychological problems result from, rather than cause, infertility.

Signs and symptoms
The inability to achieve pregnancy after having regular intercourse without contraception for at least 1 year suggests infertility.

Diagnosis

The diagnosis requires a complete physical examination and health history, including specific questions on the patient's reproductive and sexual function, past diseases, mental state, previous surgery, types of contraception used in the past, and family history. Irregular, painless menses may indicate anovulation. A history of pelvic inflammatory disease may suggest fallopian tube blockage.

Tests that assess ovulation

• *Basal body temperature graph* shows a sustained elevation in body temperature after ovulation until just before onset of menses, indicating the approximate time of ovulation.
• *Endometrial biopsy,* done on or about day 5 after the basal body temperature rises, provides histologic evidence that ovulation has occurred.
• *Progesterone blood levels,* measured when they should be highest, can show a luteal phase deficiency.

The following procedures assess structural integrity of the fallopian tubes, the ovaries, and the uterus:
• *Hysterosalpingography* provides radiologic evidence of tubal obstruction and abnormalities of the uterine cavity by injecting radiopaque contrast fluid through the cervix.
• *Endoscopy* confirms the results of hysterosalpingography and visualizes the endometrial cavity by hysteroscopy or explores the posterior surface of the uterus, fallopian tubes, and ovaries by culdoscopy. Laparoscopy allows visualization of the abdominal and pelvic areas.

Male-female interaction studies

• *Postcoital test (Sims-Huhner test)* examines the cervical mucus for motile sperm cells following intercourse that takes place at midcycle (as close to ovulation as possible).

• *Immunologic or antibody testing* detects spermicidal antibodies in the sera of the female. Further research is being conducted in this area.

Treatment

Effective treatment depends on identifying the underlying abnormality.

Functional infertility

In hyperactivity or hypoactivity of the adrenal or thyroid gland, hormone therapy is necessary; a progesterone deficiency requires progesterone replacement. Anovulation necessitates treatment with clomiphene, human menopausal gonadotropins, or human chorionic gonadotropin; ovulation usually occurs several days after such treatment.

If mucus production decreases (an adverse effect of clomiphene), small doses of estrogen to improve the quality of cervical mucus may be given concomitantly.

Anatomic infertility

Surgical restoration may correct certain anatomic causes of infertility such as fallopian tube obstruction. Surgery may also be necessary to remove tumors located in or near the hypothalamus or pituitary gland. Endometriosis requires drug therapy (danazol or medroxyprogesterone, or noncyclic administration of oral contraceptives), surgical removal of areas of endometriosis, or a combination of both.

Other options, often controversial and involving emotional and financial cost, include surrogate mothering, frozen embryos, or in-vitro fertilization.

Special considerations

• Management includes providing the infertile couple with emotional support and information about diagnostic and treatment techniques.
• Explain the procedures thoroughly.

• Encourage the patient and her partner to talk about their feelings, and listen to what they have to say with a nonjudgmental attitude.

• If the patient requires surgery, tell her what to expect postoperatively; this, of course, depends on which procedure is to be performed.

INFERTILITY, MALE

Male infertility may be suspected whenever a couple fails to achieve pregnancy after about 1 year of regular unprotected intercourse. Approximately 40% to 50% of infertility problems in the United States are totally or partially attributed to the male. (See also "Female Infertility," pages 466 to 469.)

Causes

Some of the factors that cause male infertility include:

• *varicocele,* a mass of dilated and tortuous varicose veins in the spermatic cord

• *semen disorders,* such as volume or motility disturbances or inadequate sperm density

• *proliferation of abnormal or immature sperm,* with variations in the size and shape of the head

• *systemic disease,* such as diabetes mellitus, neoplasms, hepatic and renal diseases, and viral disturbances, especially mumps orchitis

• *genital infection,* such as gonorrhea, tuberculosis, and herpes

• *disorders of the testes,* such as cryptorchidism, Sertoli-cell–only syndrome, varicocele, and ductal obstruction (caused by absence or ligation of the vas deferens or infection)

• *genetic defects,* such as Klinefelter's (chromosomal pattern XXY, eunuchoidal habitus, gynecomastia, small testes) or Reifenstein's syndrome (chromosomal pattern 46XY, reduced testosterone, azoospermia, eunuchoidism, gynecomastia, hypospadias)

• *immune disorders,* such as autoimmune infertility or allergic orchitis

• *endocrine imbalance* (rare) that disrupts pituitary gonadotropins, inhibiting spermatogenesis, testosterone production, or both; such imbalances occur in Kallmann's syndrome, panhypopituitarism, hypothyroidism, and congenital adrenal hyperplasia

• *chemicals* and *drugs* that can inhibit gonadotropins or interfere with spermatogenesis, such as arsenic, methotrexate, medroxyprogesterone acetate, nitrofurantoin, monoamine oxidase inhibitors, and some antihypertensives

• *sexual problems,* such as erectile dysfunction, ejaculatory incompetence, or low libido.

Other factors may include age, occupation, and trauma to the testes.

Signs and symptoms

The obvious indication of male infertility is failure to impregnate a fertile woman. Clinical features may include:

• atrophied testes

• empty scrotum

• scrotal edema

• varicocele or anteversion of the epididymis

• inflamed seminal vesicles

• beading or abnormal nodes on the spermatic cord and vas deferens

• penile nodes, warts, plaques, or hypospadias

• prostatic enlargement, nodules, swelling, or tenderness.

In addition, male infertility is often apt to induce troublesome negative emotions in a couple — anger, hurt, disgust, guilt, and loss of self-esteem.

Diagnosis

A detailed patient history may reveal abnormal sexual development, delayed puberty, infertility in previous relationships, and a medical history of prolonged fever, mumps, impaired nutritional status, previous surgery, or trauma to the genitalia.

After a thorough patient history and physical examination, the most conclusive test for male infertility is semen analysis. Other laboratory tests include gonadotropin assay to determine the integrity of the pituitary gonadal axis, serum testosterone levels to determine organ response to leuteinizing hormone (LH), urine 17-ketosteroid levels to measure testicular function, and a testicular biopsy to help clarify unexplained oligospermia and azoospermia. Vasography and seminal vesiculography may be necessary.

Treatment

When anatomic dysfunctions or infections cause infertility, treatment consists of correcting the underlying problem. Avaricocele requires surgical repair or removal.

For patients with sexual dysfunctions, treatment includes education, counseling or therapy (on sexual techniques, coital frequency, and reproductive physiology), and proper nutrition with vitamin supplements.

Decreased follicle-stimulating hormone levels may respond to vitamin B therapy; decreased LH levels, to chorionic gonadotropin therapy. A normal or elevated LH level requires low dosages of testosterone. Decreased testosterone levels, decreased semen motility, and volume disturbances may respond to chorionic gonadotropin.

Patients with oligospermia who have a normal history and physical examination, normal hormonal assays, and no signs of systemic disease require emotional support and counseling, adequate nutrition, multivitamins, and selective therapeutic agents, such as clomiphene, chorionic gonadotropin, and low dosages of testosterone. Obvious alternatives to such treatment are adoption and artificial insemination.

Special considerations

• Educate the couple, as necessary, regarding reproductive and sexual functions and about factors that may interfere with fertility, such as the use of lubricants and douches.
• Urge men with oligospermia to avoid habits that may interfere with normal spermatogenesis by elevating scrotal temperature, such as wearing tight underwear and athletic supporters, taking hot tub baths, or habitually riding a bicycle. Explain that cool scrotal temperatures are essential for adequate spermatogenesis.
• When possible, advise infertile couples to join group programs to share their feelings and concerns with other couples who have the same problem.
• Help prevent male infertility by encouraging patients to have regular physical examinations, to protect their testicles during athletic activity, and to receive early treatment for venereal diseases and surgical correction for anatomic defects.

INFLUENZA

Also called the grippe or the flu, influenza is an acute, highly contagious infection of the respiratory tract that results from three different types of *Myxovirus influenzae*. It occurs sporadically or in epidemics (usually during the colder months). Epidemics tend to peak within 2 to 3 weeks after initial cases and subside within a month.

Although influenza affects all age-groups, its incidence is highest in schoolchildren. However, its severity is greatest in the very young, elderly people, and those with chronic diseases. In these groups, influenza may even lead to death. The catastrophic pandemic of 1918 was responsible for an estimated 20 million deaths. The most recent pandemics—in 1957, 1968, and 1977—began in mainland China.

Causes

Transmission of influenza occurs through inhalation of a respiratory droplet from an infected person or by indirect contact, such as the use of a contaminated drinking glass. The influenza virus then invades the epithelium of the respiratory tract, causing inflammation and desquamation.

One of the remarkable features of the influenza virus is its capacity for antigenic variation. Such variation leads to infection by strains of the virus to which little or no immunologic resistance is present in the population at risk. Antigenic variation is characterized as *antigenic drift* (minor changes that occur yearly or every few years) and *antigenic shift* (major changes that lead to pandemics). Influenza viruses are classified into three groups:

• Type A, the most prevalent, strikes every year, with new serotypes causing epidemics every 3 years.

• Type B also strikes annually, but only causes epidemics every 4 to 6 years.

• Type C is endemic and causes only sporadic cases.

Signs and symptoms

Following an incubation period of 24 to 48 hours, flu symptoms begin to appear: the sudden onset of chills, a temperature of 101° to 104° F (38.3° to 40° C), headache, malaise, myalgia (particularly in the back and limbs), a nonproductive cough and, occasionally, laryngitis, hoarseness, conjunctivitis, rhinitis, and rhinorrhea.

These symptoms usually subside in 3 to 5 days, but cough and weakness may persist. Fever is usually higher in children than in adults. Also, cervical adenopathy and croup are likely to be associated with influenza in children. In some patients (especially elderly ones), lack of energy and easy fatigability may persist for several weeks.

Complications

Fever that persists longer than 3 to 5 days signals the onset of complications. The most common complication is pneumonia, which can be primary influenza viral pneumonia or secondary to bacterial infection. Influenza may also cause myositis, exacerbation of chronic obstructive pulmonary disease (COPD), Reye's syndrome and, rarely, myocarditis, pericarditis, transverse myelitis, and encephalitis.

Diagnosis

At the beginning of an influenza epidemic, early cases are usually mistaken for other respiratory disorders. Because signs and symptoms are not pathognomonic, isolation of *M. influenzae* through the inoculation of chicken embryos (with nasal secretions from infected patients) is essential at the first sign of an epidemic. In addition, nose and throat cultures and increased serum antibody titers help confirm this diagnosis.

After these measures confirm an influenza epidemic, diagnosis requires only observation of clinical signs and symptoms. Uncomplicated cases show a decreased white blood cell count with an increase in lymphocytes.

Treatment

Uncomplicated influenza is treated with bed rest, adequate fluid intake, aspirin or acetaminophen (in children) to relieve fever and muscle pain, and guaifenesin or another expectorant to relieve nonproductive coughing. Prophylactic antibiotics are not recommended because they have no effect on the influenza virus.

Amantadine (an antiviral agent) has proven to be effective in reducing the duration of signs and symptoms in influenza A infection. In influenza complicated by pneumonia, supportive care (fluid and electrolyte supplements, oxygen, assisted ventilation) and treatment of bacterial superinfection with appropriate antibiotics are necessary. No specific therapy exists for cardiac, central nervous system, or other complications.

Special considerations

• Advise the patient to use mouthwashes and increase his fluid intake. Warm baths or heating pads may relieve myalgia. Give him nonnarcotic analgesics and antipyretics as needed.

• Screen visitors to protect the patient from bacterial infection and the visitor from influenza. Use respiratory precautions.

• Teach the patient proper disposal of tissues and proper hand-washing technique to prevent the virus from spreading.

• Watch for signs and symptoms of developing pneumonia, such as crackles, another temperature rise, or coughing accompanied by purulent or bloody sputum. Assist the patient in a gradual return to his normal activities.

Educate patients about influenza immunizations. For high-risk patients and health care personnel, suggest annual inoculations at the start of the flu season (late autumn). Remember, however, that such vaccines are made from chicken embryos and must not be given to people who are hypersensitive to eggs, feathers, or chickens. The vaccine administered is based on the previous year's virus and is usually about 75% effective.

All people receiving the vaccine should be made aware of possible adverse effects (discomfort at the vacci-

nation site, fever, malaise and, rarely, Guillain-Barré syndrome). Although the vaccine has not been proven harmful to the fetus, it's not recommended for pregnant women, except those who are highly susceptible to influenza, such as those with chronic diseases. For people who are hypersensitive to eggs, amantadine is an effective alternative to the vaccine.

INGUINAL HERNIA

A hernia occurs when part of an internal organ protrudes through an abnormal opening in the containing wall of its cavity. Most hernias occur in the abdominal cavity. Although many kinds of abdominal hernias are possible, inguinal hernias are most common.

In an inguinal hernia, the large or small intestine, omentum, or bladder protrudes into the inguinal canal. Hernias can be reducible (if the hernia can be manipulated back into place with relative ease), incarcerated (if the hernia can't be reduced because adhesions have formed in the hernial sac), or strangulated (part of the herniated intestine becomes twisted or edematous, seriously interfering with normal blood flow and peristalsis, and possibly leading to intestinal obstruction and necrosis).

Causes

In males, during the seventh month of gestation, the testicle normally descends into the scrotum, preceded by the peritoneal sac. If the sac closes improperly, it leaves an opening through which the intestine can slip. In either sex, a hernia can result from weak abdominal muscles (caused by congenital malformation, trauma, or aging) or increased intra-abdominal pressure (due to heavy lifting, pregnancy, obesity, or straining). An inguinal hernia may be indirect or direct.

Indirect inguinal hernia

The more common form, an indirect inguinal hernia results from weakness in the fascial margin of the internal inguinal ring. An indirect inguinal hernia may develop at any age, is three times more common in males, and is especially prevalent in infants under age 1.

In an indirect hernia, abdominal viscera leave the abdomen through the inguinal ring and follow the spermatic cord (in males) or round ligament (in females); they emerge at the external ring and extend down the inguinal canal, often into the scrotum or labia.

Direct inguinal hernia

A direct inguinal hernia results from a weakness in the fascial floor of the inguinal canal. Instead of entering the canal through the internal ring, the hernia passes through the posterior inguinal wall, protrudes directly through the fascia transversalis of the canal (in an area known as Hesselbach's triangle), and comes out at the external ring.

Signs and symptoms

Inguinal hernia usually causes a lump to appear over the herniated area when the patient stands or strains. The lump disappears when the patient is supine. Tension on the herniated contents may cause a sharp, steady pain in the groin, which fades when the hernia is reduced.

Strangulation produces severe pain, and may lead to partial or complete bowel obstruction and even intestinal necrosis. Partial bowel obstruction may cause anorexia, vomiting, pain and tenderness in the groin, an irreducible mass, and diminished bowel sounds.

Complete obstruction may cause shock, high fever, absent bowel sounds, and bloody stools. In an infant, an inguinal hernia often coexists with an undescended testicle or a hydrocele.

Diagnosis

In a patient with a large hernia, physical examination reveals an obvious swelling or lump in the inguinal area. In the patient with a small hernia, the affected area may simply appear full. Palpation of the inguinal area while the patient is performing Valsalva's maneuver confirms the diagnosis.

To detect a hernia in a male patient, the patient is asked to stand with his ipsilateral leg slightly flexed and his weight resting on the other leg. The examiner inserts an index finger into the lower part of the scrotum and invaginates the scrotal skin so the finger advances through the external inguinal ring to the internal ring (about 1½″ to 2″ [4 to 5 cm] through the inguinal canal). The patient is then told to cough. If the examiner feels pressure against the fingertip, an indirect hernia exists; if pressure is felt against the side of the finger, a direct hernia exists.

A patient history of sharp or "catching" pain when lifting or straining may help confirm the diagnosis. A suspected bowel obstruction requires X-rays and a white blood cell count (which may be elevated).

Treatment

If the hernia is reducible, the pain may be temporarily relieved by pushing the hernia back into place. A truss may keep the abdominal contents from protruding into the hernial sac, although it won't cure the hernia. This device is especially beneficial for an elderly or debilitated patient, since any surgery is potentially hazardous to him.

Herniorrhaphy

For infants, adults, and otherwise healthy elderly patients, herniorrhaphy is the treatment of choice. Herniorrhaphy replaces the contents of the hernial sac into the abdominal cavity and closes the opening. This procedure is often performed under local anesthestic in a short-term unit, or as a single-day admission. Another effective surgical procedure for repairing hernia is hernioplasty, which reinforces the weakened area with steel mesh, fascia, or wire.

Bowel resection

A strangulated or necrotic hernia necessitates bowel resection. Rarely, an extensive resection may require temporary colostomy. In either case, bowel resection lengthens postoperative recovery and requires massive doses of antibiotics, parenteral fluids, and electrolyte replacements.

Special considerations

• Apply a truss only after a hernia has been reduced. For best results, apply it in the morning, before the patient gets out of bed.
• To prevent skin irritation, tell the patient to bathe daily and apply liberal amounts of cornstarch or baby powder. Warn against applying the truss over clothing, since this reduces the effectiveness of the truss and may make it slip.
• Watch for signs of incarceration and strangulation. Don't try to reduce an incarcerated hernia because this may perforate the bowel. If severe intestinal obstruction arises because of hernial strangulation, a nasogastric tube may be inserted promptly to empty the stomach and relieve pressure on the hernial sac.
• Before surgery, closely monitor vital signs. Administer I.V. fluids and analgesics for pain as needed. Control fever with acetaminophen or tepid

sponge baths as necessary. Place the patient in Trendelenburg's position to reduce pressure on the hernia site.
• Give special reassurance and support to a child scheduled for hernia repair. Encourage him to ask questions, and answer them as simply as possible. Offer appropriate diversions to distract him from the impending surgery.
• After surgery, make sure the patient voids within 8 to 12 hours. Check the incision and dressing at least three times a day for drainage, inflammation, or swelling. Check for normal bowel sounds and watch for fever.
• Observe carefully for postoperative scrotal swelling. To reduce such swelling, support the scrotum with a rolled towel and apply an ice bag.
• Encourage fluid intake to maintain hydration and prevent constipation. Teach deep-breathing exercises, and show the patient how to splint the incision before coughing.
• Before discharge, warn the patient against lifting or straining. In addition, tell him to watch for signs of infection (oozing, tenderness, warmth, redness) at the incision site, and to keep the incision clean and covered until the sutures are removed.

LIFE-THREATENING DISORDER

INTESTINAL OBSTRUCTION

An intestinal obstruction is a partial or complete blockage of the lumen in the small or large bowel. A small-bowel obstruction is far more common (90% of patients) and usually more serious. A complete obstruction in any part of the bowel, if untreated, can cause death within hours from shock and vascular

Paralytic (Adynamic) Ileus

Paralytic ileus is a physiologic form of intestinal obstruction that may develop in the small bowel after abdominal surgery. It causes decreased or absent intestinal motility that usually disappears spontaneously after 2 to 3 days.

Causes

This condition can develop as a response to trauma, toxemia, or peritonitis, or as a result of electrolyte deficiencies (especially hypokalemia) and the use of certain drugs, such as ganglionic blocking agents and anticholinergics. It can also result from vascular causes, such as thrombosis or embolism. Excessive air swallowing may contribute to it, but paralytic ileus brought on by this factor alone seldom lasts more than 24 hours.

Signs and symptoms

Clinical effects of paralytic ileus include severe abdominal distention, extreme distress, and possibly, vomiting. The patient may be severely constipated or may pass flatus and small, liquid stools.

Treatment

Paralytic ileus lasting longer than 48 hours necessitates intubation for decompression and nasogastric suctioning. Because of the absence of peristaltic activity, a weighted Cantor tube may be necessary in the patient with extraordinary abdominal distention. However, such procedures must be used with extreme caution, because any additional trauma to the bowel can aggravate ileus.

When paralytic ileus results from surgical manipulation of the bowel, treatment may also include cholinergic agents, such as neostigmine or bethanechol.

Special considerations

When caring for patients with paralytic ileus, warn those receiving cholinergic agents to expect certain paradoxical side effects, such as intestinal cramps and diarrhea. Remember that neostigmine produces cardiovascular side effects, usually bradycardia and hypotension. Check frequently for returning bowel sounds.

---

collapse. Intestinal obstructions are most likely to occur after abdominal surgery or in people with congenital bowel deformities.

Causes

Adhesions and strangulated hernias usually cause small-bowel obstructions; carcinomas usually cause large-bowel obstructions. A mechanical intestinal obstruction results from foreign bodies (fruit pits, gallstones, worms) or compression of the bowel wall due to stenosis, intussusception, volvulus of the sigmoid or cecum, tumors, or atresia.

A nonmechanical obstruction results from physiologic disturbances, such as paralytic ileus (see *Paralytic [adynamic] ileus*), electrolyte imbalances, toxicity (uremia, generalized infection), neurogenic abnormalities (spinal cord lesions), and thrombosis or embolism of mesenteric vessels.

The three forms of intestinal obstruction are:
• *simple:* blockage prevents intestinal contents from passing, with no other complications
• *strangulated:* blood supply to part or all of the obstructed section is cut off, in addition to blockage of the lumen

• *close-looped:* both ends of a bowel section are occluded, isolating it from the rest of the intestine.

In all three forms, the physiologic effects are similar: When intestinal obstruction occurs, fluid, air, and gas collect near the site. Peristalsis increases temporarily as the bowel tries to force its contents through the obstruction, injuring intestinal mucosa and causing distention at and above the site of the obstruction. This distention blocks the flow of venous blood and halts normal absorptive processes. As a result, the bowel begins to secrete water, sodium, and potassium into the fluid pooled in the lumen.

An obstruction in the upper intestine results in metabolic alkalosis from dehydration and loss of gastric hydrochloric acid; a lower obstruction causes slower dehydration and loss of intestinal alkaline fluids, resulting in metabolic acidosis. Ultimately, an intestinal obstruction may lead to ischemia, necrosis, and death.

Signs and symptoms
Clinical features depend on the location and extent of the obstruction.

Partial small-bowel obstruction
Colicky pain, nausea, vomiting, constipation, and abdominal distention characterize small-bowel obstruction. It may also cause drowsiness, intense thirst, malaise, and aching, and may dry up oral mucous membranes and the tongue.

Auscultation reveals bowel sounds, borborygmi, and rushes; occasionally, these are loud enough to be heard without a stethoscope. Palpation elicits abdominal tenderness, with moderate distention; rebound tenderness occurs when the obstruction has caused strangulation with ischemia. In late stages, signs of hypovolemic shock result from progressive dehydration and plasma loss.

Complete small-bowel obstruction
In a complete upper intestinal (small-bowel) obstruction, vigorous peristaltic waves propel bowel contents toward the mouth instead of the rectum. Spasms may occur every 3 to 5 minutes and last about 1 minute each, with persistent epigastric or periumbilical pain. Passage of small amounts of mucus and blood may occur. The higher the obstruction, the earlier and more severe the vomiting. Vomitus initially contains gastric juice, then bile, and finally fecal contents of the ileum.

Partial large-bowel obstruction
Symptoms of large-bowel obstruction develop more slowly because the colon can absorb fluid from its contents and distend well beyond its normal size. Constipation may be the only clinical effect for days. Colicky abdominal pain may then appear suddenly, producing spasms that last less than 1 minute each and recur every few minutes. Continuous hypogastric pain and nausea may develop, but vomiting is usually absent at first.

Large-bowel obstruction can cause dramatic abdominal distention: Loops of large bowel may become visible on the abdomen.

Complete large-bowel obstruction
Eventually, a complete large-bowel obstruction may cause fecal vomiting, continuous pain, or localized peritonitis.

Patients with a partial obstruction may display any of the above symptoms in a milder form. However, leakage of liquid stools around the obstruction is common in partial obstruction.

Diagnosis
Progressive, colicky, abdominal pain and distention, with or without nausea and vomiting, suggest bowel obstruction; X-rays confirm it.

Abdominal films show the presence and location of intestinal gas or fluid. In small-bowel obstructions, a typical "stepladder" pattern emerges, with alternating fluid and gas levels apparent in 3 to 4 hours. In large-bowel obstructions, a barium enema reveals a distended, air-filled colon or a closed loop of sigmoid with extreme distention (in sigmoid volvulus).

Laboratory results supporting this diagnosis include:
• decreased sodium, chloride, and potassium levels (due to vomiting)
• slightly elevated white blood cell count (with necrosis, peritonitis, or strangulation)
• increased serum amylase level (possibly from irritation of the pancreas by a bowel loop).

Treatment

Preoperative therapy consists of correction of fluid and electrolyte imbalances, decompression of the bowel to relieve vomiting and distention, and treatment of shock and peritonitis. A strangulated obstruction usually necessitates blood replacement as well as I.V. fluid administration. Passage of a nasogastric (NG) tube, followed by use of the longer and weighted Miller-Abbott or Cantor tube, usually accomplishes decompression, especially in small-bowel obstruction.

Close monitoring of the patient's condition determines the duration of treatment; if the patient fails to improve or if his condition deteriorates, surgery is necessary. In large-bowel obstruction, surgical resection with anastomosis, colostomy, or ileostomy commonly follows decompression with an NG tube.

Total parenteral nutrition may be appropriate if the patient suffers a protein deficit from chronic obstruction, postoperative or paralytic ileus, or infection.

Drug therapy includes analgesics, sedatives, and antibiotics for peritonitis due to bowel strangulation or infarction.

Special considerations

• Effective management of intestinal obstruction, a life-threatening condition that often causes overwhelming pain and distress, requires skillful supportive care and keen observation.
• Monitor vital signs frequently. A drop in blood pressure may indicate reduced circulating blood volume due to blood loss from a strangulated hernia. Remember, as much as 10 L of fluid can collect in the small bowel, drastically reducing plasma volume. Observe the patient closely for signs of shock (pallor, rapid pulse, and hypotension).
• Stay alert for signs of metabolic alkalosis (changes in sensorium; slow, shallow respirations; hypertonic muscles; tetany) or acidosis (shortness of breath on exertion; disorientation; and, later, deep, rapid breathing, weakness, and malaise).
• Watch for signs and symptoms of secondary infection, such as fever and chills.
• Monitor urine output carefully to assess renal function, circulating blood volume, and possible urine retention caused by bladder compression by the distended intestine. If you suspect bladder compression, catheterize the patient for residual urine immediately after he has voided. Also, measure abdominal girth frequently to detect progressive distention.
• Provide fastidious mouth and nose care if the patient has vomited or undergone decompression by intubation. Look for signs of dehydration (thick, swollen tongue; dry, cracked lips; dry oral mucous membranes).
• Record the amount and color of drainage from the decompression tube. Irrigate the tube with normal saline

solution to maintain patency. If a weighted tube has been inserted, check periodically to make sure it's advancing. Help the patient turn from side to side (or walk around, if he can) to facilitate passage of the tube.

• Keep the patient in Fowler's position as much as possible to promote pulmonary ventilation and ease respiratory distress from abdominal distention. Listen for bowel sounds, and watch for signs of returning peristalsis (passage of flatus and mucus through the rectum).

• Explain all diagnostic and therapeutic procedures to the patient, and answer any questions he may have. Make sure he understands that these procedures are necessary to relieve the obstruction and reduce pain. Tell the patient to lie on his left side for about a half hour before X-rays are taken.

• Prepare the patient and his family for the possibility of surgery, and provide emotional support and positive reinforcement afterward. Arrange for an enterostomal therapist to visit the patient who has had an ostomy.

INTUSSUSCEPTION

In intussusception, a portion of the bowel telescopes (invaginates) into an adjacent distal portion. Intussusception may be fatal, especially if treatment is delayed more than 24 hours.

Causes

Intussusception is most common in infants and occurs three times more often in males than in females; 87% of children with intussusception are under age 2; 70% of these children are between ages 4 and 11 months.

Studies suggest that intussusception may be linked to viral infections because seasonal peaks are noted—in the late spring and early summer, coinciding with the peak incidence of enteritis, and in the midwinter, coinciding with the peak incidence of respiratory tract infections.

The cause of most cases of intussusception in infants is unknown. In older children, polyps, alterations in intestinal motility, hemangioma, lymphosarcoma, lymphoid hyperplasia, or Meckel's diverticulum may trigger the process. In adults, intussusception usually results from benign or malignant tumors (65% of patients). It may also result from polyps, Meckel's diverticulum, gastroenterostomy with herniation, or an appendiceal stump.

When a bowel segment (the intussusceptum) invaginates, peristalsis propels it along the bowel, pulling more bowel along with it; the receiving segment is the intussuscipiens. This invagination produces edema, hemorrhage from venous engorgement, incarceration, and obstruction. If treatment is delayed for longer than 24 hours, strangulation of the intestine usually occurs, with gangrene, shock, and perforation.

Signs and symptoms

In an infant or child, intussusception produces four cardinal clinical effects:

• intermittent attacks of colicky pain, which cause the child to scream, draw his legs up to his abdomen, turn pale and diaphoretic, and possibly, display grunting respirations

• initially, vomiting of stomach contents; later, vomiting of bile-stained or fecal material

• "currant jelly" stools, which contain a mixture of blood and mucus

• tender, distended abdomen, with a palpable, sausage-shaped abdominal mass; often, the viscera are absent from the right lower quadrant.

In adults, intussusception produces nonspecific, chronic, and intermittent symptoms, including colicky abdominal pain and tenderness, vomiting, diarrhea (occasionally constipation), bloody stools, and weight loss. Abdominal pain usually localizes in the right lower quadrant, radiates to the back, and increases with eating. Adults with severe intussusception may develop strangulation with excruciating pain, abdominal distention, and tachycardia.

Diagnosis

The following test results confirm intussusception:
• *Barium enema* confirms colonic intussusception when it shows the characteristic coiled spring sign; it also delineates the extent of intussusception.
• *Upright abdominal X-rays* may show a soft-tissue mass and signs of complete or partial obstruction, with dilated loops of bowel.
• *White blood cell count* up to 15,000/ μl indicates obstruction; more than 15,000/μl, strangulation; more than 20,000/μl, bowel infarction should be considered.

Treatment

In children, therapy may include hydrostatic reduction or surgery. Surgery is indicated for children with recurrent intussusception, for those who show signs of shock or peritonitis, and for those in whom symptoms have been present longer than 24 hours. In adults, surgery is always the treatment of choice.

Hydrostatic reduction

During hydrostatic reduction, the radiologist drips a barium solution into the rectum from a height of not more than 3' (0.9 m); fluoroscopy traces the progress of the barium. If the procedure is successful, the barium backwashes into the ileum, and the mass disappears. If not, the procedure is stopped, and the patient is prepared for surgery.

Surgery

During surgery, manual reduction is attempted first. After compressing the bowel above the intussusception, the doctor attempts to milk the intussusception back through the bowel. However, if manual reduction fails, or if the bowel is gangrenous or strangulated, the doctor will perform a resection of the affected bowel segment. In addition, he'll probably perform a prophylactic appendectomy at this time.

Special considerations

• Monitor vital signs before and after surgery. A change in temperature may indicate sepsis; infants may become hypothermic at the onset of infection. A rising pulse rate and falling blood pressure may be signs of peritonitis.
• Check intake and output. Watch for signs of dehydration and bleeding. If the patient is in shock, give blood or plasma as necessary.
• A nasogastric (NG) tube is inserted to decompress the intestine and minimize vomiting. Monitor tube drainage, and replace lost volume as required.
• Monitor the patient who has undergone hydrostatic reduction for passage of stools and barium, a sign that the reduction was successful. Keep in mind that a few patients have a recurrence of intussusception, usually within the first 36 to 48 hours after the reduction.
• After surgery, administer broad-spectrum antibiotics as needed, and provide meticulous wound care. Most incisions heal without complications. However, closely check the incision for inflammation, drainage, or suture separation.
• Encourage the patient to deep-breathe and cough productively. Be sure to splint the incision when he coughs, or teach him to do so himself. Also, make sure he takes 10 deep breaths an hour.

• Oral fluids may be given after surgery, and the NG tube may be removed when bowel sounds and peristalsis resume. The patient's diet can be advanced as tolerated.

• Check for abdominal distention after the patient resumes a normal diet, and monitor his general condition.

• Offer special reassurance and emotional support to the child and parents. This condition is considered a pediatric emergency, and parents are often unprepared for their child's hospitalization and possible surgery; they may feel guilty for not seeking medical aid sooner. Similarly, the child is unprepared for a separation from his parents and home.

To minimize the stress of hospitalization, encourage parents to participate in their child's care as much as possible.

IRON DEFICIENCY ANEMIA

In iron deficiency anemia, an inadequate supply of iron for optimal formation of red blood cells (RBCs) results in smaller (microcytic) cells with less color on staining. Body stores of iron, including plasma iron, decrease, as does transferrin, which binds with and transports iron. Insufficient body stores of iron lead to a depleted RBC mass and, in turn, to a decreased hemoglobin concentration (hypochromia) and decreased oxygen-carrying capacity of the blood. A common disease worldwide, iron deficiency anemia affects 10% to 30% of the adult population of the United States.

Causes

Iron deficiency anemia may result from:

• inadequate dietary intake of iron (less than 1 to 2 mg/day), as in prolonged unsupplemented breast- or bottle-feeding of infants, or during periods of stress, such as rapid growth in children and adolescents

• iron malabsorption, as in chronic diarrhea, partial or total gastrectomy, and malabsorption syndromes such as celiac disease

• blood loss secondary to drug-induced GI bleeding (from anticoagulants, aspirin, steroids) or due to heavy menses, hemorrhage from trauma, GI ulcers, cancer, or varices

• pregnancy, which diverts maternal iron to the fetus for erythropoiesis

• intravascular hemolysis-induced hemoglobinuria or paroxysmal nocturnal hemoglobinuria

• mechanical erythrocyte trauma caused by a prosthetic heart valve or vena cava filters.

Iron deficiency anemia occurs most commonly in premenopausal women, infants (particularly premature or low–birth-weight infants), children, and adolescents (especially girls).

Signs and symptoms

Because of the gradual progression of iron deficiency anemia, many patients are initially asymptomatic, except for symptoms of any underlying condition. They tend not to seek medical treatment until anemia is severe.

At advanced stages, decreased hemoglobin and the consequent decrease in the blood's oxygen-carrying capacity cause the patient to develop dyspnea on exertion, fatigue, listlessness, pallor, inability to concentrate, irritability, headache, and a susceptibility to infection. Decreased oxygen perfusion causes the heart to compensate with increased cardiac output and tachycardia.

SUPPORTIVE MANAGEMENT IN ANEMIA

Follow these guidelines to help manage the patient with anemia.

Nutritional needs
• If the patient is fatigued, urge him to eat small, frequent meals throughout the day.
• If the patient has oral lesions, suggest soft, cool, bland foods.
• If the patient has dyspepsia, eliminate spicy foods, and include milk and dairy products in his diet.
• If the patient is anorexic and irritable, encourage his family to bring his favorite foods from home (unless his diet is restricted) and to keep him company during meals if possible.

Activities
• Assess the effect of a specific activity by monitoring pulse rate during the activity. If the patient's pulse accelerates rapidly and he develops hypotension with hyperpnea, diaphoresis, light-headedness, palpitations, shortness of breath, or weakness, the activity is too strenuous.
• Tell the patient to pace his activities and to allow for frequent rest periods.

Infection precautions
• Use strict aseptic technique.
• Isolate the patient from infectious persons.
• Instruct the patient to avoid crowds and other sources of infection. Encourage him to practice good handwashing technique. Stress the importance of receiving necessary immunizations and prompt medical treatment for any sign of infection.

Diagnostic tests
• Explain erythropoiesis, the function of blood, and the purpose of diagnostic and therapeutic procedures.
• Tell the patient how he can participate in diagnostic testing. Give him an honest description of the pain or discomfort he'll probably experience.
• If possible, schedule all tests to avoid disrupting the patient's meals, sleep, and visiting hours.

Complications
• Observe for signs of bleeding that may exacerbate anemia. Check stools for occult bleeding. Assess for ecchymoses, gingival bleeding, and hematuria. Monitor vital signs frequently.
• If the patient is confined to strict bed rest, assist with range-of-motion exercises and frequent turning, coughing, and deep breathing.
• If blood transfusions are needed for severe anemia (hemoglobin less than 5 g/dl), give washed RBCs as needed, in partial exchange if evidence of pump failure is present.
• Carefully monitor the patient for signs of circulatory overload or transfusion reaction. Watch for a change in pulse rate, blood pressure, or respirations, or onset of fever, chills, pruritus, or edema. If any of these signs develops, stop the transfusion.
• Warn the patient to move about or change positions slowly to minimize dizziness induced by cerebral hypoxia.

In chronic iron deficiency anemia, nails become spoon-shaped and brittle, the corners of the mouth crack, the tongue turns smooth, and the patient complains of dysphagia or may develop pica. Associated neuromuscular effects include vasomotor disturbances, numbness and tingling of the extremities, and neuralgic pain. (See *Supportive management in anemia.*)

Diagnosis

Blood studies (serum iron, total iron-binding capacity, ferritin levels) and stores in bone marrow may confirm iron deficiency anemia. However, the results of these tests can be misleading because of complicating factors, such as infection, pneumonia, blood transfusion, or iron supplements. Characteristic blood study results include:

• low hemoglobin levels (males, less than 12 g/dl; females, less than 10 g/dl)
• low hematocrit (males, less than 47 ml/dl; females, less than 42 ml/dl)
• low serum iron levels, with high binding capacity
• low serum ferritin levels
• low RBC count, with microcytic and hypochromic cells (in early stages, RBC count may be normal, except in infants and children)
• decreased mean corpuscular hemoglobin in severe anemia.

Bone marrow studies reveal depleted or absent iron stores (done by staining) and normoblastic hyperplasia.

The diagnosis must rule out other forms of anemia, such as those that result from thalassemia minor, cancer, and chronic inflammatory, hepatic, and renal disease.

Prevention

Public health professionals can play a vital role in the prevention of iron deficiency anemia by:

• teaching the basics of a nutritionally balanced diet—red meats, green vegetables, eggs, whole wheat, iron-fortified bread, and milk. (However, no food in itself contains enough iron to *treat* iron deficiency anemia; an average-sized person with anemia would have to eat at least 10 lb [4.5 kg] of steak daily to receive therapeutic amounts of iron.)
• emphasizing the need for high-risk individuals—such as premature infants, children under age 2, and pregnant women—to receive prophylactic oral iron, as ordered by a doctor. (Children under age 2 should also receive supplemental cereals and formulas high in iron.)
• assessing a family's dietary habits for iron intake and noting the influence of childhood eating patterns, cultural food preferences, and family income on adequate nutrition.
• encouraging families with deficient iron intake to eat meat, fish, or poultry; whole or enriched grain; and foods high in ascorbic acid.
• carefully assessing a patient's drug history, since certain drugs, such as pancreatic enzymes and vitamin E, may interfere with iron metabolism and absorption and since aspirin, steroids, and other drugs may cause GI bleeding. (Teach patients who must take gastric irritants to take these medications with meals or milk.)

Treatment

The first priority of treatment is to determine the underlying cause of anemia. Once this is determined, iron replacement therapy can begin. The treatment of choice is an oral preparation of iron or a combination of iron and ascorbic acid (which enhances iron absorption). However, in some cases, iron may have to be administered parenterally—for instance, if the patient is noncompliant to the oral preparation, if he needs more iron than he can take orally, if malabsorption prevents adequate iron absorption, or if a maximum rate of hemoglobin regeneration is desired. (See *Injecting iron solutions.*)

Because a total-dose I.V. infusion of supplemental iron is painless and requires fewer injections, it's usually preferred over I.M. administration. Pregnant patients and elderly patients with severe anemia, for example, should receive a total-dose infusion of iron dextran in normal saline solution over

INJECTING IRON SOLUTIONS

For deep I.M. injections of iron solutions, use the Z-track technique to avoid subcutaneous irritation and discoloration from leaking medication. Choose a 19G to 20G, 2" to 3" needle. After drawing up the solution, change to a fresh needle to avoid tracking the solution through to subcutaneous tissue. Draw 0.5 cc of air into the syringe as an "air-lock."

Displace the skin and fat at the injection site (in the upper outer quadrant of the buttocks or the ventrogluteal site only) firmly to one side. Clean the area, and insert the needle. Aspirate to check for entry into a blood vessel. Inject the solution slowly, followed by the 0.5 cc of air in the syringe. Pull the needle straight out, and release the tissues.

Apply direct pressure to the site, but don't massage it. Caution the patient against vigorous exercise for 15 to 30 minutes.

1. Displace tissues. 2. Inject.

3. Wait 10 seconds. 4. Release tissues.

8 hours. To minimize the risk of an allergic reaction to iron, an I.V. test dose of 0.5 ml should be given first.

Special considerations
• Monitor the patient's compliance with the prescribed iron supplement therapy. Advise the patient not to stop therapy, even if he feels better, because replacement of iron stores takes time.
• Advise the patient that milk or an antacid interferes with absorption but that vitamin C can increase absorption. Instruct the patient to drink liquid supplemental iron through a straw to prevent staining his teeth.

• Tell the patient to report adverse reactions, such as nausea, vomiting, diarrhea, constipation, fever, or severe stomach pain, which may require a dosage adjustment.
• If the patient receives iron I.V., monitor the infusion rate carefully, and observe for an allergic reaction. Stop the infusion and begin supportive treatment immediately if the patient shows signs of an adverse reaction. Also, watch for dizziness and headache and for thrombophlebitis around the I.V. site.
• Use the Z-track injection method when administering iron I.M. to pre-

vent skin discoloration, scarring, and irritating iron deposits in the skin.
• Because an iron deficiency may recur, advise regular checkups.

IRRITABLE BOWEL SYNDROME

Also known as spastic colon or spastic colitis, irritable bowel syndrome is a common condition marked by chronic or periodic diarrhea, alternating with constipation, and accompanied by straining and abdominal cramps. The prognosis is good. Supportive treatment or avoidance of a known irritant often relieves symptoms.

Causes
This functional disorder is generally associated with psychological stress; however, it may result from physical factors, such as diverticular disease, ingestion of irritants (coffee, raw fruits or vegetables), lactose intolerance, abuse of laxatives, food poisoning, or colon cancer.

Signs and symptoms
Irritable bowel syndrome characteristically produces lower abdominal pain (usually relieved by defecation or passage of gas) and diarrhea that typically occurs during the day. These symptoms alternate with constipation or normal bowel function. Stools are often small and contain visible mucus. Dyspepsia and abdominal distention may occur.

Diagnosis
A careful patient history is required to determine contributing psychological factors such as a recent stressful life change. The diagnosis must also rule out other disorders, such as amebiasis, diverticulitis, colon cancer, and lactose intolerance. Appropriate diagnostic procedures include sigmoidoscopy, colonoscopy, barium enema, a rectal biopsy, and stool examination for blood, parasites, and bacteria.

Treatment
Therapy aims to relieve symptoms and includes counseling to help the patient understand the relationship between stress and his illness. Strict dietary restrictions aren't beneficial, but food irritants should be investigated and the patient instructed to avoid them. Rest and heat applied to the abdomen are helpful, as is judicious use of sedatives (phenobarbital) and antispasmodics (propantheline, diphenoxylate with atropine sulfate). However, with chronic use, the patient may become dependent on these drugs. If the cause of irritable bowel syndrome is chronic laxative abuse, bowel training may help correct the condition.

Special considerations
• Because the patient with irritable bowel syndrome isn't hospitalized, focus your care on patient teaching.
• Tell the patient to avoid irritating foods, and encourage development of regular bowel habits.
• Help the patient deal with stress, and warn against dependence on sedatives or antispasmodics.
• Encourage regular checkups because irritable bowel syndrome is associated with a higher-than-normal incidence of diverticulitis and colon cancer. For patients over age 40, emphasize the need for an annual sigmoidoscopy and rectal examination.

JAW DISLOCATION OR FRACTURE

Jaw dislocation is a displacement of the temporomandibular joint. Jaw fracture is a break in one or both of the two maxillae (upper jawbones) or the mandible (lower jawbone). Treatment can usually restore jaw alignment and function.

Causes
Simple fractures or dislocations are usually caused by a manual blow along the jawline; more serious compound fractures often result from car accidents.

Signs and symptoms
Malocclusion is the most obvious sign of dislocation or fracture. Other signs include mandibular pain, swelling, ecchymosis, loss of function, and asymmetry. In addition, mandibular fractures that damage the alveolar nerve produce paresthesia or anesthesia of the chin and lower lip. Maxillary fractures produce infraorbital paresthesia and often accompany fractures of the nasal and orbital complex.

Diagnosis
Abnormal maxillary or mandibular mobility during physical examination and a history of trauma suggest fracture or dislocation; X-rays confirm it.

Treatment
As in all traumatic injuries, check first for a patent airway, adequate ventilation, and pulses; then control hemorrhage and check for other injuries. As necessary, maintain a patent airway with an oropharyngeal airway, nasotracheal intubation, or a tracheotomy. Relieve pain with analgesics as needed.

After the patient stabilizes, surgical reduction and fixation by wiring restores mandibular and maxillary alignment. Maxillary fractures may also require reconstruction and repair of soft-tissue injuries.

Teeth and bones are never removed during surgery unless unavoidable. If the patient has lost teeth from trauma, the surgeon will decide whether they can be reimplanted. If they can, he will reimplant them within 6 hours, while they're still viable. Viability is increased if the tooth is placed in milk. Dislocations are usually manually reduced under anesthesia.

Special considerations
After reconstructive surgery:
• Position the patient on his side, with his head slightly elevated. A nasogastric tube is usually in place, with low suction to remove gastric contents and prevent nausea, vomiting, and aspiration of vomitus.

• As necessary, suction the nasopharynx through the nose, or by pulling the cheek away from the teeth and inserting a small suction catheter through any natural gap between teeth.

• If the patient isn't intubated, provide nourishment through a straw. If he has a natural gap between his teeth, insert the straw there; if not, one or two teeth may have to be extracted. However, extraction is avoided when possible.

• Start the diet with clear liquids; after the patient can tolerate fluids, offer milk shakes, broth, juices, pureed foods, and nutritional supplements.

• If the patient is unable to tolerate oral fluids, I.V. therapy can maintain hydration postoperatively.

• Administer antiemetics, as needed, to minimize nausea and prevent aspiration of vomitus (a very real danger in a patient whose jaw is wired). Keep a pair of wire cutters at the bedside to snip the wires should the patient vomit.

• A dental water-pulsator may be used for mouth care while the wires are intact.

• Because the patient will have difficulty talking while his jaw is wired, provide a Magic Slate or pencil and paper, and suggest appropriate diversions.

JUVENILE RHEUMATOID ARTHRITIS

Affecting children under age 16, juvenile rheumatoid arthritis (JRA) is an inflammatory disorder of the connective tissues characterized by joint swelling and pain or tenderness. It may also involve organs such as the skin, heart, lungs, liver, spleen, and eyes, producing extra-articular signs and symptoms.

JRA has three major types: systemic (Still's disease or acute febrile type), polyarticular, and pauciarticular. Depending on the type, this disease can occur as early as age 6 weeks — although rarely before 6 months — with peaks of onset between ages 1 and 3, and 8 and 12. Considered the major chronic rheumatic disorder of childhood, JRA affects an estimated 150,000 to 250,000 children in the United States; the overall incidence is twice as high in girls, with variation among the types.

Causes

The cause of JRA remains puzzling. Research continues to test several theories, such as those linking JRA to genetic factors or to an abnormal immune response. Viral or bacterial (particularly streptococcal) infection, trauma, and emotional stress may be precipitating factors, but their relationship to JRA remains unclear.

Signs and symptoms

Signs and symptoms vary with the type of JRA.

Systemic JRA

Affecting boys and girls almost equally, systemic JRA accounts for approximately 20% to 30% of cases. The affected children may have mild, transient arthritis or frank polyarthritis associated with fever and rash. Joint involvement may not be evident at first, but the child's behavior may clearly suggest joint pain. Such a child may want to constantly sit in a flexed position, may not walk much, or may refuse to walk at all. Young children with JRA are noticeably irritable and listless.

Fever in systemic JRA occurs suddenly and spikes to 103° F (39.4° C) or higher once or twice daily, usually in the late afternoon, then rapidly returns to normal or subnormal. (This "sawtooth" or intermittent spiking fever pattern helps differentiate JRA from other inflammatory disorders.)

When fever spikes, an evanescent rheumatoid rash often appears, consisting of small, pale, or salmon pink macules, most commonly on the trunk and proximal extremities and occasionally on the face, palms, and soles.

Massaging or applying heat intensifies this rash, which is usually most conspicuous where the skin has been rubbed or subjected to pressure, such as that from underclothing.

Other signs and symptoms of systemic JRA may include hepatosplenomegaly, lymphadenopathy, pleuritis, pericarditis, myocarditis, and nonspecific abdominal pain.

Polyarticular JRA

This form of the disorder affects girls three times more often than boys and may be seronegative or seropositive for rheumatoid factor (RF). It involves five or more joints, and usually develops insidiously. Most commonly involved joints are the wrists, elbows, knees, ankles, and small joints of the hands and feet.

Polyarticular JRA can also affect larger joints, including the temporomandibular joints and those of the cervical spine, hips, and shoulders. These joints become swollen, tender, and stiff.

Usually, the arthritis is symmetrical; it may be remittent or indolent. The patient may run a low-grade fever with daily peaks. Listlessness and weight loss can occur, possibly with lymphadenopathy and hepatosplenomegaly. Other signs of polyarticular JRA include subcutaneous nodules on the elbows or heels and noticeable developmental retardation.

Seropositive polyarticular JRA, the more severe type, usually occurs late in childhood and can cause destructive arthritis that mimics adult RA.

Pauciarticular JRA

Involving few joints (usually no more than four), pauciarticular JRA most often affects the knees and other large joints. It accounts for 45% of cases. Three major subtypes exist:

• *Pauciarticular JRA with chronic iridocyclitis* most commonly strikes girls under age 6 and involves the knees, elbows, ankles, or iris. Inflammation of the iris and ciliary body is often asymptomatic but may produce pain, redness, blurred vision, and photophobia.

• *Pauciarticular JRA with sacroiliitis* usually strikes boys (9:1) over age 8, who tend to be HLA-B27–positive. This subtype is characterized by lower extremity arthritis that produces hip, sacroiliac, heel, and foot pain and Achilles tendinitis. These patients may later develop the sacroiliac and lumbar arthritis characteristic of ankylosing spondylitis. Some also experience acute iritis, but not as frequently as those with the first subtype.

• The third subtype includes patients with joint involvement who test negative for antinuclear antibody (ANA) and HLA-B27 and who don't develop iritis. These patients have a better prognosis than those with the first or second subtype.

Common to all types of JRA is joint stiffness in the morning or after periods of inactivity. Growth disturbances may also occur, resulting in overgrowth or undergrowth adjacent to inflamed joints.

Diagnosis

Persistent joint pain and the rash and fever clearly point to JRA. Laboratory tests are useful for ruling out other inflammatory or even malignant diseases that can mimic JRA and for monitoring disease activity and response to therapy.

• *Complete blood count* shows decreased hemoglobin levels, neutrophilia, and thrombocytosis.

• *Erythrocyte sedimentation rate, complement (C)-reactive protein, haptoglobin, immunoglobulins,* and *C3 levels* may be elevated.

• *ANA test* may be positive in patients who have pauciarticular JRA with chronic iridocyclitis.

• *RF* is present in 15% of JRA cases, as compared with 85% of RA cases.
• Positive *HLA-B27 test* may forecast later development of ankylosing spondylitis.
• *Early X-ray* changes include soft-tissue swelling, effusion, and periostitis in affected joints. Later, osteoporosis and accelerated bone growth may appear, followed by subchondral erosions, joint space narrowing, bone destruction, and fusion.

Treatment

Successful management of JRA usually involves administration of anti-inflammatory drugs, physical therapy, carefully planned nutrition and exercise, and regular eye examinations. Both the child and his parents must be involved in therapy.

Aspirin is the initial drug of choice, with the dosage based on the child's weight. However, other nonsteroidal anti-inflammatory drugs (NSAIDs) may also be used. If these prove ineffective, gold salts, hydroxychloroquine, and penicillamine may be tried. Because of adverse effects, steroids are generally reserved for treatment of systemic complications that are resistant to NSAIDs, such as pericarditis and iritis. Corticosteroids and mydriatic drugs are commonly used for iridocyclitis. Low-dose cytotoxic drug therapy is currently being investigated.

Physical therapy promotes regular exercise to maintain joint mobility and muscle strength, thereby preventing contractures, deformity, and disability. Good posture, gait training, and joint protection are also beneficial. Splints help reduce pain, prevent contractures, and maintain correct joint alignment.

Generally, the prognosis for JRA is good, although disabilities can occur. Surgery is usually limited to soft-tissue releases to improve joint mobility. Joint replacement is delayed until the child has matured physically and can handle vigorous rehabilitation.

Special considerations

• Encourage the child to be as independent as possible and to develop a positive attitude toward school, social development, and vocational planning.
• Schedule regular slit-lamp examinations to help ensure early diagnosis and treatment of iridocyclitis. Children with pauciarticular JRA with chronic iridocyclitis should be checked every 3 months during periods of active disease and every 6 months during remissions.

KAPOSI'S SARCOMA

Initially, this cancer of the lymphatic cell wall was described as a rare blood vessel sarcoma, occurring mostly in elderly Italian and Jewish men. In recent years, the incidence of Kaposi's sarcoma has risen dramatically along with the incidence of acquired immunodeficiency syndrome (AIDS). Currently, it's the most common AIDS-related cancer.

Kaposi's sarcoma causes structural and functional damage. When associated with AIDS, it progresses aggressively, involving the lymph nodes, the viscera and, possibly, GI structures.

Causes

The exact cause of Kaposi's sarcoma is unknown, but the disease may be related to immunosuppression. Genetic or hereditary predisposition is also suspected.

Signs and symptoms

The initial sign of Kaposi's sarcoma is one or more obvious lesions in various shapes, sizes, and colors (ranging from red-brown to dark purple) appearing most commonly on the skin, buccal mucosa, hard and soft palates, lips, gums, tongue, tonsils, conjunctiva, and sclera.

In advanced disease, the lesions may join, becoming one large plaque. Untreated lesions may appear as large, ulcerative masses.

Other signs and symptoms include:

- a health history of AIDS
- pain (if the sarcoma advances beyond the early stages or if a lesion breaks down or impinges on nerves or organs)
- edema from lymphatic obstruction
- dyspnea (in cases of pulmonary involvement), wheezing, hypoventilation, and respiratory distress from bronchial blockage.

The most common extracutaneous sites are the lungs and GI tract (esophagus, oropharynx, and epiglottis).

Signs and symptoms of disease progression and metastasis include severe pulmonary involvement and GI involvement leading to digestive problems.

Diagnosis

The diagnosis is made following a tissue biopsy that identifies the lesion's type and stage. Then, a computed tomography scan may be performed to detect and evaluate possible metastasis. (See *Laubenstein's stages in Kaposi's sarcoma,* page 490.)

Treatment

In Kaposi's sarcoma, treatment isn't indicated for all patients. Indications include cosmetically offensive, painful, or obstructive lesions of rapidly progressing disease.

Radiation therapy, chemotherapy, and biotherapy with biological response modifiers are treatment options. Radiation therapy alleviates symptoms, including pain from obstructing lesions in the oral cavity or extremities and edema caused by lym-

LAUBENSTEIN'S STAGES IN KAPOSI'S SARCOMA

The following staging system was proposed by L.J. Laubenstein for use in evaluating and treating patients who have acquired immunodeficiency syndrome and Kaposi's sarcoma:

Stage I — locally indolent cutaneous lesions

Stage II — locally aggressive cutaneous lesions

Stage III — mucocutaneous and lymph node involvement

Stage IV — visceral involvement.

Within each stage, a patient may have different symptoms classified as a stage subtype — A or B — as follows:

• Subtype A — no systemic signs or symptoms

• Subtype B — one or more systemic signs and symptoms, including 10% weight loss, fever of unknown origin that exceeds 100° F (37.8° C) for more than 2 weeks, chills, lethargy, night sweats, anorexia, and diarrhea.

---

phatic blockage. It may also be used for cosmetic improvement.

Chemotherapy includes combinations of doxorubicin, vinblastine, vincristine, and etoposide (VP-16).

Biotherapy with interferon alfa-2b may be administered for AIDS-related Kaposi's sarcoma. The treatment reduces the number of skin lesions but is ineffective in advanced disease.

Special considerations

• Listen to the patient's fears and concerns and answer his questions honestly. Stay with him during periods of severe stress and anxiety.

• The patient who's coping poorly may need a referral for psychological coun-

seling. Family members may also need help in coping with the patient's disease and with any associated demands that the disorder places upon them.

• As appropriate, allow the patient to participate in self-care decisions whenever possible, and encourage him to participate in self-care measures as much as he can.

• Inspect the patient's skin every shift. Look for new lesions and skin breakdown. If the patient has painful lesions, help him into a more comfortable position.

• Follow universal precautions when caring for the patient.

• Administer pain medications. Suggest distractions, and help the patient with relaxation techniques.

• To help the patient adjust to changes in his appearance, urge him to share his feelings and provide encouragement.

• Monitor the patient's weight daily.

• Supply the patient with high-calorie, high-protein meals. If he can't tolerate regular meals, provide him with frequent smaller meals. Consult with the dietitian, and plan meals around the patient's treatment.

• If the patient can't take food by mouth, administer I.V. fluids. Also provide antiemetics and sedatives.

• Be alert for side effects of radiation therapy or chemotherapy — such as anorexia, nausea, vomiting, and diarrhea — and take steps to prevent or alleviate them.

• Reinforce the explanation of treatments. Make sure the patient understands which adverse reactions to expect and how to manage them. For example, during radiation therapy, instruct the patient to keep irradiated skin dry to avoid possible breakdown and subsequent infection.

• Explain all prescribed medications, including any possible adverse effects and drug interactions.

• Explain infection-prevention techniques and, if necessary, demonstrate basic hygiene measures to prevent infection. Advise the patient not to share his toothbrush, razor, or other items that may be contaminated with blood. These measures are especially important if the patient also has AIDS.

• Help the patient plan daily periods of alternating activity and rest to help him cope with fatigue. Teach energy-conservation techniques. Encourage him to set priorities, accept the help of others, and delegate nonessential tasks.

• Explain the proper use of assistive devices, when appropriate, to ease ambulation and promote independence.

• Stress the need for ongoing treatment and care.

• As appropriate, refer the patient to support groups offered by the social services department.

• If the patient's prognosis is poor (less than 6 months to live), suggest immediate hospice care.

• Explain the benefits of initiating and executing advance directives and a durable power of attorney.

KERATITIS

Inflammation of the cornea (keratitis) may be acute or chronic, superficial or deep. Superficial keratitis is fairly common and may develop at any age. The prognosis is good with treatment. Untreated, recurrent keratitis may lead to blindness.

Causes
Keratitis usually results from infection by herpes simplex virus, type 1 (known as dendritic keratitis because of a characteristic branched lesion of the cornea resembling the veins of a leaf). It may also result from exposure, due to the patient's inability to close his eyelids, or from congenital syphilis (interstitial keratitis). Less commonly, it stems from bacterial and fungal infections.

Signs and symptoms
Usually unilateral, keratitis produces opacities of the cornea, mild irritation, tearing, and photophobia. If the infection is in the center of the cornea, it may produce blurred vision. When keratitis results from exposure, it usually affects the lower portion of the cornea.

Diagnosis
A slit-lamp examination confirms keratitis. If keratitis is due to herpes simplex virus, staining the eye with a fluorescein strip produces one or more small branchlike (dendritic) lesions; touching the cornea with cotton reveals reduced corneal sensation. Vision testing may show slightly decreased acuity. The patient history may reveal a recent infection of the upper respiratory tract accompanied by cold sores.

Treatment
In acute keratitis due to herpes simplex virus, treatment consists of trifluridine eye drops or vidarabine ointment. A broad-spectrum antibiotic may prevent secondary bacterial infection.

Chronic dendritic keratitis may respond more quickly to vidarabine. Long-term topical therapy may be necessary. (Corticosteroid therapy is contraindicated in dendritic keratitis or any other viral or fungal disease of the cornea.) Treatment for fungal keratitis consists of natamycin.

Keratitis due to exposure requires application of moisturizing ointment to the exposed cornea and of a plastic bubble eye shield or eye patch. Treatment for severe corneal scarring may include keratoplasty (cornea transplantation).

Special considerations
• Look for keratitis in patients predisposed to cold sores. Explain that stress, trauma, fever, colds, and overexposure to the sun may trigger flare-ups.
• Protect the exposed corneas of unconscious patients by cleaning the eyes daily, applying moisturizing ointment, or covering the eyes with an eye shield.

KIDNEY CANCER

Kidney cancer is also known as nephrocarcinoma, renal cell carcinoma, hypernephroma, and Grawitz's tumor. It usually occurs in older adults, with about 85% of tumors originating in the kidneys and others resulting from metastasis from other primary sites. Renal pelvic tumors and Wilms' tumor occur primarily in children.

Kidney tumors, which usually are large, firm, nodular, encapsulated, unilateral, and solitary, can be separated histologically into clear cell, granular, and spindle cell types. The prognosis, which sometimes seems better for the clear cell type, probably depends on the cancer stage. (See *Staging kidney cancer.*) The 5-year survival rate is about 50%; the 10-year survival rate is lower.

Causes
The causes of kidney cancer aren't known. However, the incidence of this cancer is rising, possibly as a result of exposure to environmental carcinogens as well as increased longevity. Even so, kidney cancer accounts for only about 2% of all adult cancers. It's twice as common in men as in women and usually strikes after age 40.

Signs and symptoms
Kidney cancer produces a classic clinical triad—hematuria, pain, and a palpable mass—but any one of these features may be the first sign of cancer. Microscopic or gross hematuria (which may be intermittent) suggests that the cancer has spread to the renal pelvis.

Constant abdominal or flank pain may be dull or, if the cancer causes bleeding or blood clots, acute and colicky. The mass is generally smooth, firm, and nontender. All three signs of kidney cancer coexist in only about 10% of patients.

Other symptoms include fever (perhaps from hemorrhage or necrosis); hypertension (from compression of the renal artery with renal parenchymal ischemia); rapidly progressing hypercalcemia (possibly from ectopic parathyroid hormone production by the tumor); and urine retention. Weight loss, edema in the legs, nausea, and vomiting are signs of advanced kidney cancer.

Diagnosis
Studies to identify kidney cancer usually include computed tomography scans, excretory urography and retrograde pyelography, ultrasound, cystoscopy (to rule out associated bladder cancer), and nephrotomography or renal angiography to distinguish a kidney cyst from a tumor.

Related tests include liver function studies showing increased levels of alkaline phosphatase, bilirubin, alanine aminotransferase, and aspartate aminotransferase, as well as prolonged prothrombin time. Such results may point to liver metastasis, but if metastasis hasn't occurred, these abnormalities reverse after the tumor has been resected.

Routine laboratory findings of hematuria, anemia (unrelated to blood loss), polycythemia, hypercalcemia, and increased erythrocyte sedimentation

STAGING KIDNEY CANCER

Using the TNM (tumor, node, metastasis) system, the American Joint Committee on Cancer has established the following stages for kidney cancer.

Primary tumor

TX—primary tumor can't be assessed

T0—no evidence of primary tumor

T1—tumor 2.5 cm or less in greatest dimension and limited to the kidney

T2—tumor greater than 2.5 cm in greatest dimension and limited to the kidney

T3—tumor extends into major veins or invades adrenal gland or perinephric tissues, but not beyond Gerota's fascia

T3a—tumor extends into adrenal gland or perinephric tissues, but not beyond Gerota's fascia

T3b—tumor grossly extends into renal veins or vena cava

T4—tumor extends beyond Gerota's fascia

Regional lymph nodes

NX—regional lymph nodes can't be assessed

N0—no evidence of regional lymph node metastasis

N1—metastasis in a single lymph node, 2 cm or less in greatest dimension

N2—metastasis in a single lymph node, between 2 and 5 cm in greatest dimension, or metastasis to several lymph nodes, none more than 5 cm in greatest dimension

N3—metastasis in a lymph node, more than 5 cm in greatest dimension

Distant metastasis

MX—distant metastasis can't be assessed

M0—no known distant metastasis

M1—distant metastasis

Staging categories

Kidney cancer progresses from mild to severe as follows:

Stage I—T1, N0, M0

Stage II—T2, N0, M0

Stage III—T1, N1, M0; T2, N1, M0; T3a, N0, M0; T3a, N1, M0; T3b, N0, M0; T3b, N1, M0

Stage IV—T4, any N, M0; any T, N2, M0; any T, N3, M0; any T, any N, M1

---

rate call for more testing to rule out kidney cancer.

Treatment

Radical nephrectomy, with or without regional lymph node dissection, offers the only chance of cure. Because the disease is radiation-resistant, radiation is used only if the cancer spreads to the perinephric region or the lymph nodes, or if the primary tumor or metastatic sites can't be fully excised. In these cases, high radiation doses are used.

Chemotherapy has been only erratically effective against kidney cancer. Chlorambucil, fluorouracil, cyclophosphamide, vinblastine, lomustine, vincristine, cisplatin, tamoxifen, teniposide, interferons, and hormones, such as medroxyprogesterone and testosterone, have been used, usually with poor results. Biotherapy (lymphokine-activated killer cells with recombinant interleukin-2) shows promise but causes adverse reactions. Interferon is somewhat effective in advanced disease.

Special considerations

• Meticulous postoperative care, supportive treatment during other therapy, and psychological support can hasten recovery and minimize complications.

• Before surgery, assure the patient that his body will adapt to the loss of a kidney.

• Teach the patient about such expected postoperative procedures as diaphragmatic breathing, coughing properly, splinting his incision, and others.

• After surgery, encourage diaphragmatic breathing and coughing.

• Assist the patient with leg exercises, and turn him every 2 hours.

• Check dressings often for excessive bleeding. Watch for signs of internal bleeding, such as restlessness, sweating, and increased pulse rate.

• Place the patient on the operative side to allow the pressure of adjacent organs to fill the dead space at the operative site, improving dependent drainage. If possible, help the patient walk within 24 hours after surgery.

• Maintain adequate fluid intake, and monitor intake and output. Monitor laboratory results for anemia, polycythemia, or abnormal blood values that may point to bone or liver involvement or that may result from radiation or chemotherapy.

• Treat adverse effects of medication.

• Stress the need to comply with the prescribed outpatient treatment regimen.

KYPHOSIS

Also known as roundback, kyphosis is an anteroposterior curving of the spine that causes a bowing of the back, commonly at the thoracic, but sometimes at the thoracolumbar or sacral, level. Normally, the spine displays some convexity, but excessive thoracic kyphosis is pathologic. Kyphosis occurs in children and adults.

Causes

Congenital kyphosis is rare but usually severe, with resultant cosmetic deformity and reduced pulmonary function.

Adolescent kyphosis

Also called Scheuermann's disease, juvenile kyphosis, and vertebral epiphysitis, adolescent kyphosis is the most common form of this disorder. It may result from growth retardation or a vascular disturbance in the vertebral epiphysis (usually at the thoracic level) during periods of rapid growth, or from congenital deficiency in the thickness of the vertebral plates.

Other causes include infection, inflammation, aseptic necrosis, and disk degeneration. The subsequent stress of weight-bearing on the compromised vertebrae may result in the thoracic hump often seen in adolescents with kyphosis. Symptomatic adolescent kyphosis is more prevalent in girls than in boys and occurs most often between ages 12 and 16.

Adult kyphosis

Also known as adult roundback, adult kyphosis may result from aging and associated degeneration of intervertebral disks, atrophy, and osteoporotic collapse of the vertebrae; from endocrine disorders such as hyperparathyroidism, and Cushing's disease; and from prolonged steroid therapy.

Adult kyphosis may also result from conditions such as arthritis, Paget's disease, polio, compression fracture of the thoracic vertebrae, metastatic tumor, plasma cell myeloma, or tuberculosis. In both children and adults, kyphosis may also result from poor posture.

Disk lesions called Schmorl's nodes may develop in anteroposterior curving of the spine and are localized protrusions of nuclear material through the cartilage plates and into the spongy bone of the vertebral bodies. If the anterior portions of the cartilage are destroyed, bridges of new bone may transverse the intervertebral space, causing ankylosis.

Signs and symptoms

Clinical features vary with the type of kyphosis.

Adolescent features

Development of adolescent kyphosis is usually insidious, often occurring after a history of excessive sports activity, and may be asymptomatic except for the obvious curving of the back (sometimes more than 90 degrees). In some adolescents, kyphosis may produce mild pain at the apex of the curve (about 50% of patients), fatigue, tenderness or stiffness in the involved area or along the entire spine, and prominent vertebral spinous processes at the lower dorsal and upper lumbar levels, with compensatory increased lumbar lordosis, and hamstring tightness.

Rarely, kyphosis may induce neurologic damage: spastic paraparesis secondary to spinal cord compression or herniated nucleus pulposus. In both adolescent and adult forms of kyphosis that are not due to poor posture alone, the spine won't straighten out when the patient assumes a recumbent position.

Adult features

Adult kyphosis produces a characteristic roundback appearance, possibly associated with pain, weakness of the back, and generalized fatigue. Unlike the adolescent form, adult kyphosis rarely produces local tenderness, except in senile osteoporosis with recent compression fracture.

Diagnosis

Physical examination reveals curvature of the thoracic spine in varying degrees of severity. X-rays may show vertebral wedging, Schmorl's nodes, irregular end plates and, possibly, mild scoliosis of 10 to 20 degrees.

Adolescent kyphosis must be distinguished from tuberculosis and other inflammatory or neoplastic diseases that cause vertebral collapse; the severe pain, bone destruction, or systemic symptoms associated with these diseases help to rule out a diagnosis of kyphosis. Other sites of bone disease, primary sites of cancer, and infection must also be evaluated, possibly through a vertebral biopsy.

Treatment

For kyphosis caused by poor posture alone, treatment may consist of therapeutic exercises, bed rest on a firm mattress (with or without traction), and a brace to straighten the kyphotic curve until spinal growth is complete.

Corrective exercises include pelvic tilts to decrease lumbar lordosis, hamstring stretches to overcome muscle contractures, and thoracic hyperextensions to flatten the kyphotic curve. These exercises may be performed in or out of the brace.

Lateral X-rays taken every 4 months evaluate correction. Gradual weaning from the brace can begin after maximum correction of the kyphotic curve, vertebral wedging has decreased, and the spine has reached full skeletal maturity. Loss of correction indicates that weaning from the brace has been too rapid, and time out of the brace is decreased accordingly.

Treatment for both adolescent and adult kyphosis also includes appropriate measures for the underlying cause and, possibly, spinal arthrodesis for relief of symptoms. Although rarely necessary, surgery may be recommended when kyphosis causes neurologic damage, a spinal curve greater than 60 degrees, or intractable and disabling back pain in a patient with full skeletal maturity. Preoperative measures may include halo-femoral traction.

Corrective surgery includes a posterior spinal fusion with spinal instrumentation, iliac bone grafting, and plaster immobilization. Anterior spinal fusion followed by immobilization in plaster may be necessary when kyphosis produces a spinal curve greater than 70 degrees.

Special considerations
• Effective management of kyphosis necessitates first-rate supportive care for patients in traction or a brace, skillful patient teaching, and sensitive emotional support.
• Teach the patient with adolescent kyphosis caused by poor posture alone the prescribed therapeutic exercises and the fundamentals of good posture.
• Suggest bed rest when pain is severe. Encourage use of a firm mattress, preferably with a bed board.
• If the patient needs a brace, explain its purpose and teach him how and when to wear it.
• Teach good skin care. Tell the patient not to use lotions, ointments, or powders where the brace contacts the skin.
• Warn the patient that only the doctor or orthotist should adjust the brace.
• If corrective surgery is needed, explain all preoperative tests thoroughly, as well as the need for postoperative traction or casting, if applicable.
• After surgery, check the patient's neurovascular status every 2 to 4 hours for the first 48 hours, and watch for any changes.
• Turn the patient often by logrolling him.
• Offer pain medication every 3 or 4 hours for the first 48 hours.

• Institute blood product replacement as needed.
• Accurately measure fluid intake and output, including urine specific gravity.
• Insert a nasogastric tube and an indwelling urinary catheter as needed; a rectal tube may also be necessary if paralytic ileus causes abdominal distention.
• Provide meticulous skin care. Check the skin at the cast edges several times a day; use heel and elbow protectors to prevent skin breakdown.
• Remove antiembolism stockings, if needed, at least three times a day for at least 30 minutes.
• Change dressings as necessary.
• Provide emotional support. The adolescent patient is likely to exhibit mood changes and periods of depression. Maintain communication, and offer frequent encouragement and reassurance.
• Assist during the removal of sutures and application of a new cast (usually about 10 days after surgery).
• Encourage gradual ambulation (often with the use of a tilt-table in the physical therapy department).
• At discharge, provide detailed, written cast care instructions. Tell the patient to immediately report pain, burning, skin breakdown, loss of feeling, tingling, numbness, or cast odor.
• Advise the patient to drink plenty of liquids to avoid constipation, and to report any illness (especially abdominal pain or vomiting) immediately.
• Arrange for home visits by a social worker and a home care nurse.

LABYRINTHITIS

An inflammation of the labyrinth of the inner ear, labyrinthitis frequently incapacitates the patient by producing severe vertigo that lasts for 3 to 5 days; symptoms gradually subside over a 3- to 6-week period. This disorder is rare, although viral labyrinthitis is often associated with upper respiratory tract infections.

Causes

Labyrinthitis is usually caused by viral infection. It may be a primary infection; the result of trauma; or a complication of influenza, otitis media, or meningitis. In chronic otitis media, cholesteatoma formation erodes the bone of the labyrinth, allowing bacteria to enter from the middle ear. Toxic drug ingestion is another possible cause of labyrinthitis.

Signs and symptoms

Because the inner ear controls both hearing and balance, this infection typically produces severe vertigo (with any movement of the head) and sensorineural hearing loss. Vertigo begins gradually but peaks within 48 hours, causing loss of balance and falling in the direction of the affected ear.

Other associated signs and symptoms include spontaneous nystagmus, with jerking movements of the eyes toward the unaffected ear; nausea, vomiting, and giddiness; with cholesteatoma, signs of middle ear disease; and with severe bacterial infection, purulent drainage. To minimize symptoms such as giddiness and nystagmus, the patient may assume a characteristic posture—lying on the side of the unaffected ear and looking in the direction of the affected ear.

Diagnosis

A typical clinical picture and history of upper respiratory tract infection suggest labyrinthitis. Typical diagnostic measures include culture and sensitivity testing to identify the infecting organism, if purulent drainage is present, and audiometric testing.

When an infectious etiology can't be found, additional testing must be done to rule out a brain lesion or Ménière's disease.

Treatment

Symptomatic treatment includes bed rest, with the head immobilized between pillows; oral meclizine to control vertigo; and massive doses of antibiotics to combat diffuse purulent labyrinthitis. Oral fluids can prevent dehydration from vomiting; for severe nausea and vomiting, I.V. fluids may be necessary.

When conservative management fails, treatment necessitates surgical excision of the cholesteatoma and drainage of the infected areas of the middle and inner ear. Prevention is possible by early and vigorous treatment of predisposing conditions, such as otitis media and any local or systemic infection.

Special considerations
- Keep the side rails up to prevent falls.
- If vomiting is severe, administer antiemetics. Record intake and output, and give I.V. fluids as necessary.
- Tell the patient that recovery may take as long as 6 weeks. During this time, he should limit activities that vertigo may make hazardous.
- If recovery doesn't occur within 4 to 6 weeks, a computed tomography scan should be performed to rule out an intracranial lesion.

LARYNGEAL CANCER

The most common form of laryngeal cancer is squamous cell carcinoma (95%); rare forms include adenocarcinoma, sarcoma, and others. Such cancer may be intrinsic or extrinsic.

An *intrinsic* tumor is on the true vocal cord and tends not to spread, because underlying connective tissues lack lymph nodes. An *extrinsic* tumor is on some other part of the larynx and tends to spread early. Laryngeal cancer is nine times more common in males than in females; most victims are between ages 50 and 65.

Causes
In laryngeal cancer, major predisposing factors include smoking and alcoholism; minor factors include chronic inhalation of noxious fumes and familial tendency.

Laryngeal cancer is classified according to its location:
- supraglottis (false vocal cords)
- glottis (true vocal cords)
- subglottis (downward extension from the vocal cords [rare]).

Signs and symptoms
In intrinsic laryngeal cancer, the dominant and earliest symptom is hoarseness that persists longer than 3 weeks; in extrinsic cancer, it's a lump in the throat or pain or burning in the throat when drinking citrus juice or hot liquid. Later clinical effects of metastasis include dysphagia, dyspnea, cough, enlarged cervical lymph nodes, and pain radiating to the ear.

Diagnosis
Any hoarseness that lasts longer than 2 weeks requires visualization of the larynx by laryngoscopy.

A firm diagnosis also requires xeroradiography, a biopsy, laryngeal tomography, computed tomography scan, or laryngography to define the borders of the lesion, and chest X-ray to detect metastasis. (See *Staging laryngeal cancer.*)

Treatment
Early lesions are treated with surgery or radiation; advanced lesions with surgery, radiation, and chemotherapy. The chemotherapeutic agents may include methotrexate, cisplatin, bleomycin, fluorouracil, and vincristine.

The treatment goal is to eliminate the cancer and preserve speech. If speech preservation isn't possible, speech rehabilitation may include esophageal speech or prosthetic devices; surgical techniques to construct a new voice box are still experimental. Surgical procedures vary with tumor size and can include cordectomy, partial or total laryngectomy, supraglottic laryngectomy, or total laryngectomy with laryngoplasty.

Special considerations
- Psychological support and good preoperative and postoperative care can minimize complications and speed recovery.

Staging Laryngeal Cancer

The TNM (tumor, node, metastasis) classification system developed by the American Joint Committee on Cancer describes laryngeal cancer stages and guides treatment. The T stages cover supraglottic, glottic, and subglottic tumors.

Primary tumor

TX—primary tumor unassessible
T0—no evidence of primary tumor
Tis—carcinoma in situ

Supraglottic tumor stages

T1—tumor confined to one subsite in supraglottis; vocal cords retain motion
T2—tumor extends to other sites in supraglottis or to glottis; vocal cords retain motion
T3—tumor confined to larynx, but vocal cords lose motion; or tumor extends to the postcricoid area, the pyriform sinus, or the preepiglottic space, and vocal cords lose motion; or both
T4—tumor extends through thyroid cartilage or extends to tissues beyond the larynx (such as the oropharynx or soft tissues of the neck), or both

Glottic tumor stages

T1—tumor confined to vocal cords, which retain normal motion; may involve anterior or posterior commissures
T2—tumor extends to supraglottis, subglottis, or both; vocal cords may lose motion
T3—tumor confined to larynx, but vocal cords lose motion
T4—tumor extends through thyroid cartilage, to tissues beyond the larynx (such as the oropharynx or soft tissues of the neck), or both

Subglottic tumor stages

T1—tumor confined to subglottis
T2—tumor extends to vocal cords; vocal cords may lose motion
T3—tumor confined to larynx with vocal cord fixation
T4—tumor extends through cricoid or thyroid cartilage, to tissues beyond the larynx, or both

Regional lymph nodes

NX—regional lymph nodes can't be assessed
N0—no evidence of regional lymph node metastasis
N1—metastasis in a single ipsilateral lymph node, 3 cm or less in greatest dimension
N2—metastasis in one or more ipsilateral lymph nodes, or in bilateral or contralateral nodes, larger than 3 cm but less than 6 cm in greatest dimension
N3—metastasis in a node larger than 6 cm in greatest dimension

Distant metastasis

MX—distant metastasis unassessible
M0—no evidence of distant metastasis
M1—distant metastasis

Staging categories

Laryngeal cancer progresses from mild to severe as follows:
Stage 0—Tis, N0, M0
Stage I—T1, N0, M0
Stage II—T2, N0, M0
Stage III—T3, N0, M0; T1, N1, M0; T2, N1, M0; T3, N1, M0
Stage IV—T4, N0 or N1, M0; any T, N2 or N3, M0; any T, any N, M1

Before partial or total laryngectomy:
• Instruct the patient to maintain good oral hygiene. If appropriate, instruct a male patient to shave off his beard.
• Encourage the patient to express his concerns before surgery. Help him choose a temporary nonspeaking method of communication (such as writing).
• If appropriate, arrange for a laryngectomee to visit him. Explain postoperative procedures (suctioning, nasogastric [NG] tube feeding, care of laryngectomy tube) and their results (breathing through the neck, speech alteration). Also prepare him for other functional losses: He won't be able to smell, blow his nose, whistle, gargle, sip, or suck on a straw.

After partial laryngectomy:
• Give I.V. fluids and, usually, tube feedings for the first 2 days postoperatively; then resume oral fluids. Keep the tracheostomy tube (inserted during surgery) in place until edema subsides.
• Keep the patient from using his voice until he has medical permission (usually 2 to 3 days postoperatively). Then caution him to whisper until healing is complete.

After total laryngectomy:
• As soon as the patient returns to his bed, place him on his side and elevate his head 30 to 45 degrees. When you move him, remember to support his neck.
• The patient will probably have a laryngectomy tube in place until his stoma heals (about 7 to 10 days). This tube is shorter and thicker than a tracheostomy tube but requires the same care.
• Watch for crusting and secretions around the stoma, which can cause skin breakdown. To prevent crust formation, provide adequate room humidification. Remove crusting with petrolatum, antimicrobial ointment, and moist gauze.

• Teach stoma care.
• Watch for fistula formation (redness, swelling, secretions on suture line). A fistula may form between the reconstructed hypopharynx and the skin. This eventually heals spontaneously but may take weeks or months.
• Watch for carotid artery rupture (bleeding), which usually occurs in patients who have had preoperative radiation, particularly those with a fistula that constantly bathes the carotid artery with oral secretions. If carotid rupture occurs, apply pressure to the site; call for help immediately and take the patient to the operating room for carotid ligation.
• Watch for tracheostomy stenosis (constant shortness of breath) which occurs weeks to months after laryngectomy; treatment includes fitting the patient with successively larger tracheostomy tubes until he can tolerate insertion of a large one.
• If the patient has a fistula, feed him through an NG tube; otherwise, food will leak through the fistula and delay healing.
• Monitor vital signs (be especially alert for fever, which indicates infection).
• Record fluid intake and output, and watch for dehydration.
• Give frequent mouth care.
• Suction gently unless otherwise instructed. Don't attempt deep suctioning, which could penetrate the suture line. Suction through both the tube and the patient's nose because the patient can no longer blow air through his nose; suction his mouth gently.
• After insertion of a drainage catheter (usually connected to a blood drainage system or a GI drainage system), don't stop suction until drainage is minimal. After catheter removal, check dressings for drainage.
• Give analgesics as necessary.
• If the patient has an NG feeding tube, check tube placement and elevate the patient's head to prevent aspiration.

• Reassure the patient that speech rehabilitation may help him speak again. Encourage him to contact the International Association of Laryngectomees and other sources of support.

• Support the patient through some inevitable grieving. If the depression seems severe, consider referring him for counseling.

LARYNGITIS

A common disorder, laryngitis is acute or chronic inflammation of the vocal cords. Acute laryngitis may occur as an isolated infection or as part of a generalized bacterial or viral upper respiratory tract infection. Repeated attacks of acute laryngitis cause inflammatory changes associated with chronic laryngitis.

Causes

Acute laryngitis usually results from infection (primarily viral) or excessive use of the voice, an occupational hazard in certain vocations (teaching, public speaking, singing, for example). It may also result from leisuretime activities (such as cheering at a sports event), inhalation of smoke or fumes, or aspiration of caustic chemicals. Causes of chronic laryngitis include chronic upper respiratory tract disorders (sinusitis, bronchitis, nasal polyps, allergy), mouth breathing, smoking, constant exposure to dust or other irritants, and alcohol abuse.

Signs and symptoms

Acute laryngitis typically begins with hoarseness, ranging from mild to complete loss of voice. Associated clinical features include pain (especially when swallowing or speaking), dry cough, fever, laryngeal edema, and malaise. In chronic laryngitis, persistent hoarseness is usually the only symptom.

Diagnosis

Indirect laryngoscopy confirms the diagnosis by revealing red, inflamed and, occasionally, hemorrhagic vocal cords, with rounded rather than sharp edges and exudate. Bilateral swelling may be present. In severe cases or if toxicity is a concern, a culture of the exudate is obtained.

Treatment

Primary treatment consists of resting the voice. For viral infection, symptomatic care includes analgesics and throat lozenges for pain relief. Bacterial infection requires antibiotic therapy. Severe, acute laryngitis may necessitate hospitalization. When laryngeal edema results in airway obstruction, tracheotomy may be necessary. In chronic laryngitis, effective treatment must eliminate the underlying cause.

Special considerations

• Explain to the patient why he shouldn't talk, and place a sign over the bed to remind others of this restriction. Provide a Magic Slate or a pad and pencil for communication. Mark the intercom panel so other hospital personnel are aware that the patient can't answer.

• Minimize the need to talk by trying to anticipate the patient's needs.

• Suggest that the patient maintain adequate humidification by using a vaporizer or humidifier during the winter, by avoiding air conditioning during the summer (because it dehumidifies), by using medicated throat lozenges, and by not smoking. Urge him to complete the prescribed antibiotics.

• Obtain a detailed patient history to help determine the cause of chronic laryngitis. Encourage modification of predisposing habits.

LEGIONNAIRES' DISEASE

An acute bronchopneumonia, Legionnaires' disease is produced by a fastidious, gram-negative bacillus. It derives its name and notoriety from the peculiar, highly publicized disease that struck 182 people (29 of whom died) at an American Legion convention in Philadelphia in July 1976.

This disease may occur epidemically or sporadically, usually in late summer or early fall. Its severity ranges from a mild illness, with or without pneumonitis, to multilobar pneumonia, with a mortality as high as 15%. A milder, self-limiting form (Pontiac syndrome) subsides within a few days but leaves the patient fatigued for several weeks; this form mimics Legionnaires' disease but produces few or no respiratory symptoms, no pneumonia, and no fatalities.

Causes

The causative agent of Legionnaires' disease, *Legionella pneumophila,* is an aerobic, gram-negative bacillus that's probably transmitted by an airborne route. In past epidemics, it has spread through cooling towers or evaporation condensers in air-conditioning systems. However, *Legionella* bacilli also flourish in soil and excavation sites. The disease does not spread from person to person.

Legionnaires' disease occurs more often in men than in women and is most likely to affect:

• middle-aged to elderly people
• immunocompromised patients (particularly those receiving corticosteroids, for example, after a transplant), or those with lymphoma or other disorders associated with delayed hypersensitivity
• patients with a chronic underlying disease, such as diabetes, chronic renal failure, or chronic obstructive pulmonary disease
• alcoholics
• cigarette smokers (three to four times more likely to develop Legionnaires' disease than nonsmokers).

Signs and symptoms

The multisystem clinical features of Legionnaires' disease follow a predictable sequence, although onset of the disease may be gradual or sudden.

After a 2- to 10-day incubation period, nonspecific, prodromal signs and symptoms appear, including diarrhea, anorexia, malaise, diffuse myalgias and generalized weakness, headache, recurrent chills, and an unremitting fever, which develops within 12 to 48 hours with a temperature that may reach 105° F (40.5° C). A cough then develops that initially is nonproductive but eventually may produce grayish, nonpurulent and, occasionally, blood-streaked sputum.

Other characteristic features include nausea, vomiting, disorientation, mental sluggishness, confusion, mild temporary amnesia, pleuritic chest pain, tachypnea, dyspnea, fine crackles and, in 50% of patients, bradycardia. Patients who develop pneumonia may also experience hypoxia. Other complications include hypotension, delirium, congestive heart failure, arrhythmias, acute respiratory failure, renal failure, and shock (usually fatal).

Diagnosis

The patient history focuses on possible sources of infection and predisposing conditions. In addition, a chest X-ray shows patchy, localized infiltration, which progresses to multilobar consolidation (usually involving the lower lobes), pleural effusion and, in fulminant disease, opacification of the entire lung.

Auscultation reveals fine crackles, progressing to coarse crackles as the disease advances.

Abnormal test findings include leukocytosis, an increased erythrocyte sedimentation rate, an increase in liver enzyme levels (alanine aminotransferase, aspartate aminotransferase, alkaline phosphatase), hyponatremia, decreased partial pressure of arterial oxygen, and, initially, decreased partial pressure of arterial carbon dioxide. Bronchial washings and blood, pleural fluid, and sputum tests rule out other infections.

Definitive tests include direct immunofluorescence of respiratory tract secretions and tissue, a culture of *L. pneumophila,* and indirect fluorescent antibody testing of serum comparing acute samples with convalescent samples drawn at least 3 weeks later. A convalescent serum showing a fourfold or greater rise in antibody titer for *Legionella* confirms this diagnosis.

Treatment

Antibiotic treatment begins as soon as Legionnaires' disease is suspected and diagnostic material is collected; it shouldn't await laboratory confirmation. Erythromycin is the drug of choice, but if it's not effective alone, rifampin can be added to the regimen. If erythromycin is contraindicated, rifampin or rifampin with tetracycline may be used.

Supportive therapy includes administration of antipyretics, fluid replacement, circulatory support with pressor drugs if necessary, and oxygen administration by mask, cannula, or mechanical ventilation.

Special considerations

• Closely monitor the patient's respiratory status. Evaluate chest wall expansion, depth and pattern of respirations, cough, and chest pain.

• Watch for restlessness, which may indicate that the patient is hypoxemic and requires suctioning, repositioning, or more aggressive oxygen therapy.

• Continually monitor the patient's vital signs, pulse oximetry or arterial blood gas values, level of consciousness, and dryness and color of the lips and mucous membranes. Watch for signs of shock (decreased blood pressure, thready pulse, diaphoresis, clammy skin).

• Keep the patient comfortable; avoid chills and exposure to drafts. Provide mouth care frequently. If necessary, apply soothing cream to the nostrils.

• Replace fluid and electrolytes as needed. The patient with renal failure may require dialysis.

• Provide mechanical ventilation and other respiratory therapy as needed. Teach the patient how to cough effectively, and encourage deep-breathing exercises. Stress the need to continue these measures until recovery is complete.

• Give antibiotics as necessary, and observe carefully for adverse effects.

LEUKEMIA, ACUTE

Acute leukemia is a malignant proliferation of white blood cell precursors (blasts) in bone marrow or lymph tissue and their accumulation in peripheral blood, bone marrow, and body tissues.

The most common forms are acute lymphoblastic (lymphocytic) leukemia (ALL), characterized by the abnormal growth of lymphocyte precursors (lymphoblasts); acute myeloblastic (myelogenous) leukemia (AML), in which myeloid precursors (myeloblasts) rapidly accumulate; and acute monoblastic (monocytic) leukemia, or Schilling's type, characterized by a marked increase in monocyte precursors (monoblasts). Other variants include acute myelomonocytic leukemia and acute erythroleukemia.

Untreated, acute leukemia is invariably fatal, usually because of complications that result from leukemic cell infiltration of bone marrow or vital organs. With treatment, the prognosis varies.

In ALL, treatment induces remissions in 90% of children (average survival time: 5 years) and in 65% of adults (average survival time: 1 to 2 years). Children between ages 2 and 8 have the best survival rate with intensive therapy.

In AML, the average survival time is only 1 year after diagnosis, even with aggressive treatment. In acute monoblastic leukemia, treatment induces remissions lasting 2 to 10 months in 50% of children; adults survive only about 1 year after diagnosis, even with treatment.

Causes

Research on predisposing factors isn't conclusive but points to some combination of viruses (viral remnants have been found in leukemic cells), genetic and immunologic factors, and exposure to radiation and certain chemicals.

Pathogenesis isn't clearly understood, but immature, nonfunctioning white blood cells (WBCs) appear to accumulate first in the tissue where they originate (lymphocytes in lymph tissue, granulocytes in bone marrow). These immature WBCs then spill into the bloodstream and from there infiltrate other tissues, eventually causing organ malfunction because of encroachment or hemorrhage. (See *What happens in leukemia.*)

Incidence

Acute leukemia is more common in males than in females, in whites (especially people of Jewish descent), in children between ages 2 and 5 (80% of all leukemias in this age-group are ALL), and in people who live in urban and industrialized areas. Acute leukemia ranks 20th in causes of cancer-related deaths among people of all age-groups. Among children, however, it's the most common form of cancer. In the United States, an estimated 11,000 people develop acute leukemia annually.

Signs and symptoms

Signs of acute leukemia are the sudden onset of high fever accompanied by thrombocytopenia and abnormal bleeding, such as nosebleeds, gingival bleeding, purpura, ecchymoses, petechiae, easy bruising after minor trauma, and prolonged menses. Nonspecific symptoms, such as low-grade fever, weakness, and lassitude, may persist for days or months before visible symptoms appear.

Other insidious signs include pallor, chills, and recurrent infections. In addition, ALL, AML, and acute monoblastic leukemia may cause dyspnea, anemia, fatigue, malaise, tachycardia, palpitations, systolic ejection murmur, and abdominal or bone pain. When leukemic cells cross the blood-brain barrier and thereby escape the effects of systemic chemotherapy, the patient may develop meningeal leukemia (confusion, lethargy, headache).

Diagnosis

Typical clinical findings and bone marrow aspirate showing a proliferation of immature WBCs confirm acute leukemia. An aspirate that's dry or free of leukemic cells in a patient with typ-

WHAT HAPPENS IN LEUKEMIA

This illustration shows how white blood cells (agranulocytes and granulocytes) proliferate in the bloodstream in leukemia, overwhelming red blood cells (RBCs) and platelets.

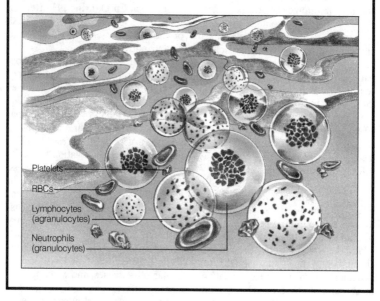

Platelets

RBCs

Lymphocytes (agranulocytes)

Neutrophils (granulocytes)

ical clinical findings requires a bone marrow biopsy, usually of the posterior superior iliac spine.

Blood counts show thrombocytopenia and neutropenia. A differential leukocyte count determines cell type. Lumbar puncture detects meningeal involvement.

Treatment

Systemic chemotherapy aims to eradicate leukemic cells and induce remission. Chemotherapy varies according to the type of leukemia:

• meningeal leukemia—intrathecal instillation of methotrexate or cytarabine with cranial radiation

• ALL—vincristine, prednisone, high-dose cytarabine, L-asparaginase, AMSA, and daunorubicin. Because

there's a 40% risk of meningeal leukemia in ALL, intrathecal methotrexate or cytarabine is given. Radiation therapy is given for testicular infiltration.

• AML—a combination of I.V. daunorubicin and cytarabine or, if these drugs fail to induce remission, a combination of cyclophosphamide, vincristine, prednisone, or methotrexate; high-dose cytarabine alone or along with other drugs; amsacrine; etoposide; and 5-azacytidine and mitoxantrone

• acute monoblastic leukemia—cytarabine and thioguanine with daunorubicin or doxorubicin.

A bone marrow transplant may be possible. Treatment also may include antibiotic, antifungal, and antiviral drugs and granulocyte injections to control infection. Transfusions may be given of platelets (to prevent bleeding) and red blood cells (to prevent anemia).

Special considerations
• For the leukemia patient, emphasize comfort, minimize the adverse effects of chemotherapy, promote preservation of veins, manage complications, and provide teaching and psychological support. Because so many of these patients are children, be especially sensitive to their emotional needs and those of their families.

Before treatment:
• Explain the course of the disease, treatments, and adverse effects of medications.
• Teach the patient and his family how to recognize infection (fever, chills, cough, sore throat) and abnormal bleeding (bruising, petechiae) and how to stop such bleeding (applying pressure and ice to the area).
• Promote good nutrition. Explain that chemotherapy may cause weight loss and anorexia, so encourage the patient to eat and drink high-calorie, high-protein foods and beverages. However, chemotherapy and adjunctive prednisone may cause weight gain, so dietary counseling and teaching are helpful.
• Help establish an appropriate rehabilitation program for the patient during remission.

For supportive care:
• Watch for signs of meningeal leukemia (confusion, lethargy, headache). If these occur, know how to manage care after intrathecal chemotherapy. After such instillation, place the patient in Trendelenburg's position for 30 minutes. Force fluids and keep the patient supine for 4 to 6 hours.
• Check the lumbar puncture site often for bleeding.
• If the patient receives cranial radiation, teach him about potential side effects, and do what you can to minimize them.
• Prevent hyperuricemia, a possible result of rapid chemotherapy-induced leukemic cell lysis. Force fluids to about 2 qt (2 L) daily, and give acetazolamide, sodium bicarbonate tablets, and allopurinol. Check urine pH often—it should be above 7.5. Watch for a rash or another hypersensitivity reaction to allopurinol.
• Watch for early signs of cardiotoxicity, such as arrhythmias, and signs of heart failure if the patient receives daunorubicin or doxorubicin.
• Control infection by placing the patient in a private room and imposing reverse isolation, if necessary. (The benefits of reverse isolation are controversial.) Coordinate patient care so the leukemic patient doesn't come in contact with staff who also care for patients with infections or infectious diseases. Avoid using indwelling urinary catheters and giving I.M. injections because they provide an avenue for infection. Screen staff and visitors for contagious diseases, and watch for any signs of infection.
• Provide thorough skin care by keeping the patient's skin and perianal area clean, applying mild lotions or creams to keep skin from drying and cracking, and thoroughly cleaning skin before all invasive skin procedures. Change I.V. tubing according to your hospital's policy. Use strict aseptic technique and a metal scalp vein needle (metal butterfly needle) when starting I.V. lines. If the patient receives total parenteral nutrition, provide scrupulous subclavian catheter care.
• Monitor the patient's temperature every 4 hours; patients with a fever over 101° F (38.3° C) and a decreased WBC count should receive prompt antibiotic therapy.

• Watch for bleeding; if it occurs, apply ice compresses and pressure, and elevate the extremity. Avoid giving I.M. injections, aspirin, and aspirin-containing drugs. Also avoid taking rectal temperatures, giving rectal suppositories, and doing digital examinations.

• Prevent constipation by providing adequate hydration, a high-residue diet, stool softeners, and mild laxatives, and by encouraging walking.

• Control mouth ulceration by checking often for obvious ulcers and gum swelling and by providing frequent mouth care and saline rinses. Tell the patient to use a soft toothbrush and to avoid hot, spicy foods and overuse of commercial mouthwashes. Also check the rectal area daily for induration, swelling, erythema, skin discoloration, or drainage.

• Provide psychological support by establishing a trusting relationship to promote communication. Allow the patient and his family to verbalize their anger and depression. Let the family participate in the patient's care as much as possible.

• Minimize stress by providing a calm, quiet atmosphere that's conducive to rest and relaxation. For children particularly, be flexible with patient care and visiting hours to promote maximum interaction with family and friends and to allow time for schoolwork and play.

• For those patients who are refractory to chemotherapy and in the terminal phase of the disease, supportive nursing care aims to provide comfort; management of pain, fever, and bleeding; and patient and family support. Provide the opportunity for religious counseling. Discuss the option of home or hospice care.

LEUKEMIA, CHRONIC GRANULOCYTIC

Chronic granulocytic leukemia (CGL) is also known as chronic myelogenous (or myelocytic) leukemia. The disease is characterized by the abnormal overgrowth of granulocytic precursors (myeloblasts, promyelocytes, metamyelocytes, and myelocytes) in bone marrow, peripheral blood, and body tissues.

CGL is most common in young and middle-aged adults and is slightly more common in men than in women; it's rare in children. In the United States, approximately 3,000 to 4,000 cases of CGL develop annually, accounting for roughly 20% of all leukemias.

CGL's clinical course proceeds in two distinct phases: the *insidious chronic phase,* with anemia and bleeding abnormalities and, eventually, the *acute phase (blastic crisis),* in which myeloblasts, the most primitive granulocytic precursors, proliferate rapidly. This disease is invariably fatal. Average survival time is 3 to 4 years after onset of the chronic phase and 3 to 6 months after onset of the acute phase.

Causes
Almost 90% of patients with CGL have the Philadelphia (Ph¹) chromosome, an abnormality discovered in 1960 in which the long arm of chromosome 22 is translocated, usually to chromosome 9. Radiation and carcinogenic chemicals may induce this chromosome abnormality. Myeloproliferative diseases also seem to increase the incidence of CGL, and some clinicians

suspect that an unidentified virus causes this disease.

Signs and symptoms

Typically, CGL induces the following clinical effects:

• anemia (fatigue, weakness, decreased exercise tolerance, pallor, dyspnea, tachycardia, and headache)

• thrombocytopenia, with resulting bleeding and clotting disorders (retinal hemorrhage, ecchymoses, hematuria, melena, bleeding gums, nosebleeds, and easy bruising)

• hepatosplenomegaly, with abdominal discomfort and pain in splenic infarction from leukemic cell infiltration.

Other symptoms include sternal and rib tenderness from leukemic infiltrations of the periosteum; low-grade fever; weight loss; anorexia; renal calculi or gouty arthritis from increased uric acid excretion; occasionally, prolonged infection and ankle edema; and, rarely, priapism and vascular insufficiency.

Diagnosis

In patients with typical clinical changes, chromosomal analysis of peripheral blood or bone marrow showing Ph[1] and low leukocyte alkaline phosphatase levels confirms CGL. Other relevant laboratory results include:

• white blood cell abnormalities: leukocytosis (leukocyte count ranging from 50,000/µl to as high as 250,000/µl), occasional leukopenia (leukocyte count less than 5,000/µl), neutropenia (neutrophil count less than 1,500/µl) despite a high leukocyte count, and increased circulating myeloblasts

• hemoglobin: often below 10 g/dl

• hematocrit: low (less than 30%)

• platelet count: thrombocytosis (more than 1 million/µl) common

• serum uric acid level: possibly greater than 8 mg/dl

• bone marrow aspirate or biopsy: hypercellular, characteristically shows bone marrow infiltration by significantly increased number of myeloid elements (a biopsy is done only if aspirate is dry); in the acute phase, myeloblasts predominate

• computed tomography scan: may identify the organs affected by leukemia.

Treatment

Aggressive chemotherapy has so far failed to produce remission in CGL. Consequently, the goal of treatment in the chronic phase is to control leukocytosis and thrombocytosis. The most commonly used oral agents are busulfan and hydroxyurea. Aspirin is commonly given to prevent stroke if the patient's platelet count is over 1 million/µl.

Ancillary CGL treatments include:

• local splenic radiation or splenectomy to increase platelet count and decrease adverse effects related to splenomegaly

• leukapheresis (selective leukocyte removal) to reduce leukocyte count

• allopurinol to prevent secondary hyperuricemia or colchicine to relieve gout caused by elevated serum uric acid levels

• prompt treatment of infections that may result from chemotherapy-induced bone marrow suppression.

During the acute phase of CGL, lymphoblastic or myeloblastic leukemia may develop. Treatment is similar to that for acute lymphoblastic leukemia. Remission, if achieved, is commonly short lived. Bone marrow transplant may produce long asymptomatic periods in the early phase of illness but has been less successful in the accelerated phase. Despite vigorous treatment, CGL usually progresses after onset of the acute phase.

For more information on treatment during the acute phase, see "Acute Leukemia," pages 503 to 507.

Special considerations
• In patients with CGL, meticulous supportive care, psychological support, and careful patient teaching help make the most of remissions and minimize complications.

• Reinforce the explanation of the disease and its treatment to the patient and his family.

Throughout the chronic phase of CGL when the patient is hospitalized:

• If the patient has persistent anemia, schedule laboratory tests and physical care with frequent rest periods in between, and assist the patient with walking if necessary.

• Regularly check the patient's skin and mucous membranes for pallor, petechiae, and bruising.

• To minimize bleeding, suggest a soft-bristled toothbrush, an electric razor, and other safety precautions.

• To minimize the abdominal discomfort of splenomegaly, provide small, frequent meals.

• For the same reason, prevent constipation with a stool softener or laxative as needed. Ask the dietary department to provide a high-bulk diet, and maintain adequate fluid intake.

• To prevent atelectasis, stress the need for coughing and deep-breathing exercises.

Because the patient with CGL often receives outpatient chemotherapy throughout the chronic phase, sound patient teaching is essential:

• Explain the usual adverse effects of chemotherapy. Pay particular attention to dangerous ones such as bone marrow suppression.

• Tell the patient to watch for and immediately report signs and symptoms of infection: any fever over 100° F (37.8° C), chills, redness or swelling, sore throat, and cough.

• Instruct the patient to watch for signs of thrombocytopenia, to immediately apply ice and pressure to any external bleeding site, and to avoid aspirin and aspirin-containing compounds because of the risk of increased bleeding.

• Emphasize the importance of adequate rest to minimize the fatigue of anemia. To minimize the toxic effects of chemotherapy, stress the importance of a high-calorie, high-protein diet.

LEUKEMIA, CHRONIC LYMPHOCYTIC

A generalized, progressive disease that's common in elderly people, chronic lymphocytic leukemia is marked by an uncontrollable spread of abnormal, small lymphocytes in lymphoid tissue, blood, and bone marrow. The prognosis is poor if anemia, thrombocytopenia, neutropenia, bulky lymphadenopathy, and severe lymphocytosis are present.

Nearly all patients with chronic lymphocytic leukemia are men over age 50. According to the American Cancer Society, chronic lymphocytic leukemia accounts for almost one-third of new leukemia cases annually.

Causes
Although the cause of chronic lymphocytic leukemia is unknown, researchers suspect hereditary factors (higher incidence has been recorded within families), still-undefined chromosome abnormalities, and certain immunologic defects (such as ataxia-telangiectasia or acquired agammaglobulinemia). The disease doesn't seem to be associated with radiation exposure.

Signs and symptoms
Chronic lymphocytic leukemia is the most benign and the most slowly progressive form of leukemia. Clinical signs derive from the infiltration of leukemic cells in bone marrow, lymphoid tissue, and organ systems.

Early stages
In early stages, patients usually complain of fatigue, malaise, fever, and nodal enlargement. They're particularly susceptible to infection.

Advanced stages
In advanced stages, patients may experience severe fatigue and weight loss, with liver or spleen enlargement, bone tenderness, and edema from lymph node obstruction. Pulmonary infiltrates may appear when lung parenchyma is involved. Skin infiltrations, manifested by macular to nodular eruptions, occur in about half the cases of chronic lymphocytic leukemia.

As the disease progresses, bone marrow involvement may lead to anemia, pallor, weakness, dyspnea, tachycardia, palpitations, bleeding, and infection. Opportunistic fungal, viral, and bacterial infections commonly occur in late stages.

Diagnosis
Typically, chronic lymphocytic leukemia is an incidental finding during a routine blood test that reveals numerous abnormal lymphocytes. In early stages, the white blood cell (WBC) count is mildly but persistently elevated. Granulocytopenia is the rule, but the WBC count climbs as the disease progresses.

Blood studies also show a hemoglobin count below 11 g, hypogammaglobulinemia, and depressed serum globulin levels. Other common findings include neutropenia (less than 1,500/μl), lymphocytosis (more than 10,000/μl), and thrombocytopenia (less than 150,000/μl). Bone marrow aspiration and biopsy show lymphocytic invasion.

Treatment
Systemic chemotherapy includes alkylating agents, usually chlorambucil or cyclophosphamide, and sometimes steroids (prednisone) when autoimmune hemolytic anemia or thrombocytopenia occurs.

When chronic lymphocytic leukemia causes obstruction or organ impairment or enlargement, local radiation treatment can be used to reduce organ size. Allopurinol can be given to prevent hyperuricemia, a relatively uncommon finding.

Special considerations
• Focus patient care on relieving symptoms and preventing infection. Clean the patient's skin daily with mild soap and water. Frequent soaks may be ordered. Watch for signs of infection: temperature over 100° F (37.8° C), chills, redness, or swelling of any body part.
• Watch for signs of thrombocytopenia (easy bruising, nosebleeds, bleeding gums, and black, tarry stools) and anemia (pale skin, weakness, fatigue, dizziness, and palpitations).
• Advise the patient to avoid aspirin and products containing aspirin. Explain that many medications contain aspirin. Teach him how to recognize aspirin variants on medication labels.
• Explain chemotherapy and its possible adverse effects. If the patient will be discharged, tell him to avoid coming in contact with obviously ill people, especially children with common contagious childhood diseases.
• Urge the patient to eat high-protein foods and drink high-calorie beverages.
• Stress the importance of follow-up care, frequent blood tests, and taking all medications exactly as prescribed.

• Teach the patient the signs of recurrence (swollen lymph nodes in the neck, axilla, and groin; increased abdominal size or discomfort), and tell him to notify his doctor immediately if he detects any of these signs.

• Provide emotional support and be a good listener. Most patients with chronic lymphocytic leukemia are elderly and many are frightened. Try to keep their spirits up by concentrating on little things like improving their personal appearance, providing a pleasant environment, and asking questions about their families. If possible, provide opportunities for their favorite activities.

LICHEN PLANUS

A benign pruritic skin eruption, lichen planus usually produces scaling, purple papules, marked by white lines or spots. Such eruptions occur most often in middle-aged persons and are uncommon in the young or elderly.

Lichen planus, a relatively rare disorder, is found in all geographic areas, with equal distribution among races. In most patients, it resolves spontaneously in 6 to 18 months; in a few, chronic lichen planus may persist for several years.

Causes
The cause of lichen planus is unknown. Eruptions similar to lichen planus have been induced by arsenic, bismuth, and gold. Exposure to developers used in color photography may likewise cause an eruption that's indistinguishable from lichen planus.

Signs and symptoms
Lichen planus may develop suddenly or insidiously. Initial lesions commonly appear on the arms or legs, and evolve into the generalized eruption of flat, glistening, purple papules, marked with white lines or spots (Wickham's striae). These lesions may be linear from scratching or may coalesce into plaques. Lesions often affect the mucous membranes (especially the buccal mucosa), male genitalia, and less often, the nails. Mild to severe pruritus is common.

Diagnosis
Although characteristic skin lesions frequently establish the diagnosis of lichen planus, confirmation may necessitate a skin biopsy.

Treatment
Essentially symptomatic, therapy aims to relieve itching with topical fluorinated steroids and occlusive dressings, intralesional injections of steroids, oatmeal baths, and antihistamines.

Erosive oral lesions and generalized severely pruritic skin lesions may be treated with systemic corticosteroids. Initially, oral prednisone (40 to 60 mg every morning for the first week) may be given; thereafter the dosage is decreased by approximately one-third each week. If the patient experiences a recurrence of itching after the drug is discontinued, he will be given a low dose every other morning. If a drug is suspected as the cause, it should be discontinued.

Special considerations
• Administer medications as necessary, and inform the patient of possible adverse effects, especially drowsiness produced by antihistamines.

• Provide emotional support, and reassure the patient that lichen planus, although annoying, is usually a benign, self-limiting condition.

LISTERIOSIS

This infection is caused by the weakly hemolytic, gram-positive bacillus *Listeria monocytogenes*. It occurs most often in fetuses, in neonates (during the first 3 weeks of life), and in older or immunosuppressed adults.

The infected fetus is usually stillborn or is born prematurely, almost always with lethal listeriosis. This infection produces milder illness in pregnant women and varying degrees of illness in older and immunosuppressed patients; their prognoses depend on the severity of underlying illness.

Causes

The primary method of person-to-person transmission is neonatal infection in utero (through the placenta) or during passage through an infected birth canal. Other possible modes of transmission include inhaling contaminated dust; drinking contaminated, unpasteurized milk; and coming in contact with infected animals, contaminated sewage or mud, or soil contaminated with feces containing *L. monocytogenes*.

Signs and symptoms

Contact with *L. monocytogenes* commonly causes a transient asymptomatic carrier state. But sometimes it produces bacteremia and a febrile, generalized illness. In a pregnant woman, especially during the third trimester, listeriosis causes a mild illness with malaise, chills, fever, and back pain. However, her fetus may suffer severe uterine infection, abortion, premature delivery, or stillbirth.

Transplacental infection may also cause early neonatal death or granulomatosis infantiseptica, which produces organ abscesses in infants.

Infection with *L. monocytogenes* commonly causes meningitis, resulting in tense fontanels, irritability, lethargy, seizures, and coma in neonates; and low-grade fever and personality changes in adults. Fulminant manifestations with coma are rare.

Diagnosis

L. monocytogenes is identified by its diagnostic tumbling motility on a wet mount of the culture. Other supportive diagnostic results include a positive culture of blood, spinal fluid, drainage from cervical or vaginal lesions, or lochia from a mother with an infected infant, but isolation of the organism from these specimens is often difficult. Listeriosis also causes monocytosis.

Treatment

The treatment of choice is ampicillin or penicillin I.V. for 3 to 6 weeks, possibly with gentamicin to increase its effectiveness. Alternate treatments include erythromycin, chloramphenicol, tetracycline, or trimethoprim sulfamethoxazole.

Ampicillin and penicillin G are best for treating meningitis due to *L. monocytogenes* because they cross the blood-brain barrier more easily. Pregnant women require prompt, vigorous treatment to combat fetal infection.

Special considerations

• Deliver specimens to the laboratory promptly. Because very few organisms may be present, take at least 10 ml of spinal fluid for culture.
• Use secretion precautions until a series of cultures are negative. Be especially careful when handling lochia from an infected mother and secretions from her infant's eyes, nose, mouth, and rectum, including meconium.

• Evaluate neurologic status at least every 2 hours. In an infant, check the fontanels for bulging. Maintain adequate I.V. fluid intake, and measure intake and output accurately.

• If the patient has central nervous system depression and becomes apneic, provide respiratory assistance, monitor respirations, and obtain frequent arterial blood gas measurements.

• Provide adequate nutrition by total parenteral nutrition, nasogastric tube feedings, or a soft diet.

• Allow parents to see and, if possible, hold their infant in the intensive care unit. Be flexible about visiting privileges. Keep parents informed of the infant's status and prognosis at all times.

• Reassure the parents of an infected neonate because they may feel guilty about the infant's illness.

• Teach pregnant women to avoid infectious materials on farms where listeriosis is endemic among livestock.

LIFE-THREATENING DISORDER

Liver Abscess

A liver abscess occurs when bacteria or protozoa destroy hepatic tissue, producing a cavity, which fills with infectious organisms, liquefied liver cells, and leukocytes. Necrotic tissue then walls off the cavity from the rest of the liver.

A liver abscess is relatively uncommon and carries a mortality of 30% to 50%. This rate soars to more than 80% with multiple abscesses and to more than 90% with complications, such as rupture into the peritoneum, pleura, or pericardium. About 70% of pyogenic liver abscesses occur among men, usually between ages 20 and 30.

Causes

In pyogenic liver abscesses, the common infecting organisms are *Escherichia coli, Klebsiella, Enterobacter* species, *Salmonella, Staphylococcus,* and *Enterococcus*. Such organisms may invade the liver directly after a liver wound, or they may spread from the lungs, skin, or other organs by the hepatic artery, portal vein, or biliary tract. Pyogenic abscesses are generally multiple and often follow cholecystitis, peritonitis, pneumonia, and bacterial endocarditis.

An amebic abscess results from infection with the protozoa *Entamoeba histolytica,* the organism that causes amebic dysentery. Amebic liver abscesses usually occur singly, in the right lobe.

Signs and symptoms

The clinical manifestations of a liver abscess depend on the degree of involvement. Some patients are acutely ill; in others, the abscess is recognized only at autopsy, after death from another illness.

The onset of symptoms of a pyogenic abscess is usually sudden; in an amebic abscess, the onset is more insidious. Common signs include right abdominal and shoulder pain, weight loss, fever, chills, diaphoresis, nausea, vomiting, and anemia. Signs of right pleural effusion, such as dyspnea and pleural pain, develop if the abscess extends through the diaphragm. Liver damage may cause jaundice.

Diagnosis

A liver scan showing filling defects at the area of the abscess more than ¾″ (2 cm) in diameter, together with characteristic clinical features, confirms this diagnosis. A liver ultrasound may indicate defects caused by the abscess but is less definitive than a liver scan. In a chest X-ray, the diaphragm on the affected side appears raised and fixed. A computed tomography scan confirms the diagnosis.

Relevant laboratory values include elevated levels of serum aspartate aminotransferase, alanine aminotransferase, alkaline phosphatase and bilirubin; an increased white blood cell count; and decreased serum albumin levels. In pyogenic abscess, a blood culture can identify the bacterial agent; in amebic abscess, a stool culture and serologic and hemagglutination tests can isolate *E. histolytica.*

Treatment
If the organism causing the liver abscess is unknown, long-term antibiotic therapy begins immediately with aminoglycosides, cephalosporins, clindamycin, or chloramphenicol.

If cultures demonstrate that the infectious organism is *E. coli,* treatment includes ampicillin; if they show *E. histolytica,* treatment includes emetine, chloroquine, or metronidazole. Drug therapy continues for 2 to 4 months. Surgery is usually avoided, but it may be done for a single pyogenic abscess or for an amebic abscess that fails to respond to antibiotics.

Special considerations
• Provide supportive care, monitor vital signs (especially temperature), and maintain fluid and nutritional intake.
• Administer anti-infectives and antibiotics, as necessary, and watch for possible adverse effects. Stress the importance of compliance with therapy.
• Explain diagnostic and surgical procedures.
• Watch carefully for complications of abdominal surgery, such as hemorrhage or infection.

LIVER CANCER

A rare form of cancer, liver cancer (primary and metastatic hepatic carcinoma) has a high mortality. It's responsible for roughly 2% of all cancers in the United States and for 10% to 50% in Africa and parts of Asia. Liver cancer is most prevalent in men (particularly over age 60); incidence increases with age. It's rapidly fatal, usually within 6 months, from GI hemorrhage, progressive cachexia, hepatic failure, or metastasis.

Most primary liver tumors (90%) originate in the parenchymal cells and are hepatomas (hepatocellular carcinoma, primary lower-cell carcinoma). Some primary tumors originate in the intrahepatic bile ducts and are known as cholangiomas (cholangiocarcinoma, cholangiocellular carcinoma). Rarer tumors include a mixed-cell type, Kupffer cell sarcoma, and hepatoblastomas (which occur almost exclusively in children and are usually resectable and curable).

The liver is one of the most common sites of metastasis from other primary cancers, particularly those of the colon, rectum, stomach, pancreas, esophagus, lung, or breast or melanoma. In the United States, metastatic liver carcinoma occurs over 20 times more often than primary carcinoma and, after cirrhosis, is the leading cause of liver-related death. At times, liver metastasis may appear as a solitary lesion, the first sign of recurrence after a remission.

Causes
The immediate cause of liver cancer is unknown, but it may be a congenital disease in children. Adult liver cancer may result from environmental exposure to carcinogens, such as the chem-

ical compound aflatoxin (a mold that grows on rice and peanuts), thorium dioxide (a contrast medium formerly used in liver radiography), *Senecio* alkaloids and, possibly, androgens and oral estrogens.

Risk factors
Roughly 30% to 70% of patients with hepatomas also have cirrhosis. (Hepatomas are 40 times more likely to develop in a cirrhotic liver than in a normal one.) Whether cirrhosis is a premalignant state, or alcohol and malnutrition predispose the liver to develop hepatomas, is still unclear. Another risk factor is exposure to the hepatitis B virus, although this risk will probably decrease with the availability of the hepatitis B vaccine.

Signs and symptoms
Clinical effects of liver cancer include:
• a mass in the right upper quadrant
• tender, nodular liver on palpation
• severe pain in the epigastrium or the right upper quadrant
• bruit, hum, or rubbing sound if the tumor involves a large part of the liver
• weight loss, weakness, anorexia, fever
• occasional jaundice or ascites
• occasional evidence of metastasis through the venous system to the lungs, from lymphatics to the regional lymph nodes, or by direct invasion of the portal veins
• dependent edema.

Diagnosis
The confirming test for liver cancer is a needle or open biopsy of the liver. Liver cancer is difficult to diagnose in the presence of cirrhosis, but several tests can help identify it:
• *Liver function studies* (aspartate aminotransferase, alanine aminotransferase, alkaline phosphatase, lactate dehydrogenase, and bilirubin) show abnormal liver function.

• *Alpha-fetoprotein level* increases above 500 μg/ml.
• *Chest X-ray* may rule out metastasis.
• *Liver scan* may show filling defects.
• *Arteriography* may define large tumors.
• *Electrolyte studies* may indicate an increased retention of sodium (resulting in functional renal failure) and hypoglycemia, leukocytosis, hypercalcemia, or hypocholesterolemia.

Treatment
Because liver cancer is often in an advanced stage at diagnosis, few hepatic tumors are resectable. A resectable tumor must be a single tumor in one lobe, without cirrhosis, jaundice, or ascites. Resection is done by lobectomy or partial hepatectomy.

Radiation therapy for unresectable tumors is usually palliative. But because of the liver's low tolerance for radiation, this therapy hasn't increased survival.

Another method of treatment is chemotherapy with I.V. fluorouracil, methotrexate, streptozocin, lomustine, or doxorubicin or with regional infusion of fluorouracil or floxuridine (catheters are placed directly into the hepatic artery or left brachial artery for continuous infusion for 7 to 21 days, or permanent implantable pumps are used on an outpatient basis for long-term infusion).

Appropriate treatment for liver metastasis may include resection by lobectomy or chemotherapy with mitomycin or fludarabine. (The results are similar to those in hepatoma.) Liver transplantation is now an alternative for some patients.

Special considerations
• Patient care should emphasize comprehensive supportive measures and emotional support.
• Control edema and ascites. Monitor the patient's diet throughout. Most pa-

tients need a special diet that restricts sodium, fluids (no alcohol allowed), and protein.

• Weigh the patient daily, and note intake and output accurately. Watch for signs of ascites — peripheral edema, orthopnea, or dyspnea on exertion. If ascites is present, measure and record abdominal girth daily.

• To increase venous return and prevent edema, elevate the patient's legs whenever possible.

• Monitor respiratory function. Note any increase in respiratory rate or shortness of breath. Bilateral pleural effusion (noted on chest X-ray) is common, as is metastasis to the lungs. Watch carefully for signs of hypoxemia from intrapulmonary arteriovenous shunting.

• Relieve fever. Administer sponge baths and aspirin suppositories if there are no signs of GI bleeding. Avoid acetaminophen because the diseased liver can't metabolize it. High fever indicates infection and requires antibiotics.

• Provide meticulous skin care. Turn the patient frequently and keep his skin clean to prevent pressure ulcers. Apply lotion to prevent chafing, and administer an antipruritic, such as diphenhydramine, for severe itching.

• Watch for encephalopathy. Many patients develop end-stage symptoms of ammonia intoxication, including confusion, restlessness, irritability, agitation, delirium, asterixis, lethargy and, finally, coma.

• Monitor the patient's serum ammonia level, vital signs, and neurologic status. Be prepared to control ammonia accumulation with sorbitol (to induce osmotic diarrhea), neomycin (to reduce bacterial flora in the GI tract), lactulose (to control bacterial elaboration of ammonia), and sodium polystyrene sulfonate (to lower the potassium level).

• If a transhepatic catheter is used to relieve obstructive jaundice, irrigate it frequently with the prescribed solution (normal saline or, sometimes, 5,000 units of heparin in 500 ml of dextrose 5% in water).

• Monitor vital signs frequently for any indication of bleeding or infection.

• After surgery, give standard postoperative care. Watch for intraperitoneal bleeding and sepsis, which may precipitate a coma. Monitor for renal failure by checking urine output, blood urea nitrogen, and creatinine levels hourly.

• Remember that throughout the course of this intractable illness, your primary concern is to keep the patient as comfortable as possible.

LIFE-THREATENING DISORDER

LUNG ABSCESS

A lung abscess is a lung infection accompanied by pus accumulation and tissue destruction. The abscess may be putrid (due to anaerobic bacteria) or nonputrid (due to anaerobes or aerobes), and often has a well-defined border. The availability of effective antibiotics has made lung abscesses much less common than they were in the past.

Causes
A lung abscess is a manifestation of necrotizing pneumonia, often the result of aspiration of oropharyngeal contents. Poor oral hygiene with dental or gingival (gum) disease is strongly associated with a putrid lung abscess. Septic pulmonary emboli commonly produce cavitary lesions. Infected cystic lung lesions and cavitating bronchial carcinoma must be distinguished from lung abscesses.

Signs and symptoms

The clinical effects of lung abscess include a cough that may produce bloody, purulent, or foul-smelling sputum; pleuritic chest pain; dyspnea; excessive sweating; chills; fever; headache; malaise; diaphoresis; and weight loss.

Complications include rupture into the pleural space, which results in empyema and, rarely, massive hemorrhage. A chronic lung abscess may cause localized bronchiectasis. Failure of an abscess to improve with antibiotic treatment suggests a possible underlying neoplasm or other causes of obstruction.

Diagnosis

The following tests are used to diagnose a lung abscess:
• *Auscultation of the chest* may reveal crackles and decreased breath sounds.
• *Chest X-ray* shows a localized infiltrate with one or more clear spaces, usually containing air-fluid levels.
• *Percutaneous aspiration of an abscess* or *bronchoscopy* may be used to obtain cultures to identify the causative organism. Bronchoscopy is only used if abscess resolution is eventful and the patient's condition permits it.
• *Blood cultures, Gram stain,* and *culture of sputum* are also used to detect the causative organism.
• *White blood cell count* commonly exceeds 10,000/µl.

Treatment

Antibiotic therapy often lasts for months until radiographic resolution or definite stability occurs. Symptoms usually disappear in a few weeks. Postural drainage may facilitate discharge of necrotic material into upper airways, where expectoration is possible; oxygen therapy may relieve hypoxemia. A poor response to therapy requires resection of the lesion or removal of the diseased section of the lung. All patients need rigorous follow-up and serial chest X-rays.

Special considerations

• Provide chest physiotherapy (including coughing and deep breathing).
• Increase fluid intake to loosen secretions, and provide a quiet, restful atmosphere.
• To prevent a lung abscess in the unconscious patient and the patient with seizures, first prevent aspiration of secretions. Do this by suctioning the patient and by positioning him to promote drainage of secretions.
• Provide good mouth care and encourage patients to practice good oral hygiene.

LUNG CANCER

Lung cancer usually develops within the wall or epithelium of the bronchial tree. Its most common types are epidermoid (squamous cell) carcinoma, small cell (oat cell) carcinoma, adenocarcinoma, and large cell (anaplastic) carcinoma.

Although the prognosis is usually poor, it varies with the extent of spread at the time of diagnosis and the growth rate of the specific cell type. Only about 13% of patients with lung cancer survive 5 years after diagnosis. Lung cancer is the most common cause of cancer death in men and is fast becoming the most common cause in women, even though it's largely preventable.

Causes

Most experts agree that lung cancer is attributable to inhalation of carcinogenic pollutants by a susceptible host. Who is most susceptible? Any smoker over age 40, especially if he began to smoke before age 15, has smoked a whole pack or more per day for 20 years, or works with or near asbestos.

Pollutants in tobacco smoke cause progressive lung cell degeneration. Lung cancer is 10 times more common in smokers than in nonsmokers; indeed, 80% of lung cancer patients are smokers.

Cancer risk is determined by the number of cigarettes smoked daily, the depth of inhalation, how early in life smoking began, and the nicotine content of cigarettes. Two other factors also increase susceptibility: exposure to carcinogenic industrial and air pollutants (asbestos, uranium, arsenic, nickel, iron oxides, chromium, radioactive dust, and coal dust), and familial susceptibility.

Signs and symptoms
Because early-stage lung cancer usually produces no symptoms, this disease is often in an advanced state at diagnosis. The following late-stage symptoms often lead to a diagnosis:
• with epidermoid and small cell carcinomas: smoker's cough, hoarseness, wheezing, dyspnea, hemoptysis, and chest pain
• with adenocarcinoma and large cell carcinoma: fever, weakness, weight loss, anorexia, and shoulder pain.

In addition to their obvious interference with respiratory function, lung tumors may also alter the production of hormones that regulate body function or homeostasis. Clinical conditions that result from such changes are known as hormonal paraneoplastic syndromes:
• *Gynecomastia* may result from large cell carcinoma.
• *Hypertrophic pulmonary osteoarthropathy* (bone and joint pain from cartilage erosion due to abnormal production of growth hormone) may result from large cell carcinoma and adenocarcinoma.

• *Cushing's* and *carcinoid syndromes* may result from small cell carcinoma.
• *Hypercalcemia* may result from epidermoid tumors.

Metastatic symptoms vary greatly, depending on the effect of tumors on intrathoracic and distant structures:
• *bronchial obstruction*: hemoptysis, atelectasis, pneumonitis, dyspnea
• *recurrent nerve invasion*: hoarseness, vocal cord paralysis
• *chest wall invasion*: piercing chest pain; increasing dyspnea; severe shoulder pain, radiating down the arm
• *local lymphatic spread*: cough, hemoptysis, stridor, pleural effusion
• *phrenic nerve involvement*: dyspnea; shoulder pain; unilateral paralyzed diaphragm, with paradoxical motion
• *esophageal compression*: dysphagia
• *vena caval obstruction*: venous distention and edema of the face, neck, chest, and back
• *pericardial involvement*: pericardial effusion, tamponade, arrhythmias
• *cervical thoracic sympathetic nerve involvement*: miosis, ptosis, exophthalmos, reduced sweating.

Distant metastasis may involve any part of the body, most commonly the central nervous system, liver, and bone.

Diagnosis
Typical clinical findings may strongly suggest lung cancer, but a firm diagnosis requires further evidence, including the following:
• *Chest X-ray* usually shows an advanced lesion, but it can detect a lesion up to 2 years before symptoms appear. It also indicates tumor size and location.
• *Sputum cytology,* which is 75% reliable, requires a specimen coughed up from the lungs and tracheobronchial tree, *not* postnasal secretions or saliva.
• *Computed tomography (CT) scan* of the chest may help to delineate the tumor's size and its relationship to surrounding structures.

• *Bronchoscopy* can locate the tumor site. Bronchoscopic washings provide material for cytologic and histologic examination. The flexible fiber-optic bronchoscope increases the test's effectiveness.

• *Needle biopsy* of the lungs uses biplane fluoroscopic visual control to detect peripherally located tumors. This allows a firm diagnosis in 80% of patients.

• *Tissue biopsy* of accessible metastatic sites includes supraclavicular and mediastinal node and pleural biopsies.

• *Thoracentesis* allows chemical and cytologic examination of pleural fluid.

Additional studies include preoperative mediastinoscopy or mediastinotomy to rule out involvement of mediastinal lymph nodes (which would preclude curative pulmonary resection).

Other tests to detect metastasis include a bone scan, bone marrow biopsy (recommended in small cell carcinoma), and a CT scan of the brain or abdomen.

After histologic confirmation, staging determines the extent of the disease and helps in planning treatment and predicting the prognosis. (See *Staging lung cancer*, page 520.)

Treatment

Various combinations of surgery, radiation, and chemotherapy may improve the prognosis and prolong survival. Nevertheless, because treatment usually begins at an advanced stage, it's largely palliative.

Surgery

Unless the tumor is nonresectable, or other conditions rule out surgery, excision is the primary treatment for stage I, stage II, or selected stage III squamous cell carcinoma, adenocarcinoma, and large cell carcinoma. Surgery may include partial removal of a lung (wedge resection, segmental resection, lobectomy, radical lobectomy) or total removal (pneumonectomy, radical pneumonectomy).

Radiation

Preoperative radiation therapy may reduce tumor bulk to allow for surgical resection. Preradiation chemotherapy helps improve response rates. Radiation therapy is ordinarily recommended for stage I and stage II lesions, if surgery is contraindicated, and for stage III lesions when the disease is confined to the involved hemithorax and the ipsilateral supraclavicular lymph nodes.

Generally, radiation therapy is delayed until 1 month after surgery, to allow the wound to heal, and is then directed to the part of the chest most likely to develop metastasis. High-dose radiation therapy or radiation implants may also be used.

Chemotherapy

Another treatment is chemotherapy including combinations of fluorouracil, vincristine, mitomycin, cisplatin, and vindesine which produce a response rate of about 40% but have a minimal effect on overall survival. Promising combinations for treating small cell carcinomas include cyclophosphamide with doxorubicin and vincristine; cyclophosphamide with doxorubicin, vincristine, and etoposide; and etoposide with cisplatin, cyclophosphamide, and doxorubicin.

Laser therapy

Still largely experimental, laser energy involves direction of laser energy through a bronchoscope to destroy local tumors.

Special considerations

Comprehensive supportive care and patient teaching can minimize complications and speed recovery from surgery, radiation, and chemotherapy.

STAGING LUNG CANCER

Using the TNM (tumor, node, metastasis) classification system, the American Joint Committee on Cancer stages lung cancer as follows.

Primary tumor
TX—primary tumor can't be assessed, or malignant tumor cells detected in sputum or bronchial washings but undetected by X-ray or bronchoscopy
T0—no evidence of primary tumor
Tis—carcinoma in situ
T1—tumor 3 cm or less in greatest dimension, surrounded by normal lung or visceral pleura; no bronchoscopic evidence of cancer closer to the center of the body than the lobar bronchus
T2—tumor larger than 3 cm; or one that involves the main bronchus and is 2 cm or more from the carina; or one that invades the visceral pleura; or one that's accompanied by atelectasis or obstructive pneumonitis that extends to the hilar region but doesn't involve the entire lung
T3—tumor of any size that extends into neighboring structures, such as the chest wall, diaphragm, or mediastinal pleura; or a tumor in the main bronchus that doesn't involve but is less than 2 cm from the carina; or a tumor that's accompanied by atelectasis or obstructive pneumonitis of the entire lung
T4—tumor of any size that invades the mediastinum, heart, great vessels, trachea, esophagus, vertebral body, or carina; or a tumor with malignant pleural effusion

Regional lymph nodes
NX—regional lymph nodes can't be assessed
N0—no detectable metastasis to lymph nodes
N1—metastasis to the ipsilateral peribronchial or hilar lymph nodes or both
N2—metastasis to the ipsilateral mediastinal or subcarinal lymph nodes or both
N3—metastasis to the contralateral mediastinal or hilar lymph nodes, the ipsilateral or contralateral scalene lymph nodes, or the supraclavicular lymph nodes

Distant metastasis
MX—distant metastasis can't be assessed
M0—no evidence of distant metastasis
M1—distant metastasis

Staging categories
Lung cancer progresses from mild to severe as follows:
Occult carcinoma—TX, N0, M0
Stage 0—Tis, N0, M0
Stage I—T1, N0, M0; T2, N0, M0
Stage II—T1, N1, M0; T2, N1, M0
Stage IIIA—T1, N2, M0; T2, N2, M0; T3, N0, M0; T3, N1, M0; T3, N2, M0
Stage IIIB—any T, N3, M0; T4, any N, M0
Stage IV—any T, any N, M1

Before surgery:
• Supplement and reinforce information about the disease and the surgical procedure.
• Explain expected postoperative procedures, such as the insertion of an indwelling urinary catheter, use of an endotracheal or chest tube (or both), dressing changes, and I.V. therapy.
• Teach the patient how to perform coughing, deep diaphragmatic breathing, and range-of-motion (ROM) exercises.

• Inform the patient that he may take nothing by mouth after midnight the night before surgery, that he'll shower with a soaplike antibacterial agent the night or morning before surgery, and that he'll be given preoperative medications, such as a sedative and an anticholinergic, to dry secretions.

After thoracic surgery:

• Maintain a patent airway, and monitor chest tubes to reestablish normal intrathoracic pressure and prevent postoperative and pulmonary complications.

• Check vital signs every 15 minutes during the first hour after surgery, every 30 minutes during the next 4 hours, and then every 2 hours. Watch for abnormal respiration and other changes.

• Suction the patient often, and encourage him to begin deep breathing and coughing as soon as possible. Check secretions often. Initially, sputum will be thick and dark with blood, but it should become thinner and grayish yellow within a day.

• Monitor and record closed chest drainage. Keep chest tubes patent and draining effectively. Fluctuation in the water seal chamber on inspiration and expiration indicates that the chest tube is patent. Watch for air leaks. Position the patient on the surgical side to promote drainage and lung reexpansion.

• Watch for and report foul-smelling discharge and excessive drainage on dressing. Usually, the dressing is removed after 24 hours, unless the wound appears infected.

• Monitor intake and output. Maintain adequate hydration.

• Watch for and treat infection, shock, hemorrhage, atelectasis, dyspnea, mediastinal shift, and pulmonary embolus.

• To prevent pulmonary embolus, apply antiembolism stockings and encourage ROM exercises.

If the patient is receiving chemotherapy and radiation:

• Explain possible adverse effects of radiation and chemotherapy. Watch for, treat, and (when possible) try to prevent them.

• Ask the dietary department to provide soft, nonirritating foods that are high in protein, and encourage the patient to eat high-calorie between-meal snacks.

• Give antiemetics and antidiarrheals as needed.

• Schedule patient care activities in a way that helps the patient conserve his energy.

• During radiation therapy, administer skin care to minimize skin breakdown. If the patient receives radiation therapy in an outpatient setting, warn him to avoid tight clothing, exposure to the sun, and harsh ointments on his chest. Teach him exercises to help prevent shoulder stiffness.

Teach high-risk patients ways to reduce their chances of developing lung cancer:

• Refer smokers who want to quit to local branches of the American Cancer Society, Smokenders, or other smoking cessation programs; or suggest group therapy, individual counseling, or hypnosis.

• Encourage patients with recurring or chronic respiratory infections and those with chronic lung disease who detect any change in the character of a cough to see their doctor promptly for evaluation.

LUPUS ERYTHEMATOSUS

A chronic inflammatory disorder of the connective tissues, lupus erythematosus appears in two forms: *discoid lupus erythematosus,* which affects only the skin, and *systemic lupus erythematosus (SLE),* which affects multiple organ systems (as well as the skin) and can be fatal. Like rheumatoid arthritis, SLE is characterized by recurring remissions and exacerbations, which are especially common during the spring and summer.

The annual incidence of SLE averages 27.5 cases per 1 million whites and 75.4 cases per 1 million blacks. SLE strikes women 8 times as often as men, increasing to 15 times as often during childbearing years. It occurs worldwide but is most prevalent among Asians and blacks. The prognosis improves with early detection and treatment but remains poor for patients who develop cardiovascular, renal, or neurologic complications or severe bacterial infections.

Causes

The exact cause of SLE remains a mystery, but available evidence points to interrelated immunologic, environmental, hormonal, and genetic factors.

Immune dysregulation

Immune dysregulation, in the form of autoimmunity, is thought to be the prime causative mechanism. In autoimmunity, the body produces antibodies against its own cells, such as the antinuclear antibody (ANA). The formed antigen-antibody complexes can suppress the body's normal immunity, and damage tissues. One significant feature in patients with SLE is their ability to produce antibodies against many different tissue components, such as red blood cells, neutrophils, platelets, lymphocytes, or almost any organ or tissue in the body.

Predisposing factors

Certain predisposing factors may make a person susceptible to SLE. Physical or mental stress, streptococcal or viral infections, exposure to sunlight or ultraviolet light, immunization, pregnancy, and abnormal estrogen metabolism may all affect the development of this disease.

SLE also may be triggered or aggravated by treatment with certain drugs — for example, procainamide, hydralazine, anticonvulsants and, less frequently, penicillins, sulfa drugs, and oral contraceptives.

Signs and symptoms

The onset of SLE may be acute or insidious and produces no characteristic clinical pattern. However, symptoms commonly include fever, weight loss, malaise, fatigue, rashes, and polyarthralgia. SLE may involve every organ system.

Joint and skin effects

In 90% of patients, joint involvement is similiar to that in rheumatoid arthritis. Skin lesions are most commonly an erythematous rash in areas exposed to light. (See *Discoid lupus erythematosus.*) The classic butterfly rash over the nose and cheeks occurs in fewer than 50% of the patients. Ultraviolet rays often provoke or aggravate skin eruptions. Vasculitis can develop (especially in the digits), possibly leading to infarctive lesions, necrotic leg ulcers, or digital gangrene. Raynaud's phenomenon appears in about 20% of patients. Patchy alopecia and painless ulcers of the mucous membranes are common.

DISCOID LUPUS ERYTHEMATOSUS

Discoid lupus erythematosus (DLE) is a form of lupus erythematosus marked by chronic skin eruptions that, if untreated, can lead to scarring and permanent disfigurement. About 1 out of 20 patients with DLE later develops systemic lupus erythematosus (SLE).

Causes
The exact cause of DLE is unknown, but some evidence suggests an autoimmune defect. An estimated 60% of patients with DLE are women in their late twenties or older. This disease is rare in children.

Clinical features
DLE lesions are raised, red, scaling plaques, with follicular plugging and central atrophy. The raised edges and sunken centers give them a coinlike appearance. Although these lesions can appear anywhere on the body, they usually erupt on the face, scalp, ears, neck, and arms or on any part of the body that's exposed to sunlight.

Such lesions can resolve completely or may cause hypopigmentation or hyperpigmentation, atrophy, and scarring. Facial plaques sometimes assume the butterfly pattern characteristic of SLE. Hair tends to become brittle or may fall out in patches.

Diagnosis
As a rule, the patient history and the appearance of the rash itself are diagnostic. A lupus erythematosus cell test is positive in fewer than 10% of patients. A skin biopsy of lesions reveals immunoglobulins or complement components. SLE must be ruled out.

Treatment
Patients with DLE should avoid prolonged exposure to the sun, fluorescent lighting, or reflected sunlight. They should wear protective clothing, use sunscreening agents, avoid engaging in outdoor activities during periods of most intense sunlight (between 10 a.m. and 2 p.m.), and report any changes in the lesions. Drug treatment consists of topical, intralesional, or systemic medication, as in SLE.

Cardiopulmonary and renal effects
About 50% of SLE patients develop signs of cardiopulmonary abnormalities, such as pleuritis, pericarditis, and dyspnea. Myocarditis, endocarditis, tachycardia, parenchymal infiltrates, and pneumonitis also may occur.

Renal effects may include hematuria, proteinuria, urine sediment, and cellular casts and may progress to total kidney failure. Urinary tract infections may result from heightened susceptibility to infection.

Neurologic effects
Seizure disorders and mental dysfunction may indicate neurologic damage. Central nervous system (CNS) involvement may produce emotional instability, psychosis, and organic brain syndrome. Headaches, irritability, and depression are common. (See *Signs of systemic lupus erythematosus*, page 524.)

Systemic effects
Constitutional symptoms of SLE include aching, malaise, fatigue, low-grade or spiking fever, chills, anorexia, and weight loss. Lymph node

SIGNS OF SYSTEMIC LUPUS ERYTHEMATOSUS

Diagnosing systemic lupus erythematosus (SLE) is difficult because SLE often mimics other diseases; symptoms may be vague and vary greatly from patient to patient.

For these reasons, the American Rheumatism Association has issued a list of criteria for classifying SLE, to be used primarily for consistency in epidemiologic surveys. Usually, four or more of these signs are present at some time during the course of the disease:

- malar or discoid rash
- photosensitivity
- oral or nasopharyngeal ulcerations
- nonerosive arthritis (of two or more peripheral joints)
- pleuritis or pericarditis
- profuse proteinuria (exceeding 0.5 g/day) or excessive cellular casts in the urine
- seizures or psychoses
- hemolytic anemia, leukopenia, lymphopenia, or thrombocytopenia
- positive lupus erythematosus cell, anti-DNA, or anti-Smith antibody test or chronic false-positive serologic test for syphilis
- abnormal titer of antinuclear antibody.

Diagnosis

Diagnostic tests for patients with SLE include a complete blood count with differential, which may show anemia and a decreased white blood cell count; platelet count, which may be decreased; erythrocyte sedimentation rate, which is often elevated; and serum electrophoresis, which may show hypergammaglobulinemia.

Specific tests for SLE include the following:

- *ANA, anti-deoxyribonucleic acid (DNA), and lupus erythematosus cell tests* are positive in active SLE; because the anti-DNA test is rarely positive in other conditions, it's the most specific test for SLE. However, if the patient is in remission, anti-DNA results may be reduced or absent (because anti-DNA correlates with disease activity, especially renal involvement, and helps monitor the patient's response to therapy).
- *Urine studies* may show red blood cells and white blood cells, urine casts and sediment, and significant protein loss (more than 0.5 g/24 hours).
- *Blood studies* reveal decreased serum complement (C3 and C4) levels, which indicate active disease.
- *Chest X-ray* may show pleurisy or lupus pneumonitis.
- *Electrocardiography* may show a conduction defect with cardiac involvement or pericarditis.
- *Kidney biopsy* determines the stage of the disease and the extent of renal involvement.

Some patients show a positive *lupus anticoagulant test* and a positive *anticardiolipin test*. Such patients are prone to antiphospholipid syndrome (thrombosis, abortion, and thrombocytopenia).

Treatment

Patients with mild disease require little or no medication. Nonsteroidal anti-inflammatory compounds, including

enlargement (diffuse or local, and nontender), abdominal pain, nausea, vomiting, diarrhea, and constipation may occur. Women may experience irregular menstrual periods or amenorrhea during the active phase of SLE.

Because SLE usually strikes women of childbearing age, questions related to pregnancy often arise. Available evidence indicates that a woman with SLE can have a safe, successful pregnancy if she has no serious renal or neurologic impairment.

aspirin, control arthritis symptoms in many patients. Skin lesions need topical treatment. Corticosteroid creams, such as flurandrenolide, are recommended for acute lesions.

Refractory skin lesions are treated with intralesional corticosteroids or antimalarials such as hydroxychloroquine. Because hydroxychloroquine can cause retinal damage, such treatment requires ophthalmologic examination every 6 months.

Corticosteroids

The treatment of choice, corticosteroids are used for systemic symptoms of SLE, for acute generalized exacerbations, or for serious disease related to vital organ systems, such as pleuritis, pericarditis, lupus nephritis, vasculitis, and CNS involvement. Initial doses equivalent to 60 mg or more of prednisone often bring noticeable improvement within 48 hours.

As soon as symptoms are under control, steroid dosage is tapered down slowly. (Rising serum complement levels and decreasing anti-DNA titers indicate that the patient is responding to the treatment.) Diffuse proliferative glomerulonephritis, a major complication of SLE, requires treatment with large doses of steroids. If renal failure occurs, dialysis or a kidney transplant may be necessary. In some patients, cytotoxic drugs — azathioprine, cyclophosphamide, or methotrexate — may delay or prevent deteriorating renal status. Antihypertensive drugs and dietary changes may also be warranted in renal disease.

Sun protection

The photosensitive patient should wear protective clothing (hat, sunglasses, long sleeves, slacks) and use a sunscreen containing para-aminobenzoic acid when outdoors.

Special considerations

• Careful assessment, supportive measures, emotional support, and patient teaching are all important parts of caring for patients with SLE.
• Watch for constitutional symptoms: joint pain or stiffness, weakness, fever, fatigue, and chills. Observe for dyspnea, chest pain, and any edema of the extremities.
• Note the size, type, and location of skin lesions.
• Check urine for hematuria, scalp for hair loss, and skin and mucous membranes for petechiae, bleeding, ulceration, pallor, and bruising.
• Provide a balanced diet. Foods high in protein, vitamins and iron help maintain optimum nutrition and prevent anemia. However, renal involvement may mandate a low-sodium, low-protein diet.
• Urge the patient to get plenty of rest. Schedule diagnostic tests and procedures to allow adequate rest.
• Explain all tests and procedures. Tell the patient that several blood samples are needed initially, then periodically, to monitor his progress.
• Apply heat packs to relieve joint pain and stiffness.
• Encourage regular exercise to maintain full range of motion (ROM) and prevent contractures. Teach ROM exercises, as well as body alignment and postural techniques. Arrange for physical therapy and occupational counseling as appropriate.
• Explain the expected benefit of prescribed medications, and watch for adverse effects, especially when the patient is taking high doses of corticosteroids.
• Advise the patient receiving cyclophosphamide to maintain adequate hydration. If prescribed, give mesna to prevent hemorrhagic cystitis and ondansetron to prevent nausea and vomiting.

- Monitor vital signs, intake and output, weight, and laboratory reports. Check pulse rates and observe for orthopnea. Check stools and GI secretions for blood.
- Observe for hypertension, weight gain, and other signs of renal involvement.
- Assess for signs of neurologic damage: personality change, paranoid or psychotic behavior, ptosis, or diplopia. Take seizure precautions. If Raynaud's phenomenon is present, warm and protect the patient's hands and feet.
- Offer cosmetic tips, such as suggesting the use of hypoallergenic makeup, and refer the patient to a hairdresser who specializes in scalp disorders.
- Advise the patient to purchase medications in quantity, if possible. Warn against "miracle" drugs for the relief of arthritis symptoms.
- Refer the patient to the Lupus Foundation of America and the Arthritis Foundation as necessary.

LYME DISEASE

A multisystemic disorder, Lyme disease is caused by the spirochete, *Borrelia burgdorferi,* which is carried by the minute tick *Ixodes dammini* or another tick in the Ixodidae family. It often begins in the summer with the classic skin lesion called erythema chronicum migrans (ECM). Weeks or months later, cardiac or neurologic abnormalities sometimes develop, possibly followed by arthritis.

Initially, Lyme disease was identified in a group of children in Lyme, Connecticut. Now Lyme disease is known to occur primarily in three parts of the United States:
- in the northeast, from Massachusetts to Maryland
- in the midwest, in Wisconsin and Minnesota
- in the west, in California and Oregon.

Although Lyme disease is endemic to these areas, cases have been reported in 43 states and 20 other countries, including Germany, Switzerland, France, and Australia.

Causes

Lyme disease occurs when a tick injects spirochete-laden saliva into the bloodstream or deposits fecal matter on the skin. After incubating for 3 to 32 days, the spirochetes migrate out to the skin, causing ECM. Then they disseminate to other skin sites or organs by the bloodstream or lymph system.

The spirochetes' life cycle isn't completely clear: They may survive for years in the joints or they may trigger an inflammatory response in the host and then die.

Signs and symptoms

Typically, Lyme disease has three stages.

Stage 1

ECM heralds stage 1 with a red macule or papule, often at the site of a tick bite. This lesion often feels hot and itchy and may grow to more than 20″ (50 cm) in diameter. Within a few days, more lesions may erupt along with a malar rash, conjunctivitis, or diffuse urticaria. In 3 to 4 weeks, lesions are replaced by small red blotches, which persist for several more weeks.

Malaise and fatigue are constant, but other findings are intermittent: headache, fever, chills, achiness, and regional lymphadenopathy. Less common effects are meningeal irritation, mild encephalopathy, migrating musculoskeletal pain, and hepatitis. A persistent sore throat and dry cough may appear several days before ECM.

Stage 2

Weeks to months later, the second stage begins with neurologic abnormalities — fluctuating meningoencephalitis with peripheral and cranial neuropathy — that usually resolve after days or months. Facial palsy is especially noticeable. Cardiac abnormalities, such as a brief, fluctuating atrioventricular heart block, may also develop.

Stage 3

Characterized by arthritis, stage 3 begins weeks or years later. Migrating musculoskeletal pain leads to frank arthritis with marked swelling, especially in the large joints. Recurrent attacks may precede chronic arthritis with severe cartilage and bone erosion.

Diagnosis

Because isolation of *B. burgdorferi* is unusual in humans and because indirect immunofluorescent antibody tests are marginally sensitive, diagnosis often rests on the characteristic ECM lesion and related clinical findings, especially in endemic areas. Mild anemia and an elevated erythrocyte sedimentation rate, leukocyte count, serum immunoglobulin M level, and aspartate aminotransferase level support the diagnosis.

Treatment

A 10- to 20-day course of oral tetracycline is the treatment of choice for adults. Penicillin and erythromycin are alternates. Oral penicillin is usually prescribed for children. When given in the early stages, these drugs can minimize later complications. When given during the late stages, high-dose penicillin I.V. may be a successful treatment.

Special considerations

- Take a detailed patient history, asking about travel to endemic areas and exposure to ticks.
- Check for drug allergies, and administer antibiotics carefully.
- For a patient with arthritis, help with range-of-motion and strengthening exercises, but avoid overexertion.
- Assess the patient's neurologic function and level of consciousness frequently. Watch for signs of increased intracranial pressure and cranial nerve involvement, such as ptosis, strabismus, and diplopia.
- Check for cardiac abnormalities, such as arrhythmias and heart block.

LYMPHOMAS, MALIGNANT

Also known as non-Hodgkin's lymphomas, and lymphosarcomas, malignant lymphomas are a heterogeneous group of malignant diseases originating in lymph glands and other lymphoid tissue. Nodular lymphomas have a better prognosis than the diffuse form of the disease, but in both, the prognosis is worse than in Hodgkin's disease.

Causes

The cause of malignant lymphomas is unknown, although some theories suggest a viral source. Up to 35,000 new cases appear annually in the United States. Malignant lymphomas are two to three times more common in males than in females and occur in all age-groups.

Although rare in children, these lymphomas occur one to three times more often and cause twice as many

CLASSIFYING MALIGNANT LYMPHOMAS

Staging and classifying systems for malignant lymphomas include the National Cancer Institute's (NCI) system, the Rappaport Histologic Classification, and the Lukes-Collins Classification.

Note: The NCI also cites a "miscellaneous" category, which includes these lymphomas: composite, mycosis fungoides, histiocytic, extramedullary plasmacytoma, and unclassifiable.

N.C.I.	RAPPAPORT	LUKES-COLLINS
LOW GRADE		
• Small lymphocytic	• Diffuse well-differentiated lymphocytic	• Small lymphocytic and plasmacytoid lymphocytic
• Follicular, predominantly small cleaved cell	• Nodular poorly differentiated lymphocytic	• Small cleaved follicular center cell, follicular only, or follicular and diffuse
• Follicular mixed, small and large cell	• Nodular mixed lymphoma	• Small cleaved follicular center cell, follicular; large cleaved follicular center cell, follicular
INTERMEDIATE GRADE		
• Follicular, predominantly large cell	• Nodular histiocytic lymphoma	• Large cleaved or noncleaved follicular center cell, or both, follicular
• Diffuse, small cleaved cell	• Diffuse poorly differentiated lymphoma	• Small cleaved follicular center cell, diffuse
• Diffuse mixed, small and large cell	• Diffuse mixed lymphocytic-histiocytic	• Small cleaved, large cleaved, or large noncleaved follicular center cell, diffuse
• Diffuse large cell, cleaved or noncleaved	• Diffuse histiocytic lymphoma	• Large cleaved or noncleaved follicular center cell, diffuse
HIGH GRADE		
• Diffuse large cell immunoblastic	• Diffuse histiocytic lymphoma	• Immunoblastic sarcoma, T-cell or B-cell type
• Large cell, lymphoblastic	• Lymphoblastic, convoluted or nonconvoluted	• Convoluted T cell
• Small noncleaved cell	• Undifferentiated, Burkitt's and non-Burkitt's diffuse undifferentiated lymphoma	• Small noncleaved follicular center cell

deaths as Hodgkin's disease in children under age 15. Incidence rises with age (median age is 50). These lymphomas seem linked to certain races and ethnic groups, with increased incidence in whites and people of Jewish ancestry.

Signs and symptoms

Usually, the first indication of malignant lymphoma is swelling of the lymph glands, enlarged tonsils and adenoids, and painless, rubbery nodes in the cervical supraclavicular areas. In children, these nodes are usually in the cervical region, and the disease causes dyspnea and coughing.

As the lymphoma progresses, the patient develops symptoms specific to the area involved and systemic complaints of fatigue, malaise, weight loss, fever, and night sweats.

Diagnosis

A positive diagnosis requires histologic evaluation of biopsied lymph nodes; of tonsils, bone marrow, liver, bowel, or skin; or of tissue removed during exploratory laparotomy. A biopsy differentiates malignant lymphoma from Hodgkin's disease. (See *Classifying malignant lymphomas.*)

Other tests include bone and chest X-rays, lymphangiography, a liver and spleen scan, computed tomography scan of the abdomen, and excretory urography. Laboratory tests include a complete blood count (which may show anemia), uric acid level (elevated or normal), serum calcium level (elevated if bone lesions are present), serum protein level (normal), and liver function studies.

Treatment

Radiation therapy is used mainly in the early localized stage of the disease. Total nodal irradiation is often effective for both nodular and diffuse histologies.

Chemotherapy is most effective with multiple combinations of antineoplastic agents. For example, cyclophosphamide, doxorubicin, vincristine (Oncovin), and prednisone (CHOP) can induce a complete remission in 70% to 80% of patients with a nodular histology and in 20% to 55% of patients with a diffuse histology. Other combinations—such as methotrexate, bleomycin, Adriamycin, Cytoxan, vincristine (Oncovin), and prednisone (M-BACOP)—induce prolonged remission and sometimes cure the diffuse form.

Special considerations

• Observe the patient who's receiving radiation or chemotherapy for anorexia, nausea, vomiting, or diarrhea. Plan small, frequent meals scheduled around treatment.

• If the patient can't tolerate oral feedings, administer I.V. fluids and, as necessary, give antiemetics and sedatives.

• Instruct the patient to keep irradiated skin dry.

• Provide emotional support by informing the patient and family about the prognosis and diagnosis and by listening to their concerns. If needed, refer the patient and family to the local chapter of the American Cancer Society for information and counseling.

• Stress the need for continued treatment and follow-up care.

MACULAR DEGENERATION

Macular degeneration, which is atrophy or degeneration of the macular disk, accounts for about 12% of all cases of blindness in the United States and for about 17% of new cases of blindness. It's one of the causes of severe irreversible loss of central vision in elderly people.

Two types of age-related macular degeneration occur. The dry, or *atrophic,* form is characterized by atrophic pigment epithelial changes and is most often associated with a slow, progressive, and mild visual loss. The wet, or *exudative,* form causes rapidly progressive and severe vision loss. It's characterized by subretinal neovascularization that causes leakage, hemorrhage, and fibrovascular scar formation, which produce significant loss of central vision.

Causes

Age-related macular degeneration results from hardening and obstruction of retinal arteries that probably reflect normal degenerative changes. No predisposing conditions have been identified. However, it may be hereditary.

Underlying pathologic changes occur primarily at the level of the retinal pigment epithelium, Bruch's membrane, and choriocapillaris in the macular region. Drusen (bumps), which are common in elderly people, appear as yellow deposits beneath the pigment epithelium and may be prominent in the macula.

Signs and symptoms

The patient notices a change in central vision; for example, he may notice a blank spot in the center of the page when reading.

Diagnosis

The following tests are used to diagnose macular degeneration:
• *indirect ophthalmoscopy:* may reveal gross macular changes
• *I.V. fluorescein angiography:* may show leaking vessels as fluorescein dye flows into the tissues from the subretinal neovascular net
• *Amsler's grid:* reveals visual field loss.

Treatment

Laser photocoagulation reduces the incidence of severe visual loss in patients with subretinal neovascularization.

Special considerations

• Inform patients who have bilateral central vision loss of the visual rehabilitation services that are available to them.
• Special devices, such as low-vision optical aids, are available to improve the quality of life in patients with good peripheral vision.

MAGNESIUM IMBALANCE

Magnesium is the second most common cation in intracellular fluid. Although its major function is to enhance neuromuscular integration, it also stimulates parathyroid hormone (PTH) secretion, thus regulating intracellular fluid calcium levels. Therefore, magnesium deficiency (hypomagnesemia) may result in transient hypoparathyroidism and may interfere with the peripheral action of PTH.

Magnesium may also regulate skeletal muscles through its influence on calcium utilization by depressing acetylcholine release at synaptic junctions. In addition, magnesium activates many enzymes for proper carbohydrate and protein metabolism, aids in cell metabolism and the transport of sodium and potassium across cell membranes, and influences sodium, potassium, calcium, and protein levels.

Approximately one-third of the magnesium taken into the body is absorbed through the small intestine and is eventually excreted in urine; the remaining unabsorbed magnesium is excreted in stools.

Because many common foods contain magnesium, a dietary deficiency is rare. Hypomagnesemia generally follows impaired absorption, too-rapid excretion, or inadequate intake during total parenteral nutrition. It frequently coexists with other electrolyte imbalances, especially low calcium and potassium levels. Magnesium excess (hypermagnesemia) is common in patients with renal failure and excessive intake of magnesium-containing antacids.

Causes

Hypomagnesemia usually results from impaired absorption of magnesium in the intestines or excessive excretion in the urine or stools. Hypermagnesemia results from the kidneys' inability to excrete magnesium that was either absorbed from the intestines or was infused.

Hypomagnesemia

Possible causes include:
- decreased magnesium intake or absorption, as in malabsorption syndrome, chronic diarrhea, or postoperative complications after bowel resection
- chronic alcoholism
- prolonged diuretic therapy, nasogastric suctioning, or administration of parenteral fluids without magnesium salts; starvation or malnutrition
- excessive loss of magnesium, as in severe dehydration and diabetic acidosis
- hyperaldosteronism and hypoparathyroidism, which result in hypokalemia and hypocalcemia
- hyperparathyroidism and hypercalcemia; excessive release of adrenocortical hormones; diuretic therapy.

Hypermagnesemia

Common causes include:
- chronic renal insufficiency
- use of laxatives (magnesium sulfate, milk of magnesia, and magnesium citrate solutions), especially with renal insufficiency
- overuse of magnesium-containing antacids
- severe dehydration (resulting oliguria can cause magnesium retention)
- overcorrection of hypomagnesemia.

SIGNS AND SYMPTOMS OF MAGNESIUM IMBALANCE

DYSFUNCTION	HYPOMAGNESEMIA	HYPERMAGNESEMIA
Neuromuscular	• Hyperirritability, tetany, leg and foot cramps, Chvostek's sign (facial muscle spasms induced by tapping the branches of the facial nerve)	• Diminished reflexes, muscle weakness, flaccid paralysis, respiratory muscle paralysis
Central nervous system	• Confusion, delusions, hallucinations, seizures	• Drowsiness, flushing, lethargy, confusion, diminished sensorium
Cardiovascular	• Arrhythmias, vasomotor changes (vasodilation and hypotension), occasionally, hypertension	• Bradycardia, weak pulse, hypotension, heart block, cardiac arrest (common with serum levels of 25 mEq/L)

Signs and symptoms

Hypomagnesemia causes neuromuscular irritability and cardiac arrhythmias. Hypermagnesemia causes central nervous system and respiratory depression in addition to neuromuscular and cardiac effects. (See *Signs and symptoms of magnesium imbalance.*)

Diagnosis

Decreased serum magnesium levels (less than 1.5 mEq/L) confirm hypomagnesemia; increased levels (greater than 2.5 mEq/L), hypermagnesemia.

Low levels of other serum electrolytes (especially potassium and calcium) often coexist with hypomagnesemia. In fact, unresponsiveness to correct treatment for hypokalemia strongly suggests hypomagnesemia. Similarly, elevated levels of other serum electrolytes are associated with hypermagnesemia.

Treatment

The aim of therapy for magnesium imbalance is identification and correction of the underlying cause.

Hypomagnesemia

Treatment of mild hypomagnesemia consists of daily magnesium supplements I.M. or by mouth; of severe hypomagnesemia, magnesium sulfate I.V. (10 to 40 mEq/L diluted in I.V. fluid). Magnesium intoxication (a possible adverse effect) requires calcium gluconate I.V.

Hypermagnesemia

Therapy for hypermagnesemia includes increased fluid intake and loop diuretics, such as furosemide, with impaired renal function; calcium gluconate (10%), a magnesium antagonist, for temporary relief of symptoms in an emergency; and peritoneal dialysis or hemodialysis if renal function fails or if excess magnesium can't be eliminated.

Special considerations

For patients with hypomagnesemia:
• Monitor serum electrolyte levels (including magnesium, calcium, and potassium) daily for mild deficits and every 6 to 12 hours during replacement therapy.

• Measure intake and output frequently. (Urine output shouldn't fall below 25 ml/hour or 600 ml/day.) Remember, the kidneys excrete excess magnesium, and hypermagnesemia could occur with renal insufficiency.

• Monitor vital signs during I.V. therapy. Infuse magnesium replacement slowly, and watch for bradycardia, heart block, and decreased respiratory rate.

• Have calcium gluconate I.V. available to reverse hypermagnesemia from overcorrection.

• Advise patients to eat foods high in magnesium, such as fish and green vegetables.

• Watch for and report signs of hypomagnesemia in patients with predisposing diseases or conditions, especially those not permitted anything by mouth or who receive I.V. fluids without magnesium.

For patients with hypermagnesemia:
• Frequently assess level of consciousness, muscle activity, and vital signs.

• Keep accurate intake and output records. Provide sufficient fluids for adequate hydration and maintenance of renal function.

• Correct abnormal serum electrolyte levels immediately.

• Be alert for electrocardiogram changes (peaked T waves, increased PR intervals, widened QRS complex).

• Watch patients receiving digitalis glycosides and calcium gluconate simultaneously because excessive calcium enhances digitalis glycoside action, predisposing the patient to digitalis toxicity.

• Advise patients not to abuse laxatives and antacids containing magnesium, particularly elderly patients or those with compromised renal function.

• Watch for signs of hypermagnesemia in predisposed patients. Observe closely for respiratory distress if serum magnesium levels exceed 10 mEq/L.

MALLORY-WEISS SYNDROME

Mild to massive and usually painless bleeding due to a tear in the mucosa or submucosa of the cardia or lower esophagus characterizes Mallory-Weiss syndrome. Such a tear, usually singular and longitudinal, results from prolonged or forceful vomiting. Sixty percent of these tears involve the cardia; 15%, the terminal esophagus; and 25%, the region across the esophagogastric junction. Mallory-Weiss syndrome is most common in men over age 40, especially alcoholics.

Causes

The direct cause of a tear in Mallory-Weiss syndrome is forceful or prolonged vomiting, probably when the upper esophageal sphincter fails to relax during vomiting. This lack of sphincter coordination seems more common after excessive intake of alcohol. Other factors and conditions that may also increase intra-abdominal pressure and predispose to esophageal tearing include coughing, straining during bowel movements, trauma, convulsions, childbirth, hiatal hernia, esophagitis, gastritis, and atrophic gastric mucosa.

Signs and symptoms

Typically, Mallory-Weiss syndrome begins with vomiting of blood or passing large amounts of blood rectally a few hours to several days after normal vomiting. This bleeding, which may be accompanied by epigastric or back pain, may range from mild to massive but is generally more profuse than in esophageal rupture.

In Mallory-Weiss syndrome, the blood vessels are only partially severed, preventing retraction and closure of the lumen. Massive bleeding—most likely when the tear is on the gastric side, near the cardia—may quickly lead to fatal shock.

Diagnosis

Identifying esophageal tears by fiberoptic endoscopy confirms Mallory-Weiss syndrome. These lesions, which usually occur near the gastroesophageal junction, appear as erythematous longitudinal cracks in the mucosa when recently produced and as raised, white streaks surrounded by erythema in older tears. Other helpful diagnostic measures include the following:

• *Angiography* (selective celiac arteriography) can determine the bleeding site but not the cause; this is used when endoscopy isn't available.

• *Gastrotomy* may be performed at the time of surgery.

• *Hematocrit* helps quantify blood loss.

Treatment

Appropriate treatment varies with the severity of bleeding. Usually, GI bleeding stops spontaneously, requiring supportive measures and careful observation but no definitive treatment. However, if bleeding continues, treatment may include:

• angiographic infusion of a vasoconstrictor (vasopressin) into the superior mesenteric artery or direct infusion into a vessel that leads to the bleeding artery

• transcatheter embolization or thrombus formation with an autologous blood clot or other hemostatic material (insertion of artificial material, such as a shredded absorbable gelatin sponge or, less often, the patient's own clotted blood through a catheter into the bleeding vessel to aid thrombus formation)

• surgery to suture each laceration (for massive recurrent or uncontrollable bleeding).

Special considerations

• Evaluate respiratory status, monitor arterial blood gas measurements, and administer oxygen as necessary.

• Assess the amount of blood loss, and record related symptoms, such as hematemesis and melena (including color, amount, consistency, and frequency).

• Monitor hematologic status (hemoglobin, hematocrit, red blood cells). Draw blood for coagulation studies (prothrombin time, partial thromboplastin time, and platelet count) and typing and crossmatching.

• Try to keep three units of matched whole blood on hand at all times. Until blood is available, insert a large-bore (14G to 18G) I.V. line, and start a temporary infusion of normal saline solution.

• Monitor the patient's vital signs, central venous pressure, urine output, and overall clinical status.

• Explain diagnostic procedures carefully.

• Keep the patient warm.

• Obtain a history of recent medications taken, dietary habits, and use of alcohol.

• Avoid giving the patient medications that may cause nausea or vomiting. Administer antiemetics, as necessary, to prevent postoperative retching and vomiting.

• Reassure the patient that bleeding will subside.

• Advise the patient to avoid alcohol, aspirin, and other irritating substances.

MASTOIDITIS

Mastoiditis is a bacterial infection and inflammation of the air cells of the mastoid antrum. Although the prognosis is good with early treatment, possible complications include meningitis, facial paralysis, brain abscess, and suppurative labyrinthitis.

Causes

Bacteria that cause mastoiditis include pneumococci, *Haemophilus influenzae, Moraxella catarrhalis,* staphylococci, beta-hemolytic streptococci, and gram-negative organisms. Mastoiditis is usually a complication of chronic otitis media; less frequently, it develops after acute otitis media.

An accumulation of pus under pressure in the middle ear cavity results in necrosis of adjacent tissue and extension of the infection into the mastoid cells. Chronic systemic diseases or immunosuppression may also lead to mastoiditis.

Signs and symptoms

Primary clinical features include a dull ache and tenderness in the area of the mastoid process, low-grade fever, and a thick, purulent discharge that gradually becomes more profuse, possibly leading to otitis externa. Postauricular erythema and edema may push the auricle out from the head; pressure within the edematous mastoid antrum may produce swelling and obstruction of the external ear canal, causing conductive hearing loss.

Diagnosis

X-rays of the mastoid area reveal hazy mastoid air cells; the bony walls between the cells appear decalcified. Examination shows a dull, thickened, and edematous tympanic membrane, if the membrane isn't concealed by obstruction. During examination, the external ear canal is cleaned; persistent oozing into the canal indicates perforation of the tympanic membrane.

Treatment

Effective treatment of mastoiditis consists of intense parenteral antibiotic therapy. If bone damage is minimal, myringotomy drains purulent fluid and provides a specimen of discharge for culture and sensitivity testing.

Recurrent or persistent infection or signs of intracranial complications necessitate simple mastoidectomy. This procedure involves removing the diseased bone and cleaning the affected area, after which a drain is inserted.

A chronically inflamed mastoid requires radical mastoidectomy (excision of the posterior wall of the ear canal, remnants of the tympanic membrane, and the malleus and incus [although these bones are usually destroyed by infection before surgery]). The stapes and facial nerve remain intact.

Radical mastoidectomy, which is seldom necessary because of antibiotic therapy, does not drastically affect the patient's hearing because significant hearing loss precedes surgery. With either surgical procedure, the patient continues oral antibiotic therapy for several weeks after surgery and hospital discharge.

Special considerations

• After simple mastoidectomy, give pain medication as needed. Check the wound drainage and reinforce the dressings. (The surgeon usually changes the dressing daily and removes the drain in 72 hours.)

• Check the patient's hearing, and watch for signs of complications, especially infection (either localized or extending to the brain); facial nerve paralysis, with unilateral facial drooping; bleeding; and vertigo, especially when the patient stands.

• After radical mastoidectomy, the wound is packed with petrolatum gauze or gauze treated with an antibiotic ointment. Give pain medication before the packing is removed, on the fourth or fifth postoperative day.

• Because of stimulation to the inner ear during surgery, the patient may feel dizzy and nauseated for several days afterward. Keep the side rails up, and assist the patient with ambulation. Also, give antiemetics as needed.

• Before discharge, teach the patient and family how to change and care for the dressing. Urge compliance with the prescribed antibiotic treatment, and promote regular follow-up care.

• If the patient is diabetic, evaluate him for malignant otitis externa.

MALIGNANT MELANOMA

A neoplasm that arises from melanocytes, malignant melanoma is relatively rare and accounts for only 1% to 2% of all types of cancer. The three types of melanomas are *superficial spreading melanoma, nodular malignant melanoma,* and *lentigo maligna melanoma.*

Melanoma is slightly more common in women than in men and is rare in children. Peak incidence occurs between ages 50 and 70, although the incidence in younger age-groups is increasing.

Melanoma spreads through the lymphatic and vascular systems and metastasizes to the regional lymph nodes, skin, liver, lungs, and central nervous system (CNS). Its course is unpredictable, however, and recurrence and metastasis may occur more than 5 years after resection of the primary lesion.

The prognosis varies with tumor thickness. Generally, superficial lesions are curable, while deeper lesions tend to metastasize. The Breslow Level Method measures tumor depth from the granular level of the epidermis to the deepest melanoma cell. Melanoma lesions less than 0.76 mm deep have an excellent prognosis, while deeper lesions (more than 0.76 mm) are at risk for metastasis. The prognosis is better for a tumor on an extremity (which is drained by one lymphatic network) than for one on the head, neck, or trunk (drained by several networks).

Causes

Several factors may influence the development of melanoma:

• *Excessive exposure to sunlight.* Melanoma is most common in sunny, warm areas and often develops on parts of the body that are exposed to the sun.

• *Skin type.* Most persons who develop melanoma have blond or red hair, fair skin, and blue eyes; are prone to sunburn; and are of Celtic or Scandinavian ancestry. Melanoma is rare among blacks; when it does develop, it usually arises in lightly pigmented areas (the palms, plantar surface of the feet, or mucous membranes).

• *Hormonal factors.* Pregnancy may increase risk and exacerbate growth.

• *Family history.* Melanoma occurs slightly more often within families.

• *Past history of melanoma.* A person who has had one melanoma is at greater risk of developing a second.

Signs and symptoms

Common sites for melanoma are on the head and neck in men, on the legs in women, and on the backs of people exposed to excessive sunlight. Up to 70% arise from a preexisting nevus. They rarely appear in the conjunctiva, choroid, pharynx, mouth, vagina, or anus.

Suspect melanoma when any skin lesion or nevus enlarges, changes color, becomes inflamed or sore, itches, ulcerates, bleeds, undergoes textural changes, or shows signs of surrounding pigment regression (halo nevus or vitiligo).

Each type of melanoma has special characteristics:

• *Superficial spreading melanoma,* the most common form, usually develops between ages 40 and 50. This lesion arises on an area of chronic irritation. In women, it's most common between the knees and ankles; in blacks and Asians, on the toe webs and soles (lightly pigmented areas subject to trauma).

Characteristically, this melanoma has a red, white, and blue color over a brown or black background and an irregular, notched margin. Its surface is irregular, with small elevated tumor nodules that may ulcerate and bleed. Horizontal growth may continue for many years; when vertical growth begins, the prognosis worsens.

• *Nodular malignant melanoma* usually develops between ages 40 and 50, grows vertically, invades the dermis, and metastasizes early. This lesion is usually a polypoidal nodule, with uniformly dark discoloration (it may be grayish), and looks like a blackberry. Occasionally, this melanoma is flesh-colored, with flecks of pigment around its base (possibly inflamed).

• *Lentigo maligna melanoma* is relatively rare. It arises from a lentigo maligna on an exposed skin surface and usually occurs between ages 60 and 70.

This lesion looks like a large (1″ to 2″ [3- to 6-cm]), flat freckle of tan, brown, black, whitish, or slate color, and has irregularly scattered black nodules on the surface. It develops slowly, usually over many years, and eventually may ulcerate. This melanoma commonly develops under the fingernails, on the face, and on the back of the hands.

Diagnosis
A skin biopsy with histologic examination can distinguish malignant melanoma from a benign nevus, seborrheic keratosis, and pigmented basal cell epithelioma; it can also determine tumor thickness. Physical examination, paying particular attention to lymph nodes, can point to metastatic involvement. (See *Staging malignant melanoma,* pages 538 and 539.)

Baseline laboratory studies include a complete blood count with differential, erythrocyte sedimentation rate, platelet count, liver function studies, and urinalysis. Depending on the depth of tumor invasion and metastasis, baseline diagnostic studies may also include a chest X-ray and computed tomography (CT) scan of the chest and abdomen. Signs of bone metastasis may call for a bone scan; CNS metastasis, a CT scan of the brain.

Treatment
A patient with malignant melanoma requires surgical resection to remove the tumor. The extent of resection depends on the size and location of the primary lesion. Closure of a wide resection may require a skin graft. Surgical treatment may also include regional lymphadenectomy.

Deep primary lesions may merit adjuvant chemotherapy and biotherapy to eliminate or reduce the number of tumor cells. Radiation therapy is usually reserved for metastatic disease; it doesn't prolong survival but may reduce tumor size and relieve pain.

Regardless of the treatment method, melanomas require close, long-term follow-up to detect metastasis and recurrences. About 13% of recurrences develop more than 5 years after the primary surgery.

Special considerations
• Management of the melanoma patient requires careful physical, psychological, and social assessment. Preoperative teaching, meticulous postoperative care, and psychological support can make the patient more comfortable, speed recovery, and prevent complications.

• After diagnosis, review the explanation of treatment options. Tell the patient what to expect before and

STAGING MALIGNANT MELANOMA

Several systems exist for staging malignant melanoma, including the TNM (tumor, node, metastasis) system, developed by the American Joint Committee on Cancer, and Clark's system, which classifies tumor progression according to skin layer penetration.

Primary tumor
TX—primary tumor can't be assessed
T0—no evidence of primary tumor
Tis—melanoma in situ (atypical melanotic hyperplasia, severe melanotic dysplasia), not an invasive lesion (Clark's level I)
T1—tumor 0.75 mm thick or less that invades the papillary dermis (Clark's level II)
T2—tumor between 0.75 and 1.5 mm thick, or tumor invades the interface between the papillary and reticular dermis (Clark's level III), or both
T3—tumor between 1.5 and 4 mm thick, or tumor invades the reticular dermis (Clark's level IV), or both
T3a—tumor between 1.5 and 3 mm thick

T3b—tumor between 3 and 4 mm thick
T4—tumor more than 4 mm thick, or tumor invades subcutaneous tissue (Clark's level V), or tumor has one or more satellites within 2 cm of the primary tumor
T4a—tumor more than 4 mm thick, or tumor invades subcutaneous tissue, or both
T4b—one or more satellites exist within 2 cm of the primary tumor

Regional lymph nodes
NX—regional lymph nodes can't be assessed
N0—no evidence of regional lymph node involvement
N1—metastasis 3 cm or less in greatest dimension in any regional lymph node
N2—metastasis greater than 3 cm in greatest dimension in any regional lymph node, or in-transit metastasis, or both

after surgery, what the wound will look like, and what type of dressing he'll have.
• Warn the patient that the donor site for a skin graft may be as painful as the tumor excision site, if not more so. Honestly answer any questions he may have about surgery, chemotherapy, and radiation.
• After surgery, be careful to prevent infection. Check dressings often for excessive drainage, foul odor, redness, or swelling.
• If surgery included lymphadenectomy, minimize lymphedema by applying an antiembolism stocking and instructing the patient to keep the extremity elevated.
• During chemotherapy, know which adverse reactions to expect and take measures to minimize them. For instance, give an antiemetic to reduce nausea and vomiting.

When preparing for discharge:
• Emphasize the need for close followup to detect recurrences early. Explain that recurrences and metastasis, if they occur, are often delayed, so follow-up must continue for years.
• Tell the patient how to recognize signs of recurrence.

Distant metastasis
MX—distant metastasis can't be assessed
M0—no evidence of distant metastasis
M1—distant metastasis
M1a—metastasis in skin, subcutaneous tissue, or lymph nodes beyond the regional nodes
M1b—visceral metastasis

Staging categories
Malignant melanoma progresses from mild to severe as follows:
Stage I—T1, N0, M0; T2, N0, M0
Stage II—T3, N0, M0
Stage III—T4, N0, M0; any T, N1, M0; any T, N2, M0
Stage IV—any T, any N, M1

Clark's levels

Level I — Epidermis
Level II — Papillary dermis
Level III
Level IV — Reticular dermis
Level V — Subcutaneous tissue

• Provide psychological support. Encourage the patient to verbalize his fears.

In advanced metastatic disease:
• Control and prevent pain with consistent, regularly scheduled administration of analgesics. *Don't* wait to relieve pain until after it occurs.
• Make referrals for home care, social services, and spiritual and financial assistance as needed.
• If the patient is dying, identify the needs of patient, family, and friends, and provide appropriate support and care.

To help prevent malignant melanoma, stress the detrimental effects of overexposure to solar radiation, especially to fair-skinned, blue-eyed patients. Recommend that they use a sunblock or sunscreen. In all physical examinations, especially in fair-skinned people, look for unusual nevi or other skin lesions.

MELASMA

A patchy, hypermelanotic skin disorder, melasma (also known as chloasma or mask of pregnancy) poses a serious cosmetic problem. Although it tends to occur equally in all races, the light-brown color characteristic of melasma is most evident in dark-skinned whites. Melasma affects females more often than males; it may be chronic but is never life-threatening.

Causes

The cause of melasma is unknown. Histologically, hyperpigmentation results from increased melanin production, although the number of melanocytes remains normal. Melasma may be related to the increased hormonal levels associated with pregnancy, ovarian carcinoma, and the use of oral contraceptives.

Progestational agents, phenytoin, and mephenytoin may also contribute to this disorder. Exposure to sunlight stimulates melasma, but it may develop without any apparent predisposing factor.

Signs and symptoms

Typically, melasma produces large, brown, irregular patches, symmetrically distributed on the forehead, cheeks, and sides of the nose. Less commonly, these patches may occur on the neck, upper lip, and temples.

Diagnosis

Observation of characteristic dark patches on the face usually confirms melasma. The patient history may reveal predisposing factors.

Treatment

Management consists primarily of application of bleaching agents containing 2% to 4% hydroquinone, to inhibit melanin synthesis. This medication is applied twice daily for up to 8 weeks. Adjunctive measures include avoidance of exposure to sunlight, use of sunscreens, and discontinuation of oral contraceptives.

Special considerations

• Advise the patient to avoid exposure by using sunscreens and wearing protective clothing. Bleaching agents may help but may require repeated treatments to maintain the desired effect. Cosmetics may help mask deep pigmentation.

• Reassure the patient that melasma is treatable. It may fade spontaneously with protection from sunlight, postpartum, and after discontinuing oral contraceptives. Serial photographs help show the patient that patches are improving.

MÉNIÈRE'S DISEASE

Also known as endolymphatic hydrops, Ménière's disease is a labyrinthine dysfunction that produces severe vertigo, sensorineural hearing loss, and tinnitus. It usually affects adults, men slightly more often than women, between ages 30 and 60. After multiple attacks over several years, this disorder leads to residual tinnitus and hearing loss.

Causes

Ménière's disease may result from overproduction or decreased absorption of endolymph, which causes endolymphatic hydrops or endolymphatic hypertension, with consequent degeneration of the vestibular and cochlear hair cells.

This condition may stem from autonomic nervous system dysfunction that produces a temporary constriction of blood vessels supplying the inner ear. In some women, premenstrual edema may precipitate attacks of Ménière's disease.

Signs and symptoms
Ménière's disease produces three characteristic effects: severe vertigo, tinnitus, and sensorineural hearing loss. Fullness or blocked feeling in the ear is also quite common. Violent paroxysmal attacks last from 10 minutes to several hours. During an acute attack, other symptoms include severe nausea, vomiting, sweating, giddiness, and nystagmus. Also, vertigo may cause loss of balance and falling to the affected side.

To lessen these symptoms, the patient may assume a characteristic posture—lying on the unaffected ear and looking in the direction of the affected ear. Initially, the patient may be asymptomatic between attacks, except for residual tinnitus that worsens during an attack.

Such attacks may occur several times a year, or remissions may last as long as several years. These attacks become less frequent as hearing loss progresses (usually unilateral); they may cease when hearing loss is total.

Diagnosis
The presence of all three typical symptoms suggests Ménière's disease. Audiometric studies indicate a sensorineural hearing loss and loss of discrimination and recruitment. Electronystagmography, electrocochleography, a computed tomography scan, magnetic resonance imaging, and X-rays of the internal meatus may be necessary for differential diagnosis.

Treatment
In Ménière's disease, treatment with atropine may stop an attack in 20 to 30 minutes. Epinephrine or diphenhydramine may be necessary in a severe attack; dimenhydrinate, meclizine, diphenhydramine, or diazepam may be effective in a milder attack.

Long-term management includes use of a diuretic or vasodilator and restricted sodium intake (less than 2 g/day). Prophylactic antihistamines or mild sedatives (phenobarbital, diazepam) may also be helpful. If Ménière's disease persists after 2 years of treatment, produces incapacitating vertigo, or resists medical management, surgery may be necessary. Destruction of the affected labyrinth permanently relieves symptoms but at the expense of irreversible hearing loss. Systemic streptomycin is reserved for patients in whom the disease is bilateral and no other treatment can be considered.

Special considerations
If the patient is in the hospital during an attack of Ménière's disease:
• Advise him against reading and exposure to glaring lights to reduce dizziness.
• Keep the side rails of the patient's bed up to prevent falls. Tell him not to get out of bed or walk without assistance.
• Instruct the patient to avoid sudden position changes and any tasks that vertigo makes hazardous because an attack can begin quite rapidly.

Before surgery:
• If the patient is vomiting, record fluid intake and output and characteristics of vomitus. Administer antiemetics, as necessary, and give small amounts of fluid frequently.

After surgery:
• Record intake and output carefully.
• Tell the patient to expect dizziness and nausea for 1 or 2 days after surgery.
• Give prophylactic antibiotics and antiemetics as required.

MENINGITIS

In meningitis, the brain and the spinal cord meninges become inflamed, usually as a result of bacterial infection. Such inflammation may involve all three meningeal membranes—the dura mater, arachnoid, and pia mater.

The prognosis is good and complications are rare, especially if the disease is recognized early and the infecting organism responds to antibiotics. However, mortality in untreated meningitis is 70% to 100%. The prognosis is poorer for infants and elderly people.

Causes

Meningitis is almost always a complication of another bacterial infection—bacteremia (especially from pneumonia, empyema, osteomyelitis, and endocarditis), sinusitis, otitis media, encephalitis, myelitis, or brain abscess—usually caused by *Neisseria meningitidis, Haemophilus influenzae, Streptococcus pneumoniae,* and *Escherichia coli.*

Meningitis may also follow skull fracture, a penetrating head wound, lumbar puncture, or ventricular shunting procedures. Aseptic meningitis may result from a virus or other organism. Sometimes no causative organism can be found.

Meningitis often begins as an inflammation of the pia-arachnoid, which may progress to congestion of adjacent tissues and destroy some nerve cells.

Signs and symptoms

Typical signs include the following features.

Cardinal signs

The cardinal signs of meningitis are those of infection (fever, chills, malaise) and of increased intracranial pressure (headache, vomiting, and, rarely, papilledema).

Meningeal irritation

Signs of meningeal irritation include nuchal rigidity, positive Brudzinski's and Kernig's signs, exaggerated and symmetrical deep tendon reflexes, and opisthotonos (a spasm in which the back and extremities arch backward so that the body rests on the head and heels).

Other manifestations

Other features of meningitis are sinus arrhythmias; irritability; photophobia, diplopia, and other visual problems; and delirium, deep stupor, and coma. An infant may show signs of infection but often is simply fretful and refuses to eat. Such an infant may vomit a great deal, leading to dehydration; this prevents a bulging fontanel and thus masks this important sign of increased intracranial pressure (ICP).

As the illness progresses, twitching, seizures (in 30% of infants), or coma may develop. Most older children have the same symptoms as adults. In subacute meningitis, onset may be insidious.

Diagnosis

A lumbar puncture showing typical findings in cerebrospinal fluid (CSF) and positive Brudzinski's and Kernig's signs usually establish this diagnosis. (See *Two telltale signs of meningitis.*) The lumbar puncture usually indicates elevated CSF pressure from obstructed CSF outflow at the arachnoid villi. The fluid may appear cloudy or milky white, depending on the number of white blood cells present. CSF protein levels tend to be high; glucose levels may be low. (In subacute menin-

Two Telltale Signs of Meningitis

To test for *Brudzinski's sign,* place the patient in a dorsal recumbent position; then put your hands behind his neck and bend it forward. Pain and resistance may indicate meningeal inflammation, neck injury, or arthritis. But if the patient also flexes the hips and knees in response to this manipulation, chances are he has meningitis.

To test for *Kernig's sign,* place the patient in a supine position. Flex his leg at the hip and knee, then straighten the knee. Pain or resistance points to meningitis.

gitis, CSF findings may vary.) CSF culture and sensitivity tests usually identify the infecting organism, unless it's a virus.

Other useful tests include the following:
• *Cultures* of blood, urine, and nose and throat secretions; a *chest X-ray; electrocardiography;* and a physical examination, with special attention to skin, ears, and sinuses, can uncover the primary infection site.
• *Blood tests* commonly reveal leukocytosis and serum electrolyte abnormalities.
• *Computed tomography scan* can rule out cerebral hematoma, hemorrhage, or tumor.

Treatment

In meningitis, treatment includes appropriate antibiotic therapy and vigorous supportive care.

Antibiotics

Usually, I.V. antibiotics are given for at least 2 weeks and are followed by oral antibiotics. Such antibiotics include penicillin G, ampicillin, or nafcillin. However, if the patient is allergic to penicillin, anti-infective therapy includes tetracycline, chloramphenicol, or kanamycin.

Other drugs include a digitalis glycoside, such as digoxin, to control arrhythmias, mannitol to decrease cerebral edema, an anticonvulsant (usually given I.V.) or a sedative to reduce restlessness, and aspirin or acetaminophen to relieve headache and fever.

Supportive care

Supportive measures include bed rest, fever reduction, and measures to prevent dehydration. Isolation is necessary if nasal cultures are positive. Of course, treatment includes appropriate therapy for any coexisting conditions, such as endocarditis or pneumonia.

To prevent meningitis, prophylactic antibiotics are sometimes used after ventricular shunting procedures, skull fracture, or penetrating head wounds, but this use is controversial.

Special considerations

• Assess neurologic function often. Observe the patient's level of consciousness, and check for signs of increased ICP (plucking at the bedcovers, vomiting, seizures, a change in motor function and vital signs). Also watch for signs of cranial nerve involvement (ptosis, strabismus, diplopia).
• Watch for deterioration in the patient's condition, which may signal an impending crisis. (See *Ominous signs in meningitis.*)
• Monitor fluid balance. Maintain adequate fluid intake to avoid dehydration, but avoid fluid overload because of the danger of cerebral edema. Measure central venous pressure and intake and output accurately.
• Watch for adverse reactions to I.V. antibiotics and other drugs. To avoid infiltration and phlebitis, check the I.V. site often, and change the site according to hospital policy.
• Position the patient carefully to prevent joint stiffness and neck pain. Turn him often, according to a planned positioning schedule. Assist with range-of-motion exercises.
• Maintain adequate nutrition and elimination. It may be necessary to provide small, frequent meals or supplement these meals with nasogastric tube or parenteral feedings.
• To prevent constipation and minimize the risk of increased ICP resulting from straining during defecation, give the patient a mild laxative or stool softener.
• Ensure the patient's comfort. Provide mouth care regularly. Maintain a quiet environment. Darkening the room may decrease photophobia.
• Relieve headache with a nonnarcotic analgesic, such as aspirin or acetamin-

ophen, as needed. (Narcotics interfere with accurate neurologic assessment.)
• Provide reassurance and support. The patient may be frightened by his illness and frequent lumbar punctures. If he's delirious or confused, attempt to reorient him often.
• Reassure the family that the delirium and behavior changes caused by meningitis usually disappear.
• If a severe neurologic deficit appears permanent, refer the patient to a rehabilitation program as soon as the acute phase of this illness has passed.
• To help prevent development of meningitis, teach patients with chronic sinusitis or other chronic infections the importance of proper medical treatment.
• Follow strict aseptic technique when treating patients with head wounds or skull fractures.

MENINGOCOCCAL INFECTIONS

Two major meningococcal infections (meningitis and meningococcemia) are caused by the gram-negative bacteria *Neisseria meningitidis,* which also causes primary pneumonia, purulent conjunctivitis, endocarditis, sinusitis, and genital infection.

Meningococcemia occurs as simple bacteremia, fulminant meningococcemia and, rarely, chronic meningococcemia. It often accompanies meningitis. (For more information on meningitis, see "Meningitis," pages 542 to 545.) Meningococcal infections may occur sporadically or in epidemics; virulent infections may be fatal within a matter of hours.

Causes
Meningococcal infections occur most often among children (ages 6 months to 1 year) and men, usually military recruits, because of overcrowding.

N. meningitidis has seven serogroups (A, B, C, D, X, Y, Z); group A causes most epidemics. These bacteria are often present in upper respiratory flora. Transmission takes place through inhalation of an infected droplet from a carrier (an estimated 2% to 38% of the population). The bacteria then localize in the nasopharynx.

Following an incubation period of approximately 3 or 4 days, the bacteria spread through the bloodstream to the joints, skin, adrenal glands, lungs, and central nervous system. The tissue damage that results (possibly due to the effects of bacterial endotoxins) produces symptoms and, in fulminant meningococcemia and meningococcal bacteremia, progresses to hemorrhage, thrombosis, and necrosis.

Signs and symptoms
Clinical features of meningococcal infection vary. Symptoms of *meningococcal bacteremia* include a sudden, spiking fever; headache; sore throat; cough; chills; myalgia (in the back and legs); arthralgia; tachycardia; tachypnea; mild hypotension; and a petechial, nodular, or maculopapular rash.

In 10% to 20% of patients, this progresses to *fulminant meningococcemia,* with extreme prostration, enlargement of skin lesions, disseminated intravascular coagulation (DIC), and shock. Unless it is treated promptly, fulminant meningococcemia results in death from respiratory or heart failure in 6 to 24 hours.

Characteristics of *chronic meningococcemia* include intermittent fever, maculopapular rash, joint pain, and enlarged spleen.

Diagnosis

Isolation of *N. meningitidis* through a positive blood culture, cerebrospinal fluid (CSF) culture, or lesion scraping confirms the diagnosis except in nasopharyngeal infections, because *N. meningitidis* exists as part of the normal nasopharyngeal flora.

Tests that support the diagnosis include counterimmunoelectrophoresis of the CSF or blood, a low white blood cell count and, in patients with skin or adrenal hemorrhages, decreased platelet and clotting levels. Diagnostic evaluation must rule out Rocky Mountain spotted fever and vascular purpuras.

Treatment

As soon as meningococcal infection is suspected, treatment begins with large doses of aqueous penicillin G, ampicillin, or a cephalosporin, such as cefoxitin and moxalactam; or, for the patient who's allergic to penicillin, chloramphenicol I.V. Therapy may also include mannitol for cerebral edema, heparin I.V. for DIC, dopamine for shock, and digoxin and a diuretic if congestive heart failure develops.

Supportive measures include fluid and electrolyte maintenance, proper ventilation (patent airway and oxygen, if necessary), insertion of an arterial or central venous pressure (CVP) line to monitor cardiovascular status, and bed rest.

Chemoprophylaxis with rifampin or minocycline is useful for hospital workers who come in close contact with the patient; minocycline can also temporarily eradicate the infection in carriers.

Special considerations

• The dosages of I.V. antibiotics should be adjusted as necessary to maintain blood and CSF drug levels.
• Enforce bed rest in early stages. Provide a dark, quiet, restful environment.
• Maintain adequate ventilation with oxygen or a ventilator, if necessary. Suction and turn the patient frequently.
• Keep accurate intake and output records to maintain proper fluid and electrolyte levels. Monitor blood pressure, pulse, arterial blood gas levels, and CVP.
• Watch for complications, such as DIC, arthritis, endocarditis, and pneumonia.
• If the patient is receiving chloramphenicol, monitor his complete blood count.
• Check the patient's drug history for allergies before giving antibiotics.

To prevent the spread of meningococcal infection:
• Impose respiratory isolation until the patient has received antibiotic therapy for 24 hours.
• Label all meningococcal specimens. Deliver them to the laboratory quickly because meningococci are very sensitive to changes in humidity and temperature.
• Report all meningococcal infections to public health department officials.

MENTAL RETARDATION

The American Association on Mental Retardation (AAMR) defines mental retardation as "significantly subaverage general intellectual function existing concurrently with deficits in adaptive behavior manifesting itself during the developmental period (before age 18)." An estimated 1% to 3% of the population is mentally retarded, demonstrating an IQ below 70 and associated difficulty in carrying out tasks required for personal independence.

Retardation commonly is accompanied by other physical and emotional disorders that may constitute handicaps in themselves. Mental retardation places a significant burden on patients and their families, resulting in stress, frustration, and family problems.

Causes

A specific cause is identifiable in only about 25% of mentally retarded people and, of these, only 10% are potentially curable. In the remaining 75%, predisposing factors, such as deficient prenatal or perinatal care, inadequate nutrition, poor social environment, and poor child-rearing practices, contribute significantly to mental retardation.

Prenatal screening for genetic defects (such as Tay-Sachs disease) and counseling for families at risk for specific defects have reduced the incidence of genetically transmitted mental retardation.

Signs and symptoms

The observable effects of mental retardation are deviations from normal adaptive behaviors, ranging from learning disabilities and uncontrollable behavior to severe cognitive and motor skill impairment. The earlier a child's adaptive deficit is recognized and he's placed in a special learning program, the more likely he is to achieve age-appropriate adaptive behaviors. If the patient is older, review his adaptation to his environment.

The family of a patient who's mentally retarded may report many problems stemming from frustration, fear, and exhaustion. These problems, such as financial difficulties, abuse, and divorce, can compromise the child's care. Physical examination may reveal signs of abuse or neglect.

People who are mentally retarded may exhibit signs and symptoms of other disorders, such as cleft lip, congenital heart defects, and cerebral palsy, as well as decreased resistance to infection.

Diagnosis

A score below 70 on a standardized IQ test confirms mental retardation. The recognized levels of mental retardation are as follows:
- mild: IQ 50–55 to approximately 70
- moderate: IQ 35–40 to 50–55
- severe: IQ 20–25 to 35–40
- profound: IQ less than 20–25.

The IQ test primarily predicts school performance and must be supplemented by other diagnostic tests, such as those described below.

Adaptive behavior evaluations

The Adaptive Behavior Scale deals with behaviors important to activities of daily living. This test evaluates self-help skills (toileting and eating), physical and social development, language, socialization, and time and number concepts. It also examines inappropriate behaviors (such as violent or destructive acts, withdrawal, and self-abusive or sexually aberrant behavior).

Age-appropriate adaptive behaviors are assessed by using developmental screening tests such as the Denver Developmental Screening test. These tests compare the subject's functional level with the normal level for the same chronologic age. The greater the discrepancy between chronologic and developmental age, the more severe the retardation.

In children, the functional level is based on sensorimotor skills, self-help skills, and socialization. In adolescents and adults, it's based on academic skills, reasoning and judgment skills, and social skills.

Treatment

Effective management requires an interdisciplinary team approach. A primary goal is to develop the patient's strengths. Another major goal is the development of social adaptive skills.

Mentally retarded children require special education and training, ideally beginning in infancy. An individualized, effective education program can optimize the quality of life for even the profoundly retarded.

The prognosis for mentally retarded people is related more to timing and aggressive treatment, personal motivation, training opportunities, and associated conditions than to the degree of mental retardation itself.

With good support systems, many mentally retarded people become productive members of society. Successful management leads to independent functioning and occupational skills for some and a sheltered environment for others.

Special considerations
• Support the parents of a child diagnosed with mental retardation. They may be overwhelmed by caretaking and financial concerns and may have difficulty accepting and bonding with their child.
• Remember that the mentally retarded child has all the ordinary needs of a normal child plus those created by his handicap. The child especially needs affection, acceptance, stimulation, and prudent, consistent discipline. He's less able to cope if rejected, overprotected, or forced beyond his abilities.
• When caring for a hospitalized retarded patient, promote continuity of care by acting as a liaison for parents and other health care professionals.
• During hospitalization, continue training programs already in place, but remember that illness may bring on some regression.
• For the parents of a severely retarded child, suggest ways to cope with the guilt, frustration, and exhaustion that often accompany caring for such a child. The parents may need an extensive teaching and discharge planning program, including physical care procedures, stress reduction techniques, support services, and referral to developmental programs.
• Ask the social services department to explore community resources.
• Teach parents how to care for the special needs of the retarded child. Suggest that they contact the AAMR.
• Teach retarded adolescents how to deal with physical changes and sexual maturation. Encourage them to participate in appropriate sex education classes. A mentally retarded person may have difficulty expressing his sexual concerns because of limited verbal skills.

LIFE-THREATENING DISORDER

METABOLIC ACIDOSIS

A physiologic state of excess acid accumulation and deficient base bicarbonate, metabolic acidosis is produced by an underlying pathologic disorder. Symptoms result from the body's attempts to correct the acidotic condition through compensatory mechanisms in the lungs, kidneys, and cells.

Metabolic acidosis is more prevalent among children, who are vulnerable to acid-base imbalance because their metabolic rates are faster and their ratios of water to total-body weight are lower. Severe or untreated metabolic acidosis can be fatal.

Causes
Metabolic acidosis usually results from excessive burning of fats in the absence of usable carbohydrates. This can be caused by diabetic ketoacidosis, chronic alcoholism, malnutrition, or a low-carbohydrate, high-fat diet—all of which produce more keto acids than the metabolic process can handle.

Other causes include:
• *anaerobic carbohydrate metabolism:* a decrease in tissue oxygenation or perfusion, as occurs with pump failure after myocardial infarction, or when pulmonary or hepatic disease, shock, or anemia forces a shift from aerobic to anaerobic metabolism, causing a corresponding rise in the lactic acid level
• *renal insufficiency and failure (renal acidosis):* underexcretion of metabolized acids or the inability to conserve base
• *diarrhea and intestinal malabsorption:* loss of sodium bicarbonate from the intestines, causing the bicarbonate buffer system to shift to the acidic side. For example, ureteroenterostomy and Crohn's disease can also induce metabolic acidosis.

Less frequently, metabolic acidosis results from salicylate intoxication (overuse of aspirin), exogenous poisoning, or Addison's disease with an increased excretion of sodium and chloride and the retention of potassium ions (due to a deficiency of glucocorticoids and mineralocorticoids).

Signs and symptoms

In mild acidosis, symptoms of the underlying disease may obscure any direct clinical evidence. Metabolic acidosis typically begins with headache and lethargy, progressing to drowsiness, central nervous system depression, Kussmaul's respirations (as the lungs attempt to compensate by "blowing off" carbon dioxide), stupor and, if the condition is severe and goes untreated, coma and death.

Associated GI distress usually produces anorexia, nausea, vomiting, and diarrhea and may lead to dehydration. Underlying diabetes mellitus may cause fruity breath from catabolism of fats and excretion of accumulated acetone through the lungs.

Diagnosis

Arterial pH below 7.35 confirms metabolic acidosis. In severe acidotic states, pH may fall to 7.10 and partial pressure of arterial carbon dioxide may be normal or less than 34 mm Hg as compensatory mechanisms take hold. The bicarbonate level may be less than 22 mEq/L. Supportive findings include:
• *urine pH:* less than 4.5 in the absence of renal disease
• *serum potassium levels:* greater than 5.5 mEq/L from chemical buffering
• *glucose:* greater than 150 mg/dl in diabetes
• *serum ketone bodies:* elevated in diabetes mellitus
• *plasma lactic acid:* elevated in lactic acidosis
• *anion gap:* greater than 14 mEq/L, indicating metabolic acidosis. These values result from increased acid production or renal insufficiency. (For more information, see *Defining the anion gap,* page 550.)

Treatment

In metabolic acidosis, treatment consists of administration of sodium bicarbonate I.V. for severe cases, evaluation and correction of electrolyte imbalances and, ultimately, correction of the underlying cause. For example, in diabetic ketoacidosis, a low-dose continuous I.V. infusion of insulin is recommended.

Special considerations

• Keep sodium bicarbonate ampules handy for emergency administration. Frequently monitor vital signs, laboratory results, and level of consciousness, since changes can occur rapidly.
• In diabetic acidosis, watch for secondary changes due to hypovolemia, such as decreasing blood pressure.
• Record intake and output accurately to monitor renal function.

DEFINING THE ANION GAP

The anion gap is the difference between concentrations of serum cations and anions — determined by measuring one cation (sodium) and two anions (chloride and bicarbonate). The normal concentration of sodium is 140 mEq/L; of chloride, 102 mEq/L; and of bicarbonate, 26 mEq/L. Thus, the anion gap between *measured* cations (actually sodium alone) and *measured* anions is about 12 mEq/L (140 minus 128).

Concentrations of potassium, calcium, and magnesium (*unmeasured* cations), or proteins, phosphate, sulfate, and organic acids (*unmeasured* anions) are not needed to measure the anion gap. Added together, the concentration of unmeasured cations would be about 11 mEq/L; of unmeasured anions, about 23 mEq/L. Thus, the normal anion gap between unmeasured cations and anions is about 12 mEq/L (23 minus 11) — give or take 2 mEq/L for normal variation.

An anion gap over 14 mEq/L indicates *metabolic acidosis*. It may result from the accumulation of excess organic acids or from retention of hydrogen ions, which chemically bond with bicarbonate and decrease bicarbonate levels.

• Watch for signs of excessive serum potassium — weakness, flaccid paralysis, and arrhythmias, possibly leading to cardiac arrest. After treatment, check for overcorrection to hypokalemia.

• Because metabolic acidosis commonly causes vomiting, position the patient to prevent aspiration.

• Prepare for possible seizures with seizure precautions.

• Provide good oral hygiene. Use sodium bicarbonate washes to neutralize mouth acids, and lubricate the patient's lips with lemon and glycerine swabs.

• To prevent metabolic acidosis, carefully observe patients receiving I.V. therapy or who have intestinal tubes in place, as well as those suffering from shock, hyperthyroidism, hepatic disease, circulatory failure, or dehydration.

• Teach the patient with diabetes how to routinely test urine for sugar and acetone, and encourage strict adherence to insulin or oral antidiabetic therapy.

LIFE-THREATENING DISORDER

METABOLIC ALKALOSIS

A clinical state marked by decreased amounts of acid or increased amounts of base bicarbonate, metabolic alkalosis causes metabolic, respiratory, and renal responses, producing characteristic symptoms — most notably, hypoventilation. This condition always occurs secondary to an underlying cause. With early diagnosis and prompt treatment, the prognosis is good; however, untreated metabolic alkalosis may lead to coma and death.

Causes
Metabolic alkalosis results from loss of acid, retention of base, or renal mechanisms associated with decreased serum levels of potassium and chloride.

Loss of acid

Causes of critical acid loss include vomiting, nasogastric tube drainage or lavage without adequate electrolyte replacement, fistulas, and the use of steroids and certain diuretics (furosemide, thiazides, and ethacrynic acid).

Hyperadrenocorticism is another cause of severe acid loss. Cushing's disease, primary hyperaldosteronism, and Bartter's syndrome, for example, all lead to retention of sodium and chloride, and urinary loss of potassium and hydrogen.

Retention of base

Excessive retention of base can result from excessive intake of bicarbonate of soda or other antacids (usually for treatment of gastritis or peptic ulcer), excessive intake of absorbable alkali (as in milk-alkali syndrome, often seen in patients with peptic ulcers), administration of excessive amounts of I.V. fluids with high concentrations of bicarbonate or lactate, or respiratory insufficiency — all of which cause chronic hypercapnia from high levels of plasma bicarbonate.

Signs and symptoms

Clinical features of metabolic alkalosis result from the body's attempt to correct the acid-base imbalance, primarily through hypoventilation. Other manifestations include irritability, picking at bedclothes (carphology), twitching, confusion, nausea, vomiting, and diarrhea (which aggravates alkalosis).

Cardiovascular abnormalities — such as atrial tachycardia — and respiratory disturbances — such as cyanosis and apnea — also occur. In the alkalotic patient, diminished peripheral blood flow during repeated blood pressure checks may provoke carpopedal spasm in the hand — a possible sign of impending tetany (Trousseau's sign). Uncorrected metabolic alkalosis may progress to seizures and coma.

Diagnosis

A blood pH greater than 7.45 and a bicarbonate level above 29 mEq/L confirm the diagnosis. A partial pressure of carbon dioxide greater than 45 mm Hg indicates attempts at respiratory compensation. Serum electrolyte levels show a potassium level of 3.5 mEq/L and a chloride level of 98 mEq/L. Other characteristic findings include:

• *urine pH* of about 7 (usually)
• *urinalysis* revealing alkalinity after the renal compensatory mechanism begins to excrete bicarbonate
• *electrocardiography* that may show a low T wave, merging with a P wave, and atrial tachycardia.

Treatment

The goal of treatment is to correct the underlying cause of metabolic alkalosis. Therapy for severe alkalosis may include cautious administration of ammonium chloride I.V. to release hydrogen chloride and restore the concentration of extracellular fluid and chloride levels.

Potassium chloride and normal saline solution (except in the presence of congestive heart failure) are usually sufficient to replace losses from gastric drainage. Electrolyte replacement with potassium chloride and discontinuing diuretics correct metabolic alkalosis resulting from potent diuretic therapy.

Special considerations

• Structure care around cautious I.V. therapy, keen observation, and strict monitoring of the patient's status.
• Dilute potassium when giving I.V. containing potassium salts. Monitor the infusion rate to prevent damage to blood vessels; watch for signs of phlebitis.

• When administering ammonium chloride 0.9%, limit the infusion rate to 1 L/4 hours; faster administration may cause hemolysis of red blood cells. Avoid overdosage because it may cause overcorrection to metabolic acidosis. Don't give ammonium chloride to a patient with signs of hepatic or renal disease.

• Watch closely for signs of muscle weakness, tetany, or decreased activity.

• Monitor vital signs frequently, and record intake and output to evaluate respiratory, fluid, and electrolyte status. Remember, respiratory rate usually decreases in an effort to compensate for alkalosis. Hypotension and tachycardia may indicate electrolyte imbalance, especially hypokalemia.

• Observe seizure precautions.

• To prevent metabolic alkalosis, warn patients against overusing alkaline agents. Irrigate nasogastric tubes with isotonic saline solution instead of plain water to prevent loss of gastric electrolytes. Monitor I.V. fluid concentrations of bicarbonate or lactate.

• Teach patients with ulcers to recognize signs of milk-alkali syndrome: a distaste for milk, anorexia, weakness, and lethargy.

MONONUCLEOSIS

Infectious mononucleosis is an acute infectious disease caused by the Epstein-Barr virus (EBV), a member of the herpes group. It primarily affects young adults and children, although in children it's usually so mild that it's often overlooked.

Characteristically, infectious mononucleosis produces fever, sore throat, and cervical lymphadenopathy (the hallmarks of the disease), as well as hepatic dysfunction, increased lymphocytes and monocytes, and devel-

opment and persistence of heterophil antibodies. The prognosis is excellent, and major complications are uncommon.

Causes

Apparently, the reservoir of EBV is limited to humans. Infectious mononucleosis probably spreads by the oropharyngeal route because about 80% of patients carry EBV in their throats during the acute infection and for an indefinite period afterward.

It can also be transmitted by blood transfusion and has been reported after cardiac surgery as the "post-pump perfusion" syndrome. Infectious mononucleosis is probably contagious from before symptoms develop until the fever subsides and oropharyngeal lesions disappear.

Infectious mononucleosis is fairly common in the United States, Canada, and Europe, and both sexes are affected equally. Incidence varies seasonally among college students (most common in the early spring and early fall) but not among the general population.

Signs and symptoms

The symptoms of mononucleosis mimic those of many other infectious diseases, including hepatitis, rubella, and toxoplasmosis. Typically, after an incubation period of about 10 days in children and from 30 to 50 days in adults, infectious mononucleosis produces prodromal symptoms, such as headache, malaise, and fatigue.

After 3 to 5 days, patients typically develop a triad of symptoms: sore throat, cervical lymphadenopathy, and temperature fluctuations, with an evening peak of 101° to 102° F (38.3° to 38.9° C). Splenomegaly, hepatomegaly, stomatitis, exudative tonsillitis, or pharyngitis may also develop.

Sometimes, early in the illness, a maculopapular rash that resembles rubella develops; also, jaundice occurs in about 5% of patients. Major complications are rare but may include splenic rupture, aseptic meningitis, encephalitis, hemolytic anemia, and Guillain-Barré syndrome. Symptoms usually subside about 6 to 10 days after onset of the disease but may persist for weeks.

Diagnosis

Physical examination demonstrating the clinical triad suggests infectious mononucleosis. The following abnormal laboratory results confirm it:

• *White blood cell (WBC) count* increases 10,000 to 20,000/µl during the second and third weeks of illness. Lymphocytes and monocytes account for 50% to 70% of the total WBC count; 10% of the lymphocytes are atypical.

• *Heterophil antibodies* (agglutinins for sheep red blood cells) in serum drawn during the acute illness and at 3- to 4-week intervals rise to four times normal.

• *Indirect immunofluorescence* shows antibodies to EBV and cellular antigens. Such testing is usually more definitive than heterophil antibodies.

• *Liver function studies* are abnormal.

Treatment

Infectious mononucleosis resists prevention and antimicrobial treatment. Thus, therapy is essentially supportive: relief of symptoms, bed rest during the acute febrile period, and aspirin or another salicylate for headache and sore throat.

If severe throat inflammation causes airway obstruction, steroids can be used to relieve swelling and avoid tracheotomy. Splenic rupture, marked by sudden abdominal pain, requires splenectomy. About 20% of patients with infectious mononucleosis will also have streptococcal pharyngotonsillitis; these patients should receive antibiotic therapy for at least 10 days.

Special considerations

Because uncomplicated infectious mononucleosis doesn't require hospitalization, patient teaching is essential. Convalescence may take several weeks, usually until the patient's WBC count returns to normal.

• During the acute illness, stress the need for bed rest. If the patient is a student, tell him he may continue less demanding school assignments and see his friends but should avoid long, difficult projects until after recovery.

• To minimize throat discomfort, encourage the patient to drink milk shakes, fruit juices, and broths, and also to eat cool, bland foods. Advise the use of saline gargles and aspirin as needed.

MOTION SICKNESS

Characterized by a loss of equilibrium, motion sickness is associated with nausea and vomiting that result from irregular or rhythmic movements or from the sensation of motion. Removal of the stimulus restores normal equilibrium.

Causes

Motion sickness may result from excessive stimulation of the labyrinthine receptors of the inner ear by certain motions, such as those experienced in a car, boat, plane, or swing. The disorder may also be caused by confusion in the cerebellum from conflicting sensory input. For example, a visual stimulus (such as a moving horizon) conflicts with labyrinthine perception.

Predisposing factors include tension or fear, offensive odors, or sights and sounds associated with a previous attack. Motion sickness from cars, elevators, trains, and swings is most common in children; from boats and airplanes, in adults. Persons who suffer from one kind of motion sickness are not necessarily susceptible to other types.

Signs and symptoms
Typically, motion sickness induces nausea, vomiting, headache, dizziness, fatigue, diaphoresis, and, occasionally, difficulty in breathing, leading to a sensation of suffocation. These symptoms usually subside when the precipitating stimulus is removed, but they may persist for several hours or days.

Treatment
The best way to treat the disorder is to stop the motion that's causing it. If this isn't possible, the patient will benefit from lying down, closing his eyes, and trying to sleep. Antiemetics, such as dimenhydrinate, cyclizine, meclizine, and scopolamine (transdermal patch), may prevent or relieve motion sickness.

Special considerations
• Tell the patient to avoid exposure to precipitating motion whenever possible. The traveler can minimize motion sickness by sitting where motion is least apparent (near the wing section in an aircraft, in the center of a boat, or in the front seat of an automobile).
• Instruct the person to keep his head still and his eyes closed or focused on a distant and stationary object. An elevated car seat may help prevent motion sickness in a child, by allowing him to see out the front window.
• Instruct the patient to avoid eating or drinking for at least 4 hours before traveling and to take an antiemetic 30 to 60 minutes before traveling or to apply a transdermal scopolamine patch at least 4 hours before traveling.
• Tell the patient with prostate enlargement or glaucoma to consult a doctor or pharmacist before taking antiemetics.

MULTIPLE ENDOCRINE NEOPLASIA

Also known as Werner's syndrome and Sipple's syndrome, multiple endocrine neoplasia (MEN) is a hereditary disorder in which two or more endocrine glands develop hyperplasia, adenoma, or carcinoma, concurrently or consecutively.

Two of the types that occur are well documented: MEN I (Werner's syndrome), the most common form, involves hyperplasia and adenomatosis of the parathyroids, islet cells of the pancreas, pituitary and, rarely, adrenals and thyroid gland; MEN II (Sipple's syndrome) involves medullary carcinoma of the thyroid, with hyperplasia and adenomatosis of the adrenal medulla (pheochromocytoma) and parathyroids.

Causes
MEN usually results from autosomal dominant inheritance, affects both males and females, and may occur at any time from adolescence to old age.

Signs and symptoms
Clinical effects of MEN may develop in various combinations and orders, depending on the glands involved.

MEN I
The most common symptom of MEN I is peptic ulceration, perhaps associated with the Zollinger-Ellison syndrome (marked by increased gastrin production from non-beta islet-cell tumors of the pancreas). Hypoglycemia may result from pancreatic beta islet

cell tumors, with increased insulin production.

When MEN I affects the parathyroids, it produces signs of hyperparathyroidism, including hypercalcemia (because the parathyroids are primarily responsible for the regulation of calcium and phosphorus levels). When MEN causes pituitary tumor, it usually triggers pituitary hyperfunction but can also result in hypofunction. MEN I rarely produces renal or skeletal complications.

MEN II

Characteristic features of MEN II with medullary carcinoma of the thyroid include enlarged thyroid mass, with resultant increased calcitonin, and, occasionally, ectopic corticotropin, causing Cushing's syndrome. With tumors of the adrenal medulla, symptoms include headache, tachyarrhythmias, and hypertension; with adenomatosis or hyperplasia of the parathyroids, symptoms result from renal calculi.

Diagnosis

Investigating symptoms of pituitary tumor, hypoglycemia, hypercalcemia, or GI hemorrhage may lead to a diagnosis of MEN.

Diagnostic tests must be used to carefully evaluate each affected endocrine gland. For example, radioimmunoassay showing increased levels of gastrin in patients with peptic ulceration and Zollinger-Ellison syndrome suggests the need for follow-up studies for MEN I because 50% of patients with Zollinger-Ellison syndrome have MEN. After confirmation of MEN, family members must also be assessed for this inherited syndrome.

Treatment

Treatment must eradicate the tumors. Subsequent therapy controls residual symptoms.

MEN I

In patients with MEN I, peptic ulceration is usually the most urgent clinical feature, so primary treatment emphasizes control of bleeding or resection of necrotic tissue. In hypoglycemia caused by insulinoma, oral administration of diazoxide or glucose can keep blood glucose levels within acceptable limits. Subtotal (partial) pancreatectomy is required to remove the tumor.

Because all parathyroid glands have the potential for neoplastic enlargement, subtotal parathyroidectomy may also be required along with transsphenoidal hypophysectomy.

MEN II

In MEN II, treatment of an adrenal medullary tumor includes antihypertensives and resection of the tumor.

Special considerations

• If MEN involves the pancreas, monitor blood glucose levels frequently. If it affects the adrenal glands, monitor blood pressure closely, especially during drug therapy.
• Manage peptic ulcers, hypoglycemia, and other complications as needed.
• If a pituitary tumor is suspected, watch for signs of pituitary trophic hormone dysfunction, which may affect any of the endocrine glands.
• Be aware that pituitary apoplexy (sudden severe headache, altered level of consciousness, visual disturbances) may occur.

MULTIPLE MYELOMA

Multiple myeloma is also known as malignant plasmacytoma, plasma cell myeloma, and myelomatosis. It's a disseminated neoplasm of marrow plasma cells that infiltrates bone to produce

BENCE JONES PROTEIN

The hallmark of multiple myeloma, this protein (a light chain of gamma globulin) was named for Henry Bence Jones, an English doctor who in 1848 noticed that patients with a curious bone disease excreted a unique protein—unique in that it coagulated at 113° to 131° F (45° to 55° C), then redissolved when heated to boiling.

It remained for Otto Kahler, an Austrian, to demonstrate in 1889 that Bence Jones protein was related to myeloma. Bence Jones protein is not found in the urine of *all* multiple myeloma patients, but it is almost never found in patients without this disease.

osteolytic lesions throughout the skeleton (flat bones, vertebrae, skull, pelvis, ribs); in late stages, it infiltrates the body organs (liver, spleen, lymph nodes, lungs, adrenal glands, kidneys, skin, and GI tract). Multiple myeloma strikes about 9,600 people yearly—mostly men over age 40.

The prognosis is usually poor because the disease is commonly diagnosed after it has already infiltrated the vertebrae, pelvis, skull, ribs, clavicles, and sternum. By then, skeletal destruction is widespread and, without treatment, leads to vertebral collapse; about 52% of patients die within 3 months of diagnosis and 90% within 2 years. Early diagnosis and treatment prolong the lives of many patients by 3 to 5 years. Death usually follows complications, such as infection, renal failure, hematologic disorders, fractures, hypercalcemia, hyperuricemia, or dehydration.

Signs and symptoms

The earliest indication of multiple myeloma is severe, constant back pain that increases with exercise. Arthritic symptoms may also occur: achiness, joint swelling, and tenderness, possibly from vertebral compression. Other effects include fever, malaise, slight evidence of peripheral neuropathy (such as peripheral paresthesia), and pathologic fractures.

As multiple myeloma progresses, symptoms of vertebral compression may become acute, accompanied by anemia, weight loss, thoracic deformities (ballooning), and loss of body height—5″ (13 cm) or more—due to vertebral collapse.

Renal complications such as pyelonephritis (caused by tubular damage from large amounts of Bence Jones protein, hypercalcemia, and hyperuricemia) may occur. (See *Bence Jones protein.*) Severe, recurrent infection, such as pneumonia, may follow damage to nerves associated with respiratory function.

Diagnosis

After a physical examination and a careful medical history, the following diagnostic tests and nonspecific laboratory abnormalities confirm the presence of multiple myeloma:

• *Complete blood count* shows moderate or severe anemia. The differential may show 40% to 50% lymphocytes but seldom more than 3% plasma cells. Rouleaux formation (often the first clue) seen on a differential smear results from an elevated erythrocyte sedimentation rate.

• *Urine studies* may show Bence Jones protein and hypercalciuria. Absence of Bence Jones protein doesn't rule out multiple myeloma; however, its presence almost invariably confirms the disease.

• *Bone marrow aspiration* detects myelomatous cells (an abnormal number of immature plasma cells).

• *Serum electrophoresis* shows an elevated globulin spike that's electrophoretically and immunologically abnormal.

• *X-rays* during early stages may show only diffuse osteoporosis. Eventually, they show multiple, sharply circumscribed osteolytic (punched-out) lesions, particularly on the skull, pelvis, and spine—the characteristic lesions of multiple myeloma.

• *Excretory urography* can assess renal involvement. To avoid precipitation of Bence Jones protein, iothalamate or diatrizoate is used instead of the usual contrast medium. And although oral fluid restriction is usually the standard procedure before excretory urography, patients with multiple myeloma receive large quantities of fluid, generally orally but sometimes I.V., before this test is done.

Treatment

Long-term treatment of multiple myeloma consists mainly of chemotherapy to suppress plasma cell growth and control pain. Some combinations include cyclophosphamide, doxorubicin, and prednisone; and carmustine, doxorubicin, and prednisone. Also, adjuvant local radiation reduces acute lesions, such as collapsed vertebrae, and relieves localized pain.

Other treatment usually includes a melphalan-prednisone combination in high intermittent doses or low continuous daily doses, and analgesics for pain. For spinal cord compression, the patient may require a laminectomy; for renal complications, dialysis.

Because the patient may have bone demineralization and may lose large amounts of calcium into blood and urine, he's a prime candidate for renal calculi, nephrocalcinosis and, eventually, renal failure due to hypercalcemia. Hypercalcemia is managed with hydration, diuretics, corticosteroids, oral phosphate, and I.V. mithramycin to decrease serum calcium levels.

Special considerations

• Push fluids; encourage the patient to drink 3,000 to 4,000 ml of fluids daily, particularly before excretory urography. Monitor his fluid intake and output. (Daily output should be at least 1,500 ml.)

• Encourage the patient to walk. (Immobilization increases bone demineralization and vulnerability to pneumonia.) Give analgesics, as needed, to lessen pain.

• Never allow the patient to walk unaccompanied; be sure that he uses a walker or other supportive aid to prevent falls. Since the patient is particularly vulnerable to pathologic fractures, he may be fearful. Give reassurance, and allow him to move at his own pace.

• Prevent complications by watching for fever or malaise, which may signal the onset of infection, and for signs of other problems, such as severe anemia and fractures.

• If the patient is bedridden, change his position every 2 hours. Give passive range-of-motion and deep-breathing exercises. When he can tolerate them, promote active exercises.

• If the patient is taking melphalan (a phenylalanine derivative of nitrogen mustard that depresses bone marrow), make sure that his blood count (platelet and white blood cell) is taken before each treatment.

• If the patient is taking prednisone, watch closely for infection because this drug often masks it.

• Whenever possible, get the patient out of bed within 24 hours after laminectomy. Check for hemorrhage, motor or sensory deficits, and loss of bowel or bladder function. Position the patient as necessary, maintain alignment, and logroll when turning.

• Provide emotional support for the patient and his family. Help relieve their anxiety by clearly explaining diagnostic tests (including painful procedures, such as bone marrow aspiration and biopsy), treatments, and the prognosis. If needed, refer them to an appropriate community resource for additional support.

MULTIPLE SCLEROSIS

This progressive disease is caused by demyelination of the white matter of the brain and spinal cord. In multiple sclerosis (MS), sporadic patches of demyelination throughout the central nervous system induce widely disseminated and varied neurologic dysfunction. Characterized by exacerbations and remissions, MS is a major cause of chronic disability in young adults.

The prognosis varies. MS may progress rapidly, disabling the patient by early adulthood or causing death within months of onset. However, 70% of patients lead active, productive lives with prolonged remissions.

Causes

The exact cause of MS is unknown, but current theories suggest a slow-acting or latent viral infection and an autoimmune response. Other theories suggest that environmental and genetic factors may also be linked to MS.

Emotional stress, overwork, fatigue, pregnancy, and acute respiratory infections may precede the onset of this illness.

MS usually begins between ages 20 and 40 (the average age of onset is 27). It affects three women for every two men and five whites for every black. Incidence is low in Japan; it's generally higher among urban populations and upper socioeconomic groups. A family history of MS and living in a cold, damp climate increase the risk.

Signs and symptoms

Clinical findings in MS depend on the extent and site of myelin destruction, the extent of remyelination, and the adequacy of subsequent restored synaptic transmission.

Signs and symptoms in MS may be transient, or they may last for hours or weeks. They may wax and wane with no predictable pattern, vary from day to day, and be bizarre and difficult for the patient to describe.

In most patients, visual problems and sensory impairment, such as paresthesia, are the first signs that something may be wrong.

Other characteristic changes include the following:

• *ocular disturbances* – optic neuritis, diplopia, ophthalmoplegia, blurred vision, and nystagmus

• *muscle dysfunction* – weakness, paralysis ranging from monoplegia to quadriplegia, spasticity, hyperreflexia, intention tremor, and gait ataxia

• *urinary disturbances* – incontinence, frequency, urgency, and frequent infections

• *emotional lability* – characteristic mood swings, irritability, euphoria, or depression.

Associated signs and symptoms include poorly articulated or scanning speech and dysphagia. Clinical effects may be so mild that the patient is unaware of them or so bizarre that he appears hysterical.

Diagnosis

Because early symptoms may be mild, years may elapse between onset of the first signs and the diagnosis. Diagnosis of this disorder requires evidence of multiple neurologic attacks and characteristic remissions and exacerbations. Periodic testing and close observation of the patient are necessary, perhaps for years, depending on the course of the disease.

The following tests may be performed:

• *Magnetic resonance imaging* may detect MS lesions.

• *EEG* is abnormal in one-third of patients.

• *Lumbar puncture* shows an elevated gamma globulin fraction of immunoglobulin G but normal total cerebrospinal fluid (CSF) protein levels. An elevated CSF gamma globulin level is significant only when serum gamma globulin levels are normal; it reflects hyperactivity of the immune system due to chronic demyelination. In addition, the WBC level in CSF may be elevated.

• *Electrophoresis* can detect oligoclonal bands of immunoglobulin in CSF. Present in most patients, they can be found even when the percentage of gamma globulin in CSF is normal.

A differential diagnosis must rule out spinal cord compression, foramen magnum tumor (which may mimic the exacerbations and remissions of MS), multiple small strokes, syphilis or another infection, and psychological disturbances.

Treatment

The aim of treatment is to shorten exacerbations and relieve neurologic deficits so that the patient can resume a normal lifestyle.

Drug therapy

Corticotropin, prednisone, or dexamethasone is used to reduce the associated edema of the myelin sheath during exacerbations. Corticotropin and corticosteroids may relieve symptoms and hasten remission, but they don't prevent future exacerbations.

Other drugs used include chlordiazepoxide to mitigate mood swings, baclofen or dantrolene to relieve spasticity, and bethanechol or oxybutynin to relieve urine retention and minimize frequency and urgency.

Interferon beta-1b may be used for ambulatory patients with relapsing and remitting MS to reduce the frequency of exacerbations. Immunosuppressants, such as azathioprine or cyclophosphamide, may suppress the immune response.

Supportive measures

During acute exacerbations, supportive measures include bed rest, comfort measures such as massages, prevention of fatigue, prevention of pressure ulcers, bowel and bladder training (if necessary), administration of antibiotics for bladder infections, physical therapy, and counseling.

Special considerations

• Assist with physical therapy. Increase the patient's comfort with massages and relaxing baths. Make sure the bathwater isn't too hot because hot water may temporarily intensify otherwise subtle symptoms.

• Assist with active, resistive, and stretching exercises to maintain muscle tone and joint mobility, decrease spasticity, improve coordination, and boost morale.

• Teach the patient and family about the chronic course of multiple sclerosis. Emphasize the need to avoid stress, infections, and fatigue and to maintain independence by developing new ways of performing daily activities.

• Be sure to tell the patient to avoid exposure to infections.

• Stress the importance of eating a nutritious, well-balanced diet that contains sufficient fiber to prevent constipation.

• Evaluate the need for bowel and bladder training during hospitalization. Encourage adequate fluid intake and regular urination. Eventually, the patient may require urinary drainage by self-catheterization or, in men, condom drainage.

• Teach the correct use of suppositories to help establish a regular bowel schedule.

• Watch for adverse reactions to drug therapy. For instance, dantrolene may cause muscle weakness and decreased muscle tone.

• Promote emotional stability. Help the patient establish a daily routine to maintain optimal functioning.

• Regulate the patient's activity level. Encourage daily physical exercise with regular rest periods to prevent fatigue.

• Inform the patient that exacerbations are unpredictable, necessitating physical and emotional adjustments in his lifestyle.

• For more information, refer the patient to the National Multiple Sclerosis Society.

MUMPS

Also known as infectious or epidemic parotitis, mumps is an acute viral disease caused by a paramyxovirus. It's most prevalent in children older than age 5 but younger than age 9. Infants under age 1 seldom get this disease because of passive immunity from maternal antibodies. Peak incidence occurs during late winter and early spring. The prognosis for complete recovery is good, although mumps sometimes causes complications.

Causes
The mumps paramyxovirus is found in the saliva of an infected person and is transmitted by droplets or by direct contact. The virus is present in the saliva 6 days before to 9 days after onset of parotid gland swelling; the 48-hour period immediately preceding onset of swelling is probably the time of highest communicability.

The incubation period ranges from 14 to 25 days (the average is 18). One attack of mumps (even if unilateral) almost always confers lifelong immunity.

Signs and symptoms
The clinical features of mumps vary widely. An estimated 30% of susceptible people have subclinical illness.

Mumps usually begins with prodromal symptoms that last for 24 hours and include myalgia, anorexia, malaise, headache, and low-grade fever, followed by an earache that's aggravated by chewing, parotid gland tenderness and swelling, a temperature of 101° to 104° F (38.3° to 40° C), and pain when chewing or when drinking sour or acidic liquids.

Simultaneously with the swelling of the parotid gland or several days later, one or more of the other salivary glands may become swollen. (See *Site of parotid inflammation in mumps.*)

Complications
Epididymo-orchitis and mumps meningitis are complications of mumps. Epididymo-orchitis, which occurs in approximately 25% of postpubertal males who contract mumps, produces abrupt onset of testicular swelling and tenderness, scrotal erythema, lower abdominal pain, nausea, vomiting, fever, and chills.

Swelling and tenderness may last for several weeks; epididymitis may precede or accompany orchitis. In 50% of men with mumps-induced orchitis, the testicles show some atrophy, but *sterility is extremely rare.*

Mumps meningitis complicates mumps in 10% of patients and affects males three to five times more often than females. Symptoms include fever, meningeal irritation (nuchal rigidity, headache, and irritability), vomiting, drowsiness, and a lymphocyte count in cerebrospinal fluid ranging from 500 to 2,000/μl.

Recovery is usually complete. Less common effects are pancreatitis, deafness, arthritis, myocarditis, encephalitis, pericarditis, oophoritis, and nephritis.

Diagnosis

In mumps, a diagnosis is usually made after the characteristic signs and symptoms develop, especially parotid gland enlargement with a history of exposure to mumps. Serologic antibody testing can verify the diagnosis when parotid or other salivary gland enlargement is absent. If comparison between a blood sample obtained during the acute phase of illness and another sample obtained 3 weeks later shows a fourfold rise in antibody titer, the patient most likely had mumps.

Treatment

Effective treatment includes analgesics for pain, antipyretics for fever, and adequate fluid intake to prevent dehydration from fever and anorexia. If the patient can't swallow, I.V. fluid replacement may be necessary.

Special considerations

• Stress the need for bed rest during the febrile period.

• Give analgesics, and apply warm or cool compresses to the neck to relieve pain.

• Give antipyretics and tepid sponge baths for fever.

• To prevent dehydration, encourage the patient to drink fluids; to minimize pain and anorexia, advise him to avoid spicy, irritating foods and those that require a lot of chewing.

• During the acute phase, observe the patient closely for signs of central nervous system involvement, such as an

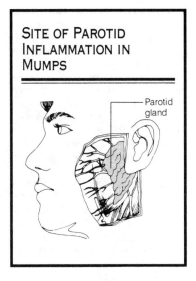

SITE OF PAROTID INFLAMMATION IN MUMPS

Parotid gland

altered level of consciousness and nuchal rigidity.

• Because the mumps virus is present in the saliva throughout the course of the disease, respiratory isolation is recommended until symptoms subside.

• Emphasize the importance of routine immunization with live attenuated mumps virus (paramyxovirus) at age 15 months and for susceptible patients (especially males) who are approaching or are past puberty.

• Remember, immunization within 24 hours of exposure may prevent or attenuate the actual disease. Immunity against mumps lasts at least 12 years.

• Report all cases of mumps to local public health authorities.

MUSCULAR DYSTROPHY

Muscular dystrophy is actually a group of congenital disorders characterized by progressive symmetric wasting of skeletal muscles without neural or sensory defects. Paradoxically, these wasted muscles tend to enlarge because of connective tissue and fat deposits, giving an erroneous impression of muscle strength.

Four main types of muscular dystrophy occur: *Duchenne's (pseudohypertrophic) muscular dystrophy,* which accounts for 50% of all cases; *Becker's (benign pseudohypertrophic) muscular dystrophy; facioscapulohumeral (Landouzy-Dejerine) dystrophy;* and *limbgirdle dystrophy.*

The prognosis varies. Duchenne's muscular dystrophy generally strikes during early childhood and usually results in death by age 20. Patients with Becker's muscular dystrophy live into their 40s. Facioscapulohumeral and limb-girdle dystrophies usually don't shorten life expectancy.

Causes

Muscular dystrophy is caused by various genetic mechanisms. Duchenne's and Becker's muscular dystrophies are X-linked recessive disorders. They result from defects in the gene coding for the muscle protein dystrophin. The defect can be mapped genetically to the Xp21 locus.

Duchenne's and Becker's muscular dystrophies affect males almost exclusively. The incidence of Duchenne's muscular dystrophy in males is 13 to 33 per 100,000. Becker's muscular dystrophy occurs in about 1 to 3 males per 100,000.

Facioscapulohumeral dystrophy is an autosomal dominant disorder. Limbgirdle dystrophy may be inherited in several ways, but it's usually an autosomal recessive trait. These two types affect both sexes about equally.

Signs and symptoms

Although the four types of muscular dystrophy cause progressive muscular deterioration, the degree of severity and the age of onset vary.

Duchenne's muscular dystrophy

Duchenne's muscular dystrophy begins insidiously, between ages 3 and 5. It affects leg and pelvic muscles initially but eventually spreads to the involuntary muscles. Muscle weakness produces a waddling gait, toe-walking, and lordosis.

Children with this disorder have difficulty climbing stairs, fall down often, can't run properly, and their scapulae flare out (or "wing") when they raise their arms. Calf muscles especially become enlarged and firm. Muscle deterioration progresses rapidly, and contractures develop. Usually, these children are confined to wheelchairs by ages 9 to 12.

Late in the disease, progressive weakening of cardiac muscle causes tachycardia, electrocardiogram abnormalities, and pulmonary complications. Death commonly results from sudden heart failure, respiratory failure, or infection.

Becker's muscular dystrophy

Signs and symptoms of Becker's muscular dystrophy resemble those of Duchenne's muscular dystrophy, but they progress more slowly. Although symptoms start around age 5, the patient can still walk well beyond age 15 — sometimes into his 40s.

Facioscapulohumeral dystrophy

This is a slowly progressive and relatively benign form of muscular dystrophy that commonly begins before age 10 but may develop during early adolescence. It weakens the muscles of the face, shoulders, and upper arms at first but eventually spreads to all voluntary muscles, producing a pendulous lower lip and absence of the nasolabial fold.

Early symptoms include inability to pucker the mouth or whistle, abnormal facial movements, and absence of facial movements when laughing or crying. Other signs consist of diffuse facial flattening that leads to a mask-like expression, winging of the scapulae, inability to raise the arms above the head, and, in infants, inability to suckle.

Limb-girdle dystrophy
This form follows a similarly slow course and often causes only slight disability. Usually, it begins between ages 6 and 10; less often, in early adulthood. Muscle weakness first appears in the upper arm and pelvic muscles. Other symptoms include winging of the scapulae, lordosis with abdominal protrusion, waddling gait, poor balance, and inability to raise the arms.

Diagnosis
Typical clinical findings, family history, and test findings are used to diagnose the disease. If another family member has muscular dystrophy, its clinical characteristics can indicate the type of dystrophy the patient has and how he may be affected.

Electromyography typically demonstrates short, weak bursts of electrical activity in affected muscles. A muscle biopsy shows variations in the size of muscle fibers and, in later stages, fat and connective tissue deposits. In Duchenne's dystrophy, a muscle biopsy reveals an absence of dystrophin.

Immunologic and molecular biological techniques now available in specialized medical centers facilitate accurate prenatal and postnatal diagnosis of Duchenne's and Becker's muscular dystrophies. These techniques also help to identify a person as a carrier.

In addition, these newer techniques are replacing muscle biopsy and serum creatine kinase tests as diagnostic procedures.

Treatment
To date, scientists have found no treatment that can stop the progressive muscle impairment of muscular dystrophy. However, orthopedic appliances, as well as exercise, physical therapy, and surgery to correct contractures can help preserve the patient's mobility and independence.

Family members who are carriers of muscular dystrophy should receive genetic counseling regarding the risk of transmitting this disease.

Special considerations
• Comprehensive long-term care and follow-up, patient and family teaching, and psychological support can help the patient and family deal with this disorder.
• When respiratory involvement occurs in Duchenne's muscular dystrophy, encourage coughing, deep-breathing exercises, and diaphragmatic breathing. Teach parents how to recognize early signs of respiratory complications.
• Encourage and assist with active and passive range-of-motion exercises to preserve joint mobility and prevent muscle atrophy.
• Advise the patient to avoid long periods of bed rest and inactivity; if necessary, limit his TV viewing and other sedentary activities.
• Refer the patient for physical therapy. Splints, braces, surgery to correct contractures, trapeze bars, overhead slings, and a wheelchair can help preserve mobility. A footboard or high-topped sneakers and a foot cradle increase comfort and prevent footdrop.
• Because inactivity may cause constipation, encourage adequate fluid intake, increase dietary bulk, and obtain an order for a stool softener.
• Because such a patient is prone to obesity because of reduced physical activity, help him and his family plan

a low-calorie, high-protein, high-fiber diet.

• Always allow the patient plenty of time to perform even simple physical tasks, because he's likely to be slow and awkward.

• Encourage communication among family members to help them deal with the emotional strain this disorder produces. Provide emotional support to help the patient cope with continual changes in body image.

• Help the child with Duchenne's muscular dystrophy maintain peer relationships and realize his intellectual potential by encouraging his parents to keep him in a regular school as long as possible.

• If necessary, refer adult patients for sexual counseling.

• Refer those who must acquire new job skills for vocational rehabilitation. (Contact the Department of Labor and Industry in your state for more information.)

• For information on social services and financial assistance, refer patients and their families to the Muscular Dystrophy Association.

• Refer family members for genetic counseling.

MYASTHENIA GRAVIS

Myasthenia gravis produces sporadic but progressive weakness and abnormal fatigability of striated (skeletal) muscles, which are exacerbated by exercise and repeated movement but improved by anticholinesterase drugs. Usually, this disorder affects muscles innervated by the cranial nerves (face, lips, tongue, neck, and throat), but it can affect any muscle group.

Myasthenia gravis follows an unpredictable course of periodic exacerbations and remissions. (See *Coping with lifelong myasthenia gravis.*) There's no known cure. Drug treatment has improved the prognosis and allows patients to lead relatively normal lives, except during exacerbations. When the disease involves the respiratory system, it may be life-threatening.

Causes
Myasthenia gravis causes a failure in transmission of nerve impulses at the neuromuscular junction. Theoretically, such impairment may result from an autoimmune response, ineffective acetylcholine release, or inadequate muscle fiber response to acetylcholine.

Myasthenia gravis affects 1 in 25,000 people at any age, but incidence peaks between ages 20 and 40. It's three times more common in women than in men in this age-group, but after age 40, the incidence is similar.

About 20% of infants born to myasthenic mothers have transient (or occasionally persistent) myasthenia. This disease may coexist with immune and thyroid disorders; about 15% of myasthenic patients have thymomas. Remissions occur in about 25% of patients.

Signs and symptoms
The dominant symptoms of myasthenia gravis are skeletal muscle weakness and fatigability. In the early stages, easy fatigability of certain muscles may appear with no other findings. Later, it may be severe enough to cause paralysis. Typically, myasthenic muscles are strongest in the morning but weaken throughout the day, especially after exercise. Short rest periods temporarily restore muscle function.

Progressive muscle weakness
More and more muscles become weak, and eventually some muscles may lose function entirely. Resulting symptoms depend on the muscle group affected; they become more intense during

COPING WITH LIFELONG MYASTHENIA GRAVIS

To help the patient deal with his condition, remember the following patient-teaching tips.

• Help the patient plan daily activities to coincide with energy peaks.

• Stress the need for frequent rest periods throughout the day. Emphasize that periodic remissions, exacerbations, and day-to-day fluctuations are common.

• Teach the patient how to recognize adverse effects and signs of toxicity of anticholinesterase drugs (headaches, weakness, sweating, abdominal cramps, nausea, vomiting, diarrhea, excessive salivation, and bronchospasm) and corticosteroids.

• Warn the patient to avoid strenuous exercise, stress, infection, and needless exposure to the sun or cold weather. All of these things may worsen signs and symptoms.

• Advise the patient with diplopia that wearing an eye patch or glasses with one frosted lens may help.

• For more information and an opportunity to meet myasthenic patients who lead full, productive lives, refer the patient to the Myasthenia Gravis Foundation.

menses and after emotional stress, prolonged exposure to sunlight or cold, or infections.

Onset may be sudden or insidious. In many patients, weak eye closure, ptosis, and diplopia are the first signs that something is wrong.

Myasthenic patients usually have blank and expressionless faces and nasal vocal tones. They experience frequent nasal regurgitation of fluids and have difficulty chewing and swallowing. Because of this, they often worry about choking. Their eyelids droop, and they may have to tilt their heads back to see. Their neck muscles may become too weak to support their heads without bobbing.

In patients with weakened respiratory muscles, decreased tidal volume and vital capacity make breathing difficult and predispose to pneumonia and other respiratory tract infections. Respiratory muscle weakness (myasthenic crisis) may be severe enough to require an emergency airway and mechanical ventilation.

Diagnosis

Muscle fatigability that improves with rest strongly suggests a diagnosis of myasthenia gravis. Tests for this neurologic condition record the effect of exercise and subsequent rest on muscle weakness. Electromyography, with repeated neural stimulation, may help confirm this diagnosis.

The classic proof of myasthenia gravis is improved muscle function after an I.V. injection of edrophonium or neostigmine. In myasthenic patients, muscle function improves within 30 to 60 seconds and lasts up to 30 minutes. Long-standing ocular muscle dysfunction may fail to respond to such testing. This test can differentiate a myasthenic crisis from a cholinergic crisis (caused by acetylcholine overactivity at the neuromuscular junction). The acetylcholine receptor antibody titer may be elevated in generalized myasthenia. Evaluation should rule out thyroid disease and thymoma.

Treatment

In myasthenia gravis, treatment is aimed at relieving symptoms. Anticholinesterase drugs, such as neostigmine and pyridostigmine, counteract fatigue and muscle weakness and allow about 80% of normal muscle function. However, these drugs become less effective as the disease worsens. Corticosteroids may relieve symptoms. Plasmapheresis is used in severe exacerbations.

Patients with thymomas require a thymectomy, which may cause remission in some cases of adult-onset myasthenia. Acute exacerbations that cause severe respiratory distress necessitate emergency treatment. Tracheotomy, positive-pressure ventilation, and vigorous suctioning to remove secretions usually produce improvement in a few days.

Because anticholinesterase drugs aren't effective in myasthenic crisis, they're stopped until respiratory function improves. Myasthenic crisis requires immediate hospitalization and vigorous respiratory support.

Special considerations

• Careful baseline assessment, early recognition and treatment of potential crises, supportive measures, and thorough patient teaching can minimize exacerbations and complications. Continuity of care is essential.

• Establish an accurate neurologic and respiratory baseline. Thereafter, monitor tidal volume and vital capacity regularly. The patient may need a ventilator and frequent suctioning to remove accumulating secretions.

• Be alert for signs of an impending crisis (increased muscle weakness, respiratory distress, difficulty in talking or chewing).

• Space administration of drugs evenly, and give them on time to prevent relapses. Be prepared to give atropine for anticholinesterase overdose or toxicity.

• Plan exercise, meals, patient care, and activities to make the most of energy peaks. For example, give medication 20 to 30 minutes before meals to facilitate chewing or swallowing. Allow the patient to participate in self-care.

• When swallowing is difficult, give soft, solid foods instead of liquids to lessen the risk of choking.

• After a severe exacerbation, try to increase social activity as soon as possible.

• Patient teaching is essential because myasthenia gravis is usually a lifelong condition.

MYCOSIS FUNGOIDES

Also known as malignant cutaneous reticulosis and granuloma fungoides, mycosis fungoides (MF) is a rare, chronic, malignant T-cell lymphoma of unknown cause that originates in the reticuloendothelial system of the skin, eventually affecting lymph nodes and internal organs. In the United States, it strikes over 1,000 people of all races annually, mostly between ages 40 and 60.

Unlike other lymphomas, MF allows an average life expectancy of 7 to 10 years after diagnosis. If correctly treated, particularly before it has spread beyond the skin, MF may go into remission for many years. However, after MF has reached the tumor stage, progression to severe disability or death is rapid.

Signs and symptoms

The first sign of MF may be generalized erythroderma, possibly associated with itching. Eventually, MF evolves into varied combinations of infiltrated, thickened, or scaly patches, tumors, or ulcerations.

Diagnosis

A clear diagnosis of MF depends on a history of multiple, varied, and progressively severe skin lesions associated with characteristic histologic evidence of lymphoma cell infiltration of the skin, with or without involvement of lymph nodes or visceral organs. Consequently, this diagnosis is often missed during the early stages until lymphoma cells are sufficiently numerous in the skin to show up in a biopsy.

The following diagnostic tests help confirm MF:
• complete blood count and differential
• a finger-stick smear for Sézary cells (abnormal circulating lymphocytes), which may be present in the erythrodermic variants of MF (Sézary syndrome)
• blood chemistry studies to screen for visceral dysfunction
• chest X-ray
• liver-spleen isotopic scanning
• lymphangiography
• lymph node biopsy to assess lymph node involvement.

These tests also help to stage the disease — a necessary prerequisite to treatment.

Treatment

Depending on the stage of the disease and its rate of progression, past treatment and results, the patient's age and overall clinical status, available treatment facilities, and other factors, treatment of MF may include:
• topical, intralesional, or systemic corticosteroid therapy
• phototherapy
• methoxsalen photochemotherapy
• radiation
• topical, intralesional, or systemic treatment with mechlorethamine hydrochloride
• other systemic chemotherapy.

Application of topical mechlorethamine hydrochloride (nitrogen mustard) is the preferred treatment for inducing remission in pretumorous stages. Plaques may also be treated with sunlight and topical steroids.

Total body electron beam radiation, which is less toxic to internal organs than standard photon beam radiation, has induced remission in some patients with early-stage MF.

Chemotherapy is used primarily for patients with advanced MF; systemic treatment with chemotherapeutic drugs (cyclophosphamide, methotrexate, doxorubicin, bleomycin, etoposide, and steroids) and interferon alfa produces transient regression.

Special considerations

• If the patient has difficulty applying nitrogen mustard to all involved skin surfaces, provide assistance. But wear gloves to prevent contact sensitization and to protect yourself from exposure to chemotherapeutic agents.
• If the patient is receiving drug treatment, report adverse reactions and infection at once.
• The patient who's receiving radiation therapy will probably develop alopecia and erythema. Suggest that he wear a wig to improve his self-image and protect his scalp until hair regrowth begins, and suggest or give medicated oil baths to ease erythema.
• Because pruritus is often worse at night, the patient may need larger bedtime doses of antipruritics or sedatives to ensure adequate sleep. When the patient's symptoms interrupt sleep, postpone early morning care to allow him more sleep.
• The patient with intense pruritus has an overwhelming need to scratch — often to the point of removing epidermis

and replacing pruritus with pain, which some patients find easier to endure. Realize that you can't keep such a patient from scratching; the best you can do is help minimize the damage.

• Advise the patient to keep his fingernails short and clean and to wear a pair of soft, white cotton gloves when itching is unbearable.

• The malignant skin lesions are likely to make the patient depressed, fearful, and self-conscious. Fully explain the disease and its stages to help the patient and his family understand and accept the disease.

MYELITIS AND ACUTE TRANSVERSE MYELITIS

Myelitis, or inflammation of the spinal cord, can result from several diseases. Poliomyelitis affects the cord's gray matter and produces motor dysfunction; leukomyelitis affects only the white matter and produces sensory dysfunction. These types of myelitis can attack any level of the spinal cord, causing partial destruction or scattered lesions.

Acute transverse myelitis, which affects the entire thickness of the spinal cord, produces both motor and sensory dysfunctions. This form of myelitis, which has a rapid onset, is the most devastating.

The prognosis depends on the severity of cord damage and prevention of complications. If spinal cord necrosis occurs, the prognosis for complete recovery is poor. Even without necrosis, residual neurologic deficits usually persist after recovery. Patients who develop spastic reflexes early in the course

of the illness are more likely to recover than those who don't.

Causes

Acute transverse myelitis has a variety of causes. It often follows acute infectious diseases, such as measles or pneumonia (the inflammation occurs after the infection has subsided), and primary infections of the spinal cord itself, such as syphilis or acute disseminated encephalomyelitis.

Acute transverse myelitis can accompany demyelinating diseases, such as acute multiple sclerosis, and inflammatory and necrotizing disorders of the spinal cord, such as hematomyelia.

Certain toxic agents (carbon monoxide, lead, and arsenic) can cause a type of myelitis in which acute inflammation (followed by hemorrhage and possible necrosis) destroys the entire circumference (myelin, axis cylinders, and neurons) of the spinal cord.

Other forms of myelitis may result from poliovirus, herpes zoster, herpesvirus B, or rabies virus; disorders that cause meningeal inflammation, such as syphilis, abscesses and other suppurative conditions, and tuberculosis; smallpox or polio vaccination; parasitic and fungal infections; and chronic adhesive arachnoiditis.

Signs and symptoms

In acute transverse myelitis, onset is rapid, with motor and sensory dysfunctions below the level of spinal cord damage appearing in 1 to 2 days.

Patients with acute transverse myelitis develop flaccid paralysis of the legs (sometimes beginning in just one leg) with loss of sensory and sphincter functions. Such sensory loss may follow pain in the legs or trunk. Reflexes disappear in the early stages but may reappear later. The extent of damage depends on which level of the spinal cord is affected; transverse myelitis rarely involves the arms. If spinal cord damage is severe, it may cause shock (hypotension and hypothermia).

Diagnosis

Paraplegia of rapid onset usually points to acute transverse myelitis. In such patients, neurologic examination confirms paraplegia or neurologic deficit below the level of the spinal cord lesion and absent or, later, hyperactive reflexes. Cerebrospinal fluid may be normal or show increased lymphocyte or protein levels.

Diagnostic evaluation must rule out a spinal cord tumor and identify the cause of any underlying infection.

Treatment

No effective treatment exists for acute transverse myelitis. However, this condition requires appropriate treatment of any underlying infection. Some patients with postinfectious or multiple sclerosis–induced myelitis have received steroid therapy, but its benefits aren't clear.

Special considerations

• Frequently assess vital signs. Watch carefully for signs of spinal shock (hypotension and excessive sweating).

• Prevent contractures with range-of-motion exercises and proper alignment.

• Watch for signs of urinary tract infections from indwelling urinary catheters.

• Prevent skin infections and pressure ulcers with meticulous skin care. Check pressure points often and keep skin clean and dry; use a water bed or another pressure-relieving device.

• Initiate rehabilitation immediately. Assist the patient with physical therapy, bowel and bladder training, and any lifestyle changes that his condition requires.

LIFE-THREATENING DISORDER

MYOCARDIAL INFARCTION

In myocardial infarction (MI), also known as heart attack, reduced blood flow through one of the coronary arteries results in myocardial ischemia and necrosis. In cardiovascular disease, the leading cause of death in the United States and Western Europe, death usually results from the cardiac damage or complications of MI.

Mortality is high when treatment is delayed; almost half of all sudden deaths due to an MI occur before hospitalization, within 1 hour of the onset of symptoms. The prognosis improves if vigorous treatment begins immediately.

Causes

Predisposing factors include:

• positive family history
• hypertension
• smoking
• elevated serum triglyceride, total cholesterol, and low-density lipoprotein levels
• diabetes mellitus
• obesity or excessive intake of saturated fats, carbohydrates, or salt
• sedentary lifestyle
• aging
• stress or a Type A personality (aggressive, ambitious, competitive, addicted to work, chronically impatient)
• drug use, especially cocaine.

Men and postmenopausal women are more susceptible to MI than premenopausal women, although incidence is rising among females, especially those who smoke and take oral contraceptives.

The site of the MI depends on the vessels involved. Occlusion of the circumflex branch of the left coronary artery causes a lateral wall infarction; occlusion of the anterior descending branch of the left coronary artery, an anterior wall infarction.

True posterior or inferior wall infarctions generally result from occlusion of the right coronary artery or one of its branches. Right ventricular infarctions can also result from right coronary artery occlusion, can accompany inferior infarctions, and may cause right heart failure. In transmural MI, tissue damage extends through all myocardial layers; in subendocardial MI, only in the innermost and possibly the middle layers.

Signs and symptoms

The cardinal symptom of MI is persistent, crushing substernal pain that may radiate to the left arm, jaw, neck, or shoulder blades. Such pain is often described as heavy, squeezing, or crushing, and may persist for 12 hours or more. However, in some MI patients — particularly older adults or diabetics — pain may not occur at all; in others, it may be mild and confused with indigestion.

In patients with coronary artery disease, angina of increasing frequency, severity, or duration (especially if not provoked by exertion, a heavy meal, or cold and wind) may signal impending infarction.

Other features

Other clinical effects include a feeling of impending doom, fatigue, nausea, vomiting, and shortness of breath. Some patients may have no symptoms. The patient may experience catecholamine responses, such as coolness in extremities, perspiration, anxiety, and restlessness. Fever is unusual at the onset of an MI, but a low-grade fever may develop during the next few days. Blood pressure varies; hypotension or hypertension may be present.

Complications

The most common post-MI complications include recurrent or persistent chest pain, arrhythmias, left ventricular failure (resulting in heart failure or acute pulmonary edema), and cardiogenic shock. Unusual but potentially lethal complications that may develop soon after infarction include thromboembolism; papillary muscle dysfunction or rupture, causing mitral insufficiency; rupture of the ventricular septum, causing ventricular septal defect; rupture of the myocardium; and ventricular aneurysm.

Up to several months after infarction, Dressler's syndrome may develop (pericarditis, pericardial friction rub, chest pain, fever, leukocytosis and, possibly, pleurisy or pneumonitis). (See *Complications of myocardial infarction*.)

Diagnosis

Persistent chest pain, ST-segment changes on the electrocardiogram (ECG), and elevated levels of total creatine kinase (CK) and the CK-MB isoenzyme over a 72-hour period usually confirm MI. Auscultation may reveal diminished heart sounds, gallops and, in papillary dysfunction, the apical systolic murmur of mitral insufficiency over the mitral valve area.

When clinical features are equivocal, assume that the patient has had an MI until tests rule it out. Diagnostic test results include the following:

• *serial 12-lead ECG:* ECG abnormalities may be absent or inconclusive during the first few hours following an MI. When present, characteristic abnormalities include serial ST-segment depression in subendocardial MI and ST-segment elevation in transmural MI.

• *serial serum enzyme levels:* CK levels are elevated, specifically, CK-MB.

COMPLICATIONS OF MYOCARDIAL INFARCTION

COMPLICATION	DIAGNOSIS	TREATMENT
Arrhythmias	• Electrocardiography (ECG) shows premature ventricular contractions, ventricular tachycardia, or ventricular fibrillation; in inferior wall myocardial infarction (MI), bradycardia and junctional rhythms or atrioventricular block; in anterior wall MI, tachycardia or heart block.	• Antiarrhythmics, atropine, cardioversion, and pacemaker
Heart failure	• In left ventricular failure, chest X-rays show venous congestion, cardiomegaly, and Kerley's B lines. • Catheterization shows increased pulmonary artery pressure (PAP) and central venous pressure.	• Diuretics, vasodilators, inotropic agents, and digitalis glycosides
Cardiogenic shock	• Catheterization shows decreased cardiac output and increased PAP and pulmonary artery wedge pressure (PAWP). • Signs include hypotension, tachycardia, S_3, S_4, decreased level of consciousness, decreased urine output, neck vein distention, and cool, pale skin.	• I.V. fluids, vasodilators, diuretics, digitalis glycosides, intra-aortic balloon pump (IABP), and beta-adrenergic stimulants
Rupture of left ventricular papillary muscle	• Auscultation reveals apical holosystolic murmur. Inspection of jugular vein pulse or hemodynamic monitoring shows increased v waves. • Dyspnea is prominent. • Color-flow and Doppler echocardiogram show mitral insufficiency. Pulmonary artery catheterization shows increased PAP and PAWP.	• Nitroprusside • IABP • Surgical replacement of the mitral valve with possible concomitant myocardial revascularization (in patients with significant coronary artery disease)
Ventricular septal rupture	• In left-to-right shunt, auscultation reveals holosystolic murmur and thrill. • Catheterization shows increased PAP and PAWP. • Confirmation by increased oxygen saturation of right ventricle and pulmonary artery	• Surgical correction, IABP, nitroglycerin, nitroprusside, low-dose inotropic agents, or pacemaker

(continued)

COMPLICATIONS OF MYOCARDIAL INFARCTION *(continued)*

COMPLICATION	DIAGNOSIS	TREATMENT
Pericarditis or Dressler's syndrome	• Auscultation reveals a friction rub. • Chest pain is relieved by sitting up.	• Nonsteroidal anti-inflammatory drugs or corticosteroids
Ventricular aneurysm	• Chest X-ray may show cardiomegaly. • ECG may show arrhythmias and persistent ST-segment elevation. • Left ventriculography shows altered or paradoxical left ventricular motion.	• Cardioversion, defibrillation, antiarrhythmics, vasodilators, anticoagulants, digitalis glycosides, and diuretics. If conservative treatment fails, surgical resection is necessary.
Thrombo-embolism	• Severe dyspnea and chest pain or neurologic changes • Nuclear scan shows ventilation-perfusion mismatch. • Angiography shows arterial blockage.	• Oxygen and heparin

• *echocardiography:* may show ventricular wall motion abnormalities in patients with a transmural MI.

Scans using I.V. technetium 99 can identify acutely damaged muscle by picking up radioactive nucleotide, which appears as a "hot spot" on the film. They are useful in localizing a recent MI.

Treatment
The goals of treatment are to relieve chest pain, to stabilize heart rhythm, to reduce cardiac workload, to revascularize the coronary artery, and to preserve myocardial tissue. Arrhythmias, the predominant problem during the first 48 hours after the infarction, may require antiarrhythmics, possibly a pacemaker and, rarely, cardioversion.

To preserve myocardial tissue, thrombolytic therapy should be started I.V. within 6 hours after the onset of symptoms (unless contraindications exist). Thrombolytic therapy includes either streptokinase, alteplase, or urokinase.

Percutaneous transluminal coronary angioplasty (PTCA) may be another option. If PTCA is performed soon after the onset of symptoms, the thrombolytic agent may be administered directly into the coronary artery.

Other treatments consist of:
• lidocaine or other drugs, such as procainamide, quinidine, bretylium, or disopyramide, for ventricular arrhythmias
• atropine I.V. or a temporary pacemaker for heart block or bradycardia
• nitroglycerin (sublingual, topical, transdermal, or I.V.); calcium channel blockers, such as nifedipine, verapamil, or diltiazem (sublingual, oral, or I.V.); or isosorbide dinitrate (sublingual, oral, or I.V.) to relieve pain by redistributing blood to ischemic areas of the myocardium, increasing cardiac output, and reducing myocardial workload

• heparin I.V. (usually follows thrombolytic therapy)

• morphine I.V. for pain and sedation

• bed rest with bedside commode to decrease cardiac workload

• oxygen administration at a modest flow rate for 24 to 48 hours (a lower concentration is necessary if the patient has chronic obstructive pulmonary disease)

• drugs to increase myocardial contractility or blood pressure

• beta-adrenergic blockers, such as propranolol or timolol, after acute MI to help prevent reinfarction

• aspirin to inhibit platelet aggregation (should be initiated within 24 hours after the onset of symptoms)

• pulmonary artery catheterization to detect left or right ventricular failure and to monitor the patient's response to treatment.

Special considerations

• Care for patients who've suffered an MI is directed toward detecting complications, preventing further myocardial damage, and promoting comfort, rest, and emotional well-being. Most MI patients receive treatment in the critical care unit (CCU), where they're under constant observation for complications.

• On admission to the CCU, monitor and record the patient's ECG, blood pressure, temperature, and heart and breath sounds.

• Assess and record the severity and duration of pain; administer analgesics. Avoid I.M. injections; absorption from the muscle is unpredictable.

• Check the patient's blood pressure after giving nitroglycerin, especially the first dose.

• Frequently monitor the ECG to detect rate changes or arrhythmias. Place rhythm strips in the patient's chart periodically for evaluation.

• During episodes of chest pain, obtain ECG, blood pressure, and pulmonary artery catheter measurements for changes.

• Watch for signs and symptoms of fluid retention (crackles, cough, tachypnea, edema), which may indicate impending heart failure. Carefully monitor daily weight, intake and output, respirations, serum enzyme levels, and blood pressure.

• Auscultate for adventitious breath sounds periodically (patients on bed rest frequently have atelectatic crackles, which may disappear after coughing) and for S_3 or S_4 gallops.

• Organize patient care and activities to maximize periods of uninterrupted rest.

• Ask the dietary department to provide a clear liquid diet until nausea subsides. A low-cholesterol, low-sodium, caffeine-free diet may be ordered.

• Provide a stool softener to prevent straining during defecation, which causes vagal stimulation and may slow the heart rate. Allow use of a bedside commode, and provide as much privacy as possible.

• Assist with range-of-motion exercises. If the patient is completely immobilized by a severe MI, turn him often.

• Antiembolism stockings help prevent venostasis and thrombophlebitis.

• Provide emotional support, and help reduce stress and anxiety; administer tranquilizers as needed.

• Explain procedures and answer questions. Explaining the CCU environment and routine can ease anxiety. Involve the patient's family in his care as much as possible.

To prepare for discharge:

• Promote compliance measures by thoroughly explaining the prescribed medication regimen and other treatment measures.

• Warn about adverse reactions to drugs, and advise the patient to watch for and report signs of toxicity (anorexia, nausea, vomiting, and yellow vision, for example, if the patient is receiving digoxin).

• Review dietary restrictions with the patient. If he must follow a low-sodium or low-fat and low-cholesterol diet, provide a list of foods that he should avoid. Ask the dietitian to speak to the patient and his family.

• Counsel the patient to resume sexual activity progressively.

• Advise the patient to report typical or atypical chest pain. Postinfarction syndrome may develop, producing chest pain that must be differentiated from recurrent MI, pulmonary infarct, or heart failure.

• If the patient has a Holter monitor in place, explain its purpose and use.

• Stress the need to stop smoking.

• Encourage participation in a cardiac rehabilitation program.

MYOCARDITIS

Myocarditis is focal or diffuse inflammation of the cardiac muscle (myocardium). It may be acute or chronic and can occur at any age. Frequently, myocarditis fails to produce specific cardiovascular symptoms or electrocardiogram (ECG) abnormalities, and recovery is usually spontaneous, without residual defects. Occasionally, myocarditis is complicated by congestive heart failure (CHF); rarely, it may lead to cardiomyopathy.

Causes

Myocarditis may result from:

• *viral infections* (most common cause in the United States and western Europe): coxsackievirus A and B strains and, possibly, poliomyelitis, influenza, rubeola, rubella, and adenoviruses and echoviruses

• *bacterial infections:* diphtheria, tuberculosis, typhoid fever, tetanus, and staphylococcal, pneumococcal, and gonococcal infections

• *hypersensitive immune reactions:* acute rheumatic fever and postcardiotomy syndrome

• *radiation therapy:* large doses of radiation to the chest in treating lung or breast cancer

• *chemical poisons:* such as chronic alcoholism

• *parasitic infections:* especially South American trypanosomiasis (Chagas' disease) in infants and immunosuppressed adults; also, toxoplasmosis

• *helminthic infections:* such as trichinosis.

Signs and symptoms

Myocarditis usually causes nonspecific symptoms — such as fatigue, dyspnea, palpitations, and fever — that reflect the accompanying systemic infection. Occasionally, it may produce mild, continuous pressure or soreness in the chest (unlike the recurring, stress-related pain of angina pectoris).

Although myocarditis is usually self-limiting, it may induce myofibril degeneration that results in right and left heart failure, with cardiomegaly, neck vein distention, dyspnea, persistent fever with resting or exertional tachycardia disproportionate to the degree of fever, and supraventricular and ventricular arrhythmias.

Sometimes myocarditis recurs or produces chronic valvulitis (when it results from rheumatic fever), cardiomyopathy, arrhythmias, and thromboembolism.

Diagnosis

The patient history commonly reveals recent febrile upper respiratory tract infection, viral pharyngitis, or tonsillitis. A physical examination shows supraventricular and ventricular arrhythmias, S_3 and S_4 gallops, a faint S_1, possibly a murmur of mitral insufficiency (from papillary muscle dysfunction) and, if pericarditis is present, a pericardial friction rub.

Electrocardiography typically shows diffuse ST-segment and T-wave abnormalities (as in pericarditis), conduction defects (prolonged PR interval), and other supraventricular arrhythmias.

Stool and throat cultures may identify the causative bacteria. An endomyocardial biopsy is used to confirm the diagnosis, but a negative biopsy doesn't exclude the diagnosis. A repeat biopsy may be needed.

Laboratory tests can't unequivocally confirm myocarditis, but the following findings support this diagnosis:

• *Cardiac enzyme levels* (creatine kinase [CK], the CK-MB isoenzyme, aspartate aminotransferase, and lactate dehydrogenase) are elevated.

• *White blood cell count* and *erythrocyte sedimentation rate* are increased.

• *Antibody titers* (such as antistreptolysin O titer in rheumatic fever) are elevated.

Treatment

In MI, treatment includes antibiotics for bacterial infection, modified bed rest to decrease the cardiac workload, and careful management of complications. CHF requires restriction of activity to minimize myocardial oxygen consumption, supplemental oxygen therapy, sodium restriction, diuretics to decrease fluid retention, and digitalis glycosides to increase myocardial contractility. However, digitalis glycosides must be administered cautiously because some patients with myocarditis show a paradoxical sensitivity to even small doses.

Arrhythmias necessitate prompt but cautious administration of antiarrhythmics, such as quinidine or procainamide, because these drugs depress myocardial contractility. Thromboembolism requires anticoagulation therapy. Treatment with corticosteroids or other immunosuppressants is controversial and therefore limited to combating life-threatening complications, such as intractable heart failure.

Special considerations

• Assess cardiovascular status frequently, watching for signs of CHF, such as dyspnea, hypotension, and tachycardia. Check for changes in cardiac rhythm or conduction.

• Observe for signs of digitalis toxicity (anorexia, nausea, vomiting, blurred vision, cardiac arrhythmias) and for complicating factors that may potentiate toxicity, such as electrolyte imbalances or hypoxia.

• Stress the importance of bed rest. Assist with bathing as necessary; provide a bedside commode, which puts less stress on the heart than using a bedpan. Reassure the patient that activity limitations are temporary.

• Offer diversional activities that are physically undemanding.

• During recovery, recommend that the patient resume normal activities slowly and avoid competitive sports.

MYRINGITIS, INFECTIOUS

Acute infectious myringitis is characterized by inflammation, hemorrhage, and effusion of fluid into the tissue at the end of the external ear canal and the tympanic membrane. This self-limiting disorder (resolving spontaneously within 3 days to 2 weeks) often follows acute otitis media or upper respiratory tract infection and frequently occurs epidemically in children.

Chronic granular myringitis, a rare inflammation of the squamous layer of the tympanic membrane, causes gradthe tympanic membrane, causes gradual hearing loss. Without specific treatment, this condition can lead to stenosis of the ear canal, as granulation extends from the tympanic membrane to the external ear.

Causes

Acute infectious myringitis usually follows viral infection but may also result from infection with bacteria (pneumococci, *Haemophilus influenzae*, beta-hemolytic streptococci, staphylococci) or any other organism that may cause acute otitis media. Myringitis is a rare sequela of atypical pneumonia caused by *Mycoplasma pneumoniae*. The cause of chronic granular myringitis is unknown.

Signs and symptoms

Acute infectious myringitis begins with severe ear pain, commonly accompanied by tenderness over the mastoid process. Small, reddened, inflamed blebs form in the canal, on the tympanic membrane, and with bacterial invasion, in the middle ear.

Fever and hearing loss are rare unless fluid accumulates in the middle ear or a large bleb totally obstructs the external auditory meatus. Spontaneous rupture of these blebs may cause bloody discharge. Chronic granular myringitis produces pruritus, purulent discharge, and gradual hearing loss.

Diagnosis

In acute infectious myringitis, the diagnosis is based on a physical examination showing characteristic blebs and on a typical patient history. Culture and sensitivity testing of exudate identifies secondary infection. In chronic granular myringitis, physical examination may reveal granulation extending from the tympanic membrane to the external ear.

Treatment

Hospitalization usually isn't required for acute infectious myringitis. Treatment consists of measures to relieve pain. Analgesics, such as aspirin or acetaminophen, and application of heat to the external ear are usually sufficient, but severe pain may necessitate the use of codeine.

Systemic or topical antibiotics prevent or treat secondary infection. Incision of the blebs and evacuation of serum and blood may relieve pressure and help drain exudate, but these measures don't speed recovery.

Treatment of chronic granular myringitis consists of systemic antibiotics or local anti-inflammatory antibiotic combination eardrops, and surgical excision and cautery. If stenosis is present, surgical reconstruction is necessary.

Special considerations

• Stress the importance of completing prescribed antibiotic therapy.
• Teach the patient how to instill topical antibiotics (eardrops). When necessary, explain incision of the blebs.
• To help prevent acute infectious myringitis, advise early treatment of acute otitis media.

Nasal Papillomas

A papilloma is a benign epithelial tissue overgrowth within the intranasal mucosa. Inverted papillomas grow into the underlying tissue, usually at the junction of the antrum and the ethmoidal sinus; they generally occur singly but sometimes are associated with squamous cell cancer.

Exophytic papillomas, which also tend to occur singly, arise from epithelial tissue, commonly on the surface of the nasal septum. Both types of papillomas are most prevalent in males. Recurrence is likely, even after surgical excision.

Causes
A papilloma may arise as a benign precursor of a neoplasm or as a response to tissue injury or viral infection, but its cause is unknown.

Signs and symptoms
Both inverted and exophytic papillomas typically produce symptoms related to unilateral nasal obstruction — stuffiness, postnasal drip, headache, shortness of breath, dyspnea, and, rarely, severe respiratory distress, nasal drainage, and infection. Epistaxis is most likely to occur with exophytic papillomas.

Diagnosis
On examination of the nasal mucosa, inverted papillomas usually appear large, bulky, highly vascular, and edematous; color varies from dark red to gray; consistency, from firm to friable. Exophytic papillomas are commonly raised, firm, and rubbery; pink to gray; and securely attached by a broad or pedunculated base to the mucous membrane. Histologic examination of excised tissue confirms the diagnosis.

Treatment
The most effective treatment is wide surgical excision or diathermy, with careful inspection of adjacent tissues and sinuses to rule out extension. The use of surgical lasers is another option. Aspirin or acetaminophen and decongestants may relieve symptoms.

Special considerations
• If bleeding occurs, have the patient sit upright, and instruct him to expectorate blood into an emesis basin. Compress both sides of the patient's nose against the septum for 10 to 15 minutes and apply ice compresses to the nose.
• Check for airway obstruction. Place your hand under the patient's nostrils to assess air exchange, and watch for signs of mild shortness of breath.
• If surgery is scheduled, tell the patient what to expect postoperatively. Instruct him not to blow his nose. (The packing is usually removed 12 to 24 hours after surgery.)
• Postoperatively, monitor vital signs and respiratory status. Use pulse oximetry to monitor oxygen saturation levels.

• As needed, administer analgesics and facilitate breathing with a cool-mist vaporizer. Provide mouth care.

• Frequently change the mustache dressing or drip pad to ensure proper absorption of drainage. Record the type and amount of drainage.

• While the nasal packing is in place, expect scant, usually bright red, clotted drainage. Remember that the amount of drainage often increases for a few hours after the packing is removed.

• Because papillomas tend to recur, tell the patient to seek medical attention at the first sign of nasal discomfort, discharge, or congestion that doesn't subside with conservative treatment.

• Encourage regular follow-up visits to detect early signs of recurrence.

NASAL POLYPS

Benign and edematous growths, nasal polyps are usually multiple, mobile, and bilateral. Nasal polyps may become large and numerous enough to cause nasal distention and enlargement of the bony framework, possibly occluding the airway. They're more common in adults than in children and tend to recur.

Causes

Nasal polyps are usually produced by the continuous pressure resulting from a chronic allergy that causes prolonged mucous membrane edema in the nose and sinuses. Other predisposing factors include chronic sinusitis, chronic rhinitis, and recurrent nasal infections.

Signs and symptoms

Nasal obstruction is the primary indication of nasal polyps. Such obstruction causes anosmia, a sensation of fullness in the face, nasal discharge, headache, and shortness of breath. Associated clinical features are usually symptomatic of allergic rhinitis.

Diagnosis

The following tests are used to diagnose nasal polyps:

• *X-rays of sinuses and nasal passages* reveal soft tissue shadows over the affected areas.

• *Examination with a nasal speculum* shows a dry, red surface, with clear or gray growths. Large growths may resemble tumors.

Nasal polyps occurring in children require further testing to rule out cystic fibrosis and Peutz-Jeghers syndrome.

Treatment

Generally, treatment consists of corticosteroids (either by direct injection into the polyps or by local spray) to temporarily reduce the polyp. Treatment of the underlying cause may include antihistamines to control allergy, and antibiotic therapy if infection is present. Local application of an astringent shrinks hypertrophied tissue. However, medical management alone is rarely effective.

Consequently, the treatment of choice is polypectomy, which is usually performed under a local anesthetic. The use of surgical lasers is becoming more popular. Continued recurrence may require surgical opening of the ethmoid and maxillary sinuses and evacuation of diseased tissue.

Special considerations

• Give antihistamines, as needed, to the patient with allergies.

• Prepare the patient for scheduled surgery by telling him what to expect postoperatively, for example, nasal packing for 1 to 2 days after surgery.

After surgery:

• Monitor for excessive bleeding or other drainage, and promote patient comfort.

• Elevate the head of the bed to facilitate breathing, reduce swelling, and promote adequate drainage.

• Change the mustache dressing or drip pad, as needed, and record the consistency, amount, and color of nasal drainage.

• Intermittently apply ice compresses over the nostrils to lessen swelling, prevent bleeding, and relieve pain.

• If nasal bleeding occurs — most likely after packing is removed — have the patient sit upright, monitor his vital signs, and advise him not to swallow blood. Compress the outside of his nose against the septum for 10 to 15 minutes. If bleeding persists, nasal packing may be necessary.

To prevent nasal polyps, instruct patients with allergies to avoid exposure to allergens and to take antihistamines at the first sign of an allergic reaction. Also, advise them to avoid overuse of nose drops and sprays.

LIFE-THREATENING DISORDER

NEAR DROWNING

Near drowning refers to surviving — temporarily, at least — the physiologic effects of hypoxemia and acidosis that result from submersion in fluid. Hypoxemia and acidosis are the primary problems in victims of near drowning.

Near drowning occurs in three forms:

• "dry" — the victim doesn't aspirate fluid but suffers respiratory obstruction or asphyxia (10% to 15% of patients)

• "wet" — the victim aspirates fluid and suffers from asphyxia or secondary changes due to fluid aspiration (about 85% of patients)

• secondary — the victim suffers recurrence of respiratory distress (usually aspiration pneumonia or pulmonary edema) within minutes or 1 to 2 days after a near-drowning incident.

Causes

In the United States, drowning claims nearly 8,000 lives annually. No statistics are available for near-drowning incidents. Near drowning results from an inability to swim or, in swimmers, from panic, a boating accident, a heart attack or a blow to the head while in the water, drinking heavily before swimming, or a suicide attempt.

Results of aspiration

Regardless of the tonicity of the fluid aspirated, hypoxemia is the most serious consequence of near drowning, followed by metabolic acidosis. Other consequences depend on the kind of water aspirated.

After fresh water aspiration, changes in the character of lung surfactant result in exudation of protein-rich plasma into the alveoli. This, plus increased capillary permeability, leads to pulmonary edema and hypoxemia.

After saltwater aspiration, the hypertonicity of sea water exerts an osmotic force, which pulls fluid from pulmonary capillaries into the alveoli. The resulting intrapulmonary shunt causes hypoxemia. Also, the pulmonary capillary membrane may be injured and induce pulmonary edema. In both kinds of near drowning, pulmonary edema and hypoxemia occur secondary to aspiration.

Signs and symptoms

Near-drowning victims can display a host of clinical problems: apnea, shallow or gasping respirations, substernal chest pain, asystole, tachycardia, bradycardia, restlessness, irritability, lethargy, fever, confusion, unconsciousness, vomiting, abdominal distention, and a cough that produces a pink, frothy fluid.

Diagnosis

A history of near drowning along with characteristic features and auscultation of crackles and rhonchi are required for a diagnosis. Supportive tests include:

• *blood tests:* may show leukocytosis

• *arterial blood gas analysis:* shows decreased oxygen content, a low bicarbonate level, and low pH

• *electrocardiography:* shows supraventricular tachycardia, occasional premature ventricular contractions, nonspecific ST segment, and T-wave abnormalities.

Treatment

• Begin emergency treatment with cardiopulmonary resuscitation (CPR) and administration of 100% oxygen.

• Stabilize the patient's neck in case he has a cervical injury.

• When the patient arrives at the hospital, assess for a patent airway. Establish one, if necessary.

• Continue CPR, intubate the patient, and provide respiratory assistance, such as mechanical ventilation with positive end-expiratory pressure, if needed.

• Assess arterial blood gas and pulse oximetry values.

• If the patient's abdomen is distended, insert a nasogastric tube. (Intubate the patient first if he's unconscious.)

• Start I.V. lines; insert an indwelling urinary catheter.

• Give medications as necessary. Much controversy exists about the benefits of drug treatment of near-drowning victims. However, such treatment may include sodium bicarbonate for acidosis, corticosteroids for cerebral edema, antibiotics to prevent infections, and bronchodilators to ease bronchospasms.

Special considerations

• Remember, all near-drowning victims should be admitted for an observation period of 24 to 48 hours because of the possibility of delayed drowning.

• Observe for pulmonary complications and signs of delayed drowning (confusion, substernal pain, adventitious breath sounds). Suction often. Pulmonary artery catheters may be useful in assessing cardiopulmonary status.

• Monitor vital signs, intake and output, and peripheral pulses. Check for skin perfusion. Watch for signs of infection.

• To facilitate breathing, raise the head of the bed slightly.

• To prevent near drowning, advise swimmers to avoid drinking alcohol before swimming, to observe water safety measures, and to take a water safety course sponsored by the Red Cross, YMCA, or YWCA.

LIFE-THREATENING DISORDER

NECROTIZING ENTEROCOLITIS

Characterized by diffuse or patchy intestinal necrosis, necrotizing enterocolitis (NEC) is accompanied by sepsis in about one-third of cases. Sepsis usually involves *Escherichia coli, Clostridium, Salmonella, Pseudomonas,* or *Klebsiella.*

Initially, necrosis is localized, occurring anywhere along the intestine, but most often it's right-sided (in the ileum, ascending colon, or rectosigmoid). With early detection, the survival rate is 60% to 80%. If diffuse bleeding occurs, NEC usually results in disseminated intravascular coagulation (DIC).

Causes

NEC occurs most often among premature infants (less than 34 weeks' gestation) and those of low birth weight (less than 5 lb [2.3 kg]). NEC is occurring more frequently, possibly because of the higher incidence and survival of premature infants and low-birth-weight neonates.

One in ten infants who develops NEC is full-term. Among premature and low-birth-weight infants in intensive care nurseries, incidence varies from 1% to 12%. NEC is associated with 2% of all infant deaths.

Possible risk factors

The exact cause of NEC is unknown. Suggested predisposing factors include birth asphyxia, postnatal hypotension, respiratory distress, hypothermia, umbilical vessel catheterization, or patent ductus arteriosus.

NEC may also be a response to significant prenatal stress, such as premature rupture of membranes, placenta previa, maternal sepsis, toxemia of pregnancy, or breech or cesarean birth.

Possible causative theory

According to current theory, NEC develops when the infant suffers perinatal hypoxemia due to shunting of blood from the gut to more vital organs. Subsequent mucosal ischemia provides an ideal medium for bacterial growth. Hypertonic formula may increase bacterial activity because—unlike maternal breast milk—it doesn't provide protective immunologic activity and because it contributes to the production of hydrogen gas. As the bowel swells and breaks down, gas-forming bacteria invade damaged areas, producing free air in the intestinal wall. This may result in fatal perforation and peritonitis.

Signs and symptoms

Any infant who has suffered from perinatal hypoxemia has the potential for developing NEC. A distended (especially tense or rigid) abdomen, with gastric retention, is the earliest and most common sign of oncoming NEC, usually appearing from 1 to 10 days after birth.

Other clinical features are increasing residual gastric contents (which may contain bile), bile-stained vomitus, and occult blood in stools. One-fourth of patients have bloody diarrhea. A red or shiny, taut abdomen may indicate peritonitis.

Nonspecific signs and symptoms include thermal instability, lethargy, metabolic acidosis, jaundice, and DIC. The major complication is perforation, which requires surgery.

Recurrence of NEC and mechanical and functional abnormalities of the intestine, especially stricture, are the usual cause of residual intestinal malfunction in any infant who survives acute NEC and may develop as late as 3 months postoperatively.

Diagnosis

Successful treatment of NEC relies on early recognition based on the following diagnostic test results:

• *Anteroposterior and lateral abdominal X-rays* confirm the diagnosis by showing nonspecific intestinal dilation and, in later stages of NEC, pneumatosis cystoides intestinalis (gas or air in the intestinal wall).

• *Platelet count* may fall below 50,000/ μl.

• *Serum sodium levels* are decreased.

• *Arterial blood gas levels* show metabolic acidosis (a result of sepsis).

• *Bilirubin levels* show infection-induced breakdown of red blood cells.

RECOGNIZING OMINOUS SIGNS IN NECROTIZING ENTEROCOLITIS

When an infant suffers perinatal hypoxemia, be alert for the following signs of gastric distention and perforation:
- apnea
- cardiovascular shock
- sudden drop in temperature
- sudden listlessness and rag-doll limpness
- bradycardia
- increasing abdominal tenderness, edema, erythema, or involuntary rigidity of the abdomen.

• *Blood and stool cultures* identify the infecting organism.
• *Clotting studies and hemoglobin levels* reveal associated DIC.
• *Guaiac test* detects occult blood in stools.

Treatment
The first signs of NEC necessitate removal of the umbilical catheter (arterial or venous) and discontinuation of oral intake for 7 to 10 days to rest the injured bowel. I.V. fluids, including hyperalimentation, maintain fluid and electrolyte balance and nutrition during this time; passage of a nasogastric (NG) tube aids bowel decompression.

If coagulation studies indicate a need for transfusion, the infant usually receives dextran to promote hemodilution, increase mesenteric blood flow, and reduce platelet aggregation.

Antibiotic therapy
Drug therapy consists of parenteral administration of an aminoglycoside or ampicillin to suppress bacterial flora and prevent bowel perforation. (These drugs can also be administered through an NG tube, if necessary.) Anteroposterior and lateral X-rays every 4 to 6 hours monitor disease progression.

Surgery
Surgery is indicated if the patient shows any of the following symptoms: signs of perforation (free intraperitoneal air on X-ray or symptoms of peritonitis), respiratory insufficiency (caused by severe abdominal distention), progressive and intractable acidosis, or DIC.

Surgery removes all necrotic and acutely inflamed bowel and creates a temporary colostomy or ileostomy. Such surgery must leave at least 12″ (30.5 cm) of bowel, or the infant may suffer from malabsorption or chronic vitamin B_{12} deficiency.

Special considerations
• Be alert for signs of gastric distention and perforation. (See *Recognizing ominous signs in necrotizing enterocolitis.*)
• Take axillary temperatures to avoid perforating the bowel.
• Prevent cross-contamination by disposing of soiled diapers properly and washing hands with povidone-iodine after diaper changes.
• Try to prepare the parents for a potential deterioration in their infant's condition. Be honest and explain all treatments, including why feedings are withheld.
• After surgery, the infant needs mechanical ventilation. Gently suction

secretions, and assess respirations often.

• Replace fluids lost through NG tube and stoma drainage. Include drainage losses in output records. Weigh the infant daily. A daily weight gain of 0.35 to 0.7 oz (9.9 to 19.8 g) indicates a good response to therapy.

• An infant with a temporary colostomy or ileostomy needs special care. Explain to the parents what a colostomy or ileostomy is and why it's necessary. Encourage them to participate in their infant's physical care after his condition is no longer critical.

• Because of the infant's small abdomen, the suture line is near the stoma; therefore, keeping the suture line clean can be a problem. Good skin care is essential because the immature infant's skin is fragile and vulnerable to excoriation and the active enzymes in bowel secretions are corrosive.

• Improvise infant-sized colostomy bags from urine collection bags, medicine cups, or condoms. Karaya gum is helpful in making a seal.

• Watch for wound disruption, infection, and excoriation — potential dangers because of severe catabolism.

• Watch for intestinal malfunction from stricture or short-bowel syndrome. Such complications usually develop 1 month after the infant resumes normal feedings.

• You may develop an attachment to infants who require intensive care, but avoid unconscious exclusion of the parents. Encourage parental visits.

• To help prevent NEC, encourage mothers to breast-feed because breast milk contains live macrophages that fight infection and has a low pH that inhibits the growth of many organisms. Also, colostrum — fluid secreted before the milk — contains high concentrations of immunoglobulin A, which directly protects the bowel from infection and which the neonate lacks for several days postpartum.

• Tell mothers that they may refrigerate their milk for 48 hours but shouldn't freeze or heat it because this destroys antibodies. Tell them to use plastic — not glass — containers, because leukocytes adhere to glass.

NEPHROTIC SYNDROME

This condition is characterized by marked proteinuria, hypoalbuminemia, hyperlipemia, and edema. Although nephrotic syndrome (NS) isn't a disease itself, it results from a specific glomerular defect and indicates renal damage. The prognosis is highly variable, depending on the underlying cause. Some forms may progress to end-stage renal failure.

Causes
About 75% of NS cases result from primary (idiopathic) glomerulonephritis. Classifications include the following:

• In *lipid nephrosis (nil lesions)* — the main cause of NS in children — the glomeruli appear normal by light microscopy. Some tubules may contain increased lipid deposits.

• *Membranous glomerulonephritis* — the most common lesion in adult idiopathic NS — is characterized by uniform thickening of the glomerular basement membrane containing dense deposits. It eventually progresses to renal failure.

• *Focal glomerulosclerosis* can develop spontaneously at any age, follow kidney transplantation, or result from heroin abuse. Reported incidence of this condition is 10% in children with NS and up to 20% in adults.

Lesions initially affect the deeper glomeruli, causing hyaline sclerosis, with later involvement of the superficial glomeruli. These lesions generally

PATHOPHYSIOLOGY OF NEPHROTIC SYNDROME

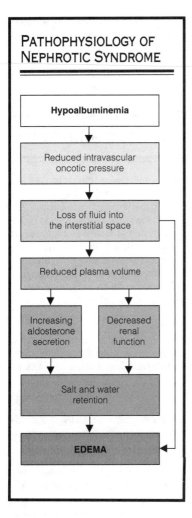

Hypoalbuminemia

↓

Reduced intravascular oncotic pressure

↓

Loss of fluid into the interstitial space

↓

Reduced plasma volume

↓

Increasing aldosterone secretion   Decreased renal function

↓

Salt and water retention

↓

EDEMA

cause slowly progressive deterioration in renal function. Remissions occur occasionally.

• In *membranoproliferative glomerulonephritis,* slowly progressive lesions develop in the subendothelial region of the basement membrane. These le-

sions may follow infection, particularly streptococcal infection. This disease occurs primarily in children and young adults.

Other causes of NS include metabolic diseases, such as diabetes mellitus; collagen-vascular disorders, such as systemic lupus erythematosus and periarteritis nodosa; circulatory diseases, such as congestive heart failure, sickle-cell anemia, and renal vein thrombosis; nephrotoxins, such as mercury, gold, and bismuth; allergic reactions; and infections, such as tuberculosis or enteritis. Other possible causes are pregnancy, hereditary nephritis, multiple myeloma, and other neoplastic diseases.

These diseases increase glomerular protein permeability, leading to increased urinary excretion of protein, especially albumin, and subsequent hypoalbuminemia.

Signs and symptoms
The dominant clinical feature of nephrotic syndrome is mild to severe dependent edema of the ankles or sacrum, or periorbital edema, especially in children. Such edema may lead to ascites, pleural effusion, and swollen external genitalia. (See *Pathophysiology of nephrotic syndrome.*)

Accompanying symptoms may include orthostatic hypotension, lethargy, anorexia, depression, and pallor. Major complications are malnutrition, infection, coagulation disorders, thromboembolic vascular occlusion, and accelerated atherosclerosis.

Diagnosis
Consistent proteinuria in excess of 3.5 g/24 hours strongly suggests NS; examination of urine also reveals an

increased number of hyaline, granular, and waxy, fatty casts, and oval fat bodies. Serum values that support the diagnosis are increased cholesterol, phospholipids, and triglycerides and decreased albumin levels. Histologic identification of the lesion requires a kidney biopsy.

Treatment

Effective treatment of NS necessitates correction of the underlying cause, if possible. Supportive treatment consists of protein replacement with a nutritional diet of 1.5 g protein/kg of body weight, with restricted sodium intake; diuretics for edema; and antibiotics for infection.

Some patients respond to an 8-week course of corticosteroid therapy (such as prednisone), followed by a maintenance dose. Others respond better to a combination course of prednisone and azathioprine or cyclophosphamide.

Special considerations

• Frequently check urine protein. (Urine containing protein appears frothy.)

• Measure blood pressure while the patient is supine and also while he's standing; be alert for a drop in blood pressure that exceeds 20 mm Hg.

• After a kidney biopsy, watch for bleeding and shock.

• Monitor intake and output and check weight at the same time each morning — after the patient voids and before he eats — and while he's wearing the same kind of clothing.

• Ask the dietitian to plan a high-protein, low-sodium diet.

• Provide good skin care because the patient with NS usually has edema.

• To avoid thrombophlebitis, encourage activity and exercise, and provide antiembolism stockings as needed.

• Watch for and teach the patient and family how to recognize adverse reactions to drug therapy, such as bone marrow toxicity from cytotoxic immunosuppressives and cushingoid symptoms (muscle weakness, mental changes, acne, moon face, hirsutism, girdle obesity, purple striae, amenorrhea) from long-term steroid therapy.

• Other steroid complications include masked infections, increased susceptibility to infections, ulcers, GI bleeding, and steroid-induced diabetes; a steroid crisis may occur if the drug is discontinued abruptly.

• To prevent GI complications, administer steroids with an antacid or with cimetidine or ranitidine.

• Explain that the adverse effects of steroids will subside when therapy stops.

• Offer the patient and family reassurance and support, especially during the acute phase, when edema is severe and the patient's body image changes.

NEURITIS, PERIPHERAL

Also known as multiple neuritis, peripheral neuropathy, and polyneuritis, peripheral neuritis is the degeneration of peripheral nerves supplying mainly the distal muscles of the extremities. It results in muscle weakness with sensory loss and atrophy, and decreased or absent deep tendon reflexes. This syndrome is associated with a noninflammatory degeneration of the axon and myelin sheaths, chiefly affecting the distal muscles of the extremities.

Although peripheral neuritis can occur at any age, its incidence is highest in men between ages 30 and 50. Because onset is usually insidious, patients may compensate by overusing unaffected muscles; however, onset is rapid with severe infection and chronic alcohol intoxication. If the cause can be identified and eliminated, the prognosis is good.

Causes

Causes of peripheral neuritis include:
• chronic intoxication (ethyl alcohol, arsenic, lead, carbon disulfide, benzene, phosphorus, and sulfonamides)
• infectious diseases (meningitis, diphtheria, syphilis, tuberculosis, pneumonia, mumps, and Guillain-Barré syndrome)
• metabolic and inflammatory disorders (gout, diabetes mellitus, rheumatoid arthritis, polyarteritis nodosa, systemic lupus erythematosus)
• nutritive diseases (beriberi and other vitamin deficiencies, and cachectic states).

Signs and symptoms

The clinical effects of peripheral neuritis develop slowly, and the disease usually affects the motor and sensory nerve fibers. Neuritis typically produces flaccid paralysis, wasting, loss of reflexes, pain of varying intensity, loss of ability to perceive vibratory sensations, and paresthesia, hyperesthesia, or anesthesia in the hands and feet.

Deep tendon reflexes are diminished or absent, and atrophied muscles are tender or hypersensitive to pressure or palpation. Footdrop may also be present. Cutaneous manifestations include glossy, red skin and decreased sweating. Patients often have a history of clumsiness and may complain of frequent vague sensations.

Diagnosis

The patient history and physical examination delineate the characteristic distribution of motor and sensory deficits. Electromyography may show a delayed action potential if this condition impairs motor nerve function.

Treatment

Effective treatment of peripheral neuritis consists of supportive measures to relieve pain, adequate bed rest, and physical therapy as needed. Most important, the underlying cause must be identified and corrected. For instance, it's essential to identify and remove the toxic agent, correct nutritional and vitamin deficiencies (the patient needs a high-calorie diet rich in vitamins, especially B complex), or counsel the patient to avoid alcohol.

Special considerations

• Relieve pain with correct positioning, analgesics, or possibly phenytoin, which has been used experimentally for neuritic pain, especially if associated with diabetic neuropathy.
• Instruct the patient to rest and refrain from using the affected extremity.
• To prevent pressure ulcers, apply a foot cradle. To prevent contractures, arrange for the patient to obtain splints, boards, braces, or other orthopedic appliances.
• After the pain subsides, passive range-of-motion exercises or massage may be beneficial. Electrotherapy is advocated for nerve and muscle stimulation.

NEUROGENIC ARTHROPATHY

Most common in men over age 40, neurogenic arthropathy (Charcot's arthropathy) is a progressively degenerative disease of peripheral and axial joints, resulting from impaired sensory innervation. The loss of sensation in the joints causes progressive deterioration, resulting from unrecognized trauma (especially repeated minor episodes) or primary disease, which leads to laxity of supporting ligaments and eventual disintegration of the affected joints.

Causes

In adults, the most common cause of neurogenic arthropathy is diabetes mellitus. Other causes include tabes dorsalis (especially among patients ages 40 to 60), syringomyelia (which progresses to neurogenic arthropathy in about 25% of patients), myelopathy of pernicious anemia, spinal cord trauma, paraplegia, hereditary sensory neuropathy, and Charcot-Marie-Tooth disease. Rarely, amyloidosis, peripheral nerve injury, myelomeningocele (in children), leprosy, or alcoholism causes neurogenic arthropathy.

Frequent intra-articular injections of corticosteroids have also been linked to neurogenic arthropathy. The analgesic effect of the corticosteroids may mask symptoms and allow continuous damaging stress to accelerate joint destruction.

Signs and symptoms

Neurogenic arthropathy begins insidiously with swelling, warmth, increased mobility, and instability in a single joint or in many joints. It can progress to deformity. The first clue to vertebral neuroarthropathy, which progresses to gross spinal deformity, may be nothing more than a mild, persistent backache. Characteristically, pain is minimal despite obvious deformity.

The specific joint that's affected varies. Diabetes usually attacks the joints and bones of the feet; tabes dorsalis attacks the large weight-bearing joints, such as the knee, hip, ankle, or lumbar and dorsal vertebrae (Charcot spine); syringomyelia, the shoulder, elbow, or

cervical intervertebral joint. Neurogenic arthropathy related to intra-articular injection of corticosteroids usually develops in the hip or knee joint.

Diagnosis

A patient history of painless joint deformity and underlying primary disease suggests neurogenic arthropathy. The physical examination may reveal bone fragmentation in advanced disease. X-rays confirm the diagnosis and assess the severity of joint damage.

In the early stage of the disease, soft-tissue swelling or effusion may be the only overt effect; in the advanced stage, articular fracture, subluxation, erosion of articular cartilage, periosteal new bone formation, and excessive growth of marginal loose bodies (osteophytosis) or resorption may be seen.

Other diagnostic measures include:
• *vertebral examination:* narrowing of disk spaces, deterioration of vertebrae, and osteophyte formation, leading to ankylosis and deforming kyphoscoliosis
• *synovial biopsy:* bony fragments and bits of calcified cartilage.

Treatment

Effective management relieves associated pain with analgesics and immobilization, using crutches, splints, braces, and restriction of weight-bearing.

In severe disease, surgery may include arthrodesis or, in severe diabetic neuropathy, amputation. However, surgery risks further damage through nonunion and infection.

Special considerations

• Assess the pattern of pain and give analgesics as needed.
• Check sensory perception, range of motion, alignment, joint swelling, and the status of underlying disease.
• Teach the patient joint protection techniques; to avoid physically stress-

ful actions that may cause pathologic fractures; and to take safety precautions, such as removing throw rugs and clutter that may cause falls.

• Advise the patient to report severe joint pain, swelling, or instability. Warm compresses may be applied to relieve local pain and tenderness.

• Teach the patient the proper technique for using crutches or other orthopedic devices. Stress the importance of proper fitting and regular professional readjustment of such devices. Warn that impaired sensation might allow damage from these aids without discomfort.

• Emphasize the need to continue regular treatment of the underlying disease.

NEUROGENIC BLADDER

Also known as neuromuscular dysfunction of the lower urinary tract, neurologic bladder dysfunction, and neuropathic bladder, neurogenic bladder refers to all types of bladder dysfunction caused by an interruption of normal bladder innervation. Subsequent complications include incontinence, residual urine retention, urinary infection, stone formation, and renal failure. A neurogenic bladder can be spastic (hypertonic, reflex, or automatic) or flaccid (hypotonic, atonic, nonreflex, or autonomous).

Causes
At one time, neurogenic bladder was thought to result primarily from spinal cord injury; now, it appears to stem from a host of underlying conditions:
• *cerebral disorders,* such as cerebrovascular accident, brain tumor (meningioma and glioma), Parkinson's

disease, multiple sclerosis, dementia, and incontinence caused by aging
• *spinal cord disease or trauma,* such as spinal stenosis (causing cord compression) or arachnoiditis (causing adhesions between the membranes covering the cord), cervical spondylosis, myelopathies from hereditary or nutritional deficiencies, and, rarely, tabes dorsalis
• *disorders of peripheral innervation,* including autonomic neuropathies resulting from endocrine disturbances such as diabetes mellitus (most common)
• *metabolic disturbances,* such as hypothyroidism, porphyria, or uremia (infrequent)
• *acute infectious diseases* such as Guillain-Barré syndrome
• *heavy metal toxicity*
• *chronic alcoholism*
• *collagen diseases* such as systemic lupus erythematosus
• *vascular diseases* such as atherosclerosis
• *distant effects of cancer,* such as primary oat cell carcinoma of the lung
• *herpes zoster*
• *sacral agenesis.*

An upper motor neuron lesion (above S2 to S4) causes spastic neurogenic bladder, with spontaneous contractions of the detrusor muscles, elevated intravesical voiding pressure, bladder wall hypertrophy with trabeculation, and urinary sphincter spasms.

A lower motor neuron lesion (below S2 to S4) causes flaccid neurogenic bladder, with decreased intravesical pressure, increased bladder capacity and large residual urine retention, and poor detrusor contraction.

Signs and symptoms
Neurogenic bladder produces a wide range of clinical signs, depending on the underlying cause and its effect on the structural integrity of the bladder. Usually, this disorder causes some de-

gree of incontinence, changes in initiation or interruption of micturition, and an inability to empty the bladder completely. Other symptoms of neurogenic bladder include vesicoureteral reflux, deterioration or infection in the upper urinary tract, and hydroureteral nephrosis.

Spastic neurogenic bladder

Depending on the site and extent of the spinal cord lesion, spastic neurogenic bladder may produce involuntary or frequent scanty urination without a feeling of bladder fullness and possibly spontaneous spasms of the arms and legs. Anal sphincter tone may be increased.

Tactile stimulation of the abdomen, thighs, or genitalia may precipitate voiding and spontaneous contractions of the arms and legs. With cord lesions in the upper thoracic (cervical) level, bladder distention can trigger hyperactive autonomic reflexes, resulting in severe hypertension, bradycardia, and headaches.

Flaccid neurogenic bladder

Features of flaccid neurogenic bladder may be associated with overflow incontinence, diminished anal sphincter tone, and a greatly distended bladder (this is evident on percussion or palpation), but without the accompanying feeling of bladder fullness due to sensory impairment.

Diagnosis

The patient's history may include a condition or disorder that can cause neurogenic bladder, incontinence, and disruptions of micturition patterns. The following tests will help evaluate the patient's bladder function:

• *Voiding cystourethrography* evaluates bladder neck function, vesicoureteral reflux, and continence.

• *Urodynamic studies* help evaluate how urine is stored in the bladder, how well

the bladder empties, and the rate of movement of urine out of the bladder during voiding. These studies consist of four components:

−*Urine flow study (uroflow)* shows diminished or impaired urine flow.

−*Cystometry* evaluates bladder nerve supply, detrusor muscle tone, and intravesical pressures during bladder filling and contraction.

−*Urethral pressure profile* determines urethral function with respect to the length of the urethra and the outlet pressure resistance.

−*Sphincter electromyelography* correlates the neuromuscular function of the external sphincter with bladder muscle function during bladder filling and contraction. This evaluates how well the bladder and urinary sphincter muscles work together.

• *Retrograde urethrography* reveals the presence of strictures and diverticula. This test may not be performed on a routine basis.

Treatment

The goals of treatment are to maintain the integrity of the upper urinary tract, control infection, and prevent urinary incontinence through evacuation of the bladder, drug therapy, surgery or, less commonly, neural blocks and electrical stimulation.

Bladder evacuation

Techniques of bladder evacuation include Credé's method, Valsalva's maneuver, and intermittent self-catheterization.

Credé's method (application of manual pressure over the lower abdomen) and Valsalva's maneuver (performing forced exhalation against a closed glottis) promote complete emptying of the bladder. (See *Dealing with neurogenic bladder,* page 590.) After appropriate instruction, most patients can perform Credé's method themselves; however, even when performed

---

TEACHING CHECKLIST

✓ DEALING WITH NEUROGENIC BLADDER

In your patient teaching for neurogenic bladder, cover the following topics:
• Explain all diagnostic tests clearly so the patient understands the procedure, the time involved, and the possible results. Assure him that the lengthy diagnostic process is necessary to identify the most effective treatment plan.
• Explain the treatment plan to the patient in detail.
• Encourage the patient to drink plenty of fluids to prevent calculus formation and infection from urinary stasis.

• Teach the patient bladder evacuation techniques, such as Credé's method, Valsalva's maneuver, and intermittent self-catheterization. Generally, a male can perform this procedure more easily, but a female can learn self-catheterization with the help of a mirror. Intermittent self-catheterization, in conjunction with a bladder-retraining program, is especially useful for patients with flaccid neurogenic bladder.
• Counsel the patient regarding sexual activities. Remember, the incontinent patient feels embarrassed and distressed. Provide emotional support.

---

properly, this method isn't always successful and doesn't always eliminate the need for catheterization.

Intermittent self-catheterization—more effective than either Credé's method or Valsalva's maneuver—has proved to be a major advance in the treatment of neurogenic bladder because it allows complete emptying of the bladder without the risks that an indwelling urinary catheter poses.

Drug therapy
In neurogenic bladder, drug therapy may include bethanechol and phenoxybenzamine to facilitate bladder emptying and propantheline, methantheline, flavoxate, dicyclomine, and imipramine to facilitate urine storage.

Surgery
When conservative treatment fails, surgery may correct the structural impairment through transurethral resection of the bladder neck, urethral dilatation, external sphincterotomy, or urinary diversion procedures. Implantation of an artificial urinary sphincter may be necessary if permanent incontinence follows surgery for neurogenic bladder.

Special considerations
Care for patients with neurogenic bladder varies according to the underlying cause and the method of treatment.
• Use strict aseptic technique during insertion of an indwelling urinary catheter (a temporary measure to drain the incontinent patient's bladder). Don't interrupt the closed drainage system for any reason.
• Obtain urine specimens with a syringe and small-bore needle inserted through the aspirating port of the catheter itself (below the junction of the balloon instillation site). Irrigate in the same manner, if necessary.
• Clean the catheter insertion site with soap and water at least twice a day.

Don't allow the catheter to become encrusted.

• Use a sterile applicator to apply antibiotic ointment around the meatus after catheter care. Keep the drainage bag below the tubing, and don't raise the bag above the level of the bladder.

• Clamp the tubing, or empty the bag before transferring the patient to a wheelchair or stretcher to prevent accidental urine reflux.

• If urine output is considerable, empty the bag more frequently than once every 8 hours because bacteria can multiply in standing urine and migrate up the catheter and into the bladder.

• Watch for signs of infection (fever, cloudy or foul-smelling urine).

• Try to keep the patient as mobile as possible. Perform passive range-of-motion exercises, if necessary.

• If urinary diversion procedure is to be performed, arrange for consultation with an enterostomal therapist, and coordinate the care.

• Before discharge, teach the patient and his family evacuation techniques as necessary (Credé's method, intermittent self-catheterization).

NOCARDIOSIS

An acute, subacute, or chronic bacterial infection, nocardiosis is caused by a weakly gram-positive species of the genus *Nocardia* — usually *Nocardia asteroides*. It's most common in men, especially those with compromised immune defense mechanisms. Its mortality in brain infection exceeds 80%; in other forms, mortality is 50%, even with appropriate therapy.

Causes

Nocardia organisms are aerobic, gram-positive bacteria with branching filaments similar in appearance to fungi.

Normally found in soil, these organisms cause occasional sporadic disease in humans and animals throughout the world. Their incubation period is unknown but is probably several weeks.

The usual mode of transmission is inhalation of organisms suspended in dust. Less often they're transmitted by direct inoculation through puncture wounds or abrasions.

Signs and symptoms

Nocardiosis originates as a pulmonary infection and causes a cough that produces thick, tenacious, purulent, mucopurulent and, possibly, blood-tinged sputum. It may also cause a fever as high as 105° F (40.6° C), chills, night sweats, anorexia, malaise, and weight loss.

This infection may lead to pleurisy, intrapleural effusions, and empyema. Other effects include tracheitis, bronchitis, pericarditis, endocarditis, peritonitis, mediastinitis, septic arthritis, and keratoconjunctivitis.

If the infection spreads through the blood to the brain, abscesses form, causing confusion, disorientation, dizziness, headache, nausea, and seizures. Rupture of a brain abscess can cause purulent meningitis. Extrapulmonary, hematogenous spread may cause endocarditis and lesions of kidneys, liver, subcutaneous tissue, and bone.

Diagnosis

Identification of *Nocardia* by culture of sputum or discharge is difficult. Special staining techniques often must be relied upon to make the diagnosis, in conjunction with a typical clinical picture (usually progressive pneumonia, despite antibiotic therapy).

Occasionally, diagnosis requires a biopsy of lung or other tissue. Chest X-rays vary and may show fluffy or interstitial infiltrates, nodules, or abscesses. Unfortunately, up to 40% of nocardial infections elude diagnosis until postmortem examination.

In brain infection with meningitis, a lumbar puncture shows nonspecific changes, such as increased pressure at the opening. Cerebrospinal fluid analysis shows an increased white blood cell count and protein levels, and decreased glucose levels compared to the serum glucose levels.

Treatment

Nocardiosis requires 12 to 18 months of treatment, preferably with co-trimoxazole or high doses of sulfonamides. Patients who don't respond to sulfonamide treatment may receive other drugs, such as ampicillin or erythromycin.

Treatment also includes surgical drainage of abscesses and excision of necrotic tissue. The acute phase requires complete bed rest; as the patient improves, activity can increase.

Special considerations

• Nocardiosis requires no isolation: It's not transmitted from person to person.

• Provide adequate nourishment through total parenteral nutrition, nasogastric tube feedings, or a balanced diet.

• Give the patient tepid sponge baths and antipyretics, as necessary, to reduce his fever.

• Monitor for allergic reactions to antibiotics.

• High-dose sulfonamide therapy (especially sulfadiazine) predisposes the patient to crystalluria and oliguria. So assess the patient frequently, force fluids, and alkalinize the urine with sodium bicarbonate, as required, to prevent these complications.

• In patients with pulmonary infection, administer chest physiotherapy. Auscultate the lungs daily, checking for increased crackles or consolidation.

Note and record the amount, color, and thickness of sputum.

• In brain infection, regularly assess neurologic function. Watch for signs of increased intracranial pressure, such as decreased level of consciousness, and respiratory abnormalities.

• In long-term hospitalization, turn the patient often, and assist with range-of-motion exercises.

Before the patient is discharged:

• Stress the need for a regular medication schedule to maintain therapeutic blood levels and continuation of drugs even after symptoms subside.

• Explain the importance of frequent follow-up examinations.

• Provide support and encouragement to help the patient and his family cope with this long-term illness.

NOSE, FRACTURED

The most common facial fracture, a fractured nose usually results from blunt injury and is often associated with other facial fractures. The severity of the fracture depends on the direction, force, and type of the blow.

A severe, comminuted fracture may cause extreme swelling or bleeding that may jeopardize the airway and require tracheotomy during early treatment. Inadequate or delayed treatment may cause permanent nasal displacement, septal deviation, and obstruction.

Signs and symptoms

Immediately after the injury, a nosebleed may occur, and soft-tissue swelling may quickly obscure the break. After several hours, pain, periorbital ecchymoses, and nasal displacement and deformity are prominent. Complications are septal hematoma, which may lead to abscess formation, resulting in avascular septic necrosis and saddle nose deformity.

Diagnosis
Palpation, X-rays, and clinical findings, such as a deviated septum, confirm a nasal fracture. The diagnosis also requires a full patient history, including the cause of the injury and the amount of nasal bleeding. Watch for clear fluid drainage, which may suggest a cerebrospinal fluid (CSF) leak and a basilar skull fracture. A computed tomography (CT) scan may be necessary.

Treatment
Treatment restores normal facial appearance and reestablishes bilateral nasal passage after swelling subsides. Reduction of the fracture corrects alignment; immobilization (intranasal packing and an external splint shaped to the nose and taped) maintains it. Reduction is best accomplished in the operating room under local anesthesia for adults and general anesthesia for children.

Severe swelling may delay treatment. In addition, CSF leakage calls for close observation, a CT scan of the basilar skull, and antibiotic therapy; septal hematoma requires incision and drainage to prevent necrosis.

Special considerations
• Start treatment immediately. While waiting for X-rays, apply ice packs to the nose to minimize swelling. Wrap the ice packs in a light towel to prevent ice from directly contacting the skin.
• To control anterior bleeding, gently apply local pressure. Posterior bleeding is rare and requires an internal tamponade applied in the emergency department.
• Because the patient will find breathing more difficult as the swelling increases, instruct him to breathe slowly through his mouth.
• To warm the inhaled air during cold weather, tell the patient to cover his mouth with a handkerchief or scarf.
• To prevent subcutaneous emphysema or intracranial air penetration (and potential meningitis), warn the patient not to blow his nose.
• After packing and splinting, apply ice in a plastic bag.
• Before discharge, tell the patient that ecchymoses should fade after about 2 weeks.

NYSTAGMUS

Nystagmus is recurring, involuntary eyeball movement. Such movement may be horizontal, vertical, rotating, or mixed; it produces blurred vision and difficulty in focusing. Nystagmus is classified according to eye movement characteristics and may be jerking or pendular. The prognosis varies with the underlying cause.

Causes
Although nystagmus may be congenital, it's usually an acquired disorder.

Jerking nystagmus
The most common type, jerking nystagmus results from excessive stimulation of the vestibular apparatus in the inner ear or from lesions of the brain stem or cerebellum.

This disorder occurs in acute labyrinthitis, Ménière's disease, multiple sclerosis, vascular lesions (especially in patients with hypertension), and any inflammation of the brain (such as encephalitis and meningitis). Jerking nystagmus may also result from drug and alcohol toxicity and congenital neurologic disorders.

Pendular nystagmus

This form results from improper transmission of visual impulses to the brain in the presence of corneal opacification, high astigmatism, congenital cataract or congenital anomalies of the optic disk, or bilateral macular lesions. Additional causes of pendular nystagmus include optic atrophy and albinism.

Signs and symptoms

In jerking nystagmus, the eyeballs oscillate faster in one direction than in the other; in pendular nystagmus, horizontal movements are approximately equal in both directions. If nystagmus results from a localized lesion, it may be unilateral; if from systemic disease, it's usually bilateral.

Diagnosis

The opticokinetic drum test is useful in diagnosing the underlying cause of nystagmus. In this test, the patient looks at a rapidly rotating, vertically striped drum—first at the stripes themselves, then quickly in the direction from which the stripes are coming, producing a normal jerking movement of the eyeballs. The absence of such a response suggests a central nervous system disturbance (such as a brain stem lesion).

Injecting warm or cold water into the external ear canal (caloric stimulation) also can precipitate nystagmus in an unaffected person. In patients with labyrinthine disorders, the response is abnormal (hypoactive or hyperactive) or absent.

Positional testing involves quickly changing the patient's position from supine to upright and turning his head from side to side, precipitating nystagmus. The direction of the nystagmus response aids in diagnosis.

Treatment

The goal of treatment is to correct the underlying cause, if possible. Unfortunately, the underlying cause often has no known cure (for example, brain stem lesions or multiple sclerosis). Eyeglasses can correct visual disturbances such as high astigmatism. The patient can help himself see by positioning his head in a certain way; if he can't focus with both eyes, he can turn his head and use only one eye.

Special considerations

• Explain testing procedures thoroughly to lessen anxiety and help ensure cooperation.

• Provide emotional support for the patient with nystagmus of rapid onset because the disorder may be caused by a brain stem lesion or some other severe neurologic disturbance.

OBSESSIVE-COMPULSIVE DISORDER

Obsessive thoughts and compulsive behaviors represent recurring efforts to control overwhelming anxiety, guilt, or unacceptable impulses that persistently enter the consciousness. The word *obsession* refers to a recurrent idea, thought, impulse, or image that is intrusive and inappropriate and causes marked anxiety or distress.

A *compulsion* is a ritualistic, repetitive, and involuntary defensive behavior. Performing a compulsive behavior reduces the patient's anxiety and increases the probability that the behavior will recur. Compulsions are often associated with obsessions.

Patients with obsessive-compulsive disorder are prone to abuse psychoactive substances, such as alcohol and anxiolytics, in an attempt to relieve their anxiety. In addition, other anxiety disorders and major depression often coexist with obsessive-compulsive disorder.

Obsessive-compulsive disorder is typically a chronic condition with remissions and flare-ups. Mild forms of the disorder are relatively common in the population at large.

Causes

The cause of obsessive-compulsive disorder is unknown. Some studies suggest the possibility of brain lesions, but the most useful research and clinical studies base an explanation on psychological theories. In addition, major depression, organic brain syndrome, and schizophrenia may contribute to the onset of obsessive-compulsive disorder.

Signs and symptoms

The psychiatric history of a patient with this disorder may reveal the presence of obsessive thoughts, words, or mental images that persistently and involuntarily invade the consciousness.

Some common obsessions include thoughts of violence (such as stabbing, shooting, maiming, or hitting), thoughts of contamination (images of dirt, germs, or feces), repetitive doubts and worries about a tragic event, and repeating or counting images, words, or objects in the environment. The patient recognizes that the obsessions are a product of his own mind and that they interfere with normal daily activities.

The patient's history also may reveal the presence of compulsions, irrational and recurring impulses to repeat a certain behavior. Common compulsions include repetitive touching, sometimes combined with counting; doing and undoing (for instance, opening and closing doors or rearranging things); washing (especially hands); and checking (to be sure no tragedy has occurred since the last time he checked). The patient's anxiety often is so strong that he will avoid the situation or the object that evokes the impulse.

When the obsessive-compulsive phenomena are mental, observation may reveal no behavioral abnormali-

DIAGNOSING OBSESSIVE-COMPULSIVE DISORDER

The diagnosis of obsessive-compulsive disorder is made when the patient's signs and symptoms meet the established criteria in the *DSM-IV*.

Either obsessions or compulsions
Obsessions are defined as all of the following:
• Recurrent and persistent thoughts, impulses, or images that are experienced, at some time during the disturbance, as intrusive and inappropriate and that cause marked anxiety or distress.
• The thoughts, impulses, or images are not simply excessive worries about real-life problems.
• The person attempts to ignore or suppress such thoughts or impulses or to neutralize them with some other thought or action.
• The person recognizes that the obsessions are the products of his mind and not externally imposed.
Compulsions are defined by all of the following:
• Repetitive behaviors or mental acts performed by the person, who feels driven to perform them in response to an obsession or according to rules that must be applied rigidly.
• The behavior or mental acts are aimed at preventing or reducing distress or preventing some dreaded event or situation. However, either

the activity is not connected in a realistic way with what it is designed to neutralize or prevent, or it is clearly excessive.
• The patient recognizes that his behavior is excessive or unreasonable (this may not be true for young children or for patients whose obsessions have evolved into overvalued ideas).

Additional criteria
• At some point, the person recognizes that the obsessions or compulsions are excessive or unreasonable.
• The obsessions or compulsions cause marked distress, are time consuming (take more than 1 hour a day), or significantly interfere with the person's normal routine, occupational functioning, or usual social activities or relationships.
• If another Axis I disorder is present, the content of the obsession is unrelated to it; for example, the ideas, thoughts, or images are not about food in the presence of an eating disorder, about drugs in the presence of a psychoactive substance abuse disorder, or about guilt in a major depressive disorder.
• The disturbance is not due to the direct physiologic effects of a substance or a general medical condition.

ties. However, compulsive acts may be observed, although feelings of shame, nervousness, or embarrassment may prompt the patient to try limiting these acts to his own private time.

You'll need to evaluate the impact of obsessive-compulsive phenomena on the patient's normal routine. He'll typically report moderate to severe impairment of social and occupational functioning.

Diagnosis
For characteristic findings in patients with this condition, see *Diagnosing obsessive-compulsive disorder*.

Treatment
Obsessive-compulsive disorder is tenacious, but with treatment, improvement occurs in 60% to 70% of patients. Current treatment usually involves a combination of medication and cognitive behavioral therapy. Other

BEHAVIORAL THERAPIES

The following behavioral therapies are used to treat the patient with obsessive-compulsive disorder.

Aversion therapy
Application of a painful stimulus creates an aversion to the obsession that leads to undesirable behavior (compulsion).

Thought stopping
This technique breaks the habit of fear-inducing anticipatory thoughts. The patient learns to stop unwanted thoughts by saying the word "stop" and then focusing his attention on achieving calmness and muscle relaxation.

Thought switching
To replace fear-inducing self-instructions with competent self-instructions, the patient learns to replace negative thoughts with positive ones

until the positive thoughts become strong enough to overcome the anxiety-provoking ones.

Flooding
This frequent, full-intensity exposure (through the use of imagery) to an object that triggers a symptom must be used with caution because it produces extreme discomfort.

Implosion therapy
A form of desensitization, implosion therapy calls for repeated exposure to a highly feared object.

Response prevention
Preventing compulsive behavior by distraction, persuasion, or redirection of activity, this form of behavioral therapy may require hospitalization or involvement of the family to be effective.

---

types of psychotherapy may also be helpful.

Effective medications include clomipramine, a tricyclic antidepressant; selective serotonin reuptake inhibitors, such as fluoxetine, paroxetine, sertraline, and fluvoxamine; and the benzodiazepine clonazepam.

Behavioral therapies—aversion therapy, thought stopping, thought switching, flooding, implosion therapy, and response prevention—have also been effective (see *Behavioral therapies*).

Special considerations
• Approach the patient unhurriedly.
• Provide an accepting atmosphere; don't appear shocked, amused, or critical of the ritualistic behavior.
• Keep the patient's physical health in mind. For example, compulsive hand washing may cause skin breakdown,

and rituals or preoccupations may cause inadequate food and fluid intake and exhaustion. Provide for basic needs, such as rest, nutrition, and grooming, if the patient becomes involved in ritualistic thoughts and behaviors to the point of self-neglect.
• Let the patient know you're aware of his behavior. For example, you might say, "I noticed you've made your bed three times today; that must be very tiring for you."
• Help the patient explore feelings associated with the behavior. For example, ask him, "What do you think about while you are performing your chores?"
• Make reasonable demands and set reasonable limits, explaining their purpose clearly. Avoid creating situations that increase frustration and provoke anger, which may interfere with treatment.

• Explore patterns leading to the behavior or recurring problems.

• Listen attentively, offering feedback.

• Encourage the use of appropriate defense mechanisms to relieve loneliness and isolation.

• Engage the patient in activities to create positive accomplishments and raise his self-esteem and confidence.

• Encourage active diversional activities, such as whistling or humming a tune, to divert attention from the unwanted thoughts and to promote a pleasurable experience.

• Help the patient develop new ways to solve problems and more effective coping skills by setting limits on unacceptable behavior (for example, by limiting the number of times per day he may indulge in compulsive behavior). Gradually shorten the time allowed. Help him focus on other feelings or problems for the remainder of the time.

• Identify insight and improved behavior (reduced compulsive behavior and fewer obsessive thoughts). Evaluate behavioral changes by your own observations and the patient's reports.

• Identify disturbing topics of conversation that reflect underlying anxiety or terror.

• When interventions do not work, re-evaluate them and recommend alternative strategies.

• Help the patient identify progress and set realistic expectations of himself and others.

• Explain how to channel emotional energy to relieve stress (for example, through sports and creative endeavors). In addition, teach the patient relaxation and breathing techniques to help reduce anxiety.

• Work with the patient and other treatment team members to establish behavioral goals and to help the patient tolerate anxiety in pursuing these goals.

OPTIC ATROPHY

Degeneration of the optic nerve, or optic atrophy, can develop spontaneously (primary) or follow inflammation or edema of the nerve head (secondary). Some forms of this condition may subside without treatment, but degeneration of the optic nerve is irreversible.

Causes

Optic atrophy usually results from central nervous system disorders, such as:

• pressure on the optic nerve from aneurysms or intraorbital or intracranial tumors

• optic neuritis, in multiple sclerosis, retrobulbar neuritis, and tabes.

Other causes include retinitis pigmentosa; chronic papilledema and papillitis; congenital syphilis; glaucoma; central retinal artery or vein occlusion that interrupts the blood supply to the optic nerve, causing degeneration of ganglion cells; trauma; ingestion of toxins, such as methanol and quinine; and deficiencies of vitamin B_{12}, amino acids, and zinc.

Symptoms and diagnosis

Optic atrophy causes abrupt or gradual painless loss of visual field or visual acuity, with subtle changes in color vision.

Slit-lamp examination and ophthalmoscopy confirm the diagnosis, although use of an opthalmoscope gives a better view.

• *Slit-lamp examination* reveals a pupil that reacts sluggishly to direct light stimulation.

• *Ophthalmoscopy* shows pallor of the nerve head from loss of microvascular circulation in the disk and deposit of fibrous or glial tissue.

• *Visual field testing* reveals a scotoma and, possibly, major visual field impairment.

Treatment

Optic atrophy is irreversible, so treatment aims to correct the underlying cause and prevent further vision loss. Steroids may be given to decrease inflammation and swelling, if a space-occupying lesion is the cause. In multiple sclerosis, optic neuritis often subsides spontaneously but may recur and improve repeatedly.

Special considerations

• Provide symptomatic care during diagnostic procedures and treatment. Assist the patient who is visually compromised to perform daily activities.
• Explain all procedures, to minimize anxiety. Offer emotional support to help the patient deal with loss of vision.

OSGOOD-SCHLATTER DISEASE

Also known as osteochondrosis, Osgood-Schlatter disease is a painful, incomplete separation of the epiphysis of the tibial tubercle from the tibial shaft. It's most common in active adolescent boys, frequently affecting one or both knees. Severe disease may cause permanent tubercle enlargement.

Causes

Osgood-Schlatter disease probably results from trauma, before the complete fusion of the epiphysis to the main bone has occurred (between ages 10 and 15). Such trauma may be a single violent action or repeated knee flexion against tight quadriceps muscle. Other causes include locally deficient blood supply and genetic factors.

Signs and symptoms

The patient complains of constant aching and pain and tenderness below the kneecap that worsens during any activity that causes forceful contraction of the patellar tendon on the tubercle, such as ascending or descending stairs. Such pain may be associated with some obvious soft-tissue swelling, localized heat, and local tenderness.

Diagnosis

Physical examination supports the diagnosis: The examiner forces the tibia into internal rotation while slowly extending the patient's knee from 90 degrees of flexion; at about 30 degrees, such flexion produces pain that subsides immediately with external rotation of the tibia.

X-rays may be normal or show epiphyseal separation and soft-tissue swelling for up to 6 months after onset; eventually, they may show bone fragmentation.

Treatment

Treatment usually consists of immobilization of the leg for 6 to 8 weeks and supportive measures. Full extension immobilization of the leg through reinforced elastic knee support, plaster cast, or splint allows revascularization and reossification of the tubercle and minimizes the pull of the quadriceps.

Supportive measures include activity restrictions, aspirin and, possibly, cortisone injections into the joint to relieve tenderness. In very mild cases, simple restriction of predisposing activities (bicycling, running) may be adequate.

Rarely, conservative measures fail, and surgery may be necessary. Such surgery includes removal or fixation of the epiphysis or drilling holes through the tubercle to the main bone to form channels for rapid revascularization.

Special considerations

• Monitor the patient's circulation, sensation, and pain, and watch for excessive bleeding after surgery.

• Assess daily for limitation of motion. Administer analgesics as needed.

• Make sure knee support or splint isn't too tight. Keep the cast dry and clean, and "petal" it around the top and bottom margins to avoid skin irritation.

• Teach proper use of crutches.

• Tell the patient to protect the injured knee with padding and to avoid trauma and repeated flexion (running, contact sports).

• Monitor for muscle atrophy.

• Give reassurance and emotional support because disruption of normal activities is difficult for an active teenager. Emphasize that restrictions are temporary.

OSTEOARTHRITIS

The most common form of arthritis, osteoarthritis is chronic, causing deterioration of the joint cartilage and formation of reactive new bone at the margins and subchondral areas of the joints. This degeneration results from a breakdown of chondrocytes, most often in the hips and knees.

Causes

Osteoarthritis is widespread, occurring equally in both sexes. Incidence is after age 40; its earliest symptoms generally begin in middle age and may progress with advancing age.

The degree of disability depends on the site and severity of involvement; it can range from minor limitation of the fingers to severe disability in persons with hip or knee involvement. The rate of progression varies, and joints may remain stable for years in an early stage of deterioration.

Causes

Primary osteoarthritis, a normal part of aging, results from many things, including metabolic, genetic, chemical, and mechanical factors. Secondary osteoarthritis usually follows an identifiable predisposing event — most commonly trauma, congenital deformity, or obesity — and leads to degenerative changes.

Signs and symptoms

The most common symptom of osteoarthritis is a deep, aching joint pain, particularly after exercise or weight bearing, usually relieved by rest. Other symptoms include:

• stiffness in the morning and after exercise (relieved by rest)

• aching during changes in weather

• "grating" of the joint during motion

• altered gait contractures

• limited movement.

These symptoms increase with poor posture, obesity, and occupational stress.

Osteoarthritis of the interphalangeal joints produces irreversible changes in the distal joints (Heberden's nodes) and proximal joints (Bouchard's nodes). These nodes may be painless at first but eventually become red, swollen, and tender, causing numbness and loss of dexterity (see *Viewing osteoarthritis*).

Diagnosis

A thorough physical examination confirms typical symptoms, and the absence of systemic symptoms rules out an inflammatory joint disorder. X-rays of the affected joint help confirm diagnosis of osteoarthritis but may be normal in the early stages. X-rays may require many views and typically show:

• narrowing of joint space or margin

• cystlike bony deposits in joint space and margins, sclerosis of the subchondral space
• joint deformity due to degeneration or articular damage
• bony growths at weight-bearing areas
• fusion of joints.

No laboratory test is specific for osteoarthritis.

Treatment

The goal of treatment is to relieve pain, maintain or improve mobility, and minimize disability. Medications include aspirin (or other nonnarcotic analgesics), phenylbutazone, indomethacin, fenoprofen, ibuprofen, propoxyphene, and, in some cases, intraarticular injections of corticosteroids. Such injections, given every 4 to 6 months, may delay the development of nodes in the hands.

Effective treatment also reduces stress by supporting or stabilizing the joint with crutches, braces, cane, walker, cervical collar, or traction. Other supportive measures include massage, moist heat, paraffin dips for hands, protective techniques for preventing undue stress on the joints, adequate rest (particularly after activity) and, occasionally, exercise when the knees are affected.

Surgical treatment, reserved for patients who have severe disability or uncontrollable pain, may include the following:
• *arthroplasty* (partial or total): replacement of deteriorated part of joint with prosthetic appliance
• *arthrodesis:* surgical fusion of bones; used primarily in spine (laminectomy)
• *osteoplasty:* scraping and lavage of deteriorated bone from joint
• *osteotomy:* change in alignment of bone to relieve stress by excision of wedge of bone or cutting of bone.

VIEWING OSTEOARTHRITIS

Involvement of the interphalangeal joints produces irreversible changes in the distal joints (Heberden's nodes) and the proximal joints (Bouchard's nodes). These nodes can be painless initially, with gradual progression to or sudden flare-ups of redness, swelling, tenderness, and impaired sensation and dexterity.

Heberden's nodes

Bouchard's nodes

Special considerations
• Promote adequate rest, particularly after activity. Plan rest periods during the day, and provide for adequate sleep at night. Moderation is the key—teach the patient to "pace" daily activities.
• Assist with physical therapy, and encourage the patient to perform gentle, isometric range-of-motion (ROM) exercises.
• If the patient needs surgery, provide appropriate preoperative and postoperative care.
• Provide emotional support and reassurance to help the patient cope with

limited mobility. Explain that osteoarthritis is *not* a systemic disease.

• Specific patient care depends on the affected joint:

—*Hand:* Apply hot soaks and paraffin dips to relieve pain, as necessary.

—*Spine (lumbar and sacral):* Recommend firm mattress (or bed board) to decrease morning pain.

—*Spine (cervical):* Check cervical collar for constriction; watch for redness with prolonged use.

—*Hip:* Use moist heat pads to relieve pain and administer antispasmodic drugs, as necessary. Assist with ROM and strengthening exercises, always making sure the patient gets the proper rest afterward. Check crutches, cane, braces, and walker for proper fit, and teach the patient how to use them correctly. For example, the patient with unilateral joint involvement should use an orthopedic appliance (such as a cane or walker) on the normal side. Advise use of cushions when sitting, as well as use of an elevated toilet seat.

—*Knee:* Twice daily, assist with prescribed ROM exercises, exercises to maintain muscle tone, and progressive resistance exercises to increase muscle strength. Provide elastic supports or braces if needed.

• To minimize the long-term effects of osteoarthritis, teach the patient to plan for adequate rest during the day, after exertion, and at night.

• Instruct the patient to take medication exactly as prescribed, and report adverse reactions immediately.

• Teach the patient to avoid overexertion. He should take care to stand and walk correctly, to minimize weight-bearing activities, and to be especially careful when stooping or picking up objects.

• Advise the patient to always wear well-fitting supportive shoes; don't allow the heels to become too worn down.

• Tell the patient to install safety devices at home, such as guard rails in the bathroom.

• Instruct the patient to do ROM exercises as gently as possible.

• Remind the patient to maintain proper body weight to lessen strain on joints and to avoid activities that require repeated impact on joints.

OSTEOMYELITIS

A pyogenic bone infection, osteomyelitis may be chronic or acute. It commonly results from a combination of local trauma — usually quite trivial but resulting in hematoma formation — and an acute infection originating elsewhere in the body. Although osteomyelitis often remains localized, it can spread through the bone to the marrow, cortex, and periosteum.

Acute osteomyelitis is usually a blood-borne disease, which most often affects rapidly growing children. Chronic osteomyelitis (rare) is characterized by multiple draining sinus tracts and metastatic lesions.

Osteomyelitis occurs more often in children than in adults — and particularly in boys — usually as a complication of an acute localized infection. The most common sites in children are the lower end of the femur and the upper end of the tibia, humerus, and radius. In adults, the most common sites are the pelvis and vertebrae, generally the result of contamination associated with surgery or trauma.

The incidence of both chronic and acute osteomyelitis is declining, except in drug abusers. With prompt treatment, the prognosis for acute osteomyelitis is very good; for chronic osteomyelitis, which is more prevalent in adults, the prognosis is still poor.

Causes

The most common pyogenic organism in osteomyelitis is *Staphylococcus aureus;* others include *Streptococcus pyogenes, Pneumococcus, Pseudomonas aeruginosa, Escherichia coli,* and *Proteus vulgaris.* Typically, these organisms find a culture site in a hematoma from recent trauma or in a weakened area, such as the site of local infection (for example, furunculosis), and spread directly to bone.

As the organisms grow and form pus within the bone, tension builds within the rigid medullary cavity, forcing pus through the haversian canals. This forms a subperiosteal abscess that deprives the bone of its blood supply and eventually may cause necrosis. In turn, necrosis stimulates the periosteum to create new bone (involucrum); the old bone (sequestrum) detaches and works its way out through an abscess or the sinuses. By the time sequestrum forms, osteomyelitis is chronic.

Signs and symptoms

Onset of acute osteomyelitis is usually rapid, with sudden pain in the affected bone, and tenderness, heat, swelling, and restricted movement over it. Associated systemic symptoms may include tachycardia, sudden fever, nausea, and malaise.

Generally, the clinical features of both chronic and acute osteomyelitis are the same, except that chronic infection can persist intermittently for years, flaring up spontaneously after minor trauma. Sometimes, however, the only symptom of chronic infection is the persistent drainage of pus from an old pocket in a sinus tract.

Diagnosis

Patient history, physical examination, and the following laboratory tests help to confirm osteomyelitis:
• *White blood cell count* shows leukocytosis.

• *Erythrocyte sedimentation rate* is elevated.
• *Blood cultures* identify the causative organism.

X-rays may not show bone involvement until the disease has been active for some time, usually 2 to 3 weeks. Bone scans can detect early infection. Diagnosis must rule out poliomyelitis, rheumatic fever, myositis, and bone fractures.

Treatment

Treatment varies for acute and chronic osteomyelitis.

Acute osteomyelitis

Acute osteomyelitis should be treated before a definitive diagnosis. Treatment includes:
• administration of large doses of I.V. antibiotics (usually a penicillinase-resistant penicillin, such as nafcillin or oxacillin) after blood cultures are taken
• early surgical drainage to relieve pressure buildup and sequestrum formation
• immobilization of the affected bone by plaster cast, traction, or bed rest
• supportive measures, such as administration of analgesics and I.V. fluids.

If an abscess forms, treatment includes incision and drainage, followed by a culture of the drainage. Antibiotic therapy to control infection may include administration of systemic antibiotics; intracavitary instillation of antibiotics through closed-system continuous irrigation with low intermittent suction; limited irrigation with blood drainage system with suction (Hemovac); or local application of packed, wet, antibiotic-soaked dressings.

Chronic osteomyelitis

In chronic osteomyelitis, surgery is usually required to remove dead bone (sequestrectomy) and to promote drainage (saucerization). The prognosis is poor even after surgery. Patients are often in great pain and require prolonged hospitalization. Resistant chronic osteomyelitis in an arm or leg may necessitate amputation.

Some centers also use hyperbaric oxygen to increase the activity of naturally occurring leukocytes.

Free tissue transfers and local muscle flaps are also used to fill in dead space and increase blood supply.

Special considerations
Your major concerns are to control infection, protect the bone from injury, and offer meticulous supportive care.
• Use strict aseptic technique when changing dressings and irrigating wounds.
• If the patient is in skeletal traction for compound fractures, cover insertion points of pin tracks with small, dry dressings, and tell him not to touch the skin around the pins and wires.
• Administer I.V. fluids to maintain adequate hydration, as necessary. Provide a diet high in protein and vitamin C.
• Assess vital signs and wound appearance daily, and monitor daily for new pain, which may indicate secondary infection.
• Carefully monitor suctioning equipment. Keep containers filled of solution being instilled. Monitor the amount of solution instilled and suctioned.
• Support the affected limb with firm pillows. Keep the limb level with the body; *don't* let it sag.
• Provide good skin care. Turn the patient gently every 2 hours and watch for signs of developing pressure ulcers.
• Provide good cast care. Support the cast with firm pillows and "petal" the edges with pieces of adhesive tape or moleskin to smooth rough edges.
• Check circulation and drainage: If a wet spot appears on the cast, circle it with a marking pen and note the time of appearance (on the cast). Be aware

of how much drainage is expected. Check the circled spot at least every 4 hours. Watch for any enlargement.
• Protect the patient from mishaps, such as jerky movements and falls, which may threaten bone integrity.
• Be alert for sudden pain, crepitus, or deformity. Watch for any sudden malposition of the limb, which may indicate fracture.
• Provide emotional support and appropriate diversions.
• Before discharge, teach the patient how to protect and clean the wound and, most importantly, how to recognize signs of recurring infection (increased temperature, redness, localized heat, and swelling).
• Stress the need for follow-up examinations.
• Instruct the patient to seek prompt treatment for possible sources of recurrence—blisters, boils, styes, and impetigo.

OSTEOPOROSIS

In osteoporosis, a metabolic bone disorder, the rate of bone resorption accelerates while the rate of bone formation slows down, causing a loss of bone mass. Bones affected by this disease lose calcium and phosphate salts and thus become porous, brittle, and abnormally vulnerable to fracture.

Osteoporosis may be primary or secondary to an underlying disease. Primary osteoporosis is often called senile or postmenopausal osteoporosis because it most commonly develops in elderly, postmenopausal women.

Causes
The cause of primary osteoporosis is unknown; however, a mild but prolonged negative calcium balance, resulting from an inadequate dietary in-

take of calcium, may be an important contributing factor — as may declining gonadal adrenal function, faulty protein metabolism due to estrogen deficiency, and a sedentary lifestyle.

Causes of secondary osteoporosis include prolonged therapy with steroids or heparin, total immobilization or disuse of a bone (as with hemiplegia, for example), alcoholism, malnutrition, malabsorption, scurvy, lactose intolerance, hyperthyroidism, osteogenesis imperfecta, and Sudeck's atrophy (localized to hands and feet, with recurring attacks).

Signs and symptoms

Osteoporosis is usually discovered when an elderly person bends to lift something, hears a snapping sound, then feels a sudden pain in the lower back. Vertebral collapse, producing a backache with pain that radiates around the trunk, is the most common presenting feature. Any movement or jarring aggravates the backache.

In another common pattern, osteoporosis can develop insidiously, with increasing deformity, kyphosis, loss of height, and a markedly aged appearance. As vertebral bodies weaken, spontaneous wedge fractures, pathologic fractures of the neck and femur, Colles' fractures after a minor fall, and hip fractures are all common.

Osteoporosis primarily affects the weight-bearing vertebrae. Only when the condition is advanced or severe, as in Cushing's syndrome or hyperthyroidism, do comparable changes occur in the skull, ribs, and long bones.

Diagnosis

Differential diagnosis must exclude other causes of rarefying bone disease, especially those affecting the spine, such as metastatic carcinoma and advanced multiple myeloma. Initial evaluation attempts to identify the specific cause of osteoporosis through the patient history. Diagnostic tests include the following:

• *X-rays* show typical degeneration in the lower thoracic and lumbar vertebrae. The vertebral bodies may appear flattened and may look denser than normal. Loss of bone mineral becomes evident in later stages.

• *Dual* or *single photon absorptiometry* allows measurement of bone mass, which helps to assess the extremities, hips, and spine.

• *Serum calcium, phosphorus,* and *alkaline phosphatase* are all within normal limits, but *parathyroid hormone* may be elevated.

• *Bone biopsy* shows thin, porous, but otherwise normal-looking bone.

Treatment

Effective treatment aims to prevent additional fractures and control pain. A physical therapy program, emphasizing gentle exercise and activity, is an important part of the treatment. Estrogen, to be started within 3 years after menopause, may be given to decrease the rate of bone resorption; sodium fluoride, to stimulate bone formation; and calcium and vitamin D, to support normal bone metabolism. However, drug therapy merely arrests osteoporosis and doesn't cure it.

Weakened vertebrae should be supported, usually with a back brace. Surgery can correct pathologic fractures of the femur by open reduction and internal fixation. Colles' fracture requires reduction with plaster immobilization for 4 to 10 weeks.

Prevention

The incidence of senile osteoporosis may be reduced through adequate intake of dietary calcium and regular exercise. Hormonal and fluoride treatments may also offer some preventive benefit.

Secondary osteoporosis can be prevented through effective treatment of the underlying disease, as well as steroid therapy, early mobilization after surgery or trauma, decreased alcohol consumption, careful observation for signs of malabsorption, and prompt treatment of hyperthyroidism.

Special considerations

• You should focus on the patient's fragility, stressing careful positioning, ambulation, and prescribed exercises.

• Check the patient's skin daily for redness, warmth, and new sites of pain, which may indicate new fractures. Encourage activity; help the patient walk several times daily.

• Perform passive range-of-motion exercises, or encourage the patient to perform active exercises. Make sure she regularly attends scheduled physical therapy sessions.

• Institute safety precautions such as keeping side rails up. Move the patient gently and carefully at all times. Explain to the patient's family and ancillary hospital personnel how easily an osteoporotic patient's bones can fracture.

• Provide a balanced diet, high in nutrients that support skeletal metabolism: vitamin D, calcium, and protein. Administer analgesics and heat to relieve pain.

• Make sure the patient and her family clearly understand the prescribed drug regimen. Tell them how to recognize significant adverse reactions and to report them immediately. Also tell the patient to report any new pain sites immediately, especially after trauma, no matter how slight.

• Advise the patient to sleep on a firm mattress and avoid excessive bed rest. Make sure she knows how to wear her back brace.

• Thoroughly explain osteoporosis to the patient and her family. If they don't understand the nature of this disease, they may feel that they could have prevented the fractures if they had been more careful.

• Teach the patient good body mechanics—to stoop before lifting anything, and to avoid twisting movements and prolonged bending.

• Instruct the female patient taking estrogen in the proper technique for self-examination of the breasts. Tell her to perform this examination at least once a month and to report any lumps immediately. Emphasize the need for regular gynecologic exams. Tell her to report abnormal bleeding promptly.

OTITIS EXTERNA

Also known as external otitis and swimmer's ear, otitis externa is an inflammation of the skin of the external ear canal and auricle. It may be acute or chronic and it is most common in the summer. With treatment, acute otitis externa usually subsides within 7 days (although it may become chronic) and tends to recur.

Causes

Otitis externa usually results from bacterial infection with an organism such as *Pseudomonas, Proteus vulgaris,* streptococci, or *Staphylococcus aureus;* sometimes it stems from a fungus, such as *Aspergillus niger* or *Candida albicans* (fungal otitis externa is most common in the tropics). Occasionally, chronic otitis externa results from dermatologic conditions, such as seborrhea or psoriasis. Predisposing factors include:

• swimming in contaminated water; cerumen creates a culture medium for the waterborne organism

• cleaning the ear canal with a cotton swab, bobby pin, finger, or other foreign objects; this irritates the ear canal

and possibly introduces the infecting microorganism
- exposure to dust, hair care products, or other irritants, which causes the patient to scratch his ear, excoriating the auricle and canal
- regular use of earphones, earplugs, or earmuffs, which trap moisture in the ear canal, creating a culture medium for infection
- chronic drainage from a perforated tympanic membrane.

Signs and symptoms

Acute otitis externa characteristically produces moderate to severe pain that is exacerbated by manipulation of the auricle or tragus, clenching the teeth, opening the mouth, or chewing. Its other clinical effects may include fever, foul-smelling aural discharge, regional cellulitis, and partial hearing loss.

Fungal otitis externa may be asymptomatic, although *A. niger* produces a black or gray blotting paper–like growth in the ear canal. In chronic otitis externa, pruritus replaces pain, which may lead to scaling and skin thickening. An aural discharge may also occur.

Diagnosis

Physical examination confirms otitis externa. In acute otitis externa, otoscopy reveals a swollen external ear canal (sometimes to the point of complete closure), periauricular lymphadenopathy (tender nodes in front of the tragus, behind the ear, or in the upper neck) and, occasionally, regional cellulitis.

In fungal otitis externa, removal of growth shows thick, red epithelium. Microscopic examination or culture and sensitivity tests can identify the causative organism and determine antibiotic treatment. Pain on palpation of the tragus or auricle distinguishes acute otitis externa from otitis media.

In chronic otitis externa, physical examination shows thick red epithelium in the ear canal. Severe chronic otitis externa may reflect underlying diabetes mellitus, hypothyroidism, or nephritis.

Treatment

Treatment varies, depending on the type of otitis externa.

Acute otitis externa

To relieve the pain of acute otitis externa, treatment includes heat therapy to the periauricular region (heat lamp; hot, damp compresses; heating pad), aspirin or acetaminophen, and codeine. Instillation of antibiotic eardrops (with or without hydrocortisone) follows cleaning of the ear and removal of debris. If fever persists or regional cellulitis develops, a systemic antibiotic is necessary.

Fungal otitis externa

As with other forms of this disorder, fungal otitis externa necessitates careful cleaning of the ear. Application of a keratolytic or 2% salicylic acid in cream containing nystatin may help treat otitis externa resulting from candidal organisms.

Instillation of slightly acidic eardrops creates an unfavorable environment in the ear canal for most fungi as well as *Pseudomonas*. No specific treatment exists for otitis externa caused by *A. niger,* except repeated cleaning of the ear canal with baby oil.

Chronic otitis externa

Primary treatment consists of cleaning the ear and removing debris. Supplemental therapy includes instillation of antibiotic eardrops or application of antibiotic ointment or cream (neomycin, bacitracin, or polymyxin, possibly combined with hydrocortisone). Another ointment contains phenol, salicylic acid, precipitated sulfur, and petrolatum and produces exfoliative and antipruritic effects.

For mild chronic otitis externa, treatment may include instilling antibiotic eardrops once or twice weekly and wearing specially fitted earplugs while showering, shampooing, or swimming.

Special considerations
If the patient has acute otitis externa:
• Monitor vital signs, particularly temperature. Watch for and record the type and amount of aural drainage.
• Remove debris and gently clean the ear canal with mild Burow's solution (aluminum acetate). Place a wisp of cotton soaked with solution into the ear, and apply a saturated compress directly to the auricle. Afterward, dry the ear gently but thoroughly. (In severe otitis externa, cleaning may be delayed until after initial treatment with antibiotic eardrops.)
• To instill eardrops in an adult, pull the pinna upward and backward to straighten the canal. To ensure that the drops reach the epithelium, insert a wisp of cotton moistened with eardrops.
• If the patient has chronic otitis externa, clean the ear thoroughly. Use wet soaks intermittently on oozing or infected skin. If the patient has a chronic fungal infection, clean the ear canal well, then apply an exfoliative ointment.

To prevent otitis externa:
• Suggest using lamb's wool earplugs coated with petrolatum, to keep water out of the ears when showering or shampooing.
• Tell the patient to wear earplugs or to keep his head above water when swimming and to instill two or three drops of 3% boric acid solution in 70% alcohol before and after swimming, to toughen the skin of the external ear canal.

• Warn against cleaning the ears with cotton swabs or other objects.
• Urge prompt treatment of otitis media to prevent perforation of the tympanic membrane.
• If the patient is diabetic, evaluate him for malignant otitis externa.

OTITIS MEDIA

Inflammation of the middle ear, otitis media may be suppurative or secretory, acute or chronic. Acute otitis media is common in children; its incidence rises during the winter months, paralleling the seasonal rise in nonbacterial respiratory tract infections.

With prompt treatment, the prognosis for acute otitis media is excellent; however, prolonged accumulation of fluid within the middle ear cavity causes chronic otitis media, with possible perforation of the tympanic membrane. Chronic suppurative otitis media may lead to scarring, adhesions, and severe structural or functional ear damage; chronic secretory otitis media, with its persistent inflammation and pressure, may cause conductive hearing loss.

Causes
Otitis media results from disruption of eustachian tube patency. (See *Site of otitis media.*)

Suppurative otitis media
In the suppurative form, respiratory tract infection, allergic reaction, nasotracheal intubation, or positional changes allow nasopharyngeal flora to reflux through the eustachian tube and colonize the middle ear. Suppurative otitis media usually results from bacterial infection with pneumococci, *Haemophilus influenzae* (the most common cause in children under age

SITE OF OTITIS MEDIA

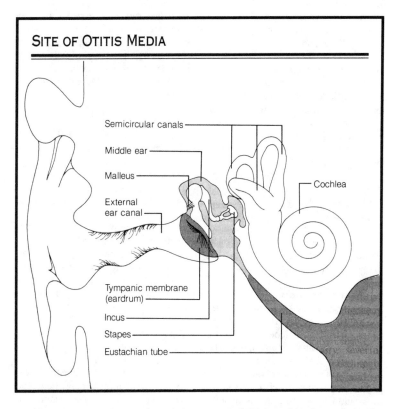

Semicircular canals

Middle ear

Malleus

External
ear canal

Cochlea

Tympanic membrane
(eardrum)

Incus

Stapes

Eustachian tube

---

6), *Moraxella catarrhalis,* beta-hemolytic streptococci, staphylococci (most common cause in children age 6 or older), or gram-negative bacteria.

Predisposing factors include the normally wider, shorter, more horizontal eustachian tubes and increased lymphoid tissue in children as well as anatomic anomalies. Chronic suppurative otitis media results from inadequate treatment of acute otitis episodes or from infection by resistant strains of bacteria or, rarely, tuberculosis.

Secretory otitis media

In this form of otitis media, obstruction of the eustachian tube causes a buildup of negative pressure in the middle ear that promotes transudation of sterile serous fluid from blood vessels in the membrane of the middle ear. Such effusion may be secondary to eustachian tube dysfunction from viral infection or allergy. It may also follow barotrauma (pressure injury caused by inability to equalize pressures between the environment and the middle ear), as can occur during rapid aircraft descent in a person with an upper respiratory tract infection or during rapid underwater ascent in scuba diving (barotitis media).

Chronic secretory otitis media follows persistent eustachian tube dysfunction from mechanical obstruction (adenoidal tissue overgrowth, tumors), edema (allergic rhinitis, chronic sinus infection), or inadequate treatment of acute suppurative otitis media.

Signs and symptoms

Clinical features vary with the specific type of the disorder.

Suppurative otitis media

Symptoms of acute suppurative otitis media include severe, deep, throbbing pain (from pressure behind the tympanic membrane); signs of upper respiratory tract infection (sneezing, coughing); mild to very high fever; hearing loss (usually mild and conductive); dizziness; nausea; and vomiting.

Other possible effects include bulging of the tympanic membrane, with concomitant erythema, and purulent drainage in the ear canal from tympanic membrane rupture. However, many patients are asymptomatic.

Secretory otitis medis

In acute secretory otitis media, a severe conductive hearing loss varies from 15 to 35 db, depending on the thickness and amount of fluid in the middle ear cavity—and, possibly, a sensation of fullness in the ear and popping, crackling, or clicking sounds on swallowing or with jaw movement. Accumulation of fluid may also cause the patient to hear an echo when he speaks and to experience a vague feeling of top-heaviness.

Chronic otitis media

The cumulative effects of chronic otitis media include thickening and scarring of the tympanic membrane, decreased or absent tympanic membrane mobility, cholesteatoma (a cystlike mass in the middle ear) and, in chronic suppurative otitis media, a painless, purulent discharge. The extent of associated conductive hearing loss varies with the size and type of tympanic membrane perforation and ossicular destruction.

If the tympanic membrane has ruptured, the patient may state that the pain has suddenly stopped. Complications may include abscesses (brain, subperiosteal, and epidural), sigmoid sinus or jugular vein thrombosis, septicemia, meningitis, suppurative labyrinthitis, facial paralysis, and otitis externa.

Diagnosis

Diagnostic tests also vary with the specific type of otitis media.

Suppurative otitis media

In acute suppurative otitis media, otoscopy reveals obscured or distorted bony landmarks of the tympanic membrane. Pneumatoscopy can show decreased tympanic membrane mobility, but this procedure is painful with an obviously bulging, erythematous tympanic membrane. The pain pattern is diagnostically significant: In acute suppurative otitis media, for example, pulling the auricle *doesn't* exacerbate the pain.

Secretory otitis media

In acute secretory otitis media, otoscopic examination reveals tympanic membrane retraction, which causes the bony landmarks to appear more prominent.

Examination also detects clear or amber fluid behind the tympanic membrane. If hemorrhage into the middle ear has occurred, as in barotrauma, the tympanic membrane appears blue-black.

Chronic otitis media

In patients with chronic otitis media, the history discloses recurrent or unresolved otitis media. Otoscopy shows thickening and sometimes scarring, and decreased mobility of the tympanic membrane; pneumatoscopy, decreased or absent tympanic membrane movement. History of recent air travel or scuba diving suggests barotitis media.

Treatment
The type of otitis media dictates the treatment guidelines.

Suppurative otitis media
In acute suppurative otitis media, antibiotic therapy includes ampicillin or amoxicillin. In areas with a high incidence of beta-lactamase–producing *H. influenzae* and in patients who are not responding to ampicillin or amoxicillin, amoxicillin/clavulanate potassium may be used.

For those who are allergic to penicillin derivatives, therapy may include cefaclor or co-trimoxazole. Severe, painful bulging of the tympanic membrane usually necessitates myringotomy. Broad-spectrum antibiotics can help prevent acute suppurative otitis media in high-risk patients. In patients with recurring otitis, antibiotics must be used with discretion to prevent development of resistant strains of bacteria.

Secretory otitis media
For patients with acute secretory otitis media, inflation of the eustachian tube by performing Valsalva's maneuver several times a day may be the only treatment required. Otherwise, nasopharyngeal decongestant therapy may be helpful. It should continue for at least 2 weeks and sometimes indefinitely, with periodic evaluation.

If decongestant therapy fails, myringotomy and aspiration of middle ear fluid are necessary, followed by insertion of a polyethylene tube into the tympanic membrane, for immediate and prolonged equalization of pressure. The tube falls out spontaneously after 9 to 12 months. Concomitant treatment of the underlying cause (such as elimination of allergens, or adenoidectomy for hypertrophied adenoids) may also be helpful in correcting this disorder.

Chronic otitis media
Treatment of chronic otitis media includes broad-spectrum antibiotics, such as amoxicillin/clavulanate potassium or cefuroxime, for exacerbations of acute otitis media; elimination of eustachian tube obstruction; treatment of otitis externa; myringoplasty and tympanoplasty to reconstruct middle ear structures when thickening and scarring are present; and, possibly, mastoidectomy. Cholesteatoma requires excision.

Special considerations
• Explain all diagnostic tests and procedures.
• After myringotomy, maintain drainage flow. Don't place cotton or plugs deep in the ear canal; however, sterile cotton may be placed loosely in the external ear to absorb drainage.
• To prevent infection, change the cotton whenever it gets damp, and wash hands before and after giving ear care. Watch for headache, fever, severe pain, or disorientation.
• After tympanoplasty, reinforce dressings, and observe for excessive bleeding from the ear canal. Administer analgesics, as needed. Warn the patient against blowing his nose or getting the ear wet when bathing.
• Encourage the patient to complete the prescribed course of antibiotic treatment. If nasopharyngeal decongestants are ordered, teach correct instillation.
• Suggest application of heat to the ear to relieve pain.
• Advise the patient with acute secretory otitis media to watch for and immediately report pain and fever—signs of secondary infection.

To prevent otitis media:
• Teach recognition of upper respiratory tract infections and encourage early treatment.
• Instruct parents not to feed their infant in a supine position or put him to

bed with a bottle. This prevents reflux of nasopharyngeal flora.

• To promote eustachian tube patency, instruct the patient to perform Valsalva's maneuver several times daily.

• Identify and treat allergies.

OTOSCLEROSIS

The most common cause of conductive deafness, otosclerosis is the slow formation of spongy bone in the otic capsule, particularly at the oval window. It occurs in at least 10% of whites and is three times as prevalent in females as in males, usually between ages 15 and 30. With surgery, the prognosis is good.

Causes

Otosclerosis appears to result from a genetic factor transmitted as an autosomal dominant trait; many patients report family histories of hearing loss (excluding presbycusis). Pregnancy may trigger the onset of this condition.

Signs and symptoms

Spongy bone in the otic capsule immobilizes the footplate of the normally mobile stapes, disrupting the conduction of vibrations from the tympanic membrane to the cochlea. This causes progressive unilateral hearing loss, which may advance to bilateral deafness. Other symptoms include tinnitus and paracusis of Willis (hearing conversation better in a noisy environment than in a quiet one).

Diagnosis

Early diagnosis is based on a Rinne test that shows bone conduction lasting longer than air conduction (normally, the reverse is true). As otosclerosis progresses, bone conduction also deteriorates.

• *Audiometric testing* reveals hearing loss ranging from 60 db, in early stages, to total loss.

• *Weber's test* detects sound lateralizing to the more affected ear.

• *Physical examination* reveals a normal tympanic membrane.

Treatment

Effective treatment consists of stapedectomy (removal of the stapes) and insertion of a prosthesis to restore partial or total hearing. This procedure is performed on only one ear at a time, beginning with the ear that has suffered greater damage. Alternative surgery includes stapedotomy (creation of a small hole in the stapes' footplate, through which a wire and piston are inserted).

Postoperatively, treatment includes hospitalization for 2 or 3 days and antibiotics to prevent infection. If surgery is not possible, a hearing aid (air conduction aid with molded ear insert receiver) enables the patient to hear conversation in normal surroundings, although this therapy isn't as effective as stapedectomy.

Special considerations

• During the first 24 hours after surgery, keep the patient lying flat, with the affected ear facing upward (to maintain the position of the graft).

• Enforce bed rest with bathroom privileges for 48 hours. Because the patient may be dizzy, keep the side rails up and assist him with ambulation.

• Assess for pain and vertigo, which may be relieved with repositioning or prescribed medication.

• Before discharge, instruct the patient to avoid loud noises and sudden pressure changes (such as those that occur while diving or flying) until healing is complete (usually 6 months).

• Advise the patient not to blow his nose for at least 1 week to prevent contaminated air and bacteria from entering the eustachian tube.

• Stress the importance of protecting the ears against cold; avoiding any activities that provoke dizziness, such as straining, bending, or heavy lifting; and, if possible, avoiding contact with anyone who has an upper respiratory tract infection.

• Teach the patient and family how to change the external ear dressing (eye pad or gauze pad) and care for the incision.

• Emphasize the need to complete the prescribed antibiotic regimen and to return for scheduled follow-up care.

OVARIAN CANCER

After cancer of the lung, breast, and colon, primary ovarian cancer ranks as the most common cause of cancer deaths among American women. In women with previously treated breast cancer, metastatic ovarian cancer is more common than cancer at any other site.

The prognosis varies with the histologic type and stage of the disease but is generally poor because ovarian tumors produce few early signs and are usually advanced at diagnosis. Although about 40% of women with ovarian cancer survive for 5 years, the overall survival rate has not improved significantly.

Three main types of ovarian cancer exist:

• *Primary epithelial tumors* account for 90% of all ovarian cancers and include serous cystoadenocarcinoma, mucinous cystoadenocarcinoma, and endometrioid and mesonephric malignancies. Serous cystoadenocarcinoma is the most common type and accounts for 50% of all cases.

• *Germ cell tumors* include endodermal sinus malignancies, embryonal carcinoma (a rare ovarian cancer that appears in children), immature teratomas, and dysgerminoma.

• *Sex cord (stromal) tumors* include granulosa cell tumors (which produce estrogen and may have feminizing effects), granulosa-theca cell tumors, and the rare arrhenoblastomas (which produce androgen and have virilizing effects).

Causes

Exactly what causes ovarian cancer isn't known, but its incidence is noticeably higher in women of upper socioeconomic levels between ages 20 and 54. However, it can occur during childhood. Other contributing factors include age at menopause; infertility; celibacy; high-fat diet; exposure to asbestos, talc, and industrial pollutants; nulliparity; familial tendency; and history of breast or uterine cancer.

Primary epithelial tumors arise in the müllerian epithelium; germ cell tumors, in the ovum itself; and sex cord tumors, in the ovarian stroma (the ovary's supporting framework).

Ovarian tumors spread rapidly intraperitoneally by local extension or surface seeding and, occasionally, through the lymphatics and the bloodstream. Generally, extraperitoneal spread is through the diaphragm into the chest cavity, which may cause pleural effusions. Other types of metastasis are rare.

Signs and symptoms

Typically, symptoms vary with the size of the tumor. Occasionally, in the early stages, ovarian cancer causes vague abdominal discomfort, dyspepsia, and other mild GI disturbances. As it progresses, it causes urinary frequency, constipation, pelvic discomfort, abdominal distention, and weight loss.

Tumor rupture, torsion, or infection may cause pain, which, in young patients, may mimic appendicitis. Granulosa cell tumors have feminizing effects (such as bleeding between periods in premenopausal women); conversely, arrhenoblastomas have virilizing effects. Advanced ovarian cancer causes ascites, rarely postmenopausal bleeding and pain, and symptoms relating to metastatic sites (most often pleural effusions).

Diagnosis

In ovarian cancer, diagosis requires clinical evaluation, a complete patient history, surgical exploration, and histologic studies. Preoperative evaluation includes a complete physical examination, including pelvic examination with Pap smear (positive in only a small number of women with ovarian cancer) and the following special tests:

• abdominal ultrasonography, computed tomography scan, or X-ray (may delineate tumor size)

• complete blood count, blood chemistries, and electrocardiography

• excretory urography for information on renal function and possible urinary tract anomalies or obstruction

• chest X-ray for distant metastasis and pleural effusions

• barium enema (especially in patients with GI symptoms) to reveal obstruction and size of tumor

• lymphangiography to show lymph node involvement

• mammography to rule out primary breast cancer

• liver function studies or a liver scan in patients with ascites

• ascites fluid aspiration for identification of typical cells by cytology

• laboratory tumor marker studies, such as ovarian carcinoma antigen, carcinoembryonic antigen, and human chorionic gonadotropin.

Despite extensive testing, accurate diagnosis and staging are impossible without exploratory laparotomy, including lymph node evaluation and tumor resection (see *Staging ovarian cancer*).

Treatment

Depending on the stage of the disease and the patient's age, treatment of ovarian cancer requires varying combinations of surgery, chemotherapy and, in some cases, radiation.

Conservative treatment

Occasionally, in girls or young women with a unilateral encapsulated tumor who wish to maintain fertility, the following conservative approach may be appropriate:

• resection of the involved ovary

• biopsies of the omentum and the uninvolved ovary

• peritoneal washings for cytologic examination of pelvic fluid

• careful follow-up, including periodic chest X-rays to rule out lung metastasis.

Aggressive treatment

Ovarian cancer usually requires more aggressive treatment, including total abdominal hysterectomy and bilateral salpingo-oophorectomy with tumor resection, omentectomy, appendectomy, lymph node biopsies with lymphadenectomy, tissue biopsies, and peritoneal washings.

Complete tumor resection is impossible if the tumor has matted around other organs or if it involves organs that can't be resected. Bilateral salpingo-oophorectomy in a prepubertal girl necessitates hormone replacement therapy, beginning at puberty, to induce the development of secondary sex characteristics.

Chemotherapy extends survival time in most ovarian cancer patients. Unfortunately, it is largely palliative in advanced disease, but prolonged remissions are being achieved in some patients.

STAGING OVARIAN CANCER

The International Federation of Gynecology and Obstetrics uses the staging system below for ovarian cancer.

Stage I — growth limited to the ovaries

Stage IA — growth limited to one ovary; no ascites; no tumor on the external surface; capsule intact

Stage IB — growth limited to both ovaries; no ascites; no tumor on the external surfaces; capsules intact

Stage IC — tumor either Stage IA or IB but on surface of one or both ovaries; or with capsule ruptured; or with ascites containing malignant cells or with positive peritoneal washings

Stage II — growth involving one or both ovaries with pelvic extension

Stage IIA — extension or metastasis, or both, to the uterus or tubes (or both)

Stage IIB — extension to pelvic tissues

Stage IIC — tumor either Stage IIA or IIB, but with tumor on surface of one or both ovaries; or with capsule (or capsules) ruptured; or with ascites present containing malignant cells or with positive peritoneal washings

Stage III — tumor involving one or both ovaries with peritoneal implants outside the pelvis or positive retroperitoneal or inguinal nodes; superficial liver metastasis equals Stage III; tumor limited to the true pelvis but with confirmed extension to small bowel or omentum

Stage IIIA — tumor grossly limited to the true pelvis with negative nodes but with confirmed microscopic seeding of abdominal peritoneal surfaces

Stage IIIB — tumor of one or both ovaries with confirmed implants of abdominal peritoneal surfaces none exceeding 2 cm in dimension; nodes are negative

Stage IIIC — abdominal implants greater than 2 cm or positive retroperitoneal or inguinal nodes or both

Stage IV — growth involving one or both ovaries with distant metastasis (such as pleural effusion and abnormal cells or parenchymal liver metastasis)

Chemotherapeutic drugs useful in ovarian cancer include melphalan, chlorambucil, thiotepa, methotrexate, cyclophosphamide, doxorubicin, vincristine, vinblastine, dactinomycin, bleomycin, paclitaxel, and cisplatin. These drugs are usually given in combination and they may be administered intraperitoneally.

Radiation therapy is generally not used for ovarian cancer because the resulting myelosuppression would limit the effectiveness of chemotherapy.

Other treatments

Radioisotopes have been used as adjuvant therapy, but they cause small-bowel obstructions and stenosis.

In addition, I.V. administration of biological response modifiers — interleukin-2, interferon, and monoclonal antibodies — is currently being investigated.

Special considerations

Because the treatment of ovarian cancer varies widely, so must the care of the patient.

Before surgery:

• Thoroughly explain all preoperative tests, the expected course of treatment, and surgical and postoperative procedures.

• Reinforce what the surgeon has told the patient about the surgical procedures listed in the surgical consent form. Explain that this form lists multiple procedures because the extent of the surgery can only be determined after the surgery itself has begun.

• In premenopausal women, explain that bilateral oophorectomy artificially induces early menopause, so they may experience hot flashes, headaches, palpitations, insomnia, depression, and excessive perspiration.

After surgery:

• Monitor vital signs frequently, and check I.V. fluids often. Monitor intake and output, while maintaining good catheter care. Check the dressing regularly for excessive drainage or bleeding, and watch for signs of infection.

• Provide abdominal support, and watch for abdominal distention. Encourage coughing and deep breathing. Reposition the patient often, and encourage her to walk shortly after surgery.

• Monitor and treat side effects of radiation and chemotherapy.

• If the patient is receiving immunotherapy, watch for flulike symptoms that may last 12 to 24 hours after drug administration. Give aspirin or acetaminophen for fever. Keep the patient well covered with blankets, and provide warm liquids to relieve chills. Administer an antiemetic as needed.

• Provide psychological support for the patient and her family. Encourage open communication, while discouraging overcompensation or "smothering" of the patient by her family. If the patient is a young woman who grieves for her lost ability to bear children, help her (and her family) overcome feelings that "there's nothing else to live for."

• If the patient is a child, find out whether or not her parents have told her she has cancer and deal with her questions accordingly.

• Enlist the help of a social worker, chaplain, and other members of the health care team for additional supportive care.

OVARIAN CYSTS

Usually ovarian cysts are nonneoplastic sacs on an ovary that contain fluid or semisolid material. Although these cysts are usually small and produce no symptoms, they require thorough investigation as possible sites of malignant change.

Common ovarian cysts include follicular cysts, lutein cysts (granulosa-lutein [corpus luteum] and theca-lutein cysts), and polycystic (or sclerocystic) ovarian disease. Ovarian cysts can develop any time between puberty and menopause, including during pregnancy. Granulosa-lutein cysts occur infrequently, usually during early pregnancy. The prognosis for nonneoplastic ovarian cysts is excellent.

Causes

Follicular cysts are generally very small and arise from follicles that overdistend instead of going through the atretic stage of the menstrual cycle. When such cysts persist into menopause, they secrete excessive amounts of estrogen in response to the hypersecretion of follicle-stimulating hormone and luteinizing hormone that normally occurs during menopause.

Granulosa-lutein cysts, which occur within the corpus luteum, are functional, nonneoplastic enlargements of the ovaries, caused by excessive accumulation of blood during the hemorrhagic phase of the menstrual cycle.

Theca-lutein cysts are commonly bilateral and filled with clear, straw-colored fluid; they are often associated with hydatidiform mole, choriocarcinoma, or hormone therapy (with human chorionic gonadotropin [HCG] or clomiphene citrate).

Polycystic ovarian disease is part of the Stein-Leventhal syndrome and stems from endocrine abnormalities.

Signs and symptoms

Small ovarian cysts (such as follicular cysts) usually don't produce symptoms unless torsion or rupture causes signs of an acute abdomen (abdominal tenderness, distention, and rigidity). Large or multiple cysts may induce mild pelvic discomfort, low back pain, dyspareunia, or abnormal uterine bleeding secondary to a disturbed ovulatory pattern. Ovarian cysts with torsion induce acute abdominal pain similar to that of appendicitis.

Granulosa-lutein cysts that appear early in pregnancy may grow as large as 2″ to 2½″ (5 to 6 cm) in diameter and produce unilateral pelvic discomfort and, if rupture occurs, massive intraperitoneal hemorrhage. In nonpregnant women, these cysts may cause delayed menses, followed by prolonged or irregular bleeding. Polycystic ovarian disease may also produce secondary amenorrhea, oligomenorrhea, or infertility.

Diagnosis

Generally, characteristic clinical features suggest ovarian cysts. Visualization of the ovaries through ultrasound, laparoscopy, or surgery (often for another condition) confirms ovarian cysts.

Extremely elevated HCG titers strongly suggest theca-lutein cysts.

In polycystic ovarian disease, physical examination demonstrates bilaterally enlarged polycystic ovaries. Tests reveal slightly elevated urinary 17-ketosteroid levels and anovulation (shown by basal body temperature graphs and endometrial biopsy). Direct visualiza-

tion must rule out paraovarian cysts of the broad ligament, salpingitis, endometriosis, and neoplastic cysts.

Treatment

The type of cyst dictates the treatment method.

Follicular cysts

This type of cyst generally doesn't require treatment because it tends to disappear spontaneously within 60 days. However, if it interferes with daily activities, administration of oral clomiphene citrate for 5 days or I.M. progesterone (also for 5 days) reestablishes the ovarian hormonal cycle and induces ovulation. Oral contraceptives may also accelerate involution of functional cysts (including both types of lutein cysts and follicular cysts).

Granulosa-lutein and theca-lutein cysts

If granulosa-lutein cysts occur during pregnancy, treatment is symptomatic because they diminish during the third trimester and rarely require surgery. Theca-lutein cysts disappear spontaneously after elimination of the hydatidiform mole, destruction of choriocarcinoma, or discontinuation of HCG or clomiphene citrate therapy.

Polycystic ovarian disease

Treatment of polycystic ovarian disease may include the administration of such drugs as clomiphene citrate to induce ovulation, medroxyprogesterone acetate for 10 days of every month for the patient who does not want to become pregnant, or low-dose oral contraceptives for the patient who needs reliable contraception.

Surgery, in the form of laparoscopy or exploratory laparotomy with possible ovarian cystectomy or oophorectomy, may become necessary if an ovarian cyst is found to be persistent or suspicious.

Special considerations

• Carefully explain the nature of the particular cyst, the type of discomfort — if any — that the patient is likely to experience, and how long the condition is expected to last.

• Preoperatively, watch for signs of cyst rupture, such as increasing abdominal pain, distention, and rigidity. Monitor vital signs for fever, tachypnea, or hypotension, which may indicate peritonitis or intraperitoneal hemorrhage. Administer sedatives, as ordered, to ensure adequate rest before surgery.

• Postoperatively, encourage frequent movement in bed and early ambulation, as ordered. Early ambulation effectively prevents pulmonary embolism.

• Provide emotional support. Offer appropriate reassurance if the patient fears cancer or infertility.

• Before discharge, advise the patient to increase her activities at home gradually — preferably over 4 to 6 weeks. Tell her to abstain from intercourse and to use tampons and douches during this period.

PAGET'S DISEASE

Also known as osteitis deformans, Paget's disease is a slowly progressive metabolic bone disease characterized by an initial phase of excessive bone resorption (osteoclastic phase), followed by a reactive phase of excessive abnormal bone formation (osteoblastic phase). The new bone structure, which is chaotic, fragile, and weak, causes painful deformities of both external contour and internal structure.

Paget's disease usually localizes in one or several areas of the skeleton (most frequently the lower torso), but occasionally, skeletal deformity is widely distributed. It can be fatal, particularly when it is associated with congestive heart failure (widespread disease creates a continuous need for high cardiac output), bone sarcoma, or giant cell tumors.

Causes

Paget's disease occurs worldwide but is extremely rare in Asia, the Middle East, Africa, and Scandinavia. In the United States, it affects approximately 2.5 million people over age 40 (mostly men).

Although its exact cause is unknown, one theory holds that early viral infection (possibly with mumps virus) causes a dormant skeletal infection that erupts many years later as Paget's disease. In 5% of the patients, the involved bone will undergo malignant changes.

Signs and symptoms

Clinical effects of Paget's disease vary.

Pain

Early stages may be asymptomatic, but when pain does develop, it is usually severe and persistent and may coexist with impaired movement resulting from impingement of abnormal bone on the spinal cord or sensory nerve root. Such pain intensifies with weight-bearing.

Other features

The patient with skull involvement shows characteristic cranial enlargement over frontal and occipital areas (hat size may increase) and may complain of headaches. Other deformities include kyphosis (spinal curvature due to compression fractures of pagetic vertebrae), accompanied by a barrel-shaped chest and asymmetric bowing of the tibia and femur, which often reduces height. Pagetic sites are warm and tender and are susceptible to pathologic fractures after minor trauma. Pagetic fractures heal slowly and often incompletely.

Complications

Bony impingement on the cranial nerves may cause blindness and hearing loss with tinnitus and vertigo. Other complications include hypertension, renal calculi, hypercalcemia, gout, congestive heart failure, and a waddling gait (from softening of pelvic bones).

Diagnosis

X-rays taken before overt symptoms develop show increased bone expansion and density. A bone scan, which is more sensitive than X-rays, clearly shows early pagetic lesions (radioisotope concentrates in areas of active disease). Bone biopsy reveals characteristic mosaic pattern. Other laboratory findings include:

• anemia

• elevated serum alkaline phosphatase levels (an index of osteoblastic activity and bone formation)

• elevated 24-hour urine levels for hydroxyproline (amino acid excreted by kidneys and an index of osteoclastic hyperactivity). Increasing use of routine chemistry screens—which include serum alkaline phosphatase—is making early diagnosis more common.

Treatment

If the patient is asymptomatic, treatment isn't needed. The patient with symptoms requires drug therapy, which may include:

• *calcitonin* (a hormone, given subcutaneously or I.M.) and *etidronate* (oral) to retard bone resorption (which relieves bone lesions) and reduce serum alkaline phosphate and urinary hydroxyproline secretion. Although calcitonin requires long-term maintenance therapy, there is noticeable improvement after the first few weeks of treatment; etidronate produces improvement after 1 to 3 months.

• *mithramycin,* a cytotoxic antibiotic, to decrease calcium, urinary hydroxyproline, and serum alkaline phosphatase levels. This drug produces remission of symptoms within 2 weeks and biochemical improvement in 1 to 2 months. However, mithramycin may destroy platelets or compromise renal function.

Self-administration of calcitonin and etidronate helps patients with Paget's disease lead near-normal lives. Nevertheless, these patients may need surgery to reduce or prevent pathologic fractures, correct secondary deformities, and relieve neurologic impairment.

To decrease the risk of excessive bleeding due to hypervascular bone, drug therapy with calcitonin and etidronate or mithramycin must precede surgery. Joint replacement is difficult because bonding material (methyl methacrylate) doesn't set properly on pagetic bone.

Other treatments vary according to symptoms. Aspirin, indomethacin, or ibuprofen usually controls pain.

Special considerations

• To evaluate the effectiveness of analgesics, assess level of pain daily. Watch for new areas of pain or restricted movements—which may indicate new fracture sites—and sensory or motor disturbances, such as difficulty in hearing, seeing, or walking.

• Monitor serum calcium and alkaline phosphatase levels.

• If the patient is confined to prolonged bed rest, prevent decubitus ulcers by providing good skin care. Reposition the patient frequently, and use a flotation mattress. Provide high-topped sneakers to prevent footdrop.

• Monitor intake and output. Encourage adequate fluid intake to minimize renal calculi formation.

• Demonstrate how to inject calcitonin properly and rotate injection sites. Warn the patient that side effects may occur (nausea, vomiting, local inflammatory reaction at injection site, facial flushing, itching of hands, and fever). Reassure him that these effects are usually mild and infrequent.

• To help the patient adjust to the changes in lifestyle imposed by this disease, teach him how to pace activities and, if necessary, how to use assistive devices.

• Encourage the patient to follow a recommended exercise program — avoiding both immobilization and excessive activity. Suggest a firm mattress or a bedboard to minimize spinal deformities.

• Warn against imprudent use of analgesics.

• To prevent falls at home, advise removal of throw rugs and other small obstacles.

• Emphasize the importance of regular checkups, including the eyes and ears.

• Tell the patient receiving etidronate to take this medication with fruit juice 2 hours before or after meals (milk or other high-calcium fluids impair absorption), to divide daily dosage to minimize side effects, and to watch for and report stomach cramps, diarrhea, fractures, and increasing or new bone pain.

• Tell the patient receiving mithramycin to watch for signs of infection, easy bruising, bleeding, and temperature elevation, and to report for regular follow-up laboratory tests.

• Help the patient and family make use of community support resources, such as a visiting nurse or home health agency. For more information, refer them to the Paget's Disease Foundation.

PAIN DISORDER

The striking feature of pain disorder is a persistent complaint of pain in the absence of appropriate physical findings. The symptoms are either inconsistent with the normal anatomic distribution of the nervous system, or they mimic a disease, such as angina, in the absence of diagnostic validation.

Although the pain has no physical cause, it is real to the patient. The disorder is more common in women than in men and frequently has an onset in the 30s and 40s. The pain usually is chronic, often interfering with interpersonal relationships or employment.

Causes
Pain disorder has no specific cause, but it may be related to severe psychological stress or conflict. The pain provides the patient with a means to cope with upsetting psychological issues. For example, a person with dependency needs may develop this disorder as an acceptable way to receive care and attention. The pain may have special significance, such as leg pain in the same leg a parent lost through amputation.

Signs and symptoms
The cardinal feature of pain disorder is a history of chronic, consistent complaints of pain without confirming physical disease. The patient may relate a long history of evaluations and procedures at multiple settings without much pain relief.

Because of frequent hospitalizations, the patient may be familiar with pain medications and tranquilizers; she may ask for a specific drug and know its correct dosage and route of administration. She may openly behave like an invalid.

Physical examination of the painful site reveals that the pain does not follow anatomic pathways. The patient may not display typical nonverbal signs of pain, such as grimacing or guarding. (Sometimes such reactions are absent in patients with chronic organic pain.)

Palpation, percussion, and auscultation may not reveal expected associated signs. Psychosocial assessment may reveal a patient who is angry at

---

DIAGNOSING PAIN DISORDER

The diagnosis of pain disorder is difficult because the perception of pain is subjective. Diagnosis is based on fulfillment of the following criteria put forth in *DSM-IV:*
• Pain in one or more body sites is the predominant focus of the patient and is sufficiently severe to warrant clinical attention.
• The pain causes clinically significant distress or impairment in social,

occupational, or other important areas of functioning.
• Psychological factors are judged to have an important role in the onset, severity, exacerbation, and maintenance of the pain.
• The symptom or deficit is not intentionally produced or feigned.
• The pain is not better accounted for by a mood, anxiety, or psychotic disorder and does not meet criteria for dyspareunia.

---

health care professionals because they've failed to relieve her pain.

Diagnosis
For characteristic findings in patients with this condition, see *Diagnosing pain disorder.*

Treatment
In pain disorder, treatment aims to ease the pain and help the patient live with it. Thus, long, invasive evaluations and surgical interventions are avoided. Treatment at a comprehensive pain center may be helpful.

Supportive measures
Such measures for pain relief may include hot or cold packs, physical therapy, distraction techniques, and cutaneous stimulation with massage or transcutaneous electrical nerve stimulation. Measures to reduce the patient's anxiety may help, as may an antidepressant medication such as a tricyclic antidepressant.

A continuing, supportive relationship with an understanding health care professional is essential for effective management; regularly scheduled follow-up appointments are helpful.

Analgesics
The patient should clearly be told what medication she will receive in addition to supportive pain-relief measures. Regularly scheduled analgesic doses can be more effective than scheduling medication as needed. Regular doses combat pain by reducing anxiety about asking for medication, and they eliminate unnecessary confrontations. The use of placebos will destroy trust when the patient discovers deceit.

Special considerations
• Observe and record characteristics of the pain: severity, duration, and any precipitating factors.
• Provide a caring atmosphere in which the patient's complaints are taken seriously and every effort is made to provide relief. This means communicating to the patient that you'll collaborate on a treatment plan, clearly stating the limitations. For example, you might say, "I can stay with you now for 15 minutes, but you can't receive another dose until 2 p.m."
• Don't tell the patient that she's imagining the pain or can wait longer for medication that's due. Assess her complaints and help her understand what's contributing to the pain.

• Provide other comfort measures, such as repositioning or massage, when possible.

• Encourage the patient to maintain independence despite her pain.

• Offer attention at times other than during the patient's complaints of pain, to weaken the link to secondary gain from attention to pain.

• Avoid confronting the patient with the somatoform nature of her pain; this seldom is helpful because such pain is her means of avoiding psychological conflict.

• Consider psychiatric referrals; however, realize that the patient may resist psychiatric intervention, and don't expect it to replace analgesic measures.

• Teach the patient noninvasive, drug-free methods of pain control, such as guided imagery, relaxation techniques, and distraction through reading or writing.

PANCREATIC CANCER

A deadly GI cancer, pancreatic cancer progresses rapidly. Pancreatic tumors are almost always adenocarcinomas and most arise in the head of the pancreas. Rarer tumors are those of the body and tail of the pancreas and islet cell tumors. The two main tissue types are cylinder cell and large, fatty, granular cell.

Causes

Pancreatic cancer occurs most commonly in men between ages 35 and 70. Geographically, the incidence is highest in Israel, the United States, Sweden, and Canada.

Evidence suggests that pancreatic cancer is linked to inhalation or absorption of the following carcinogens, which are then excreted by the pancreas:

• cigarettes
• foods high in fat and protein
• food additives
• industrial chemicals, such as beta-naphthalene, benzidine, and urea.

Possible predisposing factors are chronic pancreatitis, diabetes mellitus, and chronic alcohol abuse.

Signs and symptoms

The most common features of pancreatic carcinoma are weight loss, abdominal or low back pain, jaundice, and diarrhea (see *Types of pancreatic cancer,* page 624). Other generalized effects include fever, skin lesions (usually on the legs), and emotional disturbances, such as depression, anxiety, and premonition of fatal illness.

Diagnosis

Definitive diagnosis requires a laparotomy with a biopsy. Other tests used to detect pancreatic cancer include:

• *ultrasound* — can identify a mass but not its histology

• *computed tomography scan* — similar to ultrasound but shows greater detail

• *angiography* — shows vascular supply of tumor

• *endoscopic retrograde cholangiopancreatography* — allows visualization, instillation of contrast medium, and specimen biopsy

• *magnetic resonance imaging* — shows tumor size and location in great detail.

Laboratory tests supporting this diagnosis include serum bilirubin (increased), serum amylase and serum lipase (sometimes elevated), prothrombin time (prolonged), and aspartate aminotransferase and alanine aminotransferase (elevations indicate necrosis of liver cells).

Additional pertinent studies are alkaline phosphatase (marked elevation occurs with biliary obstruction); plasma insulin immunoassay (shows measurable serum insulin in the presence of

Types of Pancreatic Cancer

PATHOLOGY	CLINICAL FEATURES
Head of pancreas • Often obstructs ampulla of Vater and common bile duct • Directly metastasizes to duodenum • Adhesions anchor tumor to spine, stomach, and intestines.	• Jaundice (predominant symptom) — slowly progressive, unremitting; may cause skin (especially of the face and genitals) to turn olive green or black • Pruritus — often severe • Weight loss — rapid and severe (as great as 30 lb [13.6 kg]); may lead to emaciation, weakness, and muscle atrophy • Slowed digestion, gastric distention, nausea, diarrhea, and steatorrhea with clay-colored stools • Liver and gallbladder enlargement from lymph node metastasis to biliary tract and duct wall results in compression and obstruction; gallbladder may be palpable (Courvoisier's sign). • Dull, nondescript, continuous abdominal pain radiating to upper right quadrant; relieved by bending forward • GI hemorrhage and biliary infection common
Body and tail of pancreas • Large nodular masses become fixed to retropancreatic tissues and spine. • Direct invasion of spleen, left kidney, suprarenal gland, diaphragm • Involvement of celiac plexus results in thrombosis of splenic vein and spleen infarction.	*Body* • Pain (predominant symptom) — usually epigastric, develops slowly and radiates to back; relieved by bending forward or sitting up; intensified by lying supine; most intense 3 to 4 hours after eating; when celiac plexus is involved, pain is more intense and lasts longer • Venous thrombosis and thrombophlebitis — frequent; may precede other symptoms by months • Splenomegaly (from infarction), hepatomegaly (occasionally), and jaundice (rarely) *Tail* Symptoms result from metastasis: • Abdominal tumor (most common finding) produces a palpable abdominal mass; abdominal pain radiates to left hypochondrium and left chest. • Anorexia leads to weight loss, emaciation, and weakness. • Splenomegaly and upper GI bleeding

islet cell tumors); hemoglobin and hematocrit (may show mild anemia); fasting blood glucose (may indicate hypoglycemia or hyperglycemia); and stools (occult blood may signal ulceration in GI tract or ampulla of Vater).

Treatment

In pancreatic cancer, treatment is rarely successful because this disease has usually metastasized widely at diagnosis (see *Staging pancreatic cancer*).

Therapy consists of surgery and, possibly, radiation and chemotherapy.

Small advances have been made in the survival rate with surgery:

• Total pancreatectomy may increase survival time by resecting a localized tumor or by controlling postoperative gastric ulceration.

• Cholecystojejunostomy, choledochoduodenostomy, and choledochojejunostomy have partially replaced radical resection to bypass obstructing common bile duct extensions, thus decreasing the incidence of jaundice and pruritus.

• Whipple's operation, or pancreatoduodenectomy, has a high mortality but can produce wide lymphatic clearance, except with tumors located near the portal vein, superior mesenteric vein and artery, and celiac axis. This rarely used procedure removes the head of the pancreas, the duodenum, and portions of the body and tail of the pancreas, stomach, jejunum, pancreatic duct, and distal portion of the bile duct.

• Gastrojejunostomy is performed if radical resection isn't indicated and duodenal obstruction is expected to develop later.

Although pancreatic carcinoma generally responds poorly to chemotherapy, recent studies using combinations of fluorouracil, streptozocin, ifosfamide, and doxorubicin show a trend toward longer survival time. Other medications used in pancreatic cancer include:

• antibiotics (oral, I.V., or I.M.)—to prevent infection and relieve symptoms

• anticholinergics (particularly propantheline)—to decrease GI tract spasm and motility and reduce pain and secretions

• antacids (oral or by nasogastric tube)—to decrease secretion of pancreatic enzymes and suppress peptic activity, thereby reducing stress-induced damage to gastric mucosa

• diuretics—to mobilize extracellular fluid from ascites

• insulin—to provide adequate exogenous insulin supply after pancreatic resection

• narcotics—to relieve pain, but only after analgesics fail because morphine, meperidine, and codeine can lead to biliary tract spasm and increase common bile duct pressure

STAGING PANCREATIC CANCER

Using the TNM (tumor, node, metastasis) system, the American Joint Committee on Cancer has established the following stages for pancreatic cancer.

Primary tumor

TX—primary tumor can't be assessed

T0—no evidence of primary tumor

T1—tumor limited to the pancreas

T1a—tumor 2 cm or less in greatest dimension

T1b—tumor more than 2 cm in greatest dimension

T2—tumor penetrates the duodenum, bile duct, or peripancreatic tissues

T3—tumor penetrates the stomach, spleen, colon, or adjacent large vessels

Regional lymph nodes

NX—regional lymph nodes can't be assessed

N0—no evidence of regional lymph node metastasis

N1—regional lymph node metastasis

Distant metastasis

MX—distant metastasis can't be assessed

M0—no known distant metastasis

M1—distant metastasis

Staging categories

Pancreatic cancer progresses from mild to severe as follows:

Stage I—T1, N0, M0; T2, N0, M0

Stage II—T3, N0, M0

Stage III—any T, N1, M0

Stage IV—any T, any N, M1

• pancreatic enzymes (average dose is 0.5 to 1 mg with meals) — to assist in digestion of proteins, carbohydrates, and fats when pancreatic juices are insufficient because of surgery or obstruction.

Radiation therapy is usually ineffective except as an adjunct to chemotherapy or as a palliative measure.

Special considerations
Before surgery:
• Ensure that the patient is medically stable, particularly regarding nutrition (this may take 4 to 5 days). If the patient can't tolerate oral feedings, provide total parenteral nutrition and I.V. fat emulsions to correct deficiencies and maintain positive nitrogen balance.
• Give blood transfusions (to combat anemia), vitamin K (to overcome prothrombin deficiency), antibiotics (to prevent postoperative complications), and gastric lavage (to maintain gastric decompression), as necessary.
• Tell the patient about expected postoperative procedures and expected side effects of radiation and chemotherapy.
After surgery:
• Watch for and report complications, such as fistula, pancreatitis, fluid and electrolyte imbalance, infection, hemorrhage, skin breakdown, nutritional deficiency, hepatic failure, renal insufficiency, and diabetes.
• If the patient is receiving chemotherapy, treat side effects symptomatically.
Throughout this illness, provide meticulous supportive care as follows:
• Monitor fluid balance, abdominal girth, metabolic state, and weight daily. In weight loss, replace nutrients intravenously, orally, or by nasogastric tube; in weight gain (due to ascites), impose dietary restrictions, such as a low-sodium or fluid-retention diet, as required. Maintain a 2,500-calorie diet.

• Serve small, frequent nutritious meals by enlisting the dietitian's services. Administer an oral pancreatic enzyme at mealtimes, if needed. As necessary, give antacids to prevent stress ulcers.
• To prevent constipation, administer laxatives, stool softeners, and cathartics as required; modify diet; and increase fluid intake. To increase GI motility, position the patient properly at mealtime, and help him walk when he can.
• Ensure adequate rest and sleep. Assist with range-of-motion and isometric exercises, as appropriate.
• Administer pain medication, antibiotics, and antipyretics, as necessary. Note time, site (if injected), and response.
• Watch for signs of hypoglycemia or hyperglycemia; administer glucose or an antidiabetic agent as necessary. Monitor blood glucose and urine acetone levels.
• Document progression of jaundice.
• Provide meticulous skin care to avoid pruritus and necrosis. Prevent excoriation in a pruritic patient by clipping his nails and having him wear cotton gloves.
• Watch for signs of upper GI bleeding; test stools and vomitus for occult blood, and keep a flow sheet of hemoglobin and hematocrit values.
• To control active bleeding, promote gastric vasoconstriction with prescribed medication. Replace any fluid loss.
• Ease discomfort from pyloric obstruction with a nasogastric tube.
• To prevent thrombosis, apply anti-embolism stockings and assist in range-of-motion exercises. If thrombosis occurs, elevate the patient's legs, and give an anticoagulant or aspirin, as required.
• Encourage the patient to verbalize his fears. Promote family involvement, and offer the assistance of a counselor.

Help the patient and his family deal with the reality of death.

PANCREATITIS

Pancreatitis, inflammation of the pancreas, occurs in acute and chronic forms and may be due to edema, necrosis, or hemorrhage. In men, this disease is commonly associated with alcoholism, trauma, or peptic ulcer; in women, with biliary tract disease.

The prognosis is good when pancreatitis follows biliary tract disease but poor when it follows alcoholism. Mortality rises as high as 60% when pancreatitis is associated with necrosis and hemorrhage.

Causes

The most common causes of pancreatitis are biliary tract disease and alcoholism, but it can also result from pancreatic carcinoma, trauma, or certain drugs, such as glucocorticoids, sulfonamides, chlorothiazide, and azathioprine.

This disease also may develop as a complication of peptic ulcer, mumps, or hypothermia. Rarer causes are stenosis or obstruction of the sphincter of Oddi, hyperlipemia, metabolic endocrine disorders (hyperparathyroidism, hemochromatosis), vasculitis or vascular disease, viral infections, mycoplasmal pneumonia, and pregnancy.

Afro-Asian syndrome (diabetes, pancreatic insufficiency, and calcification) occurs in young people, probably from malnutrition and alcoholism, and leads to pancreatic atrophy. Regardless of the cause, pancreatitis involves autodigestion: The enzymes normally excreted by the pancreas digest pancreatic tissue.

Signs and symptoms

In many patients, the first and only symptom of mild pancreatitis is steady epigastric pain centered close to the umbilicus, radiating between the tenth thoracic and sixth lumbar vertebrae, and unrelieved by vomiting. However, a severe attack causes extreme pain, persistent vomiting, abdominal rigidity, diminished bowel activity (suggesting peritonitis), crackles at lung bases, and left pleural effusion.

Severe pancreatitis may produce extreme malaise and restlessness, with mottled skin, tachycardia, low-grade fever (100° to 102° F [37.7° to 38.8° C]), and cold, sweaty extremities. Proximity of the inflamed pancreas to the bowel may cause ileus.

If pancreatitis damages the islets of Langerhans, complications may include diabetes mellitus (see *Chronic pancreatitis,* page 628). Fulminant pancreatitis causes massive hemorrhage and total destruction of the pancreas, resulting in diabetic acidosis, shock, or coma.

Diagnosis

A careful patient history (especially for alcoholism) and physical examination are the first steps in diagnosis, but the retroperitoneal position of the pancreas makes physical assessment difficult.

Dramatically elevated serum amylase levels—frequently over 500 units—confirm pancreatitis and rule out perforated peptic ulcer, acute cholecystitis, appendicitis, and bowel infarction or obstruction.

Similarly dramatic elevations of amylase are also found in urine, ascites, or pleural fluid. Characteristically, amylase levels return to normal 48 hours after onset of pancreatitis, despite continuing symptoms. Supportive laboratory values include:
• increased serum lipase levels, which rise more slowly than serum amylase

---

CHRONIC PANCREATITIS

Usually associated with alcoholism (in over half of all patients), chronic pancreatitis can also follow hyperparathyroidism, hyperlipemia or, infrequently, gallstones, trauma, or peptic ulcer. Inflammation and fibrosis cause progressive pancreatic insufficiency and eventually destroy the pancreas.

Symptoms
Chronic pancreatitis is usually associated with constant dull pain with occasional exacerbations, malabsorption, severe weight loss, and hyperglycemia (leading to diabetic symptoms). Relevant diagnostic measures include patient history, X-rays showing pancreatic calcification, elevated erythrocyte sedimentation rate, and examination of stool for steatorrhea.

Treatment
The severe pain of chronic pancreatitis often requires large doses of analgesics or narcotics, making addiction a serious problem. Treatment also includes a low-fat diet and oral administration of pancreatic enzymes, such as pancreatin or pancrelipase to control steatorrhea, insulin or oral antidiabetic agents to curb hyperglycemia and, occasionally, surgical repair of biliary or pancreatic ducts, or the sphincter of Oddi to reduce pressure and promote the flow of pancreatic juice. The prognosis is good if the patient can avoid alcohol but poor if he can't.

• low serum calcium levels (hypocalcemia) from fat necrosis and formation of calcium soaps
• white blood cell counts that range from 8,000 to 20,000/µl, with increased polymorphonuclear leukocytes
• elevated glucose levels — as high as 500 to 900 mg/dl, indicating hyperglycemia.

The following other tests may be used to diagnose pancreatitis:
• *Electrocardiography* shows changes (prolonged QT segment but normal T wave) that help diagnose hypocalcemia.
• *Abdominal X-rays* show dilation of the small or large bowel or calcification of the pancreas.
• *GI series* indicates extrinsic pressure on the duodenum or stomach due to edema of the pancreas head.
• *Chest X-rays* show left-sided pleural effusion.

• *Ultrasonography or computed tomography scan* reveals an increased pancreatic diameter and helps distinguish acute cholecystitis from acute pancreatitis.

Treatment
The goal of therapy is to maintain circulation and fluid volume. Treatment measures must also relieve pain and decrease pancreatic secretions.

Emergency measures
Emergency treatment for shock (which is the most common cause of death in early-stage pancreatitis) consists of vigorous I.V. replacement of electrolytes and proteins.

Metabolic acidosis that develops secondary to hypovolemia and impaired cellular perfusion requires vigorous fluid volume replacement.

Drug treatment choices may include morphine sulfate for pain; diazepam for restlessness and agitation; and antibiotics, such as gentamicin, clindamycin, or chloramphenicol, for bacterial infections.

Additionally, if the patient has hypocalcemia, he will need an infusion of 10% calcium gluconate; if he has elevated serum glucose levels, he may require insulin therapy.

After the emergency

After the emergency phase, continuing I.V. therapy should provide adequate electrolytes and protein solutions that don't stimulate the pancreas (glucose or free amino acids) for 5 to 7 days.

If the patient is not ready to resume oral feedings by then, hyperalimentation may be necessary. Nonstimulating elemental gavage feedings may be safer because of the decreased risk of infection and overinfusion. In extreme cases, laparotomy to drain the pancreatic bed, 95% pancreatectomy, or a combination of cholecystostomy-gastrostomy, feeding jejunostomy, and drainage may be necessary.

Special considerations

• Acute pancreatitis is a life-threatening emergency. Provide meticulous supportive care and continuous monitoring of vital systems.
• Monitor vital signs and pulmonary artery pressure closely. If the patient has a central venous pressure line instead of a pulmonary artery catheter, monitor it closely for volume expansion (shouldn't exceed 10 cm H_2O).
• Give plasma or albumin, if necessary, to maintain blood pressure.
• Record fluid intake and output; check urine output hourly, and monitor electrolyte levels.
• Assess for crackles, rhonchi, or decreased breath sounds.
• For bowel decompression, maintain constant nasogastric suctioning, and give nothing by mouth. Perform good mouth and nose care.

• Watch for signs of calcium deficiency — tetany, cramps, carpopedal spasm, and seizures. If you suspect hypocalcemia, keep airway and suction apparatus handy and pad side rails.
• Administer analgesics, as needed, to relieve the patient's pain and anxiety. Remember that anticholinergics reduce salivary and sweat gland secretions. Warn the patient that he may experience dry mouth and facial flushing. *Caution:* Narrow-angle glaucoma contraindicates the use of atropine or its derivatives.
• Watch for adverse reactions to antibiotics: nephrotoxicity with aminoglycosides; pseudomembranous enterocolitis with clindamycin; and blood dyscrasias with chloramphenicol.
• Don't confuse thirst due to hyperglycemia (indicated by serum glucose levels up to 350 mg/dl and sugar and acetone in urine) with dry mouth due to nasogastric intubation and anticholinergics.
• Watch for complications due to hyperalimentation, such as sepsis, hypokalemia, overhydration, and metabolic acidosis.
• Watch for fever, cardiac irregularities, changes in arterial blood gas measurements, and deep respirations.
• Use strict aseptic technique when caring for the catheter insertion site.

PANIC DISORDER

Characterized by recurrent episodes of intense apprehension, terror, and impending doom, panic disorder represents anxiety in its most severe form. Initially unpredictable, these panic attacks may come to be associated with specific situations or tasks. The disorder often exists concurrently with agoraphobia. Equal numbers of men and women are affected by panic disorder alone, whereas panic disorder with agoraphobia occurs about twice as often in women.

Panic disorder typically has an onset in late adolescence or early adulthood, often in response to a sudden loss. It also may be triggered by severe separation anxiety experienced during early childhood.

Without treatment, panic disorder can persist for years, with alternating exacerbations and remissions. The patient with panic disorder is at high risk for a psychoactive substance abuse disorder: He may resort to alcohol or anxiolytics in an attempt to relieve his fear.

Causes

Like other anxiety disorders, panic disorder may stem from a combination of physiologic and psychological factors. For example, some theorists emphasize the role of stressful events or unconscious conflicts that occur early in childhood.

Recent evidence indicates that alterations in brain biochemistry, especially in norepinephrine, serotonin, and gamma-aminobutyric acid activity, may also contribute to panic disorder.

Signs and symptoms

The patient with panic disorder typically complains of repeated episodes of unexpected apprehension, fear or, rarely, intense discomfort. These panic attacks may last for minutes or hours and leave the patient shaken, fearful, and exhausted. They occur several times a week, sometimes even daily. Because the attacks occur spontaneously, without exposure to a known anxiety-producing situation, the patient often worries between attacks about when the next episode will occur.

Physical examination of the patient during a panic attack may reveal signs of intense anxiety, such as hyperventilation, tachycardia, trembling, and profuse sweating. He may also complain of difficulty breathing, digestive disturbances, and chest pain.

Diagnosis

For characteristic findings in patients with this condition, see *Diagnosing panic disorder*.

Because many medical conditions can mimic panic disorder, additional tests may be ordered to rule out an organic basis for the symptoms. For example, tests for serum glucose levels rule out hypoglycemia, studies of urine catecholamines and vanillylmandelic acid rule out pheochromocytoma, and thyroid function tests rule out hyperthyroidism.

Urine and serum toxicology tests may reveal the presence of psychoactive substances that can precipitate panic attacks, including barbiturates, caffeine, and amphetamines.

Treatment

Panic disorder may respond to behavioral therapy, supportive psychotherapy, or drug therapy, singly or in combination. Behavioral therapy works best when agoraphobia accompanies panic disorder because the identification of anxiety-inducing situations is easier.

Psychotherapy commonly uses cognitive techniques to enable the patient to view anxiety-provoking situations more realistically and to recognize panic symptoms as a misinterpretation of essentially harmless physical sensations.

Drug therapy includes antianxiety drugs, such as diazepam, alprazolam, and clonazepam, and beta blockers such as propranolol to provide symptomatic relief. Antidepressants, including tricyclic antidepressants, selective serotonin reuptake inhibitors, and monoamine oxidase inhibitors, are also effective.

DIAGNOSING PANIC DISORDER

The diagnosis of panic disorder is confirmed when the patient meets the criteria established in the *DSM-IV.*

Panic attack

A discrete period of intense fear or discomfort in which at least four of the following symptoms develop abruptly and reach a peak within 10 minutes:
• palpitations, pounding heart, or tachycardia
• sweating
• trembling or shaking
• shortness of breath or smothering sensations
• feeling of choking
• chest pain or discomfort
• nausea or abdominal distress
• dizziness or faintness
• depersonalization or derealization
• fear of losing control or going crazy
• fear of dying
• numbness or tingling sensations (paresthesia)
• hot flashes or chills.

Panic disorder without agoraphobia

• The person experiences recurrent unexpected panic attacks and at least one of the attacks has been followed by 1 month (or more) or one (or more) of the following:
—persistent concern about having additional attacks

—worry about the implications of the attack or its consequences
—a significant change in behavior related to the attacks.
• The panic attacks are not due to the direct physiologic effects of a substance or a general medical condition.
• The panic attacks are not better accounted for by another mental disorder, such as social phobia, specific phobia, obsessive-compulsive disorder, posttraumatic stress disorder, or separation anxiety disorder.

Panic disorder with agoraphobia

• The person experiences recurrent unexpected panic attacks and at least one of the attacks has been followed by 1 month (or more) or one (or more) of the following:
—persistent concern about having additional attacks
—worry about the implications of the attack or its consequences
—a significant change in behavior related to the attacks.
• The person exhibits agoraphobia.
• The panic attacks are not due to the direct physiologic effects of a substance or a general medical condition.
• The panic attacks are not better accounted for by another mental disorder, such as social phobia, specific phobia, obsessive-compulsive disorder, posttraumatic stress disorder, or separation anxiety disorder.

Special considerations
• Stay with the patient until the attack subsides. If left alone, he may become even more anxious.
• Maintain a calm, serene approach. Statements such as "I won't let anything here hurt you" and "I'll stay with you" can assure the patient that you're in control of the immediate situation.

Avoid giving him insincere expressions of reassurance.
• The patient's perceptual field may be narrowed, and excessive stimuli may cause him to feel overwhelmed. Dim bright lights or raise dim lights as necessary.
• If the patient loses control, move him to a smaller, quieter space.

• The patient may be so overwhelmed that he cannot follow lengthy or complicated instructions. Speak in short, simple sentences, and slowly give one direction at a time. Avoid giving lengthy explanations and asking too many questions.

• Allow the patient to pace around the room (provided he isn't belligerent) to help expend energy. Show him how to take slow, deep breaths if he's hyperventilating.

• Avoid touching the patient until you've established rapport. Unless he trusts you, he may be too stimulated or frightened to find touch reassuring.

• Administer medication as necessary.

• During and after a panic attack, encourage the patient to express his feelings. Discuss his fears and help him identify situations or events that trigger the attacks.

• Teach the patient relaxation techniques, and explain how he can use them to relieve stress or avoid a panic attack.

• Review with the patient any adverse effects of the drugs he'll be taking. Caution him to notify the doctor before discontinuing the medication because abrupt withdrawal could cause severe symptoms.

• Encourage the patient and his family to use community resources such as the Anxiety Disorders Association of America.

PARKINSON'S DISEASE

Named for James Parkinson, the English doctor who wrote the first accurate description of the disease in 1817, Parkinson's disease (also known as parkinsonism, paralysis agitans, shaking palsy) is a slowly progressive movement disorder that characteristically produces progressive muscle rigidity, akinesia, and involuntary tremor. The disorder is not fatal but death may result from aspiration pneumonia or some other infection.

Parkinson's disease, one of the most common crippling diseases in the United States, affects men more often than women. According to current statistics, it strikes 1 in every 100 people over age 60. Because of increased longevity, this amounts to roughly 60,000 new cases diagnosed annually in the United States alone.

Causes

Although the cause of Parkinson's disease is unknown, study of the extrapyramidal brain nuclei (corpus striatum, globus pallidus, substantia nigra) has established that a dopamine deficiency prevents affected brain cells from performing their normal inhibitory function within the central nervous system.

Signs and symptoms

The cardinal symptoms of Parkinson's disease are muscle rigidity and akinesia, and an insidious tremor that begins in the fingers (unilateral pill-roll tremor), increases during stress or anxiety, and decreases with purposeful movement and sleep.

Muscle rigidity results in resistance to passive muscle stretching, which may be uniform (lead-pipe rigidity) or jerky (cogwheel rigidity). Akinesia causes the patient to walk with difficulty (gait lacks normal parallel motion and may be retropulsive or propulsive).

Parkinson's disease also produces a high-pitched, monotone voice; drooling; a masklike facial expression; loss of posture control (the patient walks with body bent forward); and dysarthria, dysphagia, or both. Occasionally, akinesia may also cause oculogyric crises (eyes are fixed upward, with involuntary tonic movements) or blepharospasm (eyelids are completely closed). Parkinson's disease itself doesn't impair the intellect, but a co-existing disorder, such as arteriosclerosis, may.

Diagnosis

Generally, laboratory data are of little value in identifying Parkinson's disease; diagnosis is based on the patient's age and history and on the characteristic clinical picture. However, urinalysis may support the diagnosis by revealing decreased dopamine levels.

A conclusive diagnosis is possible only after ruling out other causes of tremor, involutional depression, cerebral arteriosclerosis, and, in patients under age 30, intracranial tumors, Wilson's disease, or phenothiazine or other drug toxicity.

Treatment

Because there's no cure for Parkinson's disease, the primary aim of treatment is to relieve symptoms and keep the patient functional as long as possible. Treatment consists of drugs, physical therapy and, in severe disease states unresponsive to drugs, stereotactic neurosurgery.

Drug therapy

Drug therapy usually includes levodopa, a dopamine replacement that is most effective during early stages. It's given in increasing doses until symptoms are relieved or side effects appear. Because side effects can be serious, levodopa is frequently given in combination with carbidopa to halt peripheral dopamine synthesis.

When levodopa proves ineffective or too toxic, alternative drug therapy includes anticholinergics, such as trihexyphenidyl; antihistamines, such as diphenhydramine; and amantadine, an antiviral agent. Selegiline, an enzyme-inhibiting agent, allows conservation of dopamine and enhances the therapeutic effect of levodopa.

Stereotactic neurosurgery

When drug therapy fails, stereotactic neurosurgery may be an alternative. In this procedure, electrical coagulation, freezing, radioactivity, or ultrasound destroys the ventrolateral nucleus of the thalamus to prevent involuntary movement. This is most effective in young, otherwise healthy persons with unilateral tremor or muscle rigidity. Neurosurgery can only *relieve* symptoms.

Physical therapy

Individually planned physical therapy complements drug treatment and neurosurgery to maintain normal muscle tone and function. Appropriate physical therapy includes both active and passive range-of-motion exercises, routine daily activities, walking, and baths and massage to help relax muscles.

Special considerations

• Effectively caring for the patient with Parkinson's disease requires careful monitoring of drug treatment, emphasis on teaching self-reliance, and generous psychological support.

• Monitor drug treatment so dosage can be adjusted to minimize side effects.

• If the patient has surgery, watch for signs of hemorrhage and increased intracranial pressure by frequently checking level of consciousness and vital signs.

• Encourage independence. The patient with excessive tremor may achieve partial control of his body by sitting on a chair and using its arms to steady himself. Remember that fatigue may cause him to depend more on others.

• Help the patient overcome problems related to eating and elimination. For example, if he has difficulty eating, offer supplementary or small, frequent meals to increase caloric intake.

• Help establish a regular bowel routine by encouraging the patient to drink at least 2,000 ml of liquids daily and eat high-bulk foods. He may need an elevated toilet seat to assist him from a standing to a sitting position.

• Give the patient and family emotional support. Teach them about the disease, its progressive stages, and drug side effects.

• Show the family how to prevent pressure ulcers and contractures by proper positioning. Inform them of the dietary restrictions levodopa imposes, and explain household safety measures to prevent accidents.

• Help the patient and family express their feelings and frustrations about the progressively debilitating effects of the disease.

• Establish long- and short-term treatment goals, and be aware of the patient's need for intellectual stimulation and diversion.

• To obtain more information, refer the patient and family to the National Parkinson Foundation or the United Parkinson Foundation.

PEDICULOSIS

Pediculosis is caused by parasitic forms of lice: *Pediculus humanus* var. *capitis* causes pediculosis capitis (head lice); *Pediculus humanus* var. *corporis* causes pediculosis corporis (body lice); and *Phthirus pubis* causes pediculosis pubis (crab lice). These lice feed on human blood and lay their eggs (nits) in body hairs or clothing fibers.

After the nits hatch, the lice must feed within 24 hours or die; they mature in about 2 to 3 weeks. When a louse bites, it injects a toxin into the skin that produces mild irritation and

a purpuric spot. Repeated bites cause sensitization to the toxin, leading to more serious inflammation. Treatment can effectively eliminate lice.

Causes

P. humanus var. *capitis* (most common species) feeds on the scalp and, rarely, in the eyebrows, eyelashes, and beard. This form of pediculosis is caused by overcrowded conditions and poor personal hygiene, and commonly affects children, especially girls. It spreads through shared clothing, hats, combs, and hairbrushes.

P. humanus var. *corporis* lives in the seams of clothing, next to the skin, leaving only to feed on blood. Common causes include prolonged wearing of the same clothing (which might occur in cold climates), overcrowding, and poor personal hygiene. It spreads through shared clothing and bedsheets.

P. pubis is primarily found in pubic hairs, but this species may extend to the eyebrows, eyelashes, and axillary or body hair. Pediculosis pubis is transmitted through sexual intercourse or by contact with clothes, bedsheets, or towels harboring lice.

Signs and symptoms

Clinical features vary with the cause.

Pediculosis capitis

Signs and symptoms of pediculosis capitis include itching; excoriation (with severe itching); matted, foul-smelling, lusterless hair (in severe cases); occipital and cervical lymphadenopathy; and a rash on the trunk, probably due to sensitization. Adult lice migrate from the scalp and deposit oval, gray-white nits on hair shafts.

Pediculosis corporis

Pediculosis corporis initially produces small red papules (usually on the shoulders, trunk, or buttocks). Later wheals (probably a sensitivity reaction) may develop. Untreated pediculosis corporis may lead to vertical excoriations and ultimately to dry, discolored, thickly encrusted, scaly skin, with bacterial infection and scarring. In severe cases, headache, fever, and malaise may accompany cutaneous symptoms.

Pediculosis pubis

Pediculosis pubis causes skin irritation from scratching, which is usually more obvious than the bites. Small gray-blue spots (maculae caeruleae) may appear on the thighs or upper body.

Diagnosis

Pediculosis is visible on physical examination, as follows:
• *pediculosis capitis:* oval, grayish nits that can't be shaken loose like dandruff (the closer the nits are to the end of the hair shaft, the longer the infection has been present, because the ova are laid close to the scalp)
• *pediculosis corporis:* characteristic skin lesions; nits found on clothing
• *pediculosis pubis:* nits attached to pubic hairs, which feel coarse and grainy to the touch.

Treatment

The type of pediculosis dictates the treatment.

Pediculosis capitis

Treatment consists of permethrin cream rinse rubbed into the hair and rinsed after 10 minutes. A single treatment should be sufficient. Alternatives include pyrethrins and lindane shampoo. A fine-tooth comb dipped in vinegar removes nits from hair; washing hair with ordinary shampoo removes crustations.

Pediculosis corporis

Pediculosis corporis requires bathing with soap and water to remove lice from the body; in severe infestation, treatment with lindane cream may be necessary. Lice may be removed from clothes by washing them in hot water, ironing, or dry-cleaning. Storing clothes for more than 30 days or placing them in dry heat of 140° F (60° C) kills lice. If clothes can't be washed or changed, application of 10% DDT or 10% lindane powder is effective.

Pediculosis pubis

Treatment of pediculosis pubis includes shampooing with lindane shampoo for 4 minutes. Treatment should be repeated in 1 week. Clothes and bedsheets must be laundered to prevent reinfestation.

Special considerations

• Instruct patients how to use the creams, ointments, powders, and shampoos that can eliminate lice. To prevent self-infestation, avoid prolonged contact with the patient's hair, clothing, and bedsheets.
• Ask the patient with pediculosis pubis for a history of recent sexual contacts, so that they can be examined and treated.
• To prevent the spread of pediculosis to other hospitalized persons, examine all high-risk patients on admission, especially the elderly who depend on others for care, those admitted from nursing homes, or persons living in crowded conditions.

PELVIC INFLAMMATORY DISEASE

Pelvic inflammatory disease (PID) is any acute, subacute, recurrent, or chronic infection of the oviducts and ovaries, with adjacent tissue involvement. It includes inflammation of the cervix (cervicitis), uterus (endometritis), fallopian tubes (salpingitis), and ovaries (oophoritis), which can extend to the connective tissue lying between the broad ligaments (parametritis).

Early diagnosis and treatment prevents damage to the reproductive system. Untreated PID may cause infertility and may lead to potentially fatal septicemia, pulmonary emboli, and shock.

Causes

PID can result from infection with aerobic or anaerobic organisms. The aerobic organism *Neisseria gonorrhoeae* is its most common cause because it most readily penetrates the bacteriostatic barrier of cervical mucus.

Normally, cervical secretions have a protective and defensive function. Therefore conditions or procedures that alter or destroy cervical mucus impair this bacteriostatic mechanism and allow bacteria present in the cervix or vagina to ascend into the uterine cavity; such procedures include conization or cauterization of the cervix.

Uterine infection can also follow the transfer of contaminated cervical mucus into the endometrial cavity by instrumentation. Consequently, PID can follow insertion of an intrauterine device (IUD), use of a biopsy curet or of an irrigation catheter, or tubal insufflation. Other predisposing factors include abortion, pelvic surgery, and infection during or after pregnancy.

Bacteria may also enter the uterine cavity through the bloodstream or from drainage from a chronically infected fallopian tube, a pelvic abscess, a ruptured appendix, diverticulitis of the sigmoid colon, or other infectious foci.

The most common bacteria found in cervical mucus are staphylococci, streptococci, diphtheroids, chlamydiae, and coliforms, including *Pseudomonas* and *Escherichia coli.*

Uterine infection can result from any one or several of these organisms or may follow the multiplication of normally nonpathogenic bacteria in an altered endometrial environment. Bacterial multiplication is most common during parturition, because the endometrium is atrophic, quiescent, and not stimulated by estrogen.

Signs and symptoms

Clinical features of PID vary with the affected area but generally include a profuse, purulent vaginal discharge, sometimes accompanied by low-grade fever and malaise (particularly if gonorrhea is the cause). The patient experiences lower abdomen pain; movement of the cervix or palpation of the adnexa may be extremely painful. (See *Forms of pelvic inflammatory disease.*)

Diagnosis

Diagnostic tests generally include:
• *Gram stain* of secretions from the endocervix or cul-de-sac. Culture and sensitivity testing aids selection of the appropriate antibiotic. Urethral and rectal secretions may also be cultured.
• *ultrasonography* to identify an adnexal or uterine mass. (X-rays seldom identify pelvic masses.)
• *culdocentesis* to obtain peritoneal fluid or pus for culture and sensitivity testing.

In addition, patient history is significant. In general, PID is associated with

FORMS OF PELVIC INFLAMMATORY DISEASE

Salpingooophoritis

Endometritis

Cervicitis

CAUSE AND CLINICAL FEATURES

Salpingo-oophoritis
• *Acute:* sudden onset of lower abdominal and pelvic pain, usually following menses; increased vaginal discharge; fever; malaise; lower abdominal pressure and tenderness; tachycardia; pelvic peritonitis
• *Chronic:* recurring acute episodes

Cervicitis
• *Acute:* purulent, foul-smelling vaginal discharge; vulvovaginitis, with itching or burning; red, edematous cervix; pelvic discomfort; sexual dysfunction; metrorrhagia; infertility; spontaneous abortion
• *Chronic:* cervical dystocia, laceration or eversion of the cervix, ulcerative vesicular lesion (when cervicitis results from herpes simplex virus II)

Endometritis
(generally postpartum or postabortion)
• *Acute:* mucopurulent or purulent vaginal discharge oozing from the cervix; edematous, hyperemic endometrium, possibly leading to ulceration and necrosis (with virulent organisms); lower abdominal pain and tenderness; fever; rebound pain; abdominal muscle spasm; thrombophlebitis of uterine and pelvic vessels (in severe forms)
• *Chronic:* recurring acute episodes (increasingly common because of widespread use of intrauterine devices)

DIAGNOSTIC FINDINGS

• Blood studies show leukocytosis or normal white blood cell (WBC) count.
• X-ray may show ileus.
• Pelvic exam reveals extreme tenderness.
• Smear of cervical or periurethral gland exudate shows gram-negative intracellular diplococci.

• Cultures for *N. gonorrhoeae* are positive (more than 90% of patients).
• Cytologic smears may reveal severe inflammation.
• If cervicitis is not complicated by salpingitis, WBC count normal or slightly elevated; erythrocyte sedimentation rate (ESR) elevated.
• In *acute cervicitis,* cervical palpation reveals tenderness.
• In *chronic cervicitis,* causative organisms are usually staphylococci or streptococci.

• In severe infection, palpation may reveal boggy uterus.
• Uterine and blood samples positive for causative organism, usually staphylococcus.
• WBC count and ESR are elevated.

recent sexual intercourse, IUD insertion, childbirth, or abortion.

Treatment

To prevent progression of PID, antibiotic therapy begins immediately after culture specimens are obtained. Such therapy can be reevaluated as soon as laboratory results are available (usually after 24 to 48 hours). Infection may become chronic if treated inadequately.

The guidelines of the Centers for Disease Control and Prevention (CDC) for outpatient treatment include a single dose of cefoxitin plus probenecid given concurrently or a single dose of ceftriaxone. Each of these regimens is given with doxycycline for 14 days.

The CDC guidelines for inpatient treatment include doxycycline alone or a combination of clindamycin and gentamicin.

Development of a pelvic abscess necessitates adequate drainage. A ruptured abscess is life-threatening. If this complication develops, the patient may need a total abdominal hysterectomy with bilateral salpingo-oophorectomy.

Special considerations

• After establishing that the patient has no drug allergies, administer antibiotics and analgesics, as necessary.
• Check for fever. If it persists, carefully monitor fluid intake and output for signs of dehydration.
• Watch for abdominal rigidity and distention, possible signs of developing peritonitis. Provide frequent perineal care if vaginal drainage occurs.
• To prevent a recurrence, explain the nature and seriousness of PID, and encourage the patient to comply with the treatment regimen.
• Stress the need for the patient's sexual partner to be examined and, if necessary, treated for infection.

• Because PID may cause painful intercourse, advise the patient to consult with her doctor about sexual activity.
• To prevent infection after minor gynecologic procedures, such as dilatation and curettage, tell the patient to immediately report any fever, increased vaginal discharge, or pain. After such procedures, instruct her to avoid douching and intercourse for at least 7 days.

PENILE CANCER

Penile carcinoma rarely affects circumcised men in modern cultures; when it does occur, it's usually in men over age 50. The most common form, epidermoid squamous cell carcinoma, is usually found in the glans but may also occur on the corona glandis and, rarely, in the preputial cavity.

This malignancy produces ulcerative or papillary (wartlike, nodular) lesions, which may become quite large before spreading beyond the penis; such lesions may destroy the glans prepuce and invade the corpora.

Prognosis varies according to staging at time of diagnosis. If begun early enough, radiation therapy increases the 5-year survival rate to over 60%; surgery only, to over 55%. Unfortunately, many men delay treatment of penile cancer, because they fear disfigurement and loss of sexual function.

Causes

The exact cause of penile cancer is unknown; however, it's generally associated with poor personal hygiene and phimosis in uncircumcised men. This may account for the low incidence among Jews, Muslims, and people of other cultures that practice circumcision at birth or shortly thereafter. (Incidence isn't decreased in cultures that

practice circumcision at a later date.) Early circumcision seems to prevent penile cancer by allowing for better personal hygiene and minimizing inflammatory (and often premalignant) lesions of the glans and prepuce. Such lesions include:
• *leukoplakia* — inflammation, with thickened patches that may fissure
• *balanitis* — inflammation of the penis associated with phimosis
• *erythroplasia of Queyrat* — squamous cell carcinoma in situ; velvety, erythematous lesion that becomes scaly and ulcerative
• *penile horn* — scaly, horn-shaped growth.

Signs and symptoms

In a circumcised man, early signs of penile cancer include a small circumscribed lesion, a pimple, or a sore on the penis. In an uncircumcised man, however, such early symptoms may go unnoticed, so penile cancer first becomes apparent when it causes late-stage symptoms, such as pain, hemorrhage, dysuria, purulent discharge, and obstruction of the urinary meatus. Rarely are metastases the first signs of penile cancer.

Diagnosis

Diagnosis of penile cancer requires a tissue biopsy. Preoperative baseline studies include complete blood count, urinalysis, electrocardiography, and a chest X-ray. Enlarged inguinal lymph nodes due to infection (caused by primary lesion) make detection of nodal metastasis by preoperative computed tomography scan difficult.

Treatment

Depending on the stage of progression, treatment includes surgical resection of the primary tumor and, possibly, chemotherapy and radiation. Local tumors of the prepuce only require circumcision. Invasive tumors, however, require partial penectomy (unless contraindicated because of the patient's young age); tumors of the base of the penile shaft require total penectomy and inguinal node dissection (done less often in the United States than in other countries where incidence is higher).

Radiation therapy may improve treatment effectiveness after resection of localized lesions without metastasis; it may also reduce the size of lymph nodes before nodal resection. It's not adequate primary treatment for groin metastasis, however. Bleomycin and methotrexate are generally used in chemotherapy but are not very effective.

Special considerations

Penile cancer calls for good patient teaching, psychological support, and comprehensive postoperative care. The patient with penile cancer fears disfigurement, pain, and loss of sexual function.

Before penile surgery:
• Spend time with the patient, and encourage him to talk about his fears.
• Supplement and reinforce what the doctor has told the patient about the surgery and other treatment measures, and explain expected postoperative procedures, such as dressing changes and catheterization. Show him diagrams of the surgical procedure and pictures of the results of similar surgery to help him adapt to an altered body image.
• If the patient needs urinary diversion, refer him to the enterostomal therapist.

After penile surgery:
• Constantly monitor the patient's vital signs and record his intake and output accurately.
• Provide comprehensive skin care to prevent skin breakdown from urinary diversion or suprapubic catheterization. Keep the skin dry and free from

urine. If the patient has a suprapubic catheter, make sure the catheter is patent at all times.

• Administer analgesics, as ordered. Elevate the penile stump with a small towel or pillow to minimize edema.

• Check the surgical site often for signs of infection, such as foul odor or excessive drainage on dressing.

• If the patient has had inguinal node dissection, watch for signs of lymphedema, such as decreased circulation or disproportionate swelling of a leg.

• After partial penectomy, reassure the patient that the penile stump should be sufficient for urination and sexual function. Refer him for psychological or sexual counseling if necessary.

PEPTIC ULCERS

Circumscribed lesions in the mucosal membrane, peptic ulcers can develop in the lower esophagus, stomach, pylorus, duodenum, or jejunum. About 80% of all peptic ulcers are duodenal ulcers, which affect the proximal part of the small intestine and occur most often in men between ages 20 and 50.

Gastric ulcers, which affect the stomach mucosa, are most common in middle-aged and elderly men, especially in chronic users of nonsteroidal anti-inflammatory drugs (NSAIDs) or alcohol.

Duodenal ulcers usually follow a chronic course, with remissions and exacerbations; 5% to 10% of patients develop complications that necessitate surgery.

Causes

Researchers recognize three major causes of peptic ulcer disease: infection with *Helicobacter pylori* (formerly known as *Campylobacter pylori*), use of NSAIDs, and pathologic hypersecretory states, such as Zollinger-Ellison syndrome.

How *H. pylori* produces an ulcer isn't clear, but the disorder can be cured. Gastric acid, which was considered a primary cause, now appears mainly to contribute to the consequences of infection. Ongoing studies should soon unveil the full mechanism of ulcer formation.

Other causes include use of certain drugs, for example, salicylates and other NSAIDs, which encourage ulcer formation by inhibiting the secretion of prostaglandins (the substances that suppress ulceration). Certain illnesses, such as pancreatitis, hepatic disease, Crohn's disease, preexisting gastritis, and Zollinger-Ellison syndrome, are also known causes.

Predisposing factors

Besides peptic ulcers' main causes, several predisposing factors are acknowledged. They include blood type (gastric ulcers tend to strike people with type A blood; duodenal ulcers tend to afflict people with type O blood) and other genetic factors.

Exposure to irritants, such as alcohol and tobacco, may contribute by accelerating gastric acid emptying and promoting mucosal breakdown. Physical trauma, emotional stress, and normal aging are additional predisposing conditions.

Signs and symptoms

Clinical features vary with the area affected.

Gastric ulcers

Heartburn and indigestion usually signal the beginning of a gastric ulcer attack. Eating food stretches the gastric wall and may cause or, in some cases, relieve pain and a feeling of fullness and distention. Other typical effects include weight loss and repeated episodes of massive gastrointestinal (GI) bleeding.

Duodenal ulcers

Duodenal ulcers produce heartburn, well-localized midepigastric pain (relieved by food), weight gain (because the patient eats to relieve discomfort), and a peculiar sensation of hot water bubbling in the back of the throat. Attacks usually occur about 2 hours after meals, whenever the stomach is empty, or after consumption of orange juice, coffee, aspirin, or alcohol.

Exacerbations tend to recur several times a year, then fade into remission. Vomiting and other digestive disturbances are rare.

Complications

Both kinds of ulcers may be asymptomatic or may penetrate the pancreas and cause severe back pain. Other complications of peptic ulcers include perforation, hemorrhage, and pyloric obstruction.

Diagnosis

Upper GI tract X-rays show mucosal abnormalities; gastric secretory studies show hyperchlorhydria. Upper GI endoscopy confirms an ulcer, and biopsy rules out *H. pylori* infection and cancer. Carbon-13 (^{13}C) urea breath test results can confirm *H. pylori.*

Other tests may disclose occult blood in the stools and decreased hemoglobin and hematocrit values from GI bleeding.

Treatment

Current recommendations include treating every patient at least once to eradicate *H. pylori* because the infection may occur even with other causes, such as NSAID use. Initial treatment includes tetracycline, bismuth subsalicylate, and metronidazole. Amoxicillin may be tried as an alternative treatment.

Patients taking NSAIDs may take a prostaglandin analogue (misoprostol) to suppress ulceration (or the patient may take the analogue with NSAIDs to prevent ulceration). Histamine$_2$-receptor antagonists (cimetidine or nizatidine) or omeprazole may reduce acid secretion. A coating agent may be administered to patients with duodenal ulcers.

If GI bleeding occurs, emergency treatment begins with passage of a nasogastric (NG) tube to allow for iced saline lavage, possibly containing norepinephrine. Gastroscopy allows visualization of the bleeding site and coagulation by laser or cautery to control bleeding. This type of therapy allows postponement of surgery until the patient's condition stabilizes.

Surgery is indicated for perforation, unresponsiveness to conservative treatment, and suspected malignancy. Surgical procedures for peptic ulcers include:

• *vagotomy and pyloroplasty:* severing one or more branches of the vagus nerve to reduce hydrochloric acid secretion and refashioning the pylorus to create a larger lumen and facilitate gastric emptying

• *distal subtotal gastrectomy* (with or without vagotomy): excising the antrum of the stomach, thereby removing the hormonal stimulus of the parietal cells, followed by anastomosis of the rest of the stomach to the duodenum or the jejunum.

Special considerations

Management of peptic ulcers requires careful administration of medications, thorough patient teaching, and skillful postoperative care.

• Administer medications as necessary.

• Watch for adverse reactions to histamine$_2$-receptor antagonists and omeprazole (for example dizziness, fatigue, rash, mild diarrhea).

• Advise any patient who uses antacids, who has a history of cardiac disease, or who follows a sodium-restricted diet to take only those antacids that contain low amounts of sodium.

• Warn the patient to avoid steroids and NSAIDs because they irritate the gastric mucosa.

• For the same reason, warn the patient to avoid stressful situations, excessive intake of coffee, and any ingestion of alcoholic beverages during exacerbations of peptic ulcer disease. Likewise, advise the patient to stop smoking.

• Inform the patient of the potential adverse effects of antibiotic therapy, for example, superinfection and diarrhea. Instruct him to notify the doctor if these occur.

• Describe follow-up testing that the doctor will order to confirm eradication of *H. pylori* infection.

• Tell the patient taking bismuth subsalicylate that this drug may cause constipation.

After gastric surgery:

• Keep NG tube patent. If the tube isn't functioning, don't reposition it; you may damage the suture line or anastomosis. Notify the surgeon promptly.

• Monitor intake and output, including NG tube drainage. Check for bowel sounds, and allow the patient nothing by mouth until peristalsis resumes and the NG tube is removed or clamped.

• Replace fluids and electrolytes. Assess for signs of dehydration, sodium deficiency, and metabolic alkalosis, which may occur secondary to gastric suction.

• Monitor for possible complications: hemorrhage; shock; iron, folate, or vitamin B_{12} deficiency anemia (from malabsorption or continued blood loss); and dumping syndrome (weakness, nausea, flatulence, diarrhea, distention, and palpitations within 30 minutes after a meal).

• To avoid dumping syndrome, advise the patient to lie down after meals; to drink fluids *between* meals rather than with meals; to avoid eating large amounts of carbohydrates; and to eat four to six small, high-protein, low-carbohydrate meals during the day.

PERICARDITIS

Pericarditis is an inflammation of the pericardium, the fibroserous sac that envelops, supports, and protects the heart. It occurs in both acute and chronic forms. Acute pericarditis can be fibrinous or effusive, with purulent, serous, or hemorrhagic exudate; chronic constrictive pericarditis is characterized by dense fibrous pericardial thickening. The prognosis depends on the underlying cause but is generally good in acute pericarditis, unless constriction occurs.

Causes

Common causes of this disease include:

• bacterial, fungal, or viral infection (infectious pericarditis)

• neoplasms (primary, or metastases from lungs, breasts, or other organs)

• high-dose radiation to the chest

• uremia

• hypersensitivity or autoimmune disease, such as acute rheumatic fever (most common cause of pericarditis in children), systemic lupus erythematosus, and rheumatoid arthritis

• postcardiac injury, such as myocardial infarction (MI, which later causes an autoimmune reaction [Dressler's syndrome] in the pericardium), trauma, or surgery that leaves the pericardium intact but causes blood to leak into the pericardial cavity

• drugs, such as hydralazine or procainamide
• idiopathic factors (most common in acute pericarditis).

Less common causes include aortic aneurysm with pericardial leakage and myxedema with cholesterol deposits in the pericardium.

Signs and symptoms
Clinical features vary in the acute and chronic form.

Acute pericarditis
In acute pericarditis, a sharp and often sudden pain usually starts over the sternum and radiates to the neck, shoulders, back, and arms. However, unlike the pain of MI, pericardial pain is often pleuritic, increasing with deep inspiration and decreasing when the patient sits up and leans forward, pulling the heart away from the diaphragmatic pleurae of the lungs.

Pericardial effusion, the major complication of acute pericarditis, may produce effects of heart failure — such as dyspnea, orthopnea, and tachycardia — as well as ill-defined substernal chest pain and a feeling of fullness in the chest.

If the fluid accumulates rapidly, cardiac tamponade may occur, resulting in pallor, clammy skin, hypotension, pulsus paradoxus (a decrease in systolic blood pressure ≥ 15 mm Hg during slow inspiration), neck vein distention and, eventually, cardiovascular collapse and death.

Chronic pericarditis
Chronic constrictive pericarditis causes a gradual increase in systemic venous pressure and produces symptoms similar to those of chronic right heart failure (fluid retention, ascites, hepatomegaly).

Diagnosis
Because pericarditis often coexists with other conditions, diagnosis of acute pericarditis depends on typical clinical features and elimination of other possible causes. A classic symptom, the pericardial friction rub, is a grating sound heard as the heart moves. It can usually be auscultated best during forced expiration, while the patient leans forward or is on his hands and knees in bed.

This friction rub may have up to three components, corresponding to the timing of atrial systole, ventricular systole, and the rapid-filling phase of ventricular diastole. Occasionally, it's heard only briefly or not at all. Nevertheless, its presence, together with other characteristic features, is diagnostic of acute pericarditis.

In addition, if acute pericarditis has caused very large pericardial effusions, the physical examination reveals increased cardiac dullness and diminished or absent apical impulse and distant heart sounds. In patients with chronic pericarditis, acute inflammation or effusions do not occur — only restricted cardiac filling.

Laboratory results reflect inflammation and may identify its cause:
• normal or elevated white blood cell count, especially in infectious pericarditis
• elevated erythrocyte sedimentation rate
• slightly elevated cardiac enzyme levels with associated myocarditis
• culture of pericardial fluid obtained by open surgical drainage or cardiocentesis (sometimes identifies a causative organism in bacterial or fungal pericarditis).

Electrocardiography shows the following changes in acute pericarditis: elevation of ST segments in the standard limb leads and most precordial leads without significant changes in QRS morphology that occur with MI, atrial ectopic rhythms such as atrial fibrillation, and diminished QRS voltage in pericardial effusion.

Other pertinent laboratory studies include blood urea nitrogen level to check for uremia, antistreptolysin O titers to detect rheumatic fever, and a purified protein derivative skin test to check for tuberculosis. In pericardial effusion, echocardiography is diagnostic when it shows an echo-free space between the ventricular wall and the pericardium.

Treatment
The goal of treatment is to relieve symptoms and manage underlying systemic disease.

Bed rest and drug therapy
In acute idiopathic pericarditis, post-MI pericarditis, and post-thoracotomy pericarditis, treatment consists of bed rest as long as fever and pain persist and nonsteroidal anti-inflammatory drugs, such as aspirin and indomethacin, to relieve pain and reduce inflammation.

If these drugs fail to relieve symptoms, corticosteroids may be used. Although corticosteroids produce rapid and effective relief, they must be used cautiously because episodes may recur when therapy is discontinued.

Infectious pericarditis that results from disease of the left pleural space, mediastinal abscesses, or septicemia requires antibiotics (possibly by direct pericardial injection), surgical drainage, or both. Cardiac tamponade may require pericardiocentesis. Signs of tamponade include pulsus paradoxus, neck vein distention, dyspnea, and shock.

Pericardectomy
Recurrent pericarditis may necessitate partial pericardectomy, which creates a "window" that allows fluid to drain into the pleural space. In constrictive pericarditis, total pericardectomy to permit adequate filling and contraction of the heart may be necessary. Treatment must also include management of rheumatic fever, uremia, tuberculosis, and other underlying disorders.

Special considerations
• Provide complete bed rest.
• Assess pain in relation to respiration and body position to distinguish pericardial pain from myocardial ischemic pain.
• Place the patient in an upright position to relieve dyspnea and chest pain. Provide analgesics and oxygen, and reassure the patient with acute pericarditis that his condition is temporary and treatable.
• Monitor the patient for signs of cardiac compression or cardiac tamponade, possible complications of pericardial effusion. Signs include decreased blood pressure, increased central venous pressure, and pulsus paradoxus. Because cardiac tamponade requires immediate treatment, keep a pericardiocentesis set handy whenever pericardial effusion is suspected.
• Explain tests and treatments to the patient. If surgery is necessary, he should learn deep breathing and coughing exercises beforehand. Postoperative care is similar to that given after cardiothoracic surgery.

LIFE-THREATENING DISORDER

PERITONITIS

Peritonitis is an acute or chronic inflammation of the peritoneum, the membrane that lines the abdominal cavity and covers the visceral organs. Inflammation may extend throughout the peritoneum or may be localized as an abscess.

Peritonitis commonly decreases intestinal motility and causes intestinal distention with gas. Mortality is 10%, with death usually resulting from bowel obstruction; the mortality was much higher before the introduction of antibiotics.

Causes

Although the GI tract normally contains bacteria, the peritoneum is sterile. In peritonitis, however, bacteria invade the peritoneum. Generally, such infection results from inflammation and perforation of the GI tract, allowing bacterial invasion. Usually, this is a result of appendicitis, diverticulitis, peptic ulcer, ulcerative colitis, volvulus, strangulated obstruction, abdominal neoplasm, or a stab wound.

Peritonitis may also result from chemical inflammation, as in rupture of the fallopian tube, or the bladder; perforation of a gastric ulcer; or released pancreatic enzymes.

In both chemical and bacterial inflammation, accumulated fluids containing protein and electrolytes make the transparent peritoneum opaque, red, inflamed, and edematous. Because the peritoneal cavity is so resistant to contamination, such infection is often localized as an abscess instead of disseminated as a generalized infection.

Signs and symptoms

The key symptom of peritonitis is sudden, severe, and diffuse abdominal pain that tends to intensify and localize in the area of the underlying disorder. For instance, if appendicitis causes the rupture, pain eventually localizes in the lower right quadrant. The patient often displays weakness, pallor, excessive sweating, and cold skin as a result of excessive loss of fluid, electrolytes, and protein into the abdominal cavity.

Decreased intestinal motility and paralytic ileus result from the effect of bacterial toxins on the intestinal muscles. Intestinal obstruction causes nausea, vomiting, and abdominal rigidity.

Other clinical characteristics

Typical features include hypotension, tachycardia, signs of dehydration (oliguria, thirst, dry swollen tongue, pinched skin), acutely tender abdomen associated with rebound tenderness, temperature of 103° F (39.4° C) or higher, and hypokalemia. Inflammation of the diaphragmatic peritoneum may cause shoulder pain and hiccups.

Abdominal distention and resulting upward displacement of the diaphragm may decrease respiratory capacity. Typically, the patient with peritonitis tends to breathe shallowly and move as little as possible to minimize pain.

Diagnosis

Severe abdominal pain in a person with direct or rebound tenderness suggests peritonitis. Abdominal X-rays showing edematous and gaseous distention of the small and large bowel support the diagnosis. In the case of perforation of a visceral organ, the X-ray shows air in the abdominal cavity.

Other appropriate tests include the following:

• *Chest X-ray* may show elevation of the diaphragm.

• *Blood studies* reveal leukocytosis (more than 20,000/μl).

• *Paracentesis* reveals bacteria, exudate, blood, pus, or urine.

• *Laparotomy* may be necessary to identify the underlying cause.

Treatment

Early treatment of GI inflammatory conditions and preoperative and postoperative antibiotic therapy help prevent peritonitis. After peritonitis develops, emergency treatment must combat infection, restore intestinal motility, and replace fluids and electrolytes.

Antibiotics and supplementary treatment

Massive antibiotic therapy usually includes administration of cefoxitin with an aminoglycoside or penicillin G and clindamycin with an aminoglycoside, depending on the infecting organisms. To decrease peristalsis and prevent perforation, the patient should receive nothing by mouth; he should receive supportive fluids and electrolytes parenterally.

Other supplementary measures include preoperative and postoperative administration of an analgesic, nasogastric (NG) intubation to decompress the bowel and, possibly, use of a rectal tube to facilitate passage of flatus.

Surgery

When peritonitis results from perforation, surgery is necessary as soon as the patient's condition is stable enough to tolerate it. The aim of surgery is to eliminate the source of infection by evacuating the spilled contents and inserting drains.

Occasionally, abdominocentesis may be necessary to remove accumulated fluid. Irrigation of the abdominal cavity with antibiotic solutions during surgery may be appropriate in some cases.

Special considerations

• Regularly monitor vital signs, fluid intake and output, and the amount of NG drainage or vomitus.
• Place the patient in semi-Fowler's position to help him breathe deeply with less pain and thus prevent pulmonary complications.
• Counteract mouth and nose dryness due to fever and NG intubation with regular cleaning and lubrication.

After surgery to evacuate the peritoneum:

• Maintain parenteral fluid and electrolyte administration, as ordered. Accurately record fluid intake and output, including NG and incisional drainage.
• Place the patient in Fowler's position to promote drainage (through drainage tube) by gravity. Move him carefully, because the slightest movement will intensify the pain.
• Keep the side rails up and implement other safety measures if fever and pain disorient the patient.
• Encourage and assist ambulation, as ordered, usually on the first postoperative day.
• Watch for signs of dehiscence (the patient may complain that "something gave way") and abscess formation (continued abdominal tenderness and fever).
• Frequently assess for peristaltic activity by listening for bowel sounds and checking for gas, bowel movements, and soft abdomen.
• When peristalsis returns and temperature and pulse rate are normal, the NG tube is removed.
• Gradually decrease parenteral fluids and increase oral fluids.

PERNICIOUS ANEMIA

A megaloblastic anemia, pernicious anemia is characterized by decreased gastric production of hydrochloric acid and deficiency of intrinsic factor (IF), a substance normally secreted by the parietal cells of the gastric mucosa that is essential for vitamin B_{12} absorption. The resulting deficiency of vitamin B_{12} causes serious neurologic, gastric, and intestinal abnormalities. Untreated pernicious anemia may lead to permanent neurologic disability and death.

Pernicious anemia primarily affects people of northern European ancestry; in the United States, it's most common in New England and the Great Lakes region because of ethnic concentrations. It's rare in children, blacks, and Asians. Onset typically occurs between ages 50 and 60; incidence rises with increasing age.

Causes

Familial incidence of pernicious anemia suggests a genetic predisposition. Significantly higher incidence in patients with immunologically related diseases, such as thyroiditis, myxedema, and Graves' disease, seems to support a widely held theory that an inherited autoimmune response causes gastric mucosal atrophy and, therefore, deficiency of hydrochloric acid and IF.

Deficiency of IF impairs vitamin B_{12} absorption. The resultant vitamin B_{12} deficiency inhibits cell growth, particularly of red blood cells (RBCs), leading to insufficient and deformed RBCs with poor oxygen-carrying capacity. It also impairs myelin formation, causing neurologic damage. Iatrogenic induction can follow partial gastrectomy.

Signs and symptoms

Characteristically, pernicious anemia has an insidious onset but eventually causes an unmistakable triad of symptoms: weakness, sore tongue, and numbness and tingling in the extremities. The lips, gums, and tongue appear markedly bloodless. Hemolysis-induced hyperbilirubinemia may cause faintly jaundiced sclera and pale to bright yellow skin. In addition, the patient may become highly susceptible to infection, especially of the genitourinary tract.

GI symptoms

Gastric mucosal atrophy and decreased hydrochloric acid production disturb digestion and lead to nausea, vomiting, anorexia, weight loss, flatu-

lence, diarrhea, and constipation. Gingival bleeding and tongue inflammation may hinder eating and intensify anorexia.

CNS symptoms

Demyelination caused by vitamin B_{12} deficiency initially affects the peripheral nerves but gradually extends to the spinal cord. Consequently, the neurologic effects of pernicious anemia may include neuritis, weakness in extremities, peripheral numbness and paresthesias, disturbed position sense, lack of coordination, ataxia, impaired fine finger movement, positive Babinski's and Romberg's signs, light-headedness, optic muscle atrophy, loss of bowel and bladder control, impotence (in males), and altered vision (diplopia, blurred vision), taste, and hearing (tinnitus).

The effects of pernicious anemia on the nervous system may also produce irritability, poor memory, headache, depression, and delirium. Although some of these symptoms are temporary, irreversible central nervous system changes may have occurred before treatment.

Cardiovascular symptoms

Increasingly fragile cell membranes induce widespread destruction of RBCs, resulting in low hemoglobin levels. The impaired oxygen-carrying capacity of the blood secondary to lowered hemoglobin leads to weakness, fatigue, and light-headedness. Compensatory increased cardiac output results in palpitations, wide pulse pressure, dyspnea, orthopnea, tachycardia, premature beats and, eventually, congestive heart failure.

Diagnosis

A positive family history, typical ethnic heritage, and results of blood studies, bone marrow aspiration, gastric analysis, and the Schilling test establish the diagnosis. Laboratory screening must rule out other anemias with similar symptoms, such as folic acid deficiency anemia, because treatment differs.

Diagnosis must also rule out vitamin B_{12} deficiency resulting from malabsorption due to gastrointestinal disorders, gastric surgery, radiation, or drug therapy.

Blood study results that suggest pernicious anemia include:
• decreased hemoglobin (4 to 5 g/dl) and decreased RBC count
• increased mean corpuscular volume (more than $120/\mu l$); because larger-than-normal RBCs *each* contain increased amounts of hemoglobin, mean corpuscular hemoglobin concentration is also increased
• possible low white blood cell and platelet counts and large, malformed platelets
• serum vitamin B_{12} assay levels less than 0.1 mcg/ml
• elevated serum lactate dehydrogenase levels.

Bone marrow aspiration reveals erythroid hyperplasia (crowded red bone marrow), with increased numbers of megaloblasts but few normally developing RBCs. Gastric analysis shows absence of free hydrochloric acid after histamine or pentagastrin injection.

Schilling test
In the Schilling test, the definitive test for pernicious anemia, the patient receives a small oral dose (0.5 to 2 mcg) of radioactive vitamin B_{12} after fasting for 12 hours. A larger dose (1 mg) of nonradioactive vitamin B_{12} is given I.M. 2 hours later, as a parenteral flush, and the radioactivity of a 24-hour urine specimen is measured.

About 7% of the radioactive B_{12} dose is excreted in the first 24 hours; persons with pernicious anemia excrete less than 3%. (In pernicious anemia, the vitamin remains unabsorbed and is passed in the stool.) When the Schilling test is repeated with IF added, the test shows normal excretion of vitamin B_{12}.

Serologic tests
Important serologic findings may include IF antibodies and antiparietal cell antibodies.

Treatment
Early parenteral vitamin B_{12} replacement can reverse pernicious anemia, minimize complications, and possibly prevent permanent neurologic damage.

Vitamin B_{12} replacement
An initial high dose of parenteral vitamin B_{12} causes rapid RBC regeneration. Within 2 weeks, hemoglobin should rise to normal and the patient's condition should markedly improve. Because rapid cell regeneration increases the patient's iron and folate requirements, concomitant iron and folic acid replacement is necessary to prevent iron deficiency anemia.

After the patient's condition improves, the vitamin B_{12} dosage can be decreased to maintenance levels and given monthly. Because such injections must be continued for life, patients should learn self-administration of vitamin B_{12}.

Other measures
If anemia causes extreme fatigue, the patient may require bed rest until hemoglobin rises. If hemoglobin is dangerously low, he may need blood transfusions, digoxin, a diuretic, and a low-sodium diet for congestive heart failure. Most important is the replacement of vitamin B_{12} to control the condition that led to this failure. Antibiotics help combat accompanying infections.

Special considerations

• Supportive measures minimize the risk of complications and speed recovery. Patient and family teaching can promote compliance with lifelong vitamin B_{12} replacement.

• If the patient has severe anemia, plan activities, rest periods, and necessary diagnostic tests to conserve his energy. Monitor pulse rate often; tachycardia means his activities are too strenuous.

• To ensure accurate Schilling test results, make sure that all urine over a 24-hour period is collected and that the specimens are uncontaminated.

• Warn the patient to guard against infections, and tell him to report signs of infection promptly, especially pulmonary and urinary tract infections, because the patient's weakened condition may increase susceptibility.

• Provide a well-balanced diet, including foods high in vitamin B_{12} (meat, liver, fish, eggs, and milk). Offer between-meal snacks, and encourage the family to bring favorite foods from home.

• Because a sore mouth and tongue make eating painful, ask the dietitian to avoid giving the patient irritating foods. If these symptoms make talking difficult, supply a pad and pencil or some other aid to facilitate nonverbal communication; explain this problem to the family. Provide diluted mouthwash or, with severe conditions, swab the patient's mouth with tap water or warm saline solution.

• Warn the patient with a sensory deficit not to use a heating pad, because it may cause burns.

• If the patient is incontinent, establish a regular bowel and bladder routine. After the patient is discharged, a visiting nurse should follow up on this schedule and make adjustments, as needed.

• If neurologic damage causes behavioral problems, assess mental and neurologic status often; if necessary, give tranquilizers, as ordered, and apply a jacket restraint at night.

• Stress that vitamin B_{12} replacement isn't a permanent cure and that these injections must be continued for life, even after symptoms subside.

• To prevent pernicious anemia, emphasize the importance of vitamin B_{12} supplements for patients who've had extensive gastric resections or who follow strict vegetarian diets.

PERSONALITY DISORDERS

Defined as individual traits that reflect chronic, inflexible, and maladaptive patterns of behavior, personality disorders cause social discomfort and impair social and occupational functioning. Although no statistics document the number of cases of personality disorder, these disorders are known to be widespread. Most patients with a personality disorder don't receive treatment; when they do, they're typically managed as outpatients.

According to the classification system of the *Diagnostic and Statistical Manual of Mental Disorders*, 4th edition, *(DSM-IV)*, personality disorders fall on Axis II. Knowing the features of personality disorders helps provide a fuller picture of the patient and a more accurate diagnosis. For example, many features characteristic of personality disorders are apparent during an episode of another mental disorder (such as a major depressive episode in a patient with compulsive personality features).

Personality disorders typically begin before or during adolescence and early adulthood and persist throughout adult life. The prognosis is variable.

Causes

Only recently have personality disorders been categorized in detail, and research continues to identify their causes. Various theories attempt to explain the origin of personality disorders.

• Biological theories hold that these disorders may stem from chromosomal and neuronal abnormalities or head trauma.

• Social theories hold that the disorders reflect learned responses, having much to do with reinforcement, modeling, and aversive stimuli as contributing factors.

• Psychodynamic theories hold that personality disorders reflect deficiencies in ego and superego development and are related to poor mother-child relationships that are characterized by unresponsiveness, overprotectiveness, or early separation.

Signs and symptoms

Each specific personality disorder produces characteristic signs and symptoms, which may vary among patients and within the same patient at different times. In general, the history of the patient with a personality disorder will reveal long-standing difficulties in interpersonal relationships, ranging from dependency to withdrawal, and in occupational functioning, with effects ranging from compulsive perfectionism to intentional sabotage.

The patient with a personality disorder may show any degree of self-confidence, ranging from no self-esteem to arrogance. Convinced that his behavior is normal, he avoids responsibility for its consequences, often resorting to projections and blame.

Diagnosis

For characteristic findings in patients with this condition, see *Diagnosing personality disorders*.

Treatment

Personality disorders are difficult to treat. Successful therapy requires a trusting relationship in which the therapist can use a direct approach. The type of therapy chosen depends on the patient's symptoms.

Drug therapy is ineffective but may be used to relieve acute anxiety and depression. Family and group therapy usually are effective.

Hospital inpatient milieu therapy can be effective in crisis situations and possibly for long-term treatment of borderline personality disorders. Inpatient treatment is controversial, however, because most patients with personality disorders do not comply with extended therapeutic regimens; for such patients, outpatient therapy may be more useful.

Special considerations

• Provide consistent care. Take a direct, involved approach to ensure the patient's trust. Keep in mind that many of these patients don't respond well to interviews, whereas others are charming and convincing.

• Teach the patient social skills, and reinforce appropriate behavior.

• Encourage expression of feelings, self-analysis of behavior, and accountability for actions.

Specific care measures vary with the particular personality disorder.

For paranoid personality disorder:

• Avoid situations that threaten the patient's autonomy.

• Approach the patient in a straightforward and candid manner, adopting a professional, rather than a casual or friendly, attitude. Remember that remarks intended to be humorous are easily misinterpreted by the paranoid patient.

• Provide a supportive and nonjudgmental environment in which the patient can safely explore and verbalize his feelings.

(Text continues on page 654.)

DIAGNOSING PERSONALITY DISORDERS

The diagnosis of a recognized personality disorder is made when a patient's symptoms match the following relevant diagnostic criteria put forth in the *DSM-IV.*

Paranoid personality disorder

The person must exhibit a pervasive and unwarranted tendency, beginning by early adulthood and present in various contexts, to interpret the actions of people as deliberately demeaning or threatening, as indicated by at least four of the following:

• The person suspects, without sufficient basis, that he's being exploited, deceived, or harmed by others.

• The person questions without justification the loyalty or trustworthiness of friends or associates.

• The person is reluctant to confide in others because of unwarranted fear that the information will be used against him.

• The person finds hostile or evil meanings in benign remarks.

• The person bears grudges or is unforgiving of insults or slights.

• The person is easily slighted and quick to react with anger or to counterattack.

• The person questions without justification the fidelity of a spouse or sexual partner.

The symptoms do not occur exclusively during the course of schizophrenia or other psychotic disorders and are not the direct physiologic effect of a general medical condition.

Schizoid personality disorder

The patient must exhibit a pervasive course of schizophrenia or a manic episode.

Borderline personality disorder

This pervasive pattern of instability of interpersonal relationships, self-image, and affect and marked impulsivity, beginning by early adulthood and present in various contexts, is indicated by at least five of the following features:

• The person makes frantic efforts to avoid real or imagined abandonment (excluding suicidal or self-mutilating behavior).

• The person has a pattern of unstable and intense interpersonal relationships characterized by alternating extremes of overidealization and devaluation.

• The person has an identity disturbance—a markedly and persistently unstable self-image or sense of self.

• The person shows impulsiveness in at least two areas that are potentially self-damaging, such as spending, sexual activity, substance abuse, shoplifting, reckless driving, and binge eating (excluding suicidal or self-mutilating behavior).

• The person engages in recurrent suicidal threats, gestures, or behavior or in self-mutilating behavior.

• The person has affective instability resulting from marked mood reactivity (for example, depression, irritability, or anxiety lasting usually a few hours and seldom more than a few days).

• The person has chronic feelings of emptiness or boredom.

• The person has inappropriate intense anger or difficulty controlling anger.

• The person has transient, stress-related paranoid ideation or severe dissociative symptoms.

(continued)

DIAGNOSING PERSONALITY DISORDERS *(continued)*

Histrionic personality disorder

This pervasive pattern of excessive emotionality and attention-seeking behavior, beginning by early adulthood and present in various contexts, is indicated by at least four of the following:

• The person is uncomfortable in situations in which he is not the center of attention.

• The person's interaction with others is often characterized by inappropriately sexually seductive or provocative behavior.

• The person displays rapidly shifting and shallow expression of emotions.

• The person consistently uses physical appearance to draw attention to self.

• The person has a style of speech that is excessively impressionistic and lacking in detail.

• The person shows self-dramatization, theatricality, and exaggerated emotional expression.

• The person is suggestible (easily influenced by others or circumstances).

• The person considers relationships to be more intimate than they actually are.

Narcissistic personality disorder

This pervasive pattern of grandiosity, need for admiration, and lack of empathy, beginning by early adulthood and present in various contexts, is indicated by at least five of the following:

• The person has a grandiose sense of self-importance.

• The person is preoccupied with fantasies of unlimited success, power, brilliance, beauty, or ideal love.

• The person believes that he is special and unique and can only be understood by, or should associate with, other special or high-status people (or institutions).

• The person requires excessive admiration.

• The person has a sense of entitlement (an unreasonable expectation of especially favorable treatment or automatic compliance with his expectations).

• The person is interpersonally exploitive, taking advantage of others to achieve his own ends.

• The person lacks empathy.

• The person is often envious of others or believes that others are envious of him.

• The person shows arrogant, naughty behaviors or attitudes.

Avoidant personality disorder

This pervasive pattern of social inhibition, feelings of inadequacy, and hypersensitivity to negative evaluation, beginning by early adulthood and present in a variety of contexts, is indicated by at least four of the following:

• The person avoids social or occupational activities that involve significant interpersonal contact because of fears of criticism, disapproval, or rejection.

• The person is unwilling to get involved with people unless he's certain that they will like him.

• The person shows restraint within intimate relationships because of the fear of being shamed or ridiculed.

• The person is preoccupied with being criticized or rejected in social situations.

• The person's feelings of inadequacy inhibit him in new interpersonal situations.

DIAGNOSING PERSONALITY DISORDERS   *(continued)*

• The person views himself as socially inept, personally unappealing, or inferior to others.

• The person is unusually reluctant to take personal risks or to engage in any new activities because they may prove embarrassing.

Dependent personality disorder

This pervasive and excessive need to be taken care of that leads to submissive and clinging behavior and fears of separation, beginning by early adulthood and present in a variety of contexts, is indicated by at least five of the following:

• The person has difficulty making everyday decisions without an excessive amount of advice or reassurance from others.

• The person needs others to assume responsibility for most major areas of his or her life.

• The person has difficulty expressing disagreement with others because of fear of loss of support or approval (excluding realistic fears of retribution).

• The person has difficulty initiating projects or doing things on his own (because of a lack of self-confidence in his judgment or abilities rather than a lack of motivation or energy).

• The person goes to excessive lengths to obtain nurture and support from others, to the point of volunteering to do things that are unpleasant.

• The person feels uncomfortable or helpless when alone because of exaggerated fears of inability to care for himself.

• The person urgently seeks another relationship as a source of care and support when a close relationship ends.

• The person is unrealistically preoccupied with fears of being left to take care of himself.

Obsessive-compulsive personality disorder

This pervasive pattern of preoccupation with orderliness, perfectionism, and mental and interpersonal control at the expense of flexibility, openness, and efficiency, beginning by early adulthood and present in a variety of contexts, is indicated by at least four of the following:

• The person is preoccupied with details, rules, lists, order, organization, or schedules to the extent that the core point of the activity is lost.

• The person shows perfectionism that interferes with task completion.

• The person is excessively devoted to work and productivity to the exclusion of leisure activities and friendships (not accounted for by obvious economic need).

• The person exhibits overconscientiousness, scrupulousness, and inflexibility about matters of morality, ethics, or values (not accounted for by cultural or religious identification).

• The person cannot discard worn-out or worthless objects even when they have no sentimental value.

• The person is reluctant to delegate tasks or to work with others unless they submit exactly to his way of doing things.

• The person adopts a miserly spending style toward self and others; money is viewed as something to be hoarded in preparation for future catastrophies.

• The person shows rigidity and stubborness.

For schizoid personality disorder:
- Remember that the schizoid patient needs close human contact but is easily overwhelmed. Respect the patient's need for privacy, and slowly build a trusting, therapeutic relationship so that he finds more pleasure than fear in relating to you.
- Give the patient plenty of time to express his feelings. Keep in mind that if you push him to do so before he's ready, he may retreat.

For schizotypal personality disorder:
- Recognize that the patient with this disorder is easily overwhelmed by stress. Allow him plenty of time to make difficult decisions.
- Be aware that the patient may relate unusually well to certain staff members and not at all to others.

For antisocial personality disorder:
- Be clear about your expectations and the consequences of failing to meet them.
- Use a straightforward, matter-of-fact approach to set limits on unacceptable behavior. Encourage and reinforce positive behavior.
- Expect the patient to refuse to cooperate so that he can gain control.

For borderline personality disorder:
- Encourage the patient to take responsibility for himself. Don't attempt to rescue him from the consequences of his actions.
- Don't try to solve problems that the patient can solve himself.
- Maintain a consistent approach in all interactions with the patient, and ensure that other staff members do so as well.
- Recognize that the patient may idolize some staff members and devalue others.
- Don't take sides in the patient's disputes with other staff members.

For histrionic personality disorder:
- Give the patient choices in care strategies, and incorporate his wishes into the treatment plan as much as possible. By increasing his sense of self-control, you'll reduce his anxiety.
- Deal with the patient in a professional way. He may be uncomfortable with a casual approach.

For narcissistic personality disorder:
- Respond positively to the patient's sense of entitlement. A critical attitude may cause him to become even more demanding and difficult.
- Focus on positive traits or on feelings of pain, loss, or rejection.

For avoidant personality disorder:
- Assess for signs of depression. Impaired social interaction increases the risk of affective disorders.
- Establish a trusting relationship with the patient. Be aware that he may become dependent on the few staff members whom he believes he can trust.
- Make sure that the patient has plenty of time to prepare for all upcoming procedures. This patient can't handle surprises well.
- Inform the patient when you will and will not be available if he needs assistance.

For dependent personality disorder:
- Initially, give the patient explicit directives, rather than ask him to make decisions. Later, encourage him to make easy decisions, such as what to wear or which television program to watch. Continue to provide support and reassurance as his decision-making ability improves.

For obsessive-compulsive personality disorder:
- Allow the patient to participate in his own treatment plan by offering choices whenever possible.
- Adopt a professional approach in your interactions with the patient. Avoid informality; this patient expects strict attention to detail.

PHARYNGITIS

The most common throat disorder, pharyngitis is an acute or chronic inflammation of the pharynx. It is widespread among adults who live or work in dusty or very dry environments, use their voices excessively, habitually use tobacco or alcohol, or suffer from chronic sinusitis, persistent coughs, or allergies.

Causes
Pharyngitis is usually caused by a virus. The most common bacterial cause is group A beta-hemolytic streptococci. Other common causes include *Mycoplasma* and *Chlamydia.*

Signs and symptoms
Pharyngitis produces a sore throat and slight difficulty in swallowing. Swallowing saliva is usually more painful than swallowing food. Pharyngitis may also cause the sensation of a lump in the throat as well as a constant, aggravating urge to swallow. Associated features may include mild fever, headache, muscle and joint pain, coryza, and rhinorrhea. Uncomplicated pharyngitis usually subsides in 3 to 10 days.

Diagnosis
Physical examination of the pharynx reveals generalized redness and inflammation of the posterior wall and red, edematous mucous membranes studded with white or yellow follicles. Exudate is usually confined to the lymphoid areas of the throat, sparing the tonsillar pillars. Bacterial pharyngitis usually produces a large amount of exudate.

A throat culture may be performed to identify bacterial organisms that may be the cause of the inflammation.

Treatment
The focus for treatment of acute and chronic pharyngitis varies.

Acute pharyngitis
In acute viral pharyngitis, treatment is usually symptomatic, and consists mainly of rest, warm saline gargles, throat lozenges containing a mild anesthetic, plenty of fluids, and analgesics as needed. If the patient can't swallow fluids, hospitalization may be required for I.V. hydration.

Suspected bacterial pharyngitis requires rigorous treatment with penicillin or another broad-spectrum antibiotic because *Streptococcus* is the chief infecting organism. Antibiotic therapy should continue for 48 hours until culture results are back.

If the culture (or a rapid strep test) is positive for group A beta-hemolytic streptococci, or if bacterial infection is suspected despite negative culture results, penicillin therapy should be continued for 10 days. This is to prevent the sequelae of acute rheumatic fever.

Chronic pharyngitis
In chronic pharyngitis, treatment requires the same supportive measures as acute pharyngitis but with greater emphasis on eliminating the underlying cause, such as an allergen. Preventive measures include adequate humidification and avoiding excessive exposure to air conditioning. In addition, the patient should be urged to stop smoking.

Special considerations
• Administer analgesics and warm saline gargles, as appropriate.
• Encourage the patient to drink plenty of fluids. Monitor intake and output scrupulously, and watch for signs of dehydration.
• Provide meticulous mouth care to prevent dry lips and oral pyoderma, and maintain a restful environment.

• Obtain throat cultures, and administer antibiotics as required. If the patient has acute bacterial pharyngitis, emphasize the importance of completing the full course of antibiotic therapy.

• Teach the patient with chronic pharyngitis how to minimize sources of throat irritation in the environment, such as using a bedside humidifier.

• Refer the patient to a self-help group to stop smoking, if appropriate.

PHEOCHROMOCYTOMA

A pheochromocytoma is a chromaffin-cell tumor of the adrenal medulla that secretes an excessive amount of the catecholamines epinephrine and norepinephrine, which results in severe hypertension, increased metabolism, and hyperglycemia. This disorder is potentially fatal, but the prognosis is generally good with treatment. However, pheochromocytoma-induced kidney damage is irreversible.

Causes

A pheochromocytoma may result from an inherited autosomal dominant trait. According to some estimates, about 0.5% of newly diagnosed patients with hypertension have pheochromocytoma. Although this tumor is usually benign, it may be malignant in as many as 10% of these patients. It affects all races and both sexes, occurring primarily between ages 30 and 40.

Signs and symptoms

The cardinal sign of pheochromocytoma is persistent or paroxysmal hypertension. Common clinical effects include palpitations, tachycardia, headache, diaphoresis, pallor, warmth or flushing, paresthesia, tremor, excitation, fright, nervousness, feelings of impending doom, abdominal pain, tachypnea, nausea, and vomiting.

Postural hypotension and paradoxical response to antihypertensive drugs are common, as are associated glycosuria, hyperglycemia, and hypermetabolism. Patients with hypermetabolism may show marked weight loss, but some patients with pheochromocytomas are obese.

Frequency of episodes

Symptomatic episodes may recur as seldom as once every 2 months or as often as 25 times a day. They may occur spontaneously or may follow certain precipitating events, such as postural change, exercise, laughing, smoking, induction of anesthesia, urination, or a change in environmental or body temperature.

Often, pheochromocytoma is diagnosed during pregnancy, when uterine pressure on the tumor induces more frequent attacks; such attacks can prove fatal for both mother and fetus as a result of cerebrovascular accident, acute pulmonary edema, cardiac arrhythmias, or hypoxia. In such patients, the risk of spontaneous abortion is high, but most fetal deaths occur during labor or immediately after birth.

Diagnosis

A history of acute episodes of hypertension, headache, sweating, and tachycardia—particularly in a patient with hyperglycemia, glycosuria, and hypermetabolism—strongly suggests pheochromocytoma. A patient who has intermittent attacks may have no symptoms during a latent phase.

The tumor is rarely palpable; when it is, palpation of the surrounding area may induce an acute attack and help confirm the diagnosis. Generally, diagnosis depends on laboratory findings.

Increased urinary excretion of total free catecholamines and their metabolites, vanillylmandelic acid (VMA) and metanephrine, as measured by analysis of a 24-hour urine specimen, confirms pheochromocytoma.

Labile blood pressure necessitates urine collection during a hypertensive episode and comparison of this specimen with a baseline specimen. Direct assay of total plasma catecholamines shows levels 10 to 50 times higher than normal.

Provocative tests with glucagon and phentolamine suggest the diagnosis. But they may precipitate a hypertensive crisis or induce a false-positive or false-negative result, so they're rarely used. The clonidine suppression test will cause decreased plasma catecholamine levels in normal patients but no change in those with pheochromocytoma.

Angiography demonstrates an adrenal medullary tumor (but may precipitate a hypertensive crisis). I.V. pyelography with nephrotomography, adrenal venography, or computed tomography scan helps localize the tumor.

Treatment

Surgical removal of the tumor is the treatment of choice. To decrease blood pressure, alpha-adrenergic blockers or metyrosine is given from 1 to 2 weeks before surgery. A beta-adrenergic blocker (propranolol) may also be used after achieving alpha blockade.

Postoperatively, I.V. fluids, plasma volume expanders, vasopressors and, possibly, transfusions may be required for hypotension. Persistent hypertension in the immediate postoperative period can occur.

If surgery isn't feasible, alpha- and beta-adrenergic blockers—such as phenoxybenzamine and propranolol, respectively—are beneficial in controlling catecholamine effects and preventing attacks.

Management of an acute attack or hypertensive crisis requires I.V. phen-

tolamine (push or drip) or nitroprusside to normalize blood pressure.

Special considerations

• To ensure the reliability of urine catecholamine measurements, make sure the patient avoids foods high in vanillin (such as coffee, nuts, chocolate, and bananas) for 2 days before urine collection of VMA.

• Also, be aware of possible drug therapy that may interfere with the accurate determination of VMA (such as guaifenesin and salicylates). Collect the urine in a special container, with hydrochloric acid, that has been prepared by the laboratory.

• Obtain blood pressure readings often because transient hypertensive attacks are possible. Tell the patient to report headaches, palpitations, nervousness, or other symptoms of an acute attack.

• If hypertensive crisis develops, monitor blood pressure and heart rate every 2 to 5 minutes until blood pressure stabilizes at an acceptable level.

• Check blood for glucose, and watch for weight loss from hypermetabolism.

• After surgery, blood pressure may rise or fall sharply. Keep the patient quiet; provide a private room, if possible, because excitement may trigger a hypertensive episode.

• Postoperative hypertension is common because the stress of surgery and manipulation of the adrenal gland stimulate secretion of catecholamines. Because this excess secretion causes profuse sweating, keep the room cool, and change the patient's clothing and bedding often.

• If the patient receives phentolamine, monitor blood pressure closely. Observe and record side effects: dizziness, hypotension, tachycardia. The first 24 to 48 hours immediately after surgery are the most critical, because blood pressure can drop drastically.

DIAGNOSING PHOBIAS

The diagnosis of all three types of phobias is based on criteria put forth in the *DSM-IV.*

Agoraphobia

Fear of being in places or situations from which escape might be difficult or embarrassing or in which help might be unavailable if an unexpected or situationally predisposed panic attack or paniclike symptoms occur. Agoraphobic fears typically involve characteristic clusters of situations that include being outside the home alone, being in a crowd or standing in a line, being on a bridge, or traveling in a bus, train, or automobile.

• The situations are avoided or endured with marked distress or with anxiety about having a panic attack or paniclike symptoms, or they require the presence of a companion.

• The anxiety or phobic avoidance is not better accounted for by another mental disorder, such as social phobia, specific phobia, obsessive-compulsive disorder, posttraumatic stress disorder, or separation anxiety disorder.

Social phobia

A persistent fear of one or more social or performance situations in which the person is exposed to unfa-

miliar people or possible scrutiny by others. The person fears that he may act in a way that will be humiliating or embarrassing.

• Exposure to the feared social situation almost invariably provokes anxiety, which may take the form of a situationally bound or situationally predisposed panic attack.

• The person recognizes that the fear is excessive or unreasonable.

• The feared social or performance situations are avoided or endured with intense anxiety or distress.

• The avoidance, anxious anticipation, or distress in the feared social or performance situation interferes with the person's normal routine, occupational functioning, or social activities or relationships, or there is marked distress about having the phobia.

• In individuals under age 18, the duration is at least 6 months.

• The fear or avoidance is not due to the direct physiologic effects of a substance or a general medical condition and is not better accounted for by another mental disorder.

• If the person has a general medical condition or another mental disorder, the person's social fear is unrelated to the medical or mental condition.

• If the patient is receiving vasopressors I.V., check blood pressure every 3 to 5 minutes, and regulate the drip to maintain a safe pressure. Arterial pressure lines facilitate constant monitoring.

• Watch for abdominal distention and return of bowel sounds.

• Check dressings and vital signs for indications of hemorrhage (increased

pulse rate, decreased blood pressure, cold and clammy skin, pallor, unresponsiveness).

• Give analgesics for pain, as required, but monitor blood pressure carefully, because many analgesics, especially meperidine, can cause hypotension.

• If autosomal dominant transmission of pheochromocytoma is suspected, the

Specific phobia
Marked and persistent fear that is excessive or unreasonable and cued by the presence or anticipation of a specific object or situation.
• Exposure to the phobic stimulus almost invariably provokes an immediate anxiety response, which may take the form of a situationally bound or situationally predisposed panic attack.
• The person recognizes that the fear is excessive or unreasonable.
• The person avoids the situation or endures it with intense anxiety or distress.
• The avoidance, anxious anticipation, or distress in the feared situation significantly interferes with the person's normal routine, occupational functioning, or social activities or relationships, or there is marked distress about having the phobia.
• In individuals under age 18, the duration is at least 6 months.
• The anxiety, panic attacks, or phobic avoidance associated with the specific object or situation is not better accounted for by another mental disorder, such as obsessive-compulsive disorder, posttraumatic stress disorder, separation anxiety disorder, social phobia, panic disorder with agoraphobia, or agoraphobia without a history of panic disorder.

patient's family should also be evaluated for this condition.

PHOBIAS

Defined as a persistent and irrational fear of a specific object, activity, or situation, a phobia results in a compelling desire to avoid the perceived hazard. The patient recognizes that his fear is out of proportion to any actual danger, but he can't control it or explain it away.

Three types of phobias exist: *agoraphobia,* the fear of being alone or of open space; *social,* the fear of embarrassing oneself in public; and *specific,* the fear of a single, specific object, such as animals or heights.

Seven percent of all Americans suffer from a phobic disorder. In fact, phobias are the most common psychiatric disorders in women and the second most common in men. More men than women experience social phobias, whereas agoraphobia and specific phobias are more common in women.

A social phobia typically begins in late childhood or early adolescence; a specific phobia usually begins in childhood. Most phobic patients have no family history of psychiatric illness, including phobias.

Both agoraphobia and social phobia tend to be chronic, but new treatments are improving the prognosis. A specific phobia usually resolves spontaneously as the child matures.

Causes
A phobia develops when anxiety about an object or a situation compels the patient to avoid it. The precise cause of most phobias is unknown. Psychoanalytic theory holds that the phobia is actually repression and displacement of an internal conflict. Behavior theorists view phobia as a stimulus-response reflex, avoiding a situation or object that causes anxiety.

Signs and symptoms

The phobic patient typically reports signs of severe anxiety when confronted with the feared object or situation. A patient with agoraphobia, for example, may complain of dizziness, a sensation of falling, a feeling of unreality (depersonalization), loss of bladder or bowel control, vomiting, or cardiac distress when he leaves home or crosses a bridge. Similarly, a patient who fears flying may report that he begins to sweat, his heart pounds, and he feels panicky and short of breath when he's on an airplane.

A patient who routinely avoids the object of his phobia may report a loss of self-esteem and feelings of weakness, cowardice, or ineffectiveness. If he hasn't mastered the phobia, he also may exhibit signs of mild depression.

Diagnosis

For characteristic findings in this condition, see *Diagnosing phobias*, pages 658 and 659.

Treatment

The effectiveness of treatment depends on the severity of the patient's phobia. Because phobic behavior may never be completely cured, the goal of treatment is to help the patient function effectively.

Antianxiety and antidepressant drugs may help relieve symptoms in patients with agoraphobia.

Systematic desensitization, a behavioral therapy, may be more effective than drugs, especially if it includes encouragement, instruction, and suggestion.

In some cities, phobia clinics and group therapy are available. People who have recovered from phobias can often help other phobic patients.

Special considerations

• Provide for the patient's safety and comfort, and monitor fluid and food intake as needed. Certain phobias may inhibit food or fluid intake, disturb hygiene, and disrupt the patient's ability to rest.

• No matter how illogical the patient's phobia seems, avoid the urge to trivialize his fears. Remember that this behavior represents an essential coping mechanism.

• Ask the patient how he normally copes with the fear. When he's able to face the fear, encourage him to verbalize and explore his personal strengths and resources with you.

• Don't let the patient withdraw completely. If an agoraphobic patient is being treated as an outpatient, suggest small steps to overcome his fears, such as planning a brief shopping trip with a supportive family member or friend.

• In social phobias, the patient fears criticism. Encourage him to interact with others, and provide continuous support and positive reinforcement.

• Support participation in psychotherapy, including desensitization therapy. However, don't force insight. Challenging the patient may aggravate his anxiety or lead to panic attacks.

• Teach the patient specific relaxation techniques, such as listening to music and meditating.

• Suggest ways to channel the patient's energy and relieve stress (such as running and creative activities).

PHOSPHORUS IMBALANCE

Phosphorus exists primarily in inorganic combination with calcium in teeth and bones. In extracellular fluid, the phosphate ion supports several metabolic functions: utilization of B vitamins, acid-base homeostasis, bone formation, nerve and muscle activity, cell division, transmission of hereditary traits, and metabolism of carbohydrates, proteins, and fats.

Renal tubular reabsorption of phosphate is inversely regulated by calcium levels—an increase in phosphorus causes a decrease in calcium. An imbalance causes hypophosphatemia or hyperphosphatemia. Incidence of hypophosphatemia varies with the underlying cause; hyperphosphatemia occurs most often in children, who tend to consume more phosphorus-rich foods and beverages than adults, and in children and adults with renal insufficiency. The prognosis for both conditions depends on the underlying cause.

Causes

Hypophosphatemia is usually the result of inadequate dietary intake; it is often related to malnutrition resulting from a prolonged catabolic state or chronic alcoholism. It may also stem from intestinal malabsorption, chronic diarrhea, hyperparathyroidism with resultant hypercalcemia, hypomagnesemia, or deficiency of vitamin D, which is necessary for intestinal phosphorus absorption.

Other causes include chronic use of antacids containing aluminum hydroxide, use of parenteral nutrition solution with inadequate phosphate content, renal tubular defects, tissue damage in which phosphorus is released by injured cells, and diabetic acidosis.

Hyperphosphatemia generally occurs secondary to hypocalcemia, hypervitaminosis D, hypoparathyroidism, or renal failure (often due to stress or injury). It may also result from overuse of laxatives with phosphates or phosphate enemas.

Signs and symptoms

Hypophosphatemia produces anorexia, muscle weakness, tremor, paresthesia and, when persistent, osteomalacia, causing bone pain. Impaired red blood cell function may occur in hypophosphatemia due to alterations in oxyhemoglobin dissociation, which may result in peripheral hypoxia. Hyperphosphatemia usually remains asymptomatic unless it results in hypocalcemia, with tetany and seizures.

Diagnosis

A serum phosphorus level less than 1.7 mEq/L (or 2.5 mg/dl) confirms hypophosphatemia. A urine phosphorus level more than 1.3 g/24 hours supports this diagnosis.

A serum phosphorus level exceeding 2.6 mEq/L (or 4.5 mg/dl) confirms hyperphosphatemia. Supportive values include decreased levels of serum calcium (less than 9 mg/dl) and urine phosphorus (less than 0.9 g/24 hours).

Treatment

The treatment goal is to correct the underlying cause of the phosphorus imbalance. Until this is done, management of hypophosphatemia consists of phosphorus replacement, with a high-phosphorus diet and oral administration of phosphate salt tablets or capsules.

Severe hypophosphatemia requires I.V. infusion of potassium phosphate. Severe hyperphosphatemia may require peritoneal dialysis or hemodialysis to lower the serum phosphorus level.

Special considerations

• Carefully monitor serum electrolyte, calcium, magnesium, and phosphorus levels. Report any changes immediately.

To manage hypophosphatemia:

• Record intake and output accurately. Administer potassium phosphate slow

I.V. to prevent overcorrection to hyperphosphatemia. Assess renal function, and be alert for hypocalcemia when giving phosphate supplements. If phosphate salt tablets cause nausea, use capsules instead.
• To prevent recurrence, advise the patient to follow a high-phosphorus diet containing milk and milk products, kidney, liver, turkey, and dried fruits.

To manage hyperphosphatemia:
• Monitor intake and output. If urine output falls below 25 ml/hour or 600 ml/day, notify the doctor immediately because decreased output can seriously affect renal clearance of excess serum phosphorus.
• Watch for signs of hypocalcemia, such as muscle twitching and tetany, which often accompany hyperphosphatemia.
• To prevent recurrence, advise the patient to eat foods with low phosphorus content, such as vegetables. Obtain dietary consultation if the condition results from chronic renal insufficiency.

PITUITARY TUMORS

Constituting 10% of intracranial neoplasms, pituitary tumors originate most often in the anterior pituitary (adenohypophysis). They occur in adults of both sexes, usually during the third and fourth decades of life. The three tissue types of pituitary tumors are chromophobe adenoma (90%), basophil adenoma, and eosinophil adenoma.

The prognosis is fair to good, depending on the extent to which the tumor spreads beyond the sella turcica.

Causes
Although the exact cause is unknown, a predisposition to pituitary tumors may be inherited through an autosomal dominant trait. Pituitary tumors aren't malignant in the strict sense, but because their growth is invasive, they're considered a neoplastic disease.

Chromophobe adenoma may be associated with production of corticotropin, melanocyte-stimulating hormone, growth hormone, and prolactin; basophil adenoma, with evidence of excess corticotropin production and, consequently, with signs of Cushing's syndrome; eosinophil adenoma, with excessive growth hormone.

Signs and symptoms
As pituitary adenomas grow, they replace normal glandular tissue and enlarge the sella turcica, which houses the pituitary gland. The resulting pressure on adjacent intracranial structures produces typical clinical manifestations.

Neurologic features
• Frontal headache
• Visual symptoms, beginning with blurring and progressing to field cuts (hemianopias) and then unilateral blindness
• Cranial nerve involvement (III, IV, VI) from lateral extension of the tumor, resulting in strabismus; double vision, with compensating head tilting and dizziness; conjugate deviation of gaze; nystagmus; lid ptosis; and limited eye movements
• Increased intracranial pressure (secondary hydrocephalus)
• Personality changes or dementia, if the tumor breaks through to the frontal lobes
• Seizures
• Rhinorrhea, if the tumor erodes the base of the skull
• Pituitary apoplexy secondary to hemorrhagic infarction of the adenoma. Such hemorrhage may lead to both cardiovascular and adrenocortical collapse.

Endocrine features

• Hypopituitarism, to some degree, in all patients with adenoma, becoming more obvious as the tumor replaces normal gland tissue; symptoms include amenorrhea, decreased libido and impotence in men, skin changes (waxy appearance, decreased wrinkles, and pigmentation), loss of axillary and pubic hair, lethargy, weakness, increased fatigability, intolerance to cold, and constipation (because of decreased corticotropin and thyrotropin production)

• Addisonian crisis, precipitated by stress and resulting in nausea, vomiting, hypoglycemia, hypotension, and circulatory collapse

• Diabetes insipidus, resulting from extension to the hypothalamus

• Prolactin-secreting adenomas (in 70% to 75%), with amenorrhea and galactorrhea; growth hormone-secreting adenomas, with acromegaly; and corticotropin-secreting adenomas, with Cushing's syndrome.

Diagnosis

• *Skull X-rays* with tomography show enlargement of the sella turcica or erosion of its floor; if growth hormone secretion predominates, X-rays show enlarged paranasal sinuses and mandible, thickened cranial bones, and separated teeth.

• *Carotid angiography* shows displacement of the anterior cerebral and internal carotid arteries if the tumor mass is enlarging; it also rules out intracerebral aneurysm.

• *Computed tomography scan* may confirm the existence of the adenoma and accurately depict its size.

• *Cerebrospinal fluid analysis* may show increased protein levels.

• *Endocrine function tests* may contribute helpful information, but results are often ambiguous and inconclusive.

TRANSSPHENOIDAL PITUITARY SURGERY

Placement of bivalve speculum and rongeur for pituitary gland removal.

Treatment

Surgical options include transfrontal removal of large tumors impinging on the optic apparatus and transsphenoidal resection for smaller tumors confined to the pituitary fossa (see *Transsphenoidal pituitary surgery*). Radiation is the primary treatment for small, nonsecretory tumors that don't extend beyond the sella turcica and for patients who may be poor postoperative risks; otherwise, it's an adjunct to surgery.

Postoperative treatment includes hormone replacement with cortisone, thyroid, and sex hormones; correction of electrolyte imbalance; and, as necessary, insulin therapy.

Drug therapy may include bromocriptine, an ergot derivative that shrinks prolactin-secreting and growth hormone-secreting tumors. Cyproheptadine, an antiserotonin drug, can reduce increased corticosteroid levels in the patient with Cushing's syndrome.

Adjuvant radiotherapy is used when only partial removal of the tumor is possible. Cryohypophysectomy (freezing the area with a probe inserted by

---

POSTCRANIOTOMY CARE

- Monitor vital signs (especially level of consciousness), and perform a baseline neurologic assessment from which to plan further care and assess progress.
- Maintain the patient's airway; suction as necessary.
- Monitor intake and output carefully.
- Give the patient nothing by mouth for 24 to 48 hours, to prevent aspiration and vomiting, which increases intracranial pressure.
- Observe for cerebral edema, bleeding, and cerebrospinal fluid leakage.
- Provide a restful, quiet environment.

---

transsphenoidal route) is a promising alternative to surgical dissection of the tumor.

Special considerations
- Conduct a comprehensive health history and physical assessment to establish the onset of neurologic and endocrine dysfunction and provide baseline data for later comparison.
- Establish a supportive, trusting relationship with the patient and family to assist them in coping with the diagnosis, treatment, and potential long-term changes. Make sure they understand that the patient needs lifelong evaluations and, possibly, hormone replacement.
- Reassure the patient that some of the distressing physical and behavioral signs and symptoms caused by pituitary dysfunction (for example, altered sexual drive, impotence, infertility, loss of hair, and emotional lability) will disappear with treatment.
- Maintain a safe, clutter-free environment for the visually impaired or ac-

romegalic patient. Reassure him that he'll probably recover his sight.
- Position patients who have undergone supratentorial or transsphenoidal hypophysectomy with the head of the bed elevated about 30 degrees to promote venous drainage from the head and reduce cerebral edema. (See *Postcraniotomy care.*)
- Place the patient on his side to allow drainage of secretions and prevent aspiration.
- Withhold oral fluids, which can cause vomiting and subsequent increased intracranial pressure.
- Don't allow a patient who's had transsphenoidal surgery to blow his nose.
- Watch for cerebrospinal fluid drainage from the nose. Monitor for signs of infection from the contaminated upper respiratory tract.
- Make sure the patient understands that he'll lose his sense of smell.
- Regularly compare the patient's postoperative neurologic status with your baseline assessment.
- Monitor intake and output to detect fluid and electrolyte imbalances.
- Before discharge, encourage the patient to wear a medical identification bracelet or necklace that identifies his hormone deficiencies and their proper treatment.

PLEURAL EFFUSION AND EMPYEMA

Pleural effusion is an excess of fluid in the pleural space. Normally, this space contains a small amount of extracellular fluid that lubricates the pleural surfaces. Increased production or inadequate removal of this fluid results in pleural effusion. Empyema is the accumulation of pus and necrotic tissue in the pleural space. Blood (hemothorax) and chyle (chylothorax) may also collect in this space.

Causes

The balance of osmotic and hydrostatic pressures in parietal pleural capillaries normally results in fluid movement into the pleural space. Balanced pressures in visceral pleural capillaries promote reabsorption of this fluid.

Transudative pleural effusion

Excessive hydrostatic pressure or decreased osmotic pressure can cause excessive amounts of fluid to pass across intact capillaries. The result is a transudative pleural effusion, an ultrafiltrate of plasma containing low concentrations of protein. Such effusions frequently result from congestive heart failure, hepatic disease with ascites, peritoneal dialysis, hypoalbuminemia, and disorders resulting in overexpanded intravascular volume.

Exudative pleural effusion

Exudative pleural effusions result when capillaries exhibit increased permeability with or without changes in hydrostatic and colloid osmotic pressures, allowing protein-rich fluid to leak into the pleural space.

Exudative pleural effusions occur with tuberculosis, subphrenic abscess, pancreatitis, bacterial or fungal pneumonitis or empyema, malignancy, pulmonary embolism with or without infarction, collagen disease (lupus erythematosus and rheumatoid arthritis), myxedema, and chest trauma.

Empyema

Usually associated with infection in the pleural space, empyema may be idiopathic or may be related to pneumonitis, carcinoma, perforation, or esophageal rupture.

Signs and symptoms

Patients with pleural effusion characteristically display symptoms relating to the underlying pathology. Most patients with large effusions, particularly those with underlying pulmonary disease, complain of dyspnea. Those with effusions associated with pleurisy complain of pleuritic chest pain. Other clinical features depend on the cause of the effusion. Patients with empyema also develop fever and malaise.

Diagnosis

Chest X-ray shows radiopaque fluid in dependent regions. Auscultation of the chest reveals decreased breath sounds; percussion detects dullness over the effused area, which doesn't change with respiration. These tests verify pleural effusion. However, diagnosis also requires other tests to distinguish transudative from exudative effusions and to help pinpoint the underlying disorder.

The most useful test is thoracentesis, in which analysis of aspirated pleural fluid shows:

• *transudative effusions:* lactate dehydrogenase (LD) levels < 200 IU and protein levels < 3 g/dl
• *exudative effusions:* ratio of protein in pleural fluid to serum ≥ 0.5, LD in pleural fluid ≥ 200 IU, and ratio of LD in pleural fluid to LD in serum ≥ 0.6
• *empyema:* acute inflammatory white blood cells and microorganisms
• *empyema or rheumatoid arthritis:* extremely decreased pleural fluid glucose levels.

In addition, if a pleural effusion results from esophageal rupture or pancreatitis, fluid amylase levels are usually higher than serum levels. Aspirated fluid may be tested for LE cells, antinuclear antibodies, and neoplastic cells. It may also be analyzed for color and consistency; acid-fast bacillus, fungal, and bacterial cultures; and triglycerides (in chylothorax). Cell analysis shows leukocytosis in empyema. Negative tuberculin skin test strongly rules against tuberculosis as the cause. In exudative pleural effusions in which thoracentesis is not definitive, pleural biopsy may be done; it is particularly useful for confirming tuberculosis or malignancy.

Treatment

Depending on the amount of fluid present, symptomatic effusion may require thoracentesis to remove fluid or careful monitoring of the patient's own reabsorption of the fluid. Hemothorax requires drainage to prevent fibrothorax formation.

Treatment of empyema requires insertion of one or more chest tubes after thoracentesis to allow drainage of purulent material and possibly decortication (surgical removal of the thick coating over the lung) or rib resection to allow open drainage and lung expansion. Empyema also requires parenteral antibiotics. Associated hypoxia requires oxygen administration.

Special considerations

• Explain thoracentesis to the patient. Before the procedure, tell the patient to expect a stinging sensation from the local anesthetic and a feeling of pressure when the needle is inserted.
• Instruct the patient to tell you immediately if he feels uncomfortable or has trouble breathing during the procedure.
• Reassure the patient during thoracentesis. Remind him to breathe normally and to avoid sudden movements, such as coughing or sighing. Monitor vital signs, and watch for syncope.
• If fluid is removed too quickly, the patient may suffer bradycardia, hypotension, pain, pulmonary edema, or even cardiac arrest. Watch for respiratory distress or pneumothorax (sudden onset of dyspnea, cyanosis) after thoracentesis.

• Administer oxygen and, in empyema, antibiotics.
• Encourage the patient to do deep breathing exercises to promote lung expansion. Use an incentive spirometer to promote deep breathing.
• Provide meticulous chest tube care, and use aseptic technique for changing dressings around the tube insertion site in empyema.
• Ensure chest tube patency by watching for bubbles in the underwater seal chamber. Record the amount, color, and consistency of any tube drainage.
• Because weeks of such drainage are usually necessary to obliterate the space, make visiting nurse referrals for patients who will be discharged with the tube in place.
• If pleural effusion was a complication of pneumonia or influenza, advise the patient to seek prompt medical attention for chest colds.

PLEURISY

Also known as pleuritis, pleursy is inflammation of the visceral and parietal pleurae that line the inside of the thoracic cage and envelop the lungs.

Causes

Pleurisy develops as a complication of pneumonia, tuberculosis, viruses, systemic lupus erythematosus, rheumatoid arthritis, uremia, Dressler's syndrome, cancer, pulmonary infarction, and chest trauma.

Pleuritic pain is caused by the inflammation or irritation of sensory nerve endings in the parietal pleura. As the lungs inflate and deflate, the visceral pleura covering the lungs moves against the fixed parietal pleura lining the pleural space, causing pain. This disorder usually begins suddenly.

Signs and symptoms

Sharp, stabbing pain that increases with respiration may be so severe that it limits movement on the affected side during breathing. Dyspnea also occurs. Other symptoms vary according to the underlying pathologic process.

Diagnosis

Auscultation of the chest reveals a characteristic *pleural friction rub* — a coarse, creaky sound heard during late inspiration and early expiration, directly over the area of pleural inflammation. Palpation over the affected area may reveal coarse vibration.

Treatment

Generally symptomatic treatment includes anti-inflammatory agents, analgesics, and bed rest. Severe pain may require an intercostal nerve block of two or three intercostal nerves. Pleurisy with pleural effusion calls for thoracentesis as both a therapeutic and a diagnostic measure.

Special considerations

• Stress the importance of bed rest and plan your care to allow the patient as much uninterrupted rest as possible.
• Administer antitussives and pain medication, as necessary, but be careful not to overmedicate.
• If the pain requires a narcotic analgesic, warn the patient about to be discharged to avoid overuse because such medication depresses coughing and respiration.
• Encourage the patient to cough. To minimize pain, apply firm pressure at the pain site during coughing exercises.

PNEUMOCYSTIS CARINII PNEUMONIA

Because of its association with human immunodeficiency virus (HIV) infection, *Pneumocystis carinii* pneumonia (PCP), an opportunistic infection, has increased in incidence since the 1980s. Before the advent of PCP prophylaxis, this disease was the first clue in about 60% of patients that HIV infection was present.

PCP occurs in up to 90% of HIV-infected patients in the United States at some point during their lifetime. It is the leading cause of death in these patients. Disseminated infection doesn't occur.

PCP also is associated with other immunocompromised conditions, including organ transplantation, leukemia, and lymphoma.

Causes

P. carinii, the cause of PCP, usually is classified as a protozoan, although some investigators consider it more closely related to fungi. The organism exists as a saprophyte in the lungs of humans and various animals.

Part of the normal flora in most healthy people, *P. carinii* becomes an aggressive pathogen in the immunocompromised patient. Impaired cell-mediated (T-cell) immunity is thought to be more important than impaired humoral (B-cell) immunity in predisposing the patient to PCP, but the immune defects involved are poorly understood.

The organism invades the lungs bilaterally and multiplies extracellularly. As the infestation grows, alveoli fill with organisms and exudate, impairing gas exchange. The alveoli hypertrophy and thicken progressively, eventually leading to extensive consolidation.

The primary transmission route seems to be air, although the organism is already resident in most people. The incubation period probably lasts for 4 to 8 weeks.

Signs and symptoms
The patient typically has a history of an immunocompromising condition (such as HIV infection, leukemia, or lymphoma) or procedure (such as organ transplantation).

PCP begins insidiously with increasing shortness of breath and a nonproductive cough. Anorexia, generalized fatigue, and weight loss may follow. Although the patient may have hypoxemia and hypercapnia, he may not exhibit significant symptoms. He may, however, have a low-grade, intermittent fever.

Other signs and symptoms include tachypnea, dyspnea, accessory muscle use for breathing, crackles (in about one-third of patients), and decreased breath sounds (in advanced pneumonia). Cyanosis may appear with acute illness; pulmonary consolidation develops later.

Diagnosis
• *Histologic studies* confirm *P. carinii*. In patients with HIV infection, initial examination of a first-morning sputum specimen (induced by inhaling an ultrasonically dispersed saline mist) may be sufficient; however, this technique usually is ineffective in patients without HIV infection.
• *Fiber-optic bronchoscopy* remains the most commonly used study to confirm PCP. Invasive procedures, such as transbronchial biopsy and open lung biopsy, are performed less commonly.
• *Chest X-ray* may show slowly progressing, fluffy infiltrates and occasionally nodular lesions or a spontaneous pneumothorax, but these findings must be differentiated from findings in other types of pneumonia or adult respiratory distress syndrome.
• *Gallium scan* may show increased uptake over the lungs even when the chest X-ray appears relatively normal.
• *Arterial blood gas (ABG) studies* detect hypoxia and an increased alveolar–arterial gradient.

Treatment
PCP may respond to drug therapy with co-trimoxazole or pentamidine isethionate. Because of immune system impairment, many patients who also have HIV experience severe adverse reactions to drug therapy. These reactions include bone marrow suppression, thrush, fever, hepatotoxicity, and anaphylaxis. Nausea, vomiting, and rashes are common. Diphenhydramine may be prescribed to treat the latter effects and leucovorin may reduce bone marrow suppression (and may be used prophylactically in patients with HIV infection).

Pentamidine may be administered I.V. or in aerosol form. I.V. pentamidine is associated with a high incidence of severe toxic effects. The inhaled form usually is well tolerated. However, inhaled pentamidine may not effectively reach the lung apices. Adverse reactions associated with inhalation include metallic taste, pharyngitis, cough, bronchospasm, shortness of breath, rhinitis, and laryngitis.

Supportive measures, such as oxygen therapy, mechanical ventilation, adequate nutrition, and fluid balance, are important adjunctive therapies.

Oral morphine sulfate solution may reduce the respiratory rate and anxiety, thereby enhancing oxygenation.

Special considerations

• Implement universal precautions to prevent contagion.

• Frequently assess the patient's respiratory status, and monitor ABG levels every 4 hours.

• Administer oxygen therapy as necessary. Encourage the patient to ambulate and to perform deep-breathing exercises and incentive spirometry to facilitate effective gas exchange.

• Administer antipyretics, as required, to relieve fever.

• Monitor intake and output and daily weight to evaluate fluid balance. Replace fluids as necessary.

• Give antimicrobial drugs as required. Never give pentamidine I.M. because it can cause pain and sterile abscesses. Administer the I.V. drug form slowly over 60 minutes to reduce the risk of hypotension.

• Monitor the patient for adverse reactions to antimicrobial drugs. If he's receiving co-trimoxazole, watch for nausea, vomiting, rash, bone marrow suppression, thrush, fever, hepatotoxicity, and anaphylaxis. If he's receiving pentamidine, watch for cardiac arrhythmias, hypotension, dizziness, azotemia, hypocalcemia, and hepatic disturbances.

• Provide diversional activities and coordinate health care team activities to allow adequate rest periods between procedures.

• Teach the patient energy conservation techniques as well.

• Supply nutritional supplements as needed. Encourage the patient to eat a high-calorie, protein-rich diet. Offer small, frequent meals if the patient cannot tolerate large amounts of food.

• Reduce anxiety by providing a relaxing environment, eliminating excessive environmental stimuli, and allowing ample time for meals.

• Give emotional support and help the patient identify and use meaningful support systems.

• Instruct the patient about the medication regimen, especially about possible adverse effects.

• If the patient will require oxygen therapy at home, explain that an oxygen concentrator may be most effective.

LIFE-THREATENING DISORDER

PNEUMONIA

An acute infection of the lung parenchyma, pneumonia often impairs gas exchange. The prognosis is generally good for people who have normal lungs and adequate host defenses before the onset of pneumonia; however, pneumonia is the sixth leading cause of death in the United States.

Causes

Pneumonia can be classified in several ways:

• *Microbiologic etiology* — Pneumonia can be viral, bacterial, fungal, protozoal, mycobacterial, mycoplasmal, or rickettsial in origin.

• *Location* — Bronchopneumonia involves distal airways and alveoli; lobular pneumonia, part of a lobe; and lobar pneumonia, an entire lobe.

• *Type* — Primary pneumonia results from inhalation or aspiration of a pathogen; it includes pneumococcal and viral pneumonia. Secondary pneumonia may follow initial lung damage from a noxious chemical or other insult (superinfection), or may result from hematogenous spread of bacteria from a distant focus (see *Types of pneumonia,* pages 670 to 673).

Predisposing factors

Predisposing factors to bacterial and viral pneumonia include chronic illness and debilitation, cancer (partic-

(Text continues on page 672.)

TYPES OF PNEUMONIA

TYPE	SIGNS AND SYMPTOMS
VIRAL	
Influenza (prognosis poor even with treatment; 50% mortality)	• Cough (initially nonproductive; later, purulent sputum), marked cyanosis, dyspnea, high fever, chills, substernal pain and discomfort, moist crackles, frontal headache, myalgia • Death results from cardiopulmonary collapse.
Adenovirus (insidious onset; generally affects young adults)	• Sore throat, fever, cough, chills, malaise, small amounts of mucoid sputum, retrosternal chest pain, anorexia, rhinitis, adenopathy, scattered crackles, and rhonchi
Respiratory syncytial virus (RSV) (most prevalent in infants and children)	• Listlessness, irritability, tachypnea with retraction of intercostal muscles, slight sputum production, fine moist crackles, fever, severe malaise and, possibly, cough or croup
Measles (rubeola)	• Fever, dyspnea, cough, small amounts of sputum, coryza, skin rash, and cervical adenopathy
Chickenpox (varicella) (uncommon in children, but present in 30% of adults with varicella)	• Cough, dyspnea, cyanosis, tachypnea, pleuritic chest pain, hemoptysis, and rhonchi 1 to 6 days after onset of rash
Cytomegalovirus (CMV)	• Difficult to distinguish from other nonbacterial pneumonias • Fever, cough, shaking chills, dyspnea, cyanosis, weakness, and diffuse crackles • Occurs in neonates as devastating multisystemic infection; in normal adults resembles mononucleosis; in immunocompromised hosts, varies from clinically inapparent to devastating infection
BACTERIAL	
Streptococcus (*Diplococcus pneumoniae*)	• Sudden onset of a single, shaking chill, and sustained temperature of 102° to 104° F (38.9° to 40° C); often preceded by upper respiratory tract infection

DIAGNOSIS	TREATMENT
• *Chest X-ray:* diffuse bilateral bronchopneumonia from hilus • *WBC count:* normal to slightly elevated • *Sputum smears:* no specific organisms	*Supportive:* for respiratory failure, endotracheal intubation and ventilator assistance; for fever, hypothermia blanket or antipyretics; for influenza A, amantadine or rimantadine
• *Chest X-ray:* patchy distribution of pneumonia, more severe than indicated by physical examination • *WBC count:* normal to slightly elevated	• Treat symptoms only. • Mortality low; usually clears with no residual effects
• *Chest X-ray:* patchy bilateral consolidation • *WBC count:* normal to slightly elevated	• *Supportive:* humidified air, oxygen, antimicrobials often given until viral etiology confirmed, aerosolized ribavirin • Complete recovery in 1 to 3 weeks
• *Chest X-ray:* reticular infiltrates, sometimes with hilar lymph node enlargement • *Lung tissue specimen:* characteristic giant cells	• *Supportive:* bed rest, adequate hydration, antimicrobials; assisted ventilation, if necessary
• *Chest X-ray:* shows more extensive pneumonia than indicated by physical examination, and bilateral, patchy, diffuse, nodular infiltrates • *Sputum analysis:* predominant mononuclear cells and characteristic intranuclear inclusion bodies with skin rash confirm diagnosis	• *Supportive:* adequate hydration, oxygen therapy in critically ill patients • Therapy with I.V. acyclovir
• *Chest X-ray:* in early stages, variable patchy infiltrates; later, bilateral, nodular, and more predominant in lower lobes • *Percutaneous aspiration of lung tissue, transbronchial biopsy or open lung biopsy:* microscopic examination shows intranuclear and cytoplasmic inclusions; virus can be cultured from lung tissue	• *Supportive:* adequate hydration and nutrition, oxygen therapy, bed rest • Generally, benign and self-limiting in mononucleosis-like form • In immunosuppressed patients, disease is more severe and may be fatal; ganciclovir or foscarnet treatment warranted
• *Chest X-ray:* areas of consolidation, often lobar • *WBC count:* elevated • *Sputum culture:* may show gram-positive *S. pneumoniae;* this organism not always recovered	• *Antimicrobial therapy:* penicillin G (or erythromycin, if patient's allergic to penicillin) for 7 to 10 days. Such therapy begins after obtaining culture specimen but without waiting for results. *(continued)*

TYPES OF PNEUMONIA

TYPE	SIGNS AND SYMPTOMS
BACTERIAL *(continued)*	
Klebsiella	• Fever and recurrent chills; cough producing rusty, bloody, viscous sputum (currant jelly); cyanosis of lips and nail beds due to hypoxemia; shallow, grunting respirations • Likely in patients with chronic alcoholism, pulmonary disease, and diabetes
Staphylococcus	• Temperature of 102° to 104° F (38.9° to 40° C), recurrent shaking chills, bloody sputum, dyspnea, tachypnea, and hypoxemia • Should be suspected with viral illness, such as influenza or measles, and in patients with cystic fibrosis
ASPIRATION	
Results from vomiting and aspiration of gastric or oropharyngeal contents into trachea and lungs	• Noncardiogenic pulmonary edema may follow damage to respiratory epithelium from contact with stomach acid. • Crackles, dyspnea, cyanosis, hypotension, and tachycardia • May be subacute pneumonia with cavity formation, or lung abscess may occur if foreign body is present

ularly lung cancer), abdominal and thoracic surgery, atelectasis, common colds or other viral respiratory infections, chronic respiratory disease (chronic obstructive pulmonary disease [COPD], asthma, bronchiectasis, cystic fibrosis), influenza, smoking, malnutrition, alcoholism, sickle cell disease, tracheostomy, exposure to noxious gases, aspiration, and immunosuppressant therapy.

Predisposing factors to aspiration pneumonia include old age, debilitation, nasogastric tube feedings, impaired gag reflex, poor oral hygiene, and decreased level of consciousness.

Signs and symptoms

The five cardinal symptoms of early bacterial pneumonia are coughing, sputum production, pleuritic chest pain, shaking, chills, and fever. Physical signs vary widely, ranging from diffuse, fine rales to signs of localized or extensive consolidation and pleural effusion.

Complications include hypoxemia, respiratory failure, pleural effusion, empyema, lung abscess, and bacteremia, with spread of infection to other parts of the body resulting in meningitis, endocarditis, and pericarditis.

DIAGNOSIS	TREATMENT
• *Chest X-ray:* typically, but not always, consolidation in the upper lobe that causes bulging of fissures • *WBC count:* elevated • *Sputum culture and Gram stain:* may show gram-negative cocci (*Klebsiella*)	• *Antimicrobial therapy:* an aminoglycoside and a cephalosporin
• *Chest X-ray:* multiple abscesses and infiltrates; high incidence of empyema • *WBC count:* elevated • *Sputum culture and Gram stain:* may show gram-positive staphylococci	• *Antimicrobial therapy:* nafcillin or oxacillin for 14 days if staphylococci are penicillinase producing • Chest tube drainage of empyema
Chest X-ray: locates areas of infiltrates, which suggest diagnosis	• *Antimicrobial therapy:* penicillin G or clindamycin • *Supportive:* oxygen therapy, suctioning, coughing, deep breathing, adequate hydration

Diagnosis

Clinical features, chest X-ray showing infiltrates, and sputum smear demonstrating acute inflammatory cells support this diagnosis. Positive blood cultures in patients with pulmonary infiltrates strongly suggest pneumonia produced by the organisms isolated from the blood cultures.

Pleural effusions, if present, should be tapped and fluid analyzed for evidence of infection in the pleural space. Occasionally, a transtracheal aspirate of tracheobronchial secretions or bronchoscopy with brushings or washings may be done to obtain material for smear and culture. The patient's response to antimicrobial therapy also provides important evidence of the presence of pneumonia.

Treatment

Antimicrobial therapy varies with the causative agent. Therapy should be reevaluated early in the course of treatment.

Supportive measures include humidified oxygen therapy for hypoxia, mechanical ventilation for respiratory failure, a high-calorie diet and adequate fluid intake, bed rest, and an analgesic to relieve pleuritic chest pain. Patients with severe pneumonia on mechanical ventilation may require positive end-expiratory pressure to facilitate adequate oxygenation.

Special considerations

Correct supportive care can increase patient comfort, avoid complications, and speed recovery.

Throughout the illness:
• Maintain a patent airway and adequate oxygenation. Measure arterial blood gas levels, especially in hypoxic patients. Administer supplemental oxygen if partial pressure of arterial oxygen is less than 60 mm Hg. Patients with underlying chronic lung disease should be given oxygen cautiously.
• Teach the patient how to cough and perform deep-breathing exercises to clear secretions, and encourage him to do so often.
• In severe pneumonia that requires endotracheal intubation or tracheostomy with or without mechanical ventilation, provide thorough respiratory care and suction often, using sterile technique, to remove secretions.
• Obtain sputum specimens as needed, by suction if the patient can't produce specimens independently. Collect specimens in a sterile container and deliver them promptly to the microbiology laboratory.
• Administer antibiotics, as necessary, and pain medication, as needed; record the patient's response to medications. Fever and dehydration may require I.V. fluids and electrolyte replacement.
• Maintain adequate nutrition to offset high caloric utilization secondary to infection. Ask the dietary department to provide a high-calorie, high-protein diet consisting of soft, easy-to-eat foods. Encourage the patient to eat.
• As necessary, supplement oral feedings with nasogastric tube feedings or parenteral nutrition. Monitor fluid intake and output.
• Provide a quiet, calm environment for the patient, with frequent rest periods.
• Give emotional support by explaining all procedures (especially intuba-tion and suctioning) to the patient and his family. Encourage family visits. Provide diversionary activities appropriate to the patient's age.
• To control the spread of infection, dispose of secretions properly. Tell the patient to sneeze and cough into a disposable tissue; tape a waxed bag to the side of the bed for used tissues.

To prevent pneumonia:
• Advise the patient to avoid using antibiotics indiscriminately during minor viral infections, because this may result in upper airway colonization with antibiotic-resistant bacteria. If the patient then develops pneumonia, the organisms producing the pneumonia may require treatment with more toxic antibiotics.
• Encourage annual influenza vaccination and Pneumovax for high-risk patients, such as those with COPD, chronic heart disease, or sickle cell disease.
• Urge all bedridden and postoperative patients to perform deep breathing and coughing exercises frequently. Position such patients properly to promote full aeration and drainage of secretions.
• To prevent aspiration during nasogastric tube feedings, elevate the patient's head, check the tube's position, and administer the formula slowly. Don't give large volumes at one time; this could cause vomiting. If the patient has an endotracheal tube, inflate the tube cuff.
• Keep the patient's head elevated for at least 30 minutes after the feeding. Check for residual formula at 4- to 6-hour intervals.

PNEUMOTHORAX

In peumothorax, air or gas accumulates between the parietal and visceral pleurae. The amount of air or gas trapped in the intrapleural space determines the degree of lung collapse.

In a tension pneumothorax, the air in the pleural space is under higher pressure than air in adjacent lung and vascular structures. Without prompt treatment, a tension or a large pneumothorax results in fatal pulmonary and circulatory impairment.

Causes
The type of pneumothorax varies with the cause.

Spontaneous pneumothorax
Usually occurring in otherwise healthy adults ages 20 to 40, spontaneous pneumothorax may be caused by air leakage from ruptured congenital blebs adjacent to the visceral pleural surface, near the apex of the lung. It may also result from an emphysematous bulla that ruptures during exercise or coughing or from tubercular, pneumocystic, or malignant lesions that erode into the pleural space. Spontaneous pneumothorax may also occur in interstitial lung disease, such as eosinophilic granuloma or lymphangiomyomatosis.

Traumatic pneumothorax
This type of pneumothorax may result from insertion of a central venous line, thoracic surgery, or a penetrating chest injury, such as a gunshot or knife wound, or it may follow a transbronchial biopsy. It may also occur during thoracentesis or a closed pleural biopsy. When traumatic pneumothorax follows a penetrating chest injury, it frequently coexists with hemothorax (blood in the pleural space).

Tension pneumothorax
In tension pneumothorax, positive pleural pressure develops as a result of any of the causes of traumatic pneumothorax. When air enters the pleural space through a tear in lung tissue and is unable to leave by the same vent, each inspiration traps air in the pleural space, resulting in positive pleural pressure. This in turn causes collapse of the ipsilateral lung and marked impairment of venous return, which can severely compromise cardiac output and may cause a mediastinal shift. Decreased filling of the great veins of the chest results in diminished cardiac output and lowered blood pressure.

Open or closed pneumothorax
Pneumothorax can also be classified as open or closed. In open pneumothorax (usually the result of trauma), air flows between the pleural space and the outside of the body. In closed pneumothorax, air reaches the pleural space directly from the lung.

Signs and symptoms
The cardinal features of pneumothorax are sudden, sharp, pleuritic pain (exacerbated by movement of the chest, breathing, and coughing); asymmetric chest wall movement; shortness of breath; and cyanosis. In moderate to severe pneumothorax, profound respiratory distress may develop, with signs of tension pneumothorax: weak and rapid pulse, pallor, neck vein distention, and anxiety. Tension pneumothorax produces the most severe respiratory symptoms; a spontaneous pneumothorax that releases only a small amount of air into the pleural space may cause no symptoms.

Diagnosis

Sudden, sharp chest pain and shortness of breath suggest pneumothorax. Chest X-ray showing air in the pleural space and, possibly, mediastinal shift confirms this diagnosis. In the absence of a definitive chest X-ray, physical examination occasionally reveals:

• *on inspection:* overexpansion and rigidity of the affected chest side; in tension pneumothorax, neck vein distention with hypotension and tachycardia

• *on palpation:* crackling beneath the skin, indicating subcutaneous emphysema (air in tissue) and decreased vocal fremitus

• *on percussion:* hyperresonance on the affected side

• *on auscultation:* decreased or absent breath sounds over the collapsed lung.

If the pneumothorax is significant, arterial blood gas findings include pH less than 7.35, partial pressure of arterial oxygen less than 80 mm Hg, and partial pressure of arterial carbon dioxide above 45 mm Hg.

Treatment

Treatment is conservative for spontaneous pneumothorax in which no signs of increased pleural pressure (indicating tension pneumothorax) appear, lung collapse is less than 30%, and the patient shows no signs of dyspnea or other indications of physiologic compromise.

Such treatment consists of bed rest; careful monitoring of blood pressure, pulse rate, and respirations; oxygen administration; and possibly, needle aspiration of air with a large-bore needle attached to a syringe.

If more than 30% of the lung is collapsed, treatment to reexpand the lung includes placing a thoracostomy tube in the second or third intercostal space in the midclavicular line, connected to an underwater seal or low suction pressures.

Recurring spontaneous pneumothorax requires thoracotomy and pleurectomy; these procedures prevent recurrence by causing the lung to adhere to the parietal pleura. Traumatic and tension pneumothoraces require chest tube drainage; traumatic pneumothorax may also require surgical repair.

Special considerations

• Watch for pallor, gasping respirations, and sudden chest pain. Carefully monitor vital signs at least every hour for indications of shock, increasing respiratory distress, or mediastinal shift. Listen for breath sounds over both lungs. Falling blood pressure and rising pulse and respiration rates may indicate tension pneumothorax, which could be fatal without prompt treatment.

• After the chest tube is in place, encourage the patient to cough and breathe deeply (at least once an hour) to facilitate lung expansion.

• In the patient undergoing chest tube drainage, watch for continuing air leakage (bubbling), indicating that the lung defect has failed to close; this may require surgery.

• Watch for increasing subcutaneous emphysema by checking around the neck or at the tube insertion site for crackling beneath the skin.

• If the patient is on a ventilator, watch for difficulty in breathing in time with the ventilator, as well as pressure changes on ventilator gauges.

• Change dressings around the chest tube insertion site, as necessary. Be careful not to reposition or dislodge the tube. If the tube dislodges, place a petrolatum gauze dressing over the opening immediately to prevent rapid lung collapse.

• Monitor vital signs frequently after thoracotomy. Also, for the first 24 hours, assess respiratory status by checking breath sounds hourly.

• Observe the chest tube site for leakage, and note the amount and color of drainage.
• Walk the patient, as appropriate (usually on the first postoperative day), to facilitate deep inspiration and lung expansion.
• Reassure the patient, and explain what pneumothorax is, what causes it, and all diagnostic tests and procedures.
• Make the patient as comfortable as possible. (The patient with pneumothorax is usually most comfortable sitting upright.)

LIFE-THREATENING DISORDER

POISONING

Inhalation, ingestion, or injection of, or skin contamination with, any harmful substance is a common problem. In fact, in the United States, approximately 10 million people are poisoned annually, 4,000 of them fatally. The prognosis depends on the amount of poison absorbed, its toxicity, and the time interval between poisoning and treatment.

Causes
Because of their curiosity and ignorance, children are the main victims of poisoning. Accidental poisoning — usually from ingestion of salicylates (aspirin), acetaminophen, cleaning agents, insecticides, paints, or cosmetics — is the fourth leading cause of death in children.

In adults, poisoning is most common among chemical company employees, particularly those in companies that use chlorine, carbon dioxide, hydrogen sulfide, nitrogen dioxide, and ammonia, and in companies that ignore safety standards.

Other causes of poisoning in adults include improper cooking, canning, and storage of food; ingestion of, or skin contamination from, plants; and drug overdose (usually barbiturates or tricyclic antidepressants).

Signs and symptoms
Symptoms vary according to the type of poison.

Diagnosis
A history of ingestion, inhalation, or injection of, or skin contact with, a poisonous substance and typical clinical features suggest the diagnosis. Suspect poisoning in any unconscious patient with no history of diabetes, seizure disorders, or trauma.

Toxicology studies (including drug screens) of poison levels in the mouth, vomitus, urine, feces, or blood or on the victim's hands or clothing confirm the diagnosis. If possible, have the family or patient bring the container holding the poison to the emergency room for comparable study.

In inhalation poisoning, chest X-rays may show pulmonary infiltrates or edema; in petroleum distillate inhalation, X-rays may show aspiration pneumonia.

Treatment
Effective treatment includes emergency resuscitation and support, prevention of further absorption of poison, continuing supportive or symptomatic care and, when possible, administration of a specific antidote. If barbiturate, glutethimide, or tranquilizer poisoning causes hypothermia, use a hyperthermia blanket to control the patient's temperature.

Special considerations
• Assess cardiopulmonary and respiratory function. If necessary, begin cardiopulmonary resuscitation. Care-

fully monitor vital signs and level of consciousness.

• Depending on the poison, prevent further absorption of ingested poison by inducing emesis using syrup of ipecac or by administering gastric lavage and cathartics (magnesium sulfate).

• The treatment's effectiveness depends on the speed of absorption and the time elapsed between ingestion and removal. With syrup of ipecac, give warm water (usually less than 1 quart [less than 1 liter]) until vomiting occurs, or give another dose of ipecac as needed.

• Never induce emesis if you suspect corrosive acid poisoning, if the patient is unconscious or has seizures, or if the gag reflex is impaired even in a conscious patient. Instead, neutralize the poison by instilling the appropriate antidote by nasogastric tube.

• Common antidotes include milk, magnesium salts (milk of magnesia), activated charcoal, or other chelating agents (deferoxamine, edetate disodium [EDTA]). When possible, add the antidote to water or juice. (*Note:* The removal of hydrocarbon poisoning is controversial. In the conscious patient, because the risk of aspiration with ipecac-induced emesis is lower than with lavage, emesis is becoming the preferred treatment, but some doctors still use lavage. Moreover, some believe that because of poor absorption, kerosene [a hydrocarbon] does not require removal from the gastrointestinal tract; others believe removal depends on the amount ingested.)

• When you do want to induce emesis and the patient has already taken syrup of ipecac, don't give activated charcoal to neutralize the poison until *after* emesis. Activated charcoal adsorbs ipecac.

• To perform gastric lavage, instill 30 ml of fluid by nasogastric tube; then aspirate the liquid. Repeat until aspirate is clear. Save vomitus and aspirate for analysis. (To prevent aspiration in the unconscious patient, an endotracheal tube should be in place before lavage.)

• If several hours have passed since the patient ingested the poison, use large quantities of I.V. fluids to diurese the patient. The kind of fluid you'll use depends on the patient's acid-base balance and cardiovascular status, and on the flow rate.

• Severe ingested poisoning may call for peritoneal dialysis or hemodialysis.

• To prevent further absorption of inhaled poison, remove the patient to fresh or uncontaminated air. Alert the anesthesia department and provide supplemental oxygen. Some patients may require intubation.

• To prevent further absorption from skin contamination, remove the clothing covering the contaminated skin, and immediately flush the area with large amounts of water.

• If the patient is in severe pain, give analgesics, as ordered; frequently monitor fluid intake and output, vital signs, and level of consciousness.

• Keep the patient warm, and provide support in a quiet environment.

• If the poison was ingested intentionally, refer the patient for counseling to prevent future suicide attempts.

• For more specific treatment, contact the local poison center.

• To prevent accidental poisoning, instruct patients to read the label before they take medicine. Tell them to store all medications and household chemicals properly, keep them out of reach of children, and discard old medications.

• Warn patients not to take medicines prescribed for someone else, not to transfer medicines from their original bottles to other containers without labeling them properly, and never to transfer poisons to food containers.

• Parents should not take medicine in front of their young children or call medicine "candy" to get children to take it.

• Stress the importance of using toxic sprays only in well-ventilated areas and of following instructions carefully.

• Tell patients to use pesticides carefully and to keep the number of their poison control center handy.

POLIOMYELITIS

Also known as polio and infantile paralysis, poliomyelitis is an acute communicable disease caused by the poliovirus and ranges in severity from inapparent infection to fatal paralytic illness. First recognized in 1840, poliomyelitis became epidemic in Norway and Sweden in 1905.

Outbreaks reached pandemic proportions in Europe, North America, Australia, and New Zealand during the first half of this century. Incidence peaked during the 1940s and early 1950s and led to the development of the Salk vaccine.

Minor polio outbreaks still occur, usually among nonimmunized groups, as among the Amish of Pennsylvania in 1979. The disease strikes most often during the summer and fall. Once confined mainly to infants and children, poliomyelitis occurs more often today in people over age 15. Among children, it paralyzes boys most often; adults and girls are at greater risk for infection but not for paralysis.

The prognosis depends largely on the site affected. If the central nervous system (CNS) is spared, the prognosis is excellent. However, CNS infection can cause paralysis and death. The mortality for all types of poliomyelitis is 5% to 10%.

Causes

The poliovirus has three antigenically distinct serotypes — types I, II, and III — all of which cause poliomyelitis. These polioviruses are found worldwide and are transmitted from person to person by direct contact with infected oropharyngeal secretions or feces. The incubation period ranges from 5 to 35 days — 7 to 14 days on the average.

The virus usually enters the body through the alimentary tract, multiplies in the oropharynx and lower intestinal tract, then spreads to regional lymph nodes and the blood. Factors that increase the probability of paralysis include pregnancy; old age; localized trauma, such as a recent tonsillectomy, tooth extraction, or inoculation; and unusual physical exertion at or just before clinical onset of poliomyelitis.

Signs and symptoms

Manifestations of poliomyelitis follow three basic patterns. Inapparent (subclinical) infections constitute 95% of all poliovirus infections. Abortive poliomyelitis (minor illness), which makes up between 4% and 8% of all cases, causes slight fever, malaise, headache, sore throat, inflamed pharynx, and vomiting. The patient usually recovers within 72 hours. Most inapparent and abortive cases of poliomyelitis go unnoticed.

Major poliomyelitis, however, involves the CNS and takes two forms: nonparalytic and paralytic. Children often show a biphasic course, in which the onset of major illness occurs after recovery from the minor illness stage.

Nonparalytic poliomyelitis

This form of the disease produces moderate fever, headache, vomiting, lethargy, irritability, and pains in the neck, back, arms, legs, and abdomen. It also causes muscle tenderness and spasms in the extensors of the neck and back, and sometimes in the hamstring and other muscles. (These spasms may be observed during maximum range-of-motion exercises.) Nonparalytic polio usually lasts about a week, with meningeal irritation persisting for about 2 weeks.

Paralytic poliomyelitis

The more severe paralytic poliomyelitis usually develops within 5 to 7 days of the onset of fever. The patient displays symptoms similar to those of nonparalytic poliomyelitis, with asymmetrical weakness of various muscles, loss of superficial and deep reflexes, paresthesia, hypersensitivity to touch, urine retention, constipation, and abdominal distention.

The extent of paralysis depends on the level of the spinal cord lesions, which may be cervical, thoracic, or lumbar. When the disease affects the medulla of the brain, it's called bulbar paralytic poliomyelitis, which is the most perilous type. Bulbar paralytic poliomyelitis weakens the muscles supplied by the cranial nerves (particularly the ninth and tenth) and produces symptoms of encephalitis.

Other symptoms include facial weakness, dysphasia, difficulty in chewing, inability to swallow or expel saliva, regurgitation of food through the nasal passages, dyspnea, as well as abnormal respiratory rate, depth, and rhythm, which may lead to respiratory arrest. Fatal pulmonary edema and shock are possible.

Nonparalytic and paralytic poliomyelitis

Resistance to neck flexion is characteristic in nonparalytic and paralytic poliomyelitis. The patient will "tripod" — extend his arms behind him for support — when he sits up. He'll display Hoyne's sign — his head will fall back when he is supine and his shoulders are elevated. From a supine position, he won't be able to raise his legs a full 90 degrees. Paralytic poliomyelitis also causes positive Kernig's and Brudzinski's signs.

Complications

Many complications result from prolonged immobility and respiratory muscle failure and include hypertension, urinary tract infection, urolithiasis, atelectasis, pneumonia, myocarditis, cor pulmonale, skeletal and soft-tissue deformities, and paralytic ileus.

Diagnosis

Diagnosis requires isolation of the poliovirus from throat washings early in the disease, from stools throughout the disease, and from cerebrospinal fluid (CSF) cultures in CNS infection. Coxsackievirus and echovirus infections must be ruled out. Convalescent serum antibody titers four times greater than acute titers support a diagnosis of poliomyelitis.

Routine laboratory tests are usually within normal limits, though CSF pressure and protein levels may be slightly increased and white blood cell count elevated initially, mostly due to polymorphonuclear leukocytes, which constitute 50% to 90% of the total count. Thereafter, mononuclear cells constitute most of the diminished number of cells.

Treatment

Supportive treatment includes analgesics to ease headache, back pain, and leg spasms. Morphine is contraindicated because of the danger of additional respiratory suppression. Moist heat applications may also reduce muscle spasm and pain.

Bed rest is necessary only until extreme discomfort subsides. In paralytic poliomyelitis, this may take a long time. Paralytic polio also requires long-term rehabilitation using physical therapy, braces, corrective shoes and, in some cases, orthopedic surgery.

Special considerations
• Your care must be comprehensive to help prevent complications and to assist polio patients — physically and emotionally — during their prolonged convalescence.
• Observe the patient carefully for signs of paralysis and other neurologic damage, which can occur rapidly.
• Maintain a patent airway, and watch for respiratory weakness and difficulty in swallowing. A tracheotomy is often done at the first sign of respiratory distress. Following this, the patient is then placed on a mechanical ventilator.
• Reassure the patient that his breathing is being supported. Practice strict aseptic technique during suctioning. Be sure to use only sterile solutions to nebulize medications.
• Perform a brief neurologic assessment at least once a day, but don't demand any vigorous muscle activity. Encourage a return to mild activity as soon as the patient is able.
• Check blood pressure frequently, especially with bulbar poliomyelitis, which can cause hypertension or shock because of its effect on the brain stem.
• Watch for signs of fecal impaction (due to dehydration and intestinal inactivity). To prevent this, give sufficient fluids to ensure an adequate daily urine output with low specific gravity (1.5 to 2 L/day for adults).
• Monitor the bedridden patient's food intake for an adequate, well-balanced diet. If tube feedings are required, give liquid baby foods, juices, lactose, and vitamins.
• To prevent pressure ulcers, provide good skin care, reposition the patient often, and keep the bed dry. Remember, muscle paralysis may cause bladder weakness or transient bladder paralysis.
• Apply high-top sneakers or use a footboard to prevent footdrop. To alleviate discomfort, use foam rubber pads and sandbags, as needed, and light splints.
• To control the spread of poliomyelitis, wash your hands thoroughly after contact with the patient, especially after contact with excretions. Instruct the ambulatory patient to do the same. (Only hospital personnel who have been vaccinated against poliomyelitis may have direct contact with the patient.)
• Provide emotional support to the patient and his family. Reassure the nonparalytic patient that his chances for recovery are good. Long-term support and encouragement are essential for maximum rehabilitation.
• When caring for a paralytic patient, help set up an interdisciplinary rehabilitation program. Such a program should include physical and occupational therapists, doctors and, if necessary, a psychiatrist to help manage the emotional problems that develop in a patient suddenly facing severe physical disabilities.

POLYCYSTIC KIDNEY DISEASE

An inherited disorder, polycystic kidney disease is characterized by multiple, bilateral, grapelike clusters of fluid-filled cysts that grossly enlarge the kidneys, compressing and eventually replacing functioning renal tissue. This disease appears in two distinct forms.

The infantile form causes stillbirth or early neonatal death. A few infants with this disease survive for 2 years and then develop fatal renal, congestive heart, or respiratory failure.

The adult form begins insidiously but usually becomes obvious between ages 30 and 50; rarely, it causes no symptoms until the patient is in his seventies. In the adult form, renal deterioration is more gradual but, as in the infantile form, progresses relentlessly to fatal uremia.

The prognosis in adults is extremely variable. Progression may be slow, even after symptoms of renal insufficiency appear. However, after uremic symptoms develop, polycystic kidney disease is usually fatal within 4 years unless the patient receives treatment with dialysis, a kidney transplant, or both.

Causes

Although both types of polycystic kidney disease are genetically transmitted, the incidence in two distinct age-groups and different inheritance patterns suggest two unrelated disorders. The infantile type appears to be inherited as an autosomal recessive trait; the adult type, as an autosomal dominant trait. Both types affect males and females equally.

Signs and symptoms

Clinical features vary with the form of disease.

Infantile form

The newborn with infantile polycystic disease often has pronounced epicanthal folds, a pointed nose, a small chin, and floppy, low-set ears (Potter facies). At birth, he has huge bilateral masses on the flanks that are symmetrical, tense, and cannot be transilluminated. He characteristically shows signs of respiratory distress and congestive heart failure. Eventually, he develops uremia and renal failure. Accompanying hepatic fibrosis may cause portal hypertension and bleeding varices to develop as well.

Adult form

Adult polycystic kidney disease is often asymptomatic while the patient is in his thirties and forties but may induce nonspecific symptoms, such as hypertension, polyuria, and urinary tract infection. Later, the patient develops overt symptoms related to the enlarging kidney mass, such as lumbar pain, widening girth, and a swollen or tender abdomen. Such abdominal pain is usually worsened by exertion and relieved by lying down.

In advanced stages, this disease may cause recurrent hematuria, life-threatening retroperitoneal bleeding resulting from a ruptured cyst, proteinuria, and colicky abdominal pain from the ureteral passage of clots or calculi. Generally, about 10 years after symptoms appear, progressive compression of kidney structures by the enlarging mass produces renal failure and uremia.

Diagnosis

A family history and a physical examination revealing large bilateral, irregular masses in the flanks strongly suggest polycystic kidney disease. In advanced stages, grossly enlarged and palpable kidneys make the diagnosis obvious. (See *Polycystic kidney.*) In patients with these findings, the following laboratory results are typical:

• *Excretory urography* or *retrograde uteropyelography* reveals enlarged kidneys, with elongation of pelvis, flattening of the calyces, and indentations caused by cysts. Excretory urography of the newborn shows poor excretion of contrast medium.

• *Ultrasonography, tomography,* and *radioisotope scans* show kidney enlargement and presence of cysts. *Computed tomography* and *magnetic resonance imaging* demonstrate multiple areas of cystic damage.

• *Urinalysis* and *creatinine clearance tests* — nonspecific tests that evaluate renal function — indicate abnormalities.

Diagnosis must rule out the presence of renal tumors.

Treatment
Polycystic kidney disease can't be cured. The primary goal of treatment is preserving renal parenchyma and preventing infectious complications. Management of secondary hypertension will also help prevent rapid deterioration in function. Progressive renal failure requires treatment similar to that for other types of renal disease, including dialysis or, rarely, a kidney transplant.

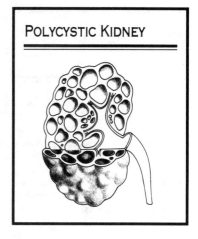

POLYCYSTIC KIDNEY

Asymptomatic stage
When adult polycystic kidney disease is discovered in the asymptomatic stage, careful monitoring is required, including urine cultures and creatinine clearance tests every 6 months. When a urine culture detects infection, prompt and vigorous antibiotic treatment is needed (even when the patient is asymptomatic).

Progressive renal impairment
As renal impairment progresses, selected patients may undergo dialysis, transplantation, or both. Cystic abscess or retroperitoneal bleeding may require surgical drainage; intractable pain (a rare symptom) may also require surgery. However, because this disease affects both kidneys, nephrectomy usually isn't recommended because it increases the risk of infection in the remaining kidney.

Special considerations
• Because polycystic kidney disease is usually relentlessly progressive, comprehensive patient teaching and emotional support are essential.
• Refer the young adult patient or the parents of infants with polycystic kidney disease for genetic counseling. Such parents will probably have many questions about the risk to other offspring.
• Provide supportive care to minimize any associated symptoms. Carefully assess the patient's lifestyle and his physical and mental status; determine how rapidly the disease is progressing. Use this information to plan individualized care.
• Acquaint yourself with all aspects of end-stage renal disease, including dialysis and transplantation, so you can provide appropriate care and patient teaching as the disease progresses.
• Explain all diagnostic procedures to the patient or to his family if the patient is an infant. Before beginning excretory urography or other procedures that use an iodine-based contrast medium, determine whether the patient has ever had an allergic reaction to iodine or shellfish. Even if the patient has no history of allergy, watch for an allergic reaction after performing the procedures.
• Administer antibiotics for urinary tract infection. Stress to the patient the need to take the medication exactly as prescribed, even if symptoms are minimal or absent.

POLYCYTHEMIA, SECONDARY

Also known as reactive polycythemia, secondary polycythemia is a disorder characterized by excessive production of circulating red blood cells (RBCs) due to hypoxia, tumor, or disease. It occurs in approximately 2 out of every 100,000 people living at or near sea level; incidence rises among persons living at high altitudes.

Causes

Secondary polycythemia may result from increased production of erythropoietin. This hormone, which is possibly produced and secreted in the kidneys, stimulates bone marrow production of RBCs. Increased production may be a compensatory physiologic response to hypoxemia, which may result from:

• chronic obstructive pulmonary disease (COPD)
• hemoglobin abnormalities (such as carboxyhemoglobinemia, which is seen in heavy smokers)
• congestive heart failure (causing a decreased ventilation-perfusion ratio)
• right-to-left shunting of blood in the heart (as in transposition of the great vessels)
• central or peripheral alveolar hypoventilation (as in barbiturate intoxication or pickwickian syndrome)
• low oxygen content at high altitudes.

Increased production of erythropoietin may also be an inappropriate (pathologic) response to renal disease (such as renal vascular impairment, renal cysts, or hydronephrosis), to central nervous system disease (such as encephalitis and parkinsonism), to neoplasms (such as renal tumors, uterine myomas, or cerebellar hemangiomas), or to endocrine disorders (such as Cushing's syndrome, Bartter's syndrome, or pheochromocytomas).

Rarely, secondary polycythemia results from a recessive genetic trait.

Signs and symptoms

In the hypoxic patient, suggestive physical findings include ruddy cyanotic skin, emphysema, hypoxemia without hepatosplenomegaly, or hypertension. Clubbing of the fingers may occur if the underlying disease is cardiovascular. When secondary polycythemia isn't caused by hypoxemia, it's usually an incidental finding during treatment for an underlying disease.

Diagnosis

Laboratory values for secondary polycythemia include increased RBC mass (increased hematocrit, hemoglobin, mean corpuscular volume, and mean corpuscular hemoglobin), urinary erythropoietin, and blood histamine, with decreased or normal arterial oxygen saturation.

Bone marrow biopsies reveal hyperplasia confined to the erythroid series. Unlike polycythemia vera, secondary polycythemia isn't associated with leukocytosis or thrombocytosis.

Treatment

The goal of treatment is correction of the underlying disease or environmental condition. In severe secondary polycythemia where altitude is a contributing factor, relocation may be advisable. If secondary polycythemia has produced hazardous hyperviscosity or if the patient doesn't respond to treatment for the primary disease, reduction of blood volume by phlebotomy or pheresis may be effective.

Emergency phlebotomy is indicated for prevention of impending vascular occlusion or before emergency surgery. In the latter case, it's usually advisable to remove excess RBCs and reinfuse the patient's plasma.

Because a patient with polycythemia has an increased risk of hemorrhage during and after surgery, elective surgery should be avoided until polycythemia is controlled. Generally, secondary polycythemia disappears when the primary disease is corrected.

Special considerations
• Keep the patient as active as possible to decrease the risk of thrombosis due to increased blood viscosity.
• Reduce calorie and sodium intake to counteract the tendency to hypertension.
• Before and after phlebotomy, check blood pressure with the patient lying down. After the procedure, give approximately 24 oz (720 ml) of water or juice. To prevent syncope, have him sit up for about 5 minutes before walking.
• Emphasize the importance of regular blood studies (every 2 to 3 months), even after the disease is controlled.
• Teach the patient and family about the underlying disorder. Help them understand its relationship to polycythemia and the measures needed to control both.
• Teach the patient to recognize symptoms of recurring polycythemia, and emphasize the importance of reporting them promptly.

POLYCYTHEMIA, SPURIOUS

Spurious polycythemia has many other names, including relative polycythemia, stress erythrocytosis, stress polycythemia, benign polycythemia, Gaisböck's syndrome, and pseudopolycythemia. Spurious polycythemia is characterized by increased hematocrit and normal or decreased red blood cell (RBC) total mass; it results from decreasing plasma volume and subsequent hemoconcentration. This disease usually affects middle-aged people and occurs more often in men than in women.

Causes
There are three possible causes of spurious polycythemia.

Dehydration
Conditions that promote severe fluid loss decrease plasma levels and lead to hemoconcentration. Such conditions include persistent vomiting or diarrhea, burns, adrenocortical insufficiency, aggressive diuretic therapy, decreased fluid intake, diabetic acidosis, and renal disease.

Hemoconcentration due to stress
Nervous stress leads to hemoconcentration by an unknown mechanism (possibly by temporarily decreasing circulating plasma volume or vascular redistribution of erythrocytes). This form of erythrocytosis (chronically elevated hematocrit) is particularly common in middle-aged men who are chronic smokers and have type A personalities (tense, hard-driving, anxious).

High-normal RBC mass and low-normal plasma volume
In many patients, an increased hematocrit merely reflects a normally high red cell mass and low plasma volume. This is particularly common in patients who are nonsmokers, are not obese, and have no history of hypertension.

Other factors that may be associated with spurious polycythemia include hypertension, thromboembolitic disease, elevated serum cholesterol and uric acid levels, and familial tendency.

Signs and symptoms

The patient with spurious polycythemia usually has no specific symptoms but may have vague complaints, such as headaches, dizziness, and fatigue. Less commonly, he may develop diaphoresis, dyspnea, and claudication.

Typically, the patient has a ruddy appearance, a short neck, slight hypertension, and a tendency to hypoventilate when recumbent. He shows no associated hepatosplenomegaly but may have cardiac or pulmonary disease.

Diagnosis

Hemoglobin and hematocrit levels and RBC count are elevated; RBC mass, arterial oxygen saturation, and bone marrow are normal. Plasma volume may be decreased or normal. Hypercholesterolemia, hyperlipemia, or hyperuricemia may be present.

Spurious polycythemia is distinguishable from polycythemia vera by its characteristic normal RBC mass, elevated hematocrit, and the absence of leukocytosis.

Treatment

The principal goals of treatment are to correct dehydration and to prevent life-threatening thromboembolism. Rehydration with appropriate fluids and electrolytes is the primary therapy for spurious polycythemia secondary to dehydration. Therapy must also include appropriate measures to prevent continuing fluid loss.

Special considerations

• During rehydration, carefully monitor intake and output to maintain fluid and electrolyte balance.
• To prevent thromboemboli in predisposed patients, suggest regular exercise and a low-cholesterol diet. Antilipemics may also be necessary. Reduced calorie intake may be required for the obese patient.

• Whenever appropriate, suggest counseling about the patient's work habits and lack of relaxation. If the patient is a smoker, make sure he understands how important it is that he stop smoking. Then, refer him to an antismoking program, if necessary.
• Emphasize the need for follow-up examinations every 3 to 4 months after leaving the hospital.
• Thoroughly explain spurious polycythemia, all diagnostic measures, and therapy. The hard-driving person predisposed to spurious polycythemia is likely to be more inquisitive and anxious than the average patient. Answer his questions honestly, but take care to reassure him that he can effectively control symptoms by complying with the prescribed treatment.

POLYCYTHEMIA VERA

Polycythemia vera (also known as primary polycythemia, erythremia, polycythemia rubra vera, splenomegalic polycythemia, Vaquez-Osler disease) is a chronic myeloproliferative disorder characterized by increased red blood cell (RBC) mass, leukocytosis, thrombocytosis, and increased hemoglobin concentration, with normal or increased plasma volume. It usually occurs between ages 40 and 60, most commonly among males of Jewish ancestry; it rarely affects children or blacks and doesn't appear to be familial.

The prognosis depends on age at diagnosis, the treatment used, and complications. Mortality is high if polycythemia is untreated or is associated with leukemia or myeloid metaplasia.

Causes

In polycythemia vera, uncontrolled and rapid cellular reproduction and maturation cause proliferation or hyperplasia of all bone marrow cells (panmyelosis). The cause of such uncontrolled cellular activity is unknown, but it is probably due to a multipotential stem cell defect.

Signs and symptoms

Increased RBC mass results in hyperviscosity and inhibits blood flow to microcirculation. Subsequently, increased viscosity, diminished velocity, and thrombocytosis promote intravascular thrombosis.

Progressive features

In early stages, polycythemia vera usually produces no symptoms. (Increased hematocrit may be an incidental finding.) However, as altered circulation secondary to increased RBC mass produces hypervolemia and hyperviscosity, the patient may complain of a feeling of fullness in the head, headache, dizziness, and other symptoms, depending on the body system affected (see *Clinical features of polycythemia vera,* page 688). Hyperviscosity may lead to thrombosis of smaller vessels with ruddy cyanosis of the nose and clubbing of the digits.

Complication

Paradoxically, hemorrhage is a complication of polycythemia vera. It may be due to defective platelet function or to hyperviscosity and the local effects from excess RBCs exerting pressure on distended venous and capillary walls.

Diagnosis

Laboratory studies confirm polycythemia vera by showing increased RBC mass and normal arterial oxygen saturation in association with splenomegaly or two of the following: thrombocytosis, leukocytosis, elevated leukocyte alkaline phosphatase level, or elevated serum vitamin B_{12} or unbound B_{12}-binding capacity.

Another common finding is increased uric acid production, leading to hyperuricemia and hyperuricuria. Other laboratory results include increased blood histamine, decreased serum iron concentration, and decreased or absent urinary erythropoietin. Bone marrow biopsy reveals panmyelosis.

Treatment

Phlebotomy can reduce RBC mass promptly. The frequency of phlebotomy and the amount of blood removed each time depend on the patient's condition. Typically, 350 to 500 ml of blood can be removed every other day until the hematocrit is reduced to the low-normal range.

After repeated phlebotomies, the patient develops iron deficiency, which stabilizes RBC production and reduces the need for phlebotomy. Pheresis permits the return of plasma to the patient, diluting the blood and reducing hypovolemic symptoms.

Phlebotomy doesn't reduce the white blood cell or platelet count and won't control the hyperuricemia associated with marrow cell proliferation.

For severe symptoms, myelosuppressive therapy may be used. In the past, radioactive phosphorus (^{32}P) or chemotherapeutic agents, such as melphalan, busulfan, or chlorambucil, could usually control the disease. But these agents may cause leukemia and should be reserved for older patients and those with problems uncontrolled by phlebotomy.

The current preferred myelosuppressive agent is hydroxyurea, which is not associated with leukemia. Patients who've had previous thrombotic problems should be considered for myelosuppressive therapy.

CLINICAL FEATURES OF POLYCYTHEMIA VERA

SYMPTOMS	CAUSES
Eye, ear, nose, and throat	
• Visual disturbances (blurring, diplopia, scotoma, engorged veins of fundus and retina) and congestion of conjunctiva, retina, retinal veins, oral mucous membrane	• Hypervolemia and hyperviscosity
• Epistaxis or gingival bleeding	• Engorgement of capillary beds
Central nervous system	
• Headache or fullness in the head, lethargy, weakness, fatigue, syncope, tinnitus, paresthesia of digits, and impaired mentation	• Hypervolemia and hyperviscosity
Cardiovascular	
• Hypertension	• Hypervolemia and hyperviscosity
• Intermittent claudication, thrombosis and emboli, angina, thrombophlebitis	• Hypervolemia, thrombocytosis, and vascular disease
• Hemorrhage	• Engorgement of capillary beds
Skin	
• Pruritus (especially after hot bath)	• Basophilia (secondary histamine release)
• Urticaria	• Altered histamine metabolism
• Ruddy cyanosis	• Hypervolemia and hyperviscosity due to congested vessels, increased oxyhemoglobin, and reduced hemoglobin
• Night sweats	• Hypermetabolism
• Ecchymosis	• Hemorrhage
Gastrointestinal and hepatic	
• Epigastric distress	• Hypervolemia and hyperviscosity
• Early satiety and fullness	• Hepatosplenomegaly
• Peptic ulcer pain	• Gastric thrombosis and hemorrhage
• Hepatosplenomegaly	• Congestion, extramedullary hemopoiesis, and myeloid metaplasia
• Weight loss	• Hypermetabolism
Respiratory	
• Dyspnea	• Hypervolemia and hyperviscosity
Musculoskeletal	
• Joint symptoms	• Increased urate production secondary to nucleoprotein turnover

Special considerations
• If the patient requires phlebotomy, explain the procedure, and reassure the patient that it will relieve distressing symptoms.

• Check blood pressure, pulse rate, and respirations.
• During phlebotomy, make sure the patient is lying down comfortably to prevent vertigo and syncope.

• Stay alert for tachycardia, clamminess, or complaints of vertigo. If these effects occur, the procedure should be stopped.

• Immediately after phlebotomy, check blood pressure and pulse rate. Have the patient sit up for about 5 minutes before allowing him to walk; this prevents vasovagal attack or orthostatic hypotension. Also, administer 24 oz (720 ml) of juice or water.

• Tell the patient to watch for and report any symptoms of iron deficiency (pallor, weight loss, asthenia, glossitis).

• Keep the patient active and ambulatory to prevent thrombosis. If bed rest is absolutely necessary, prescribe a daily program of both active and passive range-of-motion exercises.

• Watch for complications: hypervolemia, thrombocytosis, and signs of an impending cerebrovascular accident (decreased sensation, numbness, transitory paralysis, fleeting blindness, headache, and epistaxis).

• Regularly examine the patient closely for bleeding. Tell him which bleeding sites are most common (such as the nose, gingiva, and skin) so he can check for bleeding. Advise him to report any abnormal bleeding promptly.

• To compensate for increased uric acid production, give additional fluids, administer allopurinol, and alkalinize the urine to prevent uric acid calculi.

• If the patient has symptomatic splenomegaly, suggest or provide small, frequent meals, followed by a rest period, to prevent nausea and vomiting.

• Report acute abdominal pain immediately; it may signal splenic infarction, renal calculi, or abdominal organ thrombosis.

During myelosuppressive treatment:

• Monitor complete blood count (CBC) and platelet count before and during therapy. Warn an outpatient who develops leukopenia that his resistance to infection is low; advise him to avoid crowds and watch for the symptoms of infection.

• If leukopenia develops in a hospitalized patient who needs reverse isolation, follow hospital guidelines. If thrombocytopenia develops, tell the patient to watch for signs of bleeding (blood in urine, nosebleeds, black stools).

• Tell the patient about possible adverse effects (nausea, vomiting, and risk of in fection) of alkylating agents. Alopecia may follow the use of busulfan, cyclophosphamide, and uracil mustard; sterile hemorrhagic cystitis, the use of cyclophosphamide (forcing fluids can prevent it).

• Watch for adverse reactions. If nausea and vomiting occur, begin antiemetic therapy and adjust the patient's diet.

During treatment with ^{32}P:

• Explain the procedure to relieve anxiety. Tell the patient he may require repeated phlebotomies until ^{32}P takes effect.

• Take a blood sample for CBC and platelet count before beginning treatment. (*Note:* Use of ^{32}P requires radiation precautions to prevent contamination.)

• Have the patient lie down during I.V. administration (to facilitate the procedure and prevent extravasation) and for 15 to 20 minutes afterward.

POSTTRAUMATIC STRESS DISORDER

Posttraumatic stress disorder refers to a persistent psychological disturbance that occurs following a traumatic event. This disorder can follow almost any distressing event, including a natural or man-made disaster, physical or sexual abuse, or an assault or a rape.

Psychological trauma accompanies the physical trauma and involves intense fear and feelings of helplessness and loss of control. Posttraumatic stress disorder can be acute, chronic, or delayed. When the precipitating event is of human design, the disorder is more severe and more persistent. Onset can occur at any age, even during childhood.

Causes

Posttraumatic stress disorder occurs in response to an extremely distressing event, including a serious threat of harm to the patient or his family, such as war, abuse, or violent crime. It may be triggered by sudden destruction of his home or community by a bombing, fire, flood, tornado, earthquake, or similar disaster. It may also occur after the patient witnesses the death or serious injury of another person by torture, in a death camp, by natural disaster, or by a motor vehicle or airplane crash.

Preexisting psychopathology can predispose some patients to this disorder, but anyone can develop it, especially if the stressor is extreme.

Signs and symptoms

The psychosocial history of a patient with posttraumatic stress disorder may reveal early life experiences, interpersonal factors, military experiences, or other incidents that suggest the precipitating event. Typically, the patient may report that his symptoms began immediately or soon after the trauma, although they may not develop until months or years later. In such a case, avoidance symptoms usually have been present during the latency period.

Symptoms include pangs of painful emotion and unwelcome thoughts; intrusive memories; dissociative episodes (flashbacks); a traumatic reexperiencing of the event; difficulty falling or staying asleep, frequent nightmares of the traumatic event, and aggressive outbursts on awakening; emotional numbing (diminished or constricted response); and chronic anxiety or panic attacks (with physical signs and symptoms).

The patient may display rage and survivor guilt, use of violence to solve problems, depression and suicidal thoughts, and phobic avoidance of situations that arouse memories of the traumatic event (such as hot weather and tall grasses for the Vietnam veteran).

Other symptoms include memory impairment or difficulty concentrating and feelings of detachment or estrangement that destroy interpersonal relationships. Some have physical symptoms, fantasies of retaliation, and substance abuse.

Diagnosis

For characteristic findings in patients with this condition, see *Diagnosing posttraumatic stress disorder*.

Treatment

The goals of treatment for posttraumatic stress disorder include reducing the target symptoms, preventing chronic disability, and promoting occupational and social rehabilitation.

Specific treatments

Effective treatment may emphasize behavioral techniques (such as relaxation therapy to decrease anxiety and induce sleep or progressive desensitization). Antianxiety and antidepressant drugs or psychotherapy (supportive, insight, or cathartic) may minimize the risks of dependency and chronicity.

Diagnosing Posttraumatic Stress Disorder

The diagnosis of posttraumatic stress disorder is made when the patient's signs and symptoms meet the following criteria documented in the *DSM-IV:*

• The person was exposed to a traumatic event in which both of the following occurred:

– The person experienced, witnessed, or was confronted with an event or events that involved actual or threatened death or serious injury, or a threat to the physical integrity of self or others.

– The person's response involved intense fear, helplessness, or horror (in children, the response may be expressed by disorganized or agitated behavior).

• The person persistently reexperiences the traumatic event in at least one of the following ways:

– recurrent and intrusive distressing recollections of the event, including images, thoughts, or perceptions

– recurrent distressing dreams of the event

– acting or feeling as if the traumatic event were recurring (includes a sense of reliving the experience, illusions, hallucinations, and dissociative episodes that occur even when awakening or intoxicated)

– intense psychological distress at exposure to internal or external cues that symbolize or resemble an aspect of the traumatic event.

• The person persistently avoids stimuli associated with the traumatic event and experiences numbing of general responsiveness (not present before the traumatic event), as indicated by at least three of the following:

– efforts to avoid thoughts or feelings associated with the trauma

– efforts to avoid activities, places, or people that arouse recollections of the trauma

– inability to recall an important aspect of the traumatic event

– markedly diminished interest in significant activities

– feeling of detachment or estrangement from other individuals

– restricted range of affect – for example, inability to love others

– sense of foreshortened future.

• The person has persistent symptoms of increased arousal (not present before the trauma), as indicated by at least two of the following:

– difficulty falling or staying asleep

– irritability or outbursts of anger

– difficulty concentrating

– hypervigilance

– exaggerated startle response.

• The disturbance must be of at least 1 month's duration.

• The disturbance causes clinically significant distress or impairment in the patient's social, occupational, or other important areas of functioning.

Support groups

Such groups are highly effective and are provided through many Veterans Administration centers and crisis clinics. These groups provide a forum in which victims of this disorder can work through their feelings with others who have had similar conflicts.

Group settings are appropriate for most degrees of symptoms presented.

Some group programs include spouses and families in their treatment process. Rehabilitation programs in physical, social, and occupational areas also are available for victims of chronic posttraumatic stress disorder.

Many patients need treatment for depression, alcohol or drug abuse, or medical conditions before psychological healing can take place. Treatment for this disorder may be complex, and the prognosis varies.

Special considerations
• Encourage the patient with post-traumatic stress disorder to express his grief, complete the mourning process, and develop coping skills to relieve anxiety and desensitize him to the memories of the traumatic event.
• Keep in mind that such a patient tends to sharply test your commitment and interest. Therefore, first examine your feelings about the event (war or other trauma) so you won't react with disdain and shock. Such reactions hamper the working relationship with the patient and reinforce his typically poor self-image and sense of guilt.
• Know and practice crisis intervention techniques as appropriate in post-traumatic stress disorder.
• Establish trust by accepting the patient's current level of functioning and assuming a positive, consistent, honest, and nonjudgmental attitude toward the patient.
• Provide encouragement as the patient shows a commitment to work on his problem.
• Deal constructively with the patient's displays of anger.
• Encourage joint assessment of angry outbursts (identify how anger escalates and explore preventive measures that family members can take to regain control).
• Provide a safe, staff-monitored room in which the patient can safely deal with urges to commit physical violence or self-abuse through displacement (such as pounding and throwing clay or destroying selected items).
• Encourage the patient to move from physical to verbal expressions of anger.
• Help the patient relieve shame and guilt precipitated by real actions (such as killing or mutilation) that violated a consciously held moral code.

• Help the patient put his behavior into perspective, recognize his isolation and self-destructive behavior as forms of atonement, learn to forgive himself, and accept forgiveness from others.
• Refer the patient to a clergyman as appropriate.
• Provide for group therapy with other victims for peer support and forgiveness, or refer the patient to such a support group.
• Refer the patient to appropriate community resources.

POTASSIUM IMBALANCE

Potassium, a cation that is the dominant cellular electrolyte, facilitates contraction of both skeletal and smooth muscles — including myocardial contraction — and figures prominently in nerve impulse conduction, acid-base balance, enzyme action, and cell-membrane function. Because serum potassium level has such a narrow range (3.5 to 5 mEq/L), a slight deviation in either direction can produce profound clinical consequences.

Paradoxically, both hypokalemia (potassium deficiency) and hyperkalemia (potassium excess) can lead to muscle weakness and flaccid paralysis, because both create an ionic imbalance in neuromuscular tissue excitability. Both conditions also diminish excitability and conduction rate of the heart muscle, which may lead to cardiac arrest.

Causes
There are a number of possible causes of potassium imbalance.

Hypokalemia

Because many foods contain potassium, hypokalemia rarely results from a dietary deficiency. Instead, potassium loss results from:

- excessive GI or urinary losses, such as vomiting, gastric suction, diarrhea, dehydration, anorexia, or chronic laxative abuse
- trauma (injury, burns, or surgery), in which damaged cells release potassium, which enters serum or extracellular fluid, to be excreted in the urine
- chronic renal disease, with tubular potassium wasting
- certain drugs, especially potassium-wasting diuretics, steroids, and certain sodium-containing antibiotics (carbenicillin)
- acid-base imbalances, which cause potassium shifting into cells without true depletion in alkalosis
- prolonged potassium-free I.V. therapy
- hyperglycemia, causing osmotic diuresis and glycosuria
- Cushing's syndrome, primary hyperaldosteronism, excessive ingestion of licorice, and severe serum magnesium deficiency.

Hyperkalemia

Generally, hyperkalemia results from the kidneys' inability to excrete excessive amounts of potassium infused intravenously or administered orally; from decreased urine output, renal dysfunction, or renal failure; or the use of potassium-sparing diuretics, such as triamterene, by patients with renal disease. It may also result from any injuries or conditions that release cellular potassium or favor its retention, such as burns, crushing injuries, failing renal function, adrenal gland insufficiency, dehydration, or diabetic acidosis.

Signs and symptoms

See *Clinical features of potassium imbalance*, page 694.

Diagnosis

- *Hypokalemia:* serum potassium levels < 3.5 mEq/L.
- *Hyperkalemia:* serum potassium levels > 5 mEq/L.

Additional tests may be necessary to determine the underlying cause of the imbalance.

Treatment

Potassium imbalances are treated as follows.

Hypokalemia

Replacement therapy with potassium chloride (I.V. or by mouth) is the primary treatment of hypokalemia. When diuresis is necessary, spironolactone, a potassium-sparing diuretic, may be administered concurrently with a potassium-wasting diuretic to minimize potassium loss.

Hypokalemia can be prevented by giving a maintenance dose of potassium I.V. to patients who may not take anything by mouth and to others predisposed to potassium loss.

Hyperkalemia

For management of hyperkalemia, rapid infusion of 10% calcium gluconate decreases myocardial irritability and temporarily prevents cardiac arrest but doesn't correct serum potassium excess; it's also contraindicated in patients receiving a digitalis glycoside.

As an emergency measure, sodium bicarbonate I.V. increases pH and causes potassium to shift back into the cells. Insulin and 10% to 50% glucose I.V. also move potassium back into cells. Infusions should be followed by dextrose 5% in water because infusion of 10% to 15% glucose will stimulate secretion of endogenous insulin.

CLINICAL FEATURES OF POTASSIUM IMBALANCE

DYSFUNCTION	HYPOKALEMIA	HYPERKALEMIA
Cardiovascular	• Dizziness, hypotension, arrhythmias, electrocardiogram (ECG) changes (flattened T waves, elevated U waves, depressed ST segment), cardiac arrest (with serum potassium levels < 2.5 mEq/L)	• Tachycardia and later bradycardia, ECG changes (tented and elevated T waves, widened QRS, prolonged PR interval, flattened or absent P waves, depressed ST segment), cardiac arrest (with levels > 7.0 mEq/L)
Gastrointestinal	• Nausea and vomiting, anorexia, diarrhea, abdominal distention, paralytic ileus or decreased peristalsis	• Nausea, diarrhea, abdominal cramps
Musculo-skeletal	• Muscle weakness and fatigue, leg cramps	• Muscle weakness, flaccid paralysis
Genitourinary	• Polyuria	• Oliguria, anuria
CNS	• Malaise, irritability, confusion, mental depression, speech changes, decreased reflexes, respiratory paralysis	• Hyperreflexia progressing to weakness, numbness, tingling, and flaccid paralysis
Acid-base balance	• Metabolic alkalosis	• Metabolic acidosis

Sodium polystyrene sulfonate (Kayexalate) with 70% sorbitol produces exchange of sodium ions for potassium ions in the intestine. Hemodialysis or peritoneal dialysis also aids in removal of excess potassium.

Special considerations
For hypokalemia:
• Check serum potassium and other electrolyte levels in patients who are likely to develop a potassium imbalance and in those requiring potassium replacement; they risk overcorrection to hyperkalemia.
• Assess intake and output carefully. Remember, the kidneys excrete 80% to 90% of ingested potassium. Never give supplementary potassium to a patient whose urine output is less than 600 ml/day. Also, measure GI loss from suctioning or vomiting.
• Administer slow-release potassium or dilute oral potassium supplements in 4 oz (120 ml) or more of water or other fluid to reduce gastric and small-bowel irritation.
• Determine the patient's chloride level. As appropriate, give a potassium chloride supplement, if the level is low; potassium gluconate, if it's normal.
• Give I.V. potassium only after it's diluted in solution; potassium is very irritating to vascular, subcutaneous, and fatty tissues and may cause phlebitis or tissue necrosis if it infiltrates.
• Infuse potassium slowly (no more than 20 mEq/L/hour) to prevent hyperkalemia. *Never* administer it by I.V. push or bolus; it may cause cardiac arrest.

• Carefully monitor patients receiving a digitalis glycoside because hypokalemia will enhance its action and may produce signs of digitalis toxicity (anorexia, nausea, vomiting, blurred vision, and arrhythmias).

• To prevent hypokalemia, instruct patients (especially those predisposed to hypokalemia due to long-term diuretic therapy) to include in their diet foods rich in potassium — oranges, bananas, tomatoes, dark green leafy vegetables, milk, dried fruits, apricots, and peanuts.

• Monitor cardiac rhythm, and be alert for irregularities.

For hyperkalemia:

• As in hypokalemia, frequently monitor serum potassium and other electrolyte levels, and carefully record intake and output.

• Administer sodium polystyrene sulfonate orally or rectally (by retention enema). Watch for signs of hypokalemia with prolonged use and for clinical effects of hypoglycemia (muscle weakness, syncope, hunger, diaphoresis) with repeated insulin and glucose treatment.

• Watch for signs of hyperkalemia in predisposed patients, especially those with deceased urine output or those receiving oral or I.V. potassium supplements.

• Administer no more than 10 to 20 mEq/L of potassium chloride per hour; check the I.V. infusion site for signs of phlebitis or infiltration of potassium into tissues.

• Before giving a blood transfusion, check to see how long ago the blood was donated; older blood cell hemolysis releases potassium. Infuse only *fresh* blood for patients with average to high serum potassium levels.

• Watch for cardiac arrhythmias.

PREMENSTRUAL SYNDROME

Characterized by varying symptoms, premenstrual syndrome (PMS) appears 7 to 14 days before menses and usually subsides with its onset. The effects of PMS range from minimal discomfort to severe, disruptive symptoms and can include nervousness, irritability, depression, and multiple somatic complaints.

Researchers believe that 70% to 90% of women experience PMS at some time during their childbearing years, usually between ages 25 and 45.

Causes

The biological theories offered to explain the cause of PMS includes such conditions as a progesterone deficiency in the luteal phase of the menstrual cycle and vitamin deficiencies.

Failure to identify a specific disorder with a specific mechanism suggests that PMS represents a variety of manifestations triggered by normal physiologic hormonal changes.

Signs and symptoms

Clinical effects vary widely among patients and may include any combination of the following:

• *behavioral* — mild to severe personality changes, nervousness, hostility, irritability, agitation, sleep disturbances, fatigue, lethargy, and depression

• *somatic* — breast tenderness or swelling, abdominal tenderness or bloating, joint pain, headache, edema, diarrhea or constipation, and exacerbations of skin problems (such as acne or rashes), respiratory problems (such as asthma), or neurologic problems (such as seizures).

Diagnosis

The patient history shows typical symptoms related to the menstrual cycle. To help ensure an accurate history, the patient may be asked to record menstrual symptoms and body temperature on a calendar for 2 to 3 months before diagnosis.

Estrogen and progesterone blood levels may be evaluated to help rule out hormonal imbalance. A psychological evaluation is also recommended to rule out or detect an underlying psychiatric disorder.

Treatment

Education and reassurance that PMS is a real physiologic syndrome are important parts of treatment. Because treatment is predominantly symptomatic, each patient must learn to cope with her own individual set of symptoms.

Treatment may include diuretics, antidepressants, vitamins such as B complex, progestins, prostaglandin inhibitors, and nonsteroidal anti-inflammatory drugs. For effective treatment, the patient may have to maintain a diet that's low in simple sugars, caffeine, and salt.

Special considerations

• Inform the patient that self-help groups exist for women with PMS; if appropriate, help her contact such a group.
• Obtain a complete patient history to help identify any emotional problems that may contribute to PMS. If necessary, refer the patient for psychological counseling.
• If possible, discuss ways in which the patient can modify her lifestyle, such as making changes in her diet and avoiding stimulants and alcohol.
• Suggest that the patient seek further medical consultation if symptoms are severe and interfere with her normal lifestyle.

PROCTITIS

Proctitis is an acute or chronic inflammation of the rectal mucosa. The prognosis is good unless massive bleeding occurs.

Causes

Contributing factors include chronic constipation, habitual laxative use, emotional upset, radiation (especially for cancer of the cervix and of the uterus), endocrine dysfunction, rectal injury, rectal medications, bacterial infections, allergies (especially to milk), vasomotor disturbance that interferes with normal muscle control, and food poisoning.

Signs and symptoms

Key symptoms include tenesmus, constipation, a feeling of rectal fullness, and left abdominal cramps. The patient feels an intense urge to defecate, which produces a small amount of stool that may contain blood and mucus.

Diagnosis

In acute proctitis, sigmoidoscopy shows edematous, bright-red or pink rectal mucosa that's thick, shiny, friable, and possibly ulcerated. In chronic proctitis, sigmoidoscopy shows thickened mucosa, loss of vascular pattern, and stricture of the rectal lumen. Other supportive tests include biopsy to rule out carcinoma and a bacteriologic examination. A detailed patient history is essential.

Treatment

Primary treatment eliminates the underlying cause (fecal impaction, laxatives, or other medications). Soothing enemas or steroid (hydrocortisone) suppositories or enemas may be helpful if proctitis is due to radiation.

Tranquilizers may be appropriate for the patient with emotional stress.

Special considerations

• Tell the patient to watch for and report bleeding and other persistent symptoms.

• Fully explain proctitis and its treatment to help the patient understand the disorder and prevent its recurrence.

• As appropriate, offer emotional support and reassurance during rectal examinations and treatment.

PROSTATIC CANCER

Prostatic cancer is the second most common neoplasm found in men over age 50. Adenocarcinoma is its most common form; sarcoma occurs only rarely. Most prostatic carcinomas originate in the posterior prostate gland; the rest originate near the urethra.

Malignant prostatic tumors seldom result from the benign hyperplastic enlargement that commonly develops around the prostatic urethra in elderly men. Prostatic cancer seldom produces symptoms until it's advanced.

Causes

Although androgens regulate prostate growth and function and may also speed tumor growth, no definite link between increased androgen levels and prostatic cancer has been found. When primary prostatic lesions metastasize, they typically invade the prostatic capsule and spread along the ejaculatory ducts in the space between the seminal vesicles or perivesicular fascia.

Prostatic cancer accounts for about 18% of all cancers. Incidence is highest in blacks and lowest in Asians. Incidence also increases with age more rapidly than any other cancer.

Signs and symptoms

Manifestations of prostatic cancer appear only in the advanced stages (see *Staging prostatic cancer*, page 698) and include difficulty initiating a urinary stream, dribbling, urine retention, unexplained cystitis and, rarely, hematuria.

Diagnosis

A digital rectal examination that reveals a small, hard nodule may help diagnose prostatic cancer. The American Cancer Society advises a yearly digital examination for men over age 40, a yearly blood test to detect prostate-specific antigen (PSA) in men over age 50, and ultrasonography if abnormal results are found.

Biopsy confirms the diagnosis. PSA levels will be elevated in all, and serum acid phosphatase levels will be elevated in two-thirds of men with metastatic prostatic cancer. Therapy aims to return the serum acid phosphatase level to normal; a subsequent rise points to recurrence. Magnetic resonance imaging, computed tomography scan, and excretory urography may also aid the diagnosis.

Elevated alkaline phosphatase levels and a positive bone scan point to bone metastasis.

Treatment

Management of prostatic cancer depends on clinical assessment, tolerance of therapy, expected life span, and the stage of the disease. Treatment must be chosen carefully because prostatic cancer usually affects older men, who commonly have coexisting disorders, such as hypertension, diabetes, or cardiac disease.

Therapy varies with each stage of the disease and generally includes radiation, prostatectomy, orchiectomy to reduce androgen production, and hormone therapy with synthetic estrogen (diethylstilbestrol [DES]) and antian-

STAGING PROSTATIC CANCER

The American Joint Committee on Cancer recognizes the TNM (tumor, node, metastasis) cancer staging system for assessing prostatic cancer.

Primary tumor
TX—primary tumor can't be assessed

T0—no evidence of primary tumor

T1—tumor an incidental histologic finding

T1a—three or fewer microscopic foci of cancer

T1b—more than three microscopic foci of cancer

T2—tumor limited to the prostate gland

T2a—tumor less than 1.5 cm in greatest dimension, with normal tissue on at least three sides

T2b—tumor larger than 1.5 cm in greatest dimension or present in more than one lobe

T3—unfixed tumor extends into the prostatic apex or into or beyond the prostatic capsule, bladder neck, or seminal vesicle

T4—tumor fixed or invades adjacent structures not listed in T3

Regional lymph nodes
NX—regional lymph nodes can't be assessed

N0—no evidence of regional lymph node metastasis

N1—metastasis in a single lymph node, 2 cm or less in greatest dimension

N2—metastasis in a single lymph node, between 2 and 5 cm in greatest dimension, or metastasis to several lymph nodes, none more than 5 cm in greatest dimension

N3—metastasis in a lymph node more than 5 cm in greatest dimension

Distant metastasis
MX—distant metastasis can't be assessed

M0—no known distant metastasis

M1—distant metastasis

Staging categories
Prostatic cancer progresses from mild to severe as follows:

Stage 0 or Stage I—T1a, N0, M0; T2a, N0, M0

Stage II—T1b, N0, M0; T2b, N0, M0

Stage III—T3, N0, M0

Stage IV—T4, N0, M0; any T, N1, M0; any T, N2, M0; any T, N3, M0; any T, any N, M1

---

drogens such as cyproterone, megestrol, and flutamide. Radical prostatectomy is usually effective for localized lesions.

Radiation therapy is used to cure some locally invasive lesions and to relieve pain from metastatic bone involvement. A single injection of the radionuclide strontium-89 is also used to treat pain caused by bone metastasis.

If hormone therapy, surgery, and radiation therapy aren't feasible or successful, chemotherapy (using combinations of cyclophosphamide, doxorubicin, fluorouracil, cisplatin, etoposide, and vindesine) may be tried. However, current drug therapy offers limited benefit. Combining several treatment methods may be most effective.

Special considerations
Your care should emphasize psychological support, postoperative care, and treatment of radiation side effects.

Before prostatectomy:
• Explain the expected aftereffects of surgery (such as impotence and incontinence) and radiation. Discuss tube placement and dressing changes.
• Teach the patient to do perineal exercises 1 to 10 times an hour. Have him squeeze his buttocks together, hold this position for a few seconds, then relax.

After prostatectomy or suprapubic prostatectomy:
• Regularly check the dressing, incision, and drainage systems for excessive bleeding; watch the patient for signs of bleeding (pallor, falling blood pressure, rising pulse rate) and infection.
• Maintain adequate fluid intake.
• Give antispasmodics, as necessary, to control postoperative bladder spasms. Also give analgesics as needed.
• Urinary incontinence is common after surgery; keep the patient's skin clean, dry, and free of drainage and urine.
• Encourage perineal exercises within 24 to 48 hours after surgery.
• Provide meticulous catheter care — especially if a three-way catheter with a continuous irrigation system is in place. Check the tubing for kinks and blockages, especially if the patient reports pain. Warn him not to pull on the catheter.

After transurethral prostatic resection:
• Watch for signs of urethral stricture (dysuria, decreased force and caliber of urinary stream, and straining to urinate) and for abdominal distention (from urethral stricture or catheter blockage). Irrigate the catheter as needed.

After perineal prostatectomy:
• Avoid taking a rectal temperature or inserting any kind of rectal tube. Provide pads to absorb urine leakage, a rubber ring for the patient to sit on, and sitz baths for pain and inflammation.

After perineal or retropubic prostatectomy:
• Explain that urine leakage after catheter removal is normal and will subside.
• When a patient receives hormonal therapy, watch for adverse effects. Gynecomastia, fluid retention, nausea, and vomiting are common with DES. Thrombophlebitis may also occur, especially with DES.

After radiation therapy:
• Watch for common side effects: proctitis, diarrhea, bladder spasms, and urinary frequency. Internal radiation usually results in cystitis in the first 2 to 3 weeks.
• Urge the patient to drink at least 2,000 ml of fluid daily.
• Provide analgesics and antispasmodics as ordered.

PROSTATITIS

An inflammation of the prostate gland, prostatitis may be acute or chronic. Acute prostatitis most often results from gram-negative bacteria and is easy to recognize and treat. However, chronic prostatitis, the most common cause of recurrent urinary tract infection (UTI) in men, is less easy to recognize. As many as 35% of men over age 50 have chronic prostatitis.

Causes
About 80% of bacterial prostatitis cases result from infection by *Escherichia coli;* the rest, from infection by *Klebsiella, Enterobacter, Proteus, Pseudomonas, Streptococcus,* or *Staphylococcus.* These organisms probably spread to the prostate by the bloodstream or from ascending urethral infection, invasion of rectal bacteria via lymphatics, reflux of infected bladder urine into prostate ducts or, less commonly, in-

frequent or excessive sexual intercourse or such procedures as cystoscopy or catheterization. Chronic prostatitis usually results from bacterial invasion from the urethra.

Signs and symptoms

Acute prostatitis begins with fever, chills, low back pain, myalgia, perineal fullness, and arthralgia. Urination is frequent and urgent. Dysuria, nocturia, and urinary obstruction may also occur. The urine may appear cloudy. When palpated rectally, the prostate is tender, indurated, swollen, firm, and warm.

Chronic bacterial prostatitis sometimes produces no symptoms but usually elicits the same urinary symptoms as the acute form but to a lesser degree. UTI is a common complication. Other possible signs include painful ejaculation, hemospermia, persistent urethral discharge, and sexual dysfunction.

Diagnosis

Although a urine culture can often identify the causative infectious organism and characteristic rectal examination findings suggest prostatitis, firm diagnosis depends on a comparison of urine cultures of specimens obtained by the Meares and Stamey technique. This test requires four specimens:

• one collected when the patient starts voiding (voided bladder one – VB1)
• another specimen collected midstream (VB2)
• another specimen collected after the patient stops voiding and the doctor massages the prostate to produce secretions (expressed prostate secretions – EPS)
• a final voided specimen (VB3).

A significant increase in colony count in the prostatic specimens confirms prostatitis.

Treatment

Appropriate treatment includes drug therapy and support measures. Surgery may be necessary if drug therapy is unsuccessful.

Drug therapy

Systemic antibiotic therapy is the treatment of choice for acute prostatitis. Co-trimoxazole is given orally and, if the pathogen is sensitive to it, continued for about 30 days. If sepsis is likely, I.V. co-trimoxazole or I.V. gentamicin plus ampicillin may be given until sensitivity test results are known.

If test results and clinical response are favorable, parenteral therapy continues for 48 hours to 1 week; then an oral agent is substituted for 30 more days. In chronic prostatitis due to *E. coli*, co-trimoxazole is usually given for at least 6 weeks.

Support measures

Supportive therapy includes bed rest, adequate hydration, and administration of analgesics, antipyretics, sitz baths, and stool softeners as necessary. In symptomatic chronic prostatitis, regular massage of the prostate is most effective. Regular ejaculation may help promote drainage of prostatic secretions. Anticholinergics and analgesics may help relieve nonbacterial prostatitis symptoms. Alpha-adrenergic blockers and muscle relaxants may relieve prostatodynia.

Surgery

If drug therapy is unsuccessful, treatment may include transurethral resection of the prostate, which requires removal of all infected tissue. However, this procedure is usually not performed on young adults because it may cause retrograde ejaculation and sterility. Total prostatectomy is curative but may cause impotence and incontinence.

Special considerations
• Ensure bed rest and adequate hydration. Provide stool softeners and administer sitz baths, as required.
• As necessary, prepare to assist with suprapubic needle aspiration of the bladder or a suprapubic cystostomy.
• Emphasize the need for strict adherence to the prescribed drug regimen. Instruct the patient to drink at least 8 glasses of water a day. Have him report adverse drug reactions (rash, nausea, vomiting, fever, chills, and gastrointestinal irritation).

PRURITUS ANI

This disorder involves perianal itching, irritation, or superficial burning. Pruritus ani is more common in men than in women and is rare in children.

Causes
Factors that contribute to pruritus ani include:
• overcleaning of perianal area (harsh soap, vigorous rubbing with washcloth or toilet paper)
• minor trauma caused by straining to defecate
• poor hygiene
• sensitivity to spicy foods, coffee, alcohol, food preservatives, perfumed or colored toilet paper, detergents, or certain fabrics
• specific medications (antibiotics, antihypertensives, or antacids that cause diarrhea)
• excessive sweating (in occupations associated with physical labor or high stress levels)
• anal skin tags

• systemic disease, especially diabetes
• certain skin lesions, such as squamous cell carcinoma, basal cell carcinoma, Bowen's disease, Paget's disease, melanoma, syphilis, and tuberculosis
• fungus or parasite infection
• local anorectal disease (fissure, hemorrhoids, fistula).

Signs and symptoms
The key symptom of pruritus ani is perianal itching or burning after a bowel movement, during stress, or at night. In acute pruritus ani, scratching produces reddened skin, with weeping excoriations; in chronic pruritus ani, skin becomes thick and leathery, with excessive pigmentation.

Diagnosis
A detailed patient history is essential. Rectal examination rules out fissures and fistulas; biopsy rules out carcinoma. Allergy testing may also be helpful.

Treatment
After elimination of the underlying cause, treatment is symptomatic.

Special considerations
• Make sure the patient understands his condition and the causes.
• Advise the patient to avoid self-prescribed creams or powders, perfumed soaps, and colored toilet paper because they may be irritating.
• Teach the patient to keep the perianal area clean and dry. Suggest witch hazel pads for wiping and cotton balls tucked between buttocks to absorb moisture.

Pseudomembranous Enterocolitis

An acute inflammation and necrosis of the small and large intestines, pseudomembranous enterocolitis usually affects the mucosa but may extend into submucosa and, rarely, other layers. Marked by severe diarrhea, this rare condition is generally fatal in 1 to 7 days from severe dehydration and from toxicity, peritonitis, or perforation.

Causes

The exact cause of pseudomembranous enterocolitis is unknown; however, *Clostridium difficile* is thought to produce a toxin that may play a role in its development.

Pseudomembranous enterocolitis has occurred postoperatively in debilitated patients who undergo abdominal surgery or patients who have been treated with broad-spectrum antibiotics. Whatever the cause, necrosed mucosa is replaced by a pseudomembrane filled with staphylococci, leukocytes, mucus, fibrin, and inflammatory cells.

Signs and symptoms

Pseudomembranous enterocolitis begins suddenly with copious watery or bloody diarrhea, abdominal pain, and fever. Serious complications may be associated with this disorder. They include such things as severe dehydration, electrolyte imbalance, hypotension, shock, and colonic perforation.

Diagnosis

In this disorder, diagnosis is often difficult because of the abrupt onset of enterocolitis and the emergency situation it creates, so consideration of patient history is essential. A rectal biopsy through sigmoidoscopy confirms pseudomembranous enterocolitis. Stool cultures can identify *C. difficile.*

Treatment

A patient who is receiving broad-spectrum antibiotic therapy requires immediate discontinuation of the antibiotics. Effective treatment usually includes orally administered metronidazole. Oral vancomycin is usually given for severe or resistant cases.

A patient with mild pseudomembranous enterocolitis may receive anion exchange resins, such as cholestyramine, to bind the toxin produced by *C. difficile.* Supportive treatment must maintain fluid and electrolyte balance and combat hypotension and shock with pressors, such as dopamine and levarterenol.

Special considerations

• Monitor vital signs, skin color, and level of consciousness. Be alert for signs of shock.
• Record fluid intake and output, including fluid lost in stools. Watch for dehydration (poor skin turgor, sunken eyes, and decreased urine output).
• Check serum electrolyte levels daily, and watch for clinical signs of hypokalemia, especially malaise and a weak, rapid, irregular pulse.

Pseudomonas Infections

Pseudomonas is a small gram-negative bacillus that produces nosocomial infections, superinfections of various parts of the body, and a rare disease called melioidosis. This bacillus is also associated with bacteremia, endocarditis, and osteomyelitis in drug addicts.

In local *Pseudomonas* infections, treatment is usually successful and complications rare. However, in patients with poor immunologic resistance — premature infants, the elderly, or those with debilitating disease, burns, or wounds — septicemic *Pseudomonas* infections are serious and sometimes fatal.

Causes

The most common species of *Pseudomonas* is *P. aeruginosa.* Other species that typically cause disease in humans include *P. maltophilia, P. cepacia, P. fluorescens, P. testosteroni, P. acidovorans, P. alcaligenes, P. stutzeri, P. putrefaciens,* and *P. putida.*

These organisms are frequently found in hospital liquids that have been allowed to stand for a long time, such as benzalkonium chloride, hexachlorophene soap, saline solution, penicillin, water in flower vases, and fluids in incubators, humidifiers, and respiratory therapy equipment.

In elderly patients, *Pseudomonas* infection usually enters through the genitourinary tract; in infants, through the umbilical cord, skin, and GI tract.

Signs and symptoms

The most common infections associated with *Pseudomonas* include skin infections (such as burns and decubitus ulcers), urinary tract infections, infant epidemic diarrhea and other diarrheal illnesses, bronchitis, pneumonia, bronchiectasis, meningitis, corneal ulcers, mastoiditis, otitis externa, otitis media, endocarditis, and bacteremia.

Drainage in these infections has a distinct, sickly sweet odor and a greenish blue pus that forms a crust on wounds. Other symptoms depend on the site of infection. For example, when it invades the lungs, *Pseudomonas* causes pneumonia with fever, chills, and a productive cough.

Diagnosis

Diagnosis requires isolation of the *Pseudomonas* organism in blood, spinal fluid, urine, exudate, or sputum culture.

Treatment

In the debilitated or otherwise vulnerable patient with clinical evidence of *Pseudomonas* infection, treatment should begin immediately, without waiting for results of laboratory tests. Antibiotic treatment includes aminoglycosides, such as gentamicin or tobramycin, combined with a *Pseudomonas*-sensitive penicillin, such as carbenicillin disodium or ticarcillin. An alternative combination is amikacin and a similar penicillin. Such combination therapy is necessary because *Pseudomonas* quickly becomes resistant to carbenicillin alone.

In urinary tract infections, carbenicillin indanyl sodium can be used alone if the organism is susceptible and the infection doesn't have systemic effects; it is excreted in the urine and builds up high urine levels that prevent resistance.

Local *Pseudomonas* infections or septicemia secondary to wound infection requires 1% acetic acid irrigations, topical application of colistimethate sodium and polymyxin B, and debridement or drainage of the infected wound.

Special considerations

• Observe and record the character of wound exudate and sputum.

• Before administering antibiotics, ask the patient about a history of allergies, especially to penicillin. If combinations of carbenicillin or ticarcillin and an aminoglycoside are ordered, schedule the doses 1 hour apart (carbenicillin and ticarcillin may decrease the antibiotic effect of the aminoglycoside). *Don't* give both antibiotics through the same administration set.

• Monitor the patient's renal function (urine output, blood urea nitrogen, specific gravity, urinalysis, creatinine) during treatment with aminoglycosides.

• Protect immunocompromised patients from exposure to this infection. Attention to handwashing and aseptic techniques prevent further spread.

• To prevent *Pseudomonas* infection, maintain proper endotracheal and tracheostomy suctioning technique: Use strict sterile technique when caring for I.V. lines, catheters, and other tubes; dispose of suction bottle contents properly; and label and date solution bottles and change them frequently, according to policy.

PSORIASIS

This chronic, recurrent disease is marked by epidermal proliferation. Its lesions, which appear as erythematous papules and plaques covered with silver scales, vary widely in severity and distribution. Psoriasis affects about 2% of the population in the United States, and incidence is higher among whites than other races.

Although this disorder is most common in young adults, it may strike at any age, including infancy. Psoriasis is characterized by recurring partial remissions and exacerbations. Flare-ups are often related to specific systemic and environmental factors but may be unpredictable; they can usually be controlled with therapy.

Causes

The tendency to develop psoriasis is genetically determined. Researchers have discovered a significantly higher-than-normal incidence of certain human leukocyte antigens (HLA) in families with psoriasis, suggesting a possible immune disorder. Onset of the disease is also influenced by environmental factors.

Trauma can trigger the isomorphic effect or Koebner's phenomenon, in which lesions develop at sites of injury. Infections, especially those resulting from beta-hemolytic streptococci, may cause a flare-up of guttate (drop-shaped) lesions. Other contributing factors include pregnancy, endocrine changes, climate (cold weather tends to exacerbate psoriasis), and emotional stress.

Generally, a skin cell takes 14 days to move from the basal layer to the stratum corneum, where after 14 days of normal wear and tear, it's sloughed off. The life cycle of a normal skin cell is 28 days, compared to only 4 days for a psoriatic skin cell. This markedly shortened cycle doesn't allow time for the cell to mature. Consequently, the stratum corneum becomes thick and flaky, producing the cardinal manifestations of psoriasis.

Signs and symptoms

The most common complaint of the patient with psoriasis is itching and occasional pain from dry, cracked, encrusted lesions.

Plaques

Psoriatic lesions are erythematous and usually form well-defined plaques, sometimes covering large areas of the body (see *Viewing psoriasis*). Such lesions most commonly appear on the scalp, chest, elbows, knees, back, and buttocks.

The plaques consist of characteristic silver scales that either flake off easily or can thicken, covering the lesion. Removal of psoriatic scales frequently produces fine bleeding points (Auspitz sign). Occasionally, small guttate lesions appear, either alone or with plaques; these lesions are typically thin and erythematous, with few scales.

Widespread shedding of scales is common in exfoliative or erythrodermic psoriasis and may also develop in chronic psoriasis.

In about 30% of patients, psoriasis spreads to the fingernails, producing small indentations and yellow or brown discoloration. In severe cases, the accumulation of thick, crumbly debris under the nail causes it to separate from the nailbed.

Pustular psoriasis
Rarely, psoriasis becomes pustular, taking one of two forms. In localized pustular (Barber) psoriasis, pustules appear on the palms and soles and remain sterile until opened. In generalized pustular (Von Zumbusch) psoriasis, which often occurs with fever, leukocytosis, and malaise, groups of pustules coalesce to form lakes of pus on red skin. These pustules also remain sterile until opened and commonly involve the tongue and oral mucosa.

Arthritic symptoms
Some patients with psoriasis develop arthritic symptoms, usually in one or more joints of the fingers or toes, or sometimes in the sacroiliac joints, which may progress to spondylitis. Such patients may complain of morning stiffness. Joint symptoms show no consistent linkage to the course of the cutaneous manifestations of psoriasis; they demonstrate remissions and exacerbations similar to those of rheumatoid arthritis.

VIEWING PSORIASIS

In this patient with psoriasis, plaques consisting of silver scales cover a large area of the face.

Diagnosis
Diagnosis depends on patient history, appearance of the lesions and, if needed, the results of skin biopsy. Typically, serum uric acid level is elevated, due to accelerated nucleic acid degradation, but indications of gout are absent. HLA-Cw6, B-13, and B-w57 may be present in early-onset psoriasis.

Treatment
Appropriate treatment depends on the type of psoriasis, the extent of the disease and the patient's response to it, and what effect the disease has on the patient's lifestyle. No permanent cure exists, and all methods of treatment are palliative.

Removal of psoriatic scales necessitates application of occlusive ointment bases, such as petroleum jelly, salicylic acid preparations, or preparations containing urea. These medications soften the scales, which can then be removed by scrubbing them carefully with a soft brush while bathing.

UVB exposure

Methods to retard rapid cell production include exposure to ultraviolet light (UVB or natural sunlight) to the point of minimal erythema. Tar preparations or crude coal tar itself may be applied to affected areas about 15 minutes before exposure or may be left on overnight and wiped off the next morning.

A thin layer of petroleum jelly may be applied before UVB exposure (the most common treatment for generalized psoriasis). Exposure time can increase gradually. Outpatient or day treatment with UVB avoids long hospitalizations and prolongs remission.

Drug therapy

Steroid creams and ointments are useful to control psoriasis. A potent fluorinated steroid works well, except on the face and intertriginous areas. These creams require application two times a day, preferably after bathing to facilitate absorption, and overnight use of occlusive dressings, such as plastic wrap, plastic gloves or booties, or a vinyl exercise suit (under direct medical or nursing supervision).

Small, stubborn plaques may require intralesional steroid injections. Anthralin, combined with a paste mixture, may be used for well-defined plaques but must not be applied to unaffected areas because it causes injury and stains normal skin. Apply petroleum jelly around the affected skin before applying anthralin. Often used concurrently with steroids, anthralin is applied at night and steroids during the day. A new topical agent is calcipotriene ointment, a vitamin D_3 analogue.

Goeckerman, Ingram, and PUVA

In a patient with severe chronic psoriasis, the Goeckerman regimen — which combines tar baths and UVB treatments — may help achieve remission and clear the skin in 3 to 5 weeks. The Ingram technique is a variation of this treatment, using anthralin instead of tar. A therapy called PUVA combines administration of psoralens with exposure to high-intensity UVA.

Other treatments

As a last resort, a cytotoxin, usually methotrexate, may help severe, refractory psoriasis. Etretinate, a retinoid compound, is effective in treating extensive cases of psoriasis. However, because this drug is a strong teratogen, it is unsafe for use in women of childbearing age.

Low-dose antihistamines, oatmeal baths, emollients, and open wet dressings may help relieve pruritus. Aspirin and local heat help alleviate the pain of psoriatic arthritis; severe cases may require nonsteroidal anti-inflammatory drugs.

Therapy for psoriasis of the scalp consists of a tar shampoo followed by application of a steroid lotion. No effective treatment exists for psoriasis of the nails.

Special considerations

• Design your care to include patient teaching and careful monitoring for side effects of therapy.
• Make sure the patient understands his prescribed therapy; provide written instructions to avoid confusion.
• Teach correct application of prescribed ointments, creams, and lotions. A steroid cream, for example, should be applied in a thin film and rubbed gently into the skin until the cream disappears.
• Instruct the patient to apply all topical medications, especially those containing anthralin and tar, with a down-

ward motion to avoid rubbing them into the follicles. He must wear gloves because anthralin stains and injures the skin. After application, the patient may dust himself with powder to prevent anthralin from rubbing off on his clothes.

• Warn the patient never to put an occlusive dressing over anthralin. Suggest use of mineral oil, then soap and water, to remove anthralin.

• Caution the patient to avoid scrubbing his skin vigorously, to prevent Koebner's phenomenon. If a medication has been applied to the scales to soften them, suggest the patient use a soft brush to remove them.

• Watch for adverse reactions, especially allergic reactions to anthralin, atrophy and acne from steroids, and burning, itching, nausea, and squamous cell epitheliomas from PUVA.

• Initially evaluate the patient on methotrexate weekly, then monthly for red blood cell, white blood cell, and platelet counts, because cytotoxins may cause hepatic or bone marrow toxicity. Liver biopsy may be done to assess the effects of methotrexate.

• Caution the patient receiving PUVA therapy to stay out of the sun on the day of treatment, and to protect his eyes with sunglasses that screen UVA for 24 hours after treatment. Tell him to wear goggles during exposure to this light.

• Be aware that psoriasis can cause psychological problems. Assure the patient that psoriasis is not contagious, and although exacerbations and remissions occur, they're controllable with treatment. However, be sure he understands there is no cure.

• Because stressful situations tend to exacerbate psoriasis, help the patient learn to cope with these situations.

• Explain the relationship between psoriasis and arthritis, but point out that psoriasis causes no other systemic disturbances.

• Refer all patients to the National Psoriasis Foundation, which provides information and directs patients to local chapters.

PTOSIS

Drooping of the upper eyelid, ptosis may be congenital or acquired, unilateral or bilateral, constant or intermittent. Severe ptosis usually responds well to treatment; slight ptosis may require no treatment at all.

Causes
Congenital ptosis is transmitted as an autosomal dominant trait or results from a congenital anomaly in which the levator muscles of the eyelids fail to develop. This condition is usually unilateral.

Acquired ptosis may result from any of the following:

• age (involutional ptosis, the most common form)

• mechanical factors that make the eyelid heavy, such as swelling caused by a foreign body on the palpebral surface of the eyelid or by edema, inflammation produced by a tumor or pseudotumor, or an extra fatty fold

• myogenic factors, such as muscular dystrophy or myasthenia gravis (in which the defect appears to be in humoral transmission at the myoneural junction)

• neurogenic (paralytic) factors from interference in innervation of the eyelid by the oculomotor nerve (cranial nerve III), most commonly due to trauma, diabetes, or carotid aneurysm

• nutritional factors, for example, thiamine deficiency in chronic alcoholism, hyperemesis gravidarum, and other malnutrition-producing states.

Signs and symptoms

An infant with congenital ptosis has a smooth, flat upper eyelid, without the eyelid fold normally caused by the pull of the levator muscle; associated weakness of the superior rectus muscle is not uncommon.

The child with unilateral ptosis that covers the pupil can develop an amblyopic eye from disuse or lack of eye stimulation. In bilateral ptosis, the child may elevate his brow in an attempt to compensate, wrinkling his forehead in an effort to raise the upper lid. Also, the child may tilt his head backward to see.

In myasthenia gravis, ptosis results from fatigue and characteristically appears in the evening, but is relieved by rest. In addition to ptosis, oculomotor nerve damage produces a fixed, dilated pupil; divergent strabismus; and slight depression of the eyeball.

Diagnosis

A physical examination that consists of measuring palpebral fissure heights, range of lid movement, and relation of lid margin to upper border of the cornea will show the severity of ptosis. Diagnosis also includes the following tests to determine the underlying cause:
• *glucose tolerance test:* to detect diabetes
• *edrophonium test:* to reveal myasthenia gravis (in acquired ptosis with no history of trauma)
• *ophthalmologic examination:* to detect foreign bodies
• *patient history:* to reveal chronic alcoholism
• *digital subtraction angiography* or *magnetic resonance imaging:* to reveal an aneurysm.

Treatment

Slight ptosis that doesn't produce deformity or loss of vision requires no treatment. Severe ptosis that interferes with vision or is cosmetically undesirable usually necessitates resection of the weak levator muscles.

Surgery to correct congenital ptosis is usually performed at age 3 or 4, but it may be done earlier if ptosis is unilateral, because the totally occluded pupil may cause an amblyopic eye. If surgery is undesirable, special glasses with an attached suspended crutch on the frames may elevate the eyelid.

Effective treatment of ptosis also requires treatment of the underlying cause. For example, in patients with myasthenia gravis, neostigmine or steroids may be prescribed to increase the effect of acetylcholine and aid transmission of nerve impulses to muscles.

Special considerations

• Be alert for any bleeding. After surgery to correct ptosis, watch for blood on the pressure patch. (Some surgical procedures may not require a patch.)
• Apply ointment to the sutures, as necessary.
• Emphasize to the patient and family the need to prevent accidental trauma to the surgical site until healing is complete (6 weeks). Suture line damage can prompt a recurrence of ptosis.

LIFE-THREATENING DISORDER

PULMONARY EDEMA

In pulmonary edema, fluid accumulates in the extravascular spaces of the lung. In cardiogenic pulmonary edema, fluid accumulation results from elevations in pulmonary venous and capillary hydrostatic pressures. A common complication of cardiac disorders, pulmonary edema can occur as a chronic condition or develop quickly and rapidly become fatal.

Causes

Pulmonary edema usually results from left ventricular failure due to arteriosclerotic, hypertensive, cardiomyopathic, or valvular cardiac disease. In such disorders, the compromised left ventricle requires increased filling pressures to maintain adequate output; these pressures are transmitted to the left atrium, pulmonary veins, and pulmonary capillary bed.

This increased pulmonary capillary hydrostatic force promotes transudation of intravascular fluids into the pulmonary interstitium, decreasing lung compliance and interfering with gas exchange. Other factors that may predispose a person to pulmonary edema include:

• infusion of excessive volumes of I.V. fluids
• decreased serum colloid osmotic pressure as a result of nephrosis, protein-losing enteropathy, extensive burns, hepatic disease, or nutritional deficiency
• impaired lung lymphatic drainage from Hodgkin's disease or obliterative lymphangitis after radiation
• mitral stenosis and left atrial myxoma, which impair left atrial emptying
• pulmonary veno-occlusive disease.

Signs and symptoms

Symptoms vary with the stage of pulmonary edema.

Early symptoms

The early symptoms of pulmonary edema reflect interstitial fluid accumulation and diminished lung compliance: dyspnea on exertion, paroxysmal nocturnal dyspnea, orthopnea, and coughing. Clinical features include tachycardia, tachypnea, dependent crackles, neck vein distention, and a diastolic (S_3) gallop.

Later symptoms

With severe pulmonary edema, the alveoli and bronchioles may fill with fluid and intensify the early symptoms. Respiration becomes labored and rapid, with more diffuse crackles and coughing productive of frothy, bloody sputum. Tachycardia increases and arrhythmias may occur. Skin becomes cold, clammy, diaphoretic, and cyanotic. Blood pressure falls and pulse becomes thready as cardiac output falls.

Symptoms of severe heart failure with pulmonary edema may also include depressed level of consciousness and confusion.

Diagnosis

Clinical features of pulmonary edema permit a working diagnosis. The following tests are also helpful:

• *Arterial blood gas (ABG) analysis* usually shows hypoxia; partial pressure of arterial carbon dioxide varies. Both profound respiratory alkalosis and acidosis may occur. Metabolic acidosis occurs when cardiac output is low.
• *Chest X-ray* shows diffuse haziness of the lung fields and, often, cardiomegaly and pleural effusions.
• *Pulmonary artery catheterization* helps identify left ventricular failure by showing elevated pulmonary artery wedge pressures. This helps to rule out adult respiratory distress syndrome — in which pulmonary wedge pressure is usually normal.

Treatment

In pulmonary edema, treatment is designed to reduce extravascular fluid, to improve gas exchange and myocardial function and, if possible, to correct the underlying disorder.

Administration of high concentrations of oxygen by a cannula, a face mask and, if the patient fails to maintain an acceptable partial pressure of arterial oxygen, assisted ventilation improves oxygen delivery to the tissues and usually improves acid-base disturbances.

Diuretics—furosemide and bumetanide, for example—promote diuresis, which in turn helps to mobilize extravascular fluid.

Treatment of myocardial dysfunction includes a digitalis glycoside or pressor agents to increase cardiac contractility, antiarrhythmics (particularly when arrhythmias are associated with decreased cardiac output) and, occasionally, arterial vasodilators, such as nitroprusside, which decrease peripheral vascular resistance, preload, and afterload.

Other treatment includes morphine to reduce anxiety and dyspnea and to dilate the systemic venous bed, promoting blood flow from the pulmonary circulation to the periphery.

Special considerations
• Carefully monitor the vulnerable patient for early signs of pulmonary edema, especially tachypnea, tachycardia, and abnormal breath sounds. Check for peripheral edema, which may also indicate that fluid is accumulating in pulmonary tissue.
• Administer oxygen as necessary.
• Monitor vital signs every 15 to 30 minutes while administering nitroprusside in dextrose 5% in water by I.V. drip. Discard unused nitroprusside solution after 4 hours, and protect it from light by wrapping the bottle or bag with aluminum foil.
• Watch for arrhythmias in patients receiving a digitalis glycoside and for marked respiratory depression in those receiving morphine.
• Assess the patient's condition frequently, and record his response to treatment.
• Monitor ABG levels, oral and I.V. fluid intake, urine output and, in the patient with a pulmonary artery catheter, pulmonary end-diastolic and wedge pressures. Check the cardiac monitor often.
• Carefully record the time and amount of morphine given.
• Reassure the patient, who will be frightened by decreased respiratory capability, in a calm voice and explain all procedures. Provide emotional support to his family as well.

LIFE-THREATENING DISORDER

PULMONARY EMBOLISM AND INFARCTION

The most common pulmonary complication in hospitalized patients, pulmonary embolism is an obstruction of the pulmonary arterial bed by a dislodged thrombus or foreign substance. It strikes an estimated 6 million adults each year in the United States, resulting in 100,000 deaths.

Although pulmonary infarction may be so mild as to be asymptomatic, massive embolism (more than 50% obstruction of pulmonary arterial circulation) and infarction can be rapidly fatal.

Causes
Pulmonary embolism generally results from dislodged thrombi originating in the leg veins. More than half of such thrombi arise in the deep veins of the legs and are usually multiple.

Other less common sources of thrombi are the pelvic veins, renal veins, hepatic vein, right heart, and upper extremities. Such thrombus formation results directly from vascular wall damage, venostasis, or hypercoagulability of the blood.

Rare causes

Rarely, the emboli contain air, fat, amniotic fluid, talc (from drugs intended for oral administration that are injected intravenously by addicts), or tumor cells. Thrombi may embolize spontaneously during clot dissolution or may be dislodged during trauma, sudden muscular action, or a change in peripheral blood flow.

Rarely, pulmonary infarction (tissue death) may evolve from pulmonary embolism. Pulmonary infarction develops more frequently when pulmonary embolism occurs in patients with chronic cardiac or pulmonary disease. However if the embolus obstructs a large vessel, bronchial circulation may provide an inadequate oxygen supply to the lung supplied by the occluded vessel.

Risk factors

Predisposing factors to pulmonary embolism include:
- long-term immobility
- chronic pulmonary disease
- congestive heart failure or atrial fibrillation
- thrombophlebitis, polycythemia vera, thrombocytosis, autoimmune hemolytic anemia, and sickle cell disease
- varicose veins and vascular injury
- recent surgery
- advanced age
- pregnancy
- lower extremity fractures or surgery
- burns
- obesity
- malignancy
- use of oral contraceptives.

Signs and symptoms

Total occlusion of the main pulmonary artery is rapidly fatal; smaller or fragmented emboli produce symptoms that vary with the size, number, and location of the emboli. Usually, the first symptom of pulmonary embolism is dyspnea, which may be accompanied by anginal or pleuritic chest pain.

Other clinical features include tachycardia, productive cough (sputum may be blood-tinged), low-grade fever, and pleural effusion. Less common signs include massive hemoptysis, splinting of the chest, leg edema and, with a large embolus, cyanosis, syncope, and distended neck veins.

In addition, pulmonary embolism may cause pleural friction rub and signs of circulatory collapse (weak, rapid pulse; hypotension) and hypoxia (restlessness).

Diagnosis

The patient history reveals any predisposing conditions for pulmonary embolism. The following diagnostic tests are also helpful:
- *Chest X-ray* helps to rule out other pulmonary diseases; shows areas of atelectasis, elevated diaphragm and pleural effusion, prominent pulmonary artery and, occasionally, the characteristic wedge-shaped infiltrate suggestive of pulmonary infarction.
- *Lung scan* shows perfusion defects in areas beyond occluded vessels; however, it does not rule out microemboli.
- *Pulmonary angiography* is the most definitive test but requires a skilled angiographer and radiologic equipment; it also poses some risk to the patient. Its use depends on the uncertainty of the diagnosis and the need to avoid unnecessary anticoagulant therapy in high-risk patients.
- *Electrocardiography (ECG)* is inconclusive but helps distinguish pulmonary embolism from myocardial infarction. In extensive embolism, the ECG may show right axis deviation; right bundle-branch block; tall, peaked P waves; depression of ST segments and T-wave inversions (indicating right heart strain); and supraventricular tachyarrhythmias.

• *Auscultation* occasionally reveals a right ventricular S_3 gallop and increased intensity of the pulmonic component of S_2. Also, crackles and a pleural rub may be heard at the site of embolism.

• *Arterial blood gas (ABG) analysis* showing decreased partial pressure of arterial oxygen and carbon dioxide are characteristic but do not always occur.

If pleural effusion is present, thoracentesis may rule out empyema, which indicates pneumonia.

Treatment
In pulmonary embolism, treatment is designed to maintain adequate cardiovascular and pulmonary function during resolution of the obstruction and to prevent recurrence of embolic episodes.

Oxygen and anticoagulants
Because most emboli resolve within 10 to 14 days, treatment consists of oxygen therapy, as needed, and anticoagulation with heparin to inhibit new thrombus formation. Heparin therapy is monitored by daily coagulation studies (partial thromboplastin time [PTT]).

Drug therapy
Patients with massive pulmonary embolism and shock may need fibrinolytic therapy with urokinase, streptokinase, or alteplase to enhance fibrinolysis of the pulmonary emboli and remaining thrombi. Emboli that cause hypotension may require the use of vasopressors. Treatment of septic emboli requires antibiotics, not anticoagulants, and evaluation for the infection's source, particularly endocarditis.

Surgery
Interruption of the inferior vena cava is used for patients who can't take anticoagulants, who have recurrent emboli during anticoagulant therapy, or who have been treated with thrombolytic agents or pulmonary thromboendarterectomy.

Surgery (which should not be done without angiographic evidence of pulmonary embolism) consists of vena caval ligation, plication, or insertion of a device (umbrella filter) to filter blood returning to the heart and lungs. To prevent postoperative venous thromboembolism, a combination of heparin and dihydroergotamine may be given.

Special considerations
• Give oxygen by nasal cannula or mask. Check ABG levels in the event of fresh emboli or worsening dyspnea.

• Be prepared to provide endotracheal intubation with assisted ventilation if breathing is severely compromised.

• Administer heparin, as needed, through I.V. push or continuous drip. Monitor coagulation studies daily. Effective heparin therapy raises PTT to approximately 1½ to 2½ times normal.

• Watch closely for nosebleed, petechiae, and other signs of abnormal bleeding; check stools for occult blood. Tell the patient to prevent bleeding by shaving with an electric razor and by brushing his teeth with a soft toothbrush.

• After the patient is stable, encourage him to move about often, and assist with isometric and range-of-motion exercises.

• Check pedal pulses, temperature, and color of feet to detect venostasis. *Never* vigorously massage the patient's legs.

• Offer diversional activities to promote rest and relieve restlessness.

• Help the patient walk as soon as possible after surgery to prevent venostasis.

• Maintain adequate nutrition and fluid balance to promote healing.

• Note frequent pleuritic chest pain so that analgesics can be prescribed.

• Use incentive spirometry to assist in deep breathing. Provide tissues and a bag for easy disposal of expectorations.

• Warn the patient not to cross his legs; this promotes thrombus formation.

• To relieve anxiety, explain procedures and treatments. Encourage the patient's family to participate in his care.

• Most patients need treatment with an oral anticoagulant (warfarin) for 4 to 6 months after a pulmonary embolism.

• Advise patients taking anticoagulants to watch for signs of bleeding (bloody stools, blood in urine, large ecchymoses), to take the prescribed medication exactly as ordered, and to avoid taking any additional medication (even for headaches or colds) or changing doses of medication without consulting their doctors.

• Stress the importance of follow-up laboratory tests (prothrombin time) to monitor anticoagulant therapy.

• To prevent pulmonary emboli, encourage early ambulation in patients predisposed to this condition. With close medical supervision, low-dose heparin may be useful prophylactically.

PULMONARY HYPERTENSION

Pulmonary hypertension occurs when pulmonary artery pressure (PAP) rises above normal and is not attributable to the effects of aging or altitude. There is no definitive set of values used to diagnose pulmonary hypertension, but the National Institutes of Health requires that the resting mean PAP measure 25 mm Hg or more.

Primary, or *idiopathic, pulmonary hypertension* is rare, occurring most often in women between ages 20 and 40; pregnant women have the highest mortality. *Secondary pulmonary hypertension* results from existing cardiac or pulmonary disease. The prognosis depends on the severity of the underlying disorder.

Causes

Primary pulmonary hypertension begins as hypertrophy of the small pulmonary arteries. The medial and intimal muscle layers of these vessels thicken, decreasing distensibility and increasing resistance. This disorder then progresses to vascular sclerosis and obliteration of small vessels. Because this form of pulmonary hypertension occurs in association with collagen diseases, it is thought to result from altered immune mechanisms.

Usually, pulmonary hypertension is secondary to hypoxemia from an underlying disease process, including:

• *alveolar hypoventilation* from chronic obstructive pulmonary disease (most common cause in the United States), sarcoidosis, diffuse interstitial pneumonia, pulmonary metastasis, and certain diseases, such as scleroderma.

These diseases may cause pulmonary hypertension through alveolar destruction and increased pulmonary vascular resistance. Other disorders that cause alveolar hypoventilation without lung tissue damage include obesity, kyphoscoliosis, and obstructive sleep apnea.

• *vascular obstruction* from pulmonary embolism, vasculitis, and disorders that cause obstructions of small or large pulmonary veins, such as left atrial myxoma, idiopathic veno-occlusive disease, fibrosing mediastinitis, and mediastinal neoplasm.

• *primary cardiac disease,* which may be congenital or acquired. Congenital defects that cause left-to-right shunting of blood — such as patent ductus arteriosus, or atrial or ventricular septal defect — increase blood flow into the lungs and consequently raise pulmonary vascular pressure.

Acquired cardiac disease, such as rheumatic valvular disease and mitral stenosis, increases pulmonary venous pressure by restricting blood flow returning to the heart.

Signs and symptoms

Most patients complain of increasing dyspnea on exertion, weakness, syncope, and fatigability. Many also show signs of right heart failure, including peripheral edema, ascites, neck vein distention, and hepatomegaly. Other clinical effects vary according to the underlying disorder.

Diagnosis

Characteristic diagnostic findings in patients with pulmonary hypertension include the following:

• *auscultation:* abnormalities associated with the underlying disorder

• *arterial blood gas (ABG) analysis:* hypoxemia (decreased partial pressure of oxygen)

• *electrocardiography:* in right ventricular hypertrophy, shows right axis deviation and tall or peaked P waves in inferior leads

• *cardiac catheterization:* increased PAP — pulmonary systolic pressure above 30 mm Hg; pulmonary artery wedge pressure (PAWP) increased if the underlying cause is left atrial myxoma, mitral stenosis, or left ventricular failure — otherwise normal

• *pulmonary angiography:* detects filling defects in pulmonary vasculature, such as those that develop in patients with pulmonary emboli

• *pulmonary function tests:* in underlying obstructive disease, may show decreased flow rates and increased residual volume; in underlying restrictive disease, total lung capacity may decrease.

Treatment

Appropriate treatment usually includes oxygen therapy to decrease hypoxemia and resulting pulmonary vascular resistance. For patients with right heart failure, treatment also includes fluid restriction, digitalis glycosides to increase cardiac output, and diuretics to decrease intravascular volume and extravascular fluid accumulation. An important goal of treatment is correction of the underlying cause.

Special considerations

• Pulmonary hypertension requires keen observation and careful monitoring, as well as skilled supportive care.

• Administer oxygen therapy, as required, and observe the response. Be alert for signs of increasing dyspnea so that treatment can be adjusted accordingly.

• Monitor ABG levels for acidosis and hypoxemia. Watch for changes in level of consciousness.

• When caring for a patient with right heart failure, especially one receiving diuretics, record weight daily, carefully measure intake and output, and explain all medications and diet restrictions.

• Check for increasing neck vein distention, which may indicate fluid overload.

• Monitor vital signs, especially blood pressure and heart rate. Watch for hypotension and tachycardia. If the patient has a pulmonary artery catheter, check PAP and PAWP as required and watch for any changes.

• Before discharge, help the patient adjust to the limitations imposed by this disorder.

• Advise against overexertion and suggest frequent rest periods between activities.

- Refer the patient to the social services department if special equipment, such as oxygen equipment, is needed for home use.
- Make sure he understands the prescribed diet and medications.

LIFE-THREATENING DISORDER

PYELONEPHRITIS, ACUTE

One of the most common renal diseases, acute pyelonephritis (also known as acute infective tubulointerstitial nephritis) is a sudden inflammation caused by bacteria that primarily affects the interstitial area and the renal pelvis or, less often, the renal tubules. With treatment and continued follow-up, the prognosis is good and extensive permanent damage is rare.

Causes

Acute pyelonephritis results from bacterial infection of the kidneys. Infecting bacteria usually are normal intestinal and fecal flora that grow readily in urine. The most common causative organism is *Escherichia coli*, but *Proteus, Pseudomonas, Staphylococcus aureus*, and *Streptococcus faecalis* may also cause such infections.

Typically, the infection spreads from the bladder to the ureters, then to the kidneys, as in vesicoureteral reflux. Vesicoureteral reflux may result from congenital weakness at the junction of the ureter and the bladder. (See *Chronic pyelonephritis,* page 716.)

Bacteria refluxed to intrarenal tissues may create colonies of infection within 24 to 48 hours. Infection may also result from instrumentation (such as catheterization, cystoscopy, or urologic surgery), from a hematogenic infection (as in septicemia or endocarditis), or possibly from lymphatic infection.

Pyelonephritis may also result from an inability to empty the bladder (for example, in patients with neurogenic bladder), urinary stasis, or urinary obstruction due to tumors, strictures, or benign prostatic hyperplasia.

Pyelonephritis occurs more often in females, probably because of a shorter urethra and the proximity of the urinary meatus to the vagina and the rectum (both of which allow bacteria to reach the bladder more easily) and a lack of the antibacterial prostatic secretions produced in the male.

Risk factors

Incidence increases with age and is higher in the following groups:

- *sexually active women* — increased risk of bacterial contamination from intercourse.
- *pregnant women* — about 5% develop asymptomatic bacteriuria; if untreated, about 40% develop pyelonephritis.
- *diabetics* — neurogenic bladder causes incomplete emptying and urinary stasis; glycosuria may support bacterial growth in the urine.
- *people with other renal diseases* — increased susceptibility resulting from compromised renal function.

Signs and symptoms

Typical clinical features include urgency, frequency, burning during urination, dysuria, nocturia, and hematuria (usually microscopic but may be gross). Urine may appear cloudy and have an ammoniacal or fishy odor. Other common symptoms include a temperature of 102° F (38.9° C) or higher, shaking chills, flank pain, anorexia, and general fatigue.

These symptoms characteristically develop rapidly over a few hours or a few days. Although these symptoms

---

CHRONIC PYELONEPHRITIS

Chronic pyelonephritis is a persistent kidney inflammation that can scar the kidneys and may lead to chronic renal failure. Its etiology may be bacterial, metastatic, or urogenous. This disease is most common in patients who are predisposed to recurrent acute pyelonephritis, such as those with urinary obstructions or vesicoureteral reflux.

urine and, especially in late stages, hypertension. Uremia rarely develops from chronic pyelonephritis unless structural abnormalities exist in the excretory system. Bacteriuria may be intermittent. When no bacteria are found in the urine, diagnosis depends on intravenous pyelography (renal pelvis may appear small and flattened) and renal biopsy.

Clinical features
Patients with chronic pyelonephritis may have a childhood history of unexplained fevers or bed-wetting. Signs and symptoms may include flank pain, anemia, low urine specific gravity, proteinuria, leukocytes in

Treatment
Effective treatment of chronic pyelonephritis requires control of hypertension, elimination of the existing obstruction (when possible), and long-term antimicrobial therapy.

---

may disappear within days, even without treatment, residual bacterial infection is likely and may cause later recurrence of symptoms.

Diagnosis
Diagnosis requires urinalysis and culture. Typical findings include:
- *pyuria* (pus in urine) — urine sediment reveals the presence of leukocytes singly, in clumps, and in casts; and, possibly, a few red blood cells
- *significant bacteriuria* — more than 100,000 organisms/μl of urine revealed in urine culture
- *low specific gravity and osmolality* — resulting from a temporarily decreased ability to concentrate urine
- *slightly alkaline urine pH*
- *proteinuria, glycosuria, and ketonuria* — less common.

X-rays also help in the evaluation of acute pyelonephritis. X-rays of the kidneys-ureters-bladder may reveal calculi, tumors, or cysts in the kidneys and the urinary tract. Excretory urography may show asymmetrical kidneys.

Treatment
Effective treatment centers on antibiotic therapy appropriate to the specific infecting organism after identification by urine culture and sensitivity studies.

Antibiotic therapy
S. faecalis requires treatment with ampicillin, penicillin G, or vancomycin. *S. aureus* requires penicillin G or, if resistance develops, a semisynthetic penicillin, such as nafcillin, or a cephalosporin. *E. coli* may be treated with sulfisoxazole, nalidixic acid, and nitrofurantoin; *Proteus,* with ampicillin, sulfisoxazole, nalidixic acid, and a cephalosporin; and *Pseudomonas,* with gentamicin, tobramycin, and carbenicillin.

When the infecting organism cannot be identified, therapy usually consists of a broad-spectrum antibiotic, such as ampicillin or cephalexin. If the patient is pregnant, antibiotics must be prescribed cautiously. Urinary analgesics, such as phenazopyridine, are also appropriate.

Symptoms may disappear after several days of antibiotic therapy. Although urine usually becomes sterile within 48 to 72 hours, the course of such therapy is 10 to 14 days.

Follow-up treatment
Follow-up treatment includes reculturing urine 1 week after drug therapy stops, then periodically for the next year to detect residual or recurring infection. Most patients with uncomplicated infections respond well to therapy and don't suffer reinfection.

In infection from obstruction or vesicoureteral reflux, antibiotics may be less effective; treatment may then necessitate surgery to relieve the obstruction or correct the anomaly. Patients at high risk of recurring urinary tract and kidney infections—such as those with prolonged use of an indwelling catheter or maintenance antibiotic therapy—require long-term follow-up.

Special considerations
• Administer antipyretics for fever.
• Force fluids to achieve urine output of more than 2,000 ml/day. This helps to empty the bladder of contaminated urine. Don't encourage intake of more than 2 to 3 L, because this may decrease the effectiveness of the antibiotics.
• Provide an acid-ash diet to prevent calculus formation.
• Teach proper technique for collecting a clean-catch urine specimen. Be sure to refrigerate or culture a urine specimen within 30 minutes of collection to prevent overgrowth of bacteria.
• Stress the need to complete prescribed antibiotic therapy, even after symptoms subside. Encourage long-term follow-up care for high-risk patients.

To prevent acute pyelonephritis:
• Observe strict sterile technique during catheter insertion and care.
• Instruct females to prevent bacterial contamination by wiping the perineum from front to back after defecation.
• Advise routine checkups for patients with a history of urinary tract infections. Teach them to recognize signs of infection, such as cloudy urine, burning on urination, urgency, and frequency, especially when accompanied by a low-grade fever.

RABIES

Usually transmitted by an animal bite, rabies (hydrophobia) is an acute central nervous system (CNS) infection caused by a ribonucleic acid virus.

If the bite is on the face, the risk of developing rabies is about 60%; on the upper extremities, 15% to 40%; and on the lower extremities, about 10%. In the United States, dog vaccinations have reduced rabies transmission to humans. Wild animals, such as skunks, foxes, and bats, account for 70% of rabies cases.

If symptoms occur, rabies is almost always fatal. Treatment soon after a bite, however, may prevent fatal CNS invasion.

Causes

Generally, the rabies virus is transmitted to a human through the bite of an infected animal that introduces the virus through the skin or mucous membrane. The virus begins to replicate in the striated muscle cells at the bite site.

It next spreads up the nerve to the CNS and replicates in the brain. Finally, it moves through the nerves into other tissues, including the salivary glands. Occasionally, airborne droplets and infected tissue transplants can transmit the virus.

Signs and symptoms

Clinical features are progressive.

Local and prodromal symptoms

Typically, after an incubation period of 1 to 3 months, rabies produces local or radiating pain or burning, a sensation of cold, pruritus, and tingling at the bite site. It also produces prodromal symptoms, such as a slight fever (100° to 102° F [37.8° to 38.9° C]), malaise, headache, anorexia, nausea, sore throat, and persistent loose cough.

After this, the patient begins to show nervousness, anxiety, irritability, hyperesthesia, photophobia, sensitivity to loud noises, pupillary dilation, tachycardia, shallow respirations, and excessive salivation, lacrimation, and perspiration.

Excitation and hydrophobia

About 2 to 10 days after onset of prodromal symptoms, a phase of excitation begins. It's characterized by agitation, marked restlessness, anxiety and apprehension, and cranial nerve dysfunction that causes ocular palsies, strabismus, asymmetrical pupillary dilation or constriction, absence of corneal reflexes, weakness of facial muscles, and hoarseness. Severe systemic symptoms include tachycardia or bradycardia, cyclic respirations, urinary retention, and a temperature of about 103° F (39.4° C).

About 50% of affected patients exhibit hydrophobia (literally, "fear of water"), during which forceful, painful pharyngeal muscle spasms expel liquids from the mouth and cause dehydration, and possibly apnea, cyanosis, and death. Difficulty swallowing causes frothy saliva to drool from the patient's mouth.

Eventually, even the sight, mention, or thought of water causes uncontrollable pharyngeal muscle spasms and excessive salivation. Between episodes of excitation and hydrophobia, the patient commonly is cooperative and lucid.

Terminal phase

After about 3 days, excitation and hydrophobia subside and the progressively paralytic, terminal phase of this illness begins. The patient experiences gradual, generalized, flaccid paralysis that ultimately leads to peripheral vascular collapse, coma, and death.

Diagnosis

Because rabies is fatal unless treated promptly, always suspect rabies in any person who suffers an unprovoked animal bite until you can prove otherwise.

Virus isolation from the patient's saliva or throat and examination of his blood for fluorescent rabies antibody (FRA) are considered the tests that provide the most definitive diagnosis. Other results typically include an elevated white blood cell count, with increased polymorphonuclear and large mononuclear cells, and elevated urinary glucose, acetone, and protein levels.

Confinement of the suspected animal for 10 days of observation by a veterinarian also helps support this diagnosis. If the animal appears rabid, it should be killed and its brain tissue tested for FRA and Negri bodies (oval or round masses that conclusively confirm rabies).

Treatment

The patient requires wound treatment and immunization as soon as possible after exposure.

Thoroughly wash all bite wounds and scratches with soap and water. (See *First aid in animal bites.*)

First Aid in Animal Bites

- Immediately wash the bite vigorously with soap and water for at least 10 minutes to remove the animal's saliva.
- Flush the wound with a viricidal agent, followed by a clear-water rinse.
- Then apply a sterile dressing.
- If possible, don't suture the wound, and don't immediately stop the bleeding (unless it's massive), because blood flow helps to clean the wound.
- Question the patient about the bite. Ask if he provoked the animal (if so, chances are it's not rabid) and if he can identify it or its owner (the animal may be confined for observation).
- Consult local health authorities for treatment information.

Check the patient's immunization status, and administer tetanus-diphtheria prophylaxis, if needed. Take measures to control bacterial infection. If the wound requires suturing, special treatment and suturing techniques must be used to allow proper wound drainage.

After rabies exposure, a patient who hasn't been immunized before must receive passive immunization with rabies immune globulin (RIg) and active immunization with human diploid cell vaccine (HDCV). If the patient has received HDCV before and has an adequate rabies antibody titer, he doesn't need RIg immunization, just an HDCV booster.

Special considerations

- When injecting rabies vaccine, rotate injection sites on the upper arm or thigh. Watch for and treat symptoms of redness, itching, pain, and tenderness at the injection site.

• Cooperate with public health authorities to determine the vaccination status of the animal. If the animal is proven rabid, help identify others at risk.

• If rabies develops, provide aggressive supportive care (even after onset of coma) to make probable death less agonizing.

• Monitor cardiac and pulmonary function continuously.

• Isolate the patient. Wear a gown, gloves, and protection for the eyes and mouth when handling saliva and articles contaminated with saliva. Take precautions to avoid being bitten by the patient during the excitation phase.

• Keep the room dark and quiet.

• Establish communication with the patient and his family. Provide psychological support to help them cope with the patient's symptoms and probable death.

• To help prevent this dreaded disease, stress the need for vaccination of household pets that may be exposed to rabid wild animals. Warn people not to try to touch wild animals, especially if they appear ill or overly docile (a possible sign of rabies).

• Recommend prophylactic rabies vaccine to high-risk people, such as farm workers, forest rangers, spelunkers (cave explorers), and veterinarians.

RAPE TRAUMA SYNDROME

The term "rape" refers to illicit sexual intercourse without consent. It's a violent assault in which sex is used as a weapon. Rape inflicts varying degrees of physical and psychological trauma.

Rape trauma syndrome occurs during the period following the rape or attempted rape. It refers to the victim's short-term and long-term reactions and to the methods she uses to cope with this trauma.

In the United States, a rape is reported every 7 minutes (200 per day, 62,500 per year). Incidence of reported rape is highest in large cities and is rising. However, possibly over 90% of assaults are never reported.

Known victims of rape range from age 2 months to 97 years. The age-group most affected are 10- to 19-year-olds; the average victim's age is 13½. About one out of seven reported rapes involves a prepubertal child.

Over 50% of rapes occur in the home; about one-third of these involve a male intruder who forces his way into a home. Approximately half the time, the victim has some casual acquaintance with the attacker. Most rapists are ages 15 to 24. Usually, the attack is planned.

In most cases, the rapist is a man and the victim is a woman. However, rapes do occur between persons of the same sex, especially in prisons, schools, hospitals, and other institutions.

Children are also often victims of rape; most of the time these cases involve manual, oral, or genital contact with the child's genitalia. Usually, the rapist is a member of the child's family. In rare instances, a man or child is sexually abused by a woman.

The prognosis is good if the rape victim receives physical and emotional support and counseling to help her deal with her feelings. Victims who articulate their feelings are able to cope with fears, interact with others, and return to normal routines faster than those who don't.

Causes

Some of the cultural, sociological, and psychological factors that contribute to rape include increasing exposure to sex, permissiveness, cynicism about relationships, feelings of anger, and powerlessness amid social pressures.

The rapist often has feelings of violence or hatred toward women or sexual problems, such as impotence or premature ejaculation. Often he feels socially isolated and unable to form warm, loving relationships. Some rapists may be psychopaths who need violence for physical pleasure, no matter how it affects their victims; others rape to satisfy a need for power. Some were abused as children.

Signs and symptoms

A physical examination (including a pelvic examination by a gynecologist) will probably show signs of physical trauma, especially if the assault was prolonged. Depending on specific body areas attacked, a patient may have a sore throat, mouth irritation, difficulty swallowing, ecchymoses, or rectal pain and bleeding.

If additional physical violence accompanied the rape, the victim may have hematomas, lacerations, bleeding, severe internal injuries, and hemorrhage, and if the rape occurred outdoors, she may suffer from exposure. X-rays may reveal fractures. The patient may have injuries severe enough to require hospitalization.

Assessment

• When a rape victim arrives in the emergency department, assess her physical injuries. If she's not *seriously* injured, allow her to remain clothed and take her to a private room, where she can talk with you or a counselor before the necessary physical examination.

• Remember, immediate reactions to rape differ and include crying, laughing, hostility, confusion, withdrawal, or outward calm; often anger and rage don't surface until later. During the assault, the victim may have felt demeaned, helpless, and afraid for her life; afterward, she may feel ashamed, guilty, shocked, and vulnerable, and have a sense of disbelief and lowered self-esteem.

• Offer support and reassurance. Help her explore her feelings; listen, convey trust and respect, and remain nonjudgmental. Don't leave her alone unless she asks you to.

• Being careful to upset the victim as little as possible, obtain an accurate history of the rape, pertinent to physical assessment.

Remember: Your notes may be used as evidence if the rapist is tried.

• Record the victim's statements in the first person, using quotation marks. Also document objective information provided by others. Never speculate as to what may have happened or record subjective impressions or thoughts.

• Include in your notes the time the victim arrived at the hospital, the date and time of the alleged rape, and the time the victim was examined. Ask the victim about allergies to penicillin and other drugs, if she's had recent illnesses (especially venereal disease), if she was pregnant before the attack, the date of her last menstrual period, and details of her obstetric-gynecologic history.

• Thoroughly explain the examination she'll have, and tell her why it's necessary (to rule out internal injuries and obtain a specimen for venereal disease testing). Obtain her informed consent for treatment and for the police report. Allow her some control, if possible; for instance, ask her if she's ready to be examined or if she'd rather wait a bit.

• Before the examination, ask the victim whether she douched, bathed, or washed before coming to the hospital.

Note this on her chart. Have her change into a hospital gown, and place her clothing in *paper bags*. (*Never* use plastic bags, because secretions and seminal stains will mold, destroying valuable evidence.) Label each bag and its contents.

• Tell the victim she may urinate, but warn her not to wipe or otherwise clean the perineal area. If the patient wishes, ask a counselor to stay with her throughout the examination. This examination is typically very distressing for the rape victim. Reassure her and allow her as much control as possible.

• Throughout the examination, provide support and reassurance, and carefully label all possible evidence. Before the victim's pelvic area is examined, take vital signs, and if the patient is wearing a tampon, remove it, wrap it, and label it as evidence.

• During the examination, make sure all specimens collected, including those for semen and gonorrhea, receive careful labeling. Include the patient's name, the doctor's name, and the location from which the specimen was obtained. List all specimens in your notes.

• If the case comes to trial, specimens will be used for evidence, so accuracy is essential. Most emergency departments have "rape kits" with containers for specimens. Carefully collect and label fingernail scrapings and foreign material obtained by combing the victim's pubic hair; these also provide valuable evidence. Note to whom these specimens are given.

• For a male victim, be especially alert for injury to the mouth, perineum, and anus. Obtain a pharyngeal specimen for a gonorrhea culture and rectal aspirate for acid phosphatase or sperm analysis.

• Photographs of the patient's injuries will also be taken. This may be delayed for a day or repeated when bruises and ecchymoses are more apparent.

• Most states require hospitals to report rape. The patient may not press charges and may not assist the police. If the patient does *not* go to the hospital, she may not report the rape.

• If the police interview the patient in the hospital, be supportive and encourage her to recall details of the rape. Your kindness and empathy are invaluable.

• The patient may also want you to call her family. Help her to verbalize anticipation of her family's response.

Treatment

The rape victim should receive supportive care and protection against venereal disease and, if she wishes, against pregnancy.

Antibiotics are given to prevent venereal disease. To prevent pregnancy as a result of the rape, the patient may be given large doses of oral diethylstilbestrol (DES) for 5 consecutive days. Or she may wait 3 to 4 weeks and undergo a dilatation and curettage or a vacuum aspiration to abort a pregnancy.

If the patient has vulvar lacerations and hair cuts, the area will be cleaned and lacerations repaired after all the evidence is obtained. Topical use of ice packs may reduce vulvar swelling.

All victims of rape should be offered testing for human immunodeficiency virus infection and receive medical counseling and follow-up.

Recovery from rape, which may be prolonged, consists of the acute phase (immediate reaction) and the reorganization phase. During the acute phase, physical aspects include pain, loss of appetite, and wound healing; emotional reactions typically include shaking, crying, and mood swings. Feelings of grief, anger, fear, or revenge may color the victim's social interactions.

Counseling helps the victim identify her coping mechanisms. She may relate more easily to a counselor of the same sex.

During the reorganization phase, which usually begins a week after the rape and may last months or years, the victim is concerned with restructuring her life. Initially, she often has nightmares in which she's powerless; later dreams show her gradually gaining more control. When she's alone, she may also suffer from "daymares" — frightening thoughts about the rape. She may have reduced sexual desire or may develop fear of intercourse or mistrust of men.

Special considerations
• Because cultures can't detect gonorrhea or syphilis for 5 to 6 days after the rape, stress the importance of returning for follow-up venereal disease testing.
• If the patient receives DES, explain its possible adverse effects.
• Legal proceedings during this time force the victim to relive the trauma, leaving her feeling lonely and isolated, perhaps even temporarily halting her emotional recovery. To help her cope, encourage her to write her thoughts, feelings, and reactions in a daily diary, and refer her to organizations such as Women Organized Against Rape or a local rape crisis center for empathy and advice.

RAYNAUD'S DISEASE

One of several primary arteriospastic disorders, Raynaud's disease is characterized by episodic vasospasm in the small peripheral arteries and arterioles, precipitated by exposure to cold or stress. This condition occurs bilaterally and usually affects the hands or, less often, the feet.

Raynaud's disease is most prevalent in women, particularly between puberty and age 40. A benign condition, it requires no specific treatment and has no serious sequelae.

Raynaud's phenomenon, however, a condition often associated with several connective tissue disorders — such as scleroderma, systemic lupus erythematosus, and polymyositis — has a progressive course, leading to ischemia, gangrene, and amputation. Differentiating the two disorders is difficult because some patients who experience mild symptoms of Raynaud's disease for several years may later develop overt connective tissue disease — most commonly scleroderma.

Causes
Although the cause is unknown, several theories account for the reduced digital blood flow: intrinsic vascular wall hyperactivity to cold, increased vasomotor tone resulting from sympathetic stimulation, and antigen-antibody immune response (the most probable theory, because abnormal immunologic test results accompany Raynaud's phenomenon).

Signs and symptoms
After exposure to cold or stress, the skin on the fingers typically blanches, then becomes cyanotic before changing to red and before changing from cold to normal temperature. Numbness and tingling may also occur. These symptoms are relieved by warmth.

In longstanding disease, trophic changes such as sclerodactyly, ulcerations, or chronic paronychia may result. Although it's extremely uncommon, minimal cutaneous gangrene necessitates amputation of one or more phalanges.

Diagnosis

Clinical criteria that establish Raynaud's disease include skin color changes induced by cold or stress; bilateral involvement; absence of gangrene or, if present, minimal cutaneous gangrene; normal arterial pulses; and a patient history of clinical symptoms of longer than 2 years' duration. The diagnosis must also rule out secondary disease processes, such as chronic arterial occlusive or connective tissue disease.

Treatment

Initially, treatment consists of avoidance of cold, mechanical, or chemical injury; cessation of smoking; and reassurance that symptoms are benign.

Because adverse drug effects, especially from vasodilators, may be more bothersome than the disease itself, drug therapy is reserved for unusually severe symptoms. Such therapy may include phenoxybenzamine or reserpine.

When conservative treatment fails to prevent ischemic ulcers, sympathectomy may be helpful; fewer than a quarter of patients require this procedure.

Special considerations

• Warn against exposure to the cold. Tell the patient to wear mittens or gloves in cold weather or when handling cold items or defrosting the freezer.

• Advise the patient to avoid stressful situations and to stop smoking.

• Instruct the patient to inspect the skin frequently and to seek immediate care for signs of skin breakdown or infection.

• Teach the patient about drugs, their use, and their adverse effects.

• Provide psychological support and reassurance to allay the patient's fear of amputation and disfigurement.

RECTAL POLYPS

These masses of tissue rise above the mucosal membrane and protrude into the GI tract. Types of rectal polyps include common polypoid adenomas, villous adenomas, hereditary polyposis, focal polypoid hyperplasia, and juvenile polyps (hamartomas).

Villous adenomas are most prevalent in men over age 55; common polypoid adenomas, in white women between ages 45 and 60. Incidence in both sexes rises after age 70. Juvenile polyps occur most frequently among children under age 10 and are characterized by rectal bleeding.

Most rectal polyps are benign. However, villous and hereditary polyps show a marked inclination to become malignant. Indeed, a striking feature of familial polyposis is its frequent association with rectosigmoid adenocarcinoma.

Causes

Predisposing factors for developing rectal polyps include heredity, age, infection, and diet. Formation of polyps results from unrestrained cell growth in the upper epithelium.

Signs and symptoms

Because rectal polyps don't generally cause symptoms, they are usually discovered incidentally during a digital examination or rectosigmoidoscopy. Rectal bleeding is a common sign: High rectal polyps leave a streak of blood on stools; low rectal polyps bleed freely.

Rectal polyps vary in appearance:

• *Common polypoid adenomas* are small, multiple lesions that are redder than normal mucosa. They're commonly pedunculated — attached to rectal mucosa by a long, thin stalk — and granular, with a red, lobular, or eroded surface.

• *Villous adenomas* are usually sessile — attached to the mucosa by a wide base — and vary in size from 0.5 to 12 cm. They're soft, friable, and finely lobulated. They may grow large and cause painful defecation; however, because adenomas are soft, they rarely cause bowel obstruction.

Sometimes adenomas prolapse outside the anus, expelling parts of the adenoma with the feces. These polyps may cause diarrhea, bloody stools, and subsequent fluid and electrolyte depletion, with hypotension and oliguria.

• In *hereditary polyposis,* rectal polyps resemble benign adenomas but occur as hundreds of small (0.5-cm) lesions carpeting the entire mucosal surface. Associated signs include diarrhea, bloody stools, and secondary anemia. In patients with hereditary polyposis, a change in bowel habits with abdominal pain usually signals rectosigmoid cancer.

• *Juvenile polyps* are large, inflammatory lesions, often without an epithelial covering. Mucus-filled cysts cover their usually smooth surface.

• *Focal polypoid hyperplasia* produces small (less than 3 mm), granular, sessile lesions, similar to the colon in color, or gray or translucent. They usually occur at the rectosigmoid junction.

Diagnosis

A firm diagnosis of rectal polyps requires identification of the polyps through proctosigmoidoscopy or colonoscopy, and rectal biopsy. A barium enema can help identify polyps that are located high in the colon.

Supportive laboratory findings include occult blood in the stools, low hemoglobin and hematocrit (with anemia) and, possibly, serum electrolyte imbalances in patients with villous adenomas.

Treatment

Specific treatment varies according to the type and size of the polyps and their location in the colon.

Common polypoid adenomas less than 1 cm in size require polypectomy, frequently by fulguration (destruction by high-frequency electricity) during endoscopy. For common polypoid adenomas over 4 cm and all invasive villous adenomas, treatment usually consists of abdominoperineal resection or low anterior resection. Focal polypoid hyperplasia can be obliterated by a biopsy.

Depending on GI involvement, hereditary polyps necessitate total abdominoperineal resection with a permanent ileostomy, subtotal colectomy with ileoproctostomy, or ileoanal anastomosis. Juvenile polyps are prone to autoamputation; if this doesn't occur, snare removal during colonoscopy is the treatment of choice.

Special considerations

• During diagnostic evaluation, check sodium, potassium, and chloride levels daily in the patient with fluid imbalance; adjust fluid and electrolyte administration as necessary. Administer normal saline solution with potassium I.V.

• Weigh the patient daily, and record the amount of diarrhea. Watch for signs of dehydration (decreased urination, increased blood urea nitrogen levels).

• Tell the patient to watch for and report evidence of rectal bleeding.

• After biopsy and fulguration, check for signs of perforation and hemorrhage, such as sudden hypotension, a decrease in hemoglobin or hematocrit, shock, abdominal pain, and passage of red blood through the rectum.

• Watch for and record the first bowel movement, which may not occur for 2 to 3 days.

• Help the patient ambulate within 24 hours after the procedure.

- Provide sitz baths for 3 days.
- If the patient has benign polyps, stress the need for routine follow-up studies to check the polypoid growth rate.
- Prepare the patient with precancerous or familial lesions for abdominoperineal resection. Provide emotional support and preoperative instruction.
- After ileostomy or subtotal colectomy with ileoproctostomy, properly care for the abdominal dressings, I.V. lines, and indwelling urinary catheter. Record intake and output, and check vital signs for hypotension and surgical complications. Administer pain medication as needed.
- To prevent embolism, help the patient ambulate as soon as possible and apply antiembolism stockings; encourage range-of-motion exercises.
- Provide enterostomal therapy and teach stoma care.

RECTAL PROLAPSE

Defined as the circumferential protrusion of one or more layers of the mucous membrane through the anus, rectal prolapse may be complete (with displacement of the anal sphincter or bowel herniation) or partial (mucosal layer).

Rectal prolapse usually occurs in men under age 40, in women around age 45 (three times more often than men), and in children ages 1 to 3 (especially those with cystic fibrosis).

Causes

Several factors predispose the patient to rectal prolapse, especially straining during defecation, which increases intra-abdominal pressure. Other predisposing factors include conditions that affect the pelvic floor or rectum, such as weak sphincters; weak longitudinal, rectal, or levator ani muscles resulting from neurologic disorders, injury, tumors, or aging; or chronic wasting diseases, such as tuberculosis or cystic fibrosis.

Signs and symptoms

In rectal prolapse, protrusion of tissue from the rectum may occur during defecation or walking. Other indications include a persistent sensation of rectal fullness, bloody diarrhea, and pain in the lower abdomen due to ulceration. Hemorrhoids or rectal polyps may coexist with a prolapse.

Diagnosis

Typical clinical features and visual examination confirm the diagnosis. In complete prolapse, examination reveals the full thickness of the bowel wall and, possibly, the sphincter muscle protruding and mucosa falling into bulky, concentric folds.

In partial prolapse, examination reveals only partially protruding mucosa and a smaller mass of radial mucosal folds. Straining during examination may disclose the full extent of prolapse.

Treatment

The underlying cause dictates the type of treatment necessary. Sometimes eliminating this cause (straining, coughing, nutritional disorders) is the only treatment necessary.

In a child, prolapsed tissue usually diminishes as the child grows. In an older patient, injection of a sclerosing agent to cause a fibrotic reaction fixes the rectum in place.

Severe or chronic prolapse requires surgical repair by strengthening or tightening the sphincters with wire or by anterior or rectal resection of prolapsed tissue.

Special considerations

• Help the patient prevent constipation by teaching a correct diet and stool-softening regimen. Advise the patient with severe prolapse and incontinence to wear a perineal pad.

• Before surgery, explain possible complications, including permanent rectal incontinence.

• After surgery, watch for immediate complications (hemorrhage) and later ones (pelvic abscess, fever, pus drainage, pain, rectal stenosis, constipation, or pain on defecation).

• Teach perineal strengthening exercises: have the patient lie down, with his back flat on the mattress; then ask him to pull in his abdomen and squeeze while taking a deep breath; or have the patient repeatedly squeeze and relax his buttocks while sitting on a chair.

RENAL CALCULI

Although renal calculi (kidney stones) may form anywhere in the urinary tract, they usually develop in the renal pelvis or the calyces of the kidneys. Such formation follows precipitation of substances normally dissolved in the urine (calcium oxalate, calcium phosphate, magnesium ammonium phosphate or, occasionally, urate or cystine).

Renal calculi vary in size and may be solitary or multiple. They may remain in the renal pelvis or enter the ureter and may damage renal parenchyma; large calculi cause pressure necrosis. In certain locations, calculi cause obstruction, with resultant hydronephrosis, and tend to recur.

Among Americans, renal calculi develop in 1 in 1,000 people, are more common in men (especially those ages 30 to 50) than in women, and are rare in blacks and children. They're particularly prevalent in certain geographic areas, such as the southeastern United States ("stone belt"), possibly because a hot climate promotes dehydration or because of regional dietary habits.

Causes

Although the exact cause of renal calculi is unknown, predisposing factors include the following:

• *Dehydration* and resultant decreased urine production concentrates calculus-forming substances.

• *Infection* in tissue provides a site for calculus development; pH changes provide a favorable medium for calculus formation (especially for magnesium ammonium phosphate or calcium phosphate calculi); infected calculi (usually magnesium ammonium phosphate or staghorn calculi) may develop if bacteria serve as the nucleus in calculus formation. Such infections may promote destruction of renal parenchyma.

• *Obstruction* can result from urinary stasis (as in immobility from spinal cord injury), which allows calculus constituents to collect and adhere, forming calculi. Obstruction also promotes infection, which, in turn, compounds the obstruction.

• *Metabolic factors* that can predispose to renal calculi include hyperparathyroidism, renal tubular acidosis, elevated uric acid (usually with gout), defective metabolism of oxalate, genetic defect in metabolism of cystine, and excessive intake of vitamin D or dietary calcium.

Signs and symptoms

Clinical effects vary with size, location, and etiology of the calculi.

Pain

The key symptom, pain usually results from obstruction; large, rough calculi occlude the opening to the ureter and increase the frequency and force of peristaltic contractions. The pain of classic renal colic travels from the costovertebral angle to the flank, to the suprapubic region and external genitalia.

The intensity of this pain fluctuates and may be excruciating at its peak. If calculi are in the renal pelvis and calyces, pain may be more constant and dull. Back pain (from calculi that produce an obstruction within a kidney) and severe abdominal pain (from calculi traveling down a ureter) may also occur. Nausea and vomiting usually accompany severe pain.

Accompanying signs

Other associated signs include fever, chills, hematuria (when calculi abrade a ureter), abdominal distention, pyuria and, rarely, anuria (from bilateral obstruction or unilateral obstruction in the patient with one kidney).

Diagnosis

The clinical picture in conjunction with the following diagnostic tests allows a diagnosis:

• *Kidney-ureter-bladder X-rays* reveal most renal calculi.

• *Calculus analysis* shows mineral content.

• *Excretory urography* confirms the diagnosis and determines size and location of calculi.

• *Kidney ultrasonography,* an easily performed noninvasive, nontoxic test, detects obstructive changes, such as unilateral or bilateral hydronephrosis.

• *Urine culture* of midstream specimen may indicate urinary tract infection.

• *Urinalysis* may be normal, or may show increased specific gravity and acid or alkaline pH suitable for different types of stone formation. Other urinalysis findings include hematuria (gross or microscopic), crystals (urate, calcium, or cystine), casts, and pyuria with or without bacteria and white blood cells.

• A *24-hour urine collection* is evaluated for calcium oxalate, phosphorus, and uric acid excretion levels.

• *Serial blood calcium and phosphorus levels* detect hyperparathyroidism and show an increased calcium level in proportion to the normal level of serum protein.

• *Blood protein level* determines level of free calcium unbound to protein.

• *Blood chloride and bicarbonate levels* may show renal tubular acidosis.

• *Increased blood uric acid levels* may indicate gout as the cause.

Diagnosis must rule out appendicitis, cholecystitis, peptic ulcer, and pancreatitis as potential sources of pain.

Treatment

Because 90% of renal calculi are smaller than 5 mm in diameter, treatment usually consists of measures to promote their natural passage. Along with vigorous hydration, such treatment includes antimicrobial therapy (varying with the cultured organism) for infection; analgesics, such as meperidine, for pain; and diuretics to prevent urinary stasis and further calculus formation. (Thiazides decrease calcium excretion into the urine.)

Prophylaxis to prevent calculus formation includes a low-calcium diet for absorptive hypercalciuria, parathyroidectomy for hyperparathyroidism, allopurinol for uric acid calculi, and daily administration of oral ascorbic acid to acidify the urine.

Calculi too large for natural passage may require surgical removal. When a calculus is in the ureter, a cystoscope may be inserted through the urethra and the calculus manipulated with catheters or retrieval instruments. Extraction of calculi from other areas (kidney calyx, renal pelvis) may necessitate a flank or lower abdominal approach.

Percutaneous ultrasonic lithotripsy and extracorporeal shock-wave litho-

TEACHING CHECKLIST

PREVENTING RECURRENCE OF RENAL CALCULI

Before discharge, your patient needs to learn how to prevent a recurrence of renal calculi. Teach him to:
• closely follow the prescribed dietary and medication regimens
• increase fluid intake
• check his urine pH, if appropriate, and keep a daily record
• immediately report symptoms of acute obstruction (pain and inability to void).

---

tripsy shatter the calculus into fragments for removal by suction or natural passage. To prevent recurrence of calculi, the patient will also need teaching before discharge. (See *Preventing recurrence of renal calculi*.)

Special considerations

• To aid diagnosis, maintain a 24- to 48-hour record of urine pH, with nitrazine pH paper; strain all urine through gauze or a tea strainer; and save all solid material recovered for analysis.

• To facilitate spontaneous passage, encourage the patient to walk, if possible. Also promote sufficient intake of fluids to maintain a urine output of 3 to 4 L/day (urine should be very diluted and colorless).

• To help acidify urine, offer fruit juices, particularly cranberry juice. If the patient can't drink the required amount of fluid, supplemental I.V. fluids may be given. Record intake and output and daily weight to assess fluid status and renal function.

• Stress the importance of proper diet and compliance with drug therapy. For example, if the patient's stone is caused by a hyperuricemic condition, advise the patient or whoever prepares his meals which foods are high in purine.

• If surgery is necessary, provide reassurance. The patient is apt to be fearful, especially if surgery includes removal of a kidney, so emphasize that the body can adapt well to having one kidney. If he is to have an abdominal or flank incision, teach deep-breathing and coughing exercises.

• After surgery, the patient will probably have an indwelling urinary catheter or a nephrostomy tube in place. Unless one of his kidneys was removed, expect bloody drainage from the catheter.

• Check dressings regularly for bloody drainage, and know how much drainage to expect. Watch closely for signs of suspected hemorrhage (excessive drainage, rising pulse rate). Use sterile technique when changing dressings or providing catheter care.

• Watch for signs of infection (rising fever, chills), and give antibiotics as needed.

• To prevent pneumonia, encourage frequent position changes, and ambulate the patient as soon as possible. Have him hold a small pillow over the operative site to splint the incision and thereby facilitate deep-breathing and coughing exercises.

RENAL FAILURE, ACUTE

Obstruction, reduced circulation, and renal parenchymal disease can all cause the sudden interruption of kidney function. Acute renal failure is usually reversible with medical treatment; otherwise, it may progress to end-stage renal disease, uremic syndrome, and death.

Causes

Acute renal failure can be classified as prerenal, intrinsic (or parenchymal), and postrenal.

Prerenal failure

Diminished blood flow to the kidneys causes prerenal failure. Such decreased flow may result from hypovolemia, shock, embolism, blood loss, sepsis, pooling of fluid in ascites or burns, and cardiovascular disorders, such as congestive heart failure (CHF), arrhythmias, and tamponade.

Intrinsic renal failure

Parenchymal, or intrinsic, renal failure results from damage to the kidneys themselves, usually resulting from acute tubular necrosis. Such damage may also result from acute poststreptococcal glomerulonephritis, systemic lupus erythematosus, periarteritis nodosa, vasculitis, sickle-cell disease, bilateral renal vein thrombosis, nephrotoxins, ischemia, renal myeloma, and acute pyelonephritis.

Postrenal failure

Bilateral obstruction of urinary outflow results in postrenal failure. Its multiple causes include kidney stones, blood clots, papillae from papillary necrosis, tumors, benign prostatic hyperplasia, strictures, and urethral edema from catheterization.

Signs and symptoms

Acute renal failure is a critical illness. Its early signs are oliguria, azotemia and, rarely, anuria. Electrolyte imbalances, metabolic acidosis, and other severe effects follow as the patient becomes increasingly uremic and renal dysfunction disrupts other body systems:

- *GI* — anorexia, nausea, vomiting, diarrhea or constipation, stomatitis, bleeding, hematemesis, dry mucous membranes, uremic breath
- *central nervous system (CNS)* — headache, drowsiness, irritability, confusion, peripheral neuropathy, seizures, coma
- *cutaneous* — dryness, pruritus, pallor, purpura; rarely, uremic frost
- *cardiovascular* — early in the disease, hypotension; later, hypertension, arrhythmias, fluid overload, CHF, systemic edema, anemia, altered clotting mechanisms
- *respiratory* — Kussmaul's respirations, pulmonary edema.

Fever and chills indicate infection, a common complication.

Diagnosis

The patient's history may include a disorder that can cause renal failure. Blood test results indicating intrinsic acute renal failure include elevated blood urea nitrogen, serum creatinine, and potassium levels and low blood pH, bicarbonate, hematocrit, and hemoglobin levels.

Urine specimens show casts, cellular debris, decreased specific gravity and, in glomerular diseases, proteinuria and urine osmolality close to serum osmolality. The urine sodium level is less than 20 mEq/L if oliguria results from decreased perfusion, more than 40 mEq/L if it results from an intrinsic problem.

Other studies include renal ultrasonography, kidney-ureter-bladder X-rays, cautious use of excretory urography, renal scan, retrograde pyelography, and nephrotomography.

Treatment

Supportive measures include a diet high in calories and low in protein, sodium, and potassium, with supplemental vitamins and restricted fluids. Meticulous electrolyte monitoring is essential to detect hyperkalemia.

If hyperkalemia occurs, acute therapy may include dialysis, hypertonic glucose and insulin infusions, and sodium bicarbonate — all administered I.V. — and sodium polystyrene sulfonate, given orally or by enema, to remove potassium from the body.

If measures fail to control uremic symptoms, hemodialysis or peritoneal dialysis may be necessary.

Special considerations

• Measure and record intake and output, including all body fluids, such as wound drainage, nasogastric output, and diarrhea. Weigh the patient daily.
• Assess hematocrit and hemoglobin levels and replace blood components as needed. *Don't* use whole blood if the patient is prone to CHF and can't tolerate extra fluid volume.
• Monitor vital signs. Watch closely for any signs of pericarditis (pleuritic chest pain, tachycardia, pericardial friction rub), inadequate renal perfusion (hypotension), and acidosis.
• Maintain proper electrolyte balance. Strictly monitor potassium levels. Watch for symptoms of hyperkalemia (malaise, anorexia, paresthesia, or muscle weakness) and electrocardiogram changes (tall, peaked T waves; widening QRS segment; and disappearing P waves). Don't give medications containing potassium.
• Assess the patient frequently, especially during emergency treatment to lower potassium levels. If the patient receives hypertonic glucose and insulin infusions, monitor potassium levels. If you give sodium polystyrene sulfonate rectally, make sure the patient doesn't retain it and become constipated, to prevent bowel perforation.
• Maintain nutritional status. Provide a high-calorie, low-protein, low-sodium, and low-potassium diet, with vitamin supplements. Give the anorectic patient small, frequent meals.
• Use aseptic technique; the patient with acute renal failure is highly susceptible to infection. Don't allow personnel with upper respiratory tract infections to care for the patient.
• Prevent complications of immobility by encouraging frequent coughing and deep breathing and by performing passive range-of-motion exercises. Help the patient walk as soon as possible. Add lubricating lotion to the patient's bathwater to combat skin dryness.
• Provide good mouth care frequently for dry mucous membranes. If stomatitis occurs, the patient may need an antibiotic solution. Have the patient swish the solution around in his mouth before swallowing.
• Monitor for GI bleeding by applying the guaiac test to all stools. Administer medications carefully, especially antacids and stool softeners.
• Use appropriate safety measures, such as side rails and restraints; the patient with CNS involvement may be dizzy or confused.
• Provide emotional support to the patient and his family. Reassure them by clearly explaining all procedures.
• During peritoneal dialysis, position the patient carefully. Elevate the head of the bed to reduce pressure on the diaphragm and aid respiration. Be alert for signs of infection (cloudy drainage, elevated temperature) and bleeding.
• If pain occurs, reduce the amount of dialysate. Monitor the diabetic patient's blood glucose level periodically,

and administer insulin as needed. Watch for complications, such as peritonitis, atelectasis, hypokalemia, pneumonia, and shock.

• If the patient requires hemodialysis, check the blood access site (arteriovenous fistula, subclavian or femoral catheter) every 2 hours for patency and signs of clotting. Don't use the arm with the shunt or fistula for taking blood pressures or drawing blood. Weigh the patient before beginning dialysis.

• During dialysis, monitor vital signs, clotting times, blood flow, the function of the vascular access site, and arterial and venous pressures. Watch for complications, such as septicemia, embolism, hepatitis, and rapid fluid and electrolyte loss.

• After dialysis, monitor vital signs and the vascular access site, weigh the patient, and watch for signs of fluid and electrolyte imbalances.

• Follow universal precautions when handling all blood and body fluids.

LIFE-THREATENING DISORDER

RENAL FAILURE, CHRONIC

Although chronic renal failure is usually the result of a gradually progressive loss of renal function, it occasionally results from a rapidly progressive disease of sudden onset. Few symptoms develop until after more than 75% of glomerular filtration is lost; then the remaining normal parenchyma deteriorates progressively, and symptoms worsen as renal function decreases.

If this condition continues unchecked, uremic toxins accumulate and produce potentially fatal physiologic changes in all major organ systems. If

the patient can tolerate it, maintenance dialysis or kidney transplantation can sustain life.

Causes
Chronic renal failure may result from:
• *chronic glomerular disease* such as glomerulonephritis
• *chronic infections,* such as chronic pyelonephritis or tuberculosis
• *congenital anomalies* such as polycystic kidneys
• *vascular diseases,* such as renal nephrosclerosis or hypertension
• *obstructive processes* such as calculi
• *collagen diseases* such as systemic lupus erythematosus
• *nephrotoxic agents* such as long-term aminoglycoside therapy
• *endocrine diseases* such as diabetic neuropathy.

Such conditions gradually destroy the nephrons and eventually cause irreversible renal failure. Similarly, acute renal failure that fails to respond to treatment becomes chronic renal failure.

Chronic renal failure may progress through the following stages:
• reduced renal reserve (glomerular filtration rate [GFR] 40 to 70 ml/minute)
• renal insufficiency (GFR 20 to 40 ml/minute)
• renal failure (GFR 10 to 20 ml/minute)
• end-stage renal disease (GFR less than 10 ml/minute).

Signs and symptoms
Chronic renal failure produces major changes in all body systems.

Renal and urologic changes
Initially, salt-wasting and consequent hyponatremia produce hypotension, dry mouth, loss of skin turgor, listlessness, fatigue, and nausea. Later, somnolence and confusion develop.

As the number of functioning nephrons decreases, so does the kidneys' capacity to excrete sodium, resulting in salt retention and overload. Accumulation of potassium causes muscle irritability, then muscle weakness as the potassium level continues to rise.

Fluid overload and metabolic acidosis also occur. Urine output decreases; urine is very dilute and contains casts and crystals.

Cardiovascular changes
Renal failure leads to hypertension and arrhythmias, including life-threatening ventricular tachycardia or fibrillation. Other effects include cardiomyopathy, uremic pericarditis, pericardial effusion with possible cardiac tamponade, congestive heart failure (CHF), and peripheral edema.

Respiratory changes
Pulmonary changes include reduced pulmonary macrophage activity with increased susceptibility to infection, pulmonary edema, pleuritic pain, pleural friction rub and effusions, and uremic pleuritis and uremic lung (or uremic pneumonitis). Dyspnea from CHF also occurs, as do Kussmaul's respirations as a result of acidosis.

GI changes
Inflammation and ulceration of GI mucosa cause stomatitis, gum ulceration and bleeding, and, possibly, parotitis, esophagitis, gastritis, duodenal ulcers, lesions on the small and large bowel, uremic colitis, pancreatitis, and proctitis. Other GI symptoms include a metallic taste in the mouth, uremic fetor (ammonia smell to breath), anorexia, nausea, and vomiting.

Cutaneous changes
Typically, the skin is pallid, yellowish bronze, dry, and scaly. Other cutaneous symptoms include severe itching; purpura; ecchymoses; petechiae;

uremic frost (most often in critically ill or terminal patients); thin, brittle fingernails with characteristic lines; and dry, brittle hair that may change color and fall out easily.

Neurologic changes
Restless leg syndrome, one of the first signs of peripheral neuropathy, causes pain, burning, and itching in the legs and feet, which may be relieved by voluntarily shaking, moving, or rocking them. Eventually, this condition progresses to paresthesia and motor nerve dysfunction (usually bilateral footdrop) unless dialysis is initiated.

Other signs and symptoms include muscle cramping and twitching, shortened memory and attention span, apathy, drowsiness, irritability, confusion, coma, and seizures. Electroencephalogram changes indicate metabolic encephalopathy.

Endocrine changes
Common endocrine abnormalities include stunted growth patterns in children (even with elevated growth hormone levels), infertility and decreased libido in both sexes, amenorrhea and cessation of menses in women, and impotence and decreased sperm production in men. Other changes include increased aldosterone secretion (related to increased renin production) and impaired carbohydrate metabolism (causing increased blood glucose levels similar to those found in diabetes mellitus).

Hematopoietic changes
Anemia, decreased red blood cell (RBC) survival time, blood loss from dialysis and GI bleeding, mild thrombocytopenia, and platelet defects occur. Other problems include increased bleeding and clotting disorders, demonstrated by purpura, hemorrhage from body orifices, easy bruising, ecchymoses, and petechiae.

Skeletal changes

Calcium-phosphorus imbalance and consequent parathyroid hormone imbalances cause muscle and bone pain, skeletal demineralization, pathologic fractures, and calcifications in the brain, eyes, gums, joints, myocardium, and blood vessels. Arterial calcification may produce coronary artery disease. In children, renal osteodystrophy (renal rickets) may develop.

Diagnosis

Clinical assessment, a history of chronic progressive debilitation, and gradual deterioration of renal function as determined by creatinine clearance tests lead to a diagnosis of chronic renal failure.

The following laboratory findings also aid in diagnosis:
• *Blood studies* show elevated blood urea nitrogen, serum creatinine, and potassium levels; decreased arterial pH and bicarbonate; and low hemoglobin and hematocrit.
• *Urine specific gravity* becomes fixed at 1.010; urinalysis may show proteinuria, glycosuria, erythrocytes, leukocytes, and casts, depending on the etiology.
• *X-ray studies* include kidney-ureter-bladder films, excretory urography, nephrotomography, renal scan, and renal arteriography.
• *Kidney biopsy* allows histologic identification of underlying pathology.

Treatment

Conservative treatment aims to correct specific symptoms.

Diet

A low-protein diet reduces the production of end-products of protein metabolism that the kidneys can't excrete. (A patient receiving continuous peritoneal dialysis should receive a high-protein diet.)

A high-calorie diet prevents ketoacidosis and the negative nitrogen balance that results in catabolism and tissue atrophy. Such a diet also restricts sodium and potassium.

Fluid status

Maintaining fluid balance requires careful monitoring of vital signs, weight changes, and urine volume (if present). Loop diuretics such as furosemide (if some renal function remains) and fluid restriction can reduce fluid retention. Digitalis glycosides may be used to mobilize edema fluids; antihypertensives, to control blood pressure and associated edema.

Treatment for GI and blood problems

Antiemetics taken before meals may relieve nausea and vomiting; cimetidine or ranitidine may decrease gastric irritation. Methylcellulose or docusate can help prevent constipation.

Treatment may also include regular stool analysis (guaiac test) to detect occult blood and, as needed, cleansing enemas to remove blood from the GI tract.

Anemia necessitates iron and folate supplements; severe anemia requires infusion of fresh frozen packed cells or washed packed cells. However, transfusions relieve anemia only temporarily. Synthetic erythropoietin (epoetin alfa) may be given to stimulate the division and differentiation of cells within the bone marrow to produce RBCs. Androgen therapy (testosterone or nandrolone) may increase RBC production.

Drug therapy, surgery, and dialysis

Drug therapy often relieves associated symptoms: an antipruritic, such as trimeprazine or diphenhydramine, for itching and aluminum hydroxide gel to lower serum phosphate levels. The patient may also benefit from supplementary vitamins (particularly B vitamins and vitamin D) and essential amino acids.

Careful monitoring of serum potassium levels is necessary to detect hyperkalemia. Emergency treatment for severe hyperkalemia includes dialysis therapy and administration of 50% hypertonic glucose I.V., regular insulin, calcium gluconate I.V., sodium bicarbonate I.V., and cation exchange resins such as sodium polystyrene sulfonate. Cardiac tamponade resulting from pericardial effusion may require emergency pericardial tap or surgery.

Blood gas measurements may indicate acidosis; intensive dialysis and thoracentesis can relieve pulmonary edema and pleural effusions.

Hemodialysis or peritoneal dialysis (particularly continuous ambulatory peritoneal dialysis and continuous cyclic peritoneal dialysis) can help control most manifestations of endstage renal disease. (See *Continuous ambulatory peritoneal dialysis,* page 736.) Altering dialyzing bath fluids can correct fluid and electrolyte disturbances. But anemia, peripheral neuropathy, cardiopulmonary and GI complications, sexual dysfunction, and skeletal defects may persist.

Maintenance dialysis itself may produce complications, such as protein wasting, refractory ascites, and dialysis dementia. A kidney transplant may eventually be the treatment of choice for some patients with end-stage renal disease.

Special considerations

• Provide good skin care. Bathe the patient daily, using superfatted soaps, oatmeal baths, and skin lotion to ease pruritus. Give good perineal care, using mild soap and water. Pad the side rails to guard against ecchymoses. Turn the patient often, and use an egg-crate mattress to prevent skin breakdown.
• Provide good oral hygiene. Brush the patient's teeth often with a soft brush

or sponge tip to reduce breath odor. Hard candy and mouthwash minimize bad taste in the mouth and alleviate thirst.
• Offer small, palatable meals that are also nutritious; try to provide favorite foods within dietary restrictions. Encourage intake of high-calorie foods. Instruct the outpatient to avoid highsodium foods and high-potassium foods.
• Encourage adherence to fluid and protein restrictions. To prevent constipation, stress the need for exercise and sufficient dietary fiber.
• Watch for hyperkalemia. Observe for cramping of the legs and abdomen and diarrhea. As potassium levels rise, watch for muscle irritability and a weak pulse rate. Monitor the electrocardiogram for indications of hyperkalemia — tall, peaked T waves; widening QRS segment; prolonged PR interval; and disappearance of P waves.
• Assess hydration status carefully. Check for jugular vein distention, and auscultate the lungs for crackles. Measure daily intake and output carefully, including all drainage, vomitus, diarrhea, and blood loss. Record daily weight, presence or absence of thirst, axillary sweat, dryness of tongue, hypertension, and peripheral edema.
• Monitor for bone and joint complications. Prevent pathologic fractures by turning the patient carefully and ensuring his safety. Provide passive rangeof-motion exercises for the bedridden patient.
• Encourage deep breathing and coughing to prevent pulmonary congestion. Listen often for crackles, rhonchi, and decreased lung sounds. Be alert for clinical effects of pulmonary edema (dyspnea, restlessness, crackles). Administer diuretics and other medications as needed.
• Maintain strict aseptic technique. Use a micropore filter during I.V. therapy. Watch for signs of infection (listless-

CONTINUOUS AMBULATORY PERITONEAL DIALYSIS

Continuous ambulatory peritoneal dialysis is an increasingly useful alternative to hemodialysis in patients with renal failure. Using the peritoneum as a dialysis membrane, it allows almost uninterrupted exchange of dialysis solution.

With this method, four to six exchanges of fresh dialysis solution are infused each day. The approximate dwell-time for the daytime exchanges is 5 hours; for the overnight exchange, the dwell-time is 8 to 10 hours. After each dwell-time, the patient removes the dialyzing solution by gravity drainage.

This form of dialysis offers the unique advantages of a simple, easily taught procedure and allows the patient independence from a special treatment center.

In this procedure, a Tenckhoff catheter is surgically implanted in the abdomen, just below the umbilicus. A bag of dialysis solution is aseptically attached to the tube and the fluid allowed to flow into the peritoneal cavity. (This takes about 10 minutes.)

The fluid is then drained out of the peritoneal cavity through gravity flow by unrolling the bag and suspending it below the pelvis. (Drainage takes about 20 minutes.) After it drains, the patient aseptically connects a new bag of dialyzing solution and fills the peritoneal cavity again. He repeats this procedure four to six times a day.

The dialyzing fluid remains in the peritoneal cavity for about 4 to 6 hours. During this time, the bag may be rolled up and placed under a shirt or blouse, and the patient can go about normal activities while dialysis takes place.

ness, high fever, leukocytosis). Urge the outpatient to avoid contact with infected persons during the cold and flu season.

• Carefully observe and document seizure activity. Infuse sodium bicarbonate for acidosis and sedatives or anticonvulsants for seizures. Pad the side rails and keep an oral airway and suction setup at bedside. Assess neurologic status periodically, and check for Chvostek's and Trousseau's signs, indicators of low serum calcium levels.

• Observe for signs of bleeding. Watch for prolonged bleeding at puncture sites and at the vascular access site used for hemodialysis. Monitor hemoglobin and hematocrit, and check stools, urine, and vomitus for blood.

• Watch for signs of pericarditis, such as a pericardial friction rub and chest pain. Also, watch for the disappearance of friction rub, with a drop of 15 to 20 mm Hg in blood pressure during inspiration (paradoxical pulse) — an early sign of pericardial tamponade.

• Schedule medications carefully. Give iron before meals, aluminum hydroxide gels after meals, and antiemetics, as necessary, a half hour before meals. Administer antihypertensives at appropriate intervals.

• If the patient requires a rectal infusion of sodium polystyrene sulfonate for dangerously high potassium levels, apply an emollient to soothe the perianal area. Be sure the sodium polystyrene sulfonate enema is expelled; otherwise, it will cause constipation and won't lower potassium levels.

• Recommend antacid cookies as an alternative to aluminum hydroxide gels needed to bind GI phosphate.

If the patient requires dialysis:

• Prepare the patient by fully explaining the procedure. Be sure that he understands how to protect and care for the arteriovenous shunt, fistula, or other vascular access.

• Check the vascular access site every 2 hours for patency and the extremity for adequate blood supply and intact nervous function (temperature, pulse rate, capillary refill, and sensation).

• If a fistula is present, feel for a thrill and listen for a bruit. Use a gentle touch to avoid occluding the fistula. Note signs of possible clotting.

• Don't use the arm with the vascular access site to take blood pressure readings, draw blood, or give injections; these procedures may rupture the fistula or cause scarring that occludes blood flow.

• Withhold the 6 a.m. (or morning) dose of antihypertensive on the morning of dialysis, and instruct the outpatient to do the same.

• Check the patient's hepatitis antigen status. If it's positive, he is a carrier of hepatitis B, and stool, needle, blood, and excretion precautions should be instituted.

• Monitor hemoglobin and hematocrit. Assess the patient's tolerance of his levels; some individuals are more sensitive to lower levels than others. Instruct the anemic patient to conserve energy and to rest frequently.

• After dialysis, check for disequilibrium syndrome, a result of sudden correction of blood chemistry abnormalities. Symptoms range from a headache to seizures. Also, check for excessive bleeding from the dialysis site. Apply a pressure dressing or absorbable gelatin sponge, as indicated. Monitor blood pressure carefully after dialysis.

• A patient undergoing dialysis is under a great deal of stress, as is his family. Refer them to appropriate counseling agencies for assistance in coping with chronic renal failure.

SITES OF RENAL INFARCTION

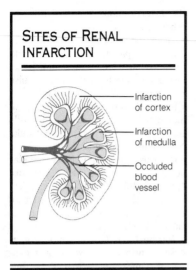

Infarction of cortex

Infarction of medulla

Occluded blood vessel

LIFE-THREATENING DISORDER

RENAL INFARCTION

Renal blood vessel occlusion results in renal infarction — the formation of a coagulated, necrotic area in one or both kidneys. The location and size of the infarction depend on the site of vascular occlusion. Most often, infarction affects the renal cortex, but it can extend into the medulla. (See *Sites of renal infarction.*) Residual renal function after infarction depends on the extent of the damage from the infarction.

Causes

In 75% of patients, renal infarction results from renal artery embolism secondary to mitral stenosis, infective endocarditis, atrial fibrillation, microthrombi in the left ventricle, rheumatic valvular disease, or recent myocardial infarction.

The embolism reduces the rate of blood flow to renal tissue and leads to ischemia. The rate and degree of blood flow reduction determine whether or not the insult will be acute or chronic as arterial narrowing progresses.

Less common causes of renal infarction are atherosclerosis, with or without thrombus formation; and thrombus from flank trauma, sickle-cell anemia, scleroderma, and arterionephrosclerosis.

Signs and symptoms

Although renal infarction may be asymptomatic, typical symptoms include severe upper abdominal pain or gnawing flank pain and tenderness, costovertebral tenderness, fever, anorexia, nausea, and vomiting. When arterial occlusion causes infarction, the affected kidney is small and not palpable.

Renovascular hypertension, a frequent complication that may occur several days after infarction, results from reduced blood flow, which stimulates the renin-angiotensin mechanism.

Diagnosis

A history of predisposing cardiovascular disease or other factors in a patient with typical clinical features strongly suggests renal infarction. A firm diagnosis requires the appropriate laboratory tests:

• *Urinalysis* reveals proteinuria and microscopic hematuria.

• *Urine enzyme levels,* especially lactate dehydrogenase (LD) and alkaline phosphatase, are often elevated as a result of tissue destruction.

• *Blood studies* may reveal elevated serum enzyme levels, especially aspartate aminotransferase, alkaline phosphatase, and LD. Blood studies may also reveal leukocytosis and an increased erythrocyte sedimentation rate.

• *Excretory urography* shows diminished or absent excretion of contrast dye, indicating vascular occlusion or urethral obstruction.

• *Isotopic renal scan,* a noninvasive technique, demonstrates absent or reduced blood flow to the kidneys.

• *Renal arteriography* provides absolute proof of an existing infarction but is used as a last resort, because it's a high-risk procedure.

Treatment

Infection in the infarcted area or significant hypertension may require surgical repair of the occlusion or nephrectomy. Surgery to establish collateral circulation to the area can relieve renovascular hypertension.

Persistent hypertension may respond to antihypertensives and a low-sodium diet. Additional treatments may include administration of intra-arterial streptokinase, lysis of blood clots, catheter embolectomy, and heparin therapy.

Special considerations

• Assess the degree of renal function and offer supportive care to maintain homeostasis.

• Monitor intake and output, vital signs (particularly blood pressure), electrolyte levels, and daily weight. Watch for signs of fluid overload, such as dyspnea, tachycardia, pulmonary edema, and electrolyte imbalances.

• Carefully explain all diagnostic procedures.

• Provide reassurance and emotional support for the patient and family.

• Encourage the patient to return for a follow-up examination, which usually includes excretory urography or a renal scan to assess regained renal function.

RENAL TUBULAR ACIDOSIS

A syndrome of persistent dehydration, hyperchloremia, hypokalemia, metabolic acidosis, and nephrocalcinosis, renal tubular acidosis (RTA) results from the kidneys' inability to conserve bicarbonate. This disorder occurs as distal RTA (Type I, or classic RTA) or proximal RTA (Type II). The prognosis is usually good but depends on the severity of renal damage that precedes treatment.

Causes

Metabolic acidosis usually results from renal excretion of bicarbonate. However, metabolic acidosis associated with RTA results from a defect in the kidneys' normal tubular acidification of urine.

Distal RTA

Type I RTA results from an inability of the distal tubule to secrete hydrogen ions against established gradients across the tubular membrane. This results in decreased excretion of titratable acids and ammonium, increased loss of potassium and bicarbonate in the urine, and systemic acidosis.

Prolonged acidosis causes mobilization of calcium from bone and eventually hypercalciuria, predisposing to the formation of renal calculi.

Distal RTA may be classified as primary or secondary:

• *Primary distal RTA* may occur sporadically or through a hereditary defect and is most prevalent in females, older children, adolescents, and young adults.

• *Secondary distal RTA* has been linked to many renal or systemic conditions, such as starvation, malnutrition, hepatic cirrhosis, and several genetically transmitted disorders.

Proximal RTA

Type II RTA results from defective reabsorption of bicarbonate in the proximal tubule. This causes bicarbonate to flood the distal tubule, which normally secretes hydrogen ions, and leads to impaired formation of titratable acids and ammonium for excretion. Ultimately, metabolic acidosis results.

Proximal RTA occurs in two forms:
• In *primary proximal RTA,* the reabsorptive defect is idiopathic and is the only disorder present.
• In *secondary proximal RTA,* the reabsorptive defect may be one of several defects and results from proximal tubular cell damage from a disease, such as Fanconi's syndrome.

Signs and symptoms

In infants, RTA produces anorexia, vomiting, occasional fever, polyuria, dehydration, growth retardation, apathy, weakness, tissue wasting, constipation, nephrocalcinosis, and rickets.

In children and adults, RTA may lead to urinary tract infection, rickets, and growth problems. Possible complications of RTA include nephrocalcinosis and pyelonephritis.

Diagnosis

Demonstration of impaired acidification of urine with systemic metabolic acidosis confirms distal RTA. Demonstration of bicarbonate wasting from impaired reabsorption confirms proximal RTA.

Other relevant laboratory results show:
• decreased serum bicarbonate, pH, potassium, and phosphorus levels

• increased serum chloride and alkaline phosphatase levels
• alkaline pH, with low titratable acids and ammonium content in urine; increased urinary bicarbonate and potassium levels, with low specific gravity.

In later stages, X-rays may show nephrocalcinosis.

Treatment

Supportive treatment for patients with RTA requires replacement of those substances being abnormally excreted, especially bicarbonate. It may include sodium bicarbonate tablets or Shohl's solution to control acidosis, oral potassium for dangerously low potassium levels, and vitamin D for bone disease. If pyelonephritis occurs, treatment may include antibiotics as well.

Treatment for renal calculi secondary to nephrocalcinosis varies and may include supportive therapy until the calculi pass or until surgery for severe obstruction is performed.

Special considerations

• Urge compliance with all medication instructions. Inform the patient and his family that the prognosis for RTA and bone lesion healing is directly related to the adequacy of treatment.
• Monitor laboratory values, especially potassium levels, for hypokalemia.
• Test urine for pH, and strain it for calculi.
• If rickets develops, explain the condition and its treatment to the patient and his family.
• Teach the patient how to recognize signs and symptoms of calculi (hematuria, low abdominal or flank pain). Advise him to immediately report any such signs and symptoms.
• Instruct the patient with low potassium levels to eat foods with a high potassium content, such as bananas and baked potatoes. Orange juice is also high in potassium.

• Because RTA may be caused by a genetic defect, encourage family members to seek genetic counseling or screening for this disorder.

RENAL VEIN THROMBOSIS

Clotting in the renal vein results in renal congestion, engorgement and, possibly, infarction. Renal vein thrombosis may affect both kidneys and may occur in an acute or chronic form.

Chronic thrombosis usually impairs renal function, causing nephrotic syndrome. Abrupt onset of thrombosis that causes extensive damage may precipitate rapidly fatal renal infarction.

If thrombosis affects both kidneys, the prognosis is poor. However, less severe thrombosis that affects only one kidney or gradual progression that allows development of collateral circulation may preserve partial renal function.

Causes

Renal vein thrombosis often results from a tumor that obstructs the renal vein (usually hypernephroma).

Other causes include thrombophlebitis of the inferior vena cava (may result from abdominal trauma) or blood vessels of the legs, congestive heart failure, and periarteritis. In infants, renal vein thrombosis usually follows diarrhea that causes severe dehydration.

Chronic renal vein thrombosis is often a complication of other glomerulopathic diseases, such as amyloidosis, systemic lupus erythematosus, diabetic nephropathy, and membranoproliferative glomerulonephritis.

Signs and symptoms

Clinical features of renal vein thrombosis vary with the speed of onset.

Rapid onset of venous obstruction produces severe lumbar pain and tenderness in the epigastric region and the costovertebral angle. Other characteristic features include fever, leukocytosis, pallor, hematuria, proteinuria, peripheral edema and, when the obstruction is bilateral, oliguria and other uremic signs. The kidneys enlarge and become easily palpable. Hypertension is unusual, but may develop.

Gradual onset causes symptoms of nephrotic syndrome. Peripheral edema is possible, but pain is generally absent. Other clinical signs include proteinuria, hypoalbuminemia, and hyperlipemia.

Infants with this disease have enlarged kidneys, oliguria, and renal insufficiency that may progress to acute or chronic renal failure.

Diagnosis

• *Excretory urography* provides reliable diagnostic evidence. In acute renal vein thrombosis, the kidneys appear enlarged and excretory function diminishes. The contrast medium seems to "smudge" necrotic renal tissue. In chronic thrombosis, this test may show ureteral indentations that result from collateral venous channels.
• *Renal arteriography* and *a biopsy* may confirm the diagnosis.
• *Urinalysis* reveals gross or microscopic hematuria, proteinuria (more than 2 g/day in chronic disease), casts, and oliguria.
• *Blood studies* show leukocytosis, hypoalbuminemia, and hyperlipidemia.
• *Venography* confirms thrombosis.
• *Magnetic resonance imaging* holds promise for diagnosis of thrombosis.

Treatment

Gradual thrombosis that affects only one kidney responds best to treatment. Anticoagulant therapy may prove helpful, especially if used long-term.

Surgery must be performed within 24 hours of thrombosis but even then has limited success, because thrombi often extend into the small veins. Extensive intrarenal bleeding may necessitate nephrectomy.

Patients who survive abrupt thrombosis with extensive renal damage develop nephrotic syndrome and require treatment for renal failure, such as dialysis and possible transplantation. Some infants with renal vein thrombosis recover completely after heparin therapy or surgery; others suffer irreversible kidney damage.

Special considerations

• Assess renal function regularly. Monitor vital signs, intake and output, daily weight, and electrolytes.

• Administer diuretics for edema, and enforce dietary restrictions, such as limited sodium and potassium intake.

• Monitor closely for signs of pulmonary emboli (chest pain, dyspnea).

• If heparin is given by constant I.V. infusion, frequently monitor partial thromboplastin time to determine the patient's response to it. Dilute the drug; administer it by infusion pump or controller so the patient receives the least amount necessary.

• During anticoagulant therapy, watch for signs of bleeding, such as tachycardia, hypotension, hematuria, bleeding from the nose or gums, ecchymoses, petechiae, and black, tarry stools.

• Instruct the patient on maintenance warfarin therapy to use an electric razor and a soft toothbrush and to avoid trauma. Suggest that he wear a medical identification bracelet, and tell him to avoid aspirin, which aggravates bleeding tendencies. Stress the need for close medical follow-up.

RENOVASCULAR HYPERTENSION

The rise in systemic blood pressure observed in renovascular hypertension results from stenosis of the major renal arteries or their branches or from intrarenal atherosclerosis. This narrowing or sclerosis may be partial or complete, and the resulting blood pressure elevation may be benign or malignant.

Approximately 5% to 10% of patients with high blood pressure display renovascular hypertension; it's most common in people under age 30 or over age 50.

Causes

Atherosclerosis (especially in older men) and fibromuscular diseases of the renal artery wall layers—such as medial fibroplasia and, less commonly, intimal and subadventitial fibroplasia—are the primary causes in 95% of all patients with renovascular hypertension. Other causes include arteritis, anomalies of the renal arteries, an embolism, trauma, a tumor, and a dissecting aneurysm.

Stenosis or occlusion of the renal artery stimulates the affected kidney to release the enzyme renin, which converts angiotensinogen—a plasma protein—to angiotensin I.

As angiotensin I circulates through the lungs and liver, it converts to angiotensin II. This causes peripheral vasoconstriction, increased arterial pressure and aldosterone secretion, and eventual hypertension.

Signs and symptoms

In addition to elevated systemic blood pressure, renovascular hypertension usually produces symptoms common to hypertensive states, such as headache, palpitations, tachycardia, anxiety, light-headedness, decreased tolerance of temperature extremes, retinopathy, and mental sluggishness.

Significant complications include congestive heart failure, myocardial infarction, cerebrovascular accident and, occasionally, renal failure.

Diagnosis

In addition to thorough patient and family histories, diagnosis requires an isotopic renal blood flow scan and rapid-sequence excretory urography to identify abnormalities of renal blood flow and discrepancies of kidney size and shape.

Renal arteriography reveals the actual arterial stenosis or obstruction; samples from both the right and left renal veins are obtained for comparison of plasma renin levels with those in the inferior vena cava. An increased renin level implicates the affected kidney and determines whether surgical correction can reverse hypertension.

Treatment

Surgery, the treatment of choice, is performed to restore adequate circulation and to control severe hypertension or severely impaired renal function by renal artery bypass, endarterectomy, arterioplasty or, as a last resort, nephrectomy.

Renal artery dilation by balloon catheter is used in selected cases to correct renal artery stenosis without the risks and morbidity of surgery. Symptomatic measures include antihypertensives, diuretics, and a sodium-restricted diet.

Special considerations

• Help the patient and family understand renovascular hypertension, and stress the importance of following prescribed treatment.

• Accurately monitor intake and output and daily weight.

• Check blood pressure in both arms regularly, with the patient lying down and standing. A drop of 20 mm Hg or more on arising may necessitate an adjustment in antihypertensive medications. Assess renal function daily.

• Administer drugs as needed. Maintain fluid and sodium restrictions. Explain the purpose of a low-sodium diet.

• Explain diagnostic tests, and prepare the patient appropriately; for example, adequately hydrate the patient before tests that use contrast media. Make sure the patient is not allergic to the dye used in diagnostic tests. After excretory urography or arteriography, watch for complications.

• If a nephrectomy is necessary, reassure the patient that the remaining kidney is adequate for renal function.

• Postoperatively, watch for bleeding and hypotension. If the sutures around the renal vessels slip, the patient can quickly go into shock, because kidneys receive 25% of cardiac output.

• Provide a quiet, stress-free environment, if possible. Urge the patient and family members to have regular blood pressure screenings.

LIFE-THREATENING DISORDER

RESPIRATORY ACIDOSIS

An acid-base disturbance characterized by reduced alveolar ventilation and manifested by hypercapnia (partial pressure of arterial carbon dioxide

[PaCO$_2$] greater than 45 mm Hg), respiratory acidosis can be acute (from a sudden failure in ventilation) or chronic (as in long-term pulmonary disease). The prognosis depends on the severity of the underlying disturbance, as well as the patient's general clinical condition.

Causes

Several factors predispose the patient to respiratory acidosis:

• *Drugs:* Narcotics, anesthetics, hypnotics, and sedatives decrease the sensitivity of the respiratory center.

• *Central nervous system (CNS) trauma:* Medullary injury may impair ventilatory drive.

• *Chronic metabolic alkalosis:* Respiratory compensatory mechanisms attempt to normalize pH by decreasing alveolar ventilation.

• *Neuromuscular disease* (such as myasthenia gravis, Guillain-Barré syndrome, and poliomyelitis): Failure of respiratory muscles to respond properly to respiratory drive reduces alveolar ventilation.

In addition, respiratory acidosis can result from airway obstruction or parenchymal lung disease, which interferes with alveolar ventilation, or from chronic obstructive pulmonary disease (COPD), asthma, severe adult respiratory distress syndrome, chronic bronchitis, large pneumothorax, extensive pneumonia, or pulmonary edema.

Hypoventilation compromises excretion of carbon dioxide produced through metabolism. The retained carbon dioxide then combines with water to form an excess of carbonic acid, decreasing the blood pH. As a result, the concentration of hydrogen ions in body fluids, which directly reflects acidity, increases.

Signs and symptoms

Acute respiratory acidosis produces CNS disturbances that reflect changes in the pH of cerebrospinal fluid rather than increased carbon dioxide levels in cerebral circulation.

Effects range from restlessness, confusion, and apprehension to somnolence, with a fine or flapping tremor (asterixis), or coma. The patient may complain of headaches and exhibit dyspnea and tachypnea with papilledema and depressed reflexes. Unless the patient is receiving oxygen, hypoxemia accompanies respiratory acidosis.

This disorder may also cause cardiovascular abnormalities, such as tachycardia, hypertension, atrial and ventricular arrhythmias and, in severe acidosis, hypotension with vasodilation (bounding pulses and warm periphery).

Diagnosis

The following arterial blood gas (ABG) levels confirm respiratory acidosis: a PaCO$_2$ exceeding the normal level of 45 mm Hg, pH usually below the normal range of 7.35 to 7.45, and a bicarbonate level that's normal in the acute stage but elevated in the chronic stage.

Treatment

Effective treatment of respiratory acidosis is designed to correct the underlying source of alveolar hypoventilation. Significantly reduced alveolar ventilation may require mechanical ventilation until the underlying condition can be treated.

In COPD, treatment includes bronchodilators, oxygen, corticosteroids and, frequently, antibiotics; drug therapy for conditions such as myasthenia gravis; removal of foreign bodies from the airway; antibiotics for pneumonia; dialysis or charcoal to remove toxic drugs; and correction of metabolic al-

---

HAZARD

 RESPIRATORY ACIDOSIS: WATCH FOR LOW pH

Be alert for dangerously low blood pH levels in a patient with respiratory acidosis. If the level drops below 7.15, profound central nervous system and cardiovascular deterioration may result, requiring administration of I.V. sodium bicarbonate.

---

kalosis. An elevated $PaCO_2$ may persist in a patient with COPD despite optimal treatment.

Special considerations
• Closely monitor the patient's blood pH level. (See *Respiratory acidosis: Watch for low pH.*)
• Be alert for critical changes in the patient's respiratory, CNS, and cardiovascular functions. Also watch closely for variations in ABG values and electrolyte status. Maintain adequate hydration.
• If acidosis requires mechanical ventilation, maintain a patent airway and provide adequate humidification. Perform tracheal suctioning regularly and vigorous chest physiotherapy if needed. Continuously monitor ventilator settings and respiratory status.
• To prevent respiratory acidosis, closely monitor patients with COPD and chronic carbon dioxide retention for signs of acidosis. Also, administer oxygen at low flow rates and closely monitor all patients who receive narcotics and sedatives.
• Instruct the patient who has received a general anesthetic to turn, cough, and perform deep-breathing exercises frequently to prevent the onset of respiratory acidosis.

LIFE-THREATENING DISORDER

RESPIRATORY ALKALOSIS

Caused by alveolar hyperventilation, respiratory alkalosis is a condition marked by a decrease in partial pressure of arterial carbon dioxide ($PaCO_2$) to below 35 mm Hg. Uncomplicated respiratory alkalosis leads to a decrease in hydrogen ion concentration, which causes elevated blood pH. Hypocapnia occurs when the elimination of carbon dioxide by the lungs exceeds the production of carbon dioxide at the cellular level.

Causes
Respiratory alkalosis can result from pulmonary or nonpulmonary causes:
• *Pulmonary* causes include pneumonia, interstitial lung disease, pulmonary vascular disease, and acute asthma.
• *Nonpulmonary* causes include anxiety, fever, aspirin toxicity, metabolic acidosis, central nervous system (CNS) disease (inflammation or tumor), sepsis, hepatic failure, and pregnancy.

Signs and symptoms

The cardinal sign of respiratory alkalosis is deep, rapid breathing, possibly exceeding 40 breaths/minute and much like the Kussmaul's respirations that characterize diabetic acidosis.

Such hyperventilation usually leads to CNS and neuromuscular disturbances, such as light-headedness or dizziness (from below-normal carbon dioxide levels that decrease cerebral blood flow), agitation, circumoral and peripheral paresthesias, carpopedal spasms, twitching (possibly progressing to tetany), and muscle weakness. Severe respiratory alkalosis may cause cardiac arrhythmias that fail to respond to conventional treatment, seizures, or both.

Diagnosis

Arterial blood gas (ABG) analysis confirms respiratory alkalosis and rules out respiratory compensation for metabolic acidosis. Findings include a $PaCO_2$ below 35 mm Hg, a pH that's elevated in proportion to the fall in $PaCO_2$ in the acute stage but that drops toward normal in the chronic stage, and a bicarbonate level that's normal in the acute stage but below normal in the chronic stage.

Treatment

The goal of treatment is to eradicate the underlying condition—for example, removal of ingested toxins, treatment of fever or sepsis, and treatment of CNS disease. In severe respiratory alkalosis, the patient may be instructed to breathe into a paper bag, which helps relieve acute anxiety and increases carbon dioxide levels.

Prevention of hyperventilation in patients receiving mechanical ventilation requires monitoring ABG values and adjusting dead space or minute ventilation volume.

Special considerations

• Watch for and report any changes in neurologic, neuromuscular, or cardiovascular functions.
• Remember that twitching and cardiac arrhythmias may be associated with alkalemia and electrolyte imbalances. Monitor ABG and serum electrolyte levels closely, watching for any variations.
• Explain all diagnostic tests and procedures to reduce anxiety.

LIFE-THREATENING DISORDER

RESPIRATORY DISTRESS SYNDROME

Also called hyaline membrane disease, respiratory distress syndrome (RDS) is the most common cause of neonatal mortality. In the United States alone, it causes the death of 40,000 neonates every year. If untreated, RDS is fatal within 72 hours of birth in up to 14% of neonates weighing less than 2,500 g (5½ lb).

RDS occurs almost exclusively in infants born before the 37th week of gestation (in 60% of those born before the 28th week). It occurs more often in infants of diabetic mothers, those delivered by cesarean section, and those delivered suddenly after antepartum hemorrhage.

Aggressive management using mechanical ventilation can improve the prognosis, but a few infants who survive have bronchopulmonary dysplasia. Mild RDS slowly subsides after 3 days.

Causes

Although the airways and alveoli of an infant's respiratory system are present by the 27th week of gestation, the intercostal muscles are weak and the alveoli and capillary blood supply are immature. In RDS, the premature infant develops widespread alveolar collapse because of lack of surfactant, a lipoprotein present in alveoli and respiratory bronchioles.

Surfactant normally lowers surface tension and aids in maintaining alveolar patency, preventing collapse, particularly at end expiration. But a deficiency results in widespread atelectasis, which leads to inadequate alveolar ventilation with shunting of blood through collapsed areas of lung, causing hypoxia and acidosis.

Signs and symptoms

Although a neonate with RDS may breathe normally at first, he usually develops rapid, shallow respirations within minutes or hours of birth, with intercostal, subcostal, or sternal retractions; nasal flaring; and audible expiratory grunting. This grunting is a natural compensatory mechanism designed to produce positive end-expiratory pressure (PEEP) and prevent further alveolar collapse.

The infant may also display hypotension, peripheral edema, and oliguria; in severe disease, apnea, bradycardia, and cyanosis (from hypoxemia, left-to-right shunting through the foramen ovale, or right-to-left shunting through atelectatic regions of the lung). Other clinical features include pallor, frothy sputum, and low body temperature as a result of an immature nervous system and the absence of subcutaneous fat.

Diagnosis

Although signs of respiratory distress in a premature infant during the first few hours of life strongly suggest RDS, the following tests are necessary to confirm the diagnosis:
• *Chest X-ray* may be normal for the first 6 to 12 hours (in 50% of neonates with RDS) but later shows a fine reticulonodular pattern.
• *ABG analysis* shows decreased partial pressure of arterial oxygen (PaO_2); normal, decreased, or increased partial pressure of arterial carbon dioxide ($PaCO_2$); and decreased pH (from respiratory or metabolic acidosis or both).
• *Chest auscultation* reveals normal or diminished air entry and crackles (rare in early stages).

When a cesarean section is necessary before the 36th week of gestation, amniocentesis allows determination of the lecithin/sphingomyelin (L/S) ratio, which helps to assess prenatal lung development and the risk of RDS.

Treatment

An infant with RDS requires vigorous respiratory support. Warm, humidified, oxygen-enriched gases are administered by oxygen hood or, if such treatment fails, by mechanical ventilation. Severe cases may require mechanical ventilation with PEEP or continuous positive airway pressure (CPAP), administered by a tightly fitting face mask or, when necessary, endotracheal (ET) intubation.

Treatment also includes:
• a radiant infant warmer or isolette for thermoregulation
• I.V. fluids and sodium bicarbonate to control acidosis and maintain fluid and electrolyte balance
• tube feedings or total parenteral nutrition if the infant is too weak to eat
• administration of surfactant by an ET tube.

Special considerations

• Closely monitor ABG levels as well as fluid intake and output. If the infant has an umbilical catheter (arterial or venous), check for arterial hypotension or abnormal central venous pressure.

• Watch for such complications as infection, thrombosis, or decreased circulation to the legs.

• If the infant has a transcutaneous PaO$_2$ monitor (an accurate method for determining PaO$_2$), change the site of the lead placement every 2 to 4 hours to avoid burning the skin.

• Weigh the infant once or twice daily. To evaluate his progress, assess skin color, rate and depth of respirations, severity of retractions, nostril flaring, frequency of expiratory grunting, frothing at the lips, and restlessness.

• Regularly assess the effectiveness of oxygen or ventilator therapy. Evaluate every change in the fraction of inspired oxygen and PEEP or CPAP by monitoring oxygen saturation or ABG levels. Be sure to adjust PEEP or CPAP as indicated, based on findings.

• When the infant is on mechanical ventilation, watch carefully for signs of barotrauma (an increase in respiratory distress, subcutaneous emphysema) and accidental disconnection from the ventilator. Check ventilator settings frequently.

Be alert for signs of complications of PEEP or CPAP therapy, such as decreased cardiac output, pneumothorax, and pneumomediastinum. Mechanical ventilation increases the risk of infection in premature infants, so preventive measures are essential.

• As needed, arrange for follow-up care with a neonatal ophthalmologist to check for retinal damage.

• Teach the parents about their infant's condition and, if possible, let them participate in his care (using aseptic technique), to encourage normal parent-infant bonding. Advise parents that full recovery may take up to 12 months. When the prognosis is poor, prepare the parents for the infant's impending death, and offer emotional support.

• Help reduce mortality in RDS by detecting respiratory distress early. Recognize intercostal retractions and grunting, especially in a premature infant, as signs of RDS, and make sure the infant receives immediate treatment.

RESPIRATORY SYNCYTIAL VIRUS INFECTION

A subgroup of the myxoviruses resembling paramyxovirus causes respiratory syncytial virus (RSV) infection. RSV is the leading cause of lower respiratory tract infections in infants and young children; it's the major cause of pneumonia, tracheobronchitis, and bronchiolitis in this age-group and a suspected cause of the fatal respiratory diseases of infancy.

Causes and incidence
Antibody titers seem to indicate that few children under age 4 escape contracting some form of RSV, even if it's mild. In fact, RSV is the only viral disease that has its maximum impact during the first few months of life (incidence of RSV bronchiolitis peaks at age 2 months).

This virus creates annual epidemics that occur during the late winter and early spring in temperate climates and during the rainy season in the tropics. The organism is transmitted from person to person by respiratory secretions and has an incubation period of 4 to 5 days.

Reinfection is common, producing milder symptoms than the primary infection. School-age children, adolescents, and young adults with mild reinfections are probably the source of infection for infants and young children.

Signs and symptoms

Clinical features of RSV infection vary in severity, ranging from mild coldlike symptoms to bronchiolitis or bronchopneumonia and, in a few patients, severe, life-threatening lower respiratory tract infections. Generally, symptoms include coughing, wheezing, malaise, pharyngitis, dyspnea, and inflamed mucous membranes in the nose and throat.

Otitis media is a common complication of RSV in infants. RSV has also been identified in patients with a variety of central nervous system disorders, such as meningitis and myelitis.

Diagnosis

The following clinical findings and epidemiologic information aid in the diagnosis:
• Cultures of nasal and pharyngeal secretions may show RSV; however, the virus is very labile, so cultures aren't always reliable.
• Serum antibody titers may be elevated, but before 6 months of age, maternal antibodies may impair test results.
• Two serologic techniques that aid in diagnosis are the indirect immunofluorescence and the enzyme-linked immunosorbent assay (ELISA) methods.
• Chest X-rays help detect pneumonia.

Treatment

Among the goals of treatment are support of respiratory function, maintenance of fluid balance, and relief of symptoms.

Special considerations

• Monitor respiratory status. Observe the rate and pattern; watch for nasal flaring or retraction, cyanosis, pallor, and dyspnea; and auscultate for wheezing, rhonchi, or other signs of respiratory distress. Monitor arterial blood gas values.

• Maintain a patent airway, and be especially watchful when the patient has periods of acute dyspnea. Perform percussion and provide drainage and suction, when necessary. Use a croup tent to provide a high-humidity atmosphere. Semi-Fowler's position may help prevent aspiration of secretions.
• Monitor intake and output carefully. Observe for signs of dehydration, such as decreased skin turgor. Encourage the patient to drink plenty of high-calorie fluids. Administer I.V. fluids as needed.
• Promote bed rest, allowing for as much uninterrupted rest as possible.
• Hold and cuddle infants; talk to and play with toddlers. Offer diversional activities suitable to the child's condition and age. Foster parental visits and cuddling. Restrain a child only as necessary.
• Impose oral secretion precautions. Enforce strict handwashing, because RSV may be transmitted from fomites.
• Staff members with respiratory illnesses shouldn't care for infants.

RETINAL DETACHMENT

When the layers of the retina become separated, creating a subretinal space, retinal detachment occurs. This space then fills with fluid, called subretinal fluid. Retinal detachment usually involves only one eye, but may involve the other eye later.

Surgical reattachment is often successful. However, the prognosis for good vision depends on the area of the retina that's been affected.

Causes

Any retinal tear or hole allows the liquid vitreous to seep between the retinal layers, separating the retina from its choroidal blood supply. In adults, retinal detachment usually results from degenerative changes of aging, which cause a spontaneous retinal hole.

Predisposing factors include myopia, cataract surgery, and trauma. Perhaps the influence of trauma explains why retinal detachment is twice as common in males.

Retinal detachment may also result from seepage of fluid into the subretinal space (because of inflammation, tumors, or systemic diseases) or from traction that's placed on the retina by vitreous bands or membranes (from proliferative diabetic retinopathy, posterior uveitis, or a traumatic intraocular foreign body).

Retinal detachment is rare in children, but occasionally can develop as a result of retinopathy of prematurity, tumors (retinoblastomas), or trauma. It can also be inherited, usually in association with myopia.

Signs and symptoms

Initially, the patient may complain of floating spots and recurrent flashes of light. But as detachment progresses, gradual, painless vision loss may be described as a veil, curtain, or cobweb that eliminates a portion of the visual field.

Diagnosis

Ophthalmoscopy after full pupil dilation allows diagnosis. Examination shows the usually transparent retina as gray and opaque; in severe detachment, it reveals folds in the retina and a ballooning out of the area. Indirect ophthalmoscopy is used to search for retinal tears. Ultrasonography is performed if the lens is opaque.

Treatment

Depending on the location and severity of the detachment, treatment may include restriction of eye movements and complete bed rest to prevent further detachment.

A hole in the peripheral retina can be treated with cryothermy; in the posterior portion, with laser therapy. Retinal detachment usually requires scleral buckling to reattach the retina and, possibly, replacement of the vitreous with silicone, oil, air, or gas.

Special considerations

• Provide emotional support; the patient may be distraught because of his loss of vision.

• To prepare for surgery, wash the patient's face with no-tears shampoo. Administer antibiotics and cycloplegic-mydriatic eyedrops.

• Postoperatively, instruct the patient to lie on his back or on his unoperated side. Discourage straining during defecation, bending down, and hard coughing, sneezing, or vomiting, which can raise intraocular pressure. Antiemetics may be indicated. Discourage activities that may cause bumping the eye.

• Observe for slight localized corneal edema and perilimbal congestion, which may follow laser treatment. To reduce edema and discomfort, apply ice packs as needed. Administer acetaminophen for headache.

• After removing the protective patch, gently clean the eye with cycloplegic eyedrops and steroid-antibiotic eyedrops. Use cold compresses to decrease swelling and pain.

• Administer analgesics as needed, noting persistent pain. Teach the patient how to properly instill eyedrops, and emphasize compliance and follow-up care. Suggest dark glasses to compensate for sensitivity to light.

REYE'S SYNDROME

An acute childhood illness, Reye's syndrome causes fatty infiltration of the liver with concurrent hyperammonemia, encephalopathy, and increased intracranial pressure (ICP). In addition, fatty infiltration of the kidneys, brain, and myocardium may occur.

Reye's syndrome affects children from infancy to adolescence and occurs equally in boys and girls. It affects whites over age 1 more often than blacks.

The prognosis depends on the severity of central nervous system depression. Previously, mortality was as high as 90%. Today, ICP monitoring and, consequently, early treatment of increased ICP, along with other treatment measures, have cut mortality to about 20%. Death is usually a result of cerebral edema or respiratory arrest. Comatose patients who survive may have residual brain damage.

Causes

Reye's syndrome almost always follows within 1 to 3 days of an acute viral infection, such as an upper respiratory infection, type B influenza, or varicella (chickenpox). Incidence often rises during influenza outbreaks and may be linked to aspirin use.

In Reye's syndrome, damaged hepatic mitochondria disrupt the urea cycle, which normally changes ammonia to urea for its excretion from the body. This results in hyperammonemia, hypoglycemia, and an increase in serum short-chain fatty acids, leading to encephalopathy. Simultaneously, fatty infiltration is found in renal tubular cells, neuronal tissue, and muscle tissue, including the heart.

Signs and symptoms

The severity of the child's signs and symptoms varies with the degree of encephalopathy and cerebral edema. In any case, Reye's syndrome develops in five stages.

After the initial viral infection, a brief recovery period follows when the child doesn't seem seriously ill. A few days later, he develops intractable vomiting, lethargy, rapidly changing mental status (mild to severe agitation, confusion, irritability, delirium), hyperactive reflexes, and rising blood pressure, respiratory rate, and pulse rate.

Reye's syndrome often progresses to coma. As the coma deepens, seizures develop, followed by decreased tendon reflexes and, frequently, respiratory failure.

Increased ICP, a serious complication, results from cerebral edema. Such edema may develop as a result of acidosis, increased cerebral metabolic rate, and an impaired autoregulatory mechanism.

Diagnosis

A history of a recent viral disorder with typical clinical features strongly suggests Reye's syndrome. An increased serum ammonia level, abnormal clotting studies, and hepatic dysfunction confirm it.

Testing the serum salicylate level rules out aspirin overdose. Absence of jaundice, despite increased liver transaminase levels, rules out acute hepatic failure and hepatic encephalopathy.

Abnormal test results may include the following:
• *Liver function studies* show aspartate aminotransferase and alanine aminotransferase elevated to twice normal levels; bilirubin is usually normal.
• *Liver biopsy* reveals fatty droplets uniformly distributed throughout cells.
• *Cerebrospinal fluid (CSF) analysis* reveals a white blood cell count of less

STAGES OF TREATMENT FOR REYE'S SYNDROME

SIGNS AND SYMPTOMS	BASELINE TREATMENT	BASELINE INTERVENTION
Stage I Vomiting, lethargy, hepatic dysfunction	• To decrease intracranial pressure (ICP) and brain edema, give I.V. fluids at two-thirds of the maintenance dose. Also give an osmotic diuretic or furosemide. • To treat hypoprothrombinemia, give vitamin K; if vitamin K is unsuccessful, give fresh frozen plasma. • Monitor serum ammonia and blood glucose levels and plasma osmolality every 4 to 8 hours to check progress.	• Monitor vital signs and check level of consciousness for increasing lethargy. Take vital signs more often as the patient's condition deteriorates. • Monitor fluid intake and output to prevent fluid overload. Maintain urine output at 1 ml/kg/hour, plasma osmolality at 290 mOsm, and blood glucose, at 150 mg/dl. (*Goal:* Keep glucose levels high, osmolality normal to high, and ammonia levels low.) Also restrict protein.
Stage II Hyperventilation, delirium, hepatic dysfunction, hyperactive reflexes	• Continue baseline treatment.	• Maintain seizure precautions. • Watch closely for any signs of coma that require invasive or supportive therapy such as intubation. • Keep head of bed at a 30-degree angle.
Stage III Coma, hyperventilation, decorticate rigidity, hepatic dysfunction	• Continue baseline and seizure treatment. • Monitor ICP with a subarachnoid screw or other invasive device. • Provide endotracheal intubation and mechanical ventilation to control partial pressure of carbon dioxide (PCO_2). A paralyzing agent, such as pancuronium I.V., may help maintain ventilation. • Give mannitol I.V. or glycerol by nasogastric tube.	• Monitor ICP (should be <20 mm Hg before suctioning) or give a barbiturate I.V. as needed; hyperventilate the patient as necessary. • When ventilating the patient, maintain PCO_2 between 25 and 30 mm Hg and PO_2 between 80 and 100 mm Hg. • Closely monitor cardiovascular status with a pulmonary artery catheter or central venous pressure line. • Give good skin and mouth care and perform range-of-motion exercises.
Stage IV Deepening coma; decerebrate rigidity; large, fixed pupils; minimal hepatic dysfunction	• Continue baseline and supportive care. • If all previous measures fail, some pediatric centers use barbiturate coma, decompressive craniotomy, hypothermia, or an exchange transfusion.	• Check patient for loss of reflexes and signs of flaccidity. • Give the family the extra support they need, considering their child's poor prognosis.

SIGNS AND SYMPTOMS	BASELINE TREATMENT	BASELINE INTERVENTION
Stage V Seizures, loss of deep tendon reflexes, flaccidity, respiratory arrest, ammonia level above 300 mg/dl	• Continue baseline and supportive care.	• Help the family to face the patient's impending death.

---

than 10/μl; with coma, CSF pressure increases.

• *Coagulation studies* result in prolonged prothrombin and partial thromboplastin times.

• *Blood values* show elevated serum ammonia levels; normal or, in 15% of cases, low serum glucose levels; and increased serum fatty acid and lactate levels.

Treatment and special considerations

The stage of the syndrome dictates the type of treatment necessary. (See *Stages of treatment for Reye's syndrome.*)

Advise parents to give nonsalicylate analgesics and antipyretics such as acetaminophen. Refer parents to the National Reye's Syndrome Foundation for more information.

RHEUMATIC FEVER AND RHEUMATIC HEART DISEASE

Often recurrent, acute rheumatic fever is a systemic inflammatory disease of childhood that follows a group A beta-hemolytic streptococcal infection. Rheumatic heart disease refers to the cardiac manifestations of rheumatic fever, and includes pancarditis (myocarditis, pericarditis, and endocarditis) during the early acute phase and chronic valvular disease later.

Long-term antibiotic therapy can minimize recurrence of rheumatic fever, reducing the risk of permanent cardiac damage and eventual valvular deformity. However, severe pancarditis occasionally produces fatal heart failure during the acute phase. Of the patients who survive this complication, about 20% die within 10 years.

Causes

Rheumatic fever appears to be a hypersensitivity reaction to a group A beta-hemolytic streptococcal infection, in which antibodies manufactured to combat streptococci react and produce characteristic lesions at specific tissue sites, especially in the heart and joints. Because very few people (about 0.3%) with streptococcal infections ever contract rheumatic fever, altered host resistance must be involved in its development or recurrence.

Although rheumatic fever tends to run in families, this may merely reflect contributing environmental factors. For example, in lower socioeconomic groups, incidence is highest in children between ages 5 and 15, probably as a result of malnutrition and crowded living conditions.

This disease strikes most often during cool, damp weather in the winter and early spring. In the United States, it's most common in the northern states.

Signs and symptoms
In 95% of patients, rheumatic fever characteristically follows a streptococcal infection that appeared a few days to 6 weeks earlier. A temperature of at least 100.4° F (38° C) occurs.

Joint pain
Most patients complain of migratory joint pain or polyarthritis. Swelling, redness, and signs of effusion usually accompany such pain, which most commonly affects the knees, ankles, elbows, or hips.

Skin lesions and nodules
In 5% of patients (generally those with carditis), rheumatic fever causes skin lesions such as erythema marginatum. This nonpruritic, macular, transient rash gives rise to red lesions with blanched centers.

Rheumatic fever may also produce firm, movable, nontender, subcutaneous nodules about 3 mm to 2 cm in diameter, usually near tendons or bony prominences of joints (especially the elbows, knuckles, wrists, and knees) and less often on the scalp and backs of the hands. These nodules persist for a few days to several weeks and, like erythema marginatum, often accompany carditis.

Chorea
Later, rheumatic fever may cause transient chorea, which develops up to 6 months after the original streptococcal infection.

Mild chorea may produce hyperirritability, a deterioration in handwriting, or inability to concentrate. Severe chorea causes purposeless, nonrepetitive, involuntary muscle spasms; poor muscle coordination; and weakness. Chorea always resolves without residual neurologic damage.

Carditis
The most destructive effect of rheumatic fever is carditis, which develops in up to 50% of patients. It may affect the endocardium, myocardium, pericardium, or the heart valves.

Pericarditis causes a pericardial friction rub and, occasionally, pain and effusion. Myocarditis produces characteristic lesions called Aschoff's bodies (in the acute stages) and cellular swelling and fragmentation of interstitial collagen, leading to formation of a progressively fibrotic nodule and interstitial scars.

Endocarditis causes valve leaflet swelling, erosion along the lines of leaflet closure, and blood, platelet, and fibrin deposits, which form beadlike vegetations. Endocarditis affects the mitral valve most often in females; the aortic valve most often in males. In both sexes, endocarditis affects the tricuspid valves occasionally and the pulmonic valve only rarely.

Severe rheumatic carditis may cause heart failure with dyspnea, upper right quadrant pain, tachycardia, tachypnea, significant mitral and aortic murmurs, and a hacking, nonproductive cough.

The most common of such murmurs include:
- a systolic murmur of mitral insufficiency (high-pitched, blowing, holosystolic, loudest at apex, possibly radiating to the anterior axillary line)
- a midsystolic murmur caused by stiffening and swelling of the mitral leaflet
- occasionally, a diastolic murmur of aortic insufficiency (low-pitched, rum-

bling, almost inaudible). Valvular disease may eventually result in chronic valvular stenosis and insufficiency, including mitral stenosis and insufficiency and aortic insufficiency. In children, mitral insufficiency remains the major sequela of rheumatic heart disease.

Diagnosis

Recognition of one or more of the classic symptoms (carditis, polyarthritis, chorea, erythema marginatum, or subcutaneous nodules) and a detailed patient history allow diagnosis. The following laboratory data support the diagnosis:

• *White blood cell count* and *erythrocyte sedimentation rate* may be elevated (during the acute phase); blood studies show slight anemia from suppressed erythropoiesis during inflammation.

• *C-reactive protein* is positive (especially during the acute phase).

• *Cardiac enzyme levels* may be increased in severe carditis.

• *Antistreptolysin O titer* is elevated in 95% of patients within 2 months of onset.

• *Electrocardiography* changes aren't diagnostic, but the PR interval is prolonged in 20% of patients.

• *Chest X-rays* show normal heart size (except with myocarditis, heart failure, or pericardial effusion).

• *Echocardiography* helps evaluate valvular damage, chamber size, and ventricular function.

• *Cardiac catheterization* evaluates valvular damage and left ventricular function in severe cardiac dysfunction.

Treatment

Effective management eradicates the streptococcal infection, relieves symptoms, and prevents recurrence, reducing the chance of permanent cardiac damage.

Treatment in acute phase

During the acute phase, treatment includes penicillin or (for patients with penicillin hypersensitivity) erythromycin. Salicylates such as aspirin relieve fever and minimize joint swelling and pain; if carditis is present or salicylates fail to relieve pain and inflammation, corticosteroids may be used.

Supportive treatment requires strict bed rest for about 5 weeks during the acute phase with active carditis, followed by a progressive increase in physical activity, depending on clinical and laboratory findings and the response to treatment.

Preventive treatment

After the acute phase subsides, a monthly I.M. injection of penicillin G benzathine or daily doses of oral sulfadiazine or penicillin G may be used to prevent recurrence. Such preventive treatment usually continues for 5 to 10 years.

Surgery and other measures

Heart failure necessitates continued bed rest and diuretics. Severe mitral or aortic valvular dysfunction causing persistent heart failure requires corrective valvular surgery, including commissurotomy (separation of the adherent, thickened leaflets of the mitral valve), valvuloplasty (inflation of a balloon within a valve), or valve replacement (with prosthetic valve). Corrective valvular surgery is rarely necessary before late adolescence.

Special considerations

• Teach the patient and family about this disease and its treatment.

• Before giving penicillin, ask the parents if the child has ever had a hypersensitivity reaction to it. Even if the patient has never had a reaction to penicillin, warn that such a reaction is possible.

• Tell the child's parents to stop the drug and immediately report the development of a rash, fever, chills, or other signs of allergy *at any time* during penicillin therapy.

• Instruct the parents to watch for and report early signs of heart failure, such as dyspnea and a hacking, nonproductive cough.

• Stress the need for bed rest during the acute phase and suggest appropriate, physically undemanding diversions.

• After the acute phase, encourage family and friends to spend as much time as possible with the child to minimize boredom. Advise the parents to secure a tutor to help the child keep up with schoolwork during his long convalescence.

• Help the parents overcome any guilt they may feel about their child's illness. Tell them that failure to seek treatment for streptococcal infection is common, because this illness often seems no worse than a cold.

• Encourage the parents and the child to vent their frustrations during the long, tedious recovery. If the child has severe carditis, help them prepare for permanent changes in the child's lifestyle.

• Warn the parents to watch for and immediately report signs of recurrent streptococcal infection — sudden sore throat, diffuse throat redness and oropharyngeal exudate, swollen and tender cervical lymph glands, pain on swallowing, a temperature of 101° to 104° F (38.3° to 40° C), headache, and nausea. Urge them to keep the child away from people with respiratory tract infections.

• Promote good dental hygiene to prevent gingival infection. Make sure the child and his family understand the need to comply with prolonged antibiotic therapy and follow-up care and the need for additional antibiotics during dental surgery. Arrange for a visiting nurse to oversee home care, if necessary.

RHEUMATOID ARTHRITIS

A chronic, systemic, inflammatory disease, rheumatoid arthritis (RA) primarily attacks peripheral joints and surrounding muscles, tendons, ligaments, and blood vessels. Spontaneous remissions and unpredictable exacerbations mark the course of this potentially crippling disease.

RA occurs worldwide, striking women three times more often than men. Although it can occur at any age, the peak onset for women occurs between ages 30 and 60. RA affects more than 6.5 million people in the United States alone.

This disease usually requires lifelong treatment and, sometimes, surgery. In most patients, it follows an intermittent course and allows normal activity, although 10% suffer total disability from severe articular deformity, associated extra-articular symptoms, or both. The prognosis worsens with the development of nodules, vasculitis, and high titers of rheumatoid factor (RF).

Causes
What causes the chronic inflammation characteristic of RA isn't known, but various theories point to infectious, genetic, and endocrine factors.

Current theory
Currently, it's believed that a genetically susceptible individual develops abnormal or altered immunoglobulin G (IgG) antibodies when exposed to an antigen. This altered IgG antibody isn't recognized as "self," and the individual forms an antibody against it — an antibody known as RF. By aggre-

gating into complexes, RF generates inflammation.

Eventually, cartilage damage by inflammation triggers additional immune responses, including activation of complement. This in turn attracts polymorphonuclear leukocytes and stimulates release of inflammatory mediators, which enhance joint destruction.

Pathogenesis

Much more is known about the pathogenesis of RA than about its causes. If unarrested, the inflammatory process within the joints occurs in four stages.

First, synovitis develops from congestion and edema of the synovial membrane and joint capsule. Formation of pannus — thickened layers of granulation tissue — marks the onset of the second stage. Pannus covers and invades cartilage, and eventually destroys the joint capsule and bone.

Progression to the third stage is characterized by fibrous ankylosis — fibrous invasion of the pannus and scar formation that occludes the joint space. Bone atrophy and malalignment cause visible deformities and disrupt the articulation of opposing bones, causing muscle atrophy and imbalance and, possibly, partial dislocations or subluxations.

In the fourth stage, fibrous tissue calcifies, resulting in bony ankylosis and total immobility.

Signs and symptoms

RA usually develops insidiously and initially produces nonspecific symptoms. These include fatigue, malaise, anorexia, persistent low-grade fever, weight loss, lymphadenopathy, and vague articular symptoms.

Specific symptoms

As the disease progresses, more specific localized articular symptoms develop, frequently in the fingers at the proximal interphalangeal (PIP), metacarpophalangeal (MCP), and metatarsophalangeal joints. These symptoms usually occur bilaterally and symmetrically and may extend to the wrists, knees, elbows, and ankles.

The affected joints stiffen after inactivity, especially on rising in the morning. The fingers may assume a spindle shape from marked edema and congestion in the joints. The joints become tender and painful, at first only when the patient moves them, but eventually even at rest. They often feel hot to the touch. Ultimately, joint function is diminished. Deformities are common if active disease continues.

PIP joints may develop flexion deformities or become hyperextended. MCP joints may swell dorsally, and volar subluxation and stretching of tendons may pull the fingers to the ulnar side ("ulnar drift").

The fingers may become fixed in a characteristic "swan's neck" appearance or "boutonnière" deformity. The hands appear foreshortened, the wrists boggy; carpal tunnel syndrome from synovial pressure on the median nerve causes paresthesia in the fingers.

Extra-articular signs

The most common extra-articular finding is the gradual appearance of rheumatoid nodules — subcutaneous, round or oval, nontender masses. These usually appear on pressure areas such as the elbows.

Vasculitis can lead to skin lesions, leg ulcers, and multiple systemic complications. Peripheral neuropathy may produce numbness or tingling in the feet or weakness and loss of sensation in the fingers. Stiff, weak, or painful muscles are common.

Other common extra-articular effects include pericarditis, pulmonary nodules or fibrosis, pleuritis, scleritis, and episcleritis.

Other complications

Another complication is destruction of the odontoid process, part of the second cervical vertebra. Rarely, spinal cord compression may occur, particularly in patients with longstanding deforming RA. Upper motor neuron signs, such as a positive Babinski's sign and muscle weakness, may also develop.

RA can also cause temporomandibular joint disease, which impairs chewing and causes earaches. Other extra-articular findings may include infection, osteoporosis, myositis, cardiopulmonary lesions, lymphadenopathy, and peripheral neuritis.

Diagnosis

Typical clinical features suggest RA, but a firm diagnosis relies on laboratory and other test results:

• *X-rays* in early stages show bone demineralization and soft-tissue swelling; later, loss of cartilage and narrowing of joint spaces; and finally, cartilage and bone destruction and erosion, subluxations, and deformities.

• *RF* is positive in 75% to 80% of patients, as indicated by a titer of 1:160 or higher.

• *Synovial fluid analysis* shows increased volume and turbidity but decreased viscosity and complement (C3 and C4) levels.

• *White blood cell count* often exceeds 10,000/µl.

• *Serum protein electrophoresis* may show elevated serum globulin levels.

• *Erythrocyte sedimentation rate* is elevated in 85% to 90% of patients (may be useful to monitor response to therapy, because elevation frequently parallels disease activity).

• *Complete blood count* usually shows moderate anemia and slight leukocytosis.

• *C-reactive protein test* can help monitor response to therapy.

Treatment

Salicylates, particularly aspirin, are the mainstay of RA therapy, because they decrease inflammation and relieve joint pain. Other useful medications include nonsteroidal anti-inflammatory agents (such as indomethacin, fenoprofen, and ibuprofen), antimalarials (hydroxychloroquine), gold salts, penicillamine, and corticosteroids (prednisone). (See *Drug therapy for arthritis.*)

Immunosuppressants, such as cyclophosphamide, methotrexate, and azathioprine, are also therapeutic. They are being used more commonly in early disease.

Supportive measures include 8 to 10 hours of sleep every night, frequent rest periods between daily activities, and splinting to rest inflamed joints. A physical therapy program, including range-of-motion exercises and carefully individualized therapeutic exercises, forestalls loss of joint function.

Application of heat relaxes muscles and relieves pain. Moist heat usually works best for patients with chronic disease. Ice packs are effective during acute episodes.

Treatment in advanced disease

Advanced disease may require synovectomy, joint reconstruction, or total joint arthroplasty. (See *When arthritis requires surgery,* page 761.)

Useful surgical procedures in RA include metatarsal head and distal ulnar resectional arthroplasty, insertion of a Silastic prosthesis between MCP and PIP joints, and arthrodesis (joint fusion). Arthrodesis sacrifices joint mobility for stability and relief of pain.

Synovectomy (removal of destructive, proliferating synovium, usually in the wrists, knees, and fingers) may halt or delay the course of this disease. Osteotomy (the cutting of bone or excision of a wedge of bone) can realign joint surfaces and redistribute stresses.

Drug Therapy for Arthritis

DRUG AND ADVERSE EFFECTS	CLINICAL CONSIDERATIONS
Aspirin • Prolonged bleeding time; GI disturbances, including nausea, dyspepsia, anorexia, ulcers, and hemorrhage; hypersensitivity reactions ranging from urticaria to anaphylaxis; salicylism (mild toxicity: tinnitus, dizziness; moderate toxicity: restlessness, hyperpnea, delirium, marked lethargy; severe toxicity: coma, seizures, severe hyperpnea)	• Don't use in patients with GI ulcers, bleeding, or hypersensitivity or in neonates. • Give with food, milk, antacid, or a large glass of water to reduce GI adverse effects. • Monitor salicylate level. Remember that toxicity can develop rapidly in febrile, dehydrated children. • Teach patient to reduce dose, one tablet at a time, if tinnitus occurs. • Teach patient to watch for signs of bleeding, such as bruising, melena, and petechiae.
Fenoprofen, ibuprofen, naproxen, piroxicam, sulindac, and tolmetin • Prolonged bleeding time; central nervous system abnormalities (headache, drowsiness, restlessness, dizziness, tremor); GI disturbances, including hemorrhage and peptic ulcer; increased blood urea nitrogen and liver enzyme levels	• Don't use in patients with renal disease, in asthmatics with nasal polyps, or in children. • Use cautiously in GI disorders and cardiac disease or when patient is allergic to other nonsteroidal anti-inflammatory drugs (NSAIDs). • Give with milk or meals to reduce GI adverse effects. • Tell patient that drugs' effect may be delayed for 2 to 3 weeks. • Monitor kidney, liver, and auditory functions in long-term therapy. Stop drugs if abnormalities develop. • Use cautiously in elderly patients; they may experience severe GI bleeding without warning.
Hydroxychloroquine • Blood dyscrasias, GI irritation, corneal opacities, and keratopathy or retinopathy	• Contraindicated in patients with retinal or visual field changes. • Use cautiously in patients with hepatic disease, alcoholism, glucose-6-phosphate dehydrogenase deficiency, or psoriasis. • Perform complete blood count (CBC) and liver function tests before therapy and during chronic therapy. Patient should also have regular ophthalmologic examination. • Tell patient to take drug with food or milk. • Warn patient that dizziness may occur.
Gold (oral and parenteral) • Dermatitis, pruritus, rash, stomatitis, nephrotoxicity, and blood dyscrasias; with oral form, GI distress and diarrhea	• Watch for adverse effects. Observe for nitritoid reaction (flushing, fainting, sweating). • Check urine for blood and albumin before each dose. If positive, drug may need to be withheld. Stress the need for regular follow-up, including blood and urine testing.

(continued)

Drug Therapy for Arthritis *(continued)*

DRUG AND ADVERSE EFFECTS	CLINICAL CONSIDERATIONS
Gold (oral and parenteral) *(continued)*	• To avoid local nerve irritation, mix drug well and give deep I.M. injection in buttock. • Advise patient not to expect improvement for 3 to 6 months. • Instruct patient to report rash, bruising, bleeding, hematuria, or oral ulcers.
Methotrexate • Tubular necrosis, bone marrow depression, leukopenia, thrombocytopenia, pulmonary interstitial infiltrates, hyperuricemia, stomatitis, rash, pruritus, dermatitis, alopecia, diarrhea, dizziness, cirrhosis, and hepatic fibrosis	• Don't give to breast-feeding or pregnant women or to alcoholic patients. • Monitor uric acid levels and CBC. • Monitor intake and output. • Warn patient to report any unusual bleeding (especially GI) or bruising promptly. • Warn patient to avoid alcohol, aspirin, and NSAIDs. • Advise patient to follow prescribed regimen.

Tendons may rupture spontaneously, requiring surgical repair. Tendon transfers may prevent deformities or relieve contractures.

Special considerations
• If the patient requires knee or hip arthroplasty, provide appropriate teaching and postoperative care.
• Assess all joints carefully. Look for deformities, contractures, immobility, and inability to perform everyday activities.
• Monitor vital signs, and note weight changes, sensory disturbances, and level of pain. Administer analgesics, and watch for adverse effects.
• Give meticulous skin care. Check for rheumatoid nodules, as well as pressure ulcers and breakdowns from immobility, vascular impairment, corticosteroid treatment, or improper splinting. Use lotion or cleansing oil, not soap, for dry skin.
• Explain all diagnostic tests and procedures. Tell the patient to expect multiple blood samples to allow a firm di-

agnosis and accurate monitoring of therapy.
• Monitor the duration, not the intensity, of morning stiffness, because duration more accurately reflects the severity of the disease. Encourage the patient to take hot showers or baths at bedtime or in the morning to reduce the need for pain medication.
• Apply splints carefully and correctly. Observe for pressure ulcers if the patient is in traction or wearing splints.
• Explain the nature of RA. Make sure the patient and his family understand that RA is a chronic disease that requires major changes in lifestyle. Emphasize that there are no miracle cures, despite claims to the contrary.
• Encourage a balanced diet, but make sure the patient understands that special diets won't cure RA. Stress the need for weight control, because obesity adds further stress to joints.
• Urge the patient to perform activities of daily living, such as dressing and feeding himself. (Supply easy-to-open cartons, lightweight cups, and unpack-

When Arthritis Requires Surgery

Arthritis severe enough to necessitate total knee or total hip arthroplasty calls for comprehensive preoperative teaching and postoperative care.

Before surgery
• Explain preoperative and surgical procedures. Show the patient the prosthesis to be used, if available.
• Teach the patient postoperative exercises (such as isometrics), and supervise his practice. Also, teach deep-breathing and coughing exercises that will be necessary after surgery.
• Explain that total hip or knee arthroplasty requires frequent range-of-motion exercises of the leg after surgery; total knee arthroplasty requires frequent leg-lift exercises.
• Show the patient how to use a trapeze to move himself about in bed after surgery, and make sure he has a fracture bedpan handy.
• Tell the patient what kind of dressings to expect after surgery. After total knee arthroplasty, the patient's knee may be placed in a constant-passive-motion device to increase postoperative mobility and prevent emboli. After total hip arthroplasty, he'll have an abduction pillow between the legs to help keep the hip prosthesis in place.

After surgery
• Closely monitor and record vital signs. Watch for complications, such as steroid crisis and shock in patients receiving steroids. Monitor distal leg pulses often, marking them

with a waterproof marker to make them easier to find.
• As soon as the patient awakens, make sure he can perform active dorsiflexion. Supervise isometric exercises every 2 hours. After total hip arthroplasty, check traction for pressure areas and keep the head of the bed raised between 30 and 45 degrees.
• Change or reinforce dressings, as needed, using aseptic technique. Check wounds for hematoma, excessive drainage, color changes, or foul odor—all possible signs of hemorrhage or infection. (Wounds on rheumatoid arthritis patients may heal slowly.) Avoid contaminating dressings while helping the patient use the urinal or bedpan.
• Administer blood replacement products, antibiotics, and pain medication as needed. Monitor serum electrolyte levels, hemoglobin, and hematocrit.
• Have the patient turn, cough, and deep-breathe every 2 hours; then percuss his chest.
• After total knee arthroplasty, keep the patient's leg extended and slightly elevated.
• After total hip arthroplasty, keep the patient's hip in abduction to prevent dislocation. Watch for any inability to rotate the hip or bear weight on it, increased pain, or a leg that appears shorter—all may indicate dislocation.
• As soon as allowed, help the patient get out of bed and sit in a chair, keeping his weight on the unaffected side. When he's ready to walk, consult with the physical therapist for walking instruction and aids.

aged silverware.) Allow the patient enough time to calmly perform these tasks.
• Provide emotional support. Remember that the patient with chronic illness easily becomes depressed, discouraged, and irritable. Encourage the RA patient to discuss his fears concerning dependency, sexuality, body image, and self-esteem. Refer him to

an appropriate social service agency as needed.

• Discuss sexual aids: alternative positions, pain medication, and moist heat to increase mobility.

• Before discharge, make sure the patient knows how and when to take his prescribed medication and how to recognize its possible adverse effects.

• Teach the patient how to stand, walk, and sit correctly: upright and erect. Tell him to sit in chairs with high seats and armrests; he'll find it easier to get up from a chair if his knees are lower than his hips. If he doesn't own a chair with a high seat, recommend putting blocks of wood under the legs of a favorite chair. Suggest an elevated toilet seat.

• Instruct the patient to pace daily activities, resting for 5 to 10 minutes out of each hour and alternating sitting and standing tasks. Adequate sleep is important, and so is correct sleeping posture. He should sleep on his back on a firm mattress and should avoid placing a pillow under his knees, which encourages flexion deformity.

• Teach the patient to avoid putting undue stress on joints and to use the largest joint available for a given task; to support weak or painful joints as much as possible; to avoid positions of flexion and promote positions of extension; to hold objects parallel to the knuckles as briefly as possible; to always use his hands toward the center of his body; and to slide—not lift—objects whenever possible.

• Enlist the aid of the occupational therapist to teach how to simplify activities and protect arthritic joints. Stress the importance of shoes with proper support.

• Suggest dressing aids—long-handled shoehorn, reacher, elastic shoelaces, zipper-pull, and buttonhook—and helpful household items, such as easy-to-open drawers, hand-held shower nozzle, handrails, and grab bars.

• Suggest wearing mittens to the patient who has trouble maneuvering fingers into gloves. Tell him to dress while in a sitting position as often as possible.

• Refer the patient to the Arthritis Foundation for more information on coping with RA.

ROSACEA

A chronic skin eruption, rosacea produces flushing and dilation of the small blood vessels in the face, especially the nose and cheeks. Papules and pustules may also occur but without the characteristic comedones of acne vulgaris.

Rosacea is most common in white women between ages 30 and 50. When it occurs in men, however, it's usually more severe and often associated with rhinophyma, which is characterized by dilated follicles and thickened, bulbous skin on the nose.

Ocular involvement may result in blepharitis, conjunctivitis, uveitis, or keratitis. Rosacea usually spreads slowly and rarely subsides spontaneously.

Causes

Although the cause of rosacea is unknown, stress, infection, vitamin deficiencies, and endocrine abnormalities can aggravate this condition. Anything that produces flushing—for example, tobacco, alcohol, spicy foods, physical activity, sunlight, extreme heat or cold, or hot beverages, such as tea or coffee—can also aggravate rosacea.

Signs and symptoms

Rosacea generally begins with periodic flushing across the central oval of the face, accompanied later by telangiectasias, papules, pustules, and nodules.

Rhinophyma is commonly associated with severe rosacea but may occur alone. It usually appears first on the lower half of the nose, and produces red, thickened skin and follicular enlargement. Related ocular lesions are uncommon.

Diagnosis

Typical vascular and acneiform lesions—without the comedones characteristically associated with acne vulgaris—and rhinophyma in severe cases confirm rosacea.

Treatment

As symptoms subside, gradually decreasing doses of oral tetracycline are given for the acneiform component of rosacea. Topical metronidazole gel helps the papules, pustules, and erythema. Topical application of 1% hydrocortisone cream reduces erythema and inflammation.

Other treatments may include electrolysis to destroy large, dilated blood vessels and removal of excess tissue in patients with rhinophyma.

Special considerations

• Instruct the patient to avoid hot beverages, alcohol, extended sun exposure, and other possible causes of flushing.

• Assess the effect of rosacea on body image. Because it's always apparent on the face, your support is essential.

ROSEOLA INFANTUM

Also called exanthema subitum, roseola infantum is an acute, benign, presumably viral infection. It usually affects infants and young children (ages 6 months to 3 years).

Roseola affects boys and girls alike. It occurs year-round but is most prevalent in the spring and fall. Overt roseola, the most common exanthem in infants under age 2, affects 30% of all children; inapparent roseola (febrile illness without a rash) may affect the rest.

Characteristically, it first causes a high fever and then a rash that accompanies an abrupt drop to normal temperature. (See *Incubation and duration of common rash-producing infections,* page 764.)

Causes and incidence

The mode of transmission isn't known. Only rarely does an infected child transmit roseola to a sibling.

Signs and symptoms

After a 10- to 15-day incubation period, the infant with roseola develops an abruptly rising, unexplainable fever and, sometimes, seizures. Temperature peaks at 103° to 105° F (39.4° to 40.6° C) for 3 to 5 days, then drops suddenly. In the early febrile period, the infant may be anorexic, irritable, and listless but doesn't seem particularly ill.

Simultaneously with an abrupt drop in temperature, a maculopapular, nonpruritic rash develops, which blanches on pressure. The rash is profuse on the infant's trunk, arms, and neck, and is mild on the face and legs. It fades within 24 hours. Although possible, complications are extremely rare.

Diagnosis

Diagnosis requires observation of the typical rash that appears about 48 hours after fever subsides.

Treatment

Because roseola is self-limiting, treatment is supportive and symptomatic: antipyretics to lower fever and, if necessary, anticonvulsants to relieve seizures.

INCUBATION AND DURATION OF COMMON RASH-PRODUCING INFECTIONS

INFECTION	INCUBATION (DAYS)	DURATION (DAYS)
Roseola	10 to 15	3 to 6
Varicella	10 to 14	7 to 14
Rubeola	13 to 17	5
Rubella	6 to 18	3
Herpes simplex	2 to 12	7 to 21

Special considerations
• Teach parents how to lower their infant's fever by giving tepid baths, keeping him in lightweight clothes, and maintaining normal room temperature. Stress the need for adequate fluid intake. Strict bed rest and isolation are unnecessary.
• Tell parents that a short febrile convulsion will not cause brain damage. Explain that convulsions will cease after fever subsides and that phenobarbital is likely to cause drowsiness; parents should call immediately if it causes stupor.

RUBELLA

Commonly called German measles, rubella is an acute, mildly contagious viral disease that produces a distinctive, 3-day rash and lymphadenopathy. It occurs most often among children ages 5 to 9, adolescents, and young adults.

Worldwide in distribution, rubella flourishes during the spring (particularly in big cities) and epidemics occur sporadically. This disease is self-limiting, and the prognosis is excellent.

Causes
The rubella virus is transmitted through contact with the blood, urine, stools, or nasopharyngeal secretions of infected persons and possibly by contact with contaminated articles of clothing. Transplacental transmission, especially in the first trimester of pregnancy, can cause serious birth defects.

Humans are the only known hosts for the rubella virus. The period of communicability lasts from about 10 days before until 5 days after the rash appears.

Signs and symptoms
In children, after an incubation period of from 16 to 18 days, an exanthematous, maculopapular rash erupts abruptly. In adolescents and adults, prodromal symptoms—headache, anorexia, malaise, low-grade fever, coryza, lymphadenopathy and, sometimes, conjunctivitis—appear first. Suboccipital, postauricular, and postcervical lymph node enlargement is a hallmark of rubella.

Short-term rash

Typically, the rubella rash begins on the face. This maculopapular eruption spreads rapidly, often covering the trunk and extremities within hours. Small, red, petechial macules on the soft palate (Forschheimer spots) may precede or accompany the rash.

By the end of the second day, the facial rash begins to fade, but the rash on the trunk may be confluent and may be mistaken for scarlet fever. The rash continues to fade in the downward order in which it appeared. The rash generally disappears on the third day, but it may persist for 4 or 5 days — sometimes accompanied by mild coryza and conjunctivitis.

The rapid appearance and disappearance of the rubella rash distinguishes it from rubeola. Rubella can occur without a rash, but this is rare. Low-grade fever (99° to 101° F [37.2° to 38.3° C]) may accompany the rash, but it usually doesn't persist after the first day of the rash; rarely, temperature may reach 104° F (40° C).

Complications

Complications seldom occur in children with rubella, but when they do, they often appear as hemorrhagic problems such as thrombocytopenia. Young women, however, often experience transient joint pain or arthritis, usually just as the rash is fading. Fever may then recur. These complications usually subside spontaneously within 5 to 30 days.

Diagnosis

The rubella rash, lymphadenopathy, other characteristic signs, and a history of exposure to infected people usually permit clinical diagnosis without laboratory tests. However, cell cultures of the throat, blood, urine, and cerebrospinal fluid can confirm the virus' presence. Convalescent serum that shows a fourfold rise in antibody titers confirms the diagnosis.

Treatment

Because the rubella rash is self-limiting and only mildly pruritic, it doesn't require topical or systemic medication. Treatment consists of aspirin for fever and joint pain. Bed rest isn't necessary, but the patient should be isolated until the rash disappears.

Immunization with live-virus vaccine RA27/3, the only rubella vaccine available in the United States, is necessary for prevention and appears to be more immunogenic than previous vaccines. The rubella vaccine should be given with measles and mumps vaccines at age 15 months to decrease the cost and the number of injections needed.

Special considerations

• Make the patient with active rubella as comfortable as possible. Give children books to read or games to play to keep them occupied.
• Explain why respiratory isolation is necessary. Make sure the patient understands how important it is to avoid exposing pregnant women to this disease.
• Report confirmed cases of rubella to local public health officials.

When giving the rubella vaccine:
• Obtain a history of allergies, especially to neomycin. If the patient has this allergy or has had a reaction to immunization in the past, check with the doctor before giving the vaccine.
• Ask women of childbearing age if they're pregnant. If they are or think they may be, *don't* give the vaccine. Warn women who receive rubella vaccine to use an effective means of birth control for at least 3 months after immunization.
• Give the vaccine at least 3 months after any administration of immune

globulin or blood, which could have antibodies that neutralize the vaccine.

• Don't vaccinate any immunocompromised patients, patients with immunodeficiency diseases, or those receiving immunosuppressive, radiation, or corticosteroid therapy. Instead, administer immune serum globulin to prevent or reduce infection in susceptible patients.

• After giving the vaccine, observe for signs of anaphylaxis for at least 30 minutes. Keep epinephrine 1:1,000 handy.

• Warn about possible mild fever, slight rash, transient arthralgia (in adolescents), and arthritis (in elderly patients). Suggest aspirin or acetaminophen for fever.

• Advise the patient to apply warmth to the injection site for 24 hours after immunization (to help the body absorb the vaccine). If swelling persists after the initial 24 hours, suggest a cold compress to promote vasoconstriction and prevent antigenic cyst formation.

RUBEOLA

Also known as measles or morbilli, rubeola is an acute, highly contagious paramyxovirus infection. It is one of the most common and the most serious of all communicable childhood diseases.

In temperate zones, incidence is highest in late winter and early spring. Before the availability of measles vaccine, epidemics occurred every 2 to 5 years in large urban areas. Use of the vaccine has reduced the occurrence of measles during childhood; as a result, measles is becoming more prevalent in adolescents and adults. (See *Administering measles vaccine.*)

In the United States, the prognosis is usually excellent. However, measles is a major cause of death in children in underdeveloped countries.

Causes

Measles is spread by direct contact or by contaminated airborne respiratory droplets. The portal of entry is the upper respiratory tract.

Signs and symptoms

Incubation is from 10 to 14 days.

Prodromal phase

Initial symptoms begin and greatest communicability occurs during a prodromal phase beginning about 11 days after exposure to the virus. This phase lasts from 4 to 5 days; symptoms include fever, photophobia, malaise, anorexia, conjunctivitis, coryza, hoarseness, and hacking cough.

At the end of the prodrome, Koplik's spots, the hallmark of the disease, appear. These spots look like tiny, bluish gray specks surrounded by a red halo. They appear on the oral mucosa opposite the molars and occasionally bleed.

Progressive symptoms

About 5 days after Koplik's spots appear, temperature rises sharply, spots slough off, and a slightly pruritic rash appears. This characteristic rash starts as faint macules behind the ears and on the neck and cheeks.

These macules become papular and erythematous, rapidly spreading over the entire face, neck, eyelids, arms, chest, back, abdomen, and thighs. When the rash reaches the feet (2 to 3 days later), it begins to fade in the same sequence it appeared, leaving a brownish discoloration that disappears in 7 to 10 days.

The disease climax occurs 2 to 3 days after the rash appears and is marked by a temperature of 103° to 105° F (39.4° to 40.6° C), severe cough, puffy red eyes, and rhinorrhea. About 5 days

Administering Measles Vaccine

Generally, one bout of measles renders immunity (a second infection is extremely rare and may represent misdiagnosis); infants under age 4 months may be immune because of circulating maternal antibodies.

Under normal conditions, measles vaccine isn't administered to children younger than age 15 months. However, during an epidemic, infants as young as 6 months may receive the vaccine; they must be reimmunized at age 15 months.

An alternative approach calls for administration of gamma globulin to infants between ages 6 and 15 months who are likely to be exposed to measles.

Special considerations
• Warn the patient or his parents that possible adverse effects of the vaccine include anorexia, malaise, rash, mild thrombocytopenia or leukopenia, and fever. Explain that the vaccine may produce slight reactions, usually within 7 to 10 days.
• Ask the patient about known allergies, especially to neomycin (each dose contains a small amount). However, a patient who's allergic to eggs may receive the vaccine, because it contains only minimal amounts of albumin and yolk components.

• Avoid giving the vaccine to a pregnant woman (ask for the date of her last menstrual period). Warn women receiving the vaccine to avoid pregnancy for at least 3 months after vaccination.
• Don't vaccinate children with untreated tuberculosis, immunodeficiencies, leukemia, or lymphoma or those receiving immunosuppressives. If such children are exposed to the virus, recommend that they receive gamma globulin. (Gamma globulin won't prevent measles but will lessen its severity.)
• Older unimmunized children who have been exposed to measles for more than 5 days may also require gamma globulin. Be sure to immunize them 3 months later.
• Delay vaccination for 8 to 12 weeks after administration of whole blood, plasma, or gamma globulin, because measles antibodies in these components may neutralize the vaccine.
• Watch for signs of anaphylaxis for 30 minutes after vaccination. Keep epinephrine 1:1,000 handy.
• Advise application of a warm compress to the vaccination site to facilitate absorption of the vaccine. If swelling occurs within 24 hours after vaccination, tell the patient to apply cold compresses to promote vasoconstriction and to prevent antigenic cyst formation.

after the rash appears, other symptoms disappear and communicability ends.

Symptoms are usually mild in patients with partial immunity (conferred by administration of gamma globulin) or infants with transplacental antibodies. More severe symptoms and complications are more likely to develop in young infants, adolescents, adults, and immunocompromised patients than in young children.

Atypical measles may appear in patients who received the killed measles vaccine. These patients are acutely ill with a fever and maculopapular rash that's most obvious in the arms and legs, or with pulmonary involvement and no skin lesions.

Complications

Severe infection may lead to secondary bacterial infection and to autoimmune reaction or organ invasion by the virus, resulting in otitis media, pneumonia, and encephalitis. Subacute sclerosing panencephalitis (SSPE), a rare and invariably fatal complication, may develop several years after measles. SSPE is less common in patients who have received the measles vaccine.

Diagnosis

Measles results in distinctive clinical features, especially the pathognomonic Koplik's spots. Mild measles may resemble rubella, roseola infantum, enterovirus infection, toxoplasmosis, and drug eruptions; laboratory tests are required for a differential diagnosis.

If necessary, measles virus may be isolated from the blood, nasopharyngeal secretions, and urine during the febrile period. Serum antibodies appear within 3 days after onset of the rash and reach peak titers 2 to 4 weeks later.

Treatment

Therapy consists of bed rest, relief of symptoms, and respiratory isolation throughout the communicable period. Vaporizers and a warm environment help reduce respiratory irritation, but cough preparations and antibiotics are generally ineffective; antipyretics can reduce fever. Treatment must also combat complications.

Special considerations

• Teach parents the importance of immunizing their children against measles, and follow appropriate procedures when giving the vaccine.
• Teach parents supportive measures, and stress the need for isolation, plenty of rest, and increased fluid intake. Advise them to cope with photophobia by darkening the room or providing sunglasses and to reduce fever with antipyretics and tepid sponge baths.
• Warn parents to watch for and report the early signs and symptoms of complications, such as encephalitis, otitis media, and pneumonia.

SALMONELLOSIS

A common infection in the United States, salmonellosis is caused by gram-negative bacilli of the genus *Salmonella,* a member of the Enterobacteriaceae family. It occurs as enterocolitis, bacteremia, localized infection, typhoid, or paratyphoid fever. (See *Clinical variants of salmonellosis,* page 770.) Nontyphoidal forms usually produce mild to moderate illness with low mortality.

Typhoid, the most severe form of salmonellosis, usually lasts from 1 to 4 weeks. Mortality is about 3% in persons who are treated and 10% in those untreated, usually as a result of intestinal perforation or hemorrhage, cerebral thrombosis, toxemia, pneumonia, or acute circulatory failure.

An attack of typhoid confers lifelong immunity, although the patient may become a carrier. Most typhoid patients are under age 30; most carriers are women over age 50. Incidence of typhoid in the United States is increasing as a result of travelers returning from endemic areas.

Enterocolitis and bacteremia are common (and more virulent) among infants, elderly people, and people already weakened by other infections; paratyphoid fever is rare in the United States.

Salmonellosis occurs 20 times more often in patients with acquired immunodeficiency syndrome. Features are increased incidence of bacteremia, inability to identify the infection source, and tendency of the infection to recur after therapy is stopped.

Causes

Of an estimated 1,700 serotypes of *Salmonella,* 10 cause the diseases most common in the United States; all 10 can survive for weeks in water, ice, sewage, or food. Nontyphoidal salmonellosis generally follows the ingestion of contaminated or inadequately processed foods, especially eggs, chicken, turkey, and duck. Proper cooking reduces the risk of contracting salmonellosis.

Other causes include contact with infected people or animals or ingestion of contaminated dry milk, chocolate bars, or drugs of animal origin. Salmonellosis may occur in children under age 5 from fecal-oral spread.

Typhoid results most frequently from drinking water contaminated by excretions of a carrier.

Signs and symptoms

Clinical manifestations of salmonellosis vary but usually include fever, abdominal pain, and severe diarrhea with enterocolitis. Headache, increasing fever, and constipation are more common with typhoidal infection.

Diagnosis

Generally, diagnosis depends on isolation of the organism in a culture, particularly blood (in typhoid, paratyphoid, and bacteremia) or feces (in enterocolitis, paratyphoid, and ty-

CLINICAL VARIANTS OF SALMONELLOSIS

VARIANT	CAUSE	CLINICAL FEATURES
Enterocolitis	Any species of nontyphoidal *Salmonella*, but usually *S. enteritidis*. Incubation period of 6 to 48 hours.	Mild to severe abdominal pain, diarrhea, sudden fever up to 102° F (38.8° C), nausea, vomiting; usually self-limiting, but may progress to enteric fever (resembling typhoid), local abscesses (usually abdominal), dehydration, septicemia
Paratyphoid	*S. paratyphi* and *S. schottmülleri* (formerly *S. paratyphi B*). Incubation period of 3 weeks or more.	Fever and transient diarrhea; generally resembles typhoid but less severe
Bacteremia	Any *Salmonella* species, but most commonly *S. choleraesuis*. Incubation period varies.	Fever, chills, anorexia, weight loss (without GI symptoms), joint pains
Localized infections	Usually follows bacteremia caused by *Salmonella* species.	Site of localization determines symptoms; localized abscesses may cause osteomyelitis, endocarditis, bronchopneumonia, pyelonephritis, and arthritis.
Typhoid fever	*S. typhi* enters GI tract and invades the bloodstream via the lymphatics, setting up intracellular sites. During this phase, infection of biliary tract leads to intestinal seeding with millions of bacilli. Involved lymphoid tissues (especially Peyer's patches in ilium) enlarge, ulcerate, and necrose, resulting in hemorrhage. Incubation period of usually 1 to 2 weeks.	Symptoms of enterocolitis may develop within hours of ingestion of *S. typhi;* they usually subside before onset of typhoid fever symptoms. *First week:* gradually increasing fever, anorexia, myalgia, malaise, headache *Second week:* remittent fever up to 104° F (40° C) usually in the evening, chills, diaphoresis, weakness, delirium, increasing abdominal pain and distention, diarrhea or constipation, cough, moist crackles, tender abdomen with enlarged spleen, maculopapular rash (especially on abdomen) *Third week:* persistent fever, increasing fatigue and weakness; usually subsides end of third week, although relapses may occur *Complications:* intestinal perforation or hemorrhage, abscesses, thrombophlebitis, cerebral thrombosis, pneumonia, osteomyelitis, myocarditis, acute circulatory failure, chronic carrier state

phoid). Other appropriate culture specimens include urine, bone marrow, pus, and vomitus.

In endemic areas, clinical symptoms of enterocolitis allow a working diagnosis before cultures are positive. Presence of *S. typhi* in stools 1 or more years after treatment indicates that the patient is a carrier, which is true of 3% of patients.

Widal's test, an agglutination reaction against somatic and flagellar antigens, may suggest typhoid with a fourfold rise in titer. However, drug use or hepatic disease can also increase these titers and invalidate test results.

Other supportive laboratory values may include transient leukocytosis during the first week of typhoidal salmonellosis, and leukopenia during the third week, and leukocytosis in local infection.

Treatment

Antimicrobial therapy for typhoid, paratyphoid, and bacteremia depends on the organism's sensitivity. It may include amoxicillin, chloramphenicol and, in severely toxemic patients, cotrimoxazole, ciprofloxacin, or ceftriaxone. Localized abscesses may also need surgical drainage.

Enterocolitis requires a short course of antibiotics only if it causes septicemia or prolonged fever. Other treatments include bed rest and replacement of fluids and electrolytes. Camphorated opium tincture, kaolin with pectin, diphenoxylate hydrochloride, codeine, or small doses of morphine may be necessary to relieve diarrhea and control cramps in patients who must remain active.

Special considerations

• Follow enteric precautions. Always wash your hands thoroughly before and after any contact with the patient, and advise other hospital personnel to do the same. Teach the patient to use proper hand-washing technique, especially after defecating and before eating or handling food. Wear gloves and a gown when disposing of feces or fecally contaminated objects.

• Continue enteric precautions until three consecutive stool cultures are negative — the first one 48 hours after antibiotic treatment ends, followed by two more at 24-hour intervals.

• Observe the patient closely for indications of bowel perforation: sudden pain in the lower right abdomen, possibly after one or more rectal bleeding episodes; sudden fall in temperature or blood pressure; and rising pulse rate.

• During acute infection, allow the patient as much rest as possible. Raise the side rails and use other safety measures because the patient may become delirious.

• The patient should have a room close to the nurses' station so he can be checked on often. Use a room deodorizer (preferably electric) to minimize odor from diarrhea and to provide a comfortable atmosphere for rest.

• Accurately record intake and output. Maintain adequate I.V. hydration. When the patient can tolerate oral feedings, encourage high-calorie fluids, such as milk shakes. Watch for constipation.

• Provide good skin and mouth care. Turn the patient frequently, and perform mild passive exercises, as indicated. Apply mild heat to the abdomen to relieve cramps.

• *Don't* administer antipyretics. These mask fever and lead to possible hypothermia. Instead, to promote heat loss through the skin without causing shivering (which keeps fever high by vasoconstriction), apply tepid, wet towels (don't use alcohol or ice) to the patient's groin and axillae. To promote heat loss by vasodilation of peripheral blood vessels, use additional wet towels on the arms and legs, wiping with long, vigorous strokes.

• After draining the abscesses of a joint, provide heat, elevation, and passive range-of-motion exercises to decrease swelling and maintain mobility.

• If the patient has positive stool cultures on discharge, tell him to use a different bathroom than other family members, if possible (while he's on antibiotics); to wash his hands afterwards; and to avoid preparing uncooked foods, such as salads, for family members.

• To prevent salmonellosis, advise prompt refrigeration of meat and cooked foods (avoid keeping them at room temperature for any prolonged period), and teach the importance of proper handwashing. Advise those at high risk of contracting typhoid (laboratory workers, travelers) to seek vaccination.

SARCOIDOSIS

A multisystemic, granulomatous disorder, sarcoidosis characteristically produces lymphadenopathy, pulmonary infiltration, and skeletal, liver, eye, or skin lesions. It occurs most often in young adults (ages 20 to 40). In the United States, sarcoidosis occurs predominantly among blacks, and affects twice as many women as men.

Acute sarcoidosis usually resolves within 2 years. Chronic, progressive sarcoidosis, which is uncommon, is associated with pulmonary fibrosis and progressive pulmonary disability.

Causes

Although the cause of sarcoidosis is unknown, the following possible causes have been considered:

• *hypersensitivity response* (possibly from a T-cell imbalance) to such agents as atypical mycobacteria, fungi, and pine pollen

• *genetic predisposition* (suggested by a slightly higher incidence of sarcoidosis within the same family)

• *chemicals* such as zirconium or beryllium can lead to illnesses resembling sarcoidosis, suggesting an extrinsic cause for this disease.

Signs and symptoms

Initial signs of sarcoidosis include arthralgia (in the wrists, ankles, and elbows), fatigue, malaise, and weight loss. Other clinical features vary according to the extent and location of the fibrosis:

• *respiratory* — breathlessness, cough (usually nonproductive), substernal pain; complications in advanced pulmonary disease include pulmonary hypertension and cor pulmonale

• *cutaneous* — erythema nodosum, subcutaneous skin nodules with maculopapular eruptions, extensive nasal mucosal lesions

• *ophthalmic* — anterior uveitis (common); glaucoma, blindness (rare)

• *lymphatic* — bilateral hilar and right paratracheal lymphadenopathy and splenomegaly

• *musculoskeletal* — muscle weakness, polyarthralgia, pain, punched-out lesions on phalanges

• *hepatic* — granulomatous hepatitis, usually asymptomatic

• *genitourinary* — hypercalciuria

• *cardiovascular* — arrhythmias (premature beats, bundle branch block, or complete heart block); cardiomyopathy (rare)

• *central nervous system (CNS)* — cranial or peripheral nerve palsies, basilar meningitis, seizures, pituitary and hypothalamic lesions producing diabetes insipidus.

Diagnosis

Typical clinical features with appropriate laboratory data and X-ray findings suggest sarcoidosis. A positive

Kveim-Siltzbach skin test supports the diagnosis.

In this test, the patient receives an intradermal injection of an antigen prepared from human sarcoidal spleen or lymph nodes from patients with sarcoidosis. If the patient has active sarcoidosis, granuloma develops at the injection site in 2 to 6 weeks. This reaction is considered positive when a biopsy of the skin at the injection site shows discrete epitheloid cell granuloma.

Other relevant findings include the following:

• *Chest X-ray* shows bilateral hilar and right paratracheal adenopathy with or without diffuse interstitial infiltrates; occasionally large nodular lesions are present in lung parenchyma.

• *Lymph node, skin, or lung biopsy* reveals noncaseating granulomas with negative cultures for mycobacteria and fungi.

• *Other laboratory data* infrequently reveal increased serum calcium, mild anemia, leukocytosis, or hyperglobulinemia.

• *Pulmonary function tests* show decreased total lung capacity and compliance and decreased diffusing capacity.

• *Arterial blood gas (ABG) analysis* shows decreased partial pressure of arterial oxygen.

Negative tuberculin skin test, fungal serologies, and sputum cultures for mycobacteria and fungi, as well as negative biopsy cultures, help rule out infection.

Treatment

Asymptomatic sarcoidosis requires no treatment. However, sarcoidosis that causes ocular, respiratory, CNS, cardiac, or systemic symptoms (such as fever and weight loss) requires treatment with systemic or topical steroids, as does sarcoidosis that produces hypercalcemia or destructive skin lesions. Such therapy is usually continued for 1 to 2 years, but some patients may need lifelong therapy.

Other treatment includes a low-calcium diet and avoidance of direct exposure to sunlight in patients with hypercalcemia.

Special considerations

• Watch for and report any complications. Be aware of any abnormal laboratory results (anemia, for example) that could alter patient care.

• For the patient with arthralgia, administer analgesics as needed. Record signs of progressive muscle weakness.

• Provide a nutritious, high-calorie diet and plenty of fluids. If the patient has hypercalcemia, suggest a low-calcium diet. Weigh the patient regularly to detect weight loss.

• Monitor respiratory function. Check chest X-rays for the extent of lung involvement; note and record any bloody sputum or increase in sputum. If the patient has pulmonary hypertension or end-stage cor pulmonale, check ABG values, watch for arrhythmias, and administer oxygen as needed.

• Because steroids may induce or worsen diabetes mellitus, perform fingerstick glucose tests at least every 12 hours at the beginning of steroid therapy. Also, watch for other adverse effects of steroids, such as fluid retention, electrolyte imbalance (especially hypokalemia), moon face, hypertension, and personality change.

• During or after steroid withdrawal (particularly in association with infection or other types of stress), watch for vomiting, orthostatic hypotension, hypoglycemia, restlessness, anorexia, malaise, and fatigue. Remember that the patient on long-term or high-dose steroid therapy is vulnerable to infection.

• When preparing the patient for discharge, stress the need for compliance with prescribed steroid therapy and regular, careful follow-up examinations and treatment.

• Refer the patient with failing vision to community support and resource groups and the American Foundation for the Blind, if necessary.

SCABIES

An age-old skin infection, scabies results from infestation with *Sarcoptes scabiei* var. *hominis* (itch mite), which provokes a sensitivity reaction. It occurs worldwide, is predisposed by overcrowding and poor hygiene, and can be endemic.

Causes

Mites can live their entire life cycles in the skin of humans, causing chronic infection. The female mite burrows into the skin to lay her eggs, from which larvae emerge to copulate and then reburrow under the skin.

Transmission of scabies occurs through skin or sexual contact. The adult mite can survive without a human host for only 2 or 3 days.

Signs and symptoms

Typically, scabies causes itching that intensifies at night. Characteristic lesions are usually excoriated and may appear as erythematous nodules.

These threadlike lesions are approximately ⅜" long and generally occur between fingers, on flexor surfaces of the wrists, on elbows, in axillary folds, at the waistline, on nipples in females, and on genitalia in males. In infants, the burrows (lesions) may appear on the head and neck.

Intense scratching can lead to severe excoriation and secondary bacterial infection. Itching may become generalized secondary to sensitization.

Diagnosis

Visual examination of the contents of the scabietic burrow may reveal the itch mite. If not, a drop of mineral oil placed over the burrow, followed by superficial scraping and examination of expressed material under a low-power microscope, may reveal ova or mite feces. However, excoriation or inflammation of the burrow often makes such identification difficult.

If diagnostic tests offer no positive identification of the mite and if scabies is still suspected (for example, close contacts of the patient also report itching), skin clearing that occurs after a therapeutic trial of a pediculicide confirms the diagnosis.

Treatment

Generally, treatment of scabies consists of application of a pediculicide — permethrin or lindane cream — in a thin layer over the entire skin surface. The pediculicide is left on for 8 to 12 hours. To make certain that all areas have been treated, this application should be repeated in approximately 1 week. Another pediculicide, crotamiton cream, may be applied on 4 consecutive nights.

Approximately 10% of a pediculicide is absorbed systemically; therefore, a 6% to 10% solution of sulfur, which is less toxic, applied for 3 consecutive days is an alternative therapy for infants and pregnant women. Widespread bacterial infections require systemic antibiotics.

Persistent pruritus (from mite sensitization or contact dermatitis) may develop from repeated use of pediculicides rather than from continued infection. An antipruritic emollient or topical steroid can reduce itching; intralesional steroids may resolve erythematous nodules.

Special considerations
• Instruct the patient to apply permethrin or lindane cream from the neck down, covering his entire body. He must wait 15 minutes before dressing and avoid bathing for 8 to 12 hours. Contaminated clothing and linens must be washed in hot water or dry-cleaned.
• Tell the patient not to apply lindane cream if his skin is raw or inflamed. Advise him that he should immediately report any skin irritation or hypersensitivity reaction, discontinue using the drug, and wash it off his skin thoroughly.
• Suggest that family members and other close contacts of the patient be checked for possible symptoms.
• If a hospitalized patient has scabies, prevent transmission to other patients: Practice good hand-washing technique or wear gloves when touching the patient, observe wound and skin precautions for 24 hours after treatment with a pediculicide, gas autoclave blood pressure cuffs before using them on other patients, isolate linens until the patient is noninfectious, and thoroughly disinfect the patient's room after discharge.

SCHIZOPHRENIA

This disorder is characterized by disturbances (for at least 6 months) in thought content and form, perception, affect, sense of self, volition, interpersonal relationships, and psychomotor behavior. The *Diagnostic and Statistical Manual of Mental Disorders,* 4th edition *(DSM-IV),* recognizes paranoid, disorganized, catatonic, undifferentiated, and residual schizophrenia.

Schizophrenia affects 1% to 2% of the U.S. population and is equally prevalent in both sexes. Onset of symptoms usually occurs during adolescence or early adulthood.

The disorder produces varying degrees of impairment. Up to one-third of patients with schizophrenia have just one psychotic episode and no more. Some patients have no disability between periods of exacerbation; others need continuous institutional care. The prognosis worsens with each episode.

Causes
Schizophrenia may result from a combination of genetic, biological, cultural, and psychological factors.

Genetic evidence
Some evidence supports a genetic predisposition. Close relatives of persons with schizophrenia are up to 50 times more likely to develop schizophrenia; the closer the degree of biological relatedness, the higher the risk.

Biochemical theory
The most widely accepted biochemical hypothesis holds that schizophrenia results from excessive activity at dopaminergic synapses. Other neurotransmitter alterations may also contribute to schizophrenic symptoms. In addition, patients with schizophrenia have structural abnormalities of the frontal and temporolimbic systems.

Other causes
Numerous psychological and sociocultural causes, such as disturbed family and interpersonal patterns, also have been proposed. Schizophrenia occurs more often among people from lower socioeconomic groups, possibly the result of downward social drift, lack of upward socioeconomic mobility, and high stress levels that may stem from poverty, social failure, illness, and inadequate social resources.

Higher incidence also is linked to low birth weight and congenital deafness.

Signs and symptoms

Schizophrenia is associated with a variety of abnormal behaviors; therefore, signs and symptoms vary widely, depending on the type and phase (prodromal, active, or residual) of the illness.

Watch for these signs and symptoms:

• ambivalence — coexisting strong positive and negative feelings, leading to emotional conflict
• apathy
• clang associations — words that rhyme or sound alike used in an illogical, nonsensical manner; for instance, "It's the rain, train, pain"
• concrete associations — inability to form or understand abstract thoughts
• delusions — false ideas or beliefs accepted as real by the patient. Delusions of grandeur, persecution, and reference (distorted belief regarding the relation between events and one's self; for example, a belief that television programs address the patient on a personal level) are common in schizophrenia. Also common are feelings of being controlled, somatic illness, and depersonalization.
• echolalia — meaningless repetition of words or phrases
• echopraxia — involuntary repetition of movements observed in others
• flight of ideas — rapid succession of incomplete and unconnected ideas
• hallucinations — false sensory perceptions with no basis in reality; usually visual or auditory but may also be olfactory, gustatory, or tactile
• illusions — false sensory perceptions with some basis in reality; for example, a car's backfiring mistaken for a gunshot
• loose associations — rapid shifts among unrelated ideas
• magical thinking — a belief that thoughts or wishes can control others or events

• neologisms — bizarre words that have meaning only for the patient
• poor interpersonal relationships
• regression — return to an earlier developmental stage
• thought blocking — sudden interruption in the patient's train of thought
• withdrawal — disinterest in objects, people, or surroundings
• word salad — illogical word groupings, such as "She had a star, barn, plant."

Diagnosis

After complete physical and psychiatric examinations rule out an organic cause of symptoms, such as an amphetamine-induced psychosis, a diagnosis of schizophrenia is made if the patient's symptoms match those in the *DSM-IV.* (See *Diagnosing schizophrenia.*)

Treatment

In schizophrenia, treatment focuses on meeting the physical and psychosocial needs of the patient, based on his previous level of adjustment and his response to various interventions. Treatment may combine drug therapy, long-term psychotherapy for the patient and his family, psychosocial rehabilitation, vocational counseling, and the use of community resources.

Antipsychotic drugs

The primary treatment for more than 30 years, antipsychotic drugs (also called neuroleptic drugs) appear to work by blocking postsynaptic dopamine receptors. These drugs reduce the incidence of psychotic symptoms, such as hallucinations and delusions, and relieve anxiety and agitation.

Other psychiatric drugs, such as antidepressants and anxiolytics, may control associated signs and symptoms.

Certain antipsychotic drugs are associated with numerous adverse reac-

DIAGNOSING SCHIZOPHRENIA

The following criteria described in the *DSM-IV* are used to diagnose a person with schizophrenia.

Characteristic symptoms

A person with schizophrenia has two or more of the following symptoms (each present for a significant time during a 1-month period—or less if successfully treated):
- delusions
- hallucinations
- disorganized speech
- grossly disorganized or catatonic behavior
- negative symptoms (such as flat affect or poverty of speech).

The diagnosis requires only one of these characteristic symptoms if the person's delusions are bizarre or if hallucinations consist of a voice issuing a running commentary on the person's behavior or thoughts, or two or more voices conversing.

Social and occupational dysfunction

For a significant period since the onset of the disturbance, one or more major areas of functioning (such as work, interpersonal relations, or self-care) are markedly below the level achieved before the onset.

When the disturbance begins in childhood or adolescence, the dysfunction takes the form of failure to achieve the expected level of interpersonal or academic development.

Duration

Continuous signs of the disturbance persist for at least 6 months. The 6-month period must include at least 1 month of symptoms (or less if signs and symptoms have been successfully treated) that match the characteristic symptoms and may include periods of prodromal or residual symptoms.

During the prodromal or residual period, signs of the disturbance may be manifested by only negative symptoms or by two or more characteristic symptoms in a less severe form.

Schizoaffective and mood disorder exclusion

Schizoaffective disorder and mood disorder with psychotic features have been ruled out for these reasons: either no major depressive, manic, or mixed episodes have occurred concurrently with the active-phase symptoms *or*, if mood disorder episodes have occurred during active-phase symptoms, their total duration has been brief relative to the duration of the active and residual periods.

Substance and general medical condition exclusion

The disturbance is not the result of the direct physiologic effects of a substance or a general medical condition.

Relationship to a pervasive developmental disorder

If the person has a history of autistic disorder or another pervasive developmental disorder, the additional diagnosis of schizophrenia is appropriate only if prominent delusions or hallucinations also are present for at least 1 month (or less if successfully treated).

tions, some of which are irreversible. Most experts agree that patients who are withdrawn, isolated, or apathetic show little improvement after antipsychotic drug treatment.

High-potency antipsychotics include fluphenazine, haloperidol, thiothixene, and trifluoperazine. Loxapine, molindone, and perphenazine are intermediate in potency, and chlorpromazine and thioridazine are low-potency agents.

Haloperidol decanoate, fluphenazine decanoate, and fluphenazine enanthate are depot formulations that are implanted I.M.; this method allows gradual release of the drug over a 30-day period, thus improving compliance. A new antipsychotic, risperidone, also is reported to be effective.

Clozapine, which differs chemically from other antipsychotic drugs, may be prescribed for severely ill patients who fail to respond to standard treatment. This agent effectively controls a wider range of psychotic signs and symptoms without the usual adverse effects. However, clozapine can cause drowsiness, sedation, excessive salivation, tachycardia, dizziness, and seizures, as well as agranulocytosis.

A potentially fatal blood disorder, agranulocytosis is characterized by a low white blood cell count and pronounced neutropenia. Routine blood monitoring is essential to detect the estimated 1% to 2% of all patients taking clozapine who develop agranulocytosis. If caught in the early stages, this disorder is reversible.

Psychotherapy

Clinicians disagree about the effectiveness of psychotherapy in treating schizophrenia. Some consider it a useful adjunct to drug therapy.

Others suggest that psychosocial rehabilitation, education, and social skills training are more effective for chronic schizophrenia. In addition to improving understanding of the disorder, these methods teach the patient and his family coping strategies, effective communication techniques, and social skills.

Because schizophrenia typically disrupts the family, family therapy may be helpful to reduce guilt and disappointment as well as improve acceptance of the patient and his bizarre behavior.

Special considerations

• Assess the patient's ability to carry out activities of daily living, paying special attention to his nutritional status. Monitor his weight if he isn't eating.

• If the patient thinks that his food is poisoned, let him fix his own food when possible or offer foods in closed containers that he can open. If you give liquid medication in a unit-dose container, allow the patient to open the container.

• Maintain a safe environment, minimizing stimuli. Administer prescribed medications to decrease symptoms and anxiety. Use physical restraints according to your hospital's policy to ensure the patient's safety and that of others.

• Adopt an accepting and consistent approach with the patient. Short, repeated contacts are best until trust has been established.

• Avoid promoting dependence. Reward positive behavior to help the patient improve his level of functioning.

• Engage the patient in reality-oriented activities that involve human contact, such as inpatient social skills training groups, outpatient day care, and sheltered workshops.

• Provide reality-based explanations for distorted body images or hypochondriacal complaints. Explain to the patient that his private language, autistic inventions, or neologisms are not understood. Set limits on inappropriate behavior.

• If the patient is hallucinating, explore the content of the hallucinations. If he hears voices, find out if he believes that he must do what they command. Explore the emotions connected with the hallucinations, but don't argue about them. If possible, change the subject.

• Teach the patient techniques that interrupt the hallucinations (listening to an audiocassette player, singing out loud, or reading out loud).

• Don't tease or joke with a schizophrenic patient. Choose words and phrases that are unambiguous and clearly understood. For instance, a patient who's told "That procedure will be done on the floor" may become frightened, thinking he'll need to lie down on the floor.

• If the patient expresses suicidal thoughts, institute suicide precautions. Document his behavior and your actions.

• If he's expressing homicidal thoughts (for example, "I have to kill my mother"), institute homicidal precautions. Notify appropriate hospital personnel and the potential victim. Document the patient's comments and the names of those who were notified.

• Don't touch the patient without telling him first exactly what you're going to do — for example, "I'm going to put this cuff on your arm so I can take your blood pressure."

• If necessary, postpone procedures that require physical contact with hospital personnel until the patient is less suspicious or agitated.

• Remember, institutionalization may produce symptoms and handicaps that are not part of the patient's illness, so evaluate symptoms carefully.

• Mobilize community resources to provide a support system for the patient. Ongoing support is essential to his mastery of social skills.

• Encourage compliance with the medication regimen to prevent a relapse. Also, monitor the patient carefully for adverse reactions to drug therapy, including drug-induced parkinsonism, acute dystonia, akathisia, tardive dyskinesia, and malignant neuroleptic syndrome. Document all such reactions.

• Help the patient explore possible connections between anxiety and stress and the exacerbation of symptoms.

For catatonic schizophrenia:

• Assess for physical illness. Remember that the mute patient won't complain of pain or physical symptoms; if he's in a bizarre posture, he's at risk for pressure ulcers or decreased circulation to a body area.

• Meet the patient's physical needs for adequate food, fluid, exercise, and elimination; provide urinary catheterization and enemas as needed.

• Provide range-of-motion exercises for the patient or help him walk every 2 hours.

• Prevent physical exhaustion and injury during periods of hyperactivity.

• Tell the patient directly, specifically, and concisely which procedures need to be done. For example, you might say to the patient, "It's time to go for a walk. Let's go." Don't offer the negativistic patient a choice.

• Spend some time with the patient even if he's mute and unresponsive. The patient is acutely aware of his environment even though he seems not to be. Your presence can be reassuring and supportive.

• Verbalize for the patient the message that his nonverbal behavior seems to convey; encourage him to do so as well.

• Offer reality orientation. You might say, "The leaves on the trees are turning colors and the air is cooler. It's fall!" Emphasize reality in all contacts to reduce distorted perceptions.

• Stay alert for violent outbursts; if they occur, get help promptly to ensure the patient's safety and your own.

For paranoid schizophrenia:

• When the patient is newly admitted, minimize his contact with the hospital staff.

• Don't crowd the patient physically or psychologically; he may strike out to protect himself.

• Be flexible; allow the patient some control. Approach him in a calm and unhurried manner. Let him talk about anything he wishes initially, but keep the conversation light and social, and avoid entering into power struggles.

• Respond to the patient's condescending attitudes (arrogance, put-downs, sarcasm, or open hostility) with neutral remarks.

• Don't let the patient put you on the defensive and don't take his remarks personally. If he tells you to leave him alone, do leave, but return soon. Brief contacts with the patient may be most useful at first.

• Don't make attempts to combat the patient's delusions with logic. Instead, respond to feelings, themes, or underlying needs—for example, "It seems you feel you've been treated unfairly" (persecution).

• Be honest and dependable. Don't threaten the patient or make promises that you can't fulfill.

• If the patient is taking clozapine, stress the importance of returning weekly to the hospital or an outpatient setting to have his blood monitored.

• Teach the patient the importance of complying with the medication regimen. Tell him to report any adverse reactions instead of discontinuing the drug. If he takes a slow-release formulation, make sure that he understands when to return for his next dose.

• Involve the patient's family in his treatment. Teach them how to recognize an impending relapse, and suggest ways to manage symptoms, such as tension, nervousness, insomnia, decreased ability to concentrate, and apathy.

SCOLIOSIS

This lateral curvature of the spine may be found in the thoracic, lumbar, or thoracolumbar spinal segment. The curve may be convex to the right (more common in thoracic curves) or to the left (more common in lumbar curves). Rotation of the vertebral column around its axis occurs and may cause rib cage deformity. Scoliosis is often associated with kyphosis (humpback) and lordosis (swayback).

Causes

Scoliosis may be functional or structural. Functional (postural) scoliosis usually results from poor posture or a discrepancy in leg lengths, not fixed deformity of the spinal column. In structural scoliosis, curvature results from a deformity of the vertebral bodies.

Structural scoliosis may be one of three types:

• *Congenital scoliosis* is usually related to a congenital defect, such as wedge vertebrae, fused ribs or vertebrae, or hemivertebrae.

• *Paralytic or musculoskeletal scoliosis* develops several months after asymmetric paralysis of the trunk muscles from polio, cerebral palsy, or muscular dystrophy

• *Idiopathic scoliosis* (the most common form) may be transmitted as an autosomal dominant or multifactorial trait. This form appears in a previously straight spine during the growing years.

Idiopathic scoliosis can be classified as infantile, which affects mostly male infants between birth and age 3 and causes left thoracic and right lumbar curves; juvenile, which affects both sexes between ages 4 and 10 and causes varying types of curvature; or adolescent, which generally affects girls between age 10 and achievement of skeletal maturity and causes varying types of curvature.

Signs and symptoms

The most common curve in functional or structural scoliosis arises in the thoracic segment, with convexity to the right, and compensatory curves (S curves) in the cervical segment above and the lumbar segment below, both with convexity to the left. As the spine curves laterally, compensatory curves develop to maintain body balance and mark the deformity.

Scoliosis rarely produces subjective symptoms until it's well established; when symptoms do occur, they include backache, fatigue, and dyspnea. Because many teenagers are shy about their bodies, their parents suspect that something is wrong only after they notice uneven hemlines, pantlegs that appear unequal in length, or subtle physical signs like one hip appearing higher than the other.

Untreated scoliosis may result in pulmonary insufficiency (curvature may decrease lung capacity), back pain, degenerative arthritis of the spine, disk disease, and sciatica.

Diagnosis

Anterior, posterior, and lateral spinal X-rays, taken with the patient standing upright and bending, confirm scoliosis and determine the degree of curvature (Cobb method) and flexibility of the spine. (See *Cobb method for measuring angle of curvature,* page 782.) A scoliometer can also be used to measure the angle of trunk rotation.

A physical examination reveals unequal shoulder heights, elbow levels, and heights of the iliac crests. Muscles on the convex side of the curve may be rounded; those on the concave side, flattened, producing asymmetry of paraspinal muscles.

Treatment

The severity of the deformity and potential spine growth determine appropriate treatment, which may include such noninvasive measures as close observation, exercise, or a brace. For more serious deformity, surgery or a combination of methods may be needed. To be most effective, treatment should begin early, when spinal deformity is still subtle.

Noninvasive measures

A curve of less than 25 degrees is mild and can be monitored by X-rays and an examination every 3 months. An exercise program that includes sit-ups, pelvic tilts, spine hyperextension, push-ups, and breathing exercises may strengthen torso muscles and prevent curve progression. A heel lift may help.

A curve of 30 to 50 degrees requires management with spinal exercises and a brace. (Transcutaneous electrical nerve stimulation may be used as an alternative.)

A brace halts progression in most patients but doesn't reverse the established curvature. Such devices passively strengthen the patient's spine by applying asymmetric pressure to skin, muscles, and ribs. Braces can be adjusted as the patient grows and can be worn until bone growth is complete.

Surgery

A curve of 40 degrees or more requires surgery (spinal fusion with instrumentation), because a lateral curve continues to progress at the rate of 1 degree a year even after skeletal maturity.

Some surgeons prescribe Cotrel dynamic traction for 7 to 10 days for preoperative preparation. This traction

Cobb Method for Measuring Angle of Curvature

The Cobb method measures the angle of curvature in scoliosis.

The top vertebra in the curve (T6 in the illustration) is the uppermost vertebra whose upper face tilts toward the curve's concave side. The bottom vertebra in the curve (T12) is the lowest vertebra whose lower face tilts toward the curve's concave side.

The angle at which perpendicular lines drawn from the upper face of the top vertebra and the lower face of the bottom vertebra intersect is the angle of the curve.

consists of a belt-pulley-weight system. While in traction, the patient should exercise for 10 minutes every hour, increasing muscle strength while keeping the vertebral column immobile.

Surgery corrects lateral curvature by posterior spinal fusion and internal stabilization with a Harrington rod. A distraction rod on the concave side of the curve "jacks" the spine into a straight position and provides an internal splint. A Cotrel-Dubousset rod system may also be used.

An alternative procedure, anterior spinal fusion with Dwyer or Zielke instrumentation, corrects curvature with vertebral staples and an anterior stabilizing cable. Some spinal fusions may require postoperative immobilization in a brace.

Postoperatively, periodic checkups are required for several months to monitor stability of the correction.

Special considerations

- Keep in mind that scoliosis often affects adolescent girls, who are likely to find activity limitations and treatment with orthopedic appliances distressing. Therefore, provide emotional support, along with meticulous skin and cast care, and patient teaching.

If the patient needs a brace:

- Enlist the help of a physical therapist, a social worker, and an orthotist (orthopedic appliance specialist). Before the patient goes home, explain what the brace does and how to care for it (how to check the screws for tightness and pad the uprights to prevent excessive wear on clothing). Suggest that loose-fitting, oversized clothes be worn for greater comfort.
- Tell the patient to wear the brace 23 hours a day and to remove it only for bathing and exercise. While she's still adjusting to the brace, tell her to lie down and rest several times a day.
- Suggest a soft mattress if a firm one is uncomfortable.
- To prevent skin breakdown, advise the patient not to use lotions, ointments, or powders on areas where the brace contacts the skin. Instead, suggest that she use rubbing alcohol or tincture of benzoin to toughen the skin. Tell her to keep the skin dry and clean and to wear a snug T-shirt under the brace.
- Advise the patient to increase activities gradually and to avoid strenuous sports. Emphasize the importance of conscientiously performing prescribed exercises. Recommend swimming during the 1 hour out of the brace but strongly warn against diving.
- Instruct the patient to turn her whole body, instead of just her head, when looking to the side. To make reading easier, tell her to hold the book so she can look straight ahead at it instead of down. If she finds this difficult, help her to obtain prism glasses.

If the patient needs traction or a cast before surgery:

- Explain these procedures to the patient and family. Remember that application of a body cast can be traumatic, because it's done on a special frame and the patient's head and face are covered throughout the procedure.
- Check the skin around the cast edge daily. Keep the cast clean and dry and edges of the cast "petaled" (padded). Warn the patient not to insert anything under the cast or let anything get under it and to immediately report cracks in the cast, pain, burning, skin breakdown, numbness, or odor.
- Before surgery, assure the patient and family that she'll have adequate pain control postoperatively. Check sensation, movement, color, and blood supply in all extremities to detect neurovascular deficit, a serious complication following spinal surgery.

After corrective surgery:

- Check neurovascular status every 2 to 4 hours for the first 48 hours, then several times a day. Logroll the patient often.
- Measure intake, output, and urine specific gravity to monitor effects of blood loss, which is often substantial.
- Monitor abdominal distention and bowel sounds.
- Encourage deep-breathing exercises to avoid pulmonary complications.
- Give analgesics, as needed, especially before any activity.
- Promote active range-of-motion (ROM) arm exercises to help maintain muscle strength. Remember that any exercise, even brushing the hair or teeth, is helpful. Encourage the patient to perform quadriceps-setting, calf-pumping, and active ROM exercises of ankles and feet.
- Watch for skin breakdown and signs of cast syndrome. Teach the patient how to recognize these signs.
- Remove antiembolism stockings for at least 30 minutes daily.

• Offer emotional support to help prevent depression, which may result from altered body image and immobility. Encourage the patient to wear her own clothes, wash her hair, and use makeup.

• If the patient is being discharged with a Harrington rod and cast and must have bed rest, arrange for a social worker and a visiting nurse to provide home care. Before discharge, make sure the patient understands activity limitations.

• If you work in a school, screen children routinely for scoliosis during physical examinations.

SEPTAL PERFORATION AND DEVIATION

A perforated septum, a hole in the nasal septum between the two air passages, usually occurs in the anterior cartilaginous septum but may occur in the bony septum.

A deviated septum, a shift from the midline, is common in most adults. This condition may be severe enough to obstruct the passage of air through the nostrils. With surgical correction, the prognosis for either a perforated or deviated septum is good.

Causes

Generally, a perforated septum is caused by traumatic irritation, most commonly from excessive nose picking; less frequently, from repeated cauterization for epistaxis or from penetrating septal injury. It may also result from perichondritis, an infection that gradually erodes the perichondrial layer and cartilage, finally forming an ulcer that perforates the septum.

Other causes of perforation include syphilis, tuberculosis, untreated septal hematoma, inhalation of irritating chemicals, snorting cocaine, chronic nasal infections, nasal carcinoma, granuloma, and chronic sinusitis.

A deviated septum commonly develops during normal growth, as the septum shifts from one side to the other. Consequently, few adults have a perfectly straight septum. Nasal trauma resulting from a fall, a blow to the nose, or surgery further exaggerates the deviation. A congenital deviated septum is rare.

Signs and symptoms

A small septal perforation is usually asymptomatic but may produce a whistle on inspiration. A large perforation causes rhinitis, epistaxis, nasal crusting, and watery discharge.

The patient with a deviated septum may develop a crooked nose, as the midline deflects to one side. The predominant symptom of severe deflection, however, is nasal obstruction. Other manifestations include a sensation of fullness in the face, shortness of breath, nasal discharge, recurring epistaxis, infection, sinusitis, and headache.

Diagnosis

Although clinical features suggest septal perforation or deviation, confirmation requires inspection of the nasal mucosa with bright light and a nasal speculum.

Treatment

Symptomatic treatment of a perforated septum includes decongestants to reduce nasal congestion by local vasoconstriction, local application of lanolin or petrolatum to prevent ulceration and crusting, and antibiotics to combat infection.

Surgery may be necessary to graft part of the perichondrial layer over the perforation. Also, a plastic or Silastic "button" prosthesis may be used to close the perforation.

Symptomatic treatment of a deviated septum usually includes analgesics to relieve headache, decongestants to minimize secretions and, as necessary, vasoconstrictors, nasal packing, or cautery to control hemorrhage. Manipulation of the nasal septum at birth can correct congenital deviated septum.

Corrective surgical options include the following:

• *Reconstruction of the nasal septum by submucous resection* repositions the nasal septal cartilage and relieves nasal obstruction.

• *Rhinoplasty* corrects nasal structure deformity by intranasal incisions.

• *Septoplasty* relieves nasal obstruction and enhances cosmetic appearance.

Special considerations

• In the patient with a perforated septum, use a cotton applicator to apply petrolatum to the nasal mucosa to minimize crusting and ulceration.

• Warn the patient with a perforation or a severe deviation against blowing his nose. To relieve nasal congestion, suggest saline nosedrops and use of a humidifier. Give decongestants as needed.

• To treat epistaxis, have the patient sit upright, provide an emesis basin, and instruct the patient to expectorate any blood. Compress the outer portion of the nose against the septum for 10 to 15 minutes and apply ice packs. Watch for persistent bleeding.

• If corrective surgery is scheduled, prepare the patient to expect postoperative facial edema, periorbital bruising, and nasal packing, which remains in place for 12 to 24 hours. The patient must breathe through his mouth.

After surgery for deviated septum, the patient may also have a splint on his nose.

• To reduce or prevent edema and promote drainage, place the patient in semi-Fowler's position and use a cool-mist vaporizer to liquefy secretions and facilitate normal breathing. To lessen facial edema and pain, place crushed ice in a rubber glove or a small ice bag and apply the glove or ice bag intermittently over the eyes and nose for 24 hours.

• Because the patient is breathing through his mouth, provide frequent and meticulous mouth care.

• Change the mustache dressing or drip pad as needed. Record the color, consistency, and amount of drainage. While nasal packing is in place, expect slight, bright red drainage, with clots. After packing is removed, watch for purulent discharge, an indication of infection.

• Watch for excessive swallowing, hematoma, or a falling or flapping septum (depressed, or soft and unstable septum). Intranasal examination is necessary to detect hematoma formation. Any of these complications requires surgical correction.

• Administer sedatives and analgesics as needed. Because of its anticoagulant properties, aspirin is contraindicated after surgery for septal deviation or perforation.

• Noseblowing may cause bruising and swelling even after nasal packing is removed. After surgery, the patient must limit physical activity for 2 or 3 days, and if he's a smoker, he must stop smoking for at least 2 days.

• Instruct the patient to sneeze with his mouth open and to avoid bending over at the waist. (Advise him to stoop to pick up fallen objects.)

SEPTIC ARTHRITIS

A medical emergency, septic (infectious) arthritis is caused by bacterial invasion of a joint, resulting in inflammation of the synovial lining. If the organisms enter the joint cavity, effusion and pyogenesis follow, with eventual destruction of bone and cartilage.

Septic arthritis can lead to ankylosis and even fatal septicemia. However, prompt antibiotic therapy and joint aspiration or drainage cures most patients.

Causes

In most cases of septic arthritis, bacteria spread from a primary site of infection, usually in adjacent bone or soft tissue, through the bloodstream to the joint.

Common infecting organisms include four strains of gram-positive cocci—*Staphylococcus aureus, Streptococcus pyogenes, Streptococcus pneumoniae,* and *Streptococcus viridans*—and two strains of gram-negative cocci—*Neisseria gonorrhoeae* and *Haemophilus influenzae.* Various gram-negative bacilli—*Escherichia coli, Salmonella,* and *Pseudomonas,* for example—also cause infection.

Anaerobic organisms such as gram-positive cocci usually infect adults and children over age 2. *H. influenzae* most often infects children under age 2.

Risk factors

Various factors can predispose a person to septic arthritis. Any concurrent bacterial infection (of the genitourinary or the upper respiratory tract, for example) or serious chronic illness (such as cancer, renal failure, rheumatoid arthritis, systemic lupus erythematosus, diabetes, or cirrhosis) heightens susceptibility. Consequently, alcoholics and elderly people run a higher risk of developing septic arthritis.

Of course, susceptibility increases with diseases that depress the auto-immune system or with prior immunosuppressive therapy. I.V. drug abuse (by heroin addicts, for example) can also cause septic arthritis.

Other predisposing factors include recent articular trauma, joint surgery, intra-articular injections, and local joint abnormalities.

Signs and symptoms

Acute septic arthritis begins abruptly, causing intense pain, inflammation, and swelling of the affected joint, with low-grade fever. It usually affects a single joint. It most often develops in the large joints but can strike any joint, including the spine and small peripheral joints.

Systemic signs of inflammation may not appear in some patients. Migratory polyarthritis sometimes precedes localization of the infection. If the bacteria invade the hip, pain may occur in the groin, upper thigh, or buttock, or may be referred to the knee.

Diagnosis

Identifying the causative organism in a Gram stain or culture of synovial fluid or a biopsy of synovial membrane confirms septic arthritis. Joint fluid analysis shows gross pus or watery, cloudy fluid of decreased viscosity, usually with $50,000/\mu l$ or more white blood cells (WBCs), primarily neutrophils.

When synovial fluid culture is negative, a positive blood culture may confirm the diagnosis. Synovial fluid glucose is often low compared with a simultaneous 6-hour postprandial blood glucose test.

Other diagnostic measures include the following:
• *X-rays* can show typical changes as early as 1 week after initial infec-

tion—distention of joint capsules, for example, followed by narrowing of joint space (indicating cartilage damage) and erosions of bone (joint destruction).

• *Radioisotope joint scan* for less accessible joints (such as spinal articulations) may help detect infection or inflammation but isn't itself diagnostic.

• *WBC count* may be elevated, with many polymorphonuclear cells; erythrocyte sedimentation rate is increased.

• *Two sets of positive culture* and *Gram stain smears* of skin exudates, sputum, urethral discharge, stools, urine, or nasopharyngeal smear confirm septic arthritis.

• *Lactic assay* can distinguish septic from nonseptic arthritis.

Treatment

Antibiotic therapy should begin promptly; it may be modified when sensitivity results become available.

Antibiotic therapy

Penicillin G is effective against infections caused by *S. aureus, S. pyogenes, S. pneumoniae, S. viridans,* and *N. gonorrhoeae.* A penicillinase-resistant penicillin, such as nafcillin, is recommended for penicillin G–resistant strains of *S. aureus;* ampicillin, for *H. influenzae;* gentamicin, for gram-negative bacilli.

Medication selection requires drug sensitivity studies of the infecting organism. Bioassays or bactericidal assays of synovial fluid and bioassays of blood may confirm clearing of the infection.

Other measures

Treatment of septic arthritis requires monitoring of progress through frequent analysis of joint fluid cultures, synovial fluid WBC counts, and glucose determinations.

Codeine or propoxyphene can be given for pain, if needed. (Aspirin causes a misleading reduction in swelling, hindering accurate monitoring of progress.) The affected joint can be immobilized with a splint or traction until movement can be tolerated.

Needle aspiration (arthrocentesis) to remove grossly purulent joint fluid should be repeated daily until fluid appears normal. If excessive fluid is aspirated or the WBC count remains elevated, open surgical drainage (usually arthrotomy with lavage of the joint) may be necessary for resistant infection or chronic septic arthritis.

Surgery

Late reconstructive surgery is warranted only for severe joint damage and only after all signs of active infection have disappeared, which usually takes several months. In some cases, the recommended procedure may be arthroplasty or joint fusion.

Prosthetic replacement remains controversial; it may exacerbate the infection. However, it has helped patients with damaged femoral heads or acetabula.

Special considerations

• Practice strict aseptic technique with all procedures. Wash hands carefully before and after giving care. Dispose of soiled linens and dressings properly. Prevent contact between immunosuppressed patients and infected patients.

• Watch for signs of joint inflammation: heat, redness, swelling, pain, or drainage. Monitor vital signs and fever pattern. Remember that corticosteroids mask signs of infection.

• Check splints or traction regularly. Keep the joint in proper alignment, but avoid prolonged immobilization. Start passive range-of-motion exercises immediately, and progress to active exercises as soon as the patient can move the affected joint and put weight on it.

• Monitor pain levels and medicate accordingly, especially before exercise (remember that the pain of septic arthritis is easy to underestimate). Administer analgesics and narcotics for acute pain and heat or ice packs for moderate pain.

• Carefully evaluate the patient's condition after joint aspiration. Provide emotional support throughout the diagnostic tests and procedures, which should be previously explained to the patient. Warn the patient before the first aspiration that it will be *extremely* painful.

• Discuss all prescribed medications with the patient. Explain why therapy must be carefully monitored.

LIFE-THREATENING DISORDER

SEPTIC SHOCK

Second only to cardiogenic shock as the leading cause of shock death, septic shock (usually a result of bacterial infection) causes inadequate blood perfusion and circulatory collapse. It occurs most often among hospitalized patients, especially men over age 40 and women ages 25 to 45.

About 25% of patients who develop gram-negative bacteremia go into shock. Unless vigorous treatment begins promptly, preferably before symptoms fully develop, septic shock rapidly progresses to death (often within a few hours) in up to 80% of these patients.

Causes

In two-thirds of patients, septic shock results from infection with gram-negative bacteria: *Escherichia coli, Klebsiella, Enterobacter, Proteus, Pseudomonas,* and *Bacteroides;* in others, from gram-positive bacteria: *Streptococcus pneumoniae, Streptococcus pyogenes,* and *Actinomyces.* Infections with viruses, rickettsiae, chlamydiae,

and protozoa may be complicated by shock.

These organisms produce septicemia in persons whose resistance is already compromised by an existing condition. Infection also results from transplantation of bacteria from other areas of the body through surgery, I.V. therapy, and catheters.

Septic shock often occurs in patients hospitalized for primary infection of the genitourinary, biliary, GI, and gynecologic tracts. Other predisposing factors include immunodeficiency, advanced age, trauma, burns, diabetes mellitus, cirrhosis, and disseminated cancer.

Signs and symptoms

Indications of septic shock vary according to the stage of the shock, the organism causing it, and the age of the patient.

• *Early stage:* oliguria, sudden fever (over 101° F [38.3° C]), chills, nausea, vomiting, diarrhea, and prostration.

• *Late stage:* restlessness, apprehension, irritability, thirst from decreased cerebral tissue perfusion, tachycardia, and tachypnea. Hypotension, altered level of consciousness, and hyperventilation may be the *only* signs among infants and elderly people.

Hypothermia and anuria are common late signs. Complications of septic shock include disseminated intravascular coagulation (DIC), renal failure, heart failure, GI ulcers, and abnormal hepatic function.

Diagnosis

Observation of one or more typical signs (fever, confusion, nausea, vomiting, hyperventilation) in a patient suspected of having an infection suggests septic shock and necessitates immediate treatment.

In the early stages, arterial blood gas (ABG) analysis indicates respiratory alkalosis (low partial pressure of carbon dioxide [PCO_2], low or normal bicarbonate [HCO_3^-] level, and high pH). As shock progresses, metabolic acidosis develops, with hypoxemia indicated by decreasing PCO_2 (which may increase as respiratory failure ensues), as well as decreasing partial pressure of oxygen, HCO_3^-, and pH levels.

The following laboratory tests support the diagnosis and determine the treatment:

• blood cultures to isolate the organism
• decreased platelet count and leukocytosis (15,000 to 30,000/μl)
• increased blood urea nitrogen and creatinine levels and decreased creatinine clearance
• abnormal prothrombin and partial thromboplastin time
• simultaneous measurement of urine and plasma osmolalities for renal failure (urine osmolality below 400 milliosmoles, with a ratio of urine to plasma below 1.5)
• decreased central venous pressure (CVP), pulmonary artery wedge pressure (PAWP), and cardiac output. (In early septic shock, cardiac output increases.)
• electrocardiogram demonstrating ST-segment depression, inverted T waves, and arrhythmias resembling myocardial infarction.

Treatment

The first goal of treatment is to monitor and reverse shock through volume expansion.

Fluid infusion

I.V. fluids are administered and a pulmonary artery catheter is inserted to check pulmonary circulation and PAWP. Administration of whole blood or plasma can then raise the PAWP to a satisfactory level of 14 to 18 mm Hg.

A respirator may be necessary for proper ventilation to overcome hypoxia. A urinary catheter allows accurate measurement of hourly urine output.

Antibiotic therapy

Treatment also requires immediate administration of I.V. antibiotics to control the infection. Depending on the organism, the antibiotic combination usually includes an aminoglycoside, such as gentamicin or tobramycin for gram-negative bacteria, combined with a penicillin, such as carbenicillin or ticarcillin.

Sometimes treatment includes a cephalosporin, such as cefazolin, and nafcillin for suspected staphylococcal infection instead of carbenicillin or ticarcillin. Therapy may also include chloramphenicol for nonsporulating anaerobes (*Bacteroides*), although it may cause bone marrow depression, and clindamycin, which may produce pseudomembranous enterocolitis.

Appropriate anti-infectives for other causes of septic shock depend on the suspected organism. Other measures to combat infections include surgery to drain and excise abscesses and debridement.

Other drug therapy

If shock persists after fluid infusion, treatment with vasopressors, such as dopamine, maintains adequate blood perfusion in the brain, liver, GI tract, kidneys, and skin. Other treatment includes I.V. bicarbonate to correct acidosis and I.V. corticosteroids, which may improve blood perfusion and increase cardiac output.

Special considerations

• Determine which of your patients are at high risk of developing septic shock. Know the signs of impending septic shock, but don't rely solely on technical aids to judge the patient's status. Consider any change in mental status and urine output as significant as a change in CVP.

- Carefully maintain the pulmonary artery catheter. Check ABG values for adequate oxygenation or gas exchange, watching for any changes.
- Keep accurate intake and output records. Maintain adequate urine output (0.5 to 1 ml/kg/hour) and systolic pressure. Be careful to avoid fluid overload.
- Monitor serum gentamicin level, and administer drugs.
- Watch closely for complications of septic shock: DIC (abnormal bleeding), renal failure (oliguria, increased specific gravity), heart failure (dyspnea, edema, tachycardia, distended neck veins), GI ulcers (hematemesis, melena), and hepatic abnormalities (jaundice, hypoprothrombinemia, and hypoalbuminemia).

LIFE-THREATENING DISORDER

SEVERE COMBINED IMMUNODEFICIENCY DISEASE

Both cell-mediated (T-cell) and humoral (B-cell) immunity are deficient or absent in severe combined immunodeficiency disease (SCID). This results in susceptibility to infection from all classes of microorganisms during infancy.

At least three types of SCID exist: reticular dysgenesis, the most severe type, in which the hematopoietic stem cell fails to differentiate into lymphocytes and granulocytes; Swiss-type agammaglobulinemia, in which the hematopoietic stem cell fails to differentiate into lymphocytes alone; and enzyme deficiency, such as adenosine deaminase (ADA) deficiency, in which the buildup of toxic products in the lymphoid tissue causes damage and subsequent dysfunction.

SCID affects more males than females; its estimated incidence is 1 in every 100,000 to 500,000 births. Most untreated patients die from infection within 1 year of birth.

Causes

SCID is usually transmitted as an autosomal recessive trait, although it may be X-linked. In most cases, the genetic defect seems associated with failure of the stem cell to differentiate into T and B lymphocytes.

Many molecular defects, such as mutation of the kinase ZAP-70, can cause SCID. X-linked SCID results from a mutation of a subunit of the interleukin-2 (IL-2), IL-4, and IL-7 receptors. Less commonly, it results from an enzyme deficiency.

Signs and symptoms

An extreme susceptibility to infection becomes obvious in the infant with SCID in the first months of life. The infant fails to thrive and develops chronic otitis, sepsis, watery diarrhea (associated with *Salmonella* or *Escherichia coli*), recurrent pulmonary infections (usually caused by *Pseudomonas*, cytomegalovirus, or *Pneumocystis carinii*), persistent oral candidiasis, (sometimes with esophageal erosions), and possibly fatal viral infections (such as chickenpox).

P. carinii pneumonia usually strikes a severely immunodeficient infant in the first 3 to 5 weeks of life. Onset is typically insidious, with gradually worsening cough, low-grade fever, tachypnea, and respiratory distress. A chest X-ray characteristically shows bilateral pulmonary infiltrates.

Diagnosis

Clinical indications point to the diagnosis. Most infants with SCID suffer recurrent overwhelming infections within 1 year of birth. Some are diagnosed after a severe reaction to vaccination.

Defective humoral immunity is difficult to detect before an infant is 5 months old. Before age 5 months, even normal infants have very small amounts of the serum immunoglobulins (Ig) IgM and IgA, and normal IgG levels merely reflect maternal IgG. However, severely diminished or absent T-cell number and function and lymph node biopsy showing absence of lymphocytes can confirm the diagnosis of SCID.

Treatment

Restoring immune response and preventing infection are the first goals of treatment. Histocompatible bone marrow transplant is the only satisfactory treatment available to correct immunodeficiency.

Because bone marrow cells must be matched according to human leukocyte antigen and mixed leukocyte culture, the most common donors are histocompatible siblings. But bone marrow transplant can produce a potentially fatal graft-versus-host (GVH) reaction, so newer methods of bone marrow transplant that eliminate GVH reaction (such as lectin separation and the use of monoclonal antibodies) are being evaluated.

Fetal thymus and liver transplants have achieved limited success. Administration of immune globulin may also play a role in treatment. Some SCID infants have received long-term protection by being isolated in a completely sterile environment. However, this approach isn't effective if the infant already has had recurring infections.

Gene therapy is being used for ADA deficiency.

Special considerations

• Constantly monitor the infant for early signs of infection; if infection develops, provide prompt and aggressive drug therapy.
• Watch for adverse effects of any medications given. Avoid vaccinations, and give only irradiated blood products if the patient needs a transfusion.
• Explain all procedures, medications, and precautions to the parents.
• Although SCID infants must remain in strict protective isolation, try to provide a stimulating atmosphere to promote growth and development. Encourage parents to visit their child often, to hold him, and to bring him toys that can be easily sterilized.
• Maintain a normal daily and nightly routine, and talk to the child as much as possible. If the parents can't visit, call them often to report on their infant's condition.
• Refer parents for genetic counseling. Refer parents and siblings for psychological and spiritual counseling to help them cope with the child's inevitable long-term illness and early death.
• For assistance in coping with the financial burden of the child's long-term hospitalization, refer the parents to social services.

SICKLE CELL ANEMIA

A congenital hemolytic anemia that occurs primarily, but not exclusively, in blacks, sickle cell anemia results from a defective hemoglobin molecule (hemoglobin S) that causes red blood cells (RBCs) to roughen and become sickle-shaped. Such cells impair circulation, resulting in chronic ill health (fatigue, dyspnea on exertion, swollen joints), periodic crises, long-term complications, and premature death.

INHERITANCE PATTERNS IN SICKLE CELL ANEMIA

■ Sickle cell anemia ■ Sickle cell trait

When both parents have sickle cell anemia, childbearing — if possible at all — is dangerous for the mother, and all offspring will have sickle cell anemia.

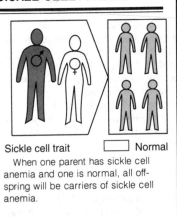

□ Normal

When one parent has sickle cell anemia and one is normal, all offspring will be carriers of sickle cell anemia.

Sickle cell anemia is most common in tropical Africans and in people of African descent; about 1 in 10 blacks carries the abnormal gene. If two such carriers have offspring, there is a 1 in 4 chance that each child will have the disease. (See *Inheritance patterns in sickle cell anemia.*) Overall, 1 in every 400 to 600 black children has sickle cell anemia.

This disease also occurs in Puerto Rico, Turkey, India, the Middle East, and the Mediterranean. The defective hemoglobin S gene may have persisted in areas where malaria is endemic because the heterozygous sickle cell trait provides resistance to malaria and is actually beneficial.

Penicillin prophylaxis can decrease morbidity and mortality from bacterial infections. Half of such patients die by their early twenties; few live to middle age.

Causes

Sickle cell anemia results from homozygous inheritance of the hemoglobin S gene, which causes substitution of the amino acid valine for glutamic

acid in the B hemoglobin chain. Heterozygous inheritance of this gene results in sickle cell trait, usually an asymptomatic condition. (See *Sickle cell trait.*)

Altered cells

The abnormal hemoglobin S found in RBCs of patients with sickle cell anemia becomes insoluble whenever hypoxia occurs. As a result, these RBCs become rigid, rough, and elongated, forming a crescent, or sickle, shape. Such sickling can produce hemolysis (cell destruction).

In addition, these altered cells tend to pile up in capillaries and smaller blood vessels, making the blood more viscous. Normal circulation is impaired, causing pain, tissue infarctions, and swelling. Such blockage causes anoxic changes that lead to further sickling and obstruction.

Signs and symptoms

Characteristically, sickle cell anemia produces tachycardia, cardiomegaly, systolic and diastolic murmurs, pulmonary infarctions (which may result in cor pulmonale), chronic fatigue, unexplained dyspnea or dyspnea on exertion, hepatomegaly, jaundice, pallor, joint swelling, aching bones, chest pains, ischemic leg ulcers (especially around the ankles), and increased susceptibility to infection.

Such symptoms usually don't develop until after age 6 months, because large amounts of fetal hemoglobin protect infants for the first few months after birth. Low socioeconomic status and related problems, such as poor nutrition and education, may delay diagnosis and supportive treatment.

Infection, stress, dehydration, and conditions that provoke hypoxia — strenuous exercise, high altitude, unpressurized aircraft, cold, and vasoconstrictive drugs — may all provoke periodic crisis. Four types of crises can occur.

Painful crisis

Also called a vaso-occlusive crisis or infarctive crisis, painful crisis is the most common crisis and the hallmark of this disease. It usually appears periodically after age 5.

A painful crisis results from blood vessel obstruction by rigid, tangled sickle cells, which causes tissue anoxia and possible necrosis. It's characterized by severe abdominal, thoracic, muscular, or bone pain and possibly increased jaundice, dark urine, or a low-grade fever.

Autosplenectomy, in which splenic damage and scarring is so extensive that the spleen shrinks and becomes impalpable, occurs in patients with long-term disease. This can lead to increased susceptibility to *Streptococcus pneumoniae* sepsis, which can be fatal without prompt treatment.

After the crisis subsides (in 4 days to several weeks), infection may develop, causing such signs as lethargy, sleepiness, fever, and apathy.

SICKLE CELL TRAIT

This relatively benign condition results from heterozygous inheritance of the abnormal hemoglobin S gene. Like sickle cell anemia, this condition is most common in blacks. Sickle cell trait *never* progresses to sickle cell anemia.

In persons with sickle cell trait (also called carriers), 20% to 40% of their total hemoglobin is hemoglobin S; the rest is normal.

Such carriers usually have no symptoms. They have normal hemoglobin and hematocrit values and can expect a normal life span. Nevertheless, they must avoid situations that provoke hypoxia, because these occasionally cause a sickling crisis similar to that in sickle cell anemia.

Genetic counseling is essential for sickle cell carriers. If two sickle cell carriers marry, each of their children has a 25% chance of inheriting sickle cell anemia.

Aplastic crisis

Also called megaloblastic crisis, aplastic crisis results from bone marrow depression and is associated with infection, usually viral. It's characterized by pallor, lethargy, sleepiness, dyspnea, possible coma, markedly decreased bone marrow activity, and RBC hemolysis.

Acute sequestration crisis

In infants between 8 months and 2 years old, an acute sequestration crisis may cause sudden massive entrapment of RBCs in the spleen and liver. This rare crisis causes lethargy and pallor; if untreated, it commonly progresses to hypovolemic shock and death.

Hemolytic crisis

Quite rare, hemolytic crisis usually occurs in patients who have glucose-6-phosphate dehydrogenase deficiency with sickle cell anemia. It probably results from complications of sickle cell anemia, such as infection, rather than from the disorder itself.

Hemolytic crisis causes liver congestion and hepatomegaly as a result of degenerative changes. It worsens chronic jaundice, although increased jaundice doesn't always point to a hemolytic crisis.

Indicators of crisis

Suspect any of these crises in a sickle cell anemia patient with pale lips, tongue, palms, or nail beds; lethargy; listlessness; sleepiness, with difficulty awakening; irritability; severe pain; temperature over 104° F (40° C); or a fever of 100° F (37.8° C) that persists for 2 days.

Long-term complications

Sickle cell anemia also causes long-term complications. Typically, such a child is small for his age, and puberty is delayed. (However, fertility isn't impaired.) If he reaches adulthood, his body build tends to be spiderlike — narrow shoulders and hips, long extremities, curved spine, barrel chest, and elongated skull.

An adult usually has complications from organ infarction, such as retinopathy and nephropathy. Premature death commonly results from infection or repeated occlusion of small blood vessels and consequent infarction or necrosis of major organs. For example, cerebral blood vessel occlusion causes cerebrovascular accident.

Diagnosis

A positive family history and typical clinical features suggest sickle cell anemia. Hemoglobin electrophoresis showing hemoglobin S or other hemoglobinopathies can confirm it. Electrophoresis should be done on umbilical cord blood samples at birth to provide sickle cell disease screening for all newborns at risk.

Additional laboratory studies show a low RBC count, elevated white blood cell and platelet counts, decreased erythrocyte sedimentation rate, increased serum iron level, decreased RBC survival, and reticulocytosis. Hemoglobin may be low or normal.

During early childhood, palpation may reveal splenomegaly, but as the child grows older, the spleen shrinks.

Treatment

Prophylactic penicillin is given before age 4 months. If the patient's hemoglobin drops suddenly or if his condition deteriorates rapidly, a transfusion of packed RBCs is needed.

In a sequestration crisis, treatment may include sedation, administration of analgesics, blood transfusion, oxygen administration, and large amounts of oral or I.V. fluids. A good antisickling agent isn't yet available; the most commonly used drug, sodium cyanate, has many adverse effects.

Special considerations

During a painful crisis:
- Apply warm compresses to painful areas, and cover the child with a blanket. (Never use cold compresses; this aggravates the condition.)
- Administer an analgesic-antipyretic, such as aspirin or acetaminophen.
- Encourage bed rest, and place the patient in a sitting position. If dehydration or severe pain occurs, hospitalization may be necessary.
- Give antibiotics when appropriate.
  During remission:
- Advise the patient to avoid tight clothing that restricts circulation.
- Warn against strenuous exercise, vasoconstricting medications, cold temperatures (including drinking large

amounts of ice water and swimming), unpressurized aircraft, high altitude, and other conditions that provoke hypoxia.

• Stress the importance of normal childhood immunizations, meticulous wound care, good oral hygiene, regular dental checkups, and a balanced diet as safeguards against infection.

• Emphasize the need for prompt treatment of infection.

• Stress the need to increase fluid intake to prevent dehydration resulting from impaired ability to concentrate urine. Tell parents to encourage such a child to drink more fluids, especially in the summer, by offering milk shakes, ice pops, and eggnog.

• To encourage normal mental and social development, warn parents against being overprotective. Although the child must avoid strenuous exercise, he can enjoy most everyday activities.

• Refer parents of children with sickle cell anemia for genetic counseling to answer their questions about the risk to future offspring. Recommend screening of other family members to determine if they're heterozygote carriers. These parents may also need psychological counseling to cope with guilt feelings. In addition, suggest they join an appropriate community support group.

During pregnancy or surgery:

• Warn women with sickle cell anemia that they're poor obstetrical risks. However, their use of oral contraceptives is also risky; refer them for birth control counseling by a gynecologist. If such women *do* become pregnant, they should maintain a balanced diet and may benefit from a folic acid supplement.

• During general anesthesia, make sure the patient has optimal ventilation to prevent hypoxic crisis. Provide a preoperative transfusion of packed RBCs as needed.

• If the patient is an adolescent or adult male, warn him that he may have sudden, painful episodes of priapism. Explain that such episodes are common and, if prolonged, can have serious reproductive consequences. Advise the patient to report the occurrence of such episodes.

SIDEROBLASTIC ANEMIAS

This group of heterogenous disorders produces a common defect—failure to use iron in hemoglobin synthesis, despite the availability of adequate iron stores. These anemias may be hereditary or acquired; the acquired form, in turn, can be primary or secondary.

Hereditary sideroblastic anemia often responds to treatment with pyridoxine. Correction of the secondary acquired form depends on the causative disorder; the primary acquired (idiopathic) form, however, resists treatment and usually proves fatal within 10 years after onset of complications or a concomitant disease.

Causes

Hereditary sideroblastic anemia appears to be transmitted by X-linked inheritance, occurring mostly in young males; females are carriers and usually show no signs of this disorder.

The acquired form may be secondary to ingestion of, or exposure to, toxins, such as alcohol and lead, or to drugs, such as isoniazid and chloramphenicol. It can also occur as a complication of other diseases, such as rheumatoid arthritis, lupus erythematosus, multiple myeloma, tuberculosis, and severe infections.

The primary acquired form, known as refractory anemia with ringed sideroblasts, is most common in elderly people. It's often associated with thrombocytopenia or leukopenia as part of a myelodysplastic syndrome.

In sideroblastic anemia, normoblasts fail to use iron to synthesize hemoglobin. As a result, iron is deposited in the mitochondria of normoblasts, which are then termed ringed sideroblasts.

Signs and symptoms
Sideroblastic anemias usually produce nonspecific clinical effects, which may exist for several years before being identified. Such effects include anorexia, fatigue, weakness, dizziness, pale skin and mucous membranes and, occasionally, enlarged lymph nodes.

Heart and liver failure may develop from excessive iron accumulation in these organs, causing dyspnea, exertional angina, slight jaundice, and hepatosplenomegaly. Hereditary sideroblastic anemia is associated with increased GI absorption of iron, causing signs of hemosiderosis. Additional symptoms in secondary sideroblastic anemia depend on the underlying cause.

Diagnosis
Ringed sideroblasts on microscopic examination of bone marrow aspirate, stained with Prussian blue or alizarin red dye, confirm the diagnosis.

Microscopic examination of blood shows hypochromic or normochromic, and slightly macrocytic erythrocytes. Red blood cell (RBC) precursors may be megaloblastic, with anisocytosis (abnormal variation in RBC size) and poikilocytosis (abnormal variation in RBC shape).

Unlike iron deficiency anemia, sideroblastic anemia lowers hemoglobin and raises serum iron and transferrin levels. In turn, faulty hemoglobin production raises urobilinogen and bilirubin levels. Platelet and leukocyte levels remain normal, but thrombocytopenia or leukopenia occasionally occurs.

Treatment
The underlying cause determines the type of treatment.

Hereditary form
Hereditary sideroblastic anemia usually responds to several weeks of treatment with high doses of pyridoxine (vitamin B_6).

Primary acquired form
Elderly patients with sideroblastic anemia — most commonly the primary acquired form — are less likely to improve quickly and are more likely to develop serious complications. Deferoxamine may be used to treat chronic iron overload in selected patients.

Carefully cross-matched transfusions (providing needed hemoglobin) or high doses of androgens are effective palliative measures for some patients with the primary acquired form of sideroblastic anemia. However, this form is essentially refractory to treatment and usually leads to death from acute leukemia or from respiratory or cardiac complications.

Some patients with sideroblastic anemia may benefit from phlebotomy to prevent hemochromatosis. Phlebotomy steps up the rate of erythropoiesis and uses up excess iron stores; thus, it reduces serum and total-body iron levels.

Secondary acquired form
The acquired secondary form generally subsides after the causative drug or toxin is removed or the underlying condition is adequately treated. Folic acid supplements may also be beneficial when concomitant megaloblastic nuclear changes in RBC precursors are present.

Special considerations

• Administer medications as needed. Teach the patient the importance of continuing prescribed therapy, even after he begins to feel better.

• Provide frequent rest periods if the patient becomes easily fatigued.

• If phlebotomy is scheduled, explain the procedure thoroughly to help reduce anxiety. If this procedure must be repeated frequently, provide a high-protein diet to help replace the protein lost during phlebotomy. Encourage the patient to follow a similar diet at home.

• Always inquire about the possibility of exposure to lead in the home (especially for children) or on the job.

• Identify patients who abuse alcohol; refer them for appropriate therapy.

SILICOSIS

A progressive disease characterized by nodular lesions, silicosis frequently progresses to fibrosis. It's the most common form of pneumoconiosis.

Silicosis can be classified according to the severity of pulmonary disease and the rapidity of its onset and progression; it usually occurs as a simple asymptomatic illness.

Acute silicosis develops after 1 to 3 years in workers (sandblasters, tunnel workers) exposed to very high concentrations of respirable silica. Accelerated silicosis appears after an average of 10 years of exposure to lower concentrations of free silica. Chronic silicosis develops after 20 or more years of exposure to lower concentrations of free silica.

The prognosis is good, unless the disease progresses into the complicated fibrotic form, which causes respiratory insufficiency and cor pulmonale and is associated with pulmonary tuberculosis.

Causes

Silicosis results from the inhalation and pulmonary deposition of respirable crystalline silica dust, mostly from quartz.

The danger to the worker depends on the concentration of dust in the atmosphere, the percentage of respirable free silica particles in the dust, and the duration of exposure. Respirable particles are less than 10 microns in diameter, but the disease-causing particles deposited in the alveolar space are usually 1 to 3 microns in diameter.

Industrial sources of silica in its pure form include the manufacture of ceramics (flint) and building materials (sandstone). It occurs in mixed form in the production of construction materials (cement); it's found in powder form (silica flour) in paints, porcelain, scouring soaps, and wood fillers and in the mining of gold, coal, lead, zinc, and iron.

Foundry workers, boiler scalers, and stonecutters are all exposed to silica dust. All are at high risk of developing silicosis.

Pathophysiology

Nodules result when alveolar macrophages ingest silica particles, which they are unable to process. As a result, the macrophages die and release proteolytic enzymes into the surrounding tissue. The subsequent inflammation attracts other macrophages and fibroblasts into the region to produce fibrous tissue and wall off the reaction.

The resulting nodule has an onion-skin appearance when viewed under a microscope. Nodules develop adjacent to terminal and respiratory bronchioles, concentrate in the upper lobes, and are frequently accompanied by bullous changes throughout both lungs.

If the disease doesn't progress, minimal physiologic disturbances occur, with no disability. Occasionally, however, the fibrotic response accelerates, engulfing and destroying large areas of the lung (progressive massive fibrosis or conglomerate lesions). Fibrosis may continue despite termination of exposure to dust.

Signs and symptoms

Silicosis initially may be asymptomatic or it may produce dyspnea on exertion, often attributed to being "out of shape" or "slowing down."

Progressive features

If the disease progresses to the chronic and complicated stage, dyspnea on exertion worsens, and other signs—usually tachypnea and an insidious, dry cough that's most pronounced in the morning—appear. Progression to the advanced stage causes dyspnea on minimal exertion, worsening cough, and pulmonary hypertension, which in turn leads to right ventricular failure and cor pulmonale.

Patients with silicosis have a high incidence of active tuberculosis, which should be considered when evaluating a patient with this disease. Central nervous system changes—confusion, lethargy, and a decrease in the rate and depth of respiration as partial pressure of carbon dioxide increases—also occur in advanced silicosis.

Other features

Other clinical features include malaise, disturbed sleep, and hoarseness.

Note: The severity of these symptoms may not correlate with chest X-ray findings or the results of pulmonary function studies.

Diagnosis

Patient history reveals occupational exposure to silica dust. Physical examination is normal in simple silicosis; in chronic silicosis with conglomerate lesions, it may reveal decreased chest expansion, diminished intensity of breath sounds, areas of hy-

poresonance and hyperresonance, fine to medium crackles, and tachypnea.

In simple silicosis, chest X-rays show small, discrete, nodular lesions distributed throughout both lung fields but typically concentrated in the upper lung zones; the hilar lung nodes may be enlarged and exhibit "eggshell" calcification. In complicated silicosis, X-rays show one or more conglomerate masses of dense tissue.

Pulmonary function studies yield the following results:

• *Forced vital capacity (FVC)* is reduced in complicated silicosis.

• *Forced expiratory volume in 1 second (FEV$_1$)* is reduced in obstructive disease (emphysematous areas of silicosis); it's also reduced in complicated silicosis, but the ratio of FEV$_1$ to FVC is normal or high.

• *Maximum voluntary ventilation* is reduced in both restrictive and obstructive diseases.

• *Diffusing capacity of the lung for carbon monoxide* is reduced when fibrosis destroys alveolar walls and obliterates pulmonary capillaries or when fibrosis thickens the alveolar capillary membrane.

In addition, arterial blood gas studies show the following:

• *Partial pressure of oxygen* is normal in simple silicosis; it may be significantly decreased when the patient breathes room air in the late stages of chronic or complicated disease.

• *Partial pressure of carbon dioxide* is normal in early stages but may decrease because of hyperventilation; it may increase as a restrictive pattern develops, particularly if the patient is hypoxic and has severe impairment of alveolar ventilation.

Treatment

The goal of treatment is to relieve respiratory symptoms, to manage hypoxia and cor pulmonale, and to prevent respiratory tract irritation and infections. Treatment also includes careful observation for the development of tuberculosis.

Respiratory symptoms may be relieved through daily use of bronchodilating aerosols and increased fluid intake (at least 3 L daily). Steam inhalation and chest physiotherapy techniques, such as controlled coughing and segmental bronchial drainage with chest percussion and vibration, help clear secretions.

In severe cases, oxygen may be administered by cannula or mask (1 to 2 L/minute) for the patient with chronic hypoxia or by mechanical ventilation if arterial oxygen can't be maintained above 40 mm Hg. Respiratory infections require prompt administration of antibiotics.

Special considerations
• Teach the patient to prevent infections by avoiding crowds and people with respiratory infections and by receiving influenza and pneumococcal vaccines.
• Increase the patient's exercise tolerance by encouraging regular activity. Advise the patient to plan his daily activities to decrease the work of breathing; he should pace himself, rest often, and generally move slowly through his daily routine.

SINUSITIS

Inflammation of the paranasal sinuses may be acute, subacute, chronic, allergic, or hyperplastic.

Acute sinusitis usually results from the common cold and lingers in subacute form in only about 10% of patients. Chronic sinusitis follows persistent bacterial infection; allergic sinusitis accompanies allergic rhinitis; hyperplastic sinusitis is a combination of purulent acute sinusitis and allergic sinusitis or rhinitis.

The prognosis is good for all types.

Causes
Sinusitis usually results from viral or bacterial infection. The bacteria responsible for acute sinusitis are usually pneumococci, other streptococci, *Haemophilus influenzae,* and *Moraxella catarrhalis.* Staphylococci and gram-negative bacteria are more likely to occur in chronic cases or in patients in intensive care.

Predisposing factors include any condition that interferes with drainage and ventilation of the sinuses, such as chronic nasal edema, deviated septum, viscous mucus, nasal polyps, allergic rhinitis, nasal intubation, or debilitation related to chemotherapy, malnutrition, diabetes, blood dyscrasias, chronic use of steroids, or immunodeficiency.

Bacterial invasion commonly occurs from the conditions listed above or after a viral infection. It may also result from swimming in contaminated water.

Signs and symptoms
Features vary with sinusitis type.

Acute sinusitis
The primary symptom of acute sinusitis is nasal congestion, followed by a gradual buildup of pressure in the affected sinus. For 24 to 48 hours after onset, nasal discharge may be present and later may become purulent. Associated symptoms include malaise, sore throat, headache, and low-grade fever (temperature of 99° to 99.5° F [37.2° to 37.5° C]).

Characteristic pain depends on the affected sinus: maxillary sinusitis causes pain over the cheeks and upper teeth; ethmoid sinusitis, pain over the eyes; frontal sinusitis, pain over the eyebrows; and sphenoid sinusitis (rare), pain behind the eyes.

Subacute sinusitis

Purulent nasal drainage that continues for longer than 3 weeks after an acute infection subsides suggests subacute sinusitis. Other clinical features of the subacute form include a stuffy nose, vague facial discomfort, fatigue, and a nonproductive cough.

Other types

The effects of chronic sinusitis are similar to those of acute sinusitis, but the chronic form causes continuous mucopurulent discharge.

The effects of allergic sinusitis are the same as those of allergic rhinitis. In both conditions, the prominent symptoms are sneezing, frontal headache, watery nasal discharge, and a stuffy, burning, itchy nose.

In hyperplastic sinusitis, bacterial growth on the diseased tissue causes pronounced tissue edema. Thickening of the mucosal lining, as well as the development of mucosal polyps, combine to produce chronic stuffiness of the nose in addition to headaches.

Diagnosis

The following measures are useful:
• *Nasal examination* reveals inflammation and pus.
• *Sinus X-rays* reveal cloudiness in the affected sinus, air and fluid, and any thickening of the mucosal lining.
• *Antral puncture* promotes drainage of purulent material. It may also be used to provide a specimen for culture and sensitivity testing of the infecting organism but is rarely done.
• *Ultrasonography* and *computed tomography (CT) scan* aid in diagnosing suspected complications. CT scans are more sensitive than routine X-rays in detecting sinusitis.

Treatment

Effective treatment depends on the type of sinusitis.

Acute sinusitis

In acute sinusitis, local decongestants usually are tried before systemic decongestants; steam inhalation may also be helpful. Local application of heat may help to relieve pain and congestion.

Antibiotics are necessary to combat purulent or persistent infection. Amoxicillin, ampicillin, and amoxicillin-clavulanate potassium are usually the antibiotics of choice. Sinusitis is a deep-seated infection, so antibiotics should be given for 2 to 3 weeks.

Subacute sinusitis

In subacute sinusitis, antibiotics and decongestants may be helpful.

Other types

Treatment of allergic sinusitis must include treatment of allergic rhinitis — administration of antihistamines, identification of allergens by skin testing, and desensitization by immunotherapy. Severe allergic symptoms may require treatment with corticosteroids and epinephrine.

In both chronic sinusitis and hyperplastic sinusitis, antihistamines, antibiotics, and a steroid nasal spray may relieve pain and congestion. If irrigation fails to relieve symptoms, one or more sinuses may require surgery. (See *Surgery for chronic and hyperplastic sinusitis.*)

Special considerations

• Enforce bed rest, and encourage the patient to drink plenty of fluids to promote drainage. Don't elevate the head of the bed more than 30 degrees.
• To relieve pain and promote drainage, apply warm compresses continuously, or four times daily for 2-hour intervals. In addition, give analgesics and antihistamines as needed.
• Watch for complications, such as vomiting, chills, fever, edema of the

SURGERY FOR CHRONIC AND HYPERPLASTIC SINUSITIS

For maxillary sinusitis
• *Nasal window procedure* creates an opening in the sinus, allowing secretions and pus to drain through the nose.
• *Caldwell-Luc procedure* removes diseased mucosa in the maxillary sinus through an incision under the upper lip.

For chronic ethmoid sinusitis
• *Ethmoidectomy* removes all infected tissue through an external or intranasal incision into the ethmoidal sinus.

For sphenoid sinusitis
• *External ethmoidectomy* removes infected ethmoidal sinus tissue through a crescent-shaped incision, beginning under the inner eyebrow and extending along the side of the nose.

For chronic frontal sinusitis
• *Frontoethmoidectomy* removes infected frontal sinus tissue through an extended external ethmoidectomy.
• *Osteoplastic flap* drains the sinuses through an incision across the skull, behind the hairline.

---

forehead or eyelids, blurred or double vision, and personality changes.
• If surgery is necessary, tell the patient what to expect postoperatively: A nasal packing will be in place for 12 to 24 hours after surgery, he'll have to breathe through his mouth, and he won't be able to blow his nose. After surgery, monitor for excessive drainage or bleeding and watch for complications.
• To prevent edema and promote drainage, place the patient in semi-Fowler's position. To relieve edema and pain and to minimize bleeding, apply ice compresses or a rubber glove filled with ice chips over the nose and iced saline gauze over the eyes. Continue these measures for 24 hours.
• Frequently change the mustache dressing or drip pad, and record the consistency, amount, and color of drainage (expect scant, bright red, and clotty drainage).
• Because the patient will be breathing through his mouth, provide meticulous mouth care.
• Tell the patient that even after the packing is removed, nose blowing may cause bleeding and swelling. If the patient is a smoker, instruct him not to smoke for at least 2 or 3 days after surgery.
• Instruct the patient to finish the prescribed antibiotics, even if his symptoms disappear.

SJÖGREN'S SYNDROME

The second most common autoimmune rheumatic disorder after rheumatoid arthritis (RA), Sjögren's syndrome (SS) is characterized by diminished lacrimal and salivary gland secretion (sicca complex). SS occurs mainly in women (90% of patients); its mean age of occurrence is 50.

SS may be a primary disorder or may be associated with a connective tissue disorder, such as RA, scleroderma, systemic lupus erythematosus, or polymyositis. In some patients, the disorder is limited to the exocrine glands (glandular SS); in others, it also involves other organs, such as the lungs and kidneys (extraglandular SS).

Causes

The cause of SS is unknown. Most likely, both genetic and environmental factors contribute to its development. Viral or bacterial infection or perhaps exposure to pollen may trigger SS in a genetically susceptible individual.

Tissue damage results from infiltration by lymphocytes or from the deposition of immune complexes. Lymphocytic infiltration may be classified as benign lymphoma, malignant lymphoma, or pseudolymphoma (nonmalignant, but tumorlike aggregates of lymphoid cells).

Signs and symptoms

About 50% of patients with SS have confirmed RA and a history of slowly developing sicca complex. However, some seek medical help for rapidly progressive and severe oral and ocular dryness, often accompanied by periodic parotid gland enlargement.

Ocular effects

Ocular dryness (xerophthalmia) leads to foreign body sensation (gritty, sandy eye), redness, burning, photosensitivity, eye fatigue, itching, and mucoid discharge. The patient may also complain of a film across his field of vision.

Oral effects

Oral dryness (xerostomia) leads to difficulty swallowing and talking; abnormal taste or smell sensation, or both; thirst; ulcers of the tongue, buccal mucosa, and lips (especially at the corners of the mouth); and severe dental caries. Dryness of the respiratory tract leads to epistaxis, hoarseness, chronic nonproductive cough, recurrent otitis media, and increased incidence of respiratory infections.

Other features

Other effects may include dyspareunia and pruritus (associated with vaginal dryness), generalized itching, fatigue, recurrent low-grade fever, and arthralgia or myalgia. Lymph node enlargement may be the first sign of malignant lymphoma or pseudolymphoma.

Specific extraglandular findings in SS include interstitial pneumonitis; interstitial nephritis, which results in renal tubular acidosis in 25% of patients; Raynaud's phenomenon (20%); and vasculitis, usually limited to the skin and characterized by palpable purpura on the legs (20%).

About 50% of patients show evidence of hypothyroidism related to autoimmune thyroid disease. A few patients develop systemic necrotizing vasculitis.

Diagnosis

A patient with SS has at least two of the following three conditions: xerophthalmia, xerostomia (with a salivary gland biopsy showing lymphocytic infiltration), and an associated autoimmune or lymphoproliferative disorder.

Tests to rule out other causes

Diagnosis must rule out other causes of oral and ocular dryness, including sarcoidosis, endocrine disorders, anxiety or depression, and effects of therapy, such as radiation to the head and neck. Over 200 commonly used drugs also produce dry mouth.

In patients with salivary gland enlargement and severe lymphoid infiltration, the diagnosis must rule out cancer.

Laboratory tests

Laboratory values include an elevated erythrocyte sedimentation rate in most patients, mild anemia and leukopenia in 30%, and hypergammaglobulinemia in 50%. Autoantibodies are also common, including SSA (anti-Ro) and SSB (anti-La), which are antinuclear and antisalivary duct antibodies. From 75% to 90% of patients test positive for rheumatoid factor; 90%, for antinuclear antibodies.

Other tests
Other tests help support this diagnosis. Schirmer's tearing test and slit-lamp examination with rose bengal dye are used to measure eye involvement. Salivary gland involvement is evaluated by measuring the volume of parotid saliva and by secretory sialography and salivary scintigraphy. A lower lip biopsy shows salivary gland infiltration by lymphocytes.

Treatment
Usually symptomatic, treatment includes conservative measures to relieve ocular or oral dryness.

Symptomatic treatment
Mouth dryness can be relieved by using a methylcellulose swab or spray and by drinking plenty of fluids, especially at meals. Meticulous oral hygiene is essential, including regular flossing, brushing, and fluoride treatment at home and frequent dental checkups.

Instillation of artificial tears as often as every half hour prevents eye damage (corneal ulcerations, corneal opacifications) from insufficient tear secretion. Some patients may also benefit from instillation of an eye ointment at bedtime, or from twice-a-day sustained-release cellulose capsules.

If an eye infection develops, antibiotics should be given immediately; topical steroids should be avoided.

Other measures
Other treatment measures vary with associated extraglandular findings. Parotid gland enlargement requires local heat and analgesics; pulmonary and renal interstitial disease, corticosteroids; accompanying lymphoma, a combination of chemotherapy, surgery, and radiation.

Special considerations
• Advise the patient to avoid drugs that decrease saliva production, such as atropine derivatives, antihistamines, anticholinergics, and antidepressants.
• If mouth lesions make eating painful, suggest high-protein, high-calorie liquid supplements to prevent malnutrition. Advise the patient to avoid sugar, which contributes to dental caries, and tobacco, alcohol, and spicy, salty, or highly acidic foods, which cause mouth irritation.
• Suggest the use of sunglasses to protect the patient's eyes from dust, wind, and strong light. Moisture chamber spectacles may also be helpful.
• Because dry eyes are more susceptible to infection, advise the patient to keep his face clean and to avoid rubbing his eyes.
• To help relieve respiratory dryness, stress the need to humidify home and work environments. Suggest normal saline solution drops or aerosolized spray for nasal dryness. Advise the patient to avoid prolonged hot showers and baths and to use moisturizing lotions to help ease dry skin. Suggest using a vaginal lubricant.
• Refer the patient to the Sjögren's Syndrome Foundation for additional information and support.

LIFE-THREATENING DISORDER

SKULL FRACTURES

Because possible damage to the brain is the first concern, rather than the fracture itself, a skull fracture is considered a neurosurgical condition. Skull fractures may be simple (closed) or compound (open) and may or may not displace bone fragments.

Skull fractures are further described as linear, comminuted, or depressed. A linear fracture is a common hairline break, without displacement of structures; a comminuted fracture splinters or crushes the bone into several fragments; a depressed fracture pushes the bone toward the brain.

In children, the skull's thinness and elasticity allow a depression without a fracture (a linear fracture across a suture line increases the possibility of epidural hematoma).

Skull fractures are also classified according to location, such as a cranial vault fracture; a basilar fracture is at the base of the skull and involves the cribriform plate and the frontal sinuses. Because of the danger of grave cranial complications and meningitis, basilar fractures are usually far more serious than vault fractures.

Causes

Like concussions and cerebral contusions or lacerations, skull fractures invariably result from a traumatic blow to the head. Motor vehicle accidents, bad falls, and severe beatings (especially in children) top the list of causes.

Signs and symptoms

Skull fractures are often accompanied by scalp wounds — abrasions, contusions, lacerations, or avulsions. If the scalp has been lacerated or torn away, bleeding may be profuse because the scalp contains many blood vessels.

Bleeding can occasionally be heavy enough to induce hypovolemic shock. The patient may also be in shock from other injuries or from medullary failure in severe head injuries.

Linear fractures that are associated only with concussion don't produce loss of consciousness. They require evaluation, but not definitive treatment.

A fracture that results in cerebral contusion or laceration, however, may cause the classic signs of brain injury: agitation and irritability, loss of consciousness, changes in respiratory pattern (labored respirations), abnormal deep tendon reflexes, and altered pupillary and motor response.

If the patient with a skull fracture remains conscious, he's apt to complain of a persistent, localized headache. A skull fracture also may result in cerebral edema, which may cause compression of the reticular activating system, cutting off the normal flow of impulses to the brain and resulting in possible respiratory distress. The patient may experience an altered level of consciousness (LOC), progressing to unconsciousness or even death.

When jagged bone fragments pierce the dura mater or the cerebral cortex, skull fractures may cause subdural, epidural, or intracerebral hemorrhage or hematoma. With the resulting space-occupying lesions, clinical findings may include hemiparesis, unequal pupils, dizziness, seizures, projectile vomiting, decreased pulse and respiratory rates, and progressive unresponsiveness.

Sphenoidal fractures may also damage the optic nerve, causing blindness. Temporal fractures may cause unilateral deafness or facial paralysis.

Symptoms reflect the severity and extent of the head injury. However, some elderly patients may have cortical brain atrophy, with more space for brain swelling under the cranium, and consequently may not show signs of increased intracranial pressure (ICP) until it's very high.

A vault fracture often produces soft-tissue swelling near the fracture, making it hard to detect without a computed tomography (CT) scan.

A basilar fracture often produces hemorrhage from the nose, pharynx, or ears; blood under the periorbital skin ("raccoon's eyes") and under the conjunctiva; and Battle's sign (supramastoid ecchymosis), sometimes with bleeding behind the eardrum. This type of fracture may also cause cerebrospinal fluid (CSF) or even brain tissue to leak from the nose or ears.

Depending on the extent of brain damage, the patient with a skull fracture may suffer residual effects, such as seizure disorders (epilepsy), hydrocephalus, and organic brain syndrome. Children may develop headaches, giddiness, easy fatigability, neuroses, and behavior disorders.

Diagnosis

Suspect brain injury in all patients with a skull fracture until clinical evaluation proves otherwise. Every suspected skull injury calls for a thorough history of the trauma and a CT scan to attempt to locate the fracture. (Keep in mind that vault fractures often aren't visible or palpable.)

A fracture also requires a neurologic examination to check cerebral function (mental status and orientation to time, place, and person), LOC, pupillary response, motor function, and deep tendon reflexes.

Using reagent strips, the draining nasal or ear fluid should be tested for CSF. The tape will turn blue if CSF is present; it won't change in the presence of blood alone. However, the tape will also turn blue if the patient is hyperglycemic.

The patient's bedsheets may show the halo sign — a blood-tinged spot surrounded by a lighter ring — from leakage of CSF.

Brain damage can be assessed through a CT scan and magnetic resonance imaging, which disclose intracranial hemorrhage from ruptured blood vessels and swelling. Expanding lesions contraindicate lumbar puncture.

Treatment

Effective treatment depends on the type and severity of the fracture.

Linear fractures

Although occasionally even a simple linear skull fracture can tear an underlying blood vessel or cause a CSF leak, linear fractures generally require only supportive treatment, including mild analgesics (such as acetaminophen), and cleaning and debridement of any wounds after injection of a local anesthetic.

If the patient with a skull fracture hasn't lost consciousness, he should be observed in the emergency room for at least 4 hours. After this observation period, if vital signs are stable and if the neurosurgeon concurs, the patient can be discharged. At this time, the patient should be given an instruction sheet to follow for 24 to 48 hours of observation at home.

Vault and basilar fractures

More severe vault fractures, especially depressed fractures, usually require a craniotomy to elevate or remove fragments that have been driven into the brain and to extract foreign bodies and necrotic tissue, thereby reducing the risk of infection and further brain damage. Other treatments for severe vault fractures include antibiotic therapy and, in profound hemorrhage, blood transfusions.

Basilar fractures call for immediate prophylactic antibiotics to prevent the onset of meningitis from CSF leaks as well as close observation for secondary hematomas and hemorrhages. Surgery may be necessary.

In addition, basilar and vault fractures often require dexamethasone I.V. or I.M. to reduce cerebral edema and minimize brain tissue damage.

Special considerations

• Establish and maintain a patent airway; nasal airways are contraindicated in patients with possible basilar skull fractures. Intubation may be necessary.

• Suction the patient through the mouth, not the nose, to prevent the introduction of bacteria in case a CSF leak is present.

• Be sure to obtain a complete history of the trauma from the patient, his family, any eyewitnesses, and ambulance personnel.

• Ask whether the patient lost consciousness and, if so, for how long. The patient will need further diagnostic tests, including a complete neurologic examination, a CT scan, and other studies.

• Check for abnormal reflexes such as Babinski's reflex.

• Look for CSF draining from the patient's ears, nose, or mouth. Check bedlinens for CSF leaks and look for a halo sign. If the patient's nose is draining CSF, wipe it — *don't let him blow it.* If an ear is draining, cover it lightly with sterile gauze — *don't pack it.*

• Position the patient with a head injury so secretions can drain properly. Elevate the head of the bed 30 degrees if intracerebral injury is suspected.

• Cover scalp wounds carefully with a sterile dressing; control any bleeding as necessary.

• Take seizure precautions, but don't restrain the patient. Agitated behavior may stem from hypoxia or increased ICP, so check for these symptoms. Speak in a calm, reassuring voice, and touch the patient gently. Don't make any sudden, unexpected moves.

• Don't give the patient narcotics or sedatives because they may depress respirations, increase carbon dioxide levels, lead to increased ICP, and mask changes in neurologic status. Give acetaminophen or another mild analgesic for pain.

When a skull fracture requires surgery:

• Obtain consent, as needed, to shave the patient's head. Explain that you're performing this procedure to provide a clean area for surgery. Type and crossmatch blood. Obtain baseline laboratory studies, such as a complete blood count, serum electrolyte studies, and urinalysis.

• After surgery, monitor vital signs and neurologic status frequently (usually every 5 minutes until the patient is stable, and then every 15 minutes for 1 hour), watching for any changes in LOC. Because skull fractures and brain injuries heal slowly, don't expect dramatic postoperative improvement.

• Monitor intake and output frequently, and maintain patency of the indwelling urinary catheter. Take special care with fluid intake. Hypotonic fluids (even dextrose 5% in water) can increase cerebral edema. Their use should be restricted; give them only as needed.

• If the patient is unconscious, provide parenteral nutrition. (Remember, the patient may regurgitate and aspirate food if you use a nasogastric tube for feedings.)

If the fracture doesn't require surgery:

• Wear sterile gloves to examine the scalp laceration. With your finger, probe the wound for foreign bodies and a palpable fracture. Gently clean lacerations and the surrounding area. Cover with sterile gauze. The patient may need suturing.

• Provide emotional support for the patient and his family. Explain the need for procedures to reduce the risk of brain injury.

• Before discharge, instruct the patient's family to watch closely for changes in mental status, LOC, or respirations and to relieve the patient's headache with acetaminophen. Tell them to return him to the hospital immediately if his LOC decreases, if his headache persists after several doses of mild analgesics, if he vomits more than once, or if weakness develops in his arms or legs.

• Teach the patient and his family how to care for his scalp wound. Emphasize the need to return for suture removal and follow-up evaluation.

SODIUM IMBALANCE

Sodium is the major cation (90%) in extracellular fluid; potassium, the major cation in intracellular fluid. During repolarization, the sodium-potassium pump continually shifts sodium into the cells and potassium out of the cells; during depolarization, it does the reverse.

Sodium cation functions include maintaining tonicity and concentration of extracellular fluid, acid-base balance (reabsorption of sodium ions and excretion of hydrogen ions), nerve conduction and neuromuscular function, glandular secretion, and water balance.

The body requires only 2 to 4 g of sodium daily. However, most Americans consume 6 to 10 g daily (mostly sodium chloride, as table salt), excreting excess sodium through the kidneys and skin.

A low-sodium diet or excessive use of diuretics may induce hyponatremia (decreased serum sodium concentration); dehydration may induce hypernatremia (increased serum sodium concentration).

Causes
Sodium imbalance can result from several causes.

Hyponatremia
One of the main causes of hyponatremia is excessive GI loss of water and electrolytes. This can result from vomiting, suctioning, or diarrhea; excessive perspiration or fever; potent diuretics; or use of tap-water enemas.

When such losses decrease circulating fluid volume, increased secretion of antidiuretic hormone (ADH) promotes maximum water reabsorption, which further dilutes serum sodium. These factors are especially likely to cause hyponatremia when combined with too much electrolyte-free water intake.

Excessive drinking of water, infusion of I.V. dextrose in water without other solutes, malnutrition or starvation, and a low-sodium diet can also cause hyponatremia, usually in combination with one of the other causes.

Trauma, surgery (wound drainage), and burns, which cause sodium to shift into damaged cells, can lead to decreased serum sodium levels, as can adrenal gland insufficiency (Addison's disease), hypoaldosteronism, and cirrhosis of the liver with ascites.

Syndrome of inappropriate antidiuretic hormone secretion (SIADH), resulting from brain tumor, cerebrovascular accident, pulmonary disease, or neoplasm with ectopic ADH production, can lead to hyponatremia also. Certain drugs, such as chlorpropamide and clofibrate, may produce a SIADH-like syndrome.

Hypernatremia
Decreased water intake can cause hypernatremia. When severe vomiting and diarrhea cause water loss that exceeds sodium loss, serum sodium levels rise, but overall extracellular fluid volume decreases.

Other causes include excess adrenocortical hormones, as in Cushing's syndrome, and ADH deficiency (diabetes insipidus). Salt intoxication—an

CLINICAL EFFECTS OF SODIUM IMBALANCE

SYSTEM	HYPONATREMIA	HYPERNATREMIA
Central nervous system	• Anxiety, headaches, muscle twitching and weakness, seizures	• Fever, agitation, restlessness, seizures
Cardiovascular	• Hypotension; tachycardia; with severe deficit, vasomotor collapse, thready pulse	• Hypertension, tachycardia, pitting edema, excessive weight gain
GI	• Nausea, vomiting, abdominal cramps	• Rough, dry tongue; intense thirst
Genitourinary	• Oliguria or anuria	• Oliguria
Respiratory	• Cyanosis with severe deficiency	• Dyspnea, respiratory arrest, and death (from dramatic rise in osmotic pressure)
Cutaneous	• Cold, clammy skin; decreased skin turgor	• Flushed skin; dry, sticky mucous membranes

uncommon cause — may result from excessive ingestion of table salt.

Signs and symptoms
Sodium imbalance has profound physiologic effects and can induce severe central nervous system, cardiovascular, and GI abnormalities. (See *Clinical effects of sodium imbalance.*)

For example, hyponatremia may result in renal dysfunction or, if serum sodium loss is abrupt or severe, seizures; hypernatremia may produce pulmonary edema, circulatory disorders, and decreased level of consciousness.

Diagnosis
Hyponatremia is defined as a serum sodium level less than 135 mEq/L; hypernatremia, as a serum sodium level greater than 145 mEq/L. However, additional laboratory studies are necessary to determine etiology and differentiate between a true deficit and an apparent deficit resulting from sodium

shift or from hypervolemia or hypovolemia.

In true hyponatremia, supportive values include urine sodium greater than 100 mEq/24 hours, with low serum osmolality; in true hypernatremia, urine sodium is less than 40 mEq/24 hours, with high serum osmolality.

Treatment
The type of treatment varies with the severity of the imbalance.

Hyponatremia
Treatment for mild hyponatremia usually consists of restricted electrolyte-free water intake when it results from hemodilution, SIADH, or conditions such as congestive heart failure, cirrhosis of the liver, and renal failure. If fluid restriction alone fails to normalize serum sodium levels, demeclocycline or lithium, which blocks ADH action in the renal tubules, can be used to promote water excretion.

In extremely rare instances of severe symptomatic hyponatremia, when the serum sodium level falls below 110 mEq/L, treatment may include an infusion of 3% or 5% saline solution.

Treatment with saline infusion requires careful monitoring of venous pressure to prevent potentially fatal circulatory overload. The aim of treatment of secondary hyponatremia is to correct the underlying disorder.

Hypernatremia
Primary treatment of hypernatremia is administration of salt-free solutions (such as dextrose in water) to return serum sodium levels to normal, followed by infusion of 0.45% sodium chloride to prevent hyponatremia.

Other measures include a sodium-restricted diet and discontinuation of drugs that promote sodium retention.

Special considerations
For hyponatremia:
• Watch for extremely low serum sodium and accompanying serum chloride levels. Monitor urine specific gravity and other laboratory results. Record fluid intake and output accurately, and weigh the patient daily.
• During administration of isosmolar or hyperosmolar saline solution, watch closely for signs of hypervolemia (dyspnea, crackles, engorged neck or hand veins). Note conditions that may cause excessive sodium loss — diaphoresis, prolonged diarrhea or vomiting, or severe burns.
• Refer the patient receiving maintenance dosage of diuretics to a dietitian for instruction about dietary sodium intake.
• To prevent hyponatremia, administer isosmolar solutions.

For hypernatremia:
• Measure serum sodium levels every 6 hours or at least daily. Monitor vital signs for changes, especially for rising pulse rate. Watch for signs of hypervolemia, especially in the patient receiving I.V. fluids.
• Record fluid intake and output accurately, checking for body fluid loss. Weigh the patient daily.
• Obtain a drug history to check for drugs that promote sodium retention.
• Explain the importance of sodium restriction, and teach the patient how to plan a low-sodium diet. Closely monitor the serum sodium levels of high-risk patients.

SOMATIZATION DISORDER

When multiple recurrent signs and symptoms of several years' duration suggest that physical disorders exist without a verifiable disease or pathophysiologic condition to account for them, somatization disorder is present.

The typical patient with somatization disorder usually undergoes repeated medical examinations and diagnostic testing that — unlike the symptoms themselves — can be potentially dangerous or debilitating. However, unlike the hypochondriac, she's not preoccupied with the belief that she has a specific disease.

Somatization disorder usually is chronic, with exacerbations during times of stress. The patient's signs and symptoms are involuntary, and she consciously wants to feel better. Nonetheless, she's seldom entirely symptom-free.

Signs and symptoms usually begin in adolescence; rarely, in the twenties. This disorder primarily affects women; it's seldom diagnosed in men.

Causes

Both genetic and environmental factors contribute to the development of somatization disorder.

Signs and symptoms

A patient with somatization disorder presents physical complaints in a dramatic, vague, or exaggerated way, often as part of a complicated medical history in which many medical diagnoses have been considered.

An important clue to this disorder is a history of multiple medical evaluations by different doctors at different institutions — sometimes simultaneously — without significant findings. The patient usually appears anxious and depressed.

Common physical complaints include:
• conversion or pseudoneurologic signs and symptoms (for example, paralysis or blindness)
• GI discomfort (abdominal pain, nausea, or vomiting)
• female reproductive difficulties (such as painful menstruation) or male reproductive difficulties (such as erectile dysfunction)
• psychosexual problems (such as sexual indifference)
• chronic pain (such as back pain)
• cardiopulmonary symptoms (chest pain, dizziness, or palpitations).

The patient typically relates her current complaints and previous evaluations in great detail. She may be quite knowledgeable about tests, procedures, and medical jargon.

Attempts to explore areas other than her medical history may cause noticeable anxiety. She tends to disparage previous health care professionals and previous treatments, often with the comment, "Everyone thinks I'm imagining these things."

Ongoing assessment should focus on new signs or symptoms or any change in old ones to avoid missing a developing physical disorder.

Diagnosis

The *Diagnostic and Statistical Manual of Mental Disorders,* 4th edition, details the characteristics of patients with this condition. (See *Diagnosing somatization disorder.*)

Diagnostic tests rule out physical disorders that cause vague and confusing symptoms, such as hyperparathyroidism, porphyria, multiple sclerosis, and systemic lupus erythematosus. In addition, multiple physical signs and symptoms that appear for the first time late in life usually stem from physical disease, rather than somatization disorder.

Treatment

The goal of treatment is to help the patient learn to live with her signs and symptoms. After diagnostic evaluation has ruled out organic causes, the patient should be told that she has no serious illness currently but will receive care for her genuine distress and ongoing medical attention for her symptoms.

The most important aspect of treatment is a continuing supportive relationship with a health care provider who acknowledges the patient's signs and symptoms and is willing to help her live with them. The patient should have regularly scheduled appointments to review her complaints and the effectiveness of her coping strategies.

The patient with somatization disorder seldom acknowledges any psychological aspect of her illness and rejects psychiatric treatment.

Special considerations

• Acknowledge the patient's symptoms, and support her efforts to function and cope despite distress. Don't characterize her signs and symptoms

DIAGNOSING SOMATIZATION DISORDER

The diagnosis of somatization disorder is made when the patient's symptoms match the diagnostic criteria in the *Diagnostic and Statistical Manual of Mental Disorders,* 4th edition, as follows:

• The patient has a history of many physical complaints, beginning before age 30 and persisting for several years, that result in the patient seeking treatment or in the patient experiencing significant social, occupational, or other impairment.

• The patient has a selection of symptoms as follows (with individual symptoms occurring at any time during the disturbance):

— *Pain:* a history of pain related to at least *four* different sites or functions (head, abdomen, back, joints, arms and legs, chest, rectum, menstruation, sexual intercourse, or urination)

— *GI upset:* a history of at least *two* GI symptoms other than pain (vomiting other than during pregnancy, nausea, bloating, diarrhea, intolerance of different foods)

— *Sexual symptoms:* a history of at least *one* sexual or reproductive symptom other than pain—for example, sexual indifference, erectile or ejaculatory dysfunction, irregular menses, excessive menstrual bleeding, vomiting throughout pregnancy

— *Pseudoneurologic symptoms:* a history of at least *one* symptom or deficit suggesting a neurologic condition not limited to pain (for example, conversion symptoms, such as impaired coordination or balance, paralysis or localized weakness, difficulty swallowing or lump in the throat, aphonia, urine retention, hallucinations, loss of touch or pain sensation, double vision, blindness, deafness, seizures; dissociative symptoms such as amnesia; or loss of consciousness other than fainting).

• A thorough investigation discloses that either the above symptoms cannot be fully explained by a known general medical condition or the direct effects of a substance or, if a related general medical condition exists, the physical complaints or resulting impairments exceed what would be expected from the history, physical examination, and diagnostic findings.

• The symptoms are not intentionally produced or feigned (as in factitious disorder or malingering).

as imaginary. Do tell her the results of tests and their significance.

• Emphasize the patient's strengths (for example, "It's good that you can still work with this pain"). Gently point out the time relationship between stress and physical symptoms.

• Help the patient manage stress. Typically, her relationships are linked to her signs and symptoms; relieving them can impair her interactions with others.

• Help the patient's family understand the patient's need for troublesome signs and symptoms.

SPINAL CORD DEFECTS

Various malformations of the spine— including spina bifida, meningocele, and myelomeningocele—result from defective embryonic neural tube closure during the first trimester of pregnancy. Generally, these defects occur in the lumbosacral area, but they are occasionally found in the sacral, thoracic, and cervical areas.

Spina bifida occulta is the most common and least severe spinal cord defect. It's characterized by incomplete closure of one or more vertebrae without protrusion of the spinal cord or meninges.

However, in more severe forms of spina bifida, incomplete closure of one or more vertebrae causes protrusion of the spinal contents in an external sac or cystic lesion.

In spina bifida with meningocele, this sac contains meninges and cerebrospinal fluid (CSF). In spina bifida with myelomeningocele (meningomyelocele), this sac contains meninges, CSF, and a portion of the spinal cord or nerve roots distal to the conus medullaris.

Spina bifida is relatively common and affects about 5% of the population. In the United States, about 12,000 infants each year are born with some form of spina bifida; spina bifida with myelomeningocele is less common than spina bifida occulta and spina bifida with meningocele. Incidence is highest in persons of Welsh or Irish ancestry.

The prognosis varies with the degree of accompanying neurologic deficit. It's worst in patients with large open lesions, neurogenic bladders (which predispose to infection and renal failure), or total paralysis of the legs.

Because such features are usually absent in spina bifida occulta and meningocele, the prognosis is better than in myelomeningocele, and many patients with these conditions can lead normal lives.

Causes
Normally, about 20 days after conception, the embryo develops a neural groove in the dorsal ectoderm. This groove rapidly deepens, and the two edges fuse to form the neural tube.

By about day 23, this tube is completely closed except for an opening at each end. Theoretically, if the posterior portion of this neural tube fails to close by the fourth week of gestation, or if it closes but then splits open from a cause such as an abnormal increase in CSF later in the first trimester, a spinal defect results.

Viruses, radiation, and other environmental factors may be responsible for such defects. However, spinal cord defects occur more often in offspring of women who have previously had children with similar defects, so genetic factors may also be responsible.

Signs and symptoms
Indications vary depending on the type of defect.

Spina bifida occulta
Although overt signs may be absent, spina bifida occulta is often accompanied by a depression or dimple, tuft of hair, soft fatty deposits, port wine nevi, or a combination of these abnormalities on the skin over the spinal defect.

Spina bifida occulta doesn't usually cause neurologic dysfunction but occasionally is associated with foot weakness or bowel and bladder disturbances. Such disturbances are especially likely during rapid growth phases, when the spinal cord's ascent within the vertebral column may be impaired by its abnormal adherence to other tissues.

Meningocele and myelomeningocele
A saclike structure protrudes over the spine in both meningocele and myelomeningocele.

Like spina bifida occulta, meningocele rarely causes neurologic deficit. But myelomeningocele, depending on the level of the defect, causes permanent neurologic dysfunction, such as flaccid or spastic paralysis and bowel and bladder incontinence.

Associated disorders include trophic skin disturbances (ulcerations, cyanosis), clubfoot, knee contractures, and hydrocephalus (in about 90% of patients). Mental retardation, Arnold-Chiari syndrome (in which part of the brain protrudes into the spinal canal), and curvature of the spine can also occur.

Diagnosis

The diagnosis varies with the type of defect.

Spina bifida occulta

Although often overlooked, spina bifida occulta is occasionally palpable, and a spinal X-ray can show the bone defect. Myelography can differentiate it from other spinal abnormalities, especially spinal cord tumors.

Meningocele and myelomeningocele

Meningocele and myelomeningocele are obvious on examination; transillumination of the protruding sac can sometimes distinguish between them. (In meningocele, it typically transilluminates; in myelomeningocele, it doesn't.)

In myelomeningocele, a pinprick examination of the legs and trunk shows the level of sensory and motor involvement; skull X-rays, cephalic measurements, and a computed tomography scan demonstrate associated hydrocephalus.

Other appropriate laboratory tests in patients with myelomeningocele include urinalysis, urine cultures, and tests for renal function starting in the neonatal period and continuing at regular intervals.

Although amniocentesis can detect only open defects, such as myelomeningocele and meningocele, this procedure is recommended for all pregnant women who have previously had children with spinal cord defects; these women are at an increased risk for having children with similar defects. If these defects are present, amniocentesis shows increased alpha-fetoprotein levels by 14 weeks' gestation.

Ultrasonography can also detect or confirm the presence and extent of neural tube defects.

Treatment

Spina bifida occulta usually requires no treatment. Treatment of meningocele consists of surgical closure of the protruding sac and continual assessment of growth and development.

Treatment of myelomeningocele requires repair of the sac and supportive measures to promote independence and prevent further complications. Surgery doesn't reverse neurologic deficits. A shunt may be needed to relieve associated hydrocephalus.

If the patient has a severe spinal defect, short- and long-term treatment will require a team approach, including a neurosurgeon, orthopedist, urologist, nurse, social worker, occupational and physical therapists, and parents.

Rehabilitation

In children or adults, rehabilitation measures may include:

• waist supports, long leg braces, walkers, crutches, and other orthopedic appliances

• diet and bowel training to manage fecal incontinence

• neurogenic bladder management to reduce urinary stasis, possibly intermittent catheterization, and antispasmodics, such as bethanechol or propantheline. In severe cases, insertion of an artificial urinary sphincter is often successful; a urinary diversion is used as a last resort to preserve kidney function.

Special considerations

Before surgery for meningocele or myelomeningocele:

• Prevent local infection by cleaning the defect gently with sterile saline solution or other solutions. Inspect the defect often for signs of infection, and cover it with sterile dressings moistened with sterile saline solution. Don't use ointments on the defect; they may cause skin maceration.

• Prevent skin breakdown by placing sheepskin or a foam pad under the infant. Keep skin clean, and apply lotion to knees, elbows, chin, and other pressure areas. Give antibiotics as needed.

• Handle the infant carefully. Hold and cuddle him, but avoid placing pressure on the sac. When holding him on your lap, position him on his abdomen, and teach the parents to do the same.

• Usually, the infant can't wear a diaper or a shirt until after surgical correction because it will irritate the sac, so keep him warm in an infant Isolette. Position him on his abdomen with the head of the bed slightly elevated to prevent contamination of the sac with urine or feces.

• Provide adequate time for parent-child bonding, if possible.

• Measure head circumference daily, and watch for signs of hydrocephalus and meningeal irritation, such as fever or nuchal rigidity. Be sure to mark the spot so you get accurate readings.

• Minimize contractures with passive range-of-motion exercises and casting. To prevent hip dislocation, abduct the hips with a pad between the knees or with sandbags and ankle rolls.

• Monitor intake and output. Watch for decreased skin turgor, dryness, or other signs of dehydration. Provide meticulous skin care to genitals and buttocks to prevent infection.

• Ensure adequate nutrition.

After surgical repair of the defect:

• Watch for hydrocephalus, which often follows such surgery. Measure the child's head circumference.

• Monitor vital signs often. Watch for signs of shock (decreased blood pressure, tachycardia, lethargy), infection (malaise, elevated temperature, alteration in feeding pattern), and increased intracranial pressure (projectile vomiting).

• Frequently assess the infant's fontanels. Remember that before age 2, infants don't show typical signs of increased intracranial pressure, because suture lines aren't fully closed. The most telling sign is bulging fontanels.

• Change the dressing regularly, and watch for any signs of drainage, wound rupture, or infection.

• If leg casts have been applied to treat deformities, watch for signs that the child is outgrowing the cast. Check distal pulses to ensure adequate circulation. Petal the edges of the cast to prevent softening and skin irritation. Use a cool-air blow-dryer to dry skin under the cast. Periodically check for foul odor and other indications of skin breakdown.

• Teach parents how to cope with their infant's problems and successfully meet long-range treatment goals.

• Teach parents how to recognize such early signs of complications as hydrocephalus, pressure ulcers, and urinary tract infections (UTIs). Also show them how to provide psychological support to the child and encourage a positive attitude.

• Help parents work through their feelings of guilt, anger, and helplessness.

• Encourage parents to begin training their child in a toileting routine by age 3. Emphasize the need for increased fluid intake to prevent UTIs. Teach intermittent catheterization and conduit hygiene as needed.

• Explain to parents how to prevent constipation and bowel obstruction. Stress the need for increased fluid intake, a high-bulk diet, exercise, and use of a stool softener (if prescribed). Teach parents to empty their child's bowel by exerting slight pressure on the abdomen, telling the child to bear down, and giving a glycerin suppository as needed.

• Teach parents to recognize developmental lags early (a possible result of hydrocephalus). If the child does fall behind, stress the importance of follow-up IQ assessment to help plan realistic educational goals. The child may need to attend a school with special facilities. Also, stress the need for stimulation to ensure maximum mental development. Help parents plan activities appropriate to their child's age and abilities.

• Refer parents for genetic counseling, and suggest that amniocentesis be performed in future pregnancies. For more information and names of support groups, refer parents to the Spina Bifida Association of America.

LIFE-THREATENING DISORDER

SPINAL INJURIES

Aside from spinal cord damage, spinal injuries include fractures, contusions, and compressions of the vertebral column, usually the result of trauma to the head or neck. The real danger lies in possible spinal cord damage. Spinal fractures most commonly occur in the fifth, sixth, and seventh cervical, twelfth thoracic, and first lumbar vertebrae.

Causes

Most serious spinal injuries result from motor vehicle accidents, falls, diving into shallow water, and gunshot wounds; less serious injuries, from lifting heavy objects and minor falls. Spinal dysfunction may also result from hyperparathyroidism and neoplastic lesions.

Signs and symptoms

The most obvious symptom of spinal injury is muscle spasm and back pain that worsens with movement. In cervical fractures, pain may produce point tenderness; in dorsal and lumbar fractures, it may radiate to other body areas such as the legs.

If the injury damages the spinal cord, clinical effects range from mild paresthesia to quadriplegia and shock. After milder injuries, such symptoms may be delayed for several days or weeks.

Diagnosis

Typically, a diagnosis is based on the patient history, the physical examination, X-rays and, possibly, lumbar puncture, computed tomography (CT) scan, and magnetic resonance imaging (MRI):

• *Patient history* may reveal trauma, a metastatic lesion, an infection that could produce a spinal abscess, or an endocrine disorder.

• *Physical examination* (including a neurologic evaluation) locates the level of injury and detects cord damage.

• *Spinal X-rays,* the most important diagnostic measure, locate the fracture.

• *Lumbar puncture* may show increased cerebrospinal fluid pressure from a lesion or trauma in spinal compression.

• *CT scan* or *MRI* can locate the spinal mass.

Treatment

The primary treatment after spinal injury is immediate immobilization to stabilize the spine and prevent cord damage; other treatment is supportive. Cervical injuries require immobilization, using sandbags on both sides of the patient's head, a hard cervical collar, or skeletal traction with skull tongs or a halo device.

Supportive treatment

Treatment of stable lumbar and dorsal fractures consists of bed rest on firm support (such as a bed board), analgesics, and muscle relaxants until the fracture stabilizes (usually 10 to 12 weeks). Later treatment includes exercises to strengthen the back muscles and a back brace or corset to provide support while walking.

An unstable dorsal or lumbar fracture requires a plaster cast, a turning frame and, in severe fracture, laminectomy and spinal fusion.

Other treatment

When the damage results in compression of the spinal column, neurosurgery may relieve the pressure. If the cause of compression is a metastatic lesion, chemotherapy and radiation may relieve it. Surface wounds accompanying the spinal injury require tetanus prophylaxis unless the patient has had recent immunization.

Special considerations

• In all spinal injuries, suspect cord damage until proven otherwise.

• During initial assessment and during X-rays, immobilize the patient on a firm surface, with sandbags on both sides of his head. Tell him not to move; avoid moving him, because hyperflexion can damage the cord.

• If you must move the patient, get at least one other member of the staff to help you logroll him to avoid disturbing body alignment.

• Throughout assessment, offer comfort and reassurance. Remember, the fear of possible paralysis will be overwhelming. Allow a family member who isn't too distraught to accompany the patient and talk to him quietly and calmly.

• If the injury requires surgery, administer prophylactic antibiotics. Catheterize the patient to avoid urine retention, and monitor defecation patterns to avoid impaction.

• Explain traction methods to the patient and his family, and reassure them that traction devices don't penetrate the brain. If the patient has a halo or skull-tong traction device, clean pin sites daily, trim hair short, and provide analgesics for persistent headaches.

• During traction, turn the patient often to prevent pneumonia, embolism, and skin breakdown; perform passive range-of-motion exercises to maintain muscle tone. If available, use a CircOlectric bed or Stryker frame to facilitate turning and to avoid spinal cord injury.

• Turn the patient on his side during feedings to prevent aspiration. Create a relaxed atmosphere at mealtimes.

• Suggest appropriate diversionary activities to fill your patient's hours of immobility.

• Watch closely for neurologic changes. Changes in skin sensation and loss of muscle strength could point to pressure on the spinal cord, possibly as a result of edema or shifting bone fragments.

• Help the patient walk as soon as his condition allows; it'll probably be necessary for him to wear a back brace.

• Before discharge, instruct the patient about continuing analgesics or other medication, and stress the importance of regular follow-up examinations.

• To help prevent a spinal injury from becoming a spinal *cord* injury, educate fire fighters, police officers, paramedics, and the general public about the proper way to handle such injuries.

SPINAL NEOPLASMS

A spinal neoplasm is any one of many tumor types that are similar to intracranial tumors and involve the spinal cord or its roots. If untreated, they can eventually cause paralysis.

Primary spinal neoplasms originate in the meningeal coverings, the parenchyma of the cord or its roots, the intraspinal vasculature, or the vertebrae. They can also occur as metastatic foci from primary tumors.

Causes

Primary spinal cord tumors may be extramedullary (occurring outside the spinal cord) or intramedullary (occurring within the cord itself). Extramedullary tumors may be intradural (meningiomas and schwannomas), which account for 60% of all primary spinal cord neoplasms, or extradural (metastatic tumors from breasts, lungs, prostate, leukemia, or lymphomas), which account for 25% of these neoplasms.

Intramedullary tumors, or gliomas (astrocytomas or ependymomas), are comparatively rare, accounting for only about 10% of tumors. In children, they're low-grade astrocytomas.

Spinal cord tumors are rare compared with intracranial tumors (ratio of 1:4). They occur with equal frequency in both men and women, with the exception of meningiomas, which occur most often in women. Spinal cord tumors can occur anywhere along the length of the cord or its roots.

Signs and symptoms

Extramedullary tumors produce symptoms by pressing on nerve roots, the spinal cord, and spinal vessels; intramedullary tumors, by destroying the parenchyma and compressing adjacent areas. Because intramedullary tumors may extend over several spinal cord segments, their symptoms are more variable than those of extramedullary tumors.

The following clinical effects are likely with all spinal cord neoplasms:
• *Pain* is most severe directly over the tumor, radiates around the trunk or down the limb on the affected side, and is unrelieved by bed rest.

• *Motor symptoms* include asymmetric spastic muscle weakness, decreased muscle tone, exaggerated reflexes, and a positive Babinski's sign. If the tumor is at the level of the cauda equina, muscle flaccidity, muscle wasting, weakness, and progressive diminution in tendon reflexes are characteristic.

• *Sensory deficits* include contralateral loss of pain, temperature, and touch sensation (Brown-Séquard syndrome). These losses are less obvious to the patient than functional motor changes. Caudal lesions invariably produce paresthesias in the nerve distribution pathway of the involved roots.

• *Bladder symptoms* vary according to the stage of the tumor. Early signs include incomplete emptying or difficulty with the urinary stream, which is usually unnoticed or ignored. Urine retention is an inevitable late sign with cord compression. Cauda equina tumors cause bladder and bowel incontinence from flaccid paralysis.

• *Constipation* can also occur.

Diagnosis

Several tests aid in diagnosis:
• *Spinal tap* shows clear yellow cerebrospinal fluid (CSF) as a result of increased protein levels if the flow is completely blocked. If the flow is partially blocked, protein levels rise, but the fluid is only slightly yellow in proportion to the CSF protein level. A Papanicolaou smear of the CSF may show malignant cells of metastatic carcinoma.

• *X-rays* show distortions of the intervertebral foramina, changes in the vertebrae, collapsed areas in the vertebral body, and localized enlargement of the spinal canal, indicating an adjacent block.

• *Myelography* identifies the level of the lesion by outlining it if the tumor is causing partial obstruction; it shows anatomic relationship of the tumor to the cord and the dura. If the obstruction is complete, the injected dye can't flow past the tumor.

Note: This study is dangerous if cord compression is nearly complete, because withdrawal or escape of CSF will actually allow the tumor to exert greater pressure against the cord.

• *Radioisotope bone scan* demonstrates metastatic invasion of the vertebrae by showing a characteristic increase in osteoblastic activity.

• *Computed tomography scan* shows cord compression and tumor location.

• *Frozen section biopsy* at surgery identifies the tissue type.

Treatment

Spinal cord tumors usually require decompression or radiation. Laminectomy is indicated for primary tumors that produce spinal cord or cauda equina compression; it's *not* usually indicated for metastatic tumors.

If the tumor is slowly progressive, or if it's treated before the cord degenerates from compression, symptoms are likely to disappear, and complete restoration of function is possible. In a patient with metastatic carcinoma or lymphoma who suddenly experiences complete transverse myelitis with spinal shock, functional improvement is unlikely, even with treatment, and his outlook is ominous.

If the patient has incomplete paraplegia of rapid onset, emergency surgical decompression may save cord function. Steroid therapy minimizes cord edema until surgery can be performed. Partial removal of intramedullary gliomas, followed by radiation, may alleviate symptoms for a short time.

Metastatic extradural tumors can be controlled with radiation, analgesics and, in the case of hormone-mediated tumors (breast and prostate), appropriate hormone therapy.

Transcutaneous electrical nerve stimulation (TENS) may control radicular pain from spinal cord tumors and is a useful alternative to narcotic analgesics. In TENS, an electrical charge is applied to the skin to stimulate large-diameter nerve fibers and thereby inhibit transmission of pain impulses through small-diameter nerve fibers.

Special considerations

• On your first contact with the patient, perform a complete neurologic evaluation to obtain baseline data for planning future care and evaluating changes in his clinical status.

• Provide psychological support. Help the patient and his family to understand and cope with the diagnosis, treatment, potential disabilities, and necessary changes in lifestyle.

• After laminectomy, check neurologic status frequently and watch for signs of infection. Administer analgesics, and aid the patient in early walking.

• Take safety precautions for the patient with impaired sensation and motor deficits. Use side rails if the patient is bedridden; if he's not, encourage him to wear flat shoes, and remove scatter rugs and clutter to prevent falls.

• Encourage the patient to be independent in performing daily activities. Avoid aggravating pain by moving the

patient slowly and by making sure his body is well aligned when giving personal care. Advise him to use TENS to block radicular pain.
• Make sure the patient receives appropriate rehabilitation, including bowel and bladder retraining.
• Administer steroids and antacids for cord edema after radiation therapy. Monitor for sensory or motor dysfunction, which indicates the need for more steroids.
• Enforce bed rest for the patient with vertebral body involvement until he can safely walk; body weight alone can cause cord collapse and cord laceration from bone fragments.
• Logroll and position the patient on his side every 2 hours to prevent pressure ulcers and other complications of immobility.
• If the patient is to wear a back brace, make sure he wears it whenever he gets out of bed.

SPOROTRICHOSIS

A chronic disease, sporotrichosis is caused by the fungus *Sporothrix schenckii*. It occurs in three forms: cutaneous-lymphatic, which produces nodular erythematous primary lesions and secondary lesions along lymphatic channels; pulmonary, a rare form that produces a productive cough and pulmonary lesions; and disseminated, another rare form, which may cause arthritis or osteomyelitis.

The course of sporotrichosis is slow, the prognosis is good, and fatalities are rare. However, untreated skin lesions may cause secondary bacterial infection.

EPIDERMAL EFFECTS OF SPOROTRICHOSIS

Ulceration, swelling, and crusting of nodules on fingers are characteristic of cutaneous-lymphatic sporotrichosis.

Causes
S. schenckii is found in soil, wood, sphagnum moss, and decaying vegetation throughout the world. Because this fungus usually enters through broken skin (the pulmonary form through inhalation), sporotrichosis is more common in horticulturists, agricultural workers, and home gardeners.

Perhaps because of occupational exposure, it's more prevalent in adult men than in women and children. The typical incubation period lasts from 1 week to 3 months.

Signs and symptoms
• Cutaneous-lymphatic sporotrichosis produces characteristic skin lesions, usually on the hands or fingers. (See *Epidermal effects of sporotrichosis.*) Each lesion begins as a small, painless, movable subcutaneous nodule but grows progressively larger, discolors, and eventually ulcerates. Later, additional lesions form along the adjacent lymph node chain.

• Pulmonary sporotrichosis causes a productive cough, lung cavities and nodules, hilar adenopathy, pleural effusion, fibrosis, and the formation of a fungus ball. It's often associated with sarcoidosis and tuberculosis.

• Disseminated sporotrichosis produces multifocal lesions that spread from the primary lesion in the skin or lungs. Onset is insidious. Typically, it causes weight loss, anorexia, synovial or bony lesions, and possibly arthritis or osteomyelitis.

Diagnosis

Typical clinical findings and culture of *S. schenckii* in sputum, pus, or bone drainage confirm this diagnosis. Histologic identification is difficult. The diagnosis must rule out tuberculosis, sarcoidosis and, in patients with the disseminated form, bacterial osteomyelitis and neoplasm.

Treatment

Sporotrichosis doesn't require isolation. The cutaneous-lymphatic form usually responds to application of a saturated solution of potassium iodide, generally continued for 1 to 2 months after lesions heal. Occasionally, cutaneous lesions must be excised or drained.

The disseminated form responds to I.V. amphotericin B but may require several weeks of treatment. Local heat application relieves pain. Cavitary pulmonary lesions may require surgery.

Special considerations

• Keep lesions clean, make the patient as comfortable as possible, and carefully dispose of contaminated dressings.

• Warn the patient about the possible adverse effects of drugs. Because amphotericin B may cause fever, chills, nausea, and vomiting, give antipyretics and antiemetics as needed.

• To help prevent sporotrichosis, advise horticulturists and home gardeners to wear gloves while working.

SPRAINS AND STRAINS

A *sprain* is a complete or incomplete tear in the supporting ligaments surrounding a joint that usually follows a sharp twist. A *strain* is an injury to a muscle or tendinous attachment. Both usually heal without surgical repair.

Signs and symptoms

Sprains and strains cause varying signs and symptoms.

Sprains

A sprain causes local pain (especially during joint movement), swelling, loss of mobility (which may not occur until several hours after the injury), and a black-and-blue discoloration from blood extravasating into surrounding tissues. A sprained ankle is the most common joint injury.

Strains

A strain may be acute (an immediate result of vigorous muscle overuse or overstress) or chronic (a result of repeated overuse).

An acute strain causes a sharp, transient pain (the patient may say he heard a snapping noise) and rapid swelling. When severe pain subsides, the muscle is tender; after several days, ecchymoses appear.

A chronic strain causes stiffness, soreness, and generalized tenderness. These conditions appear several hours after the injury.

Diagnosis

A history of recent injury or chronic overuse, clinical findings, and an X-ray to rule out fractures establish the diagnosis.

Treatment

Effective treatment differs for sprains and strains.

Sprains

Sprains call for control of pain and swelling and immobilization of the injured joint to promote healing. Immediately after the injury, elevating the joint above the level of the heart and intermittently applying ice for 12 to 48 hours controls swelling. A towel between the ice pack and the skin prevents cold injuries.

An immobilized sprain usually heals in 2 to 3 weeks, and the patient can then gradually resume normal activities. Occasionally, however, torn ligaments don't heal properly and cause recurrent dislocation, necessitating surgical repair.

Some athletes may request immediate surgical repair to hasten healing; to prevent sprains, they may tape their wrists and ankles before sports activities.

Strains

Acute strains require analgesics and application of ice for up to 48 hours, then heat. Complete muscle rupture may require surgery.

Chronic strains usually don't need treatment, but heat application, nonsteroidal anti-inflammatory drugs (such as ibuprofen), or an analgesic-muscle relaxant can relieve discomfort.

Special considerations

• For sprains, immobilize the joint, using an elastic bandage or cast or, if the sprain is severe, a soft cast or splint. Depending on the severity of the in-

jury, codeine or another analgesic may be necessary.

• If the patient has a sprained ankle, make sure he receives crutch gait training. Because patients with sprains seldom require hospitalization, provide patient teaching.

• Tell the patient with a sprain to elevate the joint for 48 to 72 hours after the injury (while sleeping, the joint can be elevated with pillows) and to apply ice intermittently for 12 to 48 hours.

• If an elastic bandage has been applied, teach the patient to reapply it by wrapping from below to above the injury, forming a figure eight. For a sprained ankle, apply the bandage from the toes to midcalf. Tell the patient to remove the bandage before going to sleep and to loosen it if it causes the leg to become pale, numb, or painful.

• Instruct the patient to call if pain worsens or persists (if so, an additional X-ray may detect a fracture originally missed).

SQUAMOUS CELL CARCINOMA

Arising from the keratinizing epidermal cells, squamous cell carcinoma of the skin is an invasive tumor with metastatic potential. It occurs most often in fair-skinned white men over age 60. Outdoor employment and residence in a sunny, warm climate (southwestern United States and Australia, for example) greatly increase the risk of developing squamous cell carcinoma.

Causes

Predisposing factors associated with squamous cell carcinoma include overexposure to the sun's ultraviolet rays and the presence of premalignant le-

STAGING SQUAMOUS CELL CARCINOMA

The American Joint Committee on Cancer uses the following TNM (tumor, node, metastasis) system for staging squamous cell carcinoma.

Primary tumor
TX—primary tumor can't be assessed
T0—no evidence of primary tumor
Tis—carcinoma in situ
T1—tumor 2 cm or less in greatest dimension
T2—tumor between 2 and 5 cm in greatest dimension
T3—tumor more than 5 cm in greatest dimension
T4—tumor invades deep extradermal structures (such as cartilage, skeletal muscle, or bone)

Regional lymph nodes
NX—regional lymph nodes can't be assessed
N0—no evidence of regional lymph node involvement

N1—regional lymph node involvement

Distant metastasis
MX—distant metastasis can't be assessed
M0—no known distant metastasis
M1—distant metastasis

Staging categories
Squamous cell carcinoma progresses from mild to severe as follows:
Stage 0—Tis, N0, M0
Stage I—T1, N0, M0
Stage II—T2, N0, M0; T3, N0, M0
Stage III—T4, N0, M0; any T, N1, M0
Stage IV—any T, any N, M1

sions (such as actinic keratosis or Bowen's disease).

Other predisposing factors include X-ray therapy, ingestion of herbicides containing arsenic, chronic skin irritation and inflammation, exposure to local carcinogens (such as tar and oil), and hereditary diseases (such as xeroderma pigmentosum and albinism). Rarely, squamous cell carcinoma may develop on the site of smallpox vaccination, psoriasis, or chronic discoid lupus erythematosus.

Signs and symptoms

Squamous cell carcinoma commonly develops on the skin of the face, the ears, the dorsa of the hands and forearms, and other sun-damaged areas. Lesions on sun-damaged skin tend to be less invasive and less likely to metastasize than lesions on unexposed skin.

Notable exceptions to this tendency are squamous cell lesions on the lower lip and the ears. These are almost invariably markedly invasive metastastic lesions with a generally poor prognosis.

Transformation from a premalignant lesion to squamous cell carcinoma may begin with induration and inflammation of the preexisting lesion. When squamous cell carcinoma arises from normal skin, the nodule grows slowly on a firm, indurated base.

If untreated, this nodule eventually ulcerates and invades underlying tissues. Metastasis can occur to the regional lymph nodes, producing characteristic systemic symptoms of pain, malaise, fatigue, weakness, and an-

TREATING ACTINIC KERATOSES

A useful drug for treating actinic keratoses, fluorouracil is available in different strengths (1%, 2%, and 5%) as a cream or solution.

Local application causes stinging and burning, followed by erythema, vesiculation, erosion, superficial ulceration, necrosis, and re-epithelialization. The 5% solution induces the most severe inflammatory response but provides complete involution of the lesions with little recurrence.

Special considerations
• Keep fluorouracil away from eyes, scrotum, or mucous membranes.

• Warn the patient to avoid excessive sun exposure during treatment, because sun intensifies the inflammatory reaction.
• Continue application of fluorouracil until the lesions reach the ulcerative and necrotic stages (2 to 4 weeks); then consider application of a corticosteroid preparation as an anti-inflammatory agent.
• Possible adverse effects include postinflammatory hyperpigmentation. Complete healing occurs within 1 to 2 months.

---

orexia. (See *Staging squamous cell carcinoma.*)

Diagnosis
An excisional biopsy provides a definitive diagnosis of squamous cell carcinoma. Other appropriate laboratory tests depend on systemic symptoms.

Treatment
The size, shape, location, and invasiveness of a squamous cell tumor and the condition of the underlying tissue determine the treatment method used.

Premalignant lesions respond well to treatment. (See *Treating actinic keratosis.*) A deeply invasive tumor may require a combination of techniques.

All the major treatment methods have excellent cure rates; the prognosis is usually better with a well-differentiated lesion than with a poorly differentiated one in an unusual location.

Depending on the lesion, treatment may consist of:
• wide surgical excision

• electrodesiccation and curettage (which offer good cosmetic results for small lesions)
• radiation therapy (generally for elderly or debilitated patients)
• chemosurgery (reserved for resistant or recurrent lesions).

Special considerations
• Establish a standard routine for changing the patient's dressing. This helps the patient and family learn how to care for the wound.
• Keep the wound dry and clean.
• Try to control odor with balsam of Peru, yogurt flakes, oil of cloves, or other odor-masking substances, even though they are often ineffective for long-term use. Topical or systemic antibiotics also temporarily control odor and eventually alter the lesion's bacterial flora.
• Be prepared for other problems that accompany a metastatic disease (pain, fatigue, weakness, anorexia).
• Help the patient and family set realistic goals and expectations.

• Disfiguring lesions are distressing to both the patient and you. Try to accept the patient as he is to increase his self-esteem and strengthen a caring relationship.

• To prevent squamous cell carcinoma, tell the patient to avoid excessive sun exposure, and wear protective clothing (hats, long sleeves).

• Instruct the patient to periodically examine the skin for precancerous lesions and have any removed promptly.

• Advise the patient to use sunblocks containing para-aminobenzoic acid, benzophenone, and zinc oxide. He should apply these agents 30 to 60 minutes before sun exposure.

• Tell the patient to use lipscreens to protect the lips from sun damage.

STAPHYLOCOCCAL SCALDED SKIN SYNDROME

A severe skin disorder, staphylococcal scalded skin syndrome (SSSS) is marked by epidermal erythema, peeling, and necrosis that give the skin a scalded appearance. SSSS is most prevalent in infants ages 1 to 3 months but may develop in children; it's uncommon in adults.

This disease follows a consistent pattern of progression, and most patients recover fully. Mortality is 2% to 3%, with death usually resulting from complications of fluid and electrolyte loss, sepsis, and involvement of other body systems.

Causes

The causative organism in SSSS is Group 2 *Staphylococcus aureus,* primarily phage type 71. Predisposing factors may include impaired immunity and renal insufficiency—present to some extent in the normal neonate because of immature development of these systems.

Signs and symptoms

SSSS can often be traced to a prodromal upper respiratory tract infection, possibly with concomitant purulent conjunctivitis. Cutaneous changes progress through three stages.

Erythema

In the first stage, erythema becomes visible, usually around the mouth and other orifices, and may spread in widening circles over the entire body surface. The skin becomes tender; Nikolsky's sign (sloughing of the skin when friction is applied) may appear.

Exfoliation

About 24 to 48 hours later, exfoliation occurs. In the more common, localized form of this disease, superficial erosions and minimal crusting develop, generally around body orifices, and may spread to exposed areas of the skin.

In the more severe forms of this disease, large, flaccid bullae erupt and may spread to cover extensive areas of the body. These bullae eventually rupture, revealing sections of denuded skin.

Desquamation

In this final stage, affected areas dry up and powdery scales form. Normal skin replaces these scales in 5 to 7 days.

Diagnosis

Careful observation of the three-stage progression of this disease allows diagnosis. Results of exfoliative cytology and a biopsy aid in the differential diagnosis, ruling out erythema multiforme and drug-induced toxic epidermal necrolysis, both of which are similar to SSSS.

Isolation of Group 2 *S. aureus* on cultures of skin lesions confirms the diagnosis. However, skin lesions sometimes appear sterile.

Treatment
Systemic antibiotics, usually penicillinase-resistant penicillin, treat the underlying infection. Replacement measures maintain fluid and electrolyte balance.

Special considerations
• Provide special care for the neonate, if required, including placement in a warming infant incubator to maintain body temperature and provide isolation.
• Carefully monitor intake and output to assess fluid and electrolyte balance. In severe cases, I.V. fluid replacement may be necessary.
• Check vital signs. Be especially alert for a sudden rise in temperature, indicating sepsis, which requires prompt, aggressive treatment.
• Maintain skin integrity. Remember to use strict aseptic technique to preclude secondary infection, especially during the exfoliative stage, because of open lesions.
• To prevent friction and sloughing of the patient's skin, leave affected areas uncovered or loosely covered. Place cotton between fingers and toes that are severely affected to prevent webbing.
• Administer warm baths and soaks during the recovery period. Gently debride exfoliated areas.
• Reassure parents that complications are rare and residual scars are unlikely.

STOMATITIS AND OTHER ORAL INFECTIONS

A common infection, stomatitis — inflammation of the oral mucosa — may extend to the buccal mucosa, lips, and palate. It may occur alone or as part of a systemic disease.

There are two main types: acute herpetic stomatitis and aphthous stomatitis. Acute herpetic stomatitis is common in children ages 1 to 3. Aphthous stomatitis is common in girls and female adolescents.

Acute herpetic stomatitis is usually self-limiting; however, it may be severe and, in neonates, may be generalized and potentially fatal. Aphthous stomatitis usually heals spontaneously, without a scar, in 10 to 14 days.

Other oral infections include gingivitis, periodontitis, Vincent's angina, and glossitis. (See *Oral infections,* page 826.)

Causes
Acute herpetic stomatitis results from herpes simplex virus. Predisposing factors for aphthous stomatitis include stress, fatigue, anxiety, febrile states, trauma, and sun overexposure.

Signs and symptoms
Acute herpetic stomatitis begins suddenly with mouth pain, malaise, lethargy, anorexia, irritability, and fever, which may persist for 1 to 2 weeks. Gums are swollen and bleed easily, and the mucous membranes are extremely tender. Papulovesicular ulcers appear in the mouth and throat and eventually become punched-out lesions with reddened areolae. Another common finding is submaxillary lymphadenitis.

Pain usually disappears from 2 to 4 days before healing of ulcers is com-

ORAL INFECTIONS

DISEASE AND CAUSES	SIGNS AND SYMPTOMS	TREATMENT
Gingivitis (inflammation of the gingiva) • Early sign of hypovitaminosis, diabetes, blood dyscrasias • Occasionally related to use of oral contraceptives	• Inflammation with painless swelling, redness, change of normal contours, bleeding, and periodontal pocket (gum detachment from teeth)	• Removal of irritating factors (calculus, faulty dentures) • Good oral hygiene; regular dental checkups; vigorous chewing • Oral or topical corticosteroids
Periodontitis (progression of gingivitis; inflammation of the oral mucosa) • Early sign of hypovitaminosis, diabetes, blood dyscrasias • Occasionally related to use of oral contraceptives • Dental factors: calculus, poor oral hygiene, malocclusion. Major cause of tooth loss after middle age	• Acute onset of bright red gum inflammation, painless swelling of interdental papillae, easy bleeding • Loosening of teeth, typically without inflammatory symptoms, progressing to loss of teeth and alveolar bone • Acute systemic infection (fever, chills)	• Scaling, root planing, and curettage for infection control • Periodontal surgery to prevent recurrence • Good oral hygiene, regular dental checkups, vigorous chewing
Vincent's angina (trench mouth, necrotizing ulcerative gingivitis) • Fusiform bacillus or spirochete infection • Predisposing factors: stress, poor oral hygiene, insufficient rest, nutritional deficiency, smoking	• Sudden onset: painful, superficial bleeding gingival ulcers (rarely, on buccal mucosa) covered with a gray-white membrane • Ulcers become punched-out lesions after slight pressure or irritation. • Malaise, mild fever, excessive salivation, bad breath, pain on swallowing or talking, enlarged submaxillary lymph nodes	• Removal of devitalized tissue with ultrasonic cavitron • Antibiotics (penicillin or oral erythromycin) for infection • Analgesics as needed • Hourly mouth rinses (equal parts hydrogen peroxide and warm water) • Soft, nonirritating diet; rest; no smoking • With treatment, improvement within 24 hours
Glossitis (tongue inflammation) • Streptococcal infection • Irritation or injury, jagged teeth, ill-fitting dentures, biting during convulsions, alcohol, spicy foods, smoking, sensitivity to toothpaste or mouthwash • Vitamin B deficiency, anemia • Skin conditions: lichen planus, erythema multiforme, pemphigus vulgaris	• Reddened ulcerated or swollen tongue (may obstruct airway) • Painful chewing and swallowing • Speech difficulty • Painful tongue without inflammation	• Treatment of underlying cause • Topical anesthetic mouthwash or systemic analgesics (aspirin and acetaminophen) for painful lesions • Good oral hygiene; regular dental checkups; vigorous chewing • Avoidance of alcohol and hot, cold, or spicy foods

plete. If the child with stomatitis sucks his thumb, these lesions spread to the hand.

A patient with aphthous stomatitis will typically report burning, tingling, and slight swelling of the mucous membrane. Single or multiple shallow ulcers with whitish centers and red borders appear and heal at one site but then appear at another.

Diagnosis
Physical examination allows diagnosis. In Vincent's angina, a smear of ulcer exudate allows identification of the causative organism.

Treatment and special considerations
For acute herpetic stomatitis, treatment is conservative. For local symptoms, management includes warm-water mouth rinses (antiseptic mouthwashes are contraindicated because they are irritating) and a topical anesthetic to relieve mouth ulcer pain. Supplementary treatment includes bland or liquid diet and, in severe cases, I.V. fluids and bed rest.

For aphthous stomatitis, primary treatment is application of a topical anesthetic. Effective long-term treatment requires alleviation or prevention of precipitating factors.

STRABISMUS

Also called squint, heterotropia, cross-eye, or walleye, strabismus is a condition of eye malalignment that results from the absence of normal, parallel, or coordinated eye movement. In children, it may be concomitant, in which the degree of deviation doesn't vary with the direction of gaze; inconcomitant, in which the degree of deviation varies with the direction of gaze; congenital (present at birth or during the first 6 months); or acquired (present during the first 2½ years).

Strabismus can also be latent (phoria), apparent when the child is tired or sick, or manifest (tropia). Tropias are categorized into four types: esotropia (eyes deviate inward), exotropia (eyes deviate outward), hypertropia (eyes deviate upward), and hypotropia (eyes deviate downward). (See *Esotropia,* page 828.)

Strabismus affects about 2% of the population. Incidence of strabismus is higher in patients with central nervous sustem (CNS) disorders, such as cerebral palsy, mental retardation, and Down syndrome.

The prognosis for correction varies with the timing of treatment and the onset of the disease. Muscle imbalances may be corrected by glasses, patching, or surgery, depending on the cause. However, residual defects in vision and extraocular muscle alignment may persist even after treatment.

Causes
Strabismus is frequently inherited, but its cause is unknown. Controversy exists over whether or not amblyopia ("lazy eye") causes or results from strabismus. In adults, strabismus may result from trauma.

Strabismic amblyopia is characterized by a loss of central vision in one eye that typically results in esotropia (from fixation in the dominant eye and suppression of images in the deviating eye). Strabismic amblyopia may result from hyperopia (farsightedness) or anisometropia (unequal refractive power).

Esotropia may result from muscle imbalance and may be congenital or acquired. In accommodative esotropia, the child's attempt to compensate for the farsightedness affects the convergent reflex, and the eyes cross.

Malalignment of the eyes leads to suppression of vision in one of the eyes.

ESOTROPIA

In esotropia, medial deviation occurs.

It causes amblyopia if it develops early in life, before bifoveal fixation is established.

Signs and symptoms

Malalignment of the eyes can be detected by external eye examination when deviation is obvious or by ophthalmoscopic observation of the corneal light reflex in the center of the pupils.

In addition, strabismus causes diplopia and other visual disturbances, which is often the reason the patient seeks medical help.

Diagnosis

Parents of children with strabismus will typically seek medical advice. Older persons with strabismus commonly seek treatment to correct double vision or to improve appearance. A careful, detailed patient history is essential not only for the diagnosis, but also for the prognosis and treatment of strabismus.

The following ophthalmologic tests help diagnose strabismus:

• *Visual acuity test* evaluates the degree of visual defect.

• *Hirschberg's method* detects malalignment. The patient fixes his gaze on a light at a distance of about 13″ (33 cm) as the examiner observes the light decentered in the deviating eye.

• *Retinoscopy* determines refractive error. This is usually done with pupils dilated.

• *Maddox rods test* assesses specific muscle involvement.

• *Convergence test* shows the distance at which convergence is sustained.

• *Duction test* reveals limitations of eye movement.

• *Cover-uncover test* demonstrates eye deviation and the rate of recovery to original alignment.

• *Alternate-cover test* shows intermittent or latent deviation.

A neurologic examination determines whether the condition is muscular or neurologic in origin. It should be performed if the onset of strabismus is sudden or if the CNS is involved.

Treatment

Initial treatment depends on the type of strabismus. For strabismic amblyopia, therapy includes patching the normal eye and prescribing corrective glasses to keep the eye straight and to counteract farsightedness (especially in accommodative esotropia).

Surgery is often necessary for cosmetic and psychological reasons to correct strabismus that results from basic esotropia or residual accommodative esotropia after correction with glasses.

Timing of surgery varies with individual circumstances. For example, a 6-month-old infant with equal visual acuity and a large esotropia will have the deviation corrected surgically. But a child with unequal visual acuity and an acquired deviation will have the affected eye patched until visual acuity is equal, *then* undergo surgery.

Surgical correction includes recession (moving the muscle posteriorly from its original insertion) or resection (shortening the muscle). A recent surgical procedure uses an adjustable suture.

Possible complications include overcorrection or undercorrection, slipped muscle, and perforation of the globe. Postoperative therapy may include patching the affected eye and applying combination antibiotic-steroid eyedrops. Eye exercises and corrective glasses may still be necessary; surgery may have to be repeated.

Special considerations
• Postoperatively, discourage the child from rubbing his eyes.
• Gently wipe the child's tears, which will be serosanguineous. Reassure his parents that this is normal.
• Administer antiemetics, if necessary.
• Apply antibiotic ointment to the affected eye. Teach the patient or his parents how to instill the ointment.
• Because this surgery is usually a one-day procedure, most children are discharged after they recover from anesthesia; encourage compliance with recommended follow-up care.

Stye

A localized, purulent staphylococcal infection, a stye (hordeolum) can occur externally (in the lumen of the smaller glands of Zeis or in Moll's glands) or internally (in the larger meibomian gland).

A stye can occur at any age. Generally, this infection responds well to treatment but tends to recur. If untreated, a stye can eventually lead to cellulitis of the eyelid.

Signs and symptoms
Typically, a stye produces redness, swelling, and pain. An abscess frequently forms at the lid margin, with an eyelash pointing outward from its center.

Diagnosis
Visual examination generally confirms this infection. Culture of purulent material from the abscess usually reveals a staphylococcal organism.

Treatment
Warm compresses applied for 10 to 15 minutes, four times a day for 3 to 4 days, facilitates drainage of the abscess, relieves pain and inflammation, and promotes suppuration. Drug therapy includes a topical sulfonamide or antibiotic eyedrops or ointment and, occasionally, a systemic antibiotic.

If conservative treatment fails, incision and drainage may be necessary.

Special considerations
• Instruct the patient to use a clean cloth for each application of warm compresses and to dispose of it or launder it separately.
• Warn against squeezing the stye; this spreads the infection and may cause cellulitis.
• Teach the patient or family members the proper technique for instilling eye drops or ointments into the cul-de-sac of the lower eyelid.

LIFE-THREATENING DISORDER

Sudden Infant Death Syndrome

A medical mystery of early infancy, sudden infant death syndrome (SIDS) — commonly called crib death — kills apparently healthy infants, usually between ages 4 weeks and 7 months, for reasons that remain unexplained, even after an autopsy. Typically, parents put the infant to bed and later find him dead, often with no indications of a struggle or distress of any kind.

Some infants may have had signs of a cold, but such symptoms are usually absent. SIDS has occurred throughout history, all over the world, and in all climates.

Causes

SIDS accounts for 7,500 to 8,000 deaths annually in the United States, making it one of the leading causes of infant death. Most of these deaths occur during the winter, in poor families, and among underweight babies and those born to mothers under age 20.

Although infants who die from SIDS often appear healthy, research suggests that many may have had undetected abnormalities such as an immature respiratory system and respiratory dysfunction. In fact, the current thinking is that SIDS may result from an abnormality in the control of ventilation, which causes prolonged apneic periods with profound hypoxemia and serious cardiac arrhythmias.

Bottle-feeding instead of breast-feeding and advanced parental age *don't* cause SIDS.

Signs and symptoms

Although parents find some victims wedged in crib corners or with blankets wrapped around their heads, autopsies rule out suffocation as the cause of death. Even when frothy, blood-tinged sputum is found around the infant's mouth or on the crib sheets, an autopsy shows a patent airway, so aspiration of vomitus is not the cause of death.

Typically, SIDS babies don't cry out and show no signs of having been disturbed in their sleep, although their positions or tangled blankets may suggest movement just before death, perhaps from terminal spasm.

Depending on how long the infant has been dead, a SIDS baby may have a mottled complexion, with extreme cyanosis of the lips and fingertips, or pooling of blood in the legs and feet that may be mistaken for bruises. Pulse and respirations are absent, and the infant's diaper is wet and full of stools.

Diagnosis

An autopsy rules out other causes of death. Characteristic histologic findings on autopsy include small or normal adrenal glands and petechiae over the visceral surfaces of the pleura, within the thymus (which is enlarged), and in the epicardium.

An autopsy also reveals extremely well-preserved lymphoid structures and certain pathologic characteristics that suggest chronic hypoxemia, such as increased pulmonary artery smooth muscle. Examination also shows edematous, congestive lungs fully expanded in the pleural cavities, liquid (not clotted) blood in the heart, and curd from the stomach inside the trachea.

Treatment

If the parents bring the infant to the emergency department, the doctor will decide whether to try to resuscitate him. An "aborted SIDS" is an infant who is found apneic and is successfully resuscitated. Such an infant, or any infant who had a sibling stricken by SIDS, should be tested for infantile apnea. If tests are positive, a home apnea monitor may be recommended.

Because most infants can't be resuscitated, however, treatment focuses on emotional support for the family.

Special considerations

• Make sure that both parents are present when the child's death is announced. The parents may lash out at emergency department personnel, the babysitter, or anyone else involved in the child's care—even at each other. Stay calm and let them express their feelings. Reassure them that they were not to blame.

• Let the parents see the baby in a private room. Allow them to express their grief in their own way. Stay in the room with them, if appropriate. Offer to call clergy, friends, or relatives.

• After the parents and family have recovered from their initial shock, explain the necessity for an autopsy to confirm the diagnosis of SIDS (in some states, this is mandatory). At this time, provide the family with some basic facts about SIDS and encourage them to give their consent for the autopsy. Make sure they receive the autopsy report promptly.

• Find out whether there's a local counseling and information program for SIDS parents. Participants in such a program will contact the parents, ensure that they receive the autopsy report promptly, put them in touch with a professional counselor, and maintain supportive telephone contact.

• Find out whether there's a local SIDS parents' group; such a group can provide significant emotional support. Contact the National Sudden Infant Death Foundation for information about such local groups.

• If your hospital's policy is to assign a public health nurse to the family, she will provide the continuing reassurance and assistance the parents will need.

• If the parents decide to have another child, make sure they receive information and counseling to help them deal with the pregnancy and the first year of the new infant's life.

SYNDROME OF INAPPROPRIATE ANTIDIURETIC HORMONE SECRETION

Excessive release of antidiuretic hormone (ADH) disturbs fluid and electrolyte balance in syndrome of inappropriate antidiuretic hormone secretion (SIADH). Such disturbances result from an inability to excrete dilute urine, retention of free water, expansion of extracellular fluid volume, and hyponatremia.

SIADH occurs secondary to diseases that affect the osmoreceptors (supraoptic nucleus) of the hypothalamus. The prognosis depends on the underlying disorder and response to treatment.

Causes

The most common cause of SIADH (80% of patients) is oat cell carcinoma of the lung, which secretes excessive levels of ADH or vasopressin-like substances. Other neoplastic diseases—such as pancreatic and prostatic cancer, Hodgkin's disease, and thymoma—may also trigger SIADH.

Less common causes include:

• *central nervous system disorders*—brain tumor or abscess, cerebrovascular accident, head injury, and Guillain-Barré syndrome

• *pulmonary disorders*—pneumonia, tuberculosis, lung abscess, and positive-pressure ventilation

• *drugs*—chlorpropamide, vincristine, cyclophosphamide, carbamazepine, clofibrate, and morphine

• *miscellaneous conditions*—psychosis and myxedema.

Signs and symptoms

SIADH may produce weight gain despite anorexia, nausea, and vomiting; muscle weakness; restlessness; and possibly seizures and coma. Edema is rare unless water overload exceeds 4 L, because much of the free-water excess is within cellular boundaries.

Diagnosis

A complete medical history revealing positive water balance may suggest SIADH. Serum osmolality less than 280 mOsm/kg of water and serum sodium less than 123 mEq/L confirm it. (Normal urine osmolality is 1½ times serum values.)

Supportive laboratory values include high urine sodium secretion (more than 20 mEq/L) without diuretics. In addition, diagnostic studies show normal renal function and no evidence of dehydration.

Treatment

Symptomatic treatment begins with restricted water intake (500 to 1,000 ml/day). With severe water intoxication, administration of 200 to 300 ml of 5% saline solution may be necessary to raise the serum sodium level.

When possible, treatment should include correction of the underlying cause of SIADH. If SIADH results from cancer, success in alleviating water retention may be obtained by surgical resection, irradiation, or chemotherapy.

If fluid restriction is ineffective, demeclocycline or lithium may be helpful by blocking the renal response to ADH.

Special considerations

• Closely monitor and record intake and output, vital signs, and daily weight. Watch for hyponatremia.
• Observe for restlessness, irritability, seizures, congestive heart failure, and unresponsiveness resulting from hyponatremia and water intoxication.
• To prevent water intoxication, explain to the patient and his family why he *must* restrict his intake.

SYPHILIS

A chronic, infectious, sexually transmitted disease, syphilis begins in the mucous membranes and quickly becomes systemic, spreading to nearby lymph nodes and the bloodstream. This disease, when untreated, is characterized by progressive stages: primary, secondary, latent, and late (formerly called tertiary).

About 34,000 cases of syphilis, in primary and secondary stages, are reported annually in the United States. Incidence is highest among urban populations, especially in persons between ages 15 and 39, drug users, and those infected with the human immunodeficiency virus (HIV).

Untreated syphilis leads to crippling or death, but the prognosis is excellent with early treatment.

Causes

Infection from the spirochete *Treponema pallidum* causes syphilis. Transmission occurs primarily through sexual contact during the primary, secondary, and early latent stages of infection. Prenatal transmission from an infected mother to her fetus is also possible. (See *Prenatal syphilis.*)

Signs and symptoms

Each stage produces distinctive signs and symptoms.

Primary syphilis

After an incubation period that generally lasts about 3 weeks, symptoms of primary syphilis develop.

Prenatal Syphilis

A woman can transmit syphilis transplacentally to her unborn child throughout pregnancy. This type of syphilis is often called congenital, but prenatal is a more accurate term. Approximately 50% of infected fetuses die before or shortly after birth. The prognosis is better for those who develop overt infection after age 2.

Signs and symptoms

The infant with prenatal syphilis may appear healthy at birth but usually develops characteristic lesions — vesicular, bullous eruptions, often on the palms and soles — 3 weeks later. Shortly afterward, a maculopapular rash similar to that in secondary syphilis may erupt on the face, mouth, genitalia, palms, or soles. Condylomata lata often occur around the anus.

Lesions may erupt on the mucous membranes of the mouth, pharynx, and nose. When the infant's larynx is affected, his cry becomes weak and forced. If the nasal mucous membranes are involved, he may also develop nasal discharge, which can be slight and mucopurulent or copious with blood-tinged pus.

Visceral and bone lesions, liver or spleen enlargement with ascites, and nephrotic syndrome may also develop.

Late prenatal syphilis becomes apparent after age 2; it may be identifiable only through blood studies or may cause unmistakable syphilitic changes: screwdriver-shaped central incisors, deformed molars or cusps, thick clavicles, saber shins, bowed tibias, nasal septum perforation, eighth cranial nerve deafness, and neurosyphilis.

Diagnosis

In the infant with prenatal syphilis, Venereal Disease Research Laboratory titer, if reactive at birth, stays the same or rises, indicating active disease. The infant's titer drops in 3 months if the mother has received effective prenatal treatment. An absolute diagnosis necessitates a darkfield examination of umbilical vein blood or lesion drainage.

Treatment

An infant with abnormal cerebrospinal fluid (CSF) may be treated with aqueous crystalline penicillin G, I.M. or I.V. (50,000 units/kg of body weight/day divided in two doses for at least 10 days), or aqueous penicillin G procaine I.M. (50,000 units/kg of body weight/day for at least 10 days). An infant with normal CSF may be treated with a single injection of penicillin G benzathine (50,000 units/kg of body weight).

When caring for a child with prenatal syphilis, record the extent of the rash, and watch for signs of systemic involvement, especially laryngeal swelling, jaundice, and decreasing urine output.

Initially, one or more chancres (small, fluid-filled lesions) erupt on the genitalia; others may erupt on the anus, fingers, lips, tongue, nipples, tonsils, or eyelids. These chancres, which are usually painless, start as papules and then erode; they have indurated, raised edges and clear bases.

Chancres typically disappear after 3 to 6 weeks, even when untreated. They are usually associated with regional lymphadenopathy (unilateral or bilateral). In women, chancres are frequently overlooked because they often develop on internal structures — the cervix or the vaginal wall.

Secondary syphilis

The development of symmetrical mucocutaneous lesions and general lymphadenopathy signals the onset of secondary syphilis, which may develop within a few days or up to 8 weeks after the onset of initial chancres.

The rash of secondary syphilis can be macular, papular, pustular, or nodular. Lesions are of uniform size, well defined, and generalized. Macules often erupt between rolls of fat on the trunk and on the arms, palms, soles, face, and scalp. In warm, moist areas (perineum, scrotum, vulva, between rolls of fat), the lesions enlarge and erode, producing highly contagious, pink, or grayish-white lesions (condylomata lata).

Mild constitutional symptoms of syphilis appear in the second stage and may include headache, malaise, anorexia, weight loss, nausea, vomiting, sore throat and, possibly, slight fever. Alopecia may occur, with or without treatment, and is usually temporary. Nails become brittle and pitted.

Latent syphilis

Although no clinical symptoms occur in latent syphilis, it produces a reactive serologic test for syphilis. Because infectious mucocutaneous lesions may reappear when infection is of less than 4 years' duration, early latent syphilis is considered contagious.

Approximately two-thirds of patients remain asymptomatic in the late latent stage until death. The rest develop characteristic late-stage symptoms.

Late syphilis

The final, destructive, but noninfectious stage of the disease, late syphilis has three subtypes, any or all of which may affect the patient: late benign syphilis, cardiovascular syphilis, and neurosyphilis.

The lesions of late benign syphilis develop between 1 and 10 years after infection. They may appear on the skin, bones, mucous membranes, upper respiratory tract, liver, or stomach.

The typical lesion is a gumma — a chronic, superficial nodule or deep, granulomatous lesion that is solitary, asymmetric, painless, and indurated. Gummas can be found on any bone — particularly the long bones of the legs — and in any organ.

If late syphilis involves the liver, it can cause epigastric pain, tenderness, enlarged spleen, and anemia; if it involves the upper respiratory tract, it may cause perforation of the nasal septum or the palate. In severe cases, late benign syphilis results in destruction of bones or organs, which eventually causes death.

Cardiovascular syphilis develops about 10 years after the initial infection in approximately 10% of patients with late, untreated syphilis. It causes fibrosis of elastic tissue of the aorta and leads to aortitis, most often in the ascending and transverse sections of the aortic arch. Cardiovascular syphilis may be asymptomatic or may cause aortic regurgitation or aneurysm.

Symptoms of neurosyphilis develop in about 8% of patients with late, untreated syphilis and appear from 5 to 35 years after infection. These clinical effects consist of meningitis and widespread CNS damage that may include general paresis, personality changes, and arm and leg weakness.

Diagnosis

Identifying *T. pallidum* from a lesion on a dark-field examination provides immediate diagnosis of syphilis. This method is most effective when moist lesions are present, as in primary, secondary, and prenatal syphilis.

The fluorescent treponemal antibody-absorption test identifies antigens of *T. pallidum* in tissue, ocular fluid, cerebrospinal fluid (CSF), tracheobronchial secretions, and exudates from lesions. This is the most sensitive test available for detecting syphilis in all stages. Once reactive, it remains so permanently.

Other appropriate procedures include the following:

• *Venereal Disease Research Laboratory (VDRL) slide test* and *rapid plasma reagin test* detect nonspecific antibodies. Both tests, if positive, become reactive within 1 to 2 weeks after the primary lesion appears or 4 to 5 weeks after the infection begins.

• *CSF examination* identifies neurosyphilis when the total protein level is above 40 mg/100 ml, VDRL slide test is reactive, and CSF cell count exceeds five mononuclear cells/μl.

Treatment

Administration of penicillin I.M. is the treatment of choice. For early syphilis, treatment may consist of a single injection of penicillin G benzathine I.M. (2.4 million units). Syphilis of more than 1 year's duration should be treated with penicillin G benzathine I.M. (2.4 million units/week for 3 weeks).

Nonpregnant patients who are allergic to penicillin may be treated with oral tetracycline or doxycycline for 15 days for early syphilis; 30 days for late infections. Nonpenicillin therapy for latent or late syphilis should be used only after neurosyphilis has been excluded. Tetracycline is contraindicated in pregnant women.

Special considerations

• Stress the importance of completing the course of therapy even after symptoms subside.

• Check for a history of drug sensitivity before administering the first dose.

• Practice universal precautions.

• In secondary syphilis, keep lesions clean and dry. If they're draining, dispose of contaminated materials properly.

• In late syphilis, provide symptomatic care during prolonged treatment.

• In cardiovascular syphilis, check for signs of decreased cardiac output (decreased urine output, hypoxia, and decreased sensorium) and pulmonary congestion.

• In neurosyphilis, regularly check level of consciousness, mood, and coherence. Watch for signs of ataxia.

• Urge patients to seek VDRL testing after 3, 6, 12, and 24 months to detect possible relapse. Patients treated for latent or late syphilis should receive blood tests at 6-month intervals for 2 years.

• Be sure to report all cases of syphilis to local public health authorities. Urge the patient to inform sexual partners of his infection so that they can receive treatment also.

• Refer the patient and his sexual partners for HIV testing.

Taeniasis

Also called tapeworm disease or cestodiasis, taeniasis is a parasitic infestation by *Taenia saginata* (beef tapeworm), *Taenia solium* (pork tapeworm), *Diphyllobothrium latum* (fish tapeworm), or *Hymenolepis nana* (dwarf tapeworm).

Taeniasis is usually a chronic, benign intestinal disease; however, infestation with *T. solium* may cause dangerous systemic and CNS symptoms if larvae invade the brain and striated muscle of vital organs.

Causes

T. saginata, *T. solium*, and *D. latum* are transmitted to humans by ingestion of beef, pork, or fish that contains tapeworm cysts. Gastric acids break down these cysts in the stomach, liberating them to mature. Mature tapeworms fasten to the intestinal wall and produce ova that are passed in the feces.

Transmission of *H. nana* is direct from person to person and requires no intermediate host; it completes its life cycle in the intestine.

Diagnosis

Tapeworm infestations are diagnosed by laboratory observation of tapeworm ova or body segments in feces. Because ova aren't excreted continuously, confirmation may require multiple specimens. A supporting dietary or travel history aids confirmation.

Treatment

Niclosamide offers a cure in up to 95% of patients. In beef, pork, and fish tapeworm infestation, the drug is given once; in severe dwarf tapeworm infestation, twice (5 to 7 days each time, spaced 2 weeks apart). Another anthelmintic agent, praziquantel, may also be effective.

After drug treatment, all types of tapeworm infestation require a follow-up laboratory examination of stool specimens during the next 3 to 5 weeks to check for any remaining ova or worm segments. Of course, persistent infestation typically requires a second course of medication.

Special considerations

• Obtain a complete history, including recent travel to endemic areas, dietary habits, and physical symptoms.

• Dispose of the patient's excretions carefully. Wear gloves when giving personal care and handling fecal excretions, bedpans, and bed linens; wash your hands thoroughly and instruct the patient to do the same.

• Tell the patient not to consume anything after midnight on the day niclosamide therapy is to start, because the drug must be given on an empty stomach. After administering the drug, document passage of strobilae.

• In pork tapeworm infestation, use enteric and secretion precautions. Avoid procedures and drugs that may cause vomiting or gagging. If the patient is a child or is incontinent, he requires a private room. Obtain a list of contacts.

• Document level of consciousness and be alert for changes. If central nervous system symptoms appear, keep an artificial airway or padded tongue blade close at hand, raise side rails, keep the bed low, and help with walking, as needed.

• To prevent reinfestation, teach proper handwashing technique and the need to cook meat and fish thoroughly. Stress the need for follow-up evaluations to monitor the success of therapy and to detect possible reinfestation.

TENDINITIS AND BURSITIS

A painful inflammation of tendons and of tendon-muscle attachments to bone, *tendinitis* usually occurs in the shoulder rotator cuff, hip, Achilles tendon, or hamstring.

Bursitis is a painful inflammation of one or more of the bursae—closed sacs that are lubricated with small amounts of synovial fluid that facilitate the motion of muscles and tendons over bony prominences. Bursitis usually occurs in the subdeltoid, olecranon, trochanteric, calcaneal, or prepatellar bursae.

Causes

• Tendinitis commonly results from trauma (such as strain during sports activity), another musculoskeletal disorder (rheumatic diseases, congenital defects), postural misalignment, abnormal body development, or hypermobility.

• Bursitis usually occurs in middle age from recurring trauma that stresses or pressures a joint or from an inflammatory joint disease (rheumatoid arthritis, gout). Chronic bursitis follows attacks of acute bursitis or repeated trauma and infection. Septic bursitis may result from wound infection or from bacterial invasion of skin over the bursa.

Signs and symptoms
Tendinitis and bursitis have characteristic signs and symptoms.

Tendinitis
The patient with tendinitis of the shoulder complains of restricted shoulder movement, especially abduction, and localized pain, which is most severe at night and often interferes with sleep. The pain extends from the acromion (the shoulder's highest point) to the deltoid muscle insertion, predominately in the so-called painful arc—that is, when the patient abducts his arm between 50 degrees and 130 degrees. Fluid accumulation causes swelling.

In calcific tendinitis, calcium deposits in the tendon cause proximal weakness and, if calcium erodes into adjacent bursae, acute calcific bursitis.

Bursitis
In bursitis, fluid accumulation in the bursae causes irritation, inflammation, sudden or gradual pain, and limited movement. Other symptoms vary according to the affected site. Subdeltoid bursitis impairs arm abduction; prepatellar bursitis (housemaid's knee) produces pain when the patient climbs stairs; hip bursitis makes crossing the legs painful.

Diagnosis
In tendinitis, X-rays may be normal at first but later show bony fragments, osteophyte sclerosis, or calcium deposits. Arthrography is usually normal, with occasional small irregularities on the undersurface of the tendon.

Diagnosis of tendinitis must rule out other causes of shoulder pain, such as myocardial infarction, cervical spondylosis, and tendon tear or rupture.

Significantly, in tendinitis, heat aggravates shoulder pain; in other painful joint disorders, heat usually provides relief.

Localized pain and inflammation and a history of unusual strain or injury 2 to 3 days before onset of pain are the bases for diagnosing bursitis. During early stages, X-rays are usually normal, except in calcific bursitis, in which X-rays may show calcium deposits.

Treatment

Therapy to relieve pain includes resting the joint (by immobilization with a sling, splint, or cast), systemic analgesics, application of cold or heat, ultrasound, or local injection of an anesthetic and corticosteroids to reduce inflammation.

A mixture of a corticosteroid and an anesthetic, such as lidocaine, generally provides immediate pain relief. Extended-release injections of a corticosteroid, such as triamcinolone or prednisolone, offer longer pain relief. Until the patient is free of pain and able to perform range-of-motion exercises easily, treatment also includes oral anti-inflammatory agents, such as sulindac and indomethacin. Short-term analgesics include codeine, propoxyphene, acetaminophen with codeine and, occasionally, oxycodone.

Supplementary treatment

Other treatment measures include fluid removal by aspiration, physical therapy to preserve motion and prevent frozen joints (improvement usually follows in 1 to 4 weeks), and heat therapy; for calcific tendinitis, ice packs. Rarely, calcific tendinitis requires surgical removal of calcium deposits.

Long-term control of chronic bursitis and tendinitis may require changes in lifestyle to prevent recurring joint irritation.

Special considerations

• Assess the severity of pain and the range of motion to determine effectiveness of the treatment.
• Before injecting corticosteroids or local anesthetics, ask the patient about drug allergies.
• Before intra-articular injection, scrub the patient's skin thoroughly with povidone-iodine or a comparable solution, and shave the injection site, if necessary. After the injection, massage the area to ensure penetration through the tissue and joint space. Apply ice intermittently for about 4 hours to minimize pain. Avoid applying heat to the area for 2 days.

Because patient teaching is essential, tell the patient to:
• take anti-inflammatory agents with milk to minimize GI distress, and to report any signs of distress immediately
• perform strengthening exercises and avoid activities that aggravate the joint
• wear a triangular sling during the first few days of an attack of subdeltoid bursitis or tendinitis to support the arm and protect the shoulder, particularly at night. Demonstrate how to wear the sling so it won't put too much weight on the shoulder. Instruct the patient's family how to pin the sling or how to tie a square knot that will lie flat on the back of the patient's neck. To protect the shoulder during sleep, a splint may be worn instead of a sling. Instruct the patient to remove the splint during the day.
• maintain joint mobility and prevent muscle atrophy by performing exercises or physical therapy when he is free of pain.

TESTICULAR CANCER

Malignant testicular tumors primarily affect young to middle-aged men and are the most common solid tumor in this group. (In children, testicular tumors are rare.) Most testicular tumors originate in gonadal cells. About 40% are seminomas — uniform, undifferentiated cells resembling primitive gonadal cells. The remainder are nonseminomas — tumor cells showing various degrees of differentiation.

The prognosis varies with the cell type and disease stage. When treated with surgery and radiation, almost all patients with localized disease survive beyond 5 years.

Causes
The cause of testicular cancer isn't known, but incidence (which peaks between ages 20 and 40) is higher in men with cryptorchidism (even when surgically corrected) and in men whose mothers used diethylstilbestrol during pregnancy. Testicular cancer is rare in nonwhite males and accounts for fewer than 1% of male cancer deaths.

Testicular cancer spreads through the lymphatic system to the iliac, para-aortic, and mediastinal lymph nodes and may metastasize to the lungs, liver, viscera, and bone.

Signs and symptoms
The first sign is usually a firm, painless, smooth testicular mass, varying in size and sometimes producing a sense of testicular heaviness. When such a tumor causes chorionic gonadotropin or estrogen production, gynecomastia and nipple tenderness may result.

In advanced stages, signs and symptoms include ureteral obstruction, abdominal mass, cough, hemoptysis, shortness of breath, weight loss, fatigue, pallor, and lethargy.

Diagnosis
• Two effective means of detecting a testicular tumor are regular self-examinations and testicular palpation during a routine physical examination.
• Transillumination can distinguish between a tumor (which doesn't transilluminate) and a hydrocele or spermatocele (which does). Follow-up measures should include an examination for gynecomastia and abdominal masses.
• Diagnostic tests include I.V. pyelography to detect ureteral deviation resulting from para-aortic node involvement, urinary or serum luteinizing hormone levels, blood tests, lymphangiography, ultrasound, and abdominal computed tomography scan.

Serum alpha-fetoprotein and beta-human chorionic gonadotropin levels — indicators of testicular tumor activity — provide a baseline for measuring response to therapy and determining the prognosis.
• Surgical excision and biopsy of the tumor and testis permits histologic verification of the tumor cell type — essential for effective treatment. Inguinal exploration determines the extent of nodal involvement. (See *Staging testicular cancer,* page 840.)

Treatment
The extent of surgery, radiation, and chemotherapy vary with tumor cell type and stage.

Surgery
Surgical procedures include orchiectomy and retroperitoneal node dissection. Most surgeons remove the testis, not the scrotum (to allow for a prosthetic implant). Hormone replacement therapy may be needed after bilateral orchiectomy.

STAGING TESTICULAR CANCER

The TNM (tumor, node, metastasis) staging system adopted by the American Joint Committee on Cancer has established the following stages for testicular cancer.

Primary tumor
TX—primary tumor can't be assessed (this stage is used in the absence of radical orchiectomy)
T0—histologic scar or no evidence of primary tumor
Tis—intratubular tumor: preinvasive cancer
T1—tumor limited to testicles, including the rete testis
T2—tumor extends beyond tunica albuginea or into epididymis
T3—tumor extends into spermatic cord
T4—tumor invades scrotum

Regional lymph nodes
NX—regional lymph nodes can't be assessed
N0—no evidence of regional lymph node metastasis
N1—metastasis in a single lymph node, 2 cm or less in greatest dimension

N2—metastasis in a single lymph node, between 2 and 5 cm in greatest dimension, or metastases to several lymph nodes, none more than 5 cm in greatest dimension
N3—metastasis in a lymph node more than 5 cm in greatest dimension

Distant metastasis
MX—distant metastasis unassessible
M0—no known distant metastasis
M1—distant metastasis

Staging categories
Testicular cancer progresses as follows:
Stage 0—Tis, N0, M0
Stage I—T1, N0, M0; T2, N0, M0
Stage II—T3, N0, M0; T4, N0, M0
Stage III—any T, N1, M0
Stage IV—any T, N2, M0; any T, N3, M0; any T, any N, M1

Radiation
The retroperitoneal and homolateral iliac nodes may receive radiation after removal of a seminoma. All positive nodes receive radiation after removal of a nonseminoma. Patients with retroperitoneal extension receive prophylactic radiation to the mediastinal and supraclavicular nodes.

Chemotherapy
Essential for tumors beyond Stage 0, chemotherapy combinations include bleomycin, etoposide, and cisplatin; cisplatin, vindesine, and bleomycin; cisplatin, vinblastine, and bleomycin; and cisplatin, vincristine, methotrexate, bleomycin, and leucovorin.

Chemotherapy and radiation followed by autologous bone marrow transplantation may help unresponsive patients.

Special considerations
• Develop a treatment plan that addresses both the patient's psychological and physical needs.

Before orchiectomy:
• Reassure the patient that sterility and impotence need not follow unilateral orchiectomy, that synthetic hormones can restore hormonal balance, and that most surgeons don't remove the scrotum. In many cases, a testicular prosthesis can correct anatomic disfigurement.

After orchiectomy:
• For the first day after surgery, apply an ice pack to the scrotum and provide analgesics.
• Check for excessive bleeding, swelling, and signs of infection.
• Provide a scrotal athletic supporter to minimize pain during ambulation.
During chemotherapy:
• Give antiemetics, as needed, for nausea and vomiting. Encourage small, frequent meals to maintain oral intake despite anorexia.
• Establish a mouth care regimen and check for stomatitis. Watch for signs of myelosuppression.
• If the patient receives vinblastine, assess for neurotoxicity (peripheral paresthesia, jaw pain, and muscle cramps). If he receives cisplatin, check for ototoxicity.
• To prevent renal damage, encourage increased fluid intake and provide I.V. fluids, a potassium supplement, and diuretics.

LIFE-THREATENING DISORDER

TETANUS

Lockjaw or tetanus is an acute exotoxin-mediated infection caused by the anaerobic, spore-forming, gram-positive bacillus *Clostridium tetani.* Usually, such infection is systemic; less often, localized.

Tetanus is fatal in up to 60% of unimmunized persons, usually within 10 days of onset. When symptoms develop within 3 days after exposure, the prognosis is poor.

Causes
Normally, transmission is through a puncture wound that is contaminated by soil, dust, or animal excreta containing *C. tetani,* or by way of burns and minor wounds. After *C. tetani* enters the body, it causes local infection and tissue necrosis. It also produces toxins that then enter the bloodstream and lymphatics and eventually spread to central nervous system tissue.

Tetanus occurs worldwide, but it's more prevalent in agricultural regions and developing countries that lack mass immunization programs. It's one of the most common causes of neonatal deaths in developing countries, where infants of unimmunized mothers are delivered under unsterile conditions. In such infants, the unhealed umbilical cord is the portal of entry.

In America, about 75% of all cases occur between April and September.

Signs and symptoms
The incubation period varies from 3 to 4 weeks in mild tetanus to under 2 days in severe tetanus. When symptoms occur within 3 days after injury, death is more likely. If tetanus remains localized, signs of onset are spasm and increased muscle tone near the wound.

If tetanus is generalized (systemic), indications include marked muscle hypertonicity, hyperactive deep tendon reflexes, tachycardia, profuse sweating, low-grade fever, and painful, involuntary muscle contractions:
• neck and facial muscles, especially cheek muscles—locked jaw (trismus) and a grotesque, grinning expression called *risus sardonicus*
• somatic muscles—arched-back rigidity (opisthotonos), boardlike abdominal rigidity
• intermittent tonic convulsions lasting several minutes, which may result in cyanosis and sudden death by asphyxiation.

Despite such pronounced neuromuscular symptoms, cerebral and sensory functions remain normal. Complications include atelectasis, pneumonia, pulmonary emboli, acute gastric ulcers, flexion contractures, and cardiac arrhythmias.

Neonatal tetanus is always generalized. The first clinical sign is difficulty in sucking, which usually appears 3 to 10 days after birth. It progresses to total inability to suck with excessive crying, irritability, and nuchal rigidity.

Diagnosis

Frequently, diagnosis must rest on clinical features and a history of trauma and no previous tetanus immunization. Blood cultures and tetanus antibody tests are often negative; only a third of patients have a positive wound culture. Cerebrospinal fluid pressure may rise above normal.

Diagnosis also must rule out meningitis, rabies, phenothiazine or strychnine toxicity, and other conditions that mimic tetanus.

Treatment

Within 72 hours after a puncture wound, a patient with no previous history of tetanus immunization first requires tetanus immune globulin (TIG) or tetanus antitoxin to confer temporary protection. Next, he needs active immunization with tetanus toxoid. A patient who has not received tetanus immunization within 5 years needs a booster injection of tetanus toxoid.

If tetanus develops despite immediate postinjury treatment, the patient will require airway maintenance and a muscle relaxant, such as diazepam, to decrease muscle rigidity and spasm. If muscle contractions aren't relieved by muscle relaxants, a neuromuscular blocker may be needed. The patient with tetanus needs high-dose antibiotics (penicillin administered I.V., if he's not allergic to it).

Special considerations

When caring for the patient with a puncture wound:

• Thoroughly debride and cleanse the injury site with 3% hydrogen peroxide, and check the patient's immunization history. Record the cause of injury. If it's a dog bite, report the case to local public health authorities.

• Before giving penicillin and TIG, antitoxin, or toxoid, obtain an accurate history of allergies to immunizations or penicillin. If the patient has a history of any allergies, keep epinephrine 1:1,000 and resuscitative equipment available.

• Stress the importance of maintaining active immunization with a booster dose of tetanus toxoid every 10 years.

After tetanus develops:

• Maintain an adequate airway and ventilation to prevent pneumonia and atelectasis. Suction often and watch for signs of respiratory distress. Keep emergency airway equipment on hand, because the patient may require artificial ventilation or oxygen administration.

• Maintain an I.V. line for medications and emergency care, if necessary.

• Monitor electrocardiography frequently for arrhythmias. Accurately record intake and output, and check vital signs often.

• Turn the patient frequently to prevent pressure sores and pulmonary stasis.

• Because even minimal external stimulation provokes muscle spasms, keep the patient's room dark and quiet. Warn visitors not to upset or overly stimulate the patient.

• If urinary retention develops, insert an indwelling catheter.

• Give muscle relaxants and sedatives, as ordered, and schedule patient care to coincide with heaviest sedation.

• Insert an artificial airway, if necessary, to prevent tongue injury and maintain airway during spasms.

• Provide adequate nutrition to meet the patient's increased metabolic needs. The patient may need nasogastric feedings or hyperalimentation.

THALASSEMIA

A hereditary group of hemolytic anemias, thalassemia is characterized by defective synthesis in the polypeptide chains necessary for hemoglobin production. Consequently, red blood cell (RBC) synthesis is also impaired. Thalassemia is most common in persons of Mediterranean ancestry (especially Italian and Greek), but also occurs in blacks and persons from southern China, southeast Asia, and India.

β-Thalassemia is the most common form of this disorder, resulting from defective beta polypeptide chain synthesis. It occurs in three clinical forms: thalassemia major, intermedia, and minor. The severity of the resulting anemia depends on whether the patient is homozygous or heterozygous for the thalassemic trait.

Prognosis for β-thalassemia varies. Patients with thalassemia major seldom survive to adulthood; children with thalassemia intermedia develop normally into adulthood, although puberty is usually delayed; persons with thalassemia minor can expect a normal life span.

Causes

Thalassemia major and *thalassemia intermedia* result from homozygous inheritance of the partially dominant autosomal gene responsible for this trait. *Thalassemia minor* results from heterozygous inheritance of the same gene.

In all these disorders, total or partial deficiency of beta polypeptide chain production impairs hemoglobin (Hb) synthesis and results in continual production of fetal hemoglobin (Hb F), lasting even past the neonatal period.

Signs and symptoms

The three clinical forms of β-thalassemia have different signs and symptoms.

Thalassemia major

In thalassemia major (also known as Cooley's anemia, Mediterranean disease, and erythroblastic anemia), the infant is well at birth but develops severe anemia, bone abnormalities, failure to thrive, and life-threatening complications. Often, the first signs are pallor and yellow skin and scleras in infants aged 3 to 6 months.

Later clinical features, in addition to severe anemia, include splenomegaly or hepatomegaly, with abdominal enlargement; frequent infections; bleeding tendencies (especially toward epistaxis); and anorexia.

Children with thalassemia major commonly have small bodies and large heads and may also be mentally retarded. Infants may have mongoloid features, because bone marrow hyperactivity has thickened the bone at the base of the nose. As these children grow older, they become susceptible to pathologic fractures, as a result of expansion of the marrow cavities with thinning of the long bones.

They are also subject to cardiac arrhythmias, heart failure, and other complications that result from iron deposits in the heart and in other tissues from repeated blood transfusions.

Thalassemia intermedia

This condition comprises moderate thalassemic disorders in homozygotes. Patients show some degree of anemia, jaundice, and splenomegaly and, possibly, signs of hemosiderosis due to increased intestinal absorption of iron.

Thalassemia minor

This form of thalassemia may cause mild anemia but usually produces no symptoms and is often overlooked.

Diagnosis

In thalassemia major:
• Laboratory results show lowered RBC count and Hb level, microcytosis, and elevated reticulocyte, bilirubin, and urinary and fecal urobilinogen levels.
• A low serum folate level indicates increased folate utilization by the hypertrophied bone marrow.
• A peripheral blood smear reveals target cells, microcytes, pale nucleated RBCs, and marked anisocytosis.
• X-rays of the skull and long bones show thinning and widening of the marrow space because of overactive bone marrow. The bones of the skull and vertebrae may appear granular; long bones may show areas of osteoporosis. The phalanges may also be deformed (rectangular or biconvex).
• Quantitative Hb studies show a significant rise in Hb F and a slight increase in Hb A_2. Diagnosis must rule out iron deficiency anemia, which also produces hypochromia (slightly lowered Hb) and microcytic (notably small) RBCs.

In thalassemia intermedia, laboratory results show hypochromia and microcytic RBCs, but the anemia is less severe than that in thalassemia major.

In thalassemia minor, laboratory results show hypochromia and microcytic RBCs. Quantitative Hb studies show a significant increase in Hb A_2 levels and a moderate rise in Hb F levels.

Treatment

Therapy for thalassemia major is essentially supportive. For example, infections require prompt treatment with appropriate antibiotics. Folic acid supplements help maintain folic acid levels in the face of increased requirements.

Transfusions of packed RBCs raise Hb levels but must be used judiciously to minimize iron overload. Splenectomy and bone marrow transplantation have been tried, but their effectiveness has not been confirmed.

Thalassemia intermedia and thalassemia minor generally don't require treatment. Iron supplements are contraindicated in all forms of thalassemia.

Special considerations

• During and after RBC transfusions for thalassemia major, watch for adverse reactions—shaking chills, fever, rash, itching, and hives.
• Stress the importance of good nutrition, meticulous wound care, periodic dental checkups, and other measures to prevent infection.
• Discuss with the parents of a young patient various options for healthy physical and creative outlets. Such a child must avoid strenuous athletic activity because of increased oxygen demand and the tendency toward pathologic fractures, but he may participate in less stressful activities.
• Teach parents to watch for signs of hepatitis and iron overload—always possible with frequent transfusions.
• Because parents may have questions about the vulnerability of future offspring, refer them for genetic counseling. Also, refer adult patients with thalassemia minor and thalassemia intermedia for genetic counseling; they need to recognize the risk of transmitting thalassemia major to their children if they marry another person with thalassemia. If such persons choose to marry and have children, all their children should be evaluated for thalassemia by age 1.
• Be sure to tell persons with thalassemia minor that their condition is benign.

Throat Abscesses

Abscess of the throat may be peritonsillar (quinsy) or retropharyngeal. Peritonsillar abscess forms in the connective tissue space between the tonsil capsule and constrictor muscle of the pharynx.

Retropharyngeal abscess, or abscess of the potential space, forms between the posterior pharyngeal wall and prevertebral fascia. With treatment, the prognosis for both types of abscesses is good.

Causes

Peritonsillar abscess is a complication of acute tonsillitis, usually after streptococcal or staphylococcal infection. It occurs more often in adolescents and young adults than in children.

Acute retropharyngeal abscess results from infection in the retropharyngeal lymph glands, which may follow an upper respiratory tract bacterial infection. Because these lymph glands, present at birth, begin to atrophy after age 2, acute retropharyngeal abscess most commonly affects infants and children under age 2.

Chronic retropharyngeal abscess may result from tuberculosis of the cervical spine (Pott's disease) and may occur at any age.

Signs and symptoms

Peritonsillar abscess and retropharyngeal abscess have different signs and symptoms.

Peritonsillar abscess

Key symptoms of peritonsillar abscess include severe throat pain, occasional ear pain on the same side as the abscess, and tenderness of the submandibular gland. Dysphagia causes drooling. Trismus may occur as a re-

sult of edema and infection spreading from the peritonsillar space to the pterygoid muscles.

Other effects include fever, chills, malaise, rancid breath, nausea, muffled speech, dehydration, cervical adenopathy, and localized or systemic sepsis.

Retropharyngeal abscess

Clinical features of retropharyngeal abscess include pain, dysphagia, fever and, when the abscess is located in the upper pharynx, nasal obstruction; with a low-positioned abscess, dyspnea, progressive inspiratory stridor (from laryngeal obstruction), neck hyperextension and, in children, drooling and muffled crying.

A very large abscess may press on the larynx, causing edema, or may erode into major vessels, causing sudden death from asphyxia or aspiration.

Diagnosis

• Diagnosing peritonsillar abscess is based on a patient history of bacterial pharyngitis. Examination of the throat shows swelling of the soft palate on the abscessed side, with displacement of the uvula to the opposite side; red, edematous mucous membranes; and tonsil displacement toward the midline. Culture may reveal streptococcal or staphylococcal infection.

• Diagnosis of retropharyngeal abscess is based on patient history of nasopharyngitis or pharyngitis and on physical examination revealing a soft, red bulging of the posterior pharyngeal wall. X-rays show the larynx pushed forward and a widened space between the posterior pharyngeal wall and vertebrae.

If neck pain or stiffness occurs, look for extension to epidural space or cervical vertebrae. Culture and sensitivity tests isolate the causative organism and determine the appropriate antibiotic.

Treatment

• For early-stage peritonsillar abscess, large doses of penicillin or another broad-spectrum antibiotic are necessary. If the patient is immunocompromised or has been repeatedly hospitalized, antibiotic therapy should include coverage for staphylococci and gram-negative organisms.

• For late-stage peritonsillar abscess, with cellulitis of the tonsillar space, primary treatment is usually incision and drainage under a local anesthetic, followed by antibiotic therapy for 7 to 10 days. Tonsillectomy, scheduled no sooner than 1 month after healing, prevents recurrence but is recommended only after several episodes.

• In acute retropharyngeal abscess, the primary treatment is incision and drainage through the pharyngeal wall.

• In chronic retropharyngeal abscess, drainage is performed through an external incision behind the sternomastoid muscle. During incision and drainage, strong, continuous mouth suction is necessary to prevent aspiration of pus. Postoperative drug therapy includes antibiotics (usually penicillin) and analgesics.

Special considerations

• Be alert for signs of respiratory obstruction (inspiratory stridor, dyspnea, increasing restlessness, or cyanosis). Keep emergency airway equipment nearby.

• Be aware that these infections can extend to the mediastinum, worsening sepsis and chest pain, and increasing breathing difficulty.

• Explain the drainage procedure to the patient or his parents. Because the procedure is generally done under a local anesthetic, the patient may be apprehensive.

• Perform incision and drainage. To allow easy expectoration and suction of pus and blood, place the patient in a semirecumbent or sitting position.

After incision and drainage:

• Give antibiotics, analgesics, and antipyretics. Stress the importance of completing the full course of prescribed antibiotic therapy.

• Monitor vital signs, and watch for any significant changes or bleeding. Assess pain and treat accordingly.

• If the patient is unable to swallow, ensure adequate hydration with I.V. therapy. Monitor fluid intake and output, and watch for dehydration.

• Provide meticulous mouth care. Apply petrolatum to the patient's lips. Promote healing with warm saline gargles or throat irrigations for 24 to 36 hours after incision and drainage. Encourage adequate rest.

THROMBOCYTOPENIA

The most common cause of hemorrhagic disorders, thrombocytopenia is characterized by deficiency of circulating platelets. Because platelets play a vital role in coagulation, this disease poses a serious threat to hemostasis.

Prognosis is excellent in drug-induced thrombocytopenia if the offending drug is withdrawn; in such cases, recovery may be immediate. Otherwise, prognosis depends on response to treatment of the cause. (See *Precautions in thrombocytopenia.*)

Causes

Thrombocytopenia may be congenital or acquired; the acquired form is more common. In either case, it usually results from the following:

• decreased or defective production of platelets in the marrow (such as occurs in leukemia, aplastic anemia, or toxicity with certain drugs)

• increased destruction outside the marrow caused by an underlying disorder (such as cirrhosis of the liver,

☑ PRECAUTIONS IN THROMBOCYTOPENIA

• Warn the patient to avoid aspirin in any form, and other drugs that impair coagulation. Teach him how to recognize aspirin or ibuprofen compounds on labels of over-the-counter remedies.

• Advise the patient to avoid straining at stool or coughing because both can lead to increased intracranial pressure, possibly causing cerebral hemorrhage in the patient with thrombocytopenia. Provide a stool softener to prevent constipation.

• If thrombocytopenia is drug-induced, stress the importance of avoiding the offending drug.

• If the patient must receive long-term steroid therapy, teach him to watch for and report cushingoid symptoms (acne, moon face, hirsutism, buffalo hump, hypertension, girdle obesity, thinning arms and legs, glycosuria, and edema). Emphasize that steroid doses must be discontinued gradually.

---

disseminated intravascular coagulation, or severe infection)

• less commonly, sequestration (hypersplenism, hypothermia) or platelet loss.

Acquired thrombocytopenia may result from certain drugs, such as nonsteroidal anti-inflammatory agents, sulfonamides, histamine blockers, alkylating agents, or antibiotic chemotherapeutic agents.

An idiopathic form of thrombocytopenia commonly occurs in children. A transient form may follow viral infection (Epstein-Barr or infectious mononucleosis).

Signs and symptoms

Thrombocytopenia typically produces a sudden onset of petechiae or ecchymoses in the skin or bleeding into any mucous membrane. Nearly all patients are otherwise asymptomatic, although some may complain of malaise, fatigue, and general weakness.

In adults, large blood-filled bullae characteristically appear in the mouth. In severe thrombocytopenia, hemorrhage may lead to tachycardia, short-

ness of breath, loss of consciousness, and death.

Diagnosis

To diagnose thrombocytopenia, obtain a patient history (especially a drug history), a physical examination, and the following laboratory tests:

• *Coagulation tests* reveal a decreased platelet count (in adults, less than 100,000/μl), prolonged bleeding time, and normal prothrombin time and partial thromboplastin time.

• If increased destruction of platelets is causing thrombocytopenia, *bone marrow studies* will reveal a greater number of megakaryocytes (platelet precursors) and shortened platelet survival (several hours or days rather than the usual 7 to 10 days).

Treatment

Effective treatment varies with the underlying cause and may include corticosteroids or immune globulin to increase platelet production. When possible, treatment consists of correction of the underlying cause or, in drug-induced thrombocytopenia, removal of the offending agents. Platelet transfusions are helpful in thrombophlebitis only in treating complications of severe hemorrhage.

Special considerations
• When caring for the patient with thrombocytopenia, take every possible precaution against bleeding.
• Protect the patient from trauma. Keep the side rails up, and pad them, if possible. Promote the use of an electric razor and a soft toothbrush. Avoid invasive procedures, such as venipuncture or urinary catheterization, if possible. When venipuncture is unavoidable, be sure to exert pressure on the puncture site for at least 20 minutes or until the bleeding stops.
• Monitor platelet count daily.
• Test stool for guaiac; dipstick urine and emesis for blood.
• Watch for bleeding (petechiae, ecchymoses, surgical or gastrointestinal bleeding, menorrhagia).
• During periods of active bleeding, maintain the patient on strict bed rest, if necessary.
• When administering platelet concentrate, remember that platelets are extremely fragile, so infuse them quickly. Do not give platelets to a patient with a fever.
• During platelet transfusion, monitor for febrile reaction (flushing, chills, fever, headache, tachycardia, hypertension). HLA-typed platelets may prevent febrile reaction. A patient with a history of minor reactions may benefit from acetaminophen and diphenhydramine before transfusion.
• During steroid therapy, monitor fluid and electrolyte balance, and watch for infection, pathologic fractures, and mood changes.
• A 1- to 2-hour postplatelet count will aid assessment of response.

THROMBOPHLEBITIS

An acute condition characterized by inflammation and thrombus formation, thrombophlebitis may occur in deep (intermuscular or intramuscular) or superficial (subcutaneous) veins.

Deep-vein thrombophlebitis affects small veins, such as the soleal venous sinuses, or large veins, such as the vena cava, and the femoral, iliac, and subclavian veins. This disorder is frequently progressive, leading to pulmonary embolism, a potentially lethal complication.

Superficial thrombophlebitis is usually self-limiting and rarely leads to pulmonary embolism. Thrombophlebitis often begins with localized inflammation alone (phlebitis), but such inflammation rapidly provokes thrombus formation. Rarely, venous thrombosis develops without associated inflammation of the vein (phlebothrombosis).

Causes
A thrombus occurs when an alteration in the epithelial lining causes platelet aggregation and consequent fibrin entrapment of red blood cells, white blood cells, and additional platelets. Thrombus formation is more rapid in areas where blood flow is slower, due to greater contact between platelets and thrombin accumulation.

The rapidly expanding thrombus initiates a chemical inflammatory process in the vessel epithelium that leads to fibrosis. The enlarging clot may occlude the vessel lumen partially or totally, or it may detach and embolize, to lodge elsewhere in the systemic circulation.

Deep-vein thrombophlebitis

This type of thrombophlebitis may be idiopathic, but it usually results from endothelial damage, accelerated blood clotting, and reduced blood flow. Predisposing factors are prolonged bed rest, trauma, surgery, childbirth, and use of oral contraceptives, such as estrogens.

Superficial thrombophlebitis

Causes of superficial thrombophlebitis include trauma, infection, I.V. drug abuse, and chemical irritation due to the extensive use of the I.V. route for medications and diagnostic tests.

Signs and symptoms

In both types of thrombophlebitis, clinical features vary with the site and length of the affected vein. Although deep-vein thrombophlebitis may occur asymptomatically, it may also produce severe pain, fever, chills, malaise and, possibly, swelling and cyanosis of the affected arm or leg.

Superficial thrombophlebitis produces visible and palpable signs, such as heat, pain, swelling, rubor, tenderness, and induration along the length of the affected vein. Extensive vein involvement may cause lymphadenitis.

Diagnosis

Some patients may display signs of inflammation and, possibly, a positive Homans' sign (pain on dorsiflexion of the foot) during physical examination; others are asymptomatic. Consequently, essential laboratory tests include:

• *Doppler ultrasonography:* to identify reduced blood flow to a specific area and any obstruction to venous flow, particularly in iliofemoral deep-vein thrombophlebitis

• *plethysmography:* to show decreased circulation distal to affected area; more sensitive than ultrasound in detecting deep-vein thrombophlebitis

• *phlebography* (usually confirms diagnosis): to show filling defects and diverted blood flow.

Diagnosis must rule out arterial occlusive disease, lymphangitis, cellulitis, and myositis.

Diagnosis of superficial thrombophlebitis is based on physical examination (redness and warmth over affected area, palpable vein, and pain during palpation or compression).

Treatment

The goals of treatment are to control thrombus development, prevent complications, relieve pain, and prevent recurrence of the disorder. Symptomatic measures include bed rest, with elevation of the affected arm or leg; warm, moist soaks to the affected area; and analgesics.

Deep-vein thrombophlebitis

After the acute episode of deep-vein thrombophlebitis subsides, the patient may resume activity while wearing antiembolism stockings that were applied before he got out of bed.

Treatment may also include anticoagulants (initially, heparin; later, warfarin) to prolong clotting time. Full anticoagulant dose must be discontinued during any operative period, due to the risk of hemorrhage.

After some types of surgery, especially major abdominal or pelvic operations, prophylactic doses of anticoagulants may reduce the risk of deep-vein thrombophlebitis and pulmonary embolism. For lysis of acute, extensive deep-vein thrombosis, treatment should include streptokinase.

Rarely, deep-vein thrombophlebitis may cause complete venous occlusion, which necessitates venous interruption through simple ligation to vein plication, or clipping. Embolectomy and insertion of a vena caval umbrella or filter may also be done.

Superficial thrombophlebitis

Therapy for severe superficial thrombophlebitis may include an anti-inflammatory drug, such as indomethacin, antiembolism stockings, warm soaks, and elevation of the leg.

Special considerations

• Patient teaching, identification of high-risk patients, and measures to prevent venostasis can prevent deepvein thrombophlebitis; close monitoring of anticoagulant therapy can prevent serious complications, such as internal hemorrhage.

• Enforce bed rest, and elevate the patient's affected arm or leg. If you plan to use pillows for elevating the leg, place them so they support the entire length of the affected leg to prevent possible compression of the popliteal space.

• Apply warm soaks to increase circulation to the affected area and to relieve pain and inflammation. Give analgesics to relieve pain.

• Measure and record the circumference of the affected arm or leg daily, and compare this measurement to the other arm or leg. To ensure accuracy and consistency of serial measurements, mark the skin over the area and measure at the same spot daily.

• Administer heparin I.V. with an infusion monitor or pump to control the flow rate, if necessary.

• Measure partial thromboplastin time regularly for the patient receiving heparin therapy and prothrombin time for the patient receiving warfarin (therapeutic anticoagulation values for both are one and a half to two times control values).

• Watch for signs and symptoms of bleeding, such as coffee-ground vomitus, ecchymoses, and black, tarry stools. Encourage the patient to use an electric razor and to avoid medications that contain aspirin.

• Be alert for signs of pulmonary emboli (rales, dyspnea, hemoptysis, sudden changes in mental status, restlessness, and hypotension).

To prepare the patient with thrombophlebitis for discharge:

• Emphasize the importance of follow-up blood studies to monitor anticoagulant therapy.

• If the patient is being discharged on heparin therapy, teach him or his family how to give subcutaneous injections. If he requires further assistance, arrange for a visiting nurse.

• Tell the patient to avoid prolonged sitting or standing to help prevent recurrence.

• Teach the patient how to properly apply and use antiembolism stockings. Tell him to report any complications, such as cold, blue toes.

• To prevent thrombophlebitis in high-risk patients, perform range-of-motion exercises while the patient is on bed rest, use intermittent pneumatic calf massage during lengthy surgical or diagnostic procedures, apply antiembolism stockings postoperatively, and encourage early ambulation.

THYROID CANCER

Cancer of the thyroid occurs in all age-groups, especially in persons who have had radiation treatment to the neck area. Papillary and follicular carcinomas are most common and are usually associated with prolonged survival.

Papillary carcinoma accounts for half of all thyroid cancers in adults; it is most common in young adult females and metastasizes slowly. It is the least virulent form of thyroid cancer. *Follicular carcinoma* is less common but more likely to recur and metastasize to the regional nodes and through blood vessels into the bones, liver, and lungs.

Medullary carcinoma originates in the parafollicular cells derived from the last branchial pouch and contains amyloid and calcium deposits. It can produce calcitonin, histaminase, corticotropin (producing Cushing's syndrome), and prostaglandin E_2 and F_3 (producing diarrhea).

This rare form of thyroid cancer is familial, associated with pheochromocytoma, and completely curable when detected before it causes symptoms. Untreated, it progresses rapidly.

Seldom curable by resection, *giant and spindle cell cancer* (anaplastic tumor) resists radiation and metastasizes rapidly.

Causes
Predisposing factors include radiation exposure, prolonged thyrotropin stimulation (through radiation or heredity), familial predisposition, or chronic goiter.

Signs and symptoms
The primary signs of thyroid cancer are a painless nodule, a hard nodule in an enlarged thyroid gland, or palpable lymph nodes with thyroid enlargement. Eventually, the pressure of such a nodule or enlargement causes hoarseness, dysphagia, dyspnea, and pain on palpation.

If the tumor is large enough to destroy the gland, hypothyroidism follows, with its typical symptoms of low metabolism (mental apathy and sensitivity to cold). However, if the tumor stimulates excess thyroid hormone production, it induces symptoms of hyperthyroidism (sensitivity to heat, restlessness, and hyperactivity).

Other clinical features include diarrhea, anorexia, irritability, vocal cord paralysis, and symptoms of distant metastasis.

Diagnosis
The first clue to thyroid cancer is usually an enlarged, palpable node in the thyroid gland, neck, lymph nodes of the neck, or vocal cords. A patient history of radiation therapy or a family history of thyroid cancer supports the diagnosis. However, tests must rule out nonmalignant thyroid enlargements, which are more common.

• *Thyroid scan* differentiates between functional nodes (rarely malignant) and hypofunctional nodes (commonly malignant) by measuring how readily nodules trap isotopes compared with the rest of the thyroid gland. In thyroid cancer, the scintiscan shows a "cold," nonfunctioning nodule.

• Other tests include needle biopsy, computed tomography scan, ultrasonic scan, chest X-ray, serum alkaline phosphatase, and serum calcitonin assay to diagnose medullary cancer. Calcitonin assay is a reliable clue to silent medullary carcinoma. (See *Staging thyroid cancer*, page 852.)

Treatment
• Total or subtotal thyroidectomy, with modified node dissection (bilateral or unilateral) on the side of the primary cancer (papillary or follicular cancer)

• Total thyroidectomy and radical neck excision (for medullary, giant, or spindle cell cancer)

• Radiation (^{131}I) with external radiation (for inoperable cancer and sometimes postoperatively in lieu of radical neck excision) or alone (for metastasis)

• Adjunctive thyroid suppression, with exogenous thyroid hormones suppressing thyrotropin production, and simultaneous administration of an adrenergic blocking agent, such as propranolol, increasing tolerance to surgery and radiation

• Chemotherapy for symptomatic, widespread metastasis is limited, but doxorubicin is sometimes beneficial.

STAGING THYROID CANCER

The classification and staging systems adopted by the American Joint Committee on Cancer describe thyroid cancer according to the tumor's (T) size and extent at its origin, its invasion of regional (cervical and upper mediastinal) lymph nodes (N), and the disease's metastasis (M) to other structures.

Primary tumor
TX—primary tumor can't be assessed
T0—no evidence of primary tumor
T1—tumor 1 cm or less in greatest dimension and limited to the thyroid
T2—tumor more than 1 cm but less than 4 cm in greatest dimension and limited to the thyroid
T3—tumor more than 4 cm and limited to the thyroid
T4—tumor (any size) extends beyond the thyroid

Regional lymph nodes
NX—regional lymph nodes can't be assessed
N0—no evidence of regional lymph node metastasis
N1—regional lymph node metastasis
N1a—metastasis in ipsilateral cervical nodes
N1b—metastasis in bilateral, midline, or contralateral cervical or mediastinal lymph nodes

Distant metastasis
MX—distant metastasis can't be assessed
M0—no evidence of distant metastasis
M1—distant metastasis

Staging categories for papillary or follicular cancer
Papillary or follicular cancer progresses from mild to severe as follows:
Stage I—any T, any N, M0 (patient under age 45); T1, N0, M0 (patient age 45 or over)
Stage II—any T, any N, M1 (patient under age 45); T2, N0, M0; T3, N0, M0 (patient age 45 or over)
Stage III—T4, N0, M0; any T, N1, M0 (patient age 45 or over)
Stage IV—any T, any N, M1 (patient age 45 or over)

Staging categories for medullary cancer
Medullary cancer progresses from mild to severe as follows:
Stage I—T1, N0, M0
Stage II—T2, N0, M0; T3, N0, M0; T4, N0, M0
Stage III—any T, N1, M0
Stage IV—any T, any N, M1

Staging categories for undifferentiated cancer
All cases are Stage IV.
Stage IV—any T, any N, any M

Special considerations
• Before surgery, tell the patient to expect temporary voice loss or hoarseness lasting several days after surgery.
   Plan meticulous postoperative care:
• When the patient regains consciousness, keep him in semi-Fowler's position, with his head neither hyperextended nor flexed, to avoid pressure on the suture line. Support his head and

neck with sandbags and pillows; when you move him, continue this support with your hands.
• After monitoring vital signs, check the patient's dressing, neck, and back for bleeding. If he complains that the dressing feels tight, loosen it.
• Check serum calcium levels daily; hypocalcemia may develop if parathyroid glands are removed.

• Watch for and report other complications: hemorrhage and shock (elevated pulse rate and hypotension), tetany (carpopedal spasm, twitching, and seizures), thyroid storm (high fever, severe tachycardia, delirium, dehydration, and extreme irritability), and respiratory obstruction (dyspnea, crowing respirations, retraction of neck tissues).

• Keep a tracheotomy set and oxygen equipment handy in case of respiratory obstruction. Use continuous steam inhalation in the patient's room until his chest is clear.

• The patient may need I.V. fluids or a soft diet, but many patients can tolerate a regular diet within 24 hours of surgery.

• Care of the patient after extensive tumor and node excision is identical to other radical neck postoperative care.

THYROIDITIS

Inflammation of the thyroid gland occurs as autoimmune thyroiditis (long-term inflammatory disease), subacute granulomatous thyroiditis (self-limiting inflammation), Riedel's thyroiditis (rare, invasive fibrotic process), and miscellaneous thyroiditis (acute suppurative, chronic infective, and chronic noninfective). Thyroiditis is more common in women than in men.

Causes

Autoimmune thyroiditis is due to antibodies to thyroid antigens in the blood. It may cause inflammation and lymphocytic infiltration (Hashimoto's thyroiditis). Glandular atrophy (myxedema) and Graves' disease are linked to autoimmune thyroiditis.

Postpartum thyroiditis (silent thyroiditis) is another autoimmune disorder associated with transient thyroiditis in women within 1 year after delivery.

Subacute granulomatous thyroiditis usually follows mumps, influenza, coxsackievirus, or adenovirus infection. *Riedel's thyroiditis* is a rare condition of unknown etiology.

Miscellaneous thyroiditis results from bacterial invasion of the gland in acute suppurative thyroiditis; tuberculosis, syphilis, actinomycosis, or other infectious agents in the chronic infective form; and sarcoidosis and amyloidosis in chronic noninfective thyroiditis.

Signs and symptoms

Autoimmune thyroiditis is usually asymptomatic and commonly occurs in women, with peak incidence in middle age. It's the most prevalent cause of spontaneous hypothyroidism.

In subacute granulomatous thyroiditis, moderate thyroid enlargement may follow an upper respiratory tract infection or a sore throat. The thyroid may be painful and tender, and dysphagia may occur.

In Riedel's thyroiditis, the gland enlarges slowly as it is replaced by hard, fibrous tissues. This fibrosis may compress the trachea or the esophagus. The thyroid feels firm.

Clinical effects of miscellaneous thyroiditis are characteristic of pyogenic infection: fever, pain, tenderness, and reddened skin over the gland.

Diagnosis

Precise diagnosis depends on the type of thyroiditis:

• *autoimmune:* high titers of thyroglobulin and microsomal antibodies present in serum

• *subacute granulomatous:* elevated erythrocyte sedimentation rate, increased thyroid hormone levels, decreased thyroidal radioactive iodine uptake

• *chronic infective and noninfective:* varied findings, depending on underlying infection or other disease.

Treatment

Appropriate treatment varies with the type of thyroiditis. Drug therapy includes levothyroxine for accompanying hypothyroidism, analgesics and anti-inflammatory drugs for mild subacute granulomatous thyroiditis, propranolol for transient hyperthyroidism, and steroids for severe episodes of acute inflammation. Suppurative thyroiditis requires antibiotic therapy.

A partial thyroidectomy may be necessary to relieve tracheal or esophageal compression in Riedel's thyroiditis.

Special considerations

• Before treatment, obtain a patient history to identify underlying diseases that may cause thyroiditis, such as tuberculosis or a recent viral infection.

• Check vital signs, and examine the patient's neck for unusual swelling, enlargement, or redness. Provide a liquid diet if the patient has difficulty swallowing, especially when due to fibrosis. If the neck is swollen, measure and record the circumference daily to monitor progressive enlargement.

• Administer antibiotics, and report and record elevations in temperature.

• Instruct the patient to watch for and report signs of hypothyroidism (lethargy, restlessness, sensitivity to cold, forgetfulness, dry skin) — especially if he has Hashimoto's thyroiditis, which often causes hypothyroidism.

• Check for signs of hyperthyroidism (nervousness, tremor, weakness), which often occur in subacute thyroiditis.

• After thyroidectomy, check vital signs every 15 to 30 minutes until the patient's condition stabilizes. Stay alert for signs of tetany secondary to accidental parathyroid injury during surgery. Keep 10% calcium gluconate available for I.V. use, if needed.

• Assess dressings frequently for excessive bleeding. Watch for signs of airway obstruction, such as difficulty in talking or increased swallowing; keep tracheotomy equipment handy.

• Explain to the patient that lifelong thyroid hormone replacement therapy is necessary if hypothyroidism occurs. Tell him to watch for signs of overdosage, such as nervousness and palpitations.

TIC DISORDERS

Including Tourette syndrome, chronic motor or vocal tic disorder, and transient tic disorder, tic disorders are similar pathophysiologically but differ in severity and prognosis. All tic disorders, commonly known simply as tics, are involuntary, spasmodic, recurrent, and purposeless motor movements or vocalizations. These disorders are classified as motor or vocal and as simple or complex.

Tics begin before age 18. All tic disorders are three times more common in boys than in girls. Transient tics usually are self-limiting, but Tourette syndrome follows a chronic course with remissions and exacerbations.

Causes

Although their exact cause is unknown, tic disorders occur more frequently in certain families, suggesting a genetic cause. Tics commonly develop when a child experiences overwhelming anxiety, usually associated with normal maturation. Tics may be precipitated or exacerbated by the use of phenothiazines or central nervous system stimulants or by head trauma.

DIAGNOSING TIC DISORDERS

The diagnosis of a tic disorder is based on *DSM-IV* criteria.

Tourette syndrome
• The patient has had multiple motor tics and one or more vocal tics at some time during the illness, although not necessarily concurrently.
• The tics occur many times a day (usually in bouts) nearly every day or intermittently for more than 1 year.
• The disturbance causes marked distress or significant impairment in social, occupational, or other important areas of functioning.
• Onset occurs before age 18.
• The disturbance isn't the direct physiologic effect of a substance or a general medical condition.

Chronic motor or vocal tic disorder
• The patient has had single or multiple motor or vocal tics, but not both, at some time during the illness.
• The tics occur many times a day nearly every day or intermittently for more than 1 year. During this time, the person never had a tic-free period exceeding 3 consecutive months.

• The disturbance causes marked distress or significant impairment in social, occupational, or other important areas of functioning.
• Onset occurs before age 18.
• The disturbance isn't the direct physiologic effect of a substance or a general medical condition.
• Criteria have never been met for Tourette syndrome.

Transient tic disorder
• The patient has single or multiple motor or vocal tics, or both.
• The tics occur many times a day nearly every day for at least 4 weeks, but for no longer than 12 consecutive months.
• The disturbance causes marked distress or significant impairment in social, occupational, or other important areas of functioning.
• Onset occurs before age 18.
• The disturbance is not the direct physiologic effect of a substance or a general medical condition.
• Criteria have never been met for Tourette syndrome or chronic motor or vocal tic disorder.

Signs and symptoms

Assessment findings vary according to the type of tic disorder. Inspection, coupled with the patient's history, may reveal the specific motor or vocal patterns that characterize the tic, as well as the frequency, complexity, and precipitating factors. The patient or his family may report that the tics occur sporadically many times a day.

Note whether certain situations exacerbate the tics. All tic disorders may be exacerbated by stress, and they usually diminish markedly during sleep. The patient also may report that they occur during activities that require concentration, such as reading or sewing.

Determine whether the patient can control the tics. Most patients can, with conscious effort, control them for short periods.

Psychosocial assessment may reveal underlying stressful factors, such as problems with social adjustment, lack of self-esteem, and depression.

Diagnosis

For characteristic findings in patients with this condition, see *Diagnosing tic disorders.*

STRESS DISORDERS WITH PHYSICAL SIGNS

Besides tic disorders, stress-related disorders that produce physical signs in children include stuttering, functional enuresis, functional encopresis, sleepwalking, and sleep terrors.

Stuttering

Characterized by abnormal speech rhythms with repetitions and hesitations at the beginning of words, stuttering may involve movements of the respiratory muscles, shoulders, and face.

It may be associated with mental dullness, poor social background, and a history of birth trauma. However, this disorder most commonly occurs in children of average or superior intelligence who fear they can't meet expectations.

Related problems may include low self-esteem, tension, anxiety, humiliation, and withdrawal from social situations. About 80% of stutterers recover after age 16. Evaluation and treatment by a speech pathologist teaches the stutterer to place equal weight on each syllable in a sentence, how to breathe properly, and how to control anxiety.

Functional enuresis

This disorder is characterized by intentional or involuntary voiding of urine, usually during the night (nocturnal enuresis). Considered normal in children until age 3 or 4, functional enuresis occurs in about 40% of children at this age and persists in 10% to age 5, in 5% to age 10, and in 1% of boys to age 18.

Causes may be related to stress, such as the birth of a sibling, the move to a new home, divorce, separation, hospitalization, faulty toilet training (inconsistent, demanding, or punitive), and unrealistic responsibilities. Associated problems include low self-esteem, social withdrawal from peers because of ostracism and ridicule, and anger, rejection, and punishment by caregivers.

Advise parents that a matter-of-fact attitude helps the child learn bladder control without undue stress. If enuresis persists into late childhood, treatment with imipramine may help. Dry-bed therapy may include the use of an alarm (wet bell pad), social motivation, self-correction of accidents, and positive reinforcement.

Functional encopresis

Denoted by evacuation of feces into the child's clothes or inappropriate receptacles, functional encopresis is associated with low intelligence, cerebral dysfunction, or other developmental symptoms such as language lag.

Some children also show inefficient, ineffective gastric motility. Related problems may include repressed anger, withdrawal from peer relationships, and loss of self-esteem.

Treatment

Behavior modification and operant conditioning help treat some tic disorders. Psychotherapy can help the patient uncover underlying conflicts and issues as well as deal with the problems caused by the tics. Tourette syndrome is best treated with medications and psychotherapy.

No medications are helpful in treating transient tics. Haloperidol is the drug of choice for Tourette syndrome.

Treatment involves encouraging the child to come to his parents when he has an "accident." Advise parents to give the child clean clothes without criticism or punishment. Medical examination should rule out any physical disorder. Child, adult, and family therapy may help reduce anger and disappointment over the child's development and improve parenting techniques.

Sleepwalking and sleep terrors
In sleepwalking, the child calmly rises from bed in a state of altered consciousness and walks around with no subsequent recollection of any dreams. In sleep terrors, he awakes terrified, in a state of clouded consciousness, often unable to recognize parents and familiar surroundings. Visual hallucinations are common.

Sleepwalking is usually a response to an emotional concern. Tell parents to gently "talk" the child back to his bed. If he wakes, they should comfort and support him, not tease him.

Sleep terrors are normal in 2 and 3-year-olds, usually occurring within 30 minutes to 3½ hours of sleep onset. Tachycardia, tachypnea, diaphoresis, dilated pupils, and piloerection are associated with sleep terrors. The child also may fear being alone.

Tell parents to make sure the child has access to them at night. Sleep terrors usually are self-limiting and subside within a few weeks.

Pimozide (an oral dopamine-blocking drug) and clonidine are alternative choices. Antianxiety agents may be useful in dealing with secondary anxiety but do not reduce the severity or frequency of the tics.

Special considerations
• Offer emotional support and help the patient prevent fatigue.
• Suggest that the patient with Tourette syndrome contact the Tourette Syndrome Association for information and support.
• Help the patient identify and eliminate any avoidable stress and learn positive new ways to deal with anxiety.
• Encourage the patient to verbalize his feelings about his illness. Help him understand that the movements are involuntary and that he shouldn't feel guilty or blame himself.
• For more information on other stress disorders, see *Stress disorders with physical signs.*

TONSILLITIS

Inflammation of the tonsils, or tonsillitis, can be acute or chronic. The uncomplicated acute form usually lasts 4 to 6 days and commonly affects children between ages 5 and 10. The presence of proven chronic tonsillitis justifies tonsillectomy, the only effective treatment. Tonsils tend to hypertrophy during childhood and atrophy after puberty.

Causes
Tonsillitis generally results from infection with group A beta-hemolytic streptococci but can result from other bacteria or viruses or from oral anaerobes.

Signs and symptoms
Acute and chronic tonsillitis have different signs and symptoms.

Acute tonsillitis
The acute form of tonsillitis commonly begins with a mild to severe sore throat. A very young child, unable to

complain about a sore throat, may stop eating. Tonsillitis may also produce dysphagia, fever, swelling and tenderness of the lymph glands in the submandibular area, muscle and joint pain, chills, malaise, headache, and pain (frequently referred to the ears).

Excess secretions may elicit the complaint of a constant urge to swallow; the back of the throat may feel constricted. Such discomfort usually subsides after 72 hours.

Chronic tonsillitis

The chronic form of tonsillitis produces a recurrent sore throat and purulent drainage in the tonsillar crypts. Frequent attacks of acute tonsillitis may also occur. Complications include obstruction from tonsillar hypertrophy and peritonsillar abscess.

Diagnosis

Diagnostic confirmation requires a thorough throat examination that reveals:
• generalized inflammation of the pharyngeal wall
• swollen tonsils that project from between the pillars of the fauces and exude white or yellow follicles
• purulent drainage when pressure is applied to the tonsillar pillars
• possible edematous and inflamed uvula.

Culture may determine the infecting organism and indicate appropriate antibiotic therapy. Leukocytosis is also usually present. Differential diagnosis rules out infectious mononucleosis and diphtheria.

Treatment

Effective treatment of acute tonsillitis requires rest, adequate fluid intake, administration of aspirin or acetaminophen and, for bacterial infection, antibiotics.

When the causative organism is group A beta-hemolytic streptococcus, penicillin is the drug of choice (another broad-spectrum antibiotic may be substituted). Most oral anaerobes will also respond to penicillin. To prevent complications, antibiotic therapy should continue for 10 to 14 days.

Chronic tonsillitis or the development of complications (obstructions from tonsillar hypertrophy, peritonsillar abscess) may require a tonsillectomy, but only after the patient has been free of tonsillar or respiratory tract infections for 3 to 4 weeks.

Special considerations

• Despite dysphagia, urge the patient to drink plenty of fluids, especially if he has a fever. Offer a child ice cream and flavored drinks and ices. Suggest gargling to soothe the throat, unless it exacerbates pain. Make sure the patient and parents understand the importance of completing the prescribed course of antibiotic therapy.
• Before tonsillectomy, explain to the adult patient that a local anesthetic prevents pain but allows a sensation of pressure during surgery. Warn the patient to expect considerable throat discomfort and some bleeding postoperatively.
• For the pediatric patient, keep your explanation simple and nonthreatening. Show the child the operating and recovery rooms, and briefly explain the hospital routine. Most hospitals allow one parent to stay with the child.
• Postoperatively, maintain a patent airway. To prevent aspiration, place the patient on his side.
• Monitor vital signs frequently, and check for bleeding. Be alert for excessive bleeding, increased pulse rate, or dropping blood pressure.
• After the patient is fully alert and the gag reflex has returned, allow him to drink water.
• Urge the patient to drink plenty of nonirritating fluids, to ambulate, and to take frequent deep breaths to pre-

vent pulmonary complications. Give pain medication as needed.

• Before discharge, provide the patient or parents with written instructions on home care. Tell them to expect a white scab to form in the throat between 5 and 10 days postoperatively and to report bleeding, ear discomfort, or a fever that lasts longer than 3 days.

TORTICOLLIS

Also called wryneck, torticollis is a neck deformity in which the sternocleidomastoid neck muscles are spastic or shortened, causing bending of the head to the affected side and rotation of the chin to the opposite side.

This disorder may be congenital or acquired. Incidence of congenital (muscular) torticollis is highest in infants after difficult delivery (breech presentation), in firstborn infants, and in girls. Acquired torticollis usually develops during the first 10 years of life or after age 40.

Causes

Possible causes of congenital torticollis include malposition of the head in utero, prenatal injury, fibroma, interruption of blood supply, or fibrotic rupture of the sternocleidomastoid muscle, with hematoma and scar formation.

The three types of acquired torticollis — acute, spasmodic, and hysterical — have differing causes.

• The acute form results from muscular damage caused by inflammatory diseases, such as myositis, lymphadenitis, and tuberculosis, and from cervical spinal injuries that produce scar tissue contracture.

• The spasmodic form results from rhythmic muscle spasms caused by an organic central nervous system disorder (probably due to irritation of the nerve root by arthritis or osteomyelitis).

• Hysterical torticollis is due to a psychogenic inability to control neck muscles.

Signs and symptoms

The following features characterize congenital torticollis and acquired torticollis.

Congenital torticollis

The first sign of congenital torticollis is often a firm, nontender, palpable enlargement of the sternocleidomastoid muscle that is visible at birth and for several weeks afterward. It slowly regresses during a period of 6 months, although incomplete regression can cause permanent contracture.

If the deformity is severe, the infant's face and head flatten from sleeping on the affected side; this asymmetry gradually worsens. The infant's chin turns away from the side of the shortened muscle, and his head tilts to the shortened side. His shoulder may be elevated on the affected side, restricting neck movement.

Acquired torticollis

The first sign of acquired torticollis is usually recurring unilateral stiffness of neck muscles, followed by a drawing sensation and a momentary twitching or contraction that pulls the head to the affected side. This type of torticollis often produces severe neuralgic pain throughout the head and neck.

Diagnosis

A history of painless neck deformity from birth suggests congenital torticollis; gradual onset of painful neck deformity suggests acquired torticollis.

However, diagnosis must rule out tuberculosis of the cervical spine, pharyngeal or tonsillar inflammations,

spinal accessory nerve damage, ruptured transverse ligaments, subdural
hematoma, dislocations and fractures,
scoliosis, congenital abnormalities of
the cervical spine, rheumatoid arthritis, and osteomyelitis.

In acquired torticollis, cervical spine
X-rays are negative for bone or joint
disease but may reveal an associated
disorder (such as tuberculosis, scar tissue formation, or arthritis).

Treatment

Congenital torticollis and acquired
torticollis are treated in different ways.

Congenital torticollis

Therapy for congenital torticollis aims
to stretch the shortened muscle. Nonsurgical treatment includes passive neck
stretching and proper positioning during sleep for an infant and active
stretching exercises for an older child—
for example, touching the ear opposite
the affected side to the shoulder and
touching the chin to the same shoulder. (See *Treating torticollis.*)

Surgical correction involves section-
ing the sternocleidomastoid muscle; this
should be done during preschool years
and only if other therapies fail.

Acquired torticollis

Treatment of acquired torticollis aims
to correct the underlying cause of the
disease. In the acute form, application
of heat, cervical traction, and gentle
massage may help relieve pain.
Stretching exercises and a neck brace
may relieve symptoms of the spasmodic and hysterical forms.

Treatment of elderly patients with
acquired torticollis may include administration of levodopa-carbidopa,
carbamazepine, and haloperidol.

Special considerations

• To aid early diagnosis of congenital
torticollis, observe the infant for limited neck movement, and thoroughly
assess his degree of discomfort.
• If surgery is necessary, prepare the
patient by shaving the neck to the hairline on the affected side.

After corrective surgery, follow these
guidelines:
• Monitor the patient closely for nausea or signs of respiratory complications, especially if he's in cervical traction. Keep suction equipment available
to prevent aspiration.
• The patient may be in a cast or in
traction day and night or at night only.
Give meticulous cast care, including the
monitoring of circulation, sensation,
and color around the cast. Protect the
cast around the patient's chin and
mouth with waterproof material. Check
for skin irritation, pressure areas, or
softening of the cast pad.
• Provide emotional support for the
patient and family to relieve their anxiety due to fear, pain, limitations from
the brace or traction, and an altered
body image.

• Begin stretching exercises as soon as the patient can tolerate them.

TOXIC SHOCK SYNDROME

An acute bacterial infection, toxic shock syndrome (TSS) is caused by toxin-producing, penicillin-resistant strains of *Staphylococcus aureus,* such as TSS toxin-1 and staphylococcal enterotoxins B and C. The disease primarily affects menstruating women under age 30 and is associated with continuous use of tampons during the menstrual period.

TSS incidence peaked in the mid-1980s and has since declined, probably because of the withdrawal of high-absorbency tampons from the market.

Causes

Although tampons are clearly implicated in TSS, their exact role is uncertain. Theoretically, tampons may contribute to development of TSS by:
• introducing *S. aureus* into the vagina during insertion
• absorbing toxin from the vagina
• traumatizing the vaginal mucosa during insertion, thus leading to infection
• providing a favorable environment for the growth of *S. aureus.*

When TSS isn't related to menstruation, it seems to be linked to *S. aureus* infections, such as abscesses, osteomyelitis, and postsurgical infections.

Signs and symptoms

Typically, TSS produces intense myalgias, fever over 104° F (40° C), vomiting, diarrhea, headache, decreased level of consciousness, rigors, conjunctival hyperemia, and vaginal hyperemia and discharge. Severe hypotension occurs with hypovolemic shock. Within a few hours of onset, a deep red rash develops — especially on the palms and soles — and later desquamates.

Major complications include persistent neuropsychological abnormalities, mild renal failure, rash, and cyanotic arms and legs.

Diagnosis

A diagnosis of TSS is based on clinical findings and the presence of at least three of the following:
• GI effects, including vomiting and profuse diarrhea
• muscular effects, with severe myalgias or a fivefold or greater increase in creatine kinase
• mucous membrane effects, such as frank hyperemia
• renal involvement with elevated blood urea nitrogen or creatinine levels (at least twice the normal levels)
• liver involvement with elevated bilirubin, alanine aminotransferase, or aspartate aminotransferase levels (at least twice the normal levels)
• blood involvement with signs of thrombocytopenia and a platelet count of less than $100,000/\mu l$
• central nervous system effects, such as disorientation without focal signs.

In addition, isolation of *S. aureus* from vaginal discharge or lesions helps support the diagnosis. Negative results on blood tests for Rocky Mountain spotted fever, leptospirosis, and measles help rule out these disorders.

Treatment

Toxic shock syndrome is treated with I.V. antistaphylococcal antibiotics that are beta-lactamase–resistant, such as oxacillin and nafcillin. To reverse shock, replace fluids with saline solution and colloids.

Special considerations
• Monitor the patient's vital signs frequently.
• Administer antibiotics slowly and strictly on time. Be sure to watch for signs of penicillin allergy.
• Check the patient's fluid and electrolyte balance.
• Obtain specimens of vaginal and cervical secretions for culture of *S. aureus*.
• Tell the patient to avoid using tampons.
• Implement universal precautions.

TOXOPLASMOSIS

One of the most common infectious diseases, toxoplasmosis results from the protozoa *Toxoplasma gondii*. Distributed worldwide, it's less common in cold or hot arid climates and at high elevations. It usually causes localized infection but may produce significant generalized infection, especially in immunodeficient patients or neonates.

Congenital toxoplasmosis, characterized by lesions in the central nervous system, may result in stillbirth or serious birth defects.

Causes
T. gondii exists in trophozoite forms in the acute stages of infection and in cystic forms (tissue cysts and oocysts) in the latent stages. Ingestion of tissue cysts in raw or undercooked meat (heating, drying, or freezing destroys these cysts) or fecal-oral contamination from infected cats transmits toxoplasmosis. (See *Avoiding toxoplasmosis.*)

However, toxoplasmosis also occurs in vegetarians who aren't exposed to cats, so other means of transmission may exist.

Congenital toxoplasmosis follows transplacental transmission from a chronically infected mother or one who acquired toxoplasmosis shortly before or during pregnancy.

Signs and symptoms
The following signs and symptoms characterize congenital toxoplasmosis and acquired toxoplasmosis.

Congenital toxoplasmosis
Toxoplasmosis acquired in the first trimester of pregnancy often results in stillbirth. About one-third of infants who survive have congenital toxoplasmosis. The later in pregnancy maternal infection occurs, the greater the risk of congenital infection in the infant.

Obvious signs of congenital toxoplasmosis include retinochoroiditis, hydrocephalus or microcephalus, cerebral calcification, seizures, lymphadenopathy, fever, hepatosplenomegaly, jaundice, and rash. Other defects, which may become apparent months or years later, include strabismus, blindness, epilepsy, and mental retardation.

Acquired toxoplasmosis
Acquired toxoplasmosis may cause localized (mild lymphatic) or generalized (fulminating, disseminated) infection. Localized infection produces fever and a mononucleosis-like syndrome (malaise, myalgia, headache, fatigue, sore throat) and lymphadenopathy.

Generalized infection produces encephalitis, fever, headache, vomiting, delirium, seizures, and a diffuse maculopapular rash (except on the palms, soles, and scalp). Generalized infection may lead to myocarditis, pneumonitis, hepatitis, and polymyositis.

Diagnosis
Identification of *T. gondii* in an appropriate tissue specimen confirms toxoplasmosis. Serologic tests may be useful, and in patients with toxoplasmosis encephalitis, computed tomography and magnetic resonance imaging scans disclose lesions.

Treatment
Acute disease is treated with sulfonamides and pyrimethamine for about 4 weeks and, possibly, folinic acid to control side effects. In patients who also have AIDS, treatment continues indefinitely. No safe, effective treatment exists for chronic toxoplasmosis or toxoplasmosis occurring in the first trimester of pregnancy.

Special considerations
• When caring for patients with toxoplasmosis, monitor drug therapy carefully and emphasize thorough patient teaching to prevent complications and control spread of the disease.
• Because sulfonamides cause blood dyscrasias and pyrimethamine depresses bone marrow, closely monitor the patient's hematologic values.

• Report all cases of toxoplasmosis to your local public health department.

TRICHINOSIS

An infection caused by larvae of the intestinal roundworm *Trichinella spiralis,* trichinosis (trichiniasis, trichinellosis) occurs worldwide, especially in populations that eat pork or bear meat. Trichinosis may produce multiple symptoms; respiratory, central nervous system (CNS), and cardiovascular complications; and, rarely, death.

Causes
Transmission is through ingestion of uncooked or undercooked meat that contains *T. spiralis* cysts. Such cysts are found primarily in swine, less often in dogs, cats, bears, foxes, wolves, and marine animals. These cysts result from the animals' ingestion of similarly contaminated flesh. In swine, such infection results from eating table scraps or raw garbage.

After gastric juices free the worm from the cyst capsule, it reaches sexual maturity in a few days. The female roundworm burrows into the intestinal mucosa and reproduces. Larvae are then transported through the lymphatic system and the bloodstream. They become embedded as cysts in striated muscle, especially in the diaphragm, chest, arms, and legs. Human-to-human transmission does not take place.

Signs and symptoms
In the United States, trichinosis is usually mild and seldom produces symptoms. When symptoms do occur, they vary with the stage and degree of infection:
• *Stage 1* — Invasion: occurs 1 week after ingestion. Release of larvae and re-

EXERCISE WARNING IN TRICHINOSIS

Emphasize the importance of bed rest. Sudden death from cardiac involvement may occur in a patient with moderate to severe trichinosis infection who has resumed activity too soon. Warn the patient to continue bed rest into the convalescent stage to avoid a serious relapse and possible death.

production of adult *T. spiralis* cause anorexia, nausea, vomiting, diarrhea, abdominal pain, and cramps.

• *Stage 2* — Dissemination: occurs 7 to 10 days after ingestion. *T. spiralis* penetrates the intestinal mucosa and begins to migrate to striated muscle.

Symptoms include edema, especially of the eyelids or face; muscle pain, particularly in extremities; and, occasionally, itching and burning skin, sweating, skin lesions, a temperature of 102° to 104° F (38.9° to 40° C), and delirium; and, in severe respiratory, cardiovascular, or CNS infections, palpitations and lethargy.

• *Stage 3* — Encystment: occurs during convalescence, generally 1 week later. *T. spiralis* larvae invade muscle fiber and become encysted.

Diagnosis

• A history of ingestion of raw or improperly cooked pork or pork products, with typical clinical features, suggests trichinosis, but infection may be difficult to prove.

• Stools may contain mature worms and larvae during the invasion stage.

• Skeletal muscle biopsies can show encysted larvae 10 days after ingestion; and, if available, analyses of contaminated meat also show larvae.

• Skin testing may show a positive histamine-like reactivity 15 minutes after intradermal injection of the antigen (within 17 to 20 days after ingestion). However, such a result may remain positive for up to 5 years after exposure.

Elevated acute and convalescent antibody titers (determined by flocculation tests 3 to 4 weeks after infection) confirm this diagnosis.

• Other abnormal results include elevated alanine aminotransferase, aspartate aminotransferase, creatine kinase, and lactate dehydrogenase levels during the acute stages and an elevated eosinophil count (up to $15,000/\mu l$). A normal or increased cerebrospinal fluid lymphocyte level (to $300/\mu l$) and increased protein levels indicate CNS involvement.

Treatment

Thiabendazole effectively combats this parasite during the intestinal stage; severe infection (especially CNS invasion) may warrant glucocorticoids to fight against possible inflammation.

Special considerations

• Question the patient about recent ingestion of pork products and the methods used to store and cook them.

• Reduce fever with alcohol rubs, tepid baths, cooling blankets, or antipyretics; relieve muscular pain with analgesics, enforced bed rest, and proper body alignment. (See *Exercise warning in trichinosis*.)

• To prevent pressure sores, frequently reposition the patient, and gently massage bony prominences.

• Tell the patient that possible adverse reactions to thiabendazole are nausea, vomiting, dizziness, dermatitis, and fever.

To help prevent trichinosis:

• Educate the public about proper cooking and storing methods not only for pork and pork products, but also for meat from carnivores. To kill trichinae, internal meat temperatures should reach 150° F (66° C) and its color should change from pink to gray unless the meat has been cured or frozen for at least 10 days at low temperatures.

• Warn travelers to foreign countries or to very poor areas in the United States to avoid eating pork; swine in these areas are often fed raw garbage.

• Report all cases of trichinosis to local public health authorities.

TRICHOMONIASIS

A protozoal infection of the lower genitourinary tract, trichomoniasis affects about 15% of sexually active females and 10% of sexually active males. Incidence is worldwide. In females, the condition may be acute or chronic. Recurrence of trichomoniasis is minimized when sexual partners are treated concurrently.

Causes

Trichomonas vaginalis—a tetraflagellated, motile protozoan—causes trichomoniasis in females by infecting the vagina, the urethra and, possibly, the endocervix, Bartholin's glands, Skene's glands, or the bladder; in males, it infects the lower urethra and, possibly, the prostate gland, seminal vesicles, or epididymis.

T. vaginalis grows best when the vaginal mucosa is more alkaline than normal (pH about 5.5 to 5.8). There-fore, factors that raise the vaginal pH—use of oral contraceptives, pregnancy, bacterial overgrowth, exudative cervical or vaginal lesions, or frequent douching, which disturbs lactobacilli that normally live in the vagina and maintain acidity—may predispose to trichomoniasis.

Trichomoniasis is usually transmitted by intercourse; less often, by contaminated douche equipment or moist washcloths. Occasionally, the neonate of an infected mother develops the condition through vaginal delivery.

Signs and symptoms

Approximately 70% of females—including those with chronic infections—and most males with trichomoniasis are asymptomatic. In females, acute infection may produce variable signs, such as a gray or greenish-yellow and possibly profuse and frothy, malodorous vaginal discharge.

Its other effects include severe itching, redness, swelling, tenderness, dyspareunia, dysuria, urinary frequency and, occasionally, postcoital spotting, menorrhagia, or dysmenorrhea.

Such symptoms may persist for a week to several months and may be more pronounced just after menstruation or during pregnancy. If trichomoniasis is untreated, symptoms may subside, although *T. vaginalis* infection persists, possibly associated with an abnormal cytologic smear of the cervix.

In males, trichomoniasis may produce mild to severe transient urethritis, possibly with dysuria and frequency.

Diagnosis

• Direct microscopic examination of vaginal or seminal discharge is decisive when it reveals *T. vaginalis,* a motile, pear-shaped organism.

• Examination of clear urine specimens may also reveal *T. vaginalis*.
• Physical examination of symptomatic females shows vaginal erythema; edema; frank excoriation; a frothy, malodorous, greenish-yellow vaginal discharge; and, rarely, a thin, gray pseudomembrane over the vagina.
• Cervical examination demonstrates punctate cervical hemorrhages, giving the cervix a strawberry appearance that is almost pathognomonic for this disorder.

Treatment

The treatment of choice for trichomoniasis is a single 2-g dose of metronidazole P.O. given to both sexual partners. Alternative treatment is 500 mg of metronidazole P.O. given b.i.d. for 7 days. Oral metronidazole has not been proven safe during the first trimester of pregnancy.

Effective alternatives are not available for patients who are allergic to metronidazole. Sitz baths may be used to help relieve symptoms.

After treatment, both sexual partners require a follow-up examination to check for residual signs of infection.

Special considerations

• Instruct the patient to refrain from douching before being examined for trichomoniasis.
• Urge abstinence from intercourse until the patient is cured. Refer partners for treatment. Tell the patient to avoid using tampons.
• Warn the patient to abstain from alcoholic beverages while taking metronidazole because alcohol consumption may provoke a disulfiram-type reaction (confusion, headache, cramps, vomiting, seizures). Also, tell the patient this drug may turn urine dark brown.
• Caution the patient to avoid over-the-counter douches and vaginal sprays, because chronic use can alter vaginal pH.
• Advise the patient to scrub the bathtub with a disinfecting cleanser before and after sitz baths.
• Tell the patient she can reduce the risk of genitourinary bacterial growth by wearing loose-fitting, cotton underwear that allows ventilation; bacteria flourish in a warm, dark, moist environment.
• To prevent neonates from contracting trichomoniasis, make sure pregnant women with this infection receive adequate treatment before delivery.
• Practice universal precautions.

TRIGEMINAL NEURALGIA

Also called tic douloureux, trigeminal neuralgia is a painful disorder of one or more branches of the fifth cranial (trigeminal) nerve that produces paroxysmal attacks of excruciating facial pain precipitated by stimulation of a trigger zone.

It occurs mostly in people over age 40, in women more often than men, and on the right side of the face more often than the left. Trigeminal neuralgia can subside spontaneously, with remissions lasting from several months to years.

Causes

Although the cause remains undetermined, trigeminal neuralgia may:
• reflect an afferent reflex phenomenon located centrally in the brain stem or more peripherally in the sensory root of the trigeminal nerve
• be related to compression of the nerve root by posterior fossa tumors, middle fossa tumors, or vascular lesions (subclinical aneurysm), although

TRIGEMINAL NERVE DISTRIBUTION AND FUNCTION

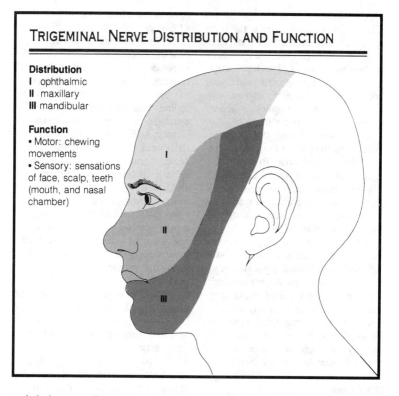

Distribution
I ophthalmic
II maxillary
III mandibular

Function
• Motor: chewing movements
• Sensory: sensations of face, scalp, teeth (mouth, and nasal chamber)

such lesions usually produce simultaneous loss of sensation
• occasionally be a manifestation of multiple sclerosis or herpes zoster.

Whatever the cause, the pain of trigeminal neuralgia is probably produced by an interaction or short-circuiting of touch and pain fibers.

Signs and symptoms
Typically, the patient reports a searing or burning pain that occurs in lightninglike jabs and lasts from 1 to 15 minutes (usually 1 to 2 minutes) in an area innervated by one of the divisions of the trigeminal nerve, primarily the superior mandibular or maxillary division.

The pain rarely affects more than one division, and seldom the first division (ophthalmic) or both sides of the face. It affects the second (maxillary) and third (mandibular) divisions of the trigeminal nerve equally. (See *Trigeminal nerve distribution and function*.)

These attacks characteristically follow stimulation of a trigger zone, usually by a light touch to a hypersensitive area, such as the tip of the nose, the cheeks, or the gums. Although attacks can occur at any time, they may follow a draft of air, exposure to heat or cold, eating, smiling, talking, or drinking hot or cold beverages.

The frequency of attacks varies greatly, from many times a day to several times a month or year. Between attacks, most patients are free of pain, although some have a constant, dull ache. No patient is ever free of the fear of the next attack.

Diagnosis

The patient's pain history is the basis for diagnosis, because trigeminal neuralgia produces no objective clinical or pathologic changes. Physical examination shows no impairment of sensory or motor function; indeed, sensory impairment implies a space-occupying lesion as the cause of pain.

Observation during the examination shows the patient favoring (splinting) the affected area. To ward off a painful attack, the patient often holds his face immobile when talking. He may also leave the affected side of his face unwashed and unshaven, or protect it with a coat or shawl.

When asked where the pain occurs, he points to — but never touches — the affected area. Witnessing a typical attack helps to confirm diagnosis. Rarely, a tumor in the posterior fossa can produce pain that is clinically indistinguishable from trigeminal neuralgia. Skull X-rays, tomography, and computed tomography scan rule out sinus or tooth infections, and tumors.

Treatment

Oral administration of carbamazepine or phenytoin may temporarily relieve or prevent pain. Narcotics may be helpful during the pain episode.

When these medical measures fail or attacks become increasingly frequent or severe, neurosurgical procedures may provide permanent relief. The preferred procedure is percutaneous electrocoagulation of nerve rootlets, under local anesthesia.

New treatments include a percutaneous radio frequency procedure, which causes partial root destruction and relieves pain, and microsurgery for vascular decompression of the trigeminal nerve.

Special considerations

• Observe and record the characteristics of each attack, including the patient's protective mechanisms.
• Provide adequate nutrition in small, frequent meals at room temperature.
• If the patient is receiving carbamazepine, watch for cutaneous and hematologic reactions (erythematous and pruritic rashes, urticaria, photosensitivity, exfoliative dermatitis, leukopenia, agranulocytosis, eosinophilia, aplastic anemia, thrombocytopenia) and, possibly, urine retention and transient drowsiness.
• For the first 3 months of carbamazepine therapy, complete blood count and liver function should be monitored weekly, then monthly thereafter. Warn the patient to immediately report fever, sore throat, mouth ulcers, easy bruising, or petechial or purpuric hemorrhage, because these may signal thrombocytopenia or aplastic anemia and may require discontinuation of drug therapy.
• If the patient is receiving phenytoin, also watch for side effects, including ataxia, skin eruptions, gingival hyperplasia, and nystagmus.
• After resection of the first division of the trigeminal nerve, tell the patient to avoid rubbing his eyes and using aerosol spray. Advise him to wear glasses or goggles outdoors and to blink often.
• After surgery to sever the second or third division, tell the patient to avoid hot foods and drinks, which could burn his mouth, and to chew carefully to avoid biting his mouth.
• Advise the patient to place food in the unaffected side of his mouth when chewing, to brush his teeth and rinse his mouth often, and to see a dentist twice a year to detect cavities. (Cavities in the area of the severed nerve won't cause pain.)

• After surgical decompression of the root or partial nerve dissection, check neurologic and vital signs often.

• Provide emotional support, and encourage the patient to express his fear and anxiety. Promote independence through self-care and maximum physical activity. Reinforce natural avoidance of stimulation (air, heat, cold) of trigger zones (lips, cheeks, gums).

LIFE-THREATENING DISORDER

TUBERCULOSIS

An acute or chronic infection caused by *Mycobacterium tuberculosis,* tuberculosis (TB) is characterized by pulmonary infiltrates, formation of granulomas with caseation, fibrosis, and cavitation. People living in crowded, poorly ventilated conditions are most likely to become infected.

In patients with strains that are sensitive to the usual antitubercular agents, the prognosis is excellent with correct treatment. However, in those with strains that are resistant to two or more of the major antitubercular agents, mortality is 50%.

Causes

After exposure to *M. tuberculosis,* roughly 5% of infected people develop active tuberculosis within 1 year; in the remainder, microorganisms cause a latent infection. The host's immune system usually controls the tubercle bacillus by killing it or walling it up in a tiny nodule (tubercle). However, the bacillus may lie dormant within the tubercle for years and later reactivate and spread.

Reactivation risk factors

Although the primary infection site is the lungs, mycobacteria commonly exist in other parts of the body. A number of factors increase the risk of infection reactivation: gastrectomy, uncontrolled diabetes mellitus, Hodgkin's disease, leukemia, silicosis, AIDS, and treatment with corticosteroids or immunosuppressives.

Mode of transmission

Tuberculosis is transmitted by droplet nuclei produced when infected persons cough or sneeze. After inhalation, if a tubercle bacillus settles in an alveolus, infection occurs. Cell-mediated immunity to the mycobacteria, which develops about 3 to 6 weeks later, usually contains the infection and arrests the disease.

Response to reactivation

If the infection reactivates, the body's response characteristically leads to caseation — the conversion of necrotic tissue to a cheeselike material. The caseum may localize, undergo fibrosis, or excavate and form cavities, the walls of which are studded with multiplying tubercle bacilli. If this happens, infected caseous debris may spread throughout the lungs by the tracheobronchial tree.

Sites of extrapulmonary TB include pleura, meninges, joints, lymph nodes, peritoneum, genitourinary tract, and bowel.

Signs and symptoms

• In primary infection, after an incubation period of from 4 to 8 weeks, TB is usually asymptomatic but may produce nonspecific symptoms, such as fatigue, weakness, anorexia, weight loss, night sweats, and low-grade fever.

• In reactivation, symptoms may include a cough that produces mucopurulent sputum, occasional hemoptysis, and chest pains.

Diagnosis

Diagnostic tests include chest X-rays, a tuberculin skin test, and sputum smears and cultures to identify *M. tuberculosis*. The following procedures aid diagnosis:

• *Auscultation* detects crepitant rales, bronchial breath sounds, wheezes, and whispered pectoriloquy.

• *Chest percussion* detects a dullness over the affected area, indicating consolidation or pleural fluid.

• *Chest X-ray* shows nodular lesions, patchy infiltrates (mainly in upper lobes), cavity formation, scar tissue, and calcium deposits; however, it may not be able to distinguish active from inactive TB.

• *Tuberculin skin test* detects TB infection. Intermediate-strength purified protein derivative (PPD) or 5 tuberculin units (0.1 ml) are injected intracutaneously on the forearm.

The test results are read in 48 to 72 hours; a positive reaction (induration of 5 to 15 mm or more, depending on risk factors) develops 2 to 10 weeks after infection in both active and inactive TB. However, severely immunosuppressed patients may never develop a positive reaction.

• *Stains and cultures* (of sputum, cerebrospinal fluid, urine, drainage from abscess, or pleural fluid) show heat-sensitive, nonmotile, aerobic, acid-fast bacilli.

Treatment

Antitubercular therapy with daily oral doses of isoniazid, rifampin, and pyrazinamide (and sometimes ethambutol) for at least 6 months usually cures tuberculosis. After 2 to 4 weeks, the disease generally is no longer infectious. The patient can resume his normal lifestyle while taking medication.

Patients with atypical mycobacterial disease or drug-resistant TB may require treatment with second-line drugs, such as capreomycin, streptomycin, para-aminosalicylic acid, cycloserine, amikacin, and quinolone drugs.

Special considerations

• Isolate the infectious patient in a quiet, well-ventilated room until he's no longer contagious.

• Teach the patient to cough and sneeze into tissues and to dispose of all secretions properly. Place a covered trash can nearby or tape a waxed bag to the side of the bed for used tissues.

• Instruct the patient to wear a mask when outside his room. Visitors and hospital personnel should wear masks when they are in the patient's room.

• Remind the patient to get plenty of rest and to eat balanced meals. If the patient is anorectic, urge him to eat small meals throughout the day. Record weight weekly.

• Be alert for side effects of medications. Because isoniazid sometimes leads to hepatitis or peripheral neuritis, monitor aspartate aminotransferase and alanine aminotransferase levels. To prevent or treat peripheral neuritis, give pyridoxine (vitamin B_6).

• If the patient receives ethambutol, watch for optic neuritis; if it develops, discontinue the drug. If he receives rifampin, watch for hepatitis and purpura. Observe the patient for other complications, such as hemoptysis.

• Emphasize the importance of regular follow-up examinations, and instruct the patient and his family concerning the signs and symptoms of recurring TB.

• Advise persons who have been exposed to infected patients to receive tuberculin tests and, if necessary, chest X-rays and prophylactic isoniazid.

ULCERATIVE COLITIS

An inflammatory, often chronic disease, ulcerative colitis affects the mucosa of the colon. It invariably begins in the rectum and sigmoid colon and often extends upward into the entire colon; it rarely affects the small intestine, except for the terminal ileum.

Ulcerative colitis produces edema (leading to mucosal friability) and ulcerations. Severity ranges from a mild, localized disorder to a fulminant disease that may cause a perforated colon, progressing to potentially fatal peritonitis and toxemia.

Causes
Although the etiology of ulcerative colitis is unknown, it is thought to be related to abnormal immune response in the gastrointestinal tract, possibly associated with food or bacteria. Stress was once thought to be a cause of ulcerative colitis, but studies show that while it isn't a cause, it does increase the severity of the attack.

Ulcerative colitis occurs primarily in young adults, especially women; it is also more prevalent among Jews and in higher socioeconomic groups. The incidence of the disease is unknown; however, some studies indicate as many as 100 out of 100,000 persons have the disease. Onset of symptoms seems to peak in the 15- to 20-year-old age-group with another peak occurring in the 55 to 60 age-group.

Signs and symptoms
The hallmark of ulcerative colitis is recurrent bloody diarrhea, often containing pus and mucus, interspersed with asymptomatic remissions. The intensity of these attacks varies with the extent of inflammation. Other symptoms include spastic rectum and anus, abdominal pain, irritability, weight loss, weakness, anorexia, nausea, and vomiting.

Ulcerative colitis may lead to complications affecting many body systems:
• *Blood:* anemia from iron deficiency, coagulation defects due to vitamin K deficiency
• *Skin:* erythema nodosum on the face and arms; pyoderma gangrenosum on the legs and ankles
• *Eye:* uveitis
• *Liver:* pericholangitis, sclerosing cholangitis, cirrhosis, possible cholangiocarcinoma
• *Musculoskeletal:* arthritis, ankylosing spondylitis, loss of muscle mass
• *Gastrointestinal:* strictures, pseudopolyps, stenosis, and perforated colon, leading to peritonitis and toxemia.

Patients with ulcerative colitis run a greater-than-normal risk of developing colorectal cancer, especially if onset of the disease occurs before age 15 or if it has persisted for longer than 10 years.

Diagnosis
• *Sigmoidoscopy* showing increased mucosal friability, decreased mucosal detail, and thick inflammatory exudate suggests this diagnosis. Biopsy can help confirm it.

- *Colonoscopy* may be used to determine the extent of the disease and also to evaluate strictured areas and pseudopolyps. (Biopsy would be done during colonoscopy.)
- *Barium enema* can assess the extent of disease and detect complications, such as strictures and carcinoma.
- *Stool specimen* should be cultured and analyzed for leukocytes, ova, and parasites.

Other supportive laboratory values include decreased serum levels of potassium, magnesium, hemoglobin, and albumin, as well as leukocytosis and prolonged prothrombin time. Elevated erythrocyte sedimentation rate correlates with the severity of the attack.

Treatment

The goals of treatment are to control inflammation, replace nutritional losses and blood volume, and prevent complications.

Supportive treatment includes bed rest, I.V. fluid replacement, and a clear-liquid diet. For patients awaiting surgery or showing signs of dehydration and debilitation from excessive diarrhea, total parenteral nutrition rests the intestinal tract, decreases stool volume, and restores positive nitrogen balance. Blood transfusions or iron supplements may be needed to correct anemia.

Drug therapy

Medications to control inflammation include corticotropin and adrenal corticosteroids, such as prednisone, prednisolone, and hydrocortisone; sulfasalazine, which has anti-inflammatory and antimicrobial properties, may also be used.

Antispasmodics, such as tincture of belladonna, and antidiarrheals, such as diphenoxylate compound, are used only for patients with frequent, troublesome diarrheal stools whose ulcerative colitis is under control. These drugs may precipitate massive dilation of the colon (toxic megacolon) and are generally contraindicated.

Surgery

If the patient has toxic megacolon, fails to respond to drugs and supportive measures, or finds symptoms unbearable, surgery is the treatment of last resort. A common surgical technique is *proctocolectomy with ileostomy.*

Another procedure, the *ileoanal pull-through,* is being performed more frequently. This procedure entails performing a total proctocolectomy and mucosal stripping, creating a pouch from the terminal ileum, and anastomosing the pouch to the anal canal. A temporary ileostomy is created to divert stools and allow the rectal anastomosis to heal.

The ileostomy is closed in 2 to 3 months, and the patient can then evacuate stools rectally. This procedure removes all the potentially malignant epithelia of the rectum and colon.

Total colectomy and ileorectal anastomosis is done less often because of its mortality rate (2% to 5%). This procedure removes the entire colon and anastomoses the rectum and the terminal ileum; it requires observation of the remaining rectal stump for any signs of cancer or colitis.

Pouch ileostomy (Kock pouch or continent ileostomy), in which the surgeon creates a pouch from a small loop of the terminal ileum and a nipple valve from the distal ileum, may be an option. The resulting stoma opens just above the pubic hairline, and the pouch empties periodically through a catheter inserted in the stoma.

A colectomy may be performed after 10 years of active ulcerative colitis because of the increased incidence of colon cancer in these patients. Performing a partial colectomy to prevent colon cancer is controversial.

Special considerations
• Accurately record intake and output, particularly the frequency and volume of stools.
• Watch for signs of dehydration and electrolyte imbalances, especially signs of hypokalemia (muscle weakness, paresthesia) and hypernatremia (fever, tachycardia, flushed skin, dry tongue).
• Monitor hemoglobin and hematocrit, and give blood transfusions.
• Provide good mouth care for the patient who is allowed nothing by mouth.
• After each bowel movement, thoroughly clean the skin around the rectum. Provide an air mattress or sheepskin to help prevent skin breakdown.
• Administer medication. Watch for adverse effects of prolonged corticosteroid therapy (moonface, hirsutism, edema, gastric irritation). Be aware that such therapy may mask infection.
• If the patient needs total parenteral nutrition, change dressings, assess for inflammation at the insertion site, and check urine every 6 hours for sugar and acetone.
• Take precautionary measures if the patient is prone to bleeding. Watch closely for signs of complications, such as a perforated colon and peritonitis (fever, severe abdominal pain, abdominal rigidity and tenderness, and cool, clammy skin), and toxic megacolon (abdominal distention, decreased bowel sounds).
• Carefully prepare the patient for surgery, and inform him about ileostomy. Do a bowel preparation.
• After surgery, provide meticulous supportive care and continue teaching correct stoma care.
• Keep the nasogastric tube patent. After removal of the tube, provide a clear-liquid diet. Gradually advance to a low-residue diet, as tolerated.
• After a proctocolectomy and ileostomy, teach good stoma care. Wash the skin around the stoma with soapy water and dry it thoroughly. Apply karaya

gum around the stoma's base to avoid irritation, and make a watertight seal. Attach the pouch over the karaya ring. Cut an opening in the ring to fit over the stoma, and secure the pouch to the skin. Empty the pouch when it's one-third full.
• After a pouch ileostomy, uncork the catheter every hour to allow contents to drain. After 10 to 14 days, gradually increase the length of time the catheter is left corked until it can be opened every 3 hours. Then remove the catheter and reinsert it every 3 to 4 hours for drainage. Teach the patient how to insert the catheter and how to take care of the stoma.
• Encourage the patient to have regular physical examinations.

URINARY TRACT INFECTION, LOWER

Cystitis and urethritis, the two forms of lower urinary tract infection (UTI), are nearly 10 times more common in women than in men and affect approximately 10% to 20% of all women at least once. Lower UTI is also a prevalent bacterial disease in children, with girls also most commonly affected.

In men and children, lower UTIs are frequently related to anatomic or physiologic abnormalities and therefore require extremely close evaluation. UTIs often respond readily to treatment, but recurrence and resistant bacterial flare-up during therapy are possible. (See *Treating and preventing UTIs,* page 874.)

Causes
Most lower UTIs result from ascending infection by a single gram-negative enteric bacteria, such as *Escherichia*

☑️ **TREATING AND PREVENTING UTIS**

Teach the female patient how to clean the perineum properly and keep the labia separated during voiding to collect a clean, midstream urine specimen. Explain that a non-contaminated midstream specimen is essential for accurate diagnosis.

Treatment
• Explain the nature and purpose of antimicrobial therapy. Emphasize the importance of completing the prescribed course of therapy or, with long-term prophylaxis, of adhering strictly to ordered dosage.
• Recommend taking nitrofurantoin macrocrystals with milk or a meal to prevent GI distress. If therapy includes phenazopyridine, warn the patient that this drug may turn urine red-orange.
• Urge the patient to drink at least eight glasses of water a day. Stress the need to maintain a consistent fluid intake of about 2,000 ml/day. More or less than this amount may alter the effect of the prescribed antimicrobial.

• Tell the patient that fruit juices, especially cranberry juice, and oral doses of vitamin C may help acidify the urine and enhance the action of the medication.
• Suggest warm sitz baths for relief of perineal discomfort.

Prevention
To prevent recurrent infections in men, urge prompt treatment of predisposing conditions such as chronic prostatitis.
  To prevent recurrent infections in women, teach the patient to:
• carefully wipe the perineum from front to back and to clean it thoroughly with soap and water after defecation
• void immediately after sexual intercourse
• drink plenty of fluids routinely
• avoid postponing urination. Recommend frequent comfort stops during long car trips, and stress the need to completely empty the bladder.

---

coli, Klebsiella, Proteus, Enterobacter, Pseudomonas, or *Serratia.* However, in a patient with neurogenic bladder, an indwelling catheter, or a fistula between the intestine and bladder, lower UTI may result from simultaneous infection with multiple pathogens.

Recent studies suggest that infection results from a breakdown in local defense mechanisms in the bladder that allow bacteria to invade the bladder mucosa and multiply. These bacteria cannot be readily eliminated by normal micturition.

Bacterial flare-up
During treatment, bacterial flare-up is generally caused by the pathogenic organism's resistance to the prescribed antimicrobial therapy. The presence of even a small number (less than 10,000/ml) of bacteria in a midstream urine sample obtained during treatment casts doubt on the effectiveness of treatment.

Recurrent UTI
In 99% of patients, recurrent lower UTI results from reinfection by the same organism or from some new pathogen; in the remaining 1%, recurrence reflects persistent infection,

usually from renal calculi, chronic bacterial prostatitis, or a structural anomaly that may become a source of infection.

High incidence in women
The high incidence of lower UTI among women may result from the shortness of the female urethra (1¼" to 2" [3 to 5 cm]), which predisposes women to infection caused by bacteria from the vagina, perineum, rectum, or a sexual partner.

Men are less vulnerable because their urethras are longer (7¾" [19.68 cm]) and their prostatic fluid serves as an antibacterial shield. In both men and women, infection usually ascends from the urethra to the bladder.

Signs and symptoms
Lower UTI usually produces urgency, frequency, dysuria, cramps or spasms of the bladder, itching, a feeling of warmth during urination, nocturia, and possibly urethral discharge in males. Inflammation of the bladder wall also causes hematuria and fever.

Other common features include low back pain, malaise, nausea, vomiting, abdominal pain or tenderness over the bladder area, chills, and flank pain.

Diagnosis
Characteristic clinical features and a microscopic urinalysis showing red blood cells and white blood cells greater than 10/high-power field suggest lower UTI.
• *A clean, midstream urine specimen* revealing a bacterial count of more than 100,000/ml confirms the diagnosis. Lower counts do not necessarily rule out infection, especially if the patient is voiding frequently, because bacteria require 30 to 45 minutes to reproduce in urine.

Careful midstream, clean-catch collection is preferred to catheterization,

which can reinfect the bladder with urethral bacteria.
• *Sensitivity testing* determines the appropriate therapeutic antimicrobial agent.
• *Voiding cystoureterography* or *excretory urography* may detect congenital anomalies that predispose the patient to recurrent UTIs.
• If patient history and physical examination warrant, a blood test or a stained smear of the discharge rules out a sexually transmitted disease.

Treatment
Appropriate antimicrobials are the treatment of choice for most initial lower UTIs. A 7- to 10-day course of antibiotic therapy is standard, but recent studies suggest that a single dose of an antibiotic or a 3- to 5-day antibiotic regimen may be sufficient to render the urine sterile. After 3 days of antibiotic therapy, urine culture should show no organisms.

If the urine is not sterile, bacterial resistance has probably occurred, making the use of a different antimicrobial necessary. Single-dose antibiotic therapy with amoxicillin or co-trimoxazole may be effective in women with acute, noncomplicated UTI. A urine culture taken 1 to 2 weeks later indicates whether or not the infection has been eradicated.

Recurrent infections due to infected renal calculi, chronic prostatitis, or structural abnormality may necessitate surgery; prostatitis also requires long-term antibiotic therapy. In patients without these predisposing conditions, long-term, low-dosage antibiotic therapy is the treatment of choice.

Special considerations
• Watch for GI disturbances from antimicrobial therapy.
• If sitz baths are not effective, apply heat sparingly to the perineum, but be careful not to burn the patient. Apply

topical antiseptics, such as povidone-iodine ointment, on the urethral meatus, as necessary.

• Collect all urine samples for culture and sensitivity testing carefully and promptly.

URTICARIA AND ANGIOEDEMA

Also called hives, *urticaria* is an episodic, usually self-limited skin reaction characterized by local dermal wheals surrounded by an erythematous flare.

Angioedema is a subcutaneous and dermal eruption that produces deeper, larger wheals (usually on the hands, feet, lips, genitalia, and eyelids) and a more diffuse swelling of loose subcutaneous tissue.

Urticaria and angioedema can occur simultaneously, but angioedema may last longer.

Causes

Urticaria and angioedema may arise from allergic reactions or may have nonallergic causes.

Allergic reactions

Urticaria and angioedema from allergies may occur in 20% of the general population at some time or other. The causes of these reactions include allergy to drugs, foods, insect stings and, occasionally, inhalant allergens (animal danders, cosmetics) that provoke an immunoglobulin E–mediated response to protein allergens. However, certain drugs may cause urticaria without an immunoglobulin E (IgE) response.

When urticaria and angioedema are part of an anaphylactic reaction, they almost always persist long after the systemic response has subsided. This occurs because circulation to the skin is the last to be restored after an allergic reaction, which results in slow histamine reabsorption at the reaction site.

Nonallergic causes

Urticaria and angioedema from nonallergic causes are probably also related to histamine release by some still-unknown mechanism. External physical stimuli, such as cold (usually in young adults), heat, water, or sunlight, may also provoke urticaria and angioedema.

Dermographic urticaria, which develops after stroking or scratching the skin, occurs in as many as 20% of the population. Such urticaria develops with varying pressure, most often under tight clothing, and is aggravated by scratching.

Mechanisms of action

Several different mechanisms and underlying disorders may provoke urticaria and angioedema. These include IgE-induced release of mediators from cutaneous mast cells, and binding of IgG or IgM to antigen, resulting in complement activation.

Disorders include localized or secondary infection (respiratory infection), neoplastic disease (Hodgkin's lymphoma), connective tissue diseases (systemic lupus erythematosus), collagen vascular disease, and psychogenic disease.

Signs and symptoms

• The characteristic features of urticaria are distinct, raised, evanescent dermal wheals surrounded by an erythematous flare. These lesions may vary in size. In cholinergic urticaria, the wheals may be tiny and blanched, surrounded by erythematous flares.

• Angioedema characteristically produces nonpitted swelling of deep subcutaneous tissue, usually on the eyelids, lips, genitalia, and mucous membranes. These swellings don't usually itch but may burn and tingle.

Diagnosis

An accurate patient history can help determine the cause of hives. Such a history should include:

• drug history, including over-the-counter preparations (vitamins, aspirin, antacids)

• frequently ingested foods (strawberries, milk products, fish)

• environmental influences (pets, carpet, clothing, soap, inhalants, cosmetics, hair dye, insect bites and stings).

Diagnosis also requires physical assessment to rule out similar conditions, and complete blood count, urinalysis, erythrocyte sedimentation rate, and chest X-ray to rule out inflammatory infections.

Skin testing, an elimination diet, and a food diary (recording time and amount of food eaten, and circumstances) can pinpoint provoking allergens. The food diary may also suggest other allergies. For instance, a patient allergic to fish may also be allergic to iodine contrast materials.

Recurrent angioedema without urticaria, along with a familial history, points to hereditary angioedema. Decreased serum levels of C4 and C1 esterase inhibitor confirm this diagnosis.

Treatment

The aim of treatment is to prevent or limit contact with triggering factors or, if this is impossible, to desensitize the patient to them and to relieve symptoms. Once the triggering stimulus has been removed, urticaria usually subsides in a few days—except for drug reactions, which may persist as long as the drug is in the bloodstream.

During desensitization, progressively larger doses of specific antigens (determined by skin testing) are injected intradermally.

Special considerations

• Tell the patient with urticaria that hydroxyzine or another antihistamine can ease itching and swelling.

• Inform the patient receiving antihistamines of the possibility of drowsiness.

• Corticosteroid therapy may be necessary for some patients. If so, explain the adverse effects.

UTERINE CANCER

Cancer of the endometrium or uterine cancer is the most common gynecologic cancer. Usually, it affects postmenopausal women between ages 50 and 60; it's uncommon between ages 30 and 40, and extremely rare before age 30. Most premenopausal women who develop uterine cancer have a history of anovulatory menstrual cycles or another hormonal imbalance.

An average of 33,000 new cases of uterine cancer are reported annually; of these, 5,500 are eventually fatal.

Causes

Uterine cancer seems linked to several predisposing factors:

• low fertility index and anovulation

• abnormal uterine bleeding

• obesity, hypertension, or diabetes

• familial tendency

• history of uterine polyps or endometrial hyperplasia

• estrogen therapy (still controversial).

Generally, uterine cancer is an adenocarcinoma that metastasizes late, usually from the endometrium to the cervix, ovaries, fallopian tubes, and other peritoneal structures. It may spread to distant organs, such as the lungs and the brain, through the blood

Signs and symptoms

Uterine enlargement and persistent and unusual premenopausal bleeding, or any postmenopausal bleeding, are the most common indications of uterine cancer. The discharge may at first be watery and blood-streaked but gradually becomes more bloody. Other symptoms, such as pain and weight loss, don't appear until the cancer is well advanced.

Diagnosis

Unfortunately, a Pap smear, so useful for detecting cervical cancer, doesn't dependably predict early-stage uterine cancer. Diagnosis of uterine cancer requires endometrial, cervical, and endocervical biopsies. (See *Staging uterine cancer.*)

Negative biopsies call for a fractional dilatation and curettage to determine diagnosis. Positive diagnosis requires the following tests for baseline data and staging:
• multiple cervical biopsies and endocervical curettage to pinpoint cervical involvement
• Schiller's test, staining the cervix and vagina with an iodine solution that turns healthy tissues brown; cancerous tissues resist the stain.
• complete physical examination
• chest X-ray or computed tomography scan
• excretory urography and, possibly, cystoscopy
• complete blood count
• electrocardiography
• proctoscopy or barium enema studies, if bladder and rectal involvement are suspected.

Treatment

Uterine cancer treatment varies, depending on the extent of the disease.

or the lymphatic system. Lymph node involvement can also occur.

Less common uterine tumors include adenoacanthoma, endometrial stromal sarcoma, lymphosarcoma, mixed mesodermal tumors (including carcinosarcoma), and leiomyosarcoma.

MANAGING PELVIC EXENTERATION

Before pelvic exenteration
• Teach the patient about ileal conduit and possible colostomy, and make sure the patient understands that her vagina will be removed.
• To minimize the risk of infection, supervise a rigorous bowel and skin preparation procedure. Decrease the residue in the patient's diet for 48 to 72 hours, then maintain a diet ranging from clear liquids to nothing by mouth. Administer oral or I.V. antibiotics, as ordered, and prep skin daily with antibacterial soap.
• Instruct the patient about postoperative procedures: I.V. therapy, central venous pressure catheter, blood drainage system, and an unsutured perineal wound with gauze packing.

After pelvic exenteration
• Check the stoma, incision, and perineal wound for drainage. Be especially careful to check the perineal wound for bleeding after the packing is removed. Expect red or serosanguineous drainage, but notify the doctor immediately if drainage is excessive, continuously bright red, foul-smelling, or purulent, or if there's bleeding from the conduit.
• Provide excellent skin care because of draining urine and feces. Use warm water and saline solution to clean the skin, because soap may be too drying and may increase skin breakdown.

Surgery
Rarely curative, surgery generally involves total abdominal hysterectomy, bilateral salpingo-oophorectomy, or possibly omentectomy with or without pelvic or para-aortic lymphadenectomy.

Total exenteration involves removal of all pelvic organs, including the vagina, and is done only when the disease is sufficiently contained to allow surgical removal of diseased parts. (See *Managing pelvic exenteration.*)

Radiation therapy
When the tumor isn't well differentiated, intracavitary or external radiation (or both), given 6 weeks before surgery, may inhibit recurrence and lengthen survival time.

Hormonal therapy
Synthetic progesterones—such as medroxyprogesterone or megestrol—may be administered for systemic disease. Tamoxifen (which produces a 20% to

40% response rate) may be given as a second-line treatment.

Chemotherapy
Varying combinations of cisplatin, doxorubicin, etoposide, and dactinomycin are usually tried when other treatments have failed.

Special considerations
• Patients with uterine cancer require teaching to help them cope with surgery, radiation, and chemotherapy. Also provide good postoperative care and psychological support.

Before surgery:
• Reinforce any previous teaching about the surgery, and explain the routine tests (e.g., repeated blood tests the morning after surgery) and postoperative care.
• If the patient is to have a lymphadenectomy *and* a total hysterectomy, explain that she'll probably have a blood drainage system for about 5 days after surgery.

• Explain indwelling urinary catheter care.

• Fit the patient with antiembolism stockings for use during and after surgery.

• Make sure the patient's blood has been typed and crossmatched.

• If the patient is premenopausal, inform her that removal of her ovaries will induce menopause.

After surgery:

• Measure fluid contents of the blood drainage system every 8 hours. Be alert for drainage that exceeds 400 ml per 8 hours.

• If the patient has received subcutaneous heparin, continue administration until the patient is fully ambulatory again. Give prophylactic antibiotics and provide good indwelling catheter care.

• Check vital signs every 4 hours. Watch for any sign of complications, such as bleeding, abdominal distention, severe pain, wheezing, or other breathing difficulties. Provide analgesics.

• Regularly encourage the patient to breathe deeply and cough to help prevent complications. Promote the use of an incentive spirometer once every waking hour to help keep lungs expanded.

• Find out if the patient is to have internal or external radiation or both. Usually, internal radiation therapy is done first.

If the patient receives internal radiation:

• Explain the internal radiation procedure, answer the patient's questions, and encourage her to express her fears and concerns.

• Explain that internal radiation usually requires a 2- to 3-day hospital stay, bowel preparation, a povidone-iodine vaginal douche, a clear liquid diet, and nothing taken by mouth the night before the implantation.

• Mention that internal radiation also requires an indwelling urinary catheter.

• Tell the patient that if the procedure is performed in the operating room, she will receive a general anesthetic. She'll be placed in a dorsal position, with her knees and hips flexed and her heels resting in footrests.

If the radioactive source isn't implanted in the operating room, it may be implanted by a member of the radiation team while the patient is in her room.

• Remember that safety precautions, including time, distance, and shielding, must be imposed immediately after the radioactive source has been implanted.

• Tell the patient that she'll require a private room.

• Encourage the patient to limit movement while the source is in place. If necessary, administer a tranquilizer to help her relax and remain still. If she prefers, elevate the head of the bed slightly. Make sure she can reach everything she needs (call bell, telephone, water) without stretching or straining.

• Assist the patient in range-of-motion *arm* exercises (leg exercises and other body movements could dislodge the source). Organize the time you spend with the patient to minimize your exposure to radiation.

• Check the patient's vital signs every 4 hours; watch for skin reaction, vaginal bleeding, abdominal discomfort, or evidence of dehydration.

• Inform visitors of safety precautions and hang a sign listing these precautions on the patient's door.

If the patient receives external radiation:

• Teach the patient and her family about the therapy before it begins. Tell the patient that treatment is usually given 5 days a week for 6 weeks. Warn her not to scrub body areas marked with indelible ink for treatment, because it's important to direct treatment to exactly the same area each time.

• Instruct the patient to maintain a high-protein, high-carbohydrate, low-residue diet to reduce bulk and yet maintain calories.

• Administer diphenoxylate with atropine to minimize diarrhea, a possible side effect of pelvic radiation.

• To minimize skin breakdown and reduce the risk of skin infection, tell the patient to keep the treatment area dry, to avoid wearing clothes that rub against the area, and to avoid using heating pads, alcohol rubs, or any skin creams.

• Teach the patient how to use a vaginal dilator to prevent vaginal stenosis and to facilitate vaginal examinations and sexual intercourse.

• Explain that except in total pelvic exenteration, the vagina remains intact and that once she recovers, sexual intercourse is possible.

UTERINE LEIOMYOMAS

Also called myomas, fibromyomas, and fibroids, uterine leiomyomas are the most common benign tumors in women. These smooth-muscle tumors usually occur in multiples in the uterine corpus, although they may appear on the cervix or on the round or broad ligament.

Uterine leiomyomas are often called fibroids, but this term is misleading because they consist of muscle cells and not fibrous tissue. Uterine leiomyomas occur in 20% to 25% of women of reproductive age and affect three times as many blacks as whites. The tumors become malignant (leiomyosarcoma) in only 0.1% of patients.

Causes

The cause of uterine leiomyomas is unknown, but steroid hormones, including estrogen and progesterone, and several growth factors, including epidermal growth factor, have been implicated as regulators of leiomyoma growth.

Leiomyomas typically arise after menarche and regress after menopause, implicating estrogen as a promoter of leiomyoma growth.

Signs and symptoms

Leiomyomas may be located within the uterine wall or may protrude into the endometrial cavity or from the serosal surface of the uterus. Most leiomyomas produce no symptoms. The most common symptom is abnormal bleeding, which typically presents clinically as menorrhagia.

Uterine leiomyomas probably do not cause pain directly except when associated with torsion of a pedunculated subserous tumor. Pelvic pressure and impingement on adjacent viscera are common indications for treatment. Various reproductive disorders, including infertility, recurrent spontaneous abortion, and preterm labor, have been attributed to uterine leiomyomas.

Diagnosis

Clinical findings and the patient history suggest uterine leiomyomas.

• *Blood studies* showing anemia from abnormal bleeding support the diagnosis.

• *Bimanual examination* may reveal an enlarged, firm, nontender, and irregularly contoured uterus.

• *Ultrasonography* allows accurate assessment of the dimensions, number, and location of tumors.

• Other diagnostic procedures include hysterosalpingography, dilatation and curettage, endometrial biopsy, and laparoscopy.

Treatment

Effective treatment depends on the severity of symptoms, the size and location of the tumors, and the patient's age, parity, pregnancy status, desire to have children, and general health. Treatment options include nonsurgical as well as surgical procedures.

Nonsurgical treatment

Conservative treatment includes taking serial histories, performing physical assessments at clinically indicated intervals, and administering gonadotropin-releasing hormone (GnRH) analogues. These drugs are capable of rapidly suppressing pituitary gonadotropin release, leading to profound hypoestrogenemia and a 50% reduction in uterine volume.

The peak effects of these GnRH analogues occur in the 12th week of therapy. The benefits are reduction in tumor size before surgery, reduction in intraoperative blood loss, and an increase in preoperative hematocrit.

Surgery

Surgery includes abdominal, laparoscopic, or hysteroscopic myomectomy — for patients who want to preserve fertility — and hysterectomy, the definitive treatment for symptomatic women who have completed childbearing.

Special considerations

• Tell the patient to report any abnormal bleeding or pelvic pain immediately.
• If a hysterectomy or oophorectomy is indicated, explain the effects of the operation on menstruation, menopause, and sexual activity to the patient.
• Reassure the patient that she won't experience premature menopause if her ovaries are left intact.
• If the patient will have a multiple myomectomy, make sure she understands pregnancy is still possible. However, if the uterine cavity is entered during surgery, explain that a cesarean delivery may be necessary.
• In a patient with severe anemia due to excessive bleeding, administer iron and blood transfusions.

VAGINAL CANCER

Cancer of the vagina accounts for approximately 2% of all gynecologic malignancies. It usually appears as squamous cell carcinoma, but occasionally as melanoma, sarcoma, or adenocarcinoma.

Vaginal cancer generally occurs in women in their early to mid-50s, but some of the rarer types do occur in younger women, and rhabdomyosarcoma appears in children.

Causes
Clear cell adenocarcinoma has an increased incidence in young women whose mothers took diethylstilbestrol. Otherwise, the cause is unknown.

Pathophysiology
Vaginal cancer varies in severity according to its location and effect on lymphatic drainage. (The vagina is a thin-walled structure with a rich lymphatic drainage.) Vaginal cancer is similar to cervical cancer in that it may progress from an intraepithelial tumor to an invasive cancer. However, it spreads more slowly than cervical cancer.

A lesion in the upper third of the vagina (the most common site) usually metastasizes to the groin nodes; a lesion in the lower third (the second most common site) usually metastasizes to the hypogastric and iliac nodes; but a lesion in the middle third metastasizes erratically.

A posterior lesion displaces and distends the vaginal posterior wall before spreading to deep layers. By contrast, an anterior lesion spreads more rapidly into other structures and deep layers, because unlike the posterior wall, the anterior vaginal wall is not flexible.

Signs and symptoms
Commonly, the patient with vaginal cancer has experienced abnormal bleeding and discharge. Also, she may have a small or large, often firm, ulcerated lesion in any part of the vagina. As the cancer progresses, it commonly spreads to the bladder (producing frequent voiding and bladder pain), the rectum (bleeding), vulva (lesion), pubic bone (pain), or other surrounding tissues.

Diagnosis
The diagnosis of vaginal cancer is based on the presence of abnormal cells on a vaginal Pap smear. Careful examination and biopsy rule out the cervix and vulva as the primary sites of the lesion. In many cases, however, the cervix contains the primary lesion that has metastasized to the vagina. Then, any visible lesion is biopsied and evaluated histologically. (See *Staging vaginal cancer,* page 884.)

The entire vagina may be difficult to visualize because the speculum blades may hide a lesion, or the patient may be uncooperative because of discomfort.

When lesions are not visible, colposcopy is used to search out abnormalities. Painting the suspected vaginal area with Lugol's solution also helps identify malignant areas by staining glycogen-containing normal tissue, while leaving abnormal tissue unstained.

Treatment

Vaginal cancer may be treated with chemotherapy, surgery, or radiation, depending on the stage of the cancer.

Early-stage cancer

In the early stages, treatment aims to preserve the normal parts of the vagina. (Preservation of a functional vagina is generally possible only in the early stages.)

Topical chemotherapy with fluorouracil and laser surgery can be used for stages 0 and I. Radiation or surgery varies with the size, depth, and location of the lesion and the patient's desire to maintain a functional vagina. Survival rates are the same for patients treated with radiation as for those with laser surgery.

Late-stage cancer

Surgery is usually recommended only when the tumor is so extensive that exenteration is needed, because close proximity to the bladder and rectum permits only minimal tissue margins around resected vaginal tissue.

Radiation therapy is the preferred treatment for advanced vaginal cancer. Most patients need preliminary external radiation treatment to shrink the tumor before internal radiation can begin. Then, if the tumor is localized to the vault and the cervix is present, radiation (using radium or cesium) can be given with an intrauterine tandem or ovoids; if the cervix is absent, a specially designed vaginal applicator is used instead.

To minimize complications, radioactive sources and filters are carefully placed away from radiosensitive tissues, such as the bladder and rectum. Internal radiation lasts 48 to 72 hours, depending on the dosage.

Special considerations

For the patient receiving internal radiation:

• Explain the internal radiation procedure, answer the patient's questions, and encourage her to express her fears and concerns.

• Because the effects of radiation are cumulative, wear a radiosensitive badge and a lead shield (if available) when you enter the patient's room.

• Check with the radiation therapist concerning the maximum recommended time that you can safely spend with the patient when giving direct care.

• While the radiation source is in place, the patient must lie flat on her back. Insert an indwelling catheter (usually done in the operating room), and do not change the patient's linens unless they are soiled. Give only partial bed baths, and make sure the patient has a call bell, phone, water, or anything else she needs within easy reach.

• The patient will be on a clear liquid or low-residue diet and an antidiarrheal drug to prevent bowel movements.

• To compensate for immobility, encourage the patient to do active range-of-motion exercises with both arms.

• Before radiation treatment, explain the necessity of immobilization, and tell the patient what it entails (such as no linen changes and the use of an indwelling catheter). Throughout therapy, encourage her to express her anxieties.

• Instruct the patient to use a stent or do prescribed exercises to prevent vaginal stenosis. Coitus is also helpful in preventing stenosis.

VAGINISMUS

Involuntary spastic constriction of the lower vaginal muscles, vaginismus usually stems from fear of vaginal penetration. This disorder may coexist with dyspareunia and, if severe, may prevent intercourse (a common cause of unconsummated marriages).

Vaginismus affects females of all ages and backgrounds. Prognosis is excellent for a motivated patient who doesn't have untreatable organic abnormalities.

Causes

Vaginismus may be physical or psychological in origin. It may occur spontaneously as a protective reflex to pain or result from organic causes, such as hymenal abnormalities, genital herpes, obstetric trauma, and atrophic vaginitis.

Psychological causes may include:

• childhood and adolescent exposure to rigid, punitive, and guilt-ridden attitudes toward sex

• fears resulting from painful or traumatic sexual experiences, such as incest or rape

• early traumatic experience with pelvic examinations

• phobias of pregnancy, venereal disease, or cancer.

Signs and symptoms

The female with vaginismus typically experiences muscle spasm with constriction and pain on insertion of any object into the vagina, such as a vaginal tampon, diaphragm, or speculum. She may profess lack of sexual interest or a normal level of sexual desire.

Diagnosis

Vaginismus is diagnosed by sexual history and pelvic examination to rule out physical disorders. The sexual history must include early childhood experiences and family attitudes toward sex, previous and current sexual responses, contraceptive practices and reproductive goals, feelings about her sexual partner, and specifics about pain on insertion of any object into the vagina.

A carefully performed pelvic examination confirms the diagnosis by showing involuntary constriction of the musculature surrounding the outer portion of the vagina.

When the disorder causes marked distress or interpersonal difficulty, it may fulfill the diagnostic criteria for a *DSM-IV* diagnosis.

Treatment

Effective treatment is designed to eliminate maladaptive muscle constriction and underlying psychological problems.

Masters and Johnson therapy

In this therapy, the patient uses a graduated series of dilators, which she inserts into her vagina while tensing and relaxing her pelvic muscles. The patient controls the time the dilator is left in place and the movement of the dilator.

Together with her sexual partner, she begins sensate focus and counseling therapy to increase sexual responsiveness, improve communication skills, and resolve any underlying conflicts.

Kaplan therapy

This therapy also uses progressive insertion of dilators or fingers (in vivo/desensitization therapy), with behavior therapy (imagining vaginal penetration until it can be tolerated) and, if necessary, psychoanalysis and hypnosis.

Both Masters and Johnson and Kaplan therapies report 100% cure; however, Kaplan states the patient and her partner may show other sexual dysfunctions that necessitate additional therapy.

Special considerations

• Because a pelvic examination may be painful for the patient with vaginismus, proceed gradually, at the patient's own pace. Support the patient throughout the pelvic examination, explaining each step before it is done. Encourage her to verbalize her feelings, and take plenty of time to answer her questions.
• Teach the patient about anatomy and physiology of the reproductive system, contraception, and human sexual response. This can be done quite naturally during the pelvic examination.
• Ask if the patient is taking any medications (antihypertensives, tranquilizers, steroids) that may affect her sexual response. If she has insufficient lubrication for intercourse, tell her about lubricating jellies and creams.

VALVULAR HEART DISEASE

In valvular heart disease, three types of mechanical disruption can occur: stenosis, or narrowing, of the valve opening; incomplete closure of the valve; or prolapse of the valve. They can result from such disorders as endocarditis (most common), congenital defects, and inflammation, and they can lead to heart failure. (For information about causes, signs and symptoms, and diagnosis, see *Forms of valvular heart disease.*)

Valvular heart disease occurs in varying forms:
• *Mitral insufficiency.* In this form, blood from the left ventricle flows back into the left atrium during systole, causing the atrium to enlarge to accommodate the backflow. As a result, the left ventricle also dilates to accommodate the increased volume of blood from the atrium and to compensate for diminishing cardiac output.

Ventricular hypertrophy and increased end-diastolic pressure result in increased pulmonary artery pressure, eventually leading to left and right ventricular failure.
• *Mitral stenosis.* Narrowing of the valve by valvular abnormalities, fibrosis, or calcification obstructs blood flow from the left atrium to the left ventricle. Consequently, left atrial volume and pressure rise and the chamber dilates.

Greater resistance to blood flow causes pulmonary hypertension, right ventricular hypertrophy, and right ventricular failure. Also, inadequate filling of the left ventricle produces low cardiac output.
• *Mitral valve prolapse (MVP).* One or both valve leaflets protrude into the left atrium. MVP is the term used when

(Text continues on page 890.)

FORMS OF VALVULAR HEART DISEASE

CAUSES AND INCIDENCE	CLINICAL FEATURES	DIAGNOSTIC MEASURES
Mitral stenosis • Results from rheumatic fever (most common cause) • Most common in females • May be associated with other congenital anomalies	• Dyspnea on exertion, paroxysmal nocturnal dyspnea, orthopnea, weakness, fatigue, palpitations • Peripheral edema, jugular vein distention, ascites, hepatomegaly (right ventricular failure in severe pulmonary hypertension) • Crackles, cardiac arrhythmias (atrial fibrillation), signs of systemic emboli • Auscultation reveals a loud S_1 or opening snap and a diastolic murmur at the apex.	• Cardiac catheterization: diastolic pressure gradient across valve; elevated left atrial and pulmonary artery wedge pressures (PAWP > 15 mm Hg) with severe pulmonary hypertension and pulmonary artery pressures; elevated right-sided heart pressure; decreased cardiac output (CO); and abnormal contraction of the left ventricle • X-ray: left atrial and ventricular enlargement, enlarged pulmonary arteries, and mitral valve calcification • Echocardiography: thickened mitral valve leaflets, left atrial enlargement • Electrocardiography: left atrial hypertrophy, atrial fibrillation, right ventricular hypertrophy, and right axis deviation
Mitral insufficiency • Results from rheumatic fever, hypertrophic cardiomyopathy, mitral valve prolapse, myocardial infarction, severe left ventricular failure, or ruptured chordae tendineae • Associated with other congenital anomalies, such as transposition of the great arteries • Rare in children without other congenital anomalies	• Orthopnea, dyspnea, fatigue, angina, palpitations • Peripheral edema, jugular vein distention, hepatomegaly (right ventricular failure) • Tachycardia, crackles, pulmonary edema • Auscultation reveals a holosystolic murmur at apex, possible split S_2, and an S_3.	• Cardiac catheterization: mitral regurgitation with increased left ventricular end-diastolic volume and pressure, increased atrial pressure and PAWP, and decreased CO • X-ray: left atrial and ventricular enlargement, pulmonary venous congestion • Echocardiography: abnormal valve leaflet motion, left atrial enlargement • Electrocardiography: may show left atrial and ventricular hypertrophy, sinus tachycardia, and atrial fibrillation

(continued)

FORMS OF VALVULAR HEART DISEASE *(continued)*

CAUSES AND INCIDENCE	CLINICAL FEATURES	DIAGNOSTIC MEASURES
Mitral valve prolapse syndrome • Cause unknown. Researchers speculate that metabolic or neuroendocrine factors cause constellation of signs and symptoms. • Most commonly affects young women but may occur in both sexes and in all age-groups	• May produce no signs • Chest pain, palpitations, headache, fatigue, exercise intolerance, dyspnea, light-headedness, syncope, mood swings, anxiety, panic attacks • Auscultation typically reveals a mobile, midsystolic click, with or without a mid-to-late systolic murmur.	• Two-dimensional echocardiography: prolapse of mitral valve leaflets into left atrium • Color-flow Doppler studies: mitral insufficiency • Resting electrocardiography: ST-segment changes, biphasic or inverted T waves in leads II, III, or AV • Exercise electrocardiography: evaluates chest pain and arrhythmias
Aortic insufficiency • Results from rheumatic fever, syphilis, hypertension, endocarditis, or may be idiopathic • Associated with Marfan syndrome • Most common in males • Associated with ventricular septal defect, even after surgical closure	• Dyspnea, cough, fatigue, palpitations, angina, syncope • Pulmonary vein congestion, congestive heart failure, pulmonary edema (left ventricular failure), "pulsating" nail beds (Quincke's sign) • Rapidly rising and collapsing pulses (pulsus biferiens), cardiac arrhythmias, wide pulse pressure in severe regurgitation • Auscultation reveals an S_3 and a diastolic blowing murmur at left sternal border. • Palpation and visualization of apical impulse in chronic disease	• Cardiac catheterization: reduction in arterial diastolic pressures, aortic regurgitation, other valvular abnormalities, and increased left ventricular end-diastolic pressure • X-ray: left ventricular enlargement, pulmonary vein congestion • Echocardiography: left ventricular enlargement, alterations in mitral valve movement (indirect indication of aortic valve disease), and mitral thickening • Electrocardiography: sinus tachycardia, left ventricular hypertrophy, and left atrial hypertrophy in severe disease

FORMS OF VALVULAR HEART DISEASE   *(continued)*

CAUSES AND INCIDENCE	CLINICAL FEATURES	DIAGNOSTIC MEASURES
Aortic stenosis • Results from congenital aortic bicuspid valve (associated with coarctation of the aorta), congenital stenosis of valve cusps, rheumatic fever, or atherosclerosis in the aged • Most common in males	• Dyspnea on exertion, paroxysmal nocturnal dyspnea, fatigue, syncope, angina, palpitations • Pulmonary vein congestion, congestive heart failure, pulmonary edema (left ventricular failure) • Diminished carotid pulses, decreased cardiac output, cardiac arrhythmias; may have pulsus alternans • Auscultation reveals systolic murmur heard at base or in carotids and, possibly, an S_4.	• Cardiac catheterization: pressure gradient across valve (indicating obstruction), increased left ventricular end-diastolic pressures • X-ray: valvular calcification, left ventricular enlargement, and pulmonary vein congestion • Echocardiography: thickened aortic valve and left ventricular wall, possibly coexistent with mitral valve stenosis • Electrocardiography: left ventricular hypertrophy
Pulmonic insufficiency • May be congenital or may result from pulmonary hypertension • May rarely result from prolonged use of pressure monitoring catheter in the pulmonary artery	• Dyspnea, weakness, fatigue, chest pain • Peripheral edema, jugular vein distention, hepatomegaly (right ventricular failure) • Auscultation reveals diastolic murmur in pulmonic area.	• Cardiac catheterization: pulmonary regurgitation, increased right ventricular pressure, and associated cardiac defects • X-ray: right ventricular and pulmonary arterial enlargement • Electrocardiography: right ventricular or right atrial enlargement
Pulmonic stenosis • Results from congenital stenosis of valve cusp or rheumatic heart disease (infrequent) • Associated with other congenital heart defects, such as tetralogy of Fallot	• Asymptomatic or symptomatic with dyspnea on exertion, fatigue, chest pain, syncope • May lead to peripheral edema, jugular vein distention, hepatomegaly (right ventricular failure) • Auscultation reveals a systolic murmur at the left sternal border, a split S_2 with a delayed or absent pulmonic component.	• Cardiac catheterization: increased right ventricular pressure, decreased pulmonary artery pressure, and abnormal valve orifice • Electrocardiography: may show right ventricular hypertrophy, right axis deviation, right atrial hypertrophy, and atrial fibrillation

(continued)

FORMS OF VALVULAR HEART DISEASE *(continued)*

CAUSES AND INCIDENCE	CLINICAL FEATURES	DIAGNOSTIC MEASURES
Tricuspid insufficiency • Results from right ventricular failure, rheumatic fever and, rarely, trauma and endocarditis • Associated with congenital disorders	• Dyspnea and fatigue • May lead to peripheral edema, jugular vein distention, hepatomegaly, and ascites (right ventricular failure) • Auscultation reveals possible S_3 and systolic murmur at lower left sternal border that increases with inspiration.	• Right heart catheterization: high atrial pressure, tricuspid regurgitation, and decreased or normal cardiac output • X-ray: right atrial dilation, right ventricular enlargement • Echocardiography: systolic prolapse of tricuspid valve, right atrial enlargement • Electrocardiography: right atrial or right ventricular hypertrophy, atrial fibrillation
Tricuspid stenosis • Results from rheumatic fever • May be congenital • Associated with mitral or aortic valve disease • Most common in women	• May be symptomatic with dyspnea, fatigue, syncope • Possibly peripheral edema, jugular vein distention, hepatomegaly, and ascites (right ventricular failure) • Auscultation reveals diastolic murmur at lower left sternal border that increases with inspiration.	• Cardiac catheterization: increased pressure gradient across valve, increased right atrial pressure, decreased cardiac output • X-ray: right atrial enlargement • Echocardiography: leaflet abnormality, right atrial enlargement • Electrocardiography: right atrial hypertrophy, right or left ventricular hypertrophy, and atrial fibrillation

the anatomic prolapse is accompanied by signs and symptoms unrelated to the valvular abnormality.

• *Aortic insufficiency.* Blood flows back into the left ventricle during diastole, causing fluid overload in the ventricle, which dilates and hypertrophies. The excess volume causes fluid overload in the left atrium and, finally, the pulmonary system. Left ventricular failure and pulmonary edema eventually result.

• *Aortic stenosis.* Increased left ventricular pressure tries to overcome the resistance of the narrowed valvular opening. The added workload increases the demand for oxygen, and diminished cardiac output causes poor coronary artery perfusion, ischemia of

the left ventricle, and left ventricular failure.

• *Pulmonic insufficiency.* Blood ejected into the pulmonary artery during systole flows back into the right ventricle during diastole, causing fluid overload in the ventricle, ventricular hypertrophy and, finally, right ventricular failure.

• *Pulmonic stenosis.* Obstructed right ventricular outflow causes right ventricular hypertrophy, eventually resulting in right ventricular failure.

• *Tricuspid insufficiency.* Blood flows back into the right atrium during systole, decreasing blood flow to the lungs and left side of the heart. Cardiac output also lessens. Fluid overload in the

right side of the heart can eventually lead to right ventricular failure.
• *Tricuspid stenosis.* Obstructed blood flow from the right atrium to the right ventricle causes the right atrium to dilate and hypertrophy. Eventually, this leads to right ventricular failure and increases pressure in the vena cava.

Treatment
Therapy depends on the nature and severity of associated symptoms. For example, heart failure requires digoxin, diuretics, a sodium-restricted diet and, in acute cases, oxygen.

Other measures may include anticoagulant therapy to prevent thrombus formation around diseased or replaced valves, prophylactic antibiotics before and after surgery or dental care, and valvuloplasty.

If the patient has severe signs and symptoms that can't be managed medically, open-heart surgery using cardiopulmonary bypass for valve replacement is indicated.

Special considerations
• Watch closely for signs of heart failure or pulmonary edema and for adverse effects of drug therapy.
• Teach the patient about diet restrictions, medications, and the importance of consistent follow-up care.
• If the patient undergoes surgery, watch for hypotension, arrhythmias, and thrombus formation. Monitor vital signs, arterial blood gases, intake, output, daily weight, blood chemistries, chest X-rays, and pulmonary artery catheter readings.

VARICELLA

Also called chickenpox, varicella is a common, acute, and highly contagious infection caused by the herpesvirus varicella-zoster (V-Z), the same virus that, in its latent stage, causes herpes zoster (shingles). It can occur at any age, but it's most common in 2- to 8-year-olds.

Varicella vaccine is effective in preventing chickenpox in up to 90% of recipients. The American Academy of Pediatrics recommends the vaccine for all children and for adolescents and adults who haven't had chickenpox. It is unknown how the vaccine affects shingles.

Causes
Congenital varicella may affect infants whose mothers had acute infections in their first or early second trimester. Neonatal infection is rare, probably due to transient maternal immunity. Second attacks are also rare.

Chickenpox is transmitted by direct contact (primarily with respiratory secretions; less often, with skin lesions) and indirect contact (air waves). The incubation period lasts from 13 to 17 days. Chickenpox is probably communicable from 1 day before lesions erupt to 6 days after vesicles form (it's most contagious in the early stages of eruption of skin lesions).

Most children recover completely. Potentially fatal complications may affect children receiving corticosteroids, antimetabolites, or other immunosuppressant agents, and those with leukemia, other neoplasms, or immunodeficiency disorders. Congenital and adult varicella may also have severe effects.

This disease occurs worldwide and is endemic in large cities. Outbreaks occur sporadically, usually in areas with large groups of susceptible children. It affects all races and both sexes equally. Seasonal distribution varies; in temperate areas, incidence is higher during late autumn, winter, and spring.

Signs and symptoms

Chickenpox produces distinctive signs and symptoms, notably a pruritic rash. During the prodromal phase, the patient has slight fever, malaise, and anorexia. Within 24 hours, the rash typically begins as crops of small, erythematous macules on the trunk or scalp that progress to papules and then clear vesicles on an erythematous base (the so-called "dewdrop on a rose petal").

The vesicles become cloudy and break easily; then scabs form. The rash spreads to the face and, rarely, to the extremities. New vesicles continue to appear for 3 or 4 days, so the rash contains a combination of red papules, vesicles, and scabs in various stages. Occasionally, chickenpox also produces shallow ulcers on mucous membranes of the mouth, conjunctivae, and genitalia.

Congenital varicella causes hypoplastic deformity and scarring of a limb, retarded growth, and central nervous system and eye manifestations. In progressive varicella, an immunocompromised patient will have lesions and a high fever for over 7 days.

Complications

Severe pruritus with this rash may provoke persistent scratching, which can lead to infection, scarring, impetigo, furuncles, and cellulitis. Rare complications include pneumonia, myocarditis, fulminating encephalitis (Reye's syndrome), bleeding disorders, arthritis, nephritis, hepatitis, and acute myositis.

Diagnosis

Chickenpox is diagnosed by characteristic clinical signs and usually doesn't require laboratory tests. However, the virus can be isolated from vesicular fluid within the first 3 or 4 days of the rash; Giemsa stain distinguishes V-Z from vaccinia-variola viruses. Serum contains antibodies 7 days after onset.

Treatment

Patients must remain in strict isolation until all the vesicles and most of the scabs disappear (usually for 1 week after the onset of the rash). Children can go back to school, however, if just a few scabs remain because, at this stage, chickenpox is no longer contagious. Congenital chickenpox requires no isolation.

Generally, treatment consists of the following:
• local or systemic antipruritics
• cool bicarbonate of soda baths
• calamine lotion
• diphenhydramine or another antihistamine
• antibiotics if bacterial infection develops.

Salicylates are contraindicated because of their link with Reye's syndrome.

Susceptible patients may need special treatment. When given up to 72 hours after exposure to varicella, varicella-zoster immune globulin may provide passive immunity. Acyclovir may slow vesicle formation, speed skin healing, and control the systemic spread of infection.

Special considerations

• Teach the child and his family how to apply topical antipruritic medications correctly. Stress the importance of good hygiene.
• Tell the patient not to scratch the lesions. However, because the need to scratch may be overwhelming, parents should trim the child's fingernails or tie mittens on his hands.
• Warn parents to watch for and immediately report signs of complications. Severe skin pain and burning may indicate a serious secondary infection and require prompt medical attention.

• To help prevent chickenpox, don't admit a child exposed to chickenpox to a unit that contains children who receive immunosuppressant agents or who have leukemia or immunodeficiency disorders. A vulnerable child who's been exposed to chickenpox should receive varicella-zoster immune globulin to lessen its severity.

VASCULAR RETINOPATHIES

Noninflammatory retinal disorders, vascular retinopathies result from interference with the blood supply to the eyes. The five distinct types of vascular retinopathy are central retinal artery occlusion, central retinal vein occlusion, diabetic retinopathy, hypertensive retinopathy, and sickle cell retinopathy.

Causes
When one of the arteries maintaining blood circulation in the retina becomes obstructed, the diminished blood flow causes visual deficits.

Central retinal artery occlusion
This form of vascular retinopathy may be idiopathic or may result from embolism, atherosclerosis, infection, or conditions that retard blood flow, such as temporal arteritis, carotid occlusion, and heart failure. Central retinal artery occlusion is rare, occurs unilaterally, and affects elderly patients.

Central retinal vein occlusion
Causes of central retinal vein occlusion include external compression of the retinal vein, trauma, diabetes, thrombosis, granulomatous diseases, generalized and localized infections, glaucoma, and atherosclerosis. This form of vascular retinopathy is most prevalent in elderly patients.

Diabetic retinopathy
This form results from juvenile or adult diabetes. Microcirculatory changes occur more rapidly when diabetes is poorly controlled. About 75% of patients with juvenile diabetes develop retinopathy within 20 years of onset of diabetes.

In adults with diabetes, incidence increases with the duration of diabetes; 80% of patients who have had diabetes for 20 to 25 years develop retinopathy. This condition is a leading cause of acquired adult blindness.

Hypertensive retinopathy
This form results from prolonged hypertensive disease, producing retinal vasospasm, and consequent damage and arteriolar narrowing.

Sickle cell retinopathy
This form results from impaired ability of the sickled cell to pass through the microvasculature, producing vasocclusion. This results in microaneurysms, chorioretinal infarction, and retinal detachment.

Signs and symptoms
The following features characterize vascular retinopathy.

Central retinal artery occlusion
This type of occlusion produces sudden, painless, unilateral loss of vision (partial or complete). It may follow amaurosis fugax or transient episodes of unilateral loss of vision lasting from a few seconds to minutes, probably due to vasospasm.

This condition typically causes permanent blindness. However, some patients experience spontaneous resolution within hours and regain partial vision.

Central retinal vein occlusion

Occlusion of this type causes reduced visual acuity, allowing perception of only hand movement and light. This condition is painless, except when it results in secondary neovascular glaucoma (uncontrolled proliferation of weak blood vessels). Prognosis is poor—5% to 20% of patients with this condition develop secondary glaucoma within 3 to 4 months after occlusion.

Diabetic retinopathy

Nonproliferative diabetic retinopathy produces changes in the lining of the retinal blood vessels that cause the vessels to leak plasma or fatty substances, which decrease or block blood flow (nonperfusion) within the retina. This disorder may also produce microaneurysms and small hemorrhages.

Although nonproliferative retinopathy causes no symptoms in some patients, in others leakage of fluid into the macular region causes significant loss of central visual acuity (necessary for reading and driving) and diminished night vision.

Proliferative diabetic retinopathy produces fragile new blood vessels on the disk and elsewhere in the fundus (neovascularization). These vessels can grow into the vitreous and then rupture, causing vitreous hemorrhage with corresponding sudden vision loss.

Scar tissue that may form along the new blood vessels can pull on the retina, causing macular distortion and even retinal detachment.

Hypertensive retinopathy

Symptoms of hypertensive retinopathy depend on the location of retinopathy. For example, mild visual disturbances, such as blurred vision, result from retinopathy located near the macula.

Without treatment, prognosis is poor (50% of patients become blind within 5 years). With treatment, prognosis varies with the severity of the disorder. Severe, prolonged disease eventually produces blindness; mild, prolonged disease, visual defects.

Diagnosis

Appropriate diagnostic tests depend on the type of vascular retinopathy. (See *Diagnosis of vascular retinopathies.*) Always include determination of visual acuity and ophthalmoscopic examination. (See *Viewing vascular retinopathies,* page 896.)

Treatment

The following measures are used to treat vascular retinopathy.

Central retinal artery occlusion

No treatment has been shown to control central retinal artery occlusion. However, an attempt is made to release the occlusion into the peripheral circulation.

To reduce intraocular pressure, therapy includes acetazolamide 500 mg I.V., eyeball massage, anterior chamber paracentesis, and inhalation of carbogen (95% oxygen and 5% carbon dioxide) to improve retinal oxygenation. Because inhalation therapy may be given hourly for up to 48 hours, the patient should be hospitalized so vital signs can be monitored.

Central retinal vein occlusion

Therapy for central retinal vein occlusion may include aspirin, which acts as a mild anticoagulant. Laser photocoagulation can reduce the risk of neovascular glaucoma for some patients whose eyes have widespread capillary nonperfusion.

Diabetic retinopathy

Treatment of *nonproliferative diabetic retinopathy* is prophylactic. Careful control of blood glucose levels during the first 5 years of the disease may re-

DIAGNOSIS OF VASCULAR RETINOPATHIES

In vascular retinopathies, diagnosis varies, depending on the type of retinopathy.

Central retinal artery occlusion

• *Ophthalmoscopy (direct or indirect)* shows emptying of retinal arterioles during transient attack.

• *Retinal examination* within 2 hours of onset shows clumps or segmentation in artery; later, milky white retina around disk due to swelling and necrosis of ganglion cells caused by reduced blood supply; also shows cherry-red spot in macula that subsides after several weeks.

• *Digital subtraction angiography (DSA)* evaluates carotid occlusion with no need for arteriography.

• *Physical examination* reveals underlying cause of vascular retinopathy, for example, diabetes or hypertension.

• *Magnetic resonance imaging and computed tomography scan (with contrast media)* may reveal carotid or other obstruction.

Central retinal vein occlusion

• *Opthalmoscopy (direct or indirect)* shows retinal hemorrhage, retinal vein engorgement, white patches among hemorrhages, and edema around the disk.

• *Ultrasonography* confirms or rules out occlusion of blood vessels.

• *Physical examination* reveals underlying cause.

Diabetic retinopathy

• *Indirect ophthalmoscopy* shows retinal changes such as microaneurysms (earliest change), retinal hemorrhages and edema, venous dilation and bending, exudates, vitreous hemorrhage, proliferation of fibrin into vitreous due to retinal holes, growth of new blood vessels, and microinfarcts of nerve fiber layer.

• *Fluorescein angiography* shows leakage of fluorescein from dilated vessels and differentiates between microaneurysms and true hemorrhages.

• *History* reveals diabetes.

Hypertensive retinopathy

• *Ophthalmoscopy (direct or indirect)* in early stages, shows hard, shiny deposits, tiny hemorrhages, silver-wire appearance of narrowed arterioles, and nicking of veins where arteries cross them (AV nicking); in late stages, cotton wool patches, exudates, retinal edema, papilledema due to ischemia and capillary insufficiency, hemorrhages, and microaneurysms.

• *Physical examination* detects elevated blood pressure.

• *History* reveals decreased vision, headache, and hypertension.

---

duce the severity of the retinopathy or delay its onset.

Patients with early symptoms of microaneurysms should have frequent eye examinations (three to four times a year); children with diabetes should have an annual eye examination.

The best treatment for *proliferative diabetic retinopathy* or severe macular edema is laser photocoagulation, which cauterizes the leaking blood vessels. Laser treatment may be focal (aimed at new blood vessels) or panretinal (placing burns throughout the peripheral retina).

Despite treatment, neovascularization doesn't always regress, and vitreous hemorrhage, with or without retinal detachment, may follow. If the

VIEWING VASCULAR RETINOPATHIES

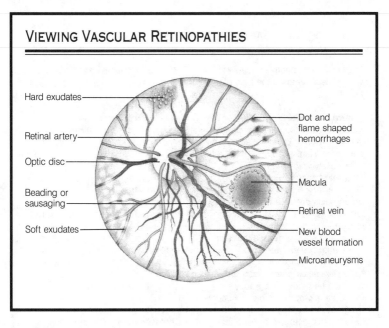

Hard exudates

Retinal artery

Optic disc

Beading or sausaging

Soft exudates

Dot and flame shaped hemorrhages

Macula

Retinal vein

New blood vessel formation

Microaneurysms

blood isn't absorbed in 3 to 6 months, vitrectomy may restore partial vision.

Hypertensive retinopathy
Treatment for hypertensive retinopathy includes control of blood pressure with appropriate drugs, diet, and exercise.

Special considerations
• Arrange for *immediate* ophthalmologic evaluation when a patient complains of sudden, unilateral loss of vision. Blindness may be permanent if treatment is delayed.
• Be sure to monitor a patient's blood pressure if he complains of occipital headache and blurred vision.
• Administer acetazolamide I.V. During inhalation therapy, monitor vital signs carefully. Discontinue therapy if blood pressure fluctuates or if patient develops arrhythmias or disorientation.
• Encourage a diabetic patient to comply with the prescribed regimen.

• For a patient with hypertensive retinopathy, stress the importance of complying with antihypertensive therapy.

VASCULITIS

A broad spectrum of disorders, vasculitis is characterized by inflammation and necrosis of blood vessels. Its clinical effects depend on the vessels involved and reflect tissue ischemia caused by blood flow obstruction.

Prognosis is also variable. For example, hypersensitivity vasculitis is usually a benign disorder limited to the skin, but more extensive polyarteritis nodosa can be rapidly fatal.

Vasculitis can occur at any age, except for mucocutaneous lymph node syndrome, which occurs only during childhood. Vasculitis may be a primary disorder or secondary to other disorders such as rheumatoid arthritis (RA) or systemic lupus erythematosus (SLE).

Causes

How vascular damage develops in vasculitis isn't well understood. It has been associated with a history of serious infectious disease, such as hepatitis B or bacterial endocarditis, and high-dose antibiotic therapy.

Excessive antigen theory

Current theory holds that vasculitis is initiated by excessive circulating antigen, which triggers the formation of soluble antigen–antibody complexes. These complexes can't be effectively cleared by the reticuloendothelial system and so are deposited in blood vessel walls (Type III hypersensitivity).

Increased vascular permeability associated with release of vasoactive amines by platelets and basophils enhances such deposition. The deposited complexes activate the complement cascade, resulting in chemotaxis of neutrophils, which release lysosomal enzymes. In turn, these enzymes cause vessel damage and necrosis, which may precipitate thrombosis, occlusion, hemorrhage, and ischemia.

Immune response

Another mechanism that may contribute to vascular damage is the cell-mediated (T cell) immune response. In this response, circulating antigen triggers the release of soluble mediators by sensitized lymphocytes, which attracts macrophages.

The macrophages release intracellular enzymes, which cause vascular damage. They can also transform into the epithelioid and multinucleated giant cells that typify the granulomatous vasculitides. Phagocytosis of immune complexes by macrophages enhances granuloma formation.

Signs and symptoms and diagnosis

Clinical effects of vasculitis and confirming laboratory procedures depend on the blood vessels involved. (For information specific to each type of vasculitis, see *Types of vasculitis*, page 898.)

Treatment

The aim of treatment is to minimize irreversible tissue damage associated with ischemia. In secondary vasculitis, treatment focuses on the underlying disorder. Primary vasculitis is mainly treated with drugs.

Treatment may involve removal of an offending antigen or use of anti-inflammatory or immunosuppressive drugs. For example, antigenic drugs, food, and other environmental substances should be identified and eliminated, if possible.

Drug therapy in primary vasculitis frequently involves low-dose cyclophosphamide (2 mg/kg P.O. daily) with daily corticosteroids. In rapidly fulminant vasculitis, cyclophosphamide dosage may be increased to 4 mg/kg daily for the first 2 to 3 days, followed by the regular dose. Prednisone should be given in a dose of 1 mg/kg daily in divided doses for 7 to 10 days, with consolidation to a single morning dose by 2 to 3 weeks.

When the vasculitis appears to be in remission or when prescribed cytotoxic drugs take full effect, corticosteroids are tapered down to a single daily dose and then to an alternate-day schedule that may continue for 3 to 6 months before steroids are slowly discontinued.

Special considerations

• Assess for dry nasal mucosa in patients with Wegener's granulomatosis. Instill nose drops to lubricate the mucosa and help diminish crusting. Or irrigate the nasal passages with warm normal saline solution.

(Text continues on page 900.)

TYPES OF VASCULITIS

TYPE	VESSELS INVOLVED
Polyarteritis nodosa	Small- to medium-sized arteries throughout body. Lesions tend to be segmental, occur at bifurcations and branchings of arteries, and spread distally to arterioles. In severe cases, lesions circumferentially involve adjacent veins.
Allergic angiitis and granulomatosis (Churg-Strauss syndrome)	Small- to medium-sized arteries and small vessels (arterioles, capillaries, and venules), mainly of the lung but also other organs
Polyangiitis overlap syndrome	Small- to medium-sized arteries and small vessels (arterioles, capillaries, venules) of lung and other organs
Wegener's granulomatosis	Small- to medium-sized vessels of the respiratory tract and kidney
Temporal arteritis	Medium- to large-sized arteries, most commonly branches of the carotid artery
Takayasu's arteritis (aortic arch syndrome)	Medium- to large-sized arteries, particularly the aortic arch and its branches and, possibly, the pulmonary artery
Hypersensitivity vasculitis	Small vessels, especially of the skin
Mucocutaneous lymph node syndrome (Kawasaki disease)	Small- to medium-sized vessels, primarily of the lymph nodes; may progress to involve coronary arteries

SIGNS & SYMPTOMS	DIAGNOSIS
Hypertension, abdominal pain, myalgias, headache, joint pain, weakness	History of symptoms. Elevated erythrocyte sedimentation rate (ESR), leukocytosis, anemia, thrombocytosis, depressed C3 complement, rheumatoid factor > 1:60, circulating immune complexes. Tissue biopsy shows necrotizing vasculitis.
Resembles polyarteritis nodosa with hallmark of severe pulmonary involvement	History of asthma. Eosinophilia; tissue biopsy shows granulomatous inflammation with eosinophilic infiltration.
Combines symptoms of polyarteritis nodosa and allergic angiitis and granulomatosis	Possible history of allergy. Eosinophilia; tissue biopsy shows granulomatous inflammation with eosinophilic infiltration.
Fever, pulmonary congestion, cough, malaise, anorexia, weight loss, mild to severe hematuria	Tissue biopsy shows necrotizing vasculitis with granulomatous inflammation. Leukocytosis; elevated ESR, IgA, and IgG; low titer rheumatoid factor; circulating immune complexes; antineutrophil cytoplasmic antibody in more than 90% of patients
Fever, myalgia, jaw claudication, visual changes, headache (associated with polymyalgia rheumatica syndrome)	Decreased hemoglobin; elevated ESR; tissue biopsy shows panarteritis with infiltration of mononuclear cells, giant cells within vessel wall, fragmentation of internal elastic lamina, and proliferation of intima.
Malaise, pallor, nausea, night sweats, arthralgias, anorexia, weight loss, pain or paresthesia distal to affected area, bruits, loss of distal pulses, syncope and, if carotid artery is involved, diplopia and transient blindness. May progress to heart failure or CVA.	Decreased hemoglobin, leukocytosis, positive LE cell preparation, and elevated ESR. Arteriography shows calcification and obstruction of affected vessels. Tissue biopsy shows inflammation of adventitia and intima of vessels and thickening of vessel walls.
Palpable purpura, papules, nodules, vesicles, bullae, ulcers, or chronic or recurrent urticaria	History of exposure to antigen, such as a microorganism or drug. Tissue biopsy shows leukocytoclastic angiitis, usually in postcapillary venules.
Fever; nonsuppurative cervical adenitis; edema; congested conjunctivae; erythema of oral cavity, lips, and palms; and desquamation of fingertips. May progress to arthritis, myocarditis, pericarditis, MI, and cardiomegaly.	History of symptoms; elevated ESR. Tissue biopsy shows intimal proliferation and infiltration of vessel walls with mononuclear cells. Echocardiography necessary.

(continued)

TYPES OF VASCULITIS *(continued)*	
TYPE	**VESSELS INVOLVED**
Behçet's disease	Small vessels, primarily of the mouth and genitalia but also of the eyes, skin, joints, GI tract, and central nervous system

• Monitor vital signs. Use a Doppler ultrasonic flowmeter, if available, to auscultate blood pressure in patients with Takayasu's arteritis, whose peripheral pulses are frequently difficult to palpate.

• Monitor intake and output. Check daily for edema. Keep the patient well-hydrated (3 L daily) to reduce the risk of hemorrhagic cystitis associated with cyclophosphamide therapy.

• Provide emotional support to help the patient and his family cope with an altered body image — the result of the disorder or its therapy. (For example, Wegener's granulomatosis may be associated with saddle nose, steroids may cause weight gain, and cyclophosphamide may cause alopecia.)

• Teach the patient how to recognize adverse reactions to drugs.

• Monitor the patient's white blood cell count during cyclophosphamide therapy to prevent severe leukopenia.

VITILIGO

Marked by stark-white skin patches that may cause a serious cosmetic problem, vitiligo results from the destruction and loss of pigment cells. This condition affects about 1% of the U.S. population, usually persons between ages 10 and 30, with peak incidence around age 20.

It shows no racial preference, but the distinctive patches are most prominent in blacks. Vitiligo doesn't favor one sex; however, women tend to seek treatment more often than men. Repigmentation therapy, which is widely used in treating vitiligo, may necessitate several summers of exposure to sunlight; the effects of this treatment may not be permanent.

Causes

Although the cause of vitiligo is unknown, inheritance seems a definite etiologic factor, because about 30% of patients with vitiligo have family members with the same condition. Other theories implicate enzymatic self-destructing mechanisms, autoimmune mechanisms, and abnormal neurogenic stimuli.

Some link exists between vitiligo and several other disorders that it often accompanies — thyroid dysfunction, pernicious anemia, Addison's disease, aseptic meningitis, diabetes mellitus, photophobia, hearing defects, alopecia areata, and halo nevi.

The most frequently reported precipitating factor is a stressful physical or psychological event — severe sunburn, surgery, pregnancy, loss of job, bereavement, or some other source of distress. Chemical agents, such as phenols and catechols, may also cause this condition.

SIGNS & SYMPTOMS	DIAGNOSIS
Recurrent oral ulcers, eye lesions, genital lesions, and cutaneous lesions	History of symptoms.

Signs and symptoms

Vitiligo produces depigmented or stark-white patches on the skin; on fair-skinned Caucasians, these are almost imperceptible. Lesions are usually bilaterally symmetric with sharp borders, which, occasionally, are hyperpigmented. (See *Depigmented skin,* page 902.)

These unique patches generally appear over bony prominences, around orifices (such as the eyes, mouth), within body folds, and at sites of trauma. The hair within these lesions may also turn white. Because hair follicles and certain parts of the eyes also contain pigment cells, vitiligo may be associated with premature gray hair and ocular pigmentary changes.

Diagnosis

Diagnosing vitiligo requires accurate history of onset and of associated illnesses, family history, and observation of characteristic lesions. Other skin disorders, such as tinea versicolor, must be ruled out.

In fair-skinned patients, Wood's light examination in a darkened room detects vitiliginous patches; depigmented skin reflects the light, and pigmented skin absorbs it. If autoimmune or endocrine disturbances are suspected, laboratory studies (thyroid indexes, for example) are appropriate.

Treatment

Two main types of treatment — repigmentation therapy and depigmentation therapy — are used for vitiligo.

Repigmentation therapy

This treatment combines systemic and topical psoralen compounds (trimethylpsoralen or 8-methoxypsoralen) with exposure to sunlight or artificial ultraviolet light, wavelength A (UVA). New pigment rises from hair follicles and appears on the skin as small freckles, which gradually enlarge and coalesce. Body parts containing few hair follicles (such as the fingertips) may resist this therapy.

Because psoralens and UVA affect the entire skin surface, systemic therapy enhances the contrast between normal skin, which turns darker than usual, and white, vitiliginous skin. Use of sunscreen on normal skin may minimize contrast while preventing sunburn.

Depigmentation therapy

Patients with vitiligo affecting over 50% of the body surface may benefit from depigmentation therapy. A cream containing 20% monobenzone permanently destroys pigment cells in unaffected areas of the skin and produces a uniform skin tone.

This medication is applied initially to a small area of normal skin once daily to test for unfavorable reactions (contact dermatitis, for example). In the absence of adverse effects, the patient

DEPIGMENTED SKIN

This illustration shows characteristic depigmented skin patches in vitiligo. These patches are usually bilaterally symmetrical, with distinct borders.

begins applying the cream twice daily to those areas he wishes to depigment first. Eventually, the entire skin may be depigmented to achieve a uniform color.

Note: Depigmentation is permanent and results in extreme photosensitivity.

Other measures

Commercial cosmetics may also help deemphasize vitiliginous skin. Some patients prefer dyes because these remain on the skin for several days, although the results are not always satisfactory.

Although often impractical, complete avoidance of exposure to sunlight through the use of screening agents and protective clothing may minimize vitiliginous lesions in whites.

Special considerations

• Instruct the patient to use psoralens medications three or four times weekly. (*Note:* Systemic psoralens should be taken 2 hours before exposure to sun; topical solutions should be applied 30 to 60 minutes before exposure.)

• Warn the patient to use a sunscreen (of highest protection factor) to protect both affected and normal skin during exposure and to wear sunglasses after taking the medication. If periorbital areas require exposure, tell the patient to keep his eyes closed during treatment.

• Suggest that the patient receiving depigmentation therapy wear protective clothing and use sunblock (SPF 15).

• Explain the therapy thoroughly, and allow the patient plenty of time to decide whether to undergo this treatment. Make sure he understands that the results of depigmentation are permanent and that he must thereafter protect his skin from the adverse effects of sunlight.

• Caution the patient about buying commercial cosmetics or dyes without trying them first, because some may not be suitable.

• Remind patients undergoing repigmentation therapy that exposure to sunlight also darkens normal skin. After being exposed to UVA for the prescribed amount of time, the patient should apply a sunscreen if he plans to be exposed to sunlight also.

If sunburn occurs, advise the patient to discontinue therapy temporarily and to apply open wet dressings (using thin sheeting) to affected areas for 15 to 20 minutes, four or five times daily or as necessary for comfort. After application of wet dressings, allow the skin to air-dry. Suggest application of a soothing lubricating cream or lotion while the skin is still slightly moist.

For the child with vitiligo:

• Modify repigmentation therapy to avoid unnecessary restrictions.

• Tell parents to give the initial dose of psoralens medication at 1 p.m. and then let the child go out to play as usual. After this, medication should be given 30 minutes earlier each day of treatment, provided the child's skin doesn't turn more than slightly pink from exposure.

• If marked erythema develops, parents should discontinue treatment and seek medical advice.

• Eventually, the child should be able to take the medication at 9:30 a.m. and play outdoors the rest of the day without adverse effects.

• Tell the parents the child should wear clothing that permits maximum exposure of vitiliginous areas to the sun.

• Reinforce patient teaching with written instructions.

• Be sensitive to the patient's emotional needs, but avoid promoting unrealistic hope for a total cure.

VOCAL CORD NODULES AND POLYPS

Nodules on the vocal cord result from hypertrophy of fibrous tissue and form at the point where the cords come together forcibly. Vocal cord polyps are swellings on the true vocal cord caused by edema in the lamina propria of the mucous membrane. Both nodules and polyps have good prognoses, unless continued voice abuse causes recurrence, with subsequent scarring and permanent hoarseness.

Causes
Vocal cord nodules and polyps usually result from voice abuse, especially in the presence of infection. Consequently, they're most common in teachers, singers, and sports fans, and in energetic children (ages 8 to 12) who continually shout while playing. Polyps are common in adults who smoke, live in dry climates, or have allergies.

Signs and symptoms
Nodules and polyps inhibit the approximation of vocal cords and produce painless hoarseness. The voice may also develop a breathy or husky quality.

Diagnosis
Persistent hoarseness suggests vocal cord nodules and polyps; visualization by indirect laryngoscopy confirms it.

• In the patient with vocal cord nodules, laryngoscopy initially shows small red nodes; later, white solid nodes on one or both cords.

• In the patient with polyps, laryngoscopy reveals unilateral or, occasionally, bilateral, sessile or pedunculated polyps of varying size, anywhere on the vocal cords. (See *How nodules cause hoarseness,* page 904.)

Treatment
Conservative management of small vocal cord nodules and polyps includes humidification, speech therapy (voice rest, training to reduce the intensity and duration of voice production), and treatment of any underlying allergies.

When conservative treatment fails to relieve hoarseness, nodules or polyps require removal under direct laryngoscopy. Microlaryngoscopy may be done for small lesions, to avoid injuring the vocal cord surface.

If nodules or polyps are bilateral, excision may be performed in two stages: one cord is allowed to heal before excision of polyps on the other cord. Two-stage excision prevents laryngeal web, which occurs when epithelial tissue is removed from adjacent cord surfaces, and these surfaces grow together.

For children, treatment consists of speech therapy. If possible, surgery should be delayed until the child is old enough to benefit from voice training, or until he can understand the need to abstain from voice abuse.

How Nodules Cause Hoarseness

Vocal cord nodules cause hoarseness by inhibiting proper closure of the vocal cords during phonation. The most common site of vocal cord nodules is the point of maximal vibration and impact (junction of the anterior one-third and the posterior two-thirds of the vocal cord).

Anterior one-third

Posterior two-thirds

Nodules

Special considerations

• Postoperatively, stress the importance of resting the voice for 10 days to 2 weeks while the vocal cords heal. Provide an alternative means of communication — Magic Slate, pad and pencil, or alphabet board.

• Place a sign over the bed to remind visitors that the patient shouldn't talk. Mark the intercom so other hospital personnel are aware the patient can't answer.

• Minimize the need to speak by trying to anticipate the patient's needs.

• If the patient is a smoker, encourage him to stop smoking entirely or, at the very least, to refrain from smoking during recovery from surgery.

• Use a vaporizer to increase humidity and decrease throat irritation.

• Make sure the patient receives speech therapy after healing, if necessary, because continued voice abuse causes recurrence of growths.

Vocal Cord Paralysis

Paralysis of the vocal cords results from disease of or injury to the superior or, most often, the recurrent laryngeal nerve.

Causes

Vocal cord paralysis commonly results from the accidental severing of the recurrent laryngeal nerve or of one of its extralaryngeal branches during thyroidectomy.

Other causes include pressure from an aortic aneurysm or from an enlarged atrium (in patients with mitral stenosis), bronchial or esophageal carcinoma, hypertrophy of the thyroid gland, trauma (such as neck injuries) and intubation, and neuritis due to infections or metallic poisoning. Vocal cord paralysis can also result from hysteria and, rarely, lesions of the central nervous system.

Signs and symptoms

Unilateral paralysis, the most common form, may cause vocal weakness and hoarseness. Bilateral paralysis typically produces vocal weakness and incapacitating airway obstruction if the cords become paralyzed in the adducted position.

Diagnosis

Patient history and characteristic features suggest vocal cord paralysis. Visualization by indirect laryngoscopy shows one or both cords fixed in an adducted or partially abducted position and confirms the diagnosis.

Treatment

In unilateral vocal cord paralysis, treatment consists of injection of Teflon into the paralyzed cord, under direct laryngoscopy. This procedure enlarges the cord and brings it closer to the other cord, which usually strengthens the voice and protects the airway from aspiration.

Thyroplasty also serves to medialize the vocal cord, but in this procedure an implant is placed through a neck incision. The ansa cervicalis nerve transfer allows for reinnervation of the muscles of the vocal cord. Bilateral cord paralysis in an adducted position necessitates tracheotomy.

Alternative treatments for adults include endoscopic arytenoidectomy to open the glottis, and lateral fixation of the arytenoid cartilage through an external neck incision. Excision or fixation of the arytenoid cartilage improves airway patency but produces residual voice impairment. Treatment of hysterical aphonia may include psychotherapy and hypnosis.

Special considerations

• If the patient chooses direct laryngoscopy and Teflon injection, explain these procedures thoroughly. Tell him these measures will improve his voice but won't restore it to normal. Patients are sometimes placed on voice rest for 24 to 48 hours to reduce stress on the vocal cords, which would increase the edema and might lead to airway obstruction.

• Many patients with bilateral cord paralysis prefer to keep a tracheostomy instead of having an arytenoidectomy; their voices are generally better with a tracheostomy alone than after corrective surgery.

• If the patient is scheduled to undergo a tracheotomy, explain the procedure thoroughly, and offer reassurance. Because the procedure is performed under a local anesthetic, the patient may be apprehensive.

• Teach the patient how to suction, clean, and change the tracheostomy tube.

• Reassure the patient that he can still speak by covering the lumen of the tracheostomy tube with his finger or a tracheostomy plug.

• If the patient elects to have an arytenoidectomy, explain the procedure thoroughly. Advise the patient that the tracheostomy will remain in place until the edema has subsided and the airway is patent.

VOLVULUS

A twisting of the intestine at least 180 degrees on its mesentery, volvulus results in blood vessel compression and ischemia.

Causes

In volvulus, twisting may result from an anomaly of rotation, an ingested foreign body, or an adhesion; in some cases, however, the cause is unknown. Volvulus usually occurs in a bowel segment with a mesentery long enough to twist.

The most common area, particularly in adults, is the sigmoid; the small bowel is a common site in children. Other common sites include the stomach and cecum. Volvulus secondary to meconium ileus may occur in patients with cystic fibrosis.

Signs and symptoms

Vomiting and rapid, marked abdominal distention follow sudden onset of severe abdominal pain. Without immediate treatment, volvulus can lead to strangulation of the twisted bowel loop, ischemia, infarction, perforation, and fatal peritonitis.

Diagnosis

Sudden onset of severe abdominal pain and physical examination that may reveal a palpable mass suggest volvulus. Appropriate special tests include:
• *X-rays.* Abdominal X-rays may show obstruction and abnormal air-fluid levels in the sigmoid and cecum; in midgut volvulus, abdominal X-rays may be normal.
• *Barium enema.* In cecal volvulus, barium fills the colon distal to the section of cecum; in sigmoid volvulus in children, barium may twist to a point, and, in adults, barium may take on an "ace of spades" configuration.
• *Upper GI series.* In midgut volvulus, obstruction and possibly a twisted contour show in a narrow area near the duodenojejunal junction, where barium will not pass.
• *White blood cell count.* In strangulation, the count is greater than 15,000/μl; in bowel infarction, greater than 20,000/μl.

Treatment

Therapy varies according to the severity and location of the volvulus. For children with midgut volvulus, treatment is surgical. For adults with sigmoid volvulus, a proctoscopic examination is performed to check for infarction, and nonsurgical treatment includes reduction by careful insertion of a sigmoidoscope or a long rectal tube to deflate the bowel.

Success of nonsurgical reduction is indicated by expulsion of gas and immediate relief of abdominal pain. If the bowel is distended but viable, surgery consists of detorsion (untwisting); if the bowel is necrotic, surgery includes resection and anastomosis.

Special considerations

• After surgical correction of volvulus, monitor vital signs, watching for temperature changes (a sign of sepsis), and a rapid pulse rate and falling blood pressure (signs of shock and peritonitis).
• Carefully monitor fluid intake and output (including stools), electrolyte values, and complete blood count. Be sure to measure and record drainage from the nasogastric tube and drains.
• Encourage frequent coughing and deep breathing.
• Reposition the patient often, and suction him as needed.
• Keep dressings clean and dry. Record any excessive or unusual drainage.
• Later, check for incisional inflammation and separation of sutures.
• When bowel sounds and peristalsis return, begin oral feedings with clear liquids, as ordered. Before removing the nasogastric tube, clamp it for a trial period, and watch for abdominal distention. When solid food can be tolerated, gradually expand the diet.
• Reassure the patient and family, and explain all diagnostic procedures. If the patient is a child, encourage parents to participate in their child's care to minimize the stress of hospitalization.

VON WILLEBRAND'S DISEASE

A hereditary bleeding disorder, von Willebrand's disease is characterized by prolonged bleeding time, moderate deficiency of clotting Factor VIII_{AHF} (antihemophilic factor), and impaired platelet function.

This disease commonly causes bleeding from the skin or mucosal surfaces and, in females, excessive uterine bleeding. Bleeding may range from mild and asymptomatic to severe, potentially fatal hemorrhage. Prognosis, however, is usually good.

Causes

Unlike hemophilia, von Willebrand's disease is inherited as an autosomal dominant trait and occurs more often in females. One theory of pathophysiology holds that mild to moderate deficiency of Factor VIII and defective platelet adhesion prolong coagulation time.

Specifically, this results from a deficiency of the von Willebrand factor (VWF), which stabilizes the Factor VIII molecule and is needed for proper platelet function.

Defective platelet function is characterized by:
• decreased agglutination and adhesion at the bleeding site
• reduced platelet retention when filtered through a column of packed glass beads
• diminished ristocetin-induced platelet aggregation.

Recently, an acquired form has been identified in patients with cancer and immune disorders.

Signs and symptoms

Von Willebrand's disease produces easy bruising, epistaxis, and bleeding from the gums. Severe forms of this disease may cause hemorrhage after laceration or surgery, menorrhagia, and gastrointestinal bleeding. Excessive postpartum bleeding is uncommon, because Factor VIII levels and bleeding time abnormalities become less pronounced during pregnancy.

Massive soft-tissue hemorrhage and bleeding into joints rarely occur. Severity of bleeding may lessen with age, and bleeding episodes occur sporadically — a patient may bleed excessively after one dental extraction but not after another.

Diagnosis

Diagnosing this disease is difficult, because symptoms are mild, laboratory values are borderline, and Factor VIII levels fluctuate. However, a positive family history and characteristic bleeding patterns and laboratory values help establish diagnosis. Typical laboratory data include:
• prolonged bleeding time (less than 6 minutes)
• slightly prolonged partial thromboplastin time (more than 45 seconds)
• absent or reduced levels of Factor VIII-related antigens (VIII_{AGN}), and low Factor VIII activity level
• defective in vitro platelet aggregation (using the ristocetin coagulation factor assay test)
• normal platelet count and normal clot retraction.

Treatment

The aims of treatment are to shorten bleeding time by local measures and to replace Factor VIII (and, consequently, VWF) by infusion of cryoprecipitate or blood fractions that are rich in Factor VIII.

During bleeding and before surgery, I.V. infusion of cryoprecipitate or fresh-frozen plasma (in quantities sufficient to raise Factor VIII levels to 50% of normal) shortens bleeding time. Desmopressin given parenterally or intranasally is effective in raising serum levels of VWF.

Special considerations

• Care should include local measures to control bleeding and patient teaching to prevent bleeding, unnecessary trauma, and complications.

• After surgery, monitor bleeding time for 24 to 48 hours, and watch for signs of new bleeding.

• During a bleeding episode, elevate and apply cold compresses and gentle pressure to the bleeding site.

• Refer parents of affected children for genetic counseling.

• Advise the patient to seek medical attention after even minor trauma and before all surgery, to determine if replacement of blood components is necessary.

• Tell the patient to watch for signs of hepatitis within 6 weeks to 6 months after transfusion.

• Warn against using aspirin and other drugs that impair platelet function.

• Advise the patient who has a severe form to avoid contact sports.

VULVOVAGINITIS

Inflammation of the vulva (vulvitis) and vagina (vaginitis) is called vulvovaginitis. Because of the proximity of these two structures, inflammation of one usually precipitates inflammation of the other. Vulvovaginitis may occur at any age and affects most females at some time. Prognosis is good with treatment.

Causes

Common causes of vaginitis (with or without consequent vulvitis) include:

• infection with *Trichomonas vaginalis,* a protozoan flagellate, usually transmitted through sexual intercourse

• infection with *Candida albicans (Monilia),* a fungus that requires glucose for growth. Incidence rises during the secretory phase of the menstrual cycle. Such infection occurs twice as often in pregnant females as in nonpregnant females. It also commonly affects users of oral contraceptives, diabetics, and patients receiving systemic therapy with broad-spectrum antibiotics (incidence may reach 75%).

• infection with *Gardnerella vaginitis,* a gram-negative bacillus

• venereal infection with *Neisseria gonorrhoeae* (gonorrhea), a gram-negative diplococcus

• viral infection with venereal warts (condylomata acuminata) or herpesvirus Type II, usually transmitted by sexual intercourse

• vaginal mucosa atrophy in menopausal women due to decreasing levels of estrogen, which predisposes to bacterial invasion.

Common causes of vulvitis include:

• parasitic infection (*Phthirus pubis* [crab louse])

• trauma (skin breakdown may lead to secondary infection)

• poor personal hygiene

• chemical irritations, or allergic reactions to hygiene sprays, douches, detergents, clothing, or toilet paper

• vulval atrophy in menopausal women due to decreasing estrogen levels

• retention of a foreign body such as a tampon or diaphragm.

Signs and symptoms

• In trichomonal vaginitis, vaginal discharge is thin, bubbly, green-tinged, and malodorous. This infection causes marked irritation and itching, and urinary symptoms, such as burning and frequency.

• Monilia vaginitis produces a thick, white, cottage-cheese–like discharge and red, edematous mucous membranes, with white flecks adhering to the vaginal wall, and is often accompanied by intense itching.

• Hemophilus vaginitis produces a gray, foul-smelling discharge.

• Gonorrhea may produce no symptoms at all, or a profuse, purulent discharge and dysuria.

• Acute vulvitis causes a mild to severe inflammatory reaction, including edema, erythema, burning, and pruritus. Severe pain on urination and dyspareunia may necessitate immediate treatment.

• Herpes infection may cause painful ulceration or vesicle formation during the active phase.

• Chronic vulvitis generally causes relatively mild inflammation, possibly associated with severe edema that may involve the entire perineum.

Diagnosis

Vaginitis is diagnosed by identification of the infectious organism during microscopic examination of vaginal exudate on a wet slide preparation (a drop of vaginal exudate placed in normal saline solution).

• In trichomonal infections, the presence of motile, flagellated trichomonads confirms the diagnosis.

• In monilia vaginitis, 10% potassium hydroxide is added to the slide, and microscopic examination seeks "clue cells" (granular epithelial cells); however, diagnosis requires identification of *C. albicans* fungi.

• Gonorrhea necessitates culture of vaginal exudate on Thayer-Martin or Transgrow medium to confirm diagnosis.

Diagnosis of vulvitis or suspected venereal disease may require complete blood count, urinalysis, cytology screening, biopsy of chronic lesions to rule out malignancy, and culture of exudate from acute lesions.

Treatment

Common therapeutic measures include the following:

• oral metronidazole for the patient with trichomonal vaginitis and for all sexual partners

• topical miconazole 2% or clotrimazole 1% for candidal infection

• metronidazole for *Gardnerella*

• systemic antibiotic therapy for the patient with gonorrhea and for all sexual partners

• doxycycline or erythromycin for chlamydial infection.

Cold compresses or cool sitz baths may provide relief from pruritus in acute vulvitis; severe inflammation may require warm compresses. Other therapy includes avoiding drying soaps, wearing loose clothing to promote air circulation, and applying topical corticosteroids to reduce inflammation.

Chronic vulvitis may respond to topical hydrocortisone or antipruritics and good hygiene (especially in elderly or incontinent patients). Topical estrogen ointments may be used to treat atrophic vulvovaginitis.

No cure currently exists for herpesvirus infections; however, oral and topical acyclovir (Zovirax) decreases the duration and symptoms of active lesions.

Special considerations

Ask the patient if she has any drug allergies. Stress the importance of taking the medication for the length of time prescribed, even if symptoms subside.

WHOOPING COUGH

Pertussis or whooping cough is a highly contagious respiratory infection usually caused by the nonmotile, gramnegative coccobacillus *Bordetella pertussis* and, occasionally, by the related similar bacteria *Bordetella parapertussis* and *Bordetella bronchiseptica*.

Characteristically, whooping cough produces an irritating cough that becomes paroxysmal and often ends in a high-pitched inspiratory whoop.

Since the 1940s, immunization and aggressive diagnosis and treatment have significantly reduced mortality from whooping cough in the United States.

Causes

Whooping cough is usually transmitted by the direct inhalation of contaminated droplets from a patient in the acute stage; it may also be spread indirectly through soiled linen and other articles contaminated by respiratory secretions.

Whooping cough is endemic throughout the world, and usually occurs in early spring and late winter. About half the time it strikes unimmunized children under age 2.

Signs and symptoms

After an incubation period of about 7 to 10 days, *B. pertussis* enters the tracheobronchial mucosa, where it produces progressively tenacious mucus. Whooping cough follows a classic 6-week course that includes three stages, each of which lasts about 2 weeks.

Catarrhal stage

First, the catarrhal stage characteristically produces an irritating hacking nocturnal cough, anorexia, sneezing, listlessness, infected conjunctiva and, occasionally, a low-grade fever. This stage is highly communicable.

Paroxysmal stage

After 7 to 14 days, the paroxysmal stage produces spasmodic and recurrent coughing that may expel tenacious mucus. Each cough characteristically ends in a loud, crowing inspiratory whoop, and choking on mucus causes vomiting. (Infants might not develop the typical whoop.)

Paroxysmal coughing may induce complications, such as increased venous pressure, nosebleed, periorbital edema, conjunctival hemorrhage, hemorrhage of the anterior chamber of the eye, detached retina (and blindness), rectal prolapse, inguinal or umbilical hernia, seizures, atelectasis, and pneumonitis.

In infants, choking spells may cause apnea, anoxia, and disturbed acid-base balance. During this stage, patients are highly vulnerable to fatal secondary bacterial or viral infections. Suspect such secondary infection (usually otitis media or pneumonia) in any whooping cough patient with a fever during this stage, because whooping cough itself seldom causes fever.

Convalescent stage

During the convalescent stage, paroxysmal coughing and vomiting gradually subside. However, for months afterward, even a mild upper respiratory infection may trigger paroxysmal coughing.

Diagnosis

Classic clinical findings, especially during the paroxysmal stage, suggest this diagnosis; laboratory studies confirm it.

• *Nasopharyngeal swabs and sputum cultures* show *B. pertussis* only in the early stages of this disease.

• *Fluorescent antibody screening* of nasopharyngeal smears provides quicker results than cultures but is less reliable.

• *White blood cell (WBC) count* is usually increased, especially in children older than age 6 months and early in the paroxysmal stage. The WBC count may reach 175,000 to 200,000/μl, with 60% to 90% lymphocytes.

Treatment

Vigorous supportive therapy requires hospitalization of infants (often in the ICU), and fluid and electrolyte replacement. Other treatment includes adequate nutrition, codeine and mild sedation to decrease coughing, oxygen therapy in apnea, and antibiotics, such as erythromycin and, possibly, ampicillin, to shorten the period of communicability and prevent secondary infections.

Immunization

Because very young infants are particularly susceptible to pertussis, immunization — usually with diphtheria and tetanus toxoids (DPT) — begins at age 2, 4, and 6 months. Boosters follow at age 18 months and at age 4 to 6 years.

Special considerations

• Whooping cough calls for aggressive, supportive care and respiratory isolation (masks only) for 5 to 7 days after initiation of antibiotic therapy.

• Monitor acid-base, fluid, and electrolyte balances.

• Carefully suction secretions, and monitor oxygen therapy. Remember: Suctioning removes oxygen as well as secretions.

• Create a quiet environment to decrease coughing stimulation. Provide small, frequent meals, and treat constipation or nausea caused by codeine.

• To decrease exposure to organisms, change soiled linen, empty the suction bottle, and change the trash bag at least once each shift.

SELECTED REFERENCES

Antonucci, G. et al. "Risk Factors for Tuberculosis in HIV-Infected Persons: A Prospective Cohort Study," *JAMA* 274(2):143-48, July 12, 1995.

Chernow, B., ed. *Essentials of Critical Care Pharmacology.* Abridged from *The Pharmacologic Approach to the Critically Ill Patient,* 3rd ed. Baltimore: Williams & Wilkins Co., 1994.

Cotran, R.S., et al. *Robbins Pathologic Basis of Disease,* 5th ed. Philadelphia: W.B. Saunders Co., 1994.

Davidson, T., et al. "Implantable Cardioverter Defibrillators: A Guide for Clinicians," *Heart and Lung* 23(3):205-17, May-June 1994.

Deresinski, S.C., et al. "Emerging Infections: Beyond the Media Hype," *Patient Care* 29(9):29-55, May 15, 1995.

Diabetes Control and Complications Trial Research Group. "The Effect of Intensive Treatment of Diabetes on the Development and Progression of Long-Term Complications in Insulin-Dependent Diabetes Mellitus," *New England Journal of Medicine* 329(14):977-86, Sept. 30, 1993.

Diagnostic and Statistical Manual of Mental Disorders, 4th ed. Washington D.C.: American Psychiatric Association, 1994.

Duchin, J.S., et al. "Hantavirus Pulmonary Syndrome: A Clinical Description of 17 Patients with a Newly Recognized Disease," *New England Journal of Medicine* 330(14):949-55, April 7, 1994.

Grant, C., ed. *Psychiatric Nursing.* Albany, N.Y.: Delmar Publishers, 1994.

Guberman, A. *An Introduction to Clinical Neurology: Pathophysiology, Diagnosis, and Treatment.* Boston: Little, Brown & Co., 1994.

Horne, M., and Swearingen, P. *Pocket Guide to Fluids, Electrolytes, and Acid-Base Balance,* 2nd ed. St. Louis: Mosby-Year Book, Inc., 1993.

Isselbacher, K.J., et al., eds. *Harrison's Principles of Internal Medicine,* 13th ed. New York: McGraw-Hill Book Co., 1994.

Kinzler, K., et al. "Cancer Genes: What We Know Today," *Patient Care* 29(8):13-20, April 30, 1995.

McKennis, A.T., and Waddington, C. "Unilateral Vocal Cord Paralysis," *ORL Head and Neck Nursing* 12(1):9-13, Winter 1994.

Murphy, M.C., et al. "Differences in Symptoms During and Post PTCA Versus Rotational Ablation," *Progress in Cardiovascular Nursing* 9(2):4-9, Spring 1994.

Rakel, R.E., ed. *Conn's Current Therapy 1995.* Philadelphia: W.B. Saunders Co., 1995.

Sleisenger, M.H., and Fordtran, J.S., eds. *Gastrointestinal Disease: Pathophysiology, Diagnosis, Management,* 5th ed. Philadelphia: W.B. Saunders Co., 1993.

Swaiman, K.F. *Pediatric Neurology: Principles and Practice,* 2nd ed. St. Louis: Mosby-Year Book, Inc., 1994.

Vidt, D.G. "Hypertension: A New Classification System Helps You Better Define Risk," *Consultant* 33(5):53-61, May 1993.

Weiss, M.K., et al. "Diagnosis and Management of Bipolar II Disorder," *Comprehensive Therapy* 20(2):121-24, February 1994.

INDEX

i indicates illustration; *t* indicates table.